BASIC
NEUROLOGY

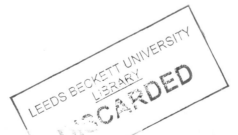

NOTICE

Medicine is an ever-changing science. As new research and clinical experience broaden our knowledge, changes in treatment and drug therapy are required. The authors and the publisher of this work have checked with sources believed to be reliable in their efforts to provide information that is complete and generally in accord with the standards accepted at the time of publication. However, in view of the possibility of human error or changes in medical sciences, neither the authors nor the publisher nor any other party who has been involved in the preparation or publication of this work warrants that the information contained herein is in every respect accurate or complete, and they are not responsible for any errors or omissions or for the results obtained from use of such information. Readers are encouraged to confirm the information contained herein with other sources. For example and in particular, readers are advised to check the product information sheet included in the package of each drug they plan to administer to be certain that the information contained in this book is accurate and that changes have not been made in the recommended dose or in the contraindications for administration. This recommendation is of particular importance in connection with new or infrequently used drugs.

BASIC
NEUROLOGY
THIRD EDITION

John Gilroy, M.D., F.R.C.P. (Can), F.A.C.P.

Clinical Professor of Neurology, Wayne State University, Detroit, Michigan
Chairman of Neurology, William Beaumont Hospital, Royal Oak, Michigan
Former Professor and Chairman, Department of Neurology, Wayne State University,
Detroit, Michigan

INTERNATIONAL EDITION

McGraw-Hill
HEALTH PROFESSIONS DIVISION

New York   St. Louis   San Francisco   Auckland   Bogotá
Caracas   Lisbon   London   Madrid   Mexico City   Milan   Montreal
New Delhi   San Juan   Singapore   Sydney   Tokyo   Toronto

McGraw-Hill

*A Division of The **McGraw·Hill** Companies*

BASIC NEUROLOGY, 3/e

1234567890   DOC DOC   99

INTERNATIONAL EDITION

Copyright © 2000
Exclusive rights by The McGraw-Hill Companies, Inc., for manufacture and export. This book cannot be re-exported from the country to which it is consigned by The McGraw-Hill Companies.

When ordering this title, use ISBN 0-07-115289-X.

This book was set in Times Roman by Progressive Information Technologies, Inc.
The editors were Joseph A. Hefta, Martin J. Wonsiewicz, and Peter J. Boyle.
The production supervisor was Richard C. Ruzycka.
The cover designer was Alexander Tsiaras.
The indexer was Kathrin Unger.
R. R. Donnelley and Sons Company was printer and binder.

This book is printed on acid-free paper.

Cataloging-in-publication data is on file for this title at the Library of Congress.

CONTENTS

PREFACE

The third edition of *Basic Neurology* is the product of more than four years of work generated in response to the flood of new material published in the last ten years. Indeed, I am keenly aware that we have experienced "a decade of the brain" with a magnificent explosion of knowledge in the neurosciences. This has placed the neurosciences in the forefront of medicine and should be a source of pride to all who are associated with this specialty. While *Basic Neurology* is primarily directed to the neurologist, the complete neurologist cannot function in isolation and must have close contact with neurosurgery, neurophysiology, neuroradiology, neuropathology, and the many other subspecialties that contribute to the neurosciences. This has been emphasized in this book, but at the same time there is a reiteration of the tradition of the practice of neurology and the care of the patient which remains the prime concern of the good physician.

The first chapter is essentially unchanged with the exception of the section on speech and language, largely rewritten following suggestions from the Department of Speech Pathology, William Beaumont Hospital. The remainder of the chapter continues to emphasize the orderly approach to the neurological evaluation which remains the key to accurate diagnosis or differential diagnosis, leading, when necessary, to the appropriate choice of ancillary studies.

The remaining chapters contain an abundance of new material selected to emphasize the dynamic changes in neurology and the neurosciences.

The majority of the illustrations are new and reflect the improvement in MRI scanning with some reference to innovated techniques available to neuroradiologists. There are minor changes in the line drawings originally produced by the medical illustrator, Mr. William Loecher. All new illustrations were produced by the personnel of the Department of Medical Photography, William Beaumont Hospital, to whom I am most grateful for their cooperation, patience, and prompt service. The manuscript was prepared by Karen Richardson, Merrill Evans, and Bonnie Abbott, who, in addition to transcription and the orderly running of a busy neurological practice, kept manuscripts in order and maintained an efficient contact with the publisher.

The medical library at William Beaumont Hospital, under Nancy Bulgarelli, M.S.L.S., the director of library information services, and her dedicated staff performed in their usual efficient manner with prompt responses to my many requests for references, copies, or computer searches.

I am also indebted to many colleagues at William Beaumont Hospital for advice, criticism, and support during the rewriting of this edition of *Basic Neurology*.

Edward M. Cohn, M.D.
Chief, Section of Neuro-ophthalmology
William Beaumont Hospital

Ay Ming Wang, M.D.
Chief of Neuroradiology
William Beaumont Hospital

William Sanders, M.D.
Staff Neuroradiologist
William Beaumont Hospital

Samir Noujaim, M.D.
Chief, Head and Neck Radiology and
  Neuroradiologist
William Beaumont Hospital

Michael Rolnick, Ph.D.
Chief, Speech Pathology
William Beaumont Hospital

Richard Merson, Ph.D.
Deputy Chief, Speech Pathology
William Beaumont Hospital

A. Martin Lerner, M.D.
Division of Infectious Diseases
William Beaumont Hospital

Carl Lauter, M.D.
Division of Infectious Diseases
William Beaumont Hospital

Bishara Freij, M.D.
Pediatric Infectious Diseases
William Beaumont Hospital

Darlene Fink-Bennett, M.D.
Department of Nuclear Medicine
William Beaumont Hospital

Kamalesh Lahiri, M.D.
Cardiologist
William Beaumont Hospital

Barbara Joyce, Ph.D.
Neuropsychologist
Michigan State University

Barbara Coslow, R.N., M.S.
Neurology Nurse Practitioner

Rebecca Sexton, M.D.
Resident in Ophthalmology
Kresge Eye Institute
Wayne State University
Detroit, Michigan

Jodi Ganley, D.O.
Neurologist
William Beaumont Hospital

All references were checked by:
Alex Chasnis, transitional resident
Oakwood Hospital
Dearborn, Michigan
and
Suzanne Eddy, fourth-year student
Syracuse University
Now a public relations specialist
Lucent Technologies, New Jersey

And finally, my wife, Marsha K. Gilroy, Ph.D., Assistant Professor of Psychology, University of Detroit Mercy, who advised me on many of the psychology aspects of neurological disease and who showed an enduring patience and fortitude during the more than four years of preparation of this edition.

The Health Professions Division of McGraw-Hill has been the most supportive of publishers, ever patient and never critical of missed deadlines. My immediate contact, Joe Hefta, never wavered in his positive approach to my complaints and excuses. I am deeply indebted to him for his patience and understanding. I also wish to thank Peter Boyle, Editing Supervisor, who helped mold the present edition into its present form. I am also indebted to Martin J. Wonsiewicz, Publisher, Health Professions Division.

BASIC
NEUROLOGY

Chapter 1

THE NEUROLOGICAL EVALUATION

The neurological evaluation (Table 1-1) should be conducted in a relaxed atmosphere. The examiner should face the patient, who may be accompanied by relatives or close friends, and all should be seated comfortably. Children aged 6 or older usually feel most secure when seated between parents; younger children are less apprehensive when seated on the lap of one of the parents.

HISTORY

The history begins with the identification of the chief complaint. The patient may be asked, "Mr. X, why have you come to see me?" If the patient cannot answer the question through apparent failure of comprehension or lack of insight, the query should be addressed to those accompanying the patient. The individual answering can then be asked to supply the remainder of the history.

The chief complaint is the focal point of the history and is the key to the subsequent analysis of information leading to a differential diagnosis. Once the chief complaint has been identified, the examiner should record the history of the present illness in chronological order up to the time of the interview. This provides an excellent opportunity to analyze the information associated with the chief complaint and develop an appropriate differential diagnosis. The examiner must learn to encourage the flow of information and at the same time minimize the interjection of valueless statements made by the patient or relatives. The experienced examiner is polite, firm, and tactful in maintaining control of the interview and keeping the history "on track" so that the maximum amount of relevant information is obtained. It is important to realize that patients and their relatives are usually incorrect in their interpretation of symptoms. Their tendency is to misconstrue statements made by other

physicians and to misinterpret the results of diagnostic studies performed in the past.

It is often possible to obtain additional information by observing the patient during the interview. The patient may appear to be comfortable, apprehensive, alert, or drowsy. The facial expression is important in assessing appropriate or inappropriate affect. Lack of facial expression may indicate depression, early parkinsonism, or failure of comprehension. Ptosis, involuntary eye movements, tics, myokymia, hemifacial spasm, or facial asymmetry may be observed during the interview. The examiner may see intermittent involuntary movements or tremors affecting the limbs, head, or trunk, or may observe abnormal posture as the interview proceeds. The interplay between the patient and spouse, relatives, or friends is important in determining closeness or conflict in their relationships and is apparent only on continuing observation.

The next step in the history is the neurological review, which supplies additional information and is a logical extension of the history of the present illness. The neurological review consists of a series of questions about the presence of common neurological symptoms (Table 1-2). If the answer is affirmative, the examiner must decide whether to continue interrogating the patient until the maximum amount of information is obtained or to discontinue questioning if the symptom adds little to the total picture. The decision to disregard or pursue a positive response to a question is often a matter of experience or may be based on information already obtained from the patient. For example, the question "Do you suffer from headaches?" is likely to receive the answer "Yes" in the majority of cases. However, the examiner will benefit from additional questioning about headache if the headache is the chief complaint when the headache is of recent origin or if there has been a recent change in the frequency or severity of chronic

Table 1-1
Outline for the neurological evaluation

History
  Chief complaint
  History of the present illness
  Neurological review
  Past medical history
  Social history
General physical examination
Neurological examination
  Mental status examination
    Speech, orientation, current events, judgment, insight,
    abstraction, vocabulary, perception, emotional
    response, memory, calculation, object recognition,
    praxis
  Cranial nerve examination
    I. Olfaction
    II. Visual acuity, ophthalmoscopic exam, visual fields
    III, IV, VI. Pupils, eye movements
    V. Corneal reflex; sensation—face, scalp; motor
       function—muscles of mastication: jaw jerk
    VII. Motor function—facial muscles; taste—anterior
       ⅔ tongue
    VIII. Hearing, equilibrium
    IX, X. Motor function, palate and pharynx, phonation,
       taste, posterior third of tongue
    XI. Motor function—sternocleidomastoid and
       trapezius
    XII. Motor function—tongue
  Motor
    Inspection, posture, tone, and power
  Coordination
    Rapid alternating movements, finger-to-nose and
    heel-to-shin tests
  Gait and station
    Gait testing, tandem gait, walking on heels and toes,
    Romberg test
  Sensory
    Touch, pinprick, vibration, position, and temperature
    senses
  Reflexes
    Tendon reflexes, plantar response, abdominal reflexes,
    release phenomena

cides that the headache is relevant to the neurological complaint, a series of subsidiary questions must be posed to the patient to obtain the maximum information about the headache. This includes such questions as: "How often does the headache occur? What factors precipitate the headache? When does it occur? Are there any early warning symptoms? Where is the pain? What kind of pain is it? How long does it last? Does anything relieve the pain? Does anything make it worse? Are there any associated symptoms during the headache such as nausea, photophobia, phonophobia, or osmophobia? What do you prefer to do when the headache is severe? How do you feel after the headache has resolved?"

The question regarding visual symptoms is related to sudden dimness or blurring of vision that may occur in neurological conditions such as transient cerebral ischemia or multiple sclerosis. For example, transient visual loss in one eye (amaurosis fugax) is a feature of internal carotid artery disease. The next series of questions on diplopia, hearing, tinnitus, and vertigo are related to the function of other cranial nerves and their central connections (the third, fourth, and sixth nerves, and the acoustic and vestibular divisions of the eighth nerve). The examiner is advised to avoid the use of the term "dizzy" and to seek clarification of the term if it is used by the patient. "Dizzy" or "dizziness" may be used to describe vertigo, ataxia, light-headedness, transient impairment of consciousness, or minor seizure activity. These conditions are unrelated pathophysiologically, and the term "dizzy" is meaningless without clear definition.

There are several reasons for ataxia, including weakness, poor coordination, sensory loss, or transient impairment of consciousness. Focal weakness is a condition that alarms patients, and a history of recent focal weakness is usually obtained as one of the initial complaints. However, transient episodes may not be remembered unless the patient is asked about this symptom. Paradoxically, transient numbness or paresthesias affecting a limb or part of the trunk are often tolerated without seeking medical opinion and frequently forgotten if they resolve. Impairment of bladder function is not unusual with lesions at almost all levels of the central nervous system (CNS) and in many peripheral neuropathies. Urgency, frequency, and incontinence frequently indicate impairment of

headaches. A headache pattern that has been present and unchanged for many years, and is not the primary complaint, is unlikely to be related to the chief neurological complaint. Conversely, if the examiner de-

Table 1-2
Neurological review

Subject	Question
Headache	Do you suffer from headaches?
Visual symptoms	Have you experienced sudden dimness or sudden loss of vision in one or both eyes?
Diplopia	Have you had any double vision?
Hearing	Has there been any change in your hearing?
Tinnitus	Do you get any buzzing or ringing in your ears at any time?
Vertigo	Do you ever get a sensation that objects are moving around you or feel that you are moving or spinning?
Ataxia	Are you unsteady when you walk or are you clumsy when using your hands?
Focal weakness	Have you ever had weakness of an arm, hand, or leg on one side?
Focal numbness	Has there been any numbness or tingling involving an arm, hand, leg, or any part of your body at any time?
Sphincter problems	Do you ever get a sensation that you may suddenly lose control of your bladder? Do you have to rush to the bathroom to empty your bladder? Have you ever lost control of your bladder?
Speech	Have you noticed any slurring of speech recently? Do you find that you are unable to understand other people or that you cannot produce the right word in conversation?
Writing	Has your writing changed recently?
Reading	Do you have any difficulty in reading or understanding what you have read?
Memory	Have you had any difficulty with memory recently?
Walking	Do you feel unsteady when you walk? Have you fallen recently?
Loss of consciousness	Have you ever lost consciousness, fainted, or felt that you were not aware of what was going on around you?
Sleeping	Do you sleep well or do you awaken during the night?

neurological control of the bladder in patients with suspected neurological disease. However, the symptoms are often misinterpreted by patients and their physicians as bladder infections.

Obvious language problems are readily recognized as the patient communicates with the examiner, but many patients can recognize subtle changes in speech or recent difficulties in communication that may only be revealed by direct questioning. Writing is usually affected by any condition involving the function of the dominant hand. Deterioration in writing may be due to dysgraphia secondary to a lesion in the frontal or parietal lobe in the dominant hemisphere or may indicate weakness, tremor, ataxia, sensory loss, spasticity, or rigidity of the hand and upper limb. Thus, a change in writing is a nonspecific complaint but is often an early indication of impairment of the neuromuscular control of the hand. A problem with reading may occur in patients with visual failure or diplopia, or when there is a failure of comprehension of printed or written material. This latter condition is not uncommon in early dementia but will be uncovered only if the question is posed to the patient. Many patients with failing memory recognize this problem but are reluctant to disclose the symptom unless asked directly by the examiner. Thus, patients with early dementia frequently resort to writing notes to compensate for this situation. These notes are often produced during the interview, and the patient uses them as a guide when giving the history.

The last question in the neurological review is concerned with impairment or loss of consciousness. The cause is apparent in the great majority of cases if the examiner listens carefully to the description of the syncopal episode and obtains a total picture of the event by direct questioning. The examiner should adopt the same approach to this problem whether the symptom is disclosed as the chief complaint, during the history of the present illness, or in the neurological review. The patient must describe the attack, or each attack if there seem to be several types of syncopal episodes, from the time there was a sensation of something abnormal to loss of consciousness. If there appears to be some difficulty, the examiner might begin the process by saying: "I want you to describe the last attack for me. Can we go back to the time when you felt perfectly normal? I would like you to describe every event as it occurred until you lost consciousness." Having obtained the preictal history, the examiner should obtain as much information as possible about events after return of consciousness: "How did you feel? Were you confused? Now tell me everything you remember from that moment until you felt absolutely normal." The examiner now has a complete description of the preictal and postictal symptoms. The patient cannot, of course, describe events during loss of consciousness, and this gap should be closed by questioning an observer. However, the observer may augment the information already given by the patient regarding the preictal and postictal states. Therefore, the observer should be asked to describe the state of the patient from the moment that there seemed to be some abnormality up to the loss of consciousness. This is followed by observations during loss of consciousness, and finally a description of events that occurred from the moment the patient recovered consciousness up to the time that the patient appeared to be functioning normally. In the great majority of cases the combined description by the patient and observer should give the examiner a clear history of the attack and provide sufficient information for diagnosis.

The interview now continues with the recording of the past medical history, family history, and social history.

The past medical history should be recorded in chronological order beginning with any unusual diseases during childhood. A history of systemic disease such as diabetes mellitus, hypertension, or heart disease is important.

The family history is important for two reasons. A number of neurological conditions are inherited, and there will be a strong family history of neurological problems when the condition is inherited as an autosomal dominant trait. A sex-linked recessive form of inheritance is apparent when only males are affected. Many patients with cerebrovascular disease have a family history of stroke, diabetes, hypertension, and ischemic heart disease. The examiner should inquire about the presence of these conditions in family members.

The social history includes questions about the patient's occupation. The physician should learn something about the activities of people in the community and show an interest in the patient's occupation. This helps to form a rapport with the patient and may provide useful information. Questions about smoking, alcohol consumption, and the use of illicit drugs are routine during the social history. Patients should be asked about exposure to any unusual chemical or toxic substances. The examiner should record the marital status of the patient, the number of children, and the health of the children.

Finally, a list of all medications used in the preceding 2 years, the reason for prescription, and possible adverse effects to the drugs should be obtained.

GENERAL PHYSICAL EXAMINATION

Many neurological problems are associated with systemic diseases, and the patient should have a general physical examination either before or after the neurological examination. During this examination the blood pressure should be measured with the patient lying prone, immediately followed by measuring the blood pressure with the patient standing erect, to detect any tendency toward postural hypotension. This procedure should be routine in all examinations, but it is particularly important to look for postural hypotension in patients with cerebrovascular disease or Parkinson disease, in patients taking antihypertensive medication, and in all elderly patients.

NEUROLOGICAL EXAMINATION

The neurological examination begins with the assessment of mental status.

Mental Status Examination

Speech, Language, and Communication

Verbal communication consists of four distinctive and complex neurophysiological processes: voice, speech, language, and cognition (mentation). Disorders of voice are known as dysphonias, speech and voice disorders secondary to neuromuscular dysfunction as dysarthrias, and the production or comprehension of language as dysphasia or aphasia; cognitive impairment is a primary symptom of dementia. Neurological diseases often include one or more of these four areas of communication as well as swallowing disorders termed dysphagia.

The several types of dysarthria are listed in Table 1-3, dysphasia and aphasia in Table 1-4, and a screening test for all facets of verbal communication in Table 1-5. An accurate assessment of verbal communication, swallowing, and cognition can make a significant contribution to the differential diagnosis of neurological disorders and identify the type and management in the development of a rehabilitation program.[1–3]

Dysphonia   Any disorder of the laryngeal tone (voice) and its resonance in the oronasal pharyngeal tract is a *dysphonia.* Voice disorders can occur in congenital disorders or after trauma, behavioral abuse, surgical procedures, or medication reactions that affect the larynx, voice apparatus, or the neuromuscular physiology of phonation. Dysphonias of local organic origin occur in juvenile papilloma, laryngeal web, laryngeal carcinoma, and craniofacial abnormalities. Functional dysphonias without an organic cause are treated behaviorally by speech/language pathologists. Dysphonias owing to central or peripheral

Table 1-3

Dysarthrias: neuropathology and speech-voice symptomatology

Dysarthria	Neuropathology	Prominent speech voice symptoms
Spastic dysarthria	Upper motor neuron (Pseudobulbar palsy) Hypertonia, reduced range	Harsh voice, imprecise and strained speech sound production with reduced rate of speech Slow consonant-vowel syllable repetition
Flaccid dysarthria	Lower motor neuron (Bulbar palsy) Hypotonia	Hypernasal and breathy voice quality with nasal air escape on speech sound production Weak pressure consonant-vowel syllable repetition
Ataxic dysarthria	Cerebellum (Ataxia) Reduced timing, accuracy	Dysrhythmic speech timing, random speech sound prolongation Reduced speech rate
Hypokinetic dysarthria	Extrapyramidal (Bradykinesia) Rigidity, reduced range of motion	Reduced voice loudness, absence of voice intonation, fast rushes of speech production, and inappropriate speech silences
Hyperkinetic dysarthria	Extrapyramidal (Dystonia) Myoclonus, dyskinesias	Highly random-intermittent speech or voice strain, imprecision or sudden speech tics, grimaces

Neurological disorders can present with mixed combinations of the dysarthrias described above as in amyotrophic lateral sclerosis.

Source: Darley and colleagues,[5] with permission.

Table 1-4

Receptive and expressive language abnormalities in aphasia[a]

Left hemisphere area	Primary language deficit	Language retained	Aphasia synonym(s)
Zone 1 (connection B, C)	Expressive language, speech repetition, naming, reading aloud Nonfluent speech and writing	Functional comprehension of spoken and read language	Nonfluent aphasia: Broca aphasia[b] Anterior type aphasia Expressive aphasia Transcortical motor aphasia
(connection C)	Speech repetition, naming, reading aloud Nonfluent speech	Comprehension of spoken and read language is normal Functional writing	Apraxia of speech[c] Broca aphasia[b]
Zone 2 (connection A, E)	Comprehension of verbal and read language Speech and writing will have some neologisms or jargon utterances	Some spontaneous speech, naming objects and fluent speech syllable productions	Fluent aphasia: Wernicke aphasia Receptive aphasia Posterior-type aphasia Word deafness Transcortical sensory aphasia
(connection D)	Comprehension of written language, reading aloud	All other language intact	Alexia without agraphia
Zone 3 (connection F, G)	Naming and writing objects, nouns (salient words)	Visual and auditory comprehension functional Verbal circumlocution	Anomic aphasia
(connection H)	Naming objects, colors, nouns, reading aloud, comprehension of written language	Comprehension of spoken language, spontaneous speech	Visual agnosia

[a] All aphasias exhibit some degree of expressive and receptive language abnormalities in speaking, reading, writing, and listening.

[b] Broca aphasia as originally documented by P. Broca is considered an apraxia of speech and not an aphasia syndrome.

[c] Apraxia of speech is a motor programming disorder and not a type of aphasia or a language disorder. It is listed here because it is commonly confused or may coexist with aphasia.

neurological diseases are the result of intrinsic or extrinsic laryngeal muscle paralysis, paresis, or dyscoordination.[4]

Dysarthria *Dysarthria* is a difficulty in articulation caused by paralysis, paresis, or incoordination of speech and voice production.[5] Patterns of dysarthria can be specific to certain neurological abnormalities (see Table 1-3), (i.e., parkinsonism—hypokinetic dysarthria, myasthenia gravis—flaccid dysarthria, cerebellar ataxia—ataxic dysarthria). Dysarthrias may affect the oral-facial muscles of the tongue, lips, cheeks,

soft palate, or mandible and cause speech articulation to be imprecise, slurred, weak in consonant air pressure, reduced in range or dysrhythmic in tempo, as in the ataxic dysarthria of multiple sclerosis. Dysarthrias may also affect the pharyngeal and laryngeal musculature, creating a dysphonia as in parkinsonism, cerebral palsy, or laryngeal dystonia (spasmodic dysphonia). Finally, dysarthrias may result from impairment of respiratory muscles that deliver the air power for production of voice and speech. Such conditions are seen in the Guillain-Barré syndrome, myasthenia gravis, or amyotrophic lateral sclerosis.

Table 1-5

Screening test for communication disorders

Communication area	Screen procedure	Rule out/in
1. Language	Request: Naming of objects Sentence repetition Define: Bird, island, courage Write/Read: Word/sentence	Aphasia Anomia, agnosia, dyslexia, dysgraphia, agrammatism, word errors, jargon
2. Speech	Repeat: Words: Tornado, catastrophe Sentence: Joe took father's shoebench out. Syllables: Pa^3-ta^3-ka^3	Dysarthria Spastic, flaccid, ataxic, hypokinetic, hyperkinetic Apraxia Laryngeal, oral, verbal
3. Voice	Imitate: Sustain vowel: /ah/ Pitch glides: High to low tone Intonation: We were away where were you?	Dysphonias Breathy, harsh, nasal pitch, loudness, tremor
4. Cognitive	Describe: Time, space Define: Proverbs "The grass is always greener on the other side of the fence." "Don't cry over spilled milk."	Dementia high-level language disorders
5. Swallowing	Test: Tongue and lip strength Laryngeal elevation Liquid delay/aspiration	Dysphagia Oral, pharyngeal, esophageal

This chart lists a series of five communication screening tasks that physicians may use to differentiate the communication pathologies of aphasia, dysarthria, apraxia, dysphonia, dementia, and dysphagia.

Dysphasia Dysphasias are disorders of language due primarily to dysfunction or damage in the dominant cerebral hemisphere (Fig. 1-1). A dysphasia can affect all components of verbal reception and expression, that is, oral expression, auditory comprehension, visual reading, and visuomotor writing tasks.[6] A variety of isolated language symptoms can be identified in the dysphasias (anomia—naming and word finding; auditory agnosia—word recognition; dysgraphia—writing; dyslexia—reading; paraphasia—word substitution; agrammatism—grammatical errors). These symptoms may appear in isolation or in combinations of varying severity.[7] Some dysphasias are identified as nonfluent because of predominantly expressive language difficulties with milder receptive deficits (see Table 1-4). Fluent dysphasias exhibit more receptive language problems with secondary expressive disturbances.

Nondominant Hemisphere Dysfunction Patients with lesions in the nondominant hemisphere present with a unique pattern of dysfunction. Although speech or language impairment may not be present, these individuals will often experience impaired judgment and reasoning, memory problems, extinction or neglect of stimuli on the opposite side to the nondominant hemisphere, visual perception disorders, a lack of insight, attention deficits, loss of organizational skills, poor task initiation, rambling or off-topic remarks, and denial of problems. Dysarthria and

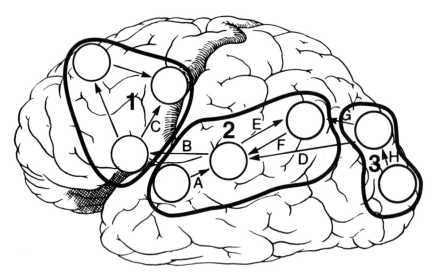

Figure 1-1
A simplified illustration of the concept of general cerebral localization for language abnormalities in aphasia or apraxia of speech. Zone 1 outlines the cerebral area most frequently responsible for nonfluent aphasias and apraxia of speech syndromes, zone 2 for the fluent aphasias, and zone 3 for visual agnosias.

dysphagia are also common impairments in nondominant hemisphere dysfunction.

Cerebral Integration of Language All auditory stimuli are transmitted from the periphery through the auditory system to the primary auditory areas of Heschl's gyrus in both temporal lobes (see Fig. 1-1, zone 2, connection A). In the dominant hemisphere, the information is directed from the primary auditory area directly to the auditory association areas in the posterior aspect of the superior temporal lobe (see Fig. 1-1, connections E and F). Information from the nondominant hemisphere is transmitted through the corpus callosum to the auditory association area in the dominant hemisphere. This area can be regarded as a word identification center and has long been termed Wernicke's area. Once the word has been identified as a language symbol, information is transmitted to a word recognition area that probably lies in the inferior portion of the parietal lobe in the dominant hemisphere. Recognition of the language symbol is based on past experience, and the function of the language recognition area is not only the recognition of language symbols but also the relationship of one symbol to another. When this function has been accomplished, information is transmitted back to or through Wernicke's area to areas of the brain concerned with encoding of or response to the language input. The generation of ex-

pressive language (Fig. 1-1, zone 1, connection C) by an individual is probably mediated through the word recognition area (see Fig. 1-1, zone 1, connection B) followed by a passage of information to the word identification area. Communication is established between the word identification area and the motor encoding area via association fibers that connect the posterior portion of the superior temporal gyrus to the opercular area of the frontal lobe. The motor encoding area (Broca's area, see Fig. 1-1, connection C) is responsible for the preliminary conversion of language symbols into motor activity. Information from the motor encoding area is then transmitted to the primary motor area of the dominant hemisphere to be converted into the necessary speech-motor movements (speech respiration, phonation, and oral articulation), which produce audible, grammatically acceptable, and meaningful verbal output. At the same time, there is communication from the Broca's area to the supplementary motor area that lies on the medial aspect of the superior frontal gyrus. There is further communication from the supplementary motor area to the primary motor area. This reflex loop from Broca's area through the supplementary motor area to the primary motor area seems to be responsible for the smooth conversion of information in the primary motor area into impulses that generate speech.

Visual language symbols are received as visual impulses in the primary visual center in the occipital lobes of both hemispheres (see Fig. 1-1, zone 3). Information is then passed to the visual association areas where object recognition and identification of language symbols occur (Fig. 1-1, zone 3, connection H). There are two main pathways from the visual association area concerned with language. In the first pathway, information from the dominant visual association area passes directly to the word identification area (see Fig. 1-1, connections G and D). Information from the nondominant visual association area crosses to the dominant hemisphere via the corpus callosum. Information concerned with object naming passes from both visual association areas to the word recognition area in the dominant hemisphere. At the same time, impulses concerned with object naming enter the language system and are transmitted forward through Wernicke's area (see Fig. 1-1, connection G).

Dyspraxia Apraxia of speech is a central neuromotor speech programming disorder.[1,6] It was first described in literature by Paul Broca in 1861 as an "aphemia" or difficulty in articulate speech in a person with a lesion in the left prefrontal lobe.[8] The symptoms of this disorder are seen in Table 1-4 (i.e., disorder of speech repetition, naming and reading without difficulties in comprehension of spoken or read language) are not aphasic symptoms. It is, however, commonly and erroneously referred to as Broca aphasia although language is not impaired.[2,6] Some patients, depending on the location or severity of the cerebral lesion, may exhibit isolated forms of oromotor or laryngeal apraxia.

Dysphagia Disorders of swallowing are identified as *dysphagia*. These swallowing disorders may occur in advanced dementia, other neurological diseases particularly brainstem infarction or multiple cerebral infarction, structural anomalies, or after surgery. Neurological dysfunction may affect any phase of the swallowing process, with oral, pharyngeal, laryngeal, or esophageal muscle weakness, paralysis, or incoordination. Cerebral or brainstem infarction and postsurgery conditions are the commonest cause of oropharyngeal dysphagias. These patients are assessed with a fluoroscopic modified barium swallow procedure to examine the site and type of oropharyngeal dysfunction. The speech/language

pathologist will often provide swallowing rehabilitation, which restores function, nutrition, and hydration while minimizing the risk of aspiration. Although oropharyngeal dysphagias are often rehabilitative with behavioral management, esophageal dysphagias require more direct medical surgical management.

Dementia Dementia is an impairment in cognitive or intellectual functioning. These functions are typical: orientation to time and space, short- and long-term memory, verbal abstraction, calculation, and abnormal personality characteristics. These are mental functions distinctly different from the receptive and expressive language disorders of aphasia, or the productive speech disorders of dysarthria or apraxia of speech. Dementias are often referred to as cognitive impairments of neuropsychological dysfunctions. Whereas patients with Alzheimer disease and other forms of dementia have a poor rehabilitative prognosis, individuals with posttraumatic head injury are more responsive to cognitive rehabilitation.

Testing for Communication Disorders The physician may easily detect an obvious aphasia in a stroke patient during the first few words of the interview. However, accompanying communication deficits are usually less distinctive. Table 1-5 provides a series of screening tests that the physician may use to examine for the presence of language, speech, voice, cognitive, or swallowing dysfunctions.

Using Table 1-5 to examine language, the physician would ask the patient to point to several common objects (e.g., pen, watch, blanket), name them, and then put them in a sentence (verbally and written). For more abstract expressive and receptive language skills, the patient is asked to define the words bird, island, and courage. This type of screening procedure will identify expressive and receptive language symptoms and point to the presence of aphasia, agnosia, dyslexia, or dysgraphias. In this same manner, speech, voice, cognitive, and swallowing symptoms may be identified using the screening test listed in column two of Table 1-5 and differential diagnostic impressions can be obtained from column three. Although these screening tests are important to the attending physician, assessment by a speech/language pathologist should be obtained when complex communication disorders are present or rehabilitation is anticipated.

Orientation   Orientation to time, place, and person indicates an ability to correlate environmental clues with past experience. The patient should be asked:

1. The day of the week
2. The date
3. The name of the building where the examination is taking place
4. The occupation of the examiner

Current Events   A knowledge of current events requires intact orientation, recent memory, and the ability to think in an abstract fashion. The patient should be asked to give the name of the President of the United States, the governor of the state, and the mayor of the city. This is followed by a request for information on current events anywhere in the world with an interpretation of these events.

Judgment   The ability to give a reasonable assessment of the situation or a failure to do so may be apparent from the examiner's contact with the patient up to this point. Judgment may, however, be tested by asking the patient to interpret a simple story requiring judgment.

   Example 1.   What would you do if you were walking along a street and saw an envelope lying on the sidewalk? The envelope is sealed, addressed, and has an unused stamp in the corner.

   Correct Answer. Pick it up and mail it.

   Incorrect Answer. Pick it up, open it, and read it or leave it alone.

   Example 2.   What would you do if you were sitting in the middle of a crowded theater and you were the first person to notice that smoke was pouring out of a ventilator?

   Correct Answer. Get up quietly, find an usher or the manager and inform him that this was occurring and request immediate action.

   Incorrect Answer. Stand up and shout "Fire."

Insight   *Insight* may be defined as the awareness of a reason for a given situation. An experienced examiner can usually tell whether insight is intact on ob-

taining the history from the patient. When there is doubt, the patient may be asked to give an explanation for consulting the examiner.

Abstraction   *Abstraction* is an intellectual function of high order requiring comprehension, understanding, and judgment. This can usually be tested by asking the patient to interpret proverbs such as:

1. Don't put all of your eggs in one basket.
2. People in glass houses should not throw stones.
3. The grass is always greener on the other side of the fence.

   The patient may fail to interpret the proverb, give a concrete interpretation such as "It might break the glass" in response to proverb 2, or make a correct abstract interpretation of the proverb.

   Another way of testing abstract thinking is to ask for similarities and differences. Example: "What is similar about a bicycle and an airplane?"

Vocabulary   The examiner is now in a position to assess the patient's vocabulary, which is one of the best methods of assessing the patient's premorbid intellectual capacity. Patients with progressive dementia tend to retain a premorbid vocabulary, which often gives a false impression of their intellectual abilities. When dementia is suspected, the patient should be asked to give the definition of words presented at increasing levels of difficulty, for example, dog, winter, assemble, reluctant, tangible, and abstruse.

Perception   Perceptual difficulties are often experienced by patients with neurological problems. The following may be encountered:

   1. *Delusion*—a false belief

   2. *Illusion*—a false interpretation of a sensory perception

   3. *Hallucination*—a false sensory perception that does not result from an external stimulus

   4. *Déjà vu phenomenon*—a sudden feeling by the patient that he or she has experienced an event in the past identical to the event that is occurring at the time of the experience (e.g., the patient suddenly has an intense feeling that he or she has been in the ex-

aminer's office in the past, having never done so). The déjà vu phenomenon is not unusual in patients with disease involving the temporal lobes, particularly in partial complex seizures (psychomotor seizures).

Emotional Response   It is not unusual to obtain a history of change in mood when a patient has a neurological problem. In addition, chronic diseases and ill health often result in depression that may be obvious to the examiner. Nevertheless, it is useful to inquire whether there has been a change of mood and to assess this change in terms of depression, elation, irritability, anger, or anxiety. At the same time an estimate of the patient's affect should also be made. *Affect* may be defined as an emotional response to a situation. The response may be appropriate or flat. An example of an inappropriate response would be laughter while discussing an obviously sad situation or spontaneous laughter during the interview, suggesting hypomania or euphoria. A patient who fails to show an appropriate emotional response is said to have inappropriate affect. A patient with flat affect has little or no emotional response. Patients with bilateral damage to the cerebral hemispheres lose finer control of emotional response. Their response may be said to be "all or none." Usually this takes the form of crying in a situation that would normally produce only a mild emotional response. Inappropriate laughing is less frequently encountered. These types of emotional responses are usually associated with pseudo-bulbar palsy, with bilateral spasticity and rigidity indicating damage to both cerebral hemispheres.

Memory   A number of the tests used in the mental status examination evaluate a function mediated through a well-recognized anatomical site in the brain. Abnormalities in a specific test may therefore indicate some abnormality in a focal area of the brain.

Both recent and remote memory depend on the integrity of the hippocampal complex in the temporal lobes. Progressive disease involving the temporal lobes usually results in loss of recent memory with retention of remote memory. Loss of memory for remote events indicates severe involvement of both cerebral hemispheres. The formation of a memory re-

quires the retention of information. The ability to retain information may be tested by asking the patient to remember the names of three objects, two similar and one dissimilar, for a fixed period of time (e.g., 3 min) and then asking the patient to recall the names of those objects. This test should not present any difficulty. If the patient fails to recall the names, an assessment of the deficit of retention and recall can be gauged by presenting the patient with the names of three additional objects, continuing the examination, and then asking the patient to recall the names of the objects after $2\frac{1}{2}$ min. The time scale is reduced progressively by 30 s when the patient fails to answer correctly, until an assessment of the period of time taken to retain and recall the information is obtained. The most severe failure of retention and recall occurs in acute lesions involving the temporal lobes such as *Herpes simplex* encephalitis or Korsakoff psychosis.

Calculation   Recognition and intellectual manipulation of mathematical symbols depend on the integrity of the angular gyrus in the dominant hemisphere. This faculty can be tested by asking the patient to perform simple arithmetic problems such as subtracting seven from 100, then subtracting seven from the result and continuing to do this in serial fashion (reversed serial sevens). If the patient fails to perform serial sevens, the patient should be asked to perform simple addition. Difficulty with subtraction or simple addition is called dyscalculia. Failure to use mathematical symbols constitutes acalculia.

Object Recognition   The individual may recognize an object by use of one or more of the primary senses. Agnosia may be defined as a failure to recognize objects in the presence of adequate primary sensation. A number of agnosias are recognized in clinical practice.

Visual Agnosia   *Visual agnosia* is the failure to recognize an object visually in the presence of adequate vision and suggests that the patient may be suffering from a lesion involving the visual association areas of the brain. In this condition the patient can see the object but cannot recognize or name it. It is possible to exclude nominal aphasia if the patient can name the object by tactile contact. There are a number of subtypes of visual agnosia, including failure to recognize familiar surroundings and failure to maintain orientation in a previously known environment *(visual spatial agnosia).*

Finger Agnosia   *Finger agnosia* is a condition in which the patient shows inability to identify fingers on request (e.g., "Show me your right index finger; now show me your left thumb"). Finger agnosia is often associated with right-left disorientation *(allochiria),* agraphia, and acalculia. These symptoms constitute Gerstmann syndrome and are associated with lesions involving the angular gyrus in the dominant hemisphere.

Autotopagnosia   *Autotopagnosia* is a failure to recognize a body part. The patient with this affliction may fail to recognize his own hand or arm and may readily accept the examiner's hand or arm as a substitute. This condition occurs in lesions of the nondominant parietal lobe.

Anosognosia   *Anosognosia* is denial of disease and is a condition in which the patient will deny loss of function of a body part. The loss of function is usually severe and the patient may, for example, deny paralysis in the presence of an obvious hemiplegia. Anosognosia is a feature of disease of the posterior frontal and parietal lobes of the brain and is more often seen when the lesion involves the nondominant hemisphere.

Tactile Agnosia   *Tactile agnosia* is a condition in which there is failure to recognize an object by palpation in the absence of a primary sensory deficit. The condition is sometimes called *astereognosis* and occurs with lesions involving the nondominant parietal lobe.

Auditory Agnosia   *Auditory agnosia* is a failure to identify the meaning of sounds in the presence of adequate hearing. Auditory agnosia occurs when there is bilateral damage to the primary auditory cortex.

Praxis   *Dyspraxia* may be defined as difficulty or absence (apraxia) of ability to perform a planned motor activity in the absence of paralysis of the muscles normally used in the performance of that act.

A number of dyspraxic states are recognized.

Ideational Apraxia   In this condition the patient is unable to formulate a plan of action. The request to perform the act is clearly understood, but the patient is unable to develop a sequence of activities that will result in the movement necessary to complete the requested action. This condition is said to resemble absentmindedness. The patient is asked to pour water from a jug into a glass and then drink the water from the glass. The patient may fail to pour the water into the glass and attempt to lift the empty glass to his lips or may lift the jug and take a drink of water directly from the jug.

Ideomotor Apraxia   This condition occurs when there is failure to transmit the plan of action and convert the plan into motor movement in the frontal lobes of the brain. Patients with ideomotor apraxia may be unable to close the eyes on request, yet are seen to blink spontaneously; they may be unable to protrude the tongue on request yet tongue movements are adequate in conversation. Patients with ideomotor apraxia have great difficulty in performing simple tasks such as dressing, combing the hair, and using eating utensils.

Motor Apraxia   Motor apraxia is an inability to perform finely coordinated skilled movements in the absence of weakness or paralysis of the involved muscles. This presents as a loss of dexterity in handling small objects, particularly in the performance of rapid finger movements.

Constructional Apraxia   Constructional apraxia is an inability to construct simple models or simple designs, although visual perception and object recognition are intact and there is no apparent paralysis of muscles of the hands. Patients with constructional apraxia cannot copy simple designs or copy simple models with wooden blocks. The condition appears to be a failure of revisualization of the task and occurs in the presence of lesions affecting the visual association areas in the posterior portion of the parietal lobe. Constructional apraxia is often considered indicative of involvement of the visual association areas in the nondominant hemisphere, but it is probable that the condition is more apparent with nondominant hemisphere involvement because of the preservation of language.

Cranial Nerve Examination

The cranial nerve examination should be carried out in an orderly and efficient manner. Table 1-6 lists the cranial nerves, their components, their function, and the clinical findings with lesions. Figures 1-2 and 1-3 illustrate the sensory and motor cranial nerve nuclei and their approximate location in the brainstem.

The First Nerve (Olfactory Nerve)

Anatomy   The peripheral portion of the olfactory system consists of nerve endings that arise from

bipolar cells located in the mucous membrane of the upper portion of the nasal cavity. The central processes of the bipolar cells pass in bundles through the cribriform plate of the ethmoid bone to enter the olfactory bulb on the floor of the anterior cranial fossa. These afferent fibers synapse with the dendrites of the mitral and tufted cells in the olfactory bulb, and the axons of the mitral cells pass through the olfactory bulb and divide into medial and lateral olfactory striae. Fibers in the medial olfactory striae terminate in the paraolfactory area, subcallosal gyrus, and the inferior portion of the cingulate gyrus. Fibers from the lateral olfactory striae enter the gyriform area, which contains the uncus and the anterior portion of the hippocampal gyrus.

The rhinencephalon (olfactory bulbs, olfactory tracts, olfactory striae, and central connections) constitutes one of the phylogenetically oldest portions of

Figure 1-2
Cranial nerve sensory nuclei.

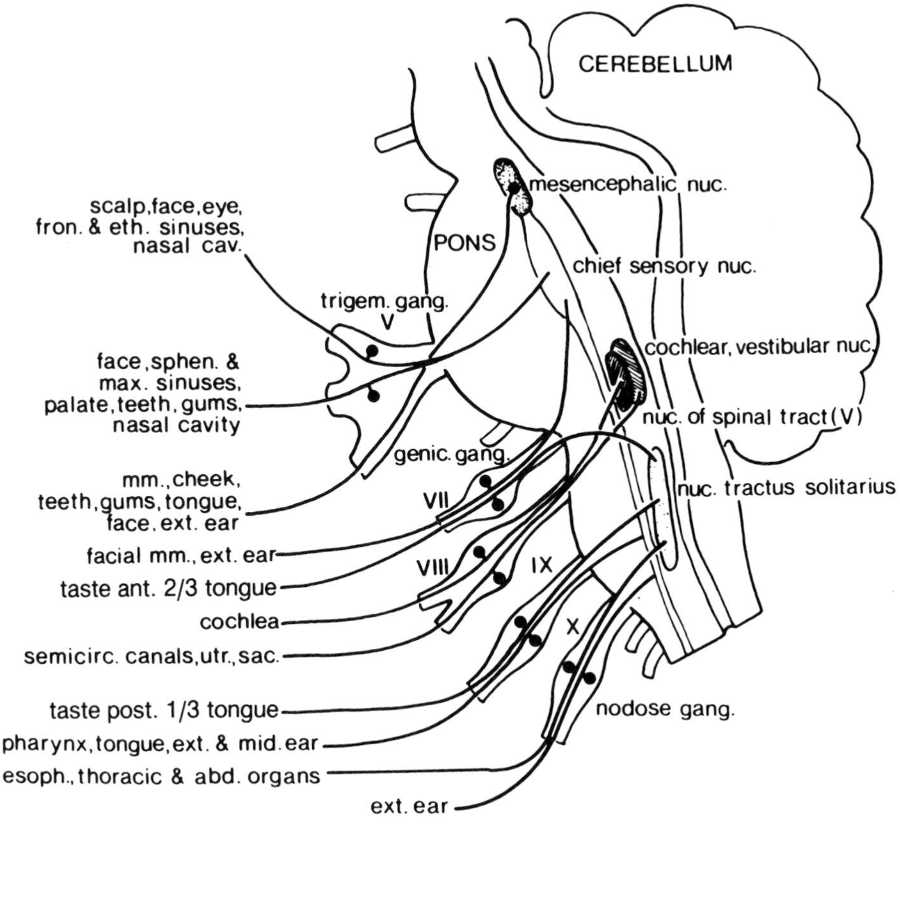

Table 1-6
Components and functions of cranial nerves

Cranial nerve		Component and location	Function	Clinical findings with lesion
Olfactory (I)	SVA	Neurosensory cells of sup. nasal concha and upper ⅓ of nasal septum → bipolar cells of olfactory epithelium → olfactory bulb	Smell	Anosmia
Optic (II)	SSA	Bipolar cells of retina → ganglion cell layer of retina → lateral geniculate → visual cortex	Vision	Amaurosis, anopia
Oculomotor (III)	GSE	Oculomotor nucleus → levator palpebrae; medial, sup., inf. recti; inf. oblique	Eye movements	Diplopia, ptosis
	GVE	Edinger-Westphal nucleus → ciliary and episcleral ganglia to sphincter pupillae and ciliary muscle	Pupillary constriction, accommodation	Mydriasis, loss of accommodation
Trochlear (IV)	GSE	Trochlear nucleus → superior oblique	Eye movement	Diplopia
Trigeminal (V)	GSA	Sensory endings of skin of face, mucous membranes, teeth, orbital contents, supratentorial meninges → trigeminal ganglion → spinal trigeminal and chief sensory nucleus	General sensation	Numbness of face
	GSA	Muscles of mastication and ext. ocular muscles → mesencephalic nucleus	Proprioception	_____
	SVE	Motor nucleus → masseters, temporalis, pterygoids, mylohyoid, tensor tympani, ant. belly digastric	Mastication	Weakness, wasting
Abducens (VI)	GSE	Abducens nucleus → lateral rectus	Eye movement	Diplopia
Facial (VII)	SVA	Taste buds of ant. ⅔ tongue → chorda tympani → geniculate ganglion → rostral tractus solitarius	Taste	Loss of taste ant. ⅔ tongue
	GVA	Sensory receptors of tonsil, soft palate and middle ear to geniculate ganglion → caudal tractus solitarius	General sensation	_____
	GSA	Sensory receptors of ext. auditory meatus and ext. ear → geniculate ganglion → spinal trigeminal nucleus	General sensation	_____

Table 1-6

(Continued)

Cranial nerve		Component and location	Function	Clinical findings with lesion
	GVE	Sup. salivatory nucleus → greater petrosal n. → Sphenopalatine ganglion → maxillary n. → lacrimal gland, nasal and palatal mucosa: chorda tympani to lingual → submandibular post. gang. to submandibular and sublingual glands	Secretion	Dry mouth, loss of lacrimation
	SVE	Motor nucleus → facial muscles, stylohyoid, and post. belly digastric	Facial expression	Paralysis of upper and lower facial muscles
Vestibulocochlear (VIII)	SSA	Hair cells or organ of Corti → bipolar cells of spiral ganglion → dorsal and ventral cochlear nucleus	Hearing	Hearing impairment, tinnitus
	SSA	Hair cells of crista ampullae, semicircular canal and maculae of saccule and utricle → vestibular nuclei and cerebellum	Equilibrium	Vertigo, dysequilibrium, nystagmus
Glossopharyngeal (IX)	SVA	Taste buds post. ⅓ tongue → inf. petrosal ganglion → rostral tractus solitarius	Taste	Loss taste post. ⅓ tongue
	GVA	Sensory receptors of ant. surface epiglottis, root of tongue, border of soft palate, uvula, tonsil, pharynx, eustachian tube, carotid sinus and body → caudal tractus solitarius	General sensation	Anesthesia of pharynx
	GSA	Sensory receptors of middle and external ear → geniculate ganglion → spinal trigeminal nucleus	General sensation	—
	SVE	Nucleus ambiguus → stylopharyngeus	Elev	
	GVE	Inf. salivatory nucleus → tympani nerve to → less petrosal nerve → → auriculotem parotid gland		...rtial dry mouth
Vagus (X)	SVA	Taste buds in re epiglottis → ganglion → solitarius		

(Continued)

Table 1-6
(Continued)

Cranial nerve		Component and location	Function	Clinical findings with lesion
	GVA	Sensory receptors post. surface epiglottis, larynx, trachea, bronchi, esophagus, stomach, small intestine, ascending and transverse colon → inf. (nodose) ganglion → caudal tractus solitarius	General sensation	————
	GSA	Sensory receptors in ext. ear and meatus → sup. (jugular) ganglion → spinal trigeminal nucleus	General sensation	————
	SVE	Nucleus ambiguus → pharyngeal constrictor and intrinsic muscles of larynx, palatal muscles	Deglutition, phonation	Dysphagia, hoarseness, palatal paralysis
	GVE	Dorsal motor nucleus → thoracic and abdominal viscera	Cardiac depress., visceral movement, secretion	————
Spinal accessory (XI)	SVE	Caudal nucleus ambiguus → vagus → muscles of larynx	Phonation	Hoarseness
	GSE	Ant. horn cells C1–C5 → sternocleidomastoid and trapezius	Head and shoulder movement	Weakness, wasting
Hypoglossal (XII)	GSE	Hypoglossal nucleus → muscles of tongue	Tongue movements	Weakness, wasting

GSA, general somatic afferent; GSE, general somatic efferent; GVA, general visceral afferent; GVE, general visceral efferent; SSA, special somatic afferent; SVA, special visceral afferent; SVE, special visceral efferent

[text partially obscured] ... ral hemisphere, and olfaction plays a major ... ctional response of many animals. Con- ... re several anatomic pathways that ... areas of the frontal and tempo- ... mus, thalamus, and brain- ... timuli give rise to auto- ... veloped and often ... t are less essen-

Examination ... tient is asked to ... pa-

nostril occluded as the examiner brings the test substance close to the nonoccluded side. Test substances, which must be nonirritating, include, freshly ground coffee or volatile oil solutions such as oil of lavender, oil of cloves, or oil of lemon. Each nostril is tested separately, and the examiner notes that inhalation is adequate, then requests the patient to identify the test substance. A consistent loss of sense of smell on one side, unilateral anosmia, is usually more significant than a bilateral loss, unless the patient's chief complaint is of sudden total anosmia. Unilateral anosmia is indicative of a lesion involving the olfactory

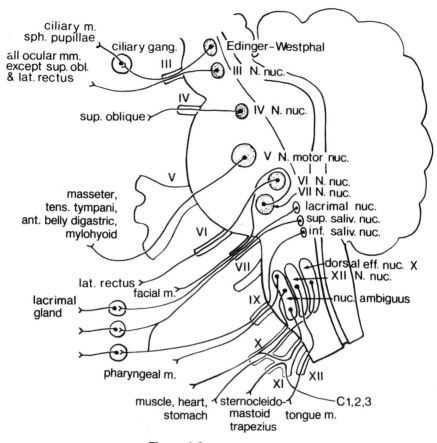

Figure 1-3
Cranial nerve motor nuclei.

nerves, olfactory bulb, or olfactory tract. Central lesions in the hemispheres do not produce anosmia because of the decussation of olfactory fibers in the anterior commissure.

Many neurologists omit tests of olfaction unless the clinical examination is abnormal and indicates that examination for loss of the sense of smell might give a positive result. A unilateral anosmia suggests compression of the olfactory bulb or olfactory tract by a frontal lobe abscess or glioma, olfactory groove meningioma, sphenoid ridge meningioma, and pituitary and parasellar tumors. Tumors may extend posterolaterally to involve the ipsilateral optic nerve causing optic atrophy. The same tumor mass may also cause increased intracranial pressure with pap-

illedema of the opposite optic nerve. The combination of unilateral anosmia with ipsilateral optic atrophy and contralateral papilledema is known as the Foster-Kennedy syndrome.

The Second Nerve (Optic Nerve) and Visual System

Anatomy of the Visual System

RETINA The receptors for visual stimuli are of two types—rods and cones—and are the outer segments of the cells in the outer nuclear cell layer. The rods and cones are specialized photosensitive receptors. The cell bodies of the rods and cones are located in the outer nuclear layer of the retina and the afferent

processes synapse with dendrites of bipolar cells lying in the bipolar cell layer. The bipolar cells in turn
synapse with dendrites of ganglion cells lying in the
ganglion cell layer of the retina. The unmyelinated
axons of the ganglion cells converge in centripetal
fashion in the superficial, nerve fiber layer of the
retina and form the optic nerve.

OPTIC NERVE The optic nerve is situated
slightly to the nasal side of the retina. The fibers that
compose the optic nerve become myelinated as they
pierce the lamina cribrosa of the sclera. The optic
nerve courses caudally and medially, surrounded by a
sheath of dura, arachnoid, and pia. It traverses the optic foramen of the orbit accompanied by the ophthalmic artery and is joined by the central artery of
the retina. The course within the cranial cavity is
short and the optic nerve is closely related to the olfactory tract, internal carotid, and anterior cerebral arteries as it terminates in the optic chiasm.

OPTIC CHIASM The optic chiasm is located superior and slightly anterior to the pituitary fossa, pituitary gland, and infundibulum. The anterior communicating artery lies superior and just anterior to the
optic chiasm, and the lamina terminalis and hypothalamus are immediately superior to the chiasm.

Nerve fibers from the nasal half of each retina
decussate in the optic chiasm and enter the opposite
optic tract. Fibers from the inferior nasal quadrant of
the retina loop forward into the opposite optic nerve
just before they turn into the optic tract (Fig. 1-4).

OPTIC TRACT The optic tract receives fibers
from the temporal half of the ipsilateral retina and the
nasal half of the contralateral retina (see Fig. 1-4).
The optic tract passes posterolaterally around the
cerebral peduncle and terminates in the lateral geniculate body of the thalamus. The infundibulum and tuber cinereum of the hypothalamus lie between the
two optic tracts anteriorly, and each optic tract is
closely related to the posterior communicating and
posterior cerebral arteries.

OPTIC RADIATION The optic radiation arises
from the lateral geniculate body and passes laterally

in the retrolenticular portion of the internal capsule
anterior to the descending portion of the lateral ventricle. Fibers that arise in the medial portion of the
lateral geniculate body, which represent the lower visual fields, pass dorsally along the lateral wall of the
posterior horn of the lateral ventricle and terminate in
the superior lip of the calcarine fissure. Fibers from
the lateral portion of the lateral geniculate body,
which represent the upper visual fields, pass forward
in the roof of the temporal horn of the lateral ventricle. They then loop backward (Meyer's loop) and
pass inferiorly into the parietal lobe in the lateral wall
of the posterior horn of the lateral ventricle and terminate in the inferior lip of the calcarine fissure.

Examination of the Visual System Examination and interpretation of abnormalities of the visual
system can be performed satisfactorily only if the examiner has an adequate knowledge of the anatomy
and physiology of the optic nerve and its peripheral
and central connections. The examination is divided
into three parts:

1. Visual acuity
2. Ophthalmoscopic examination
3. Plotting of visual fields

VISUAL ACUITY The examination of visual acuity involves evaluation of distant vision and near vision.

DISTANT VISION The patient is seated 20 feet
from a well-illuminated Snellen test chart. Each eye is
tested separately, followed by testing of binocular vision. Visual acuity is expressed as a fraction. The nu-
merator is the distance between the patient and the
chart (i.e., 20 feet). The denominator is obtained by
finding the smallest type read without error. The number printed at the side of this type is the maximum
distance at which a person with normal vision can
read the type. Normal vision is usually expressed as
20/20 or as a fraction with denominator below 20,
(i.e., 20/15). Impaired distant vision might be measured as 20/60 when the subject is only able to read
material at 20 feet that a normal individual could read
at 60 feet.

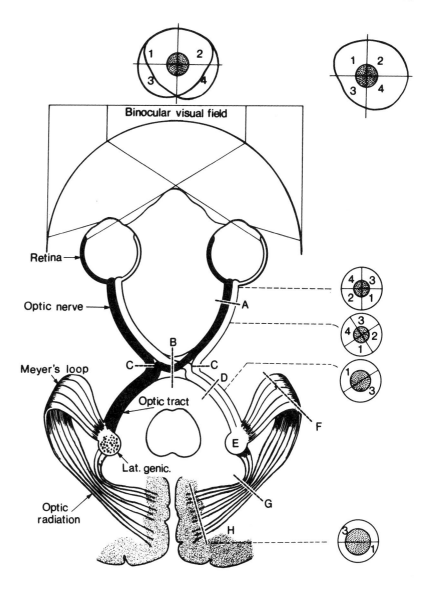

Figure 1-4
Commonly encountered visual field defects and the loci of their corresponding lesions. A, right anopsia; B, bitemporal hemianopia; C, binasal hemianopia; D, left homonymous hemianopia; E, left homonymous hemianopia; F, left homonymous superior quadrantanopia; G, left homonymous inferior or superior homonymous quadrantopia; H, left homonymous hemianopia.

NEAR VISION   The reading card published by the American Medical Association is probably the best of the many test cards available. This card is read at 14 inches from the eyes and gives a measure of near vision expressed in fractional form similar to the Snellen type. The patient should always wear his or her glasses or bifocals when near vision is being evaluated. Impaired visual acuity may occur under the following conditions:

1. A structural lesion involving the cornea, lens, or vitreous humor
2. A refractive error in which the object is not projected or "focused" sharply onto the fovea of the retina
3. A structural lesion involving the visual pathways from the retina to the occipital cortex
4. Conversion (hysterical) reaction (hysterical blindness)
5. One amblyopic eye from an old squint or asymmetrical refractive error.

Determination of the cause of impaired visual acuity requires an adequate ophthalmological and neurological examination. A number of findings suggest the presence of a conversion reaction. These include:

1. Good visual acuity is a function of the fovea and is represented by the central 5° of visual field; a complaint of poor visual acuity without loss of this small central field suggests a conversion reaction.
2. The presence of stereopsis when visual acuity is impaired in one or both eyes suggests a conversion reaction because stereopsis requires good binocular visual acuity.
3. The presence of optokinetic nystagmus in one eye with greatly reduced visual acuity or blindness in that eye is also a feature of a conversion reaction because optokinetic nystagmus depends on appreciation of and accurate pursuit of moving stripes on a rotating drum.
4. The presence of tubular (cylindric) fields in patients who demonstrate no difficulty in ambulation is strongly suggestive of a conversion reaction.

OPHTHALMOSCOPIC EXAMINATION The patient is asked to fix the gaze on a distant object at approximately eye level. The examiner focuses the light from the ophthalmoscope onto the cornea using a 10+ lens and examines the cornea for abrasions or opacities. The aqueous humor, iris, lens, vitreous humor, and retina are then examined by interposing lenses of decreasing power between the light source and the patient's eye. When a clear outline of the retina is obtained, the examiner evaluates the optic nerve head, the blood vessels, and the retina.

The optic nerve head or optic disc is a yellowish white structure situated slightly to the nasal side of the optic axis. The temporal margin of the disc is clearly outlined in the majority of cases but may be blurred in myopic subjects. The nasal margin is often indistinct, but this finding is of no significance. The optic disc contains a smaller, whitish, eccentric depression known as the optic cup, where the central retinal artery enters and the retinal veins leave the optic nerve. Careful examination will reveal venous pulsation in the majority of cases. Venous pulsation is present in about 80 percent of individuals and is indicative of normal intracranial pressure (ICP). Conversely, absence of venous pulsation does not invariably indicate increased ICP. Occasionally the optic cup is enlarged and occupies most of the surface of the optic disc. Because the cup has a whiter appearance, enlargement may lead to a spurious impression of optic atrophy.

PAPILLEDEMA *Papilledema* is defined as edema of the optic disc. The pathogenesis of papilledema is uncertain but is believed to be the result of increased ICP, venous stasis, and lymphatic stasis. The rate of development depends on the degree of increased ICP or venous stasis and the consistency of elevated ICP. There are two forms of papilledema—noninflammatory and inflammatory.

In *noninflammatory papilledema* the patient may report transient 5- to 10-s episodes of grayness or blackouts of vision. Sudden standing or excitement may precipitate these visual difficulties. Chronic papilledema may eventually result in blindness. Symptoms of increased ICP such as headache, nausea and vomiting, sixth nerve palsies, or alteration of consciousness may be present. Noninflammatory papilledema is characterized on ophthalmologic examination by cylindric elevation of the nerve head, obliteration of the disc margins, hyperemia of the disc, venous distention, absence of venous pulsations, loss of optic cup, and the appearance of concentric ripples of the retina on the temporal side of the disc (Paton's lines) (Fig. 1-5). Noninflammatory papilledema may be difficult to distinguish in its early stages of development. Hemorrhages associated with papilledema due to increased ICP are usually located in the peripapillary area; hemorrhages that occur in papilledema due to hypertension are widespread and accompanied by hypertensive retinopathy. Examination of the visual fields in noninflammatory papilledema usually reveals enlargement of the blind spot and constriction of peripheral visual fields. Noninflammatory papilledema may be seen with mass lesions of the intracranial cavity (e.g., tumor, abscess, or subdural hematoma), in subarachnoid hemorrhage, in various infectious diseases, and in metabolic conditions (e.g., hypertension, anemia, emphysema, and benign intracranial hypertension [pseudo-tumor cerebri, otitic hydrocephalus]).

Inflammatory papilledema (optic neuritis) (Fig. 1-6) is characterized by sudden unilateral amaurosis, ocular pain, particularly on eye movement, and palpable globe tenderness. Ophthalmologic examination

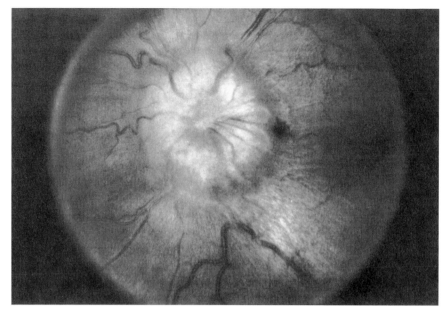

Figure 1-5
Papilledema.

may reveal findings similar to those of noninflammatory papilledema plus inflammatory cells in the vitreous. The elevation of the nerve head may appear more gradual rather than cylindric. Examination of the visual fields may reveal a central, paracentral, or cecocentral scotoma of the involved eye. An afferent pupil defect is likely to be present. Optic neuritis is a frequent occurrence in demyelinating diseases, particularly multiple sclerosis. It may also be seen when an infection involves the nerve (e.g., meningitis, encephalitis), in metabolic diseases (e.g., diabetes mellitus, thyroid dysfunction, vitamin B_1 or B_{12} deficiency), in toxic conditions (e.g., methylalcohol poisoning), and in vascular disorders (e.g., giant cell [temporal] arteritis).

RETROBULBAR NEURITIS *Retrobulbar neuritis* is a form of inflammatory edema of the optic nerve in which the edema remains confined to the retrobulbar portion of the optic nerve and does not extend into the optic nerve head. The clinical features are those of optic neuritis, but the optic disc has a normal ophthalmologic appearance.

OPTIC ATROPHY *Optic atrophy* is defined as pallor of the optic disc due to demyelination and axonal degeneration of the optic nerve. Primary optic atrophy occurs without evidence of preceding papilledema. The disc typically appears uniformly white with a clearly outlined margin. Secondary optic atrophy follows papilledema and the disc is white, but the margins are grayish and indistinct.

Optic atrophy may occur in hereditary cerebral degenerations, for example, cerebral lipidoses, metachromatic leukodystrophy, and Leber's optic atrophy. It may follow inflammatory or noninflammatory papilledema, or it may be associated with compressive lesions of the nerve, trauma, glaucoma, vascular disorders, or exposure to toxins.

EXAMINATION OF THE VISUAL FIELDS The method used in office practice or at the bedside is called *confrontation* and compares the examiner's field of vision with that of the patient. The patient should be seated facing the examiner at eye level. The patient is instructed to look at the examiner's nose and the examiner looks at the patient's nose.

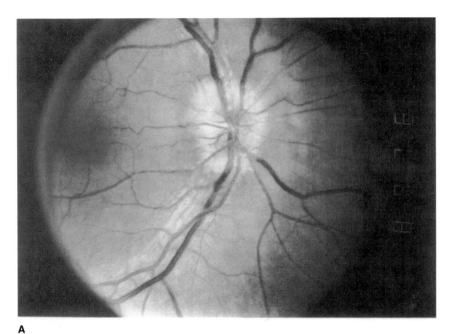

A

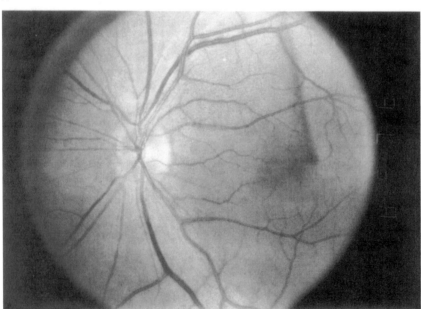

B

Figure 1-6
A. *Optic neuritis. There was retrobulbar pain on eye movement. Visual acuity 20/80.*
B. *Normal opposite fundus and disc.*

The examiner extends his arms to each side in a position roughly midway between patient and examiner so that the fingers are beyond the periphery of the examiner's visual field. The patient is instructed to indicate when he sees the examiner's finger move, and the examiner begins to rhythmically move his right index finger and at the same time advances it slowly toward the center of his own visual field. The patient with a normal peripheral visual field will indicate that the moving finger is visible at the same time as it appears at the periphery of the examiner's visual field. The process is then repeated with the left index finger. The test should be carried out in the following order: patient's left upper quadrant, right upper quadrant, left lower quadrant, and right lower quadrant. The examiner then brings his fingers to the periphery of the midfield (equivalent to three o'clock and nine o'clock) and moves both index fingers simultaneously. The movement (bilateral simultaneous stimulation) should be appreciated in the right and left visual fields by the patient. Failure to appreciate movement of one finger in an intact visual field on bilateral simultaneous stimulation is termed *visual extinction* (Fig. 1-7). This

phenomenon occurs in the presence of an early lesion of the opposite parietal lobe that has not developed sufficiently to produce a homonymous visual field defect.

Testing of binocular visual fields should be followed by testing of the visual fields in each eye. This is accomplished by asking the patient to close one eye or cover one eye with a hand. The examiner closes the opposite eye and instructs the patient to gaze into the examiner's open eye. The examiner then maps the periphery of the visual fields for each eye using the method previously described.

The following abnormalities may be observed during the examination of the visual fields:

1. Immediately after the examiner has instructed the patient to look at the examiner's nose and has extended his arms laterally, the patient moves his gaze from the examiner's nose to the hand on one side. This suggests the presence of a homonymous hemianopia on the side opposite to the patient's eye movement.

2. The patient changes his gaze from the examiner's nose to the moving finger on either side

Figure 1-7
Visual fields by confrontation. Bilateral simultaneous stimulation.

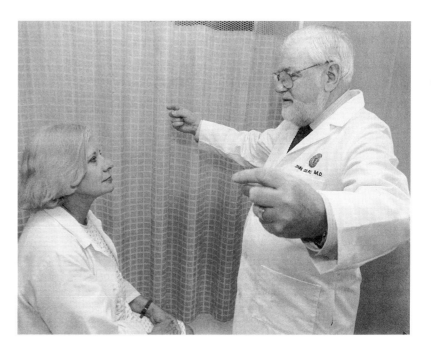

despite repeated instructions to continue looking at the examiner's nose. This condition is called impersistence and represents an inability to maintain gaze on a designated object when another stimulus enters the visual field. Impersistence suggests the presence of degenerative disease of the brain.

3. The visual fields appear to be intact by confrontation when binocular testing is performed. However, a partial superior temporal quadrantanopsia is observed on one side only when the eyes are tested individually. This defect would not be apparent unless the eyes were tested individually because the intact field on one side compensates for the partial loss of the temporal field on the other side. The reason for this partial visual field loss is illustrated in Figure 1-4.

TESTING FOR SCOTOMATA Patients with inflammatory papilledema, retrobulbar neuritis, or optic atrophy may develop scotomata. These scotomata may be central, involving the central portion of the visual field; paracentral, involving an area near the central field; or cecocentral, involving the central portion of the visual field and extending to the blind spot.

Scotomata are usually detected by using a tangent screen, but it is possible to test for the presence of a scotoma in the office. The patient is instructed to maintain a steady gaze into the pupil of the examiner's eye. The examiner brings a small white object, such as the head of a corsage pin, from the periphery across the visual field, moving steadily from the temporal to the nasal side (Fig. 1-8). Under normal conditions the patient and examiner will observe that the object disappears momentarily in the physiological blind spot but remains clearly visible in the central area of the field. However, the patient will report that the object disappears again if there is a central or paracentral field defect. The boundaries of the scotoma can be defined by bringing the object from the periphery in vertical diagonal and horizontal planes. Scotomata are usually larger when measured with colored objects, particularly red objects.

The Third, Fourth, and Sixth Nerves (Oculomotor, Trochlear, and Abducens)

Anatomy   The motor fibers of the third nerve supply extraocular muscles, which control eye move-

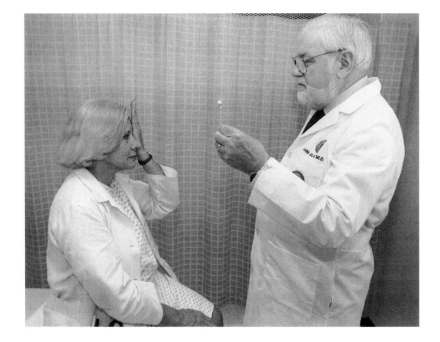

Figure 1-8
Testing for central or paracentral scotoma.

ment, and instrinsic muscles, which control accommodation and pupilloconstriction.

The third nerve arises from a compound nucleus located in the midbrain immediately ventral to the cerebral aqueduct. The fibers pass through the tegmentum of the midbrain and emerge as a series of rootlets in the sulcus oculomotorius on the medial aspect of the cerebral peduncle. The rootlets unite to form the oculomotor nerve, which passes between the posterior cerebral artery and the superior cerebellar artery to enter the lateral wall of the cavernous sinus. The oculomotor nerve is situated immediately above the fourth, fifth, and sixth nerves in the lateral wall of the cavernous sinus and emerges anteriorly to enter the orbit through the superior orbital fissure. At this point the nerve divides into a superior branch, which supplies the levator palpebrae and the superior rectus, and an inferior branch, which supplies the medial rectus, inferior rectus, and inferior oblique muscles. The inferior branch also contains the parasympathetic fibers, which have their origin in the most superior portion of the third nerve nucleus (Edinger-Westphal nucleus). These fibers synapse in the ciliary ganglion, and a series of postganglionic fibers pass through several short ciliary nerves to supply the ciliary and sphincter pupillae muscles of the eye.

The nucleus of the fourth nerve lies ventral to the cerebral aqueduct in the midbrain at the level of the inferior colliculus. Fibers emerging from the nucleus pass dorsally and decussate in the anterior medullary velum immediately below the inferior colliculus on the dorsal surface of the midbrain. The trochlear nerve then passes ventrally around the cerebral peduncle and pierces the dura to enter the lateral wall of the cavernous sinus. The nerve passes through the superior orbital fissure to innervate the superior oblique muscle.

The sixth nerve arises from the abducens nucleus, which lies in the dorsal pons ventral to the floor of the fourth ventricle. The nerve has an anteroventral course through the pons and emerges close to the midline at the junction of the pons and medulla. There is a relatively long course in the posterior fossa where the nerve is in contact with the ventral surface of the pons. The nerve crosses the apex of the petrous temporal bone and enters the lateral wall of the cavernous sinus to lie below and me-

dial to the third and fourth cranial nerves and ophthalmic and maxillary divisions of the fifth cranial nerve and lateral to the internal carotid artery. The sixth nerve then enters the orbit through the superior orbital fissure and supplies the lateral rectus muscle.

Pupillary Reflexes

TYPES There are three pupillary reflexes: the light reflex, near-vision reflex, and reflex dilatation.

LIGHT REFLEX The afferent pathway for the pupillary light reflex is activated by light, which stimulates the rods and cones in the retina. The afferent pathway passes via the optic nerve with partial decussation in the optic chiasm and then continues bilaterally through both optic tracts and the brachium of the superior colliculi to the pretectal region of the midbrain. From the pretectal region the fibers pass forward close to the aqueduct to enter the Edinger-Westphal nucleus on the same side or pass through the posterior commissure to enter the nucleus on the opposite side. The efferent side of the reflex is completed by fibers that pass from the neurons in the Edinger-Westphal nucleus through the oculomotor nerve to the ciliary ganglion, and thereafter by short ciliary nerves to the constrictor muscles of the iris.

NEAR-VISION REFLEX Afferent impulses for the pupillary constrictor reflex for near vision are transmitted through the visual pathway to the visual cortex. Impulses then pass from cortical neurons through the corticotectal tract to synapse with neurons in the pretectal area of the midbrain. The connections from the pretectal area to the Edinger-Westphal nucleus on either side pass ventrally to the fibers for the pupillary light reflex to reach the Edinger-Westphal nucleus. The remainder of the efferent pathway for the near-vision reflex is similar to that for the pupillary light reflex.

PUPILLARY DILATATION Almost any emotional or sensory stimulus (with the exception of light and near vision) may produce pupillary dilatation in man. One well-known example is the ciliospinal reflex in which there is pupillary dilatation on pinching the skin on the side of the neck. The pupillary dilatation reflex is probably mediated through the posterior hypothalamus with activation of sympathetic fibers, which pass down through the brainstem to the superior cervical ganglion and via the carotid plexus to the radially arranged dilator muscle fibers of the iris. The reflex activity also includes a simultaneous inhibition of the Edinger-Westphal nucleus through hypothalamic connections via the reticular activating system to the Edinger-Westphal nucleus in the midbrain.

EXAMINATION OF PUPIL In the majority of cases, the pupils will appear to be equal, round, and centrally placed in relation to the cornea. It is not unusual to see some mild inequality of pupils, "anisocoria," and observation will show that this difference in size may fluctuate over a relatively short period of time.

The pupillary light reflex is tested by flashing a bright light into each eye and quickly swinging the light between the two eyes. Under normal conditions there is an immediate constriction of the pupil in the eye stimulated by light and an immediate constriction of the pupil on the other side (consensual response). When the light is swung to the other side, the pupil dilates momentarily and then constricts when the stimulus is perceived. Occasionally there may be a sustained dilatation followed by delayed constriction after the light is directed into the eye. This suggests some delay in the afferent pathway of the light reflex and is commonly seen in optic neuritis, retrobulbar neuritis, and optic atrophy. This delay in pupillary constriction on stimulation, erroneously called the Marcus-Gunn phenomenon, is often present in multiple sclerosis. The Marcus-Gunn sign consists of a pupillary reaction to light with failure to sustain the reaction and a slow dilatation of the pupil, a phenomenon seen in optic neuritis, optic atrophy, or retrobulbar neuritis.

It is not unusual to see a brisk pupillary constriction to the light stimulus, followed by rhythmic relaxation and contraction of the iris. This condition, which is called *hippus,* is a normal response and is also said to be more common in multiple sclerosis and in barbiturate poisoning.

ABNORMALITIES OF PUPILLARY LIGHT REFLEX
The pupillary reaction to light may be absent or impaired if there is a lesion involving the reflex pathway at any site. These include:

1. Failure of light to reach the retina—local diseases of the eye (e.g., vitreous opacities, as in diabetes), cataract
2. Diseases of the retina—retinitis pigmentosa, macular hemorrhage or scar
3. Diseases of the optic nerve—severe inflammatory papilledema, retrobulbar neuritis, optic atrophy
4. Diseases involving the optic tracts and the connections to the midbrain
5. Diseases of the midbrain
6. Diseases involving the third nerve or ciliary ganglion

ARGYLL ROBERTSON PUPIL The Argyll Robertson pupil is said to occur when there is impairment or failure of the pupils to react to light but preservation of reaction to near vision. It should be noted that the classical description of the Argyll Robertson pupil, as an irregular miotic pupil that fails to react to light, is only a partial description of this abnormality. In fact, the Argyll Robertson pupil may be present when:

1. The pupil shows absence of response to light with preservation of constriction to near vision.
2. The pupil shows some response to light, but this response is reduced and is much less than the pupillary response to near vision.
3. In early cases the pupil may be normal in size because the development of miosis is a late feature of the Argyll Robertson pupil.
4. The pupils are often round, and it is only later when they become scarred by synechiae and atrophy from inflammatory iris disease that they appear irregular and unequal.

The Argyll Robertson pupil is the result of a lesion involving fibers that pass from the pretectal area of the midbrain to the Edinger-Westphal nucleus. However, only the rostrally placed fibers subserving the light reflex are involved, while the more caudally located fibers responsible for the near-vision reflex are unaffected. The Argyll Robertson pupil was first described in neurosyphilis, in which neuronal destruction and gliosis occurred in the periaqueductal area of the midbrain with destruction of fibers involved in the light reflex. Consequently, the Argyll Robertson pupil is a feature of tabes dorsalis, general paresis, and meningovascular syphilis. Other causes of the Argyll Robertson pupil are rare and include viral encephalitis, Wernicke encephalopathy, cerebrovascular disease and infarction of the midbrain, multiple sclerosis with demyelination of the midbrain, and neoplasm involving the rostral midbrain. This pupillary abnormality may also be seen in advanced cases of chronic degenerative diseases involving the central nervous system, including Alzheimer disease, spinocerebellar degeneration, and hereditary neuropathy with liability to pressure palsy.

SPASTIC MIOTIC PUPIL   This condition can be regarded as a variant of the Argyll Robertson pupil. In the spastic miotic pupil the reaction to light and to near vision is poor or absent. This condition indicates the presence of a lesion in the midbrain involving nerve fibers serving both light and near vision.

LESIONS OF THE THIRD NERVE   Pupillary constrictor fibers form an outer sheath on the third nerve and surround the inner core of nerve fibers, which supply the extraocular muscles. Therefore, pressure on the third nerve will produce pupillary dilatation, which may occur before paralysis of extraocular movement. This is commonly seen:

1. When the third nerve is stretched over the free edge of the tentorium cerebelli during herniation of the medial aspect of the temporal lobe
2. When the third nerve is compressed by a mass such as a posterior communicating artery aneurysm

LESIONS OF THE CILIARY GANGLION: THE TONIC PUPIL (HOLMES-ADIE OR ADIE SYNDROME)   Injury to the cells of the ciliary ganglion or to the short ciliary nerves may result in denervation of the pupil. The subsequent reinnervation from surviving ganglion cells is such that the majority of regenerating nerve fibers reach the ciliary muscle. This leaves the iris relatively denervated and produces a condition known as the tonic pupil. The condition is usually unilateral. The pupil is large and fails to contract, or shows a

very slow, delayed contraction to light and to near vision. In each case the pupil contracts slowly and then remains small for some time before returning to normal size with an equally slow movement. The tonic pupil is exquisitely sensitive to local application of 0.125% fresh solution of pilocarpine with prompt constriction. A similar application would not affect a normal pupil.

Disorders of Eye Movement   Eye movements are tested by asking the patient to look to the right, look to the left, look upward, and look downward. The patient is then instructed to follow a moving object, which is moved by the examiner in the same fashion.

Three types of eye movement disorder can be recognized. The patient may have a disturbance of conjugate eye movements, nystagmus, or paralysis of individual extraocular muscles.

CONJUGATE EYE MOVEMENTS   Fibers arising in the frontal cortex, the occipital cortex, the vestibular system, and the cerebellum converge in the pons and terminate in the paramedian pontine reticular formation (PPRF). The PPRF is the center for coordinating nerve impulses concerned with conjugate gaze. Fibers from the PPRF pass to the ipsilateral abducens nucleus and terminate on neurons in that nucleus. The abducens nucleus gives rise to fibers that enter the sixth nerve and terminate in the lateral rectus muscle. A second pathway from the abducens nucleus enters the contralateral medial longitudinal fasciculus and terminates in the oculomotor nucleus. Abnormalities of conjugate eye movement include:

1. Conjugate deviation of the eyes at rest. This may be due to:
   a. A destructive lesion involving one hemisphere. This produces conjugate deviation of the eyes toward the side of the destructive lesion. A destructive lesion produces imbalance of cortical activity transmitted to the PPRF, and conjugate movement is influenced only by the intact hemisphere with deviation of the eyes toward the destructive lesion.
   b. An irritative lesion involving one hemisphere. This results in deviation of the eyes away from the side of the irritative lesion. In this case the irritative influ-

ence is stronger than the normal activity generated in the opposite hemisphere.
   c. A destructive lesion in the brainstem below the decussation of the corticobulbar fibers. This produces deviation of the eyes away from the side of the lesion.
   d. An irritative lesion of the frontal lobe. This results in conjugate vertical deviation of the eyes. Prolonged tonic deviation of the eyes in an upward direction, "oculogyric crisis," has been described in postencephalitic parkinsonism.
2. Dysconjugate deviation of the eyes at rest. This may be the result of:
   a. A destructive lesion of one oculomotor nucleus or oculomotor nerve. This results in outward deviation of the eye on the affected side due to unopposed activity of the abducens nerve and the lateral rectus muscle.
   b. Destruction of one abducens nucleus or abducens nerve. This results in inward deviation of the eye on the affected side due to the unopposed activity of the oculomotor nerve and medial rectus muscle.
   c. A destructive lesion involving the tectooculomotor pathway on one side. This produces vertical deviation of the eye on the opposite side.
   d. A destructive lesion involving the medial longitudinal fasciculus on one side in the pons. This lesion results in skew deviation of the eyes with one eye elevated and the other eye depressed.

VOLUNTARY CONJUGATE EYE MOVEMENTS   Abnormalities of voluntary conjugate eye movements may be due to:

1. Disease of one frontal lobe. This causes paralysis of voluntary conjugate gaze to one side. There is an inability to direct the gaze away from the side of the lesion on command.
2. Diffuse disease involving both hemispheres. This results in impairment of smooth pursuit conjugate eye movements. These are replaced by coarse, interrupted, conjugate saccadic movements and occur when the patient attempts to follow a moving object in a horizontal plane.
3. Diffuse degenerative processes involving both hemispheres. This may result in ocular impersistence. The patient cannot sustain gaze on an object once movement of it ceases.
4. Bilateral involvement of corticobulbar tracts, which enter the brainstem at the level of the midbrain. This can

produce loss of gaze in any direction on command or in following a moving object. Initial impairment is usually in upward gaze.

Reflex conjugate eye movements occur:

1. In response to a moving visual stimulus
2. In response to tonic neck and vestibular reflexes in the absence of a visual stimulus

In reflex conjugate eye movements, which depend on the integrity of the visual cortex, afferent stimuli are received in the primary visual cortex, which is located on the upper and lower borders of the calcarine fissure, and are then transmitted to the visual association areas. The visual association areas project to the brainstem via internal corticotectal fibers, which pass to the tectum of the midbrain, and via corticotegmental fibers, which pass through the pons and terminate in the PPRF.

Abnormalities can occur when there are:

1. Lesions involving the internal corticotectal pathway or tectooculomotor connections in the midbrain. This results in impairment of upward gaze. The most common cause of this phenomenon is compression of the middle of the superior colliculi by a pineal tumor resulting in loss of upward gaze (Parinaud syndrome).
2. Lesions involving the pons. This produces paralysis of reflex conjugate horizontal gaze. This commonly occurs in multiple sclerosis infarction and tumors of the pons, which impair the function of the PPRF and its immediate connections.

In the absence of visual stimulation, reflex mechanisms, such as tonic neck reflexes and vestibular reflexes, can produce reflex conjugate eye movements. These movements can be elicited in unconscious patients in the absence of visual stimuli. When the head is turned in one direction reflex conjugate movement of the eyes occurs in the opposite direction. These movements have been termed *doll's-eye movements*. Reflex conjugate eye movements are impaired or lost in bilateral destructive lesions of the brainstem, which interrupt impulses from cortical and subcortical structures that inhibit input from the vestibular nuclei to the third, fourth, and sixth nerve nuclei. Consequently, loss of doll's-eye movements is usually an indication of bilateral pontine dysfunction.

NYSTAGMUS Nystagmus is an involuntary rhythmic movement of the eyes, which may be present at rest or occur with eye movement. In the latter case it persists for an interval after eye movement has ceased. Nystagmus may be bilateral or unilateral, although unilateral nystagmus is rare.

Nystagmus may result from imbalance of coordinated reflex activity involving the labyrinth, vestibular nuclei, cerebellum, medial longitudinal fasciculus, or nuclei of the third, fourth, and sixth nerves. It may also occur from remote influences that affect this reflex system. These include disease of the retina; disease of the third, fourth, and sixth cranial nerves; and disease of the cervical cord. Drugs may also act as a remote influence on the central reflex mechanism and produce nystagmus. Nystagmus may be horizontal, vertical, oblique, or rotatory (clockwise to the right, counterclockwise to the left) in nature. Nystagmus may be pendular or jerk.

PENDULAR NYSTAGMUS This is characterized by a regular to-and-fro movement of the eyes in which both phases are equal in duration. In jerk nystagmus one phase of eye movement is faster than the other. Jerk nystagmus may result from loss of central vision. Pendular nystagmus occurs in:

1. Spasmus nutans. Spasmus nutans is a benign condition that appears in infants between 3 and 8 months of age and lasts months to years. The onset is thought to be related to a viral illness. It is characterized by pendular nystagmus, usually horizontal, occasionally vertical, and often monocular; rhythmic head nodding, usually up and down; and head tilting.

2. Patients with defective vision since birth. Infants with congenital cataracts, central corneal opacities, or chorioretinitis may develop pendular nystagmus, which is coarse, slow, and usually horizontal.

3. Occupational nystagmus. Miners' nystagmus occurs in individuals who work in poorly illuminated surroundings. Rods are required for vision under these conditions, and there are no rods in the macula. Consequently, there is constant movement of the eye in an attempt to project the image on more peripheral parts of the retina.

4. Congenital nystagmus. Congenital nystagmus is inherited as an autosomal dominant or sex-linked recessive trait. It appears at birth, persists throughout life, and is occasionally accompanied by titubation of the head. On deviation of the eyes it may become jerk in nature.

JERK NYSTAGMUS   This occurs in:

1. Optokinetic nystagmus. Optokinetic nystagmus is a normal physiological response to a series of objects moving in the same direction across the visual field. The eyes follow one object to the edge of the visual field, then rapidly return to the central fixation point to focus the next object. Optokinetic nystagmus can be produced by rotation of a drum with alternating vertical black and white stripes before the patient's eyes. There is a slow movement in the direction of the movement of the drum with a quick return in the opposite direction. Testing is usually carried out in a horizontal or vertical plane but can be carried out in any direction of gaze. Optokinetic nystagmus is a reflex phenomenon dependent on the integrity of the cortical visual pathways. It may be absent or reduced in deep parietal lobe lesions and infrequently in temporal and frontal lobe lesions.

2. Vestibular nystagmus. Vestibular nystagmus is the result of asymmetric impulses from the semicircular canals. It is independent of visual stimuli and is inhibited by fixation. It may be elicited by rotation in a Barany chair, by caloric irrigation of the external auditory canals, or by galvanic stimulation of the labyrinth or vestibular nerve. Abnormal occurrence of vestibular nystagmus may occur when there is disease of the labyrinth, such as labyrinthitis, hemorrhage, or hydrops (Ménière disease). Peripheral disease is usually associated with spontaneous nystagmus (horizontal and rotary) and is accompanied by vertigo. When the brainstem is involved, the spontaneous nystagmus may be horizontal, rotary, or vertical, and vertigo is not a prominent feature. Rotary nystagmus is characteristic of vestibular nystagmus.

3. Nystagmus of neuromuscular origin. This occurs with:

a. Fatigue. It is not unusual to see irregular jerking movements of the eyes on extreme lateral gaze during fatigue. This is of no significance.
b. Paresis. Contraction of paretic extraocular muscle will produce irregular nystagmoid movements. This condition can occur in myopathies, in myasthenia gravis, and in partial lesions of the oculomotor nerves.

4. Cerebellar nystagmus. Although cerebellar nystagmus can occur with lesions involving the cerebellum, the majority of cases are due to involvement of cerebellar connections in the brainstem including the vestibular nuclei, vestibular cerebellar tracts, cerebellar pathways in the brainstem, and medial longitudinal fasciculus. The nystagmus is horizontal and more pronounced on looking to the side of the lesion.

5. Nystagmus due to lesions of the medial longitudinal fasciculus.

a. The nystagmus of internuclear ophthalmoplegia is described below.
b. Nystagmus occurs with involvement of the medial longitudinal fasciculus in any portion of the brainstem and also occurs with involvement of the medial longitudinal fasciculus in the upper portion of the cervical cord by demyelinization in multiple sclerosis or by an intramedullary tumor.

6. Miscellaneous forms of nystagmus. These include:

a. Drug-induced nystagmus. Many drugs can cause nystagmus, the most common being barbiturates and phenytoin. Other causes include alcohol, nonbarbiturate sedatives, and quinine. This is typically a horizontal nystagmus.
b. Seesaw nystagmus. Seesaw nystagmus is a rare condition usually associated with a parasellar lesion such as a craniopharyngioma. It is characterized by a seesaw displacement of the eyes in the horizontal plane with intorsion of the globe on depression and extorsion on elevation.
c. Retraction convergence nystagmus. This is a rare type of nystagmus associated with tectal and pretectal lesions of the midbrain. The eyes jerk back into the orbits with simultaneous adduction of both eyes. The optokinetic drum is an excellent way of eliciting this condition.
d. Vertical nystagmus. Vertical nystagmus that occurs when the eyes are in the primary position is indicative of a le-

sion involving the anterior vermis of the cerebellum or medulla. Vertical nystagmus that occurs on downward gaze is found with lesions of the cervical medullary junctions such as basilar impression or the Arnold-Chiari malformation.
e. Ocular bobbing. Ocular bobbing consists of brisk, downward conjugate movements of both eyes followed by a slow return to position of rest, and occurs in destructive lesions of the caudal pons and cerebellar hemorrhage.
f. Ocular flutter. Ocular flutter, consisting of rapid, rhythmical eye movements of decreasing amplitude when the eyes fix on an object, is characteristic of cerebellar disease, and is a form of ocular dysmetria.
g. Irregular jerking of one eye in the presence of coma. This can occur in lateral vertical, or rotary form and is indicative of severe destructive lesions involving the pons.
h. Opsoclonus. Opsoclonus consists of totally random clonic conjugate movements of the eyes in any direction and occurs in diffuse bilateral brainstem disease.

PARALYSIS OF EXTRAOCULAR MUSCLES Actions of the extraocular muscles are illustrated in Figure 1-9 and outlined in Table 1-7. The eye findings in individual muscle paralysis are listed in Table 1-8. There are several rules for determining the cause of diplopia and determining paralysis of extraocular muscles:

1. Diplopia will be present at rest and there will be an apparent ocular deviation at rest when one or more of the extraocular muscles is paralyzed on one side.
2. Diplopia will increase when gaze is attempted in the direction of pull of the paralyzed muscle.
3. The ocular deviation will increase when the eyes are moved in the direction of action of the paralyzed muscle.
4. When the paretic eye attempts to look at any object in the field of action of the paralyzed muscle, there is overaction or secondary deviation of the sound eye. Central neuronal discharges are enhanced in this situation, and because of reciprocal innervation a stronger impulse is received by the nonparalyzed muscles producing reciprocal movement of the eye. The secondary deviation is always greater than primary deviation in paralytic squint, whereas the deviation remains the same in all directions of gaze in nonparalytic or concomitant squint.
5. When an attempt is made to fix an object on the macula in the direction of pull of the paralyzed muscle, the image is projected onto the retina outside of the macular

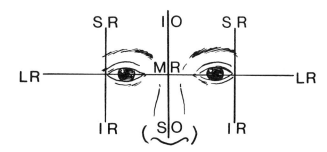

Figure 1-9
Clinical actions of the extraocular muscles.

area. This produces a false projection of the image, incorrect localization, and past pointing by the patient.

6. If the affected eye is occluded, then the occlusion quickly removed, the eye will have deviated in the direction opposite to the pull of the paretic muscle.

7. If the sound eye is occluded and the affected eye is made to fix on an object in the direction of pull of a paretic muscle, the sound eye will seem to deviate excessively in the same direction (secondary deviation) when the occlusion is removed.

SUMMARY OF DISORDERS OF EYE MOVEMENT SEEN WITH PONTINE LESIONS These include:

1. Lesions of the sixth nerve in the pons produce internal strabismus at rest due to paralysis of the lateral rectus muscle, diplopia at rest, and increased diplopia on attempted gaze toward the side of the lesion.

2. Destruction of the sixth nerve nucleus produces all of #1 and in addition is usually associated with seventh nerve paralysis on the same side because of close association of seventh nerve to the sixth nerve nucleus in the pons.

3. Lesion of the medial longitudinal fasciculus in the pons produces double vision or oscillopsia. The patient is unable to adduct the eye on the side of the lesion because of paralysis of the connections to the medial rectus muscle. In addition, there is nystagmus of the abducting eye, which is occasionally accompanied by slight skew deviation. In midbrain lesions there is an additional failure of convergence (anterior internuclear ophthalmoplegia), whereas in pontine lesions (posterior internuclear ophthalmoplegia) the ability to converge the eyes is maintained. Bilateral internuclear ophthalmoplegia occurs most frequently in multiple sclerosis.

Table 1-7
Clinical actions of extraocular muscles

Muscle	Cranial nerve	Action
Medial rectus	III	Adduction
Superior rectus	III	Elevates when eye abducted
Inferior oblique	III	Elevates when eye adducted
Inferior rectus	III	Depresses when eye abducted
Superior oblique	IV	Depresses when eye adducted
Lateral rectus	VI	Abduction
Levator palpebrae	III	Elevates upper lid
Müller's muscle	Sympathetic	Elevates upper lid
Orbicularis oculi	VII	Closure of eyelids

The Fifth Nerve (Trigeminal Nerve) The trigeminal nerve supplies sensation to the face, the buccal and nasal mucosa, sinuses, contents of the orbit, teeth, gums, and part of the scalp. The motor root supplies the muscles of mastication.

Anatomy The trigeminal (gasserian) ganglion is located on the floor of the middle fossa and contains the unipolar cells subserving touch, pain, and temperature sensation. The peripheral fibers leaving the ganglion enter the three major subdivisions of the trigeminal nerve, the ophthalmic, maxillary, and mandibular nerves. The proximal fibers enter the lateral pons at the junction of the pons and middle cerebellar peduncle. Fibers that carry discriminatory touch information ascend and synapse in the chief sensory nucleus of the trigeminal complex. The mesencephalic nucleus contains the cells of origin subserving proprioception.

Table 1-8

Eye findings in cases of individual muscle paralysis

Paralyzed muscle	Upper lid	Eye at rest	Movements	Images	Head
Superior rectus	Ptosis	Normal position	Limited elevation particularly on abduction	Oblique, false above true—diplopia increases on attempted elevation and abduction	
Inferior oblique	Normal	Normal position	Limited elevation when eye adducted	Oblique, false above and lateral to true—diplopia increases on attempted elevation and adduction	
Medial rectus	Normal	Abducted	Limited adduction	Crossed, parallel, diplopia increasing on attempted adduction	
Inferior rectus	Normal	Normal position	Limited depression particularly on abduction	Oblique, false image below and medial to true image—diplopia increases on attempted depression and abduction	
Superior oblique	Normal	Normal position	Limited depression when eye adducted	Oblique, false image below and lateral to true—diplopia increases on attempted depression and adduction	Head tilted toward sound side
Lateral rectus	Normal	Adducted	Limited abduction	Parallel, uncrossed—diplopia increases on attempted abduction and distance vision	Head turned toward affected side

The peripheral fibers are located in the maxillary division and carry proprioceptive information from the muscles of mastication. Fibers that carry pain, temperature, and crude touch descend and synapse in the nucleus of the spinal tract of the trigeminal nerve, which extends to the upper cervical portion of the spinal cord. The nucleus of the tract is divided into three portions: the oralis, which extends from the midpons to olive; the interpolaris, which extends from the olive to the pyramidal decussation; and the caudalis, which extends from the decussation to the C2 level. Axons carrying pain information synapse in the caudalis, while axons carrying temperature information synapse in all three portions. Fibers carrying crude touch information synapse in the oralis and interpolaris. Fibers from the mandibular portion of the nerve are most dorsal in the tract; fibers from the ophthalmic portion are most ventral. The maxillary fibers occupy an intermediate position. The dorsal trigeminothalamic tract arises from the chief sensory nucleus, contains crossed and uncrossed fibers, and ascends to the posteromedial ventral nucleus of the thalamus. Tertiary neurons send fibers through the posterior limb of the internal capsule to the lower one-third to one-half of the postcentral gyrus. Fibers arising in the spinal nucleus decussate and form the ventral trigeminothalamic tract, which ascends in the medial aspect of the medial lemniscus to synapse in the posteromedial ventral nucleus of the thalamus. Pain, temperature, and crude touch sensations are then relayed through the posterior limbs of the internal capsule to the postcentral portion of the parietal lobe.

The motor neurons of the motor nucleus of the trigeminal nerve lie in the midpons, central and slightly medial to the chief sensory nucleus. Axons of the motor neurons pass in the motor portion of the trigeminal nerve to exit from the pons and pass beneath the trigeminal ganglion to join the mandibular division.

The three divisions of the trigeminal nerve are distributed as follows:

1. The ophthalmic division passes along the lateral wall of the cavernous sinus, enters the orbit through the superior orbital fissure, and divides into a number of branches which supply the frontal and ethmoid sinuses, the conjunctiva, cornea, upper lid, bridge of nose, forehead, and the scalp posteriorly as far as the vertex of the skull.

2. The maxillary division enters the lateral wall of the cavernous sinus and leaves the middle cranial fossa through the foramen rotundum to enter the sphenomaxillary fossa. The nerve enters the orbit through the inferior orbital fissure, passes through the floor of the orbit in the inferior orbital canal, and emerges below the orbit through the inferior orbital foramen. The maxillary division supplies sensation to the skin of the cheek, the sphenoid and maxillary sinuses, the lateral aspect of the nose, the upper teeth, and the mucous membrane covering the nasal pharynx, hard palate, uvula, and inferior part of the nasal cavity.

3. The mandibular division leaves the middle cranial fossa through the foramen ovale accompanied by the motor branch of the trigeminal nerve. Sensory fibers are distributed to the skin over the chin and lower jaw, extending as far back as the pinna of the ear; the anterior portion of the external auditory meatus; the anterior two-thirds of the tongue; the lower teeth; the gums and floor of the mouth; and the buccal surface of the cheek. The motor fibers supply the muscles of mastication, tensor tympani, anterior belly of the digastric, and mylohyoid.

Examination of the Trigeminal Nerve Examination of the trigeminal nerve includes evaluation of the corneal reflex, sensation over the face and scalp, motor function, and the jaw jerk.

CORNEAL REFLEX This reflex is tested by the light application of cotton to the cornea. The examiner takes a cotton applicator and pulls the cotton head into a fine point. The patient is asked to look upward, and the cotton is brought toward the eye from a lateral position and gently applied to the cornea (Fig. 1-10). Application should produce a prompt bilateral reflex closure of the eyelids. The response is compared on the two sides, and the patient is asked whether the sensation appears to be equal on the two sides. The afferent loop of this reflex is via the ophthalmic division of the trigeminal nerve. The efferent side of the reflex is conducted through the facial nerve.

SENSATION OVER THE FACE AND SCALP The patient is asked to close the eyes and to respond if touched. The cotton is applied to the forehead on one side, followed by application to the forehead in a similar position on the other side, then to the cheeks on the two sides, then to the jaws on the two sides. The patient's responses are monitored, and the patient is asked whether the sensation appears to be equal on the two sides of the face. The same test is then repeated using a sharp pin with gentle application in the ophthalmic, maxillary, and mandibular area, alternating between the two sides. The examiner then touches each cheek simultaneously with a sharp pin (Fig. 1-11) and asks the patient to identify the site of pinpricks. The correct answer—both sides. There may be failure of appreciation of pinprick on one side even though the patient has appreciated pinprick when

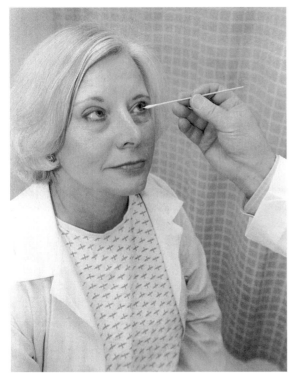

Figure 1-10
Testing the corneal reflex.

applied unilaterally to the face. The phenomenon termed extinction occurs occasionally in early lesions affecting the opposite parietal lobe or the thalamo-parietal connections.

MOTOR FUNCTION The examiner places the fingers over the temporalis muscles and asks the patient to clench the teeth or bite. The temporalis muscles will be felt to contract under the examiner's hands on both sides. A similar maneuver is performed with the fingers over the masseter muscles (Fig. 1-12). The pterygoids can be tested by having the patient deviate the jaw to one side against resistance. In unilateral lesions the jaw deviates toward the side of the lesion.

JAW JERK The jaw jerk is tested by lightly tapping the anterior, lower jaw with the reflex hammer (Fig. 1-13). Normally, there is a slight upward movement of the mandible. The jaw jerk is increased in destructive or compressive lesions involving the corticopontine pathways and is discussed in more detail below.

Figure 1-11
Bilateral simultaneous stimulation of the face.

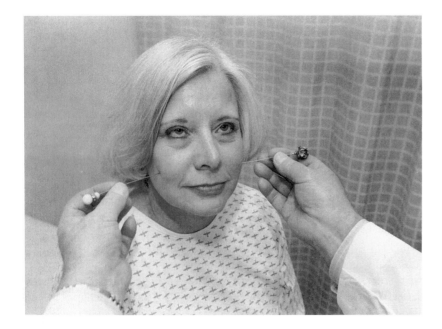

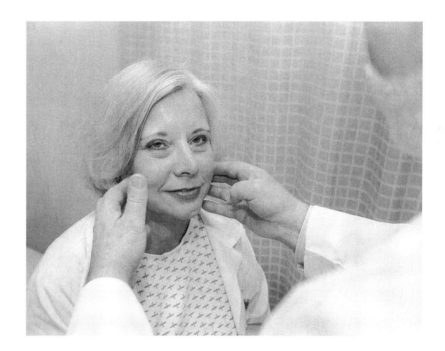

Figure 1-12
Examination for contraction of masseter muscles. Patient is asked to clench teeth.

Figure 1-13
The jaw jerk. Patient is asked to open the mouth partially. Examiner places index finger on the chin and taps finger lightly with reflex hammer.

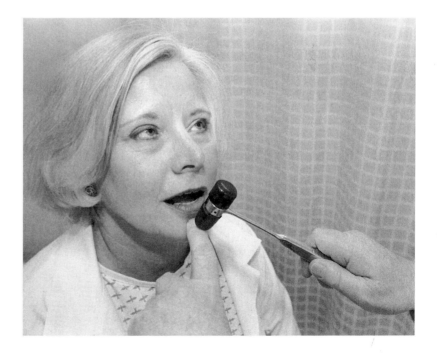

The Seventh Nerve (Facial Nerve) The seventh nerve innervates the facial muscles and supplies taste sensation to the anterior two-thirds of the tongue and general sensation to a small portion of the external ear.

Anatomy The motor neurons of the seventh nerve are located in the facial nucleus in the tegmentum of the pons. The motor fibers pass dorsally and medially from the nucleus, loop around the nucleus of the sixth cranial nerve, and then proceed in a ventro-lateral and caudal direction to emerge at the lateral pontomedullary junction. The facial nerve immediately enters the internal auditory meatus in association with the eighth cranial nerve. The seventh nerve leaves the internal auditory canal, enters the facial canal, and passes through the facial canal to emerge through the stylomastoid foramen at the inferior border of the temporal bone. The nerve then penetrates the parotid gland and divides into several branches, which supply the muscles of the face, the stylohyoid, the buccinator, the posterior belly of the digastric muscle, and the platysma. The facial nerve also gives off a branch to the stapedius muscle in the facial canal.

The facial nerve carries parasympathetic motor fibers that arise from the superior salivatory nucleus in the pons. These fibers leave the facial nerve via the greater superficial petrosal nerve and pass to the sphenopalatine ganglion. The postganglionic fibers innervate the glands and mucous membranes of the palate, nasopharynx, and paranasal sinuses. The remaining parasympathetic fibers leave the facial nerve via the chorda tympani and terminate in the submaxillary ganglion. Postganglionic fibers innervate the sublingual and submaxillary salivary glands.

The sensory neurons of the seventh nerve are located in the geniculate ganglion, which is situated in the proximal portion of the facial canal. The peripheral branches of these nerve cells transmit taste sensation from the anterior two-thirds of the tongue and reach the geniculate ganglion via the lingual nerve, chorda tympani, and a short portion of the facial nerve. The central branches pass from the geniculate ganglion, form a separate bundle called the nerve of Wrisberg, enter the pons, and terminate in the nucleus of the tractus solitarius.

The facial nerve has a relatively small general somatic sensory component. These sensory fibers supply sensation to a small portion of the external ear, and the impulses are transmitted to the unipolar cells in the geniculate ganglion and through the facial nerve into the pons.

Examination of the Facial Nerve The patient is asked to contract the facial muscles and show the teeth. The contraction should be symmetrical on the two sides and simultaneously performed. The patient is then asked to close the eyes tightly and the examiner attempts to open the lids (Fig. 1-14). Normally this is not possible even when the examiner uses considerable force. Finally, the patient is asked to wrinkle the forehead in an upward direction. Again, this should be symmetrical on the two sides.

Two types of facial weakness may be observed:

1. Upper motor neuron lesions involving the corticobulbar pathways will produce weakness of the lower portion of the face with normal function when the patient is asked to wrinkle the forehead. The lower portion of the face has unilateral innervation from cortical centers, while the forehead is bilaterally innervated from cortical centers.

2. Involvement of the facial nucleus in the pons or the facial nerve will produce total involvement of the facial muscles on the same side, and the lower facial muscles and forehead are equally involved in the process.

There are three forms of taste sensation: sweet, sour, and bitter. The sense of taste is tested by placing a test substance, sugar (sweet), vinegar (sour), or quinine (bitter), on the tongue. The test is best conducted by asking the patient to protrude the tongue, exposing one side. The side of the tongue is then dried and the test substance that has been prepared in solution is gently applied with a cotton applicator. The patient signals when the test substance is identified and can then draw the tongue back into the mouth and verbally identify the solution.

The Eighth Nerve (Acoustic Nerve) The eighth nerve, or acoustic nerve, is a compound nerve

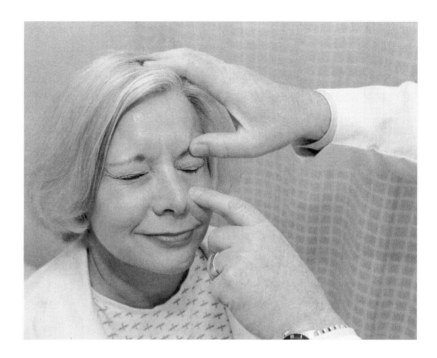

Figure 1-14
Testing for weakness of facial muscles—orbicularis oculi— patient is asked to close the eyes tightly, and examiner attempts to open the eyelids.

with two divisions: the cochlear, subserving hearing, and the vestibular, subserving motion, balance, and an awareness of position in space.

Anatomy

THE COCHLEAR NERVE The ganglion cells in the spiral ganglia of the cochlea have short peripheral and long central processes. The peripheral processes terminate around the hair cells of the organ of Corti, while the central processes pass to the cochlear nuclei in the brainstem. The cochlear nerve and the vestibular nerve form a common trunk, the acoustic nerve, which is closely related to the facial nerve in the internal auditory meatus. The two divisions of the acoustic nerve separate, and the cochlear nerve enters the brainstem lateral to the vestibular nerve at the junction of the pons and medulla. On entering the pons, the cochlear nerve divides, and fibers synapse in the dorsal and ventral cochlear nuclei.

Axons from cells in the ventral cochlear nucleus enter the trapezoid body and pass to the contralateral lateral lemniscus and medial longitudinal

fasciculus and to the ipsilateral superior olivary nucleus and then to the medial longitudinal fasciculus and the nucleus of the sixth cranial nerve.

Axons from neurons in the dorsal cochlear nucleus cross the midline immediately below the fourth ventricle and enter the contralateral lateral lemniscus. The lateral lemniscus is a multisynaptic pathway, and the fibers within the structure may synapse as they pass through the pons and lower midbrain and ascend to the inferior colliculus. Several commissural connections cross between the two lateral lemnisci. The inferior colliculus is a relay station in the auditory pathway, which may also be concerned with the interpretation of sound stimuli. Consequently, the majority of fibers from the lateral lemniscus enter and synapse with cells in the inferior colliculus, while a few fibers bypass the inferior colliculus and enter the brachium of the medial geniculate to terminate in neurons within this latter structure. Fibers arising from neurons in the inferior colliculus also terminate in the medial geniculate body.

The axons of neurons within the medial geniculate body form the auditory radiation, which passes through the sublenticular portion of the posterior limb of the internal capsule to the superior transverse temporal gyri. These structures constitute the primary auditory reception areas of the cerebral cortex and are located on the opercular surface of the superior temporal gyrus.

THE VESTIBULAR NERVE The vestibular ganglion is attached to the vestibular nerve and is situated just within the internal auditory meatus. The ganglion contains bipolar cells with peripheral processes distributed to the maculae of the utricle and saccule and to the ampullae of the superior, lateral, and posterior semicircular canals. The central processes form the vestibular nerve, which accompanies the cochlear nerve and enters the brainstem. The vestibular nerve then passes dorsomedially between the inferior cerebellar peduncle and the spinal tract of the fifth cranial nerve to reach the vestibular nuclei. The vestibular nuclei consist of four separate structures: the medial vestibular nucleus, which extends from mid medulla to the inferior pons forming the vestibular area of the fourth ventricle; the lateral vestibular nucleus, which extends from the medulla, caudally, to the level of the sixth cranial nerve in the pons; the inferior (spinal) vestibular nucleus, located almost entirely within the medulla; and the superior vestibular nucleus, which is situated in the floor of the fourth ventricle and extends through the pons into the lower portion of the midbrain.

Efferent fibers from the vestibular nuclei pass to the medial longitudinal fasciculus, which brings the vestibular system into communication with other cranial nerve nuclei. Other fibers enter the pontine reticular formation or descend into the upper spinal cord to communicate with motor neurons. There are additional connections to the cerebellum and an ascending fiber system, which takes an unknown course and terminates in the temporal cortex in the posterior aspects of the superior temporal gyrus.

Tests of Auditory Function Testing for hearing at the bedside is inaccurate. Audiograms should be obtained in all cases where there is doubt about the patient's ability to hear properly.

Conduction tests are useful, however, because in the normal state, air conduction is much more sen-

sitive than bone conduction. Testing is carried out by placing a tuning fork over the mastoid process and asking the patient to indicate when the sound is no longer audible (Fig. 1-15). At this point the fork is placed at the level of the external auditory meatus and the patient is asked whether the sound is audible. Under normal circumstances this will be so, because air conduction is better than bone conduction. This test, the *Rinné* test, is said to be positive when air conduction is more sensitive than bone conduction. In conditions where bone conduction is more sensitive than air conduction, the Rinné test is negative. This indicates some obstruction of transmission of sound by disease involving the external auditory meatus, such as foreign bodies or wax, some malfunction of the drum, or some malfunction of the middle ear. Diseases of the cochlea or cochlear nerve produce impairment of hearing, and both air and bone conduction are diminished, but the Rinné test remains positive.

The examination continues with the performance of the *Weber test*, in which the tuning fork is placed on the center of the forehead and the patient is asked to indicate the location of the sound (Fig. 1-16). This will usually be heard equally in both ears or appreciated at the site of the tuning fork on the forehead. When there is impairment of air conduction on one side, the Weber lateralizes to that ear. On the other hand, if there is disease of the cochlea or cochlear nerve, the Weber will lateralize to the side opposite the diseased ear.

Test of Vestibular Function The vestibular system is an extremely sensitive system, and disturbances of function of the vestibular system or the vestibular division of the eighth nerve are accompanied by vertigo. *Vertigo* is a sensation of movement in which objects seem to be moving in a rotating fashion around the subject or when the subject has an illusion of rotation. Occasionally vertigo may present with an illusion of tilting of objects in a horizontal or vertical plane without a rotary component. Vertigo is always accompanied by nystagmus because of the connections between the vestibular system and third, fourth, and sixth nerves via the medial longitudinal fasciculus. This anatomical pathway can be tested as follows.

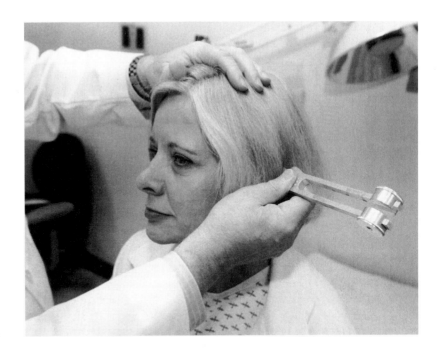

Figure 1-15
The Rinné test.

BARANY TEST Labyrinthine nystagmus may be induced by rotating the subject in a Barany chair. The patient's eyes are closed and the head is inclined forward 30° to test the lateral semicircular canal, or extended backward 60° to test the anterior canal. Under these circumstances, the canal to be tested is in the horizontal plane. The chair is then rotated 10 times in 20 s, which produces stimulation of the cristae in the

Figure 1-16
The Weber test.

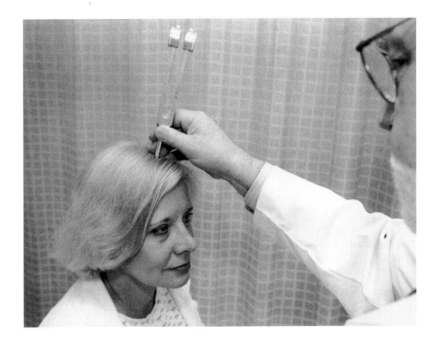

canal. When the movement of the chair is stopped, the inertia of the endolymph continues to stimulate the cristae, producing a sensation of vertigo in the direction opposite to the previous rotation of the chair. This is accompanied by nystagmus, past-pointing, and deviation of the eyes in the direction of the previous rotation. The sensation of vertigo usually lasts about 35 s under normal circumstances. Vertigo is reduced in disease of the stimulated canal or vestibular nerve. The vertigo may be increased in certain conditions that produce dysfunction of the vestibular system.

CALORIC TESTING Caloric testing can be performed by tilting the head of a supine patient forward 30° and irrigating the external auditory canal of one side with 10 to 15 mL of iced water or warm water for 30 s. The larger volume should be used in testing comatose individuals for presence or absence of brainstem function. The effect of caloric stimulation is reduced in disease of the external auditory canal, the vestibular apparatus or the vestibular nerve, and the central connections.

The Ninth Nerve (Glossopharyngeal Nerve)
This nerve supplies motor fibers to the stylopharyngeus muscle; sensation to the pharynx, tonsillar fossa, posterior third of the tongue, ear canal, and tympanic membrane; secretomotor fibers to the parotid gland; and taste sensation to the posterior third of the tongue.

Anatomy Motor fibers to the stylopharyngeus muscle arise from a rostral extension of the nucleus ambiguus in the upper medulla. Secretomotor fibers arise from the inferior salivatory nucleus in the medulla.

Both motor and secretomotor fibers leave the medulla in the groove between the inferior olive and the inferior cerebellar peduncle in a series of rootlets lying rostral to the rootlets of the vagus nerve. The rootlets unite to form the glossopharyngeal nerve, which passes from the skull through the jugular foramen. The nerve descends between the internal jugular vein and the internal carotid artery, crosses the styloid process, enters the pharynx between the middle and inferior constrictors, and is distributed to the pharyn-

geal structures. The majority of the secretomotor fibers leave the glossopharyngeal nerve as it emerges from the jugular foramen and form the tympanic nerve, which passes into the middle ear to join the tympanic plexus. The lesser superficial petrosal nerve arises from the tympanic plexus and passes to the otic ganglion. Postganglionic fibers from the otic ganglion enter the auricular temporal branch of the fifth cranial nerve and are distributed to the parotid gland.

Fibers that carry sensation from the pharynx, tonsils, and posterior third of the tongue arise from neurons in the petrosal ganglion, which is situated in the jugular foramen. The central fibers enter the brainstem and terminate in the nucleus of the tractus solitarius. Taste sensation from the posterior one-third of the tongue is transmitted by neurons in the petrosal ganglion, which have central fibers terminating in the nucleus of the tractus solitarius in the brainstem.

The glossopharyngeal nerve also carries impulses from the carotid sinus and the carotid body. The fibers arise from ganglion cells in the petrosal ganglion and enter the nucleus solitarius.

Examination of the Glossopharyngeal Nerve
Examination of the glossopharyngeal nerve includes evaluation of:

1. Taste sensation. The taste sensation of the posterior third of the tongue is tested in the same manner as taste over the anterior two-thirds of the tongue.
2. Gag reflex. The glossopharyngeal nerve forms the afferent loop of the gag reflex, which can be tested by stimulation of the pharyngeal wall. The efferent part of this reflex is served by the vagus nerve.

The Tenth Nerve (Vagus Nerve)
The vagus nerve supplies autonomic fibers to viscera of the thorax and abdomen, motor fibers to the pharynx and larynx, sensation to viscera of the thorax and abdomen, and sensation to the external ear and dura of the posterior fossa.

Anatomy Autonomic (parasympathetic) fibers arise from neurons in the dorsal nucleus of the vagus, which lies immediately beneath the floor of the fourth ventricle in the dorsal medulla. The fibers pass between the nucleus ambiguus and tractus solitarius and emerge in the ventral medulla between the inferior olive and inferior cerebellar peduncle. The emerging fibers form a series of rootlets, which unite to form the vagus nerve, which leaves the skull through the jugular foramen. The vagus nerve then passes between the carotid artery and internal jugular vein to the root of the neck and enters the thorax. The vagus nerves supply branches to the heart, bronchi, and esophagus in the chest and to all of the abdominal viscera.

Motor fibers to the pharynx and larynx arise from neurons in the nucleus ambiguus, which extends through the whole length of the medulla. The fibers form a dorsal loop, then turn ventrally and laterally to join with other fibers of the vagus complex and emerge as a series of rootlets on the ventral surface of the medulla. The motor fibers are distributed to:

1. The pharynx through a series of pharyngeal branches, which supply the muscles of the pharynx and soft palate
2. The inferior constrictor of the pharynx and cricothyroid muscle through the superior laryngeal nerve
3. The intrinsic muscles of the larynx except the cricothyroideus through the recurrent laryngeal nerve. The recurrent laryngeal nerve arises from the vagus nerve at the level of the anterior aspect of the subclavian artery on the right side and at the level of the aortic arch on the left side. Both nerves wind around the vessels and ascend between the esophagus and the trachea to enter the larynx.

Sensory fibers arising in the viscera have cell bodies located in the inferior ganglion. The peripheral processes are distributed with the vagus nerve to thoracic and abdominal viscera. The central processes terminate in the tractus solitarius.

Cutaneous sensation fibers arise from neurons situated in the superior jugular ganglion. The peripheral processes are distributed to the external auditory meatus, the skin on the back of the auricle, and the dura of the posterior fossa. The central processes join the spinal tract of the fifth cranial nerve in the medulla.

Examination of the Vagus

CHANGES IN SPEECH Paralysis of the vagus nerve or its branches may give rise to dysphonia or dysarthria.

Dysphonia may be defined as difficulty in phonation and occurs when there is paralysis of the larynx or vocal cords due to a lesion of one or both recurrent laryngeal nerves. The voice is hoarse and the volume reduced. Bilateral recurrent laryngeal paralysis produces stridor due to unrestricted activity of the cricothyroid muscles, causing the partially paralyzed cords to lie close to the midline.

Dysarthria, or difficulty in articulation, has many causes, but unilateral or bilateral vagal paralysis results in weakness of the soft palate and imparts a nasal quality to the voice.

EXAMINATION OF THE SOFT PALATE The patient is asked to open the mouth and say "Ah." Under normal circumstances the soft palate elevates symmetrically and the uvula remains in the midline. Unilateral vagal paralysis results in a failure of palatal movement on one side. The palate does not elevate on the affected side, and the uvula is drawn to the opposite side by the contraction and arching of the palate on the nonaffected side.

DYSPHAGIA Dysphagia, or difficulty in swallowing, occurs when vagal nerve paralysis produces weakness of the pharyngeal muscles. This weakness can be demonstrated during phonation as the pharynx fails to contract.

The Eleventh Nerve (Accessory Nerve) The accessory nerve is a purely motor nerve supplying the sternocleidomastoid and trapezius muscles.

Anatomy The motor neurons of the accessory nerve lie in the intermediate column of gray matter in the upper five segments of the cervical cord. Fibers that emerge from these motor neurons pass dorsolaterally and emerge midway between the anterior and posterior roots and unite to form an ascending trunk, which passes through the foramen magnum into the posterior fossa. The spinal portion of the accessory nerve then joins the bulbar accessory nerve, which is the lowest portion of the vagus nerve, and leaves the posterior fossa through the jugular foramen. The bulbar portion then joins the vagus nerve while the spinal portion descends in the neck to terminate in the sternocleidomastoid and trapezius muscles on the same side.

Evidence suggests that the motor neurons in the upper cervical cord supplying the sternocleidomastoid and trapezius muscles have a segmental distribution, the more rostral cells supplying the sternocleidomastoid and the caudal neurons supplying the trapezius.

Examination of the Accessory Nerve The sternocleidomastoid is examined by asking the patient to turn the head to one side against resistance by the examiner's hand. The belly of the sternocleidomastoid can be felt to contract firmly if the examiner palpates the opposite side of the neck (Fig. 1-17). The trapezius is tested by the examiner placing both hands on the patient's shoulders and palpating the muscle on each side between the thumb and forefinger. The patient is then asked to elevate the shoulders against the examiner's resistance; equal contraction of the trapezius should occur on the two sides.

The Twelfth Nerve (Hypoglossal Nerve) The
hypoglossal nerve is a purely motor nerve that supplies motor fibers to the muscles of the tongue.

Anatomy The motor neurons are contained in the hypoglossal nucleus, which lies in the dorsal and inferior portion of the medulla immediately below the floor of the lateral ventricle. The nerve passes ventrally through the substance of the medulla to emerge between the medullary pyramid and the inferior olive as a series of rootlets, which unite to form the hypoglossal nerve. The nerve leaves the posterior fossa through the anterior condyloid foramen and traverses the neck to terminate in a series of branches, which supply the ipsilateral muscles of the tongue.

Examination of the Tongue The tongue should be inspected with the mouth open and the tongue lying quietly on the floor of the mouth. This is the only way to see involuntary movements, particularly fasciculations, because the protruded tongue always has some involuntary movement. The tongue should also be inspected for asymmetry indicating wasting and scarring. The latter condition is not infrequent in a patient with a generalized seizure disorder. The examiner then places a wooden tongue blade edged upward in the midline, immediately below the lower lip, and the patient is asked to protrude the tongue. Under normal circumstances the tongue is

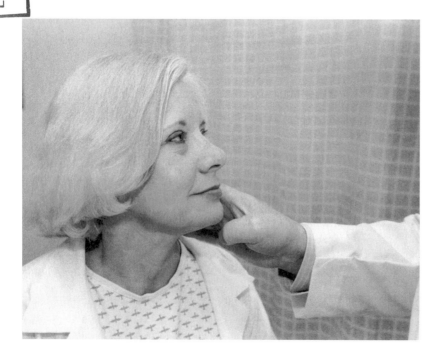

Figure 1-17
Contraction of the sternocleidomastoid muscle. Patient turns head to one side against resistance.

protruded and lies symmetrically on the edge of the tongue blade (Fig. 1-18). This method allows the examiner to detect slight deviations of the tongue that otherwise might not be noticeable if the patient is simply allowed to protrude the tongue without a clear indication of the midline. The paralyzed tongue deviates toward the side of a lower motor neuron lesion.

When the tongue is protruded, the examiner should take the opportunity to examine the tongue more closely for the presence of scars and the state of the mucous membrane. Glossitis is not unusual in patients suffering from vitamin deficiency. An atrophic membrane can occur in long-standing pernicious anemia due to vitamin B_{12} deficiency.

The examiner then removes the tongue blade, and the patient is asked to move the tongue back and forth in rhythmic fashion as rapidly as possible. Rapid alternating movements of the tongue should be smoothly performed and rhythmic in character. Slowing or dysrhythmia can occur in the presence of weakness and in cerebellar dysfunction. Cerebellar difficulties can also be recognized by asking the patient to repeat syllables such as "mi-mi-mi" or "la-la-la." Again, this should be performed rhythmically, without any irregularity.

The remainder of the neurological examination consists of evaluation of the motor system, coordination, gait and station, sensation, and reflexes. In the ambulatory patient it is most convenient to evaluate the upper extremities completely, and then evaluate the gait and station and lower limbs.

Examination of Motor Function

The examination of motor function begins by inspection. The examiner stands in front of the patient who is seated and suitably clothed to expose the upper limbs, shoulders, and lower limbs. The contours and muscle development of the two sides should be equal. It is important to observe the limbs from the front and sides and to walk behind the patient and inspect all muscle groups. During this inspection, which is primarily directed toward the detection of muscle wasting, the presence of muscle fasciculations or involuntary movements of the limbs should be noted.

Muscle tone is tested by passively moving the joints and comparing the two sides. The examiner quickly learns to appreciate the smooth sensations of normal tone, and experience permits the detection of even a slight increase in tone when it is present. Pal-

Figure 1-18
Deviation of the tongue. The tongue blade is placed in the midline; the patient is asked to protrude the tongue.

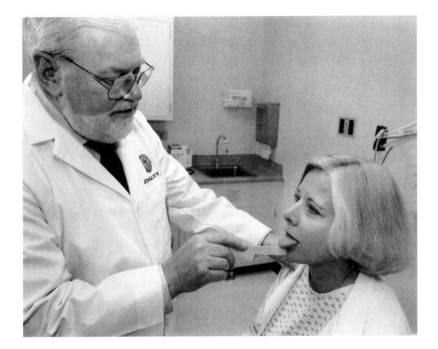

pation of the proximal muscle with one hand during passive movement will detect the presence of cogwheeling, which is a ratchety jerkiness associated with extrapyramidal disease. In the lower extremities, the examiner should grasp the foot and perform several passive dorsiflexion and plantar flexion movements followed by sudden forced dorsiflexion of the foot. The presence of involuntary rhythmic dorsiflexion/plantar flexion movements is termed ankle clonus and occurs only in the presence of increased tone. Ankle clonus is occasionally present in healthy athletic individuals but is not sustained. The presence of sustained clonus or unilateral clonus with absence on the other side is abnormal.

Strength is tested by asking the patient to contract a muscle group against resistance applied by the examiner. It is important to compare the two sides. As a minimum the examiner should evaluate: abduction, arm at 70°, testing deltoid muscle contraction and avoiding contribution from the trapezius muscle which occurs at 90°; flexion and extension, forearm; flexion and extension, wrist; grip; flexion and extension, thigh; flexion and extension, leg; dorsi and plantar flexion, foot; inversion and eversion, foot; extension, great toe (Fig. 1-19); flexion, toes. A more

detailed evaluation is indicated when the history suggests the presence of a spinal cord or peripheral nerve lesion (Table 1-9).

The differentiation of lower motor neuron lesions from upper motor neuron lesions is listed in Table 1-10.

Muscle strength can be graded on a scale of 0 to 5: 5, normal strength; 4, slight weakness; 3, marked weakness; 2, ability to contract against gravity; and 0, total paralysis.

Examination of Coordination

While cerebellar dysfunction is often the source of impaired coordination, other factors including muscle weakness, lack of sensory (proprioceptive) input, and dyspraxia can affect coordination. The cerebellum, located in the posterior cranial fossa, coordinates muscle movement and maintains body equilibrium and muscle tone. The main anatomical divisions of the cerebellum consist of two large lateral hemispheres, an anterior lobe, and a flocculonodular lobe. There are connections to the midbrain, pons, and medulla by the superior, middle, and inferior cerebellar peduncles. Disease of the cerebellum produces

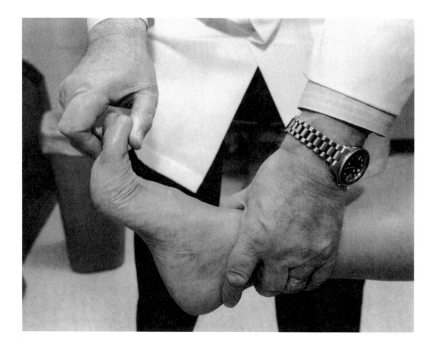

Figure 1-19
Testing extension of the great toe by the extensor hallucis. Patient is asked to resist attempts to flex the toe.

Table 1-9

Muscle innervation—action

Muscle	Nerve root level	Action
Rhomboids	Dorsal scapular N C4–C5	Adduction—scapula
Supraspinatus	Suprascapular N C4–C5	Abduction—arm
Infraspinatus	Suprascapular N C4–C6	Lateral rotation—arm
Serratus anterior	Long thoracic N C5–C7	Draws scapula forward during pushing
Subscapularis	Subscapular N C5–C6	Medial rotation—arm
Latissimus dorsi	Thoracodorsal N C6–C8	Adduction, medial rotation—arm
Teres major	Lateral subscapular N C5–C7	Adduction, extension, medial rotation—arm
Deltoid	Axillary N C5–C6	Abduction—arm
Biceps brachii	Musculocutaneous N C5–C6	Flexion—forearm Supination—hand
Triceps	Radial N C6–C8	Extension—forearm
Brachioradialis	Radial N C5–C6	Flexion—forearm
Extensor carpi radialis	Radial N C5–C7	Extension, abduction—hand
Supinator	Radial N C5–C7	Supination—hand
Extensor digitorum	Radial N C6–C8	Extension—wrist, phalanges
Extensor carpi ulnaris	Radial N C6–C8	Extension adduction—hand
Abductor pollicis longus	Radial N C6–C8	Abduction—thumb
Extensor pollicis longus	Radial N C6–C8	Extension—second phalanx thumb
Extensor pollicis brevis	Radial N C7–T1	Extension—first phalanx thumb
Pronator teres	Median N C6–C7	Pronation—hand
Flexor carpi radialis	Median N C6–C7	Flexion, abduction—hand
Flexor digitorum sublimis	Median N C7–T1	Flexion—second phalanx—fingers
Flexor digitorum profundus	Median N C7–T1	Flexion—terminal phalanx—fingers
Flexor pollicis longus	Median N C6–C8	Flexion—second phalanx thumb
Abductor pollicis brevis	Median N C7–T1	Abduction—thumb
Opponens pollicis	Median N C7–T1	Abduction, flexion—thumb
Flexor pollicis brevis	Median N C7–T1	Adduction, flexion—thumb
Flexor carpi ulnaris	Ulnar N C7–T1	Flexion, adduction—hand
Abductor digiti quinti brevis	Ulnar N C8–T1	Abduction—little finger
Flexor digiti quinti brevis	Ulnar N C8–T1	Flexion—little finger
Opponens digiti quinti	Ulnar N C8–T1	Abduction, flexion—little finger
Abductor pollicis	Ulnar N C8–T1	Adduction—thumb
Interossei	Ulnar N C8–T1	Dorsal—abduction fingers from middle finger
Lumbricals	1,2–median 3,4–ulnar C8–T1	Palmar—adduction fingers toward middle finger
Neck flexors	C1–C6	Flexion—neck
Neck extensors	C1–T1	Extension—neck

(Continued)

Table 1-9
(Continued)

Muscle	Nerve root level	Action
Diaphragm	Phrenic N C3–C5	Diaphragmatic breathing
Abdominal muscles		
upper	T5–T9	
lower	T10–L3	
Iliopsoas	Femoral N L2–L4	Flexion—thigh at hip
Adductor magnus, longus, brevis	Obturator N L2–L4	Adduction—thigh
Gluteus medius minimus	Superior gluteal N L4–S1	Abduction, medial rotation—thigh
Gluteus maximus	Inferior gluteal N L4–S2	Extension, lateral rotation—thigh
Quadriceps femoris	Femoral N L4–S1	Extension—leg at knee
Hamstrings	Sciatic N L4–S1	Flexion—leg at knee
Tibialis anterior	Deep peroneal N L4–L5	Dorsiflexion, inversion—foot
Extensor hallucis longus	Deep peroneal N L4–S1	Extension—great toe dorsiflexion—foot
Extensor dig. longus	Deep peroneal N L4–S1	Extension—lat. 4 toes dorsiflexion—foot
Extensor dig. brevis	Deep peroneal N L4–S1	Extension—all toes except little toe
Peroneus longus brevis	Sup. peroneal N L5–S1	Eversion—foot
Gastrocnemius soleus	Tibial N L5–S2	Plantar flexion—foot
Tibialis posterior	Posterior tibial N L5–S1	Inversion—foot
Flexor dig. longus	Posterior tibial L5–S2	Plantar flexion—toes
Flexor hallucis longus	Posterior tibial L5–S2	Plantar flexion—great toe
Foot intrinsics	Posterior tibial L5–S2	

ataxia, intention tremor, nystagmus, dysmetria (disturbed ability to gauge distances), dysdiadochokinesia (disturbed ability to perform rapid alternating movements), hypotonia, and rebound. See Table 1-11 for correlation of areas of cerebellum involved and symptoms and signs produced.

Testing for abnormalities of coordinated movements of the upper limbs is carried out by asking the patient to extend the arms forward 90° with the forearms and hands supinated. The patient is then asked to close the eyes and maintain the limbs in the extended position without movement. There may be a very slow "drift" of one of the upper limbs (Fig. 1-20). This usually takes the form of very slow pronation of the affected limb and then gradual descent. Drifting may be seen with minimal weakness of the affected limb or sensory (proprioceptive) impairment of the limb. Upward or lateral drifting is seen occa-

sionally in the presence of impaired proprioception or cerebellar disease. Rebound may be tested by depressing one of the extended limbs and releasing it rapidly. The extended arm in the intact individual will immediately reassume the initial position, but the arm of the patient with cerebellar disease will make several oscillations of decreasing amplitude before it assumes the resting position.

The patient is then asked to rapidly pronate and supinate the extended forearms and hands. These rapid alternating movements should be of equal rate and amplitude on the two sides. Slowing may be present on one side in the presence of weakness, increased tone, dyspraxia, disturbed sensation, or cerebellar impairment. Cerebellar ataxia produces slowing and overflinging, which is an increased amplitude of the supination/pronation movement. The patient is next asked to hold one hand in a pronated

Table 1-10
Differentiation of upper motor and lower motor neuron lesions

	Tone	Muscle bulk	Reflexes	Fasciculations
Upper motor neuron lesion	Spastic—may be flaccid early	Min. atrophy only after long period of disuse	Increased—may be clonus, plantar extensor	Absent
Lower motor neuron lesion	Flaccid	Decrease in bulk	Decreased or absent, plantar flexor	Present

position and to tap the back of the hand rhythmically with the fingers of the other hand as rapidly as possible. This is normally performed in a rhythmic fashion, but the rhythm is variable and the amplitude inconsistent in cerebellar disease. The patient is then instructed alternately to supinate and pronate one hand on the dorsal surface of the other hand as rapidly as possible. Again, the rate is slowed, the rhythm is abnormal, and there is overflinging in the presence of cerebellar disease. The dyspraxic patient is unable to perform this complex movement and usually substitutes a simple tapping movement or alternatively taps one hand on the dorsal surface of the other hand. The activity on the two sides is compared in each of these maneuvers.

Testing is continued by asking the patient to perform the finger-to-nose test. The examiner holds his extended index finger at arm's length from the patient. The patient is asked to touch the finger then touch his nose (Fig. 1-21*A* and *B*). This should be performed slowly. In many cases a patient will reach out and tap the examiner's finger and then rapidly return his finger to the nose. This will effectively block a mild degree of tremor. Cerebellar disease is characterized by past-pointing, with the patient's index finger repeatedly overshooting the target, and intention tremor, a terminal tremor that increases as the finger approaches the target.

Cerebellar function of the lower limbs is evaluated by the heel-to-shin test, in which the patient

Table 1-11
Signs and symptoms of cerebellar disease[a]

	Cerebellar hemisphere (posterior lobe-neocerebellum)	Rostral cerebellum (anterior lobe-paleocerebellum)	Caudal cerebellum (flocculonodular lobe-archicerebellum)
Ataxia	+	Truncal ataxia + upper extremity ataxia	Truncal ataxia + lower extremity ataxia
Nystagmus	+	0	±
Intention tremor	+	0	0
Hypotonia	+	+	±
Rebound	+	±	0
⎰ Dysmetria ⎨ Dysdiadochokinesia ⎱ Dysarthria	+	0	0

[a] It is important to remember that cerebellar lesions tend to produce ipsilateral symptoms and signs.

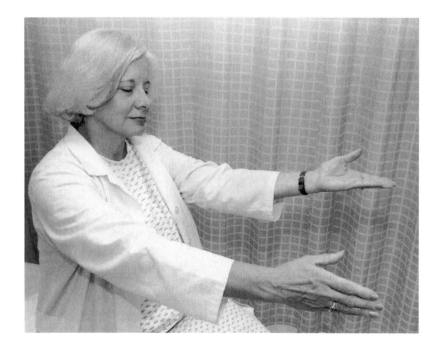

Figure 1-20
Drift and pronation of the weak upper limb.

slides the heel of one lower extremity down the anterior tibial surface of the other. This should be a smooth movement, and the heel should remain on the tibial crest without ataxia. Other tests include the toe tap test, in which the patient taps the patella of one extremity with the toes of the other; and foot tapping test, where the patient stands with one foot placed forward and slightly to the side, rests the heel on the floor, and rapidly taps the floor with the toes.

Examination of Gait and Station

The patient is asked to walk across the examining room while the examiner observes the gait. The patient should have normal posture. The feet should be a normal distance apart, and there should be good associated movement of the arms. A loss of associated movement of the arm on one side indicates the early development of either spasticity or rigidity in that limb. Particular attention should be given as the patient turns; this movement is likely to produce slight ataxia or a shuffle indicating early dyspraxia of gait. After the patient has walked back and forth several times, the examiner demonstrates tandem gait and asks the patient to walk toward the examiner, with one foot placed in front of the other, the heel touching the toes at each step (Fig. 1-22). This is normally performed without any undue unsteadiness or sudden lateral placement of one foot to maintain balance, which would indicate the presence of ataxia. The patient is then asked to walk across the examining room on his heels and return on the toes. These maneuvers not only tend to accentuate ataxia but can also disclose unexpected weakness in the lower limbs. The ability to perform heel walking and toe walking indicates good strength in the dorsiflexors and plantar flexors of the feet.

The examiner then requests the patient to stand with the feet together and parallel so that the heels and toes are touching. The examiner stands at the side of the patient and extends one arm in front of and one arm behind the patient at chest height. The patient is now ready to perform the Romberg test and is requested to close the eyes. The examiner maintains the arms in an extended position ready to give support to the patient should the patient fall (Fig. 1-23). The patient should be able to maintain posture without movement of the feet with the eyes closed indefi-

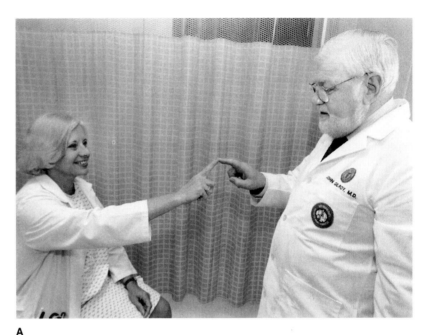

A

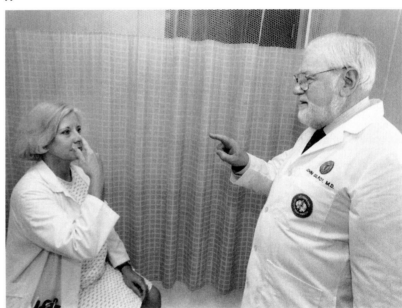

Figure 1-21
A, B. *Finger-to-nose test.*   B

nitely. The Romberg test is then said to be negative. The Romberg test is positive if the patient has to move one or both feet to maintain balance. When there is marked loss of proprioception due to periph-eral neuropathy or posterior column disease, the patient with a positive Romberg test may fall suddenly on closing the eyes and the examiner must always be prepared to give support to the patient.

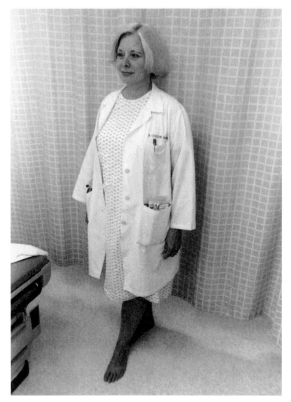

Figure 1-22
Tandem gait.

Examination of Sensory Function

Tests of sensory function are concerned with appreciation of primary or cutaneous sensation and evaluation of cortical integration of sensory impulses.

The examination of *cutaneous sensation* begins with an evaluation of light touch. The examiner takes a wisp of cotton and applies it lightly to the skin. The patient closes the eyes and is instructed to answer yes when the stimulus is appreciated. The examiner alternates between the two sides, examining the homotopic areas. The patient sits with the hands supinated, and the cotton is applied to the skin of the neck beginning in the C3 dermatome on each side and passing down the neck to the shoulder and the lateral aspect of the arm and forearm to the hand. The fingers are tested individually and the cotton is then applied up the medial aspect of the forearm and upper limb to the chest. Sensation in the lower limbs is examined in

a similar fashion with an alternating application of the cotton down the lateral aspect of the thigh, leg, and foot and up the medial aspect of the foot, leg, and thigh.

Pain sensation is tested with a corsage pin or pinwheel. The examiner begins distally on the index finger and progresses to the lateral border of the hand, forearm, upper arm, and across the shoulder to the neck, up to the angle of the jaw. The two sides are compared and the patient is asked whether there is any difference between the two sides and whether there is any change as the pin is moved between the distal and proximal areas. The examiner then applies the pin to the middle finger, progressing to the palm and forearm, which tests sensation in the C7 dermatome. Again, the two sides are compared. Finally,

Figure 1-23
Romberg test. Feet together, eyes closed. Examiner must stand with arms extended in front of and behind patient, ready to give support if there is a sudden fall (Romberg positive).

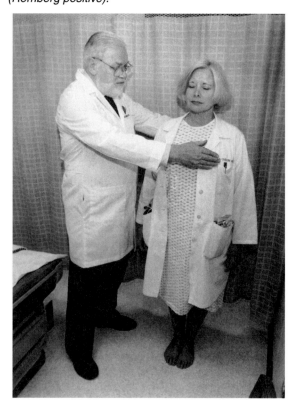

the pin is applied to the little finger, the medial aspect of the hand, the medial forearm, and the upper arm as high as the axilla. Once more the patient is asked to compare the two sides and to indicate whether there is any change as the pin is moved from distal to proximal areas. In testing pain over the lower limbs, the examiner begins distally at the level of the little toe and moves the pin up the lateral border of the foot and lower limb as high as the inguinal area. The two sides are compared, and the medial aspects of the foot, leg, and thigh are tested in similar fashion. Once again the patient is asked to compare the two sides and to indicate whether there is any change in pin sensation as it is moved from distal to proximal areas. When there is an indication of possible spinal cord lesion, it is important to test pinprick over the abdomen and thorax as high as the neck, again comparing the two sides (Fig. 1-24).

Figure 1-24
Distribution of peripheral nerves and dermatomes.

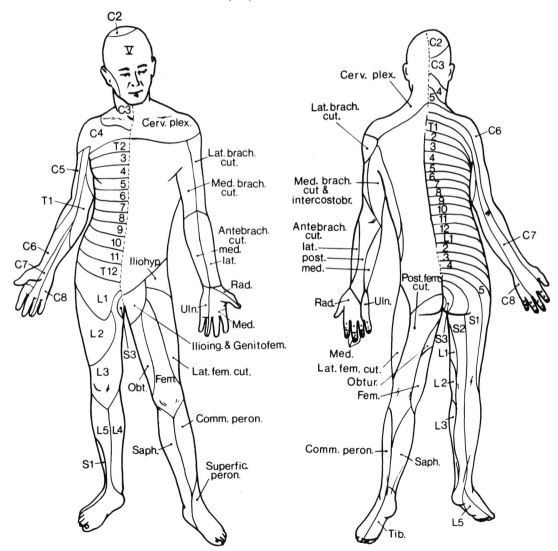

Vibration sense is tested by placing the base of the tuning fork over a bony prominence and instructing the patient to indicate when the sensation of vibration is no longer appreciated. Tests of vibration should be carried out over the terminal phalanx of the index finger bilaterally and over the terminal phalanx of the hallux bilaterally. If vibration is not appreciated at these sites then the examination is conducted more proximally at the level of the wrist and ankle. Under normal circumstances the patient indicates that vibration sense is no longer appreciated at the same time as the examiner loses the sense of vibration from the tuning fork. Vibration is decreased when the examiner appreciates the continuation of vibration that is no longer appreciated by the patient. Vibration sense should be equal on the two sides of the body.

Position sense or proprioception is tested by gently moving a terminal phalanx. The examiner grasps the terminal phalanx at the sides and gently moves it a few degrees in an upward or downward direction while the patient is instructed to close the eyes and indicate whether the digit is moved up or down. It is important that the examiner grasp the digit only on the sides so that the patient does not obtain indication of movement by alteration of pressure from above and below (Fig. 1-25). It is customary to

test movement at the terminal phalanx of the index finger and the terminal phalanx of the hallux and compare the two sides. Loss of position sense at these sites is an indication for testing movement of the finger at the metacarpal phalangeal joint and the hallux at the metatarsal phalangeal joint. Position sense will be lost at these joints only when this modality is severely impaired.

Temperature sensation is evaluated by application of glass tubes filled with hot or iced water to the skin. The examiner applies the two tubes in a random fashion and alternates to each side of the body as described under light touch (Fig. 1-26). The patient, who is sitting or lying supine with eyes closed, is asked to identify whether the stimulus is hot or cold. The use of the flat surface of a tuning fork to test for appreciation of a cold stimulus is erroneous since the object is clearly exhibiting room temperature.

Discrimination of tactile stimuli is a cortical function sometimes termed cortical sensation, which may be evaluated by testing for tactile localization, extinction, two-point discrimination, graphism, and stereognosis.

Tactile localization is tested by asking the patient to close the eyes and to name the body part that is touched with a piece of cotton. This is a complex

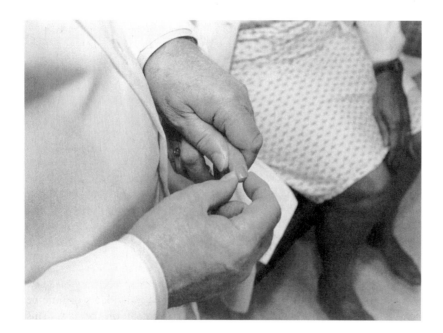

Figure 1-25
Position sense terminal phalanx fingers.

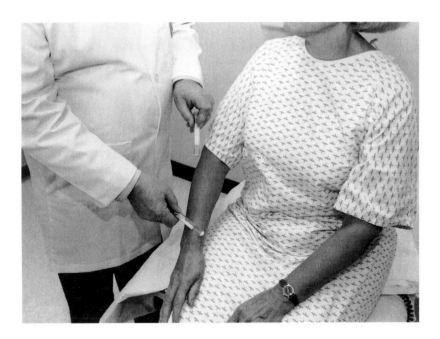

Figure 1-26
Temperature sensation using hot and cold stimuli.

sensory task requiring cortical integration. The patient is then touched at an identical site on both sides of the body at the same time. Under normal circumstances the patient will appreciate both stimuli. However, if there is an early lesion involving the parietal lobe, the patient will appreciate only one stimulus and will fail to appreciate the stimulus applied to the side opposite the parietal lobe lesion. This failure is termed *extinction.*

Two-point discrimination tests the ability of the patient to differentiate one stimulus from two. The ability to appreciate two stimuli shows great variation; the fingertips have the most sensitivity and are able to differentiate two points 2 mm apart. The test is carried out by asking the patient to close the eyes and applying either one or two points over the fingertips (Fig. 1-27). The patient is asked to indicate whether one or two points were applied. The fingertips over the right and left hand are compared. Two-point discrimination is impaired in parietal lobe lesions.

Stereognosis is an integrative function of parieto-occipital location in which the patient attempts to identify familiar objects placed in the palm of the hand when the eyes are closed. *Astereognosis,* the inability to identify the object, is associated with pari-

eto-occipital lobe lesions and is usually easy to identify when the nondominant lobe is involved. *Graphism* is tested by asking the patient to close the eyes and extend the hand in a supine position. Using a sharp pencil, the examiner then constructs numbers in random fashion from zero to nine over the finger pad of the terminal phalanx (Fig. 1-28). The patient is asked to identify each number. The number of incorrect responses can be compared on the two sides. *Graphesthesia* or impaired graphism is a sensitive indicator of parietal lobe damage.

Examination of Reflexes

Reflexes are of three types: tendon reflexes, superficial reflexes, and release reflexes.

The *jaw jerk* is obtained by placing the examining index finger in the midline on the patient's jaw and asking the patient to open the mouth about 30° and then relax. The examiner then strikes the index finger with the tendon hammer (Fig. 1-13). This produces stretching of the masseter and pterygoid muscles, followed by reflex contraction of these muscles, and the jaw jerks toward a closed position. The jaw jerk is often absent in normal individuals or may be present with minimal movement of the jaw. This

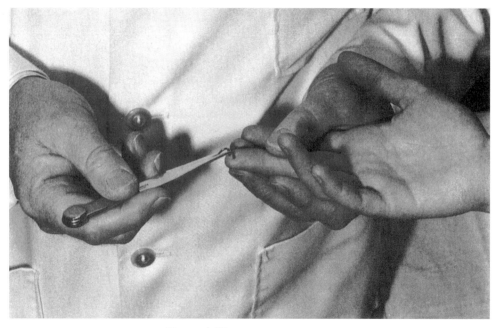

Figure 1-27
Testing two-point discrimination.

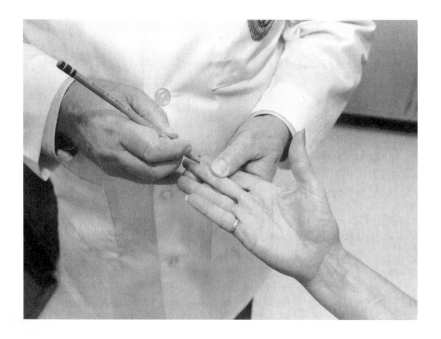

Figure 1-28
Graphism. Examiner uses sharp point of pencil and writes random numbers between zero and nine on finger pad, terminal phalanx.

movement is exaggerated in corticobulbar tract lesions above the midpons. The jaw jerk is important because it is the highest stretch reflex that can be elicited in the neurological examination. An increased jaw jerk means that the lesion is above the midpons. A normal jaw jerk with increase in the tendon reflexes in the upper limbs indicates that the lesion lies below the pons but above C5.

The *tendon reflexes* of the upper limb are tested with the patient seated and the hands in a supine position on the thighs. The patient is instructed to relax. The examiner tests the brachioradialis reflex by percussion of the radius proximal to the wrist joint (Fig. 1-29). The stimulus causes contraction of the brachioradialis (C5–C6) with a flexion movement at the elbow. The response on the two sides is compared. The examiner then places his index finger on the patient's biceps tendon and gently strikes the finger with the tendon hammer (Fig. 1-30). This produces contraction of the biceps (C5–C6) and flexion at the elbow. The two sides are compared. To test the triceps reflex, the elbow is flexed to 90° and the wrist is supported by the examiner's left arm. The triceps tendon is percussed by the tendon hammer just above the elbow, producing extension of the elbow (Fig. 1-31). The triceps reflex (C6–C7) is compared on the two sides. Finally, the finger jerk (C7–C8) is tested by flexing the patient's fingers over the examiner's index and middle finger (Fig. 1-32). The examiner then strikes his index and middle fingers with the tendon hammer. This produces flexion of the fingers.

The tendon reflexes in the lower limbs are tested with the patient seated and the legs relaxed and flexed at right angles to the thighs. The examiner then strikes the patellar tendon and notes the response. The patellar reflexes should be symmetrical (Fig. 1-33). When these reflexes (L2–L4) are depressed, the patient is asked to perform the Jendrassik maneuver by hooking the fingers of the two hands together and attempting to pull the hands apart (Fig. 1-33). This often suffices to accentuate or reinforce the patellar reflexes. In testing the ankle jerks (S1–S2) the patient is asked to apply gentle plantar flexion onto the palmar surface of the examiner's hand. The examiner notes the pressure on the hand and using the tendon hammer in his other hand strikes the Achilles tendon (Fig. 1-34). The degree of plantar flexion is noted. The examiner then asks the patient to apply the same pressure on the examiner's hand on the other side and once again strikes the Achilles tendon with the tendon hammer. The response should be symmetrical.

Figure 1-29
Brachioradialis reflex.

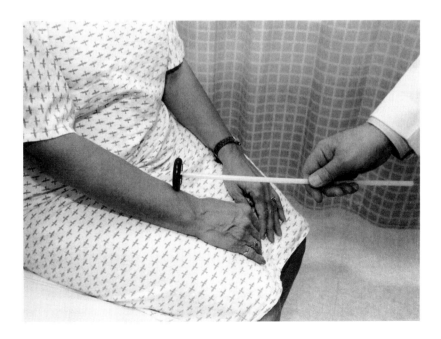

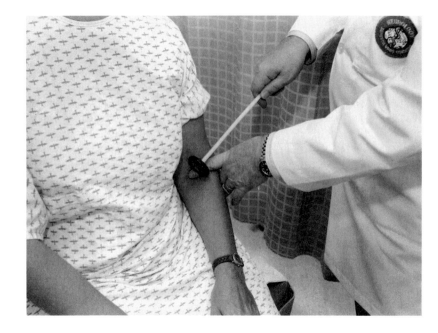

Figure 1-30
The biceps reflex.

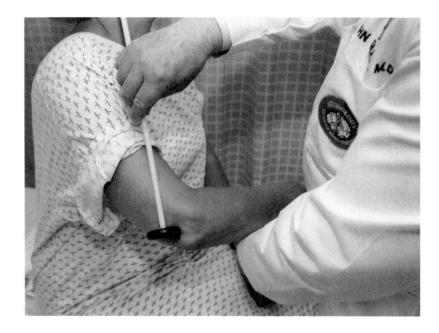

Figure 1-31
The triceps reflex.

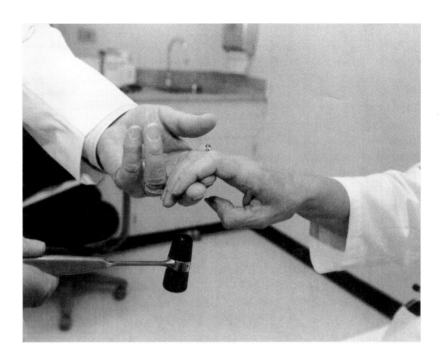

Figure 1-32
Testing the finger jerk.

Tendon reflexes should be graded as follows: 0, absent; 1+, diminished; 2+, normal; 3+, increased; and 4+, clonic.

Superficial reflexes are elicited by applying gentle pressure to the skin in a specific area. The abdominal reflexes can be elicited by stroking the skin of the abdomen gently with a blunt object such as the wooden end of a cotton applicator. The skin is stroked in a diagonal fashion moving downward lateral to medial toward the midline. The sites stimulated are above the umbilicus, at the level of the umbilicus, and below the umbilicus. The abdominal muscles contract beneath the stimulus under normal circumstances. The abdominal reflexes are absent on the side of the corticospinal tract lesion but also may be absent if the innervation of the stimulated quadrant is interfered with for any reason. It is often difficult to observe abdominal reflexes in obese individuals.

The plantar response is elicited by stimulation of the lateral aspect of the sole of the foot with a blunt object. The movement is carried along the lateral aspect of the sole and then across the head of the metatarsal bones. This gentle stimulus should produce flexion of the hallux, which is a normal plantar flexor response. Not a "negative Babinski" an inaccurate term that is used so frequently now. One cannot replace a normal response with a negative abnormality. Any extension movement is abnormal and should be recorded as an extensor plantar response. The Babinski response, which is rare, is a dual response consisting of extension of the hallux and extension of the other toes, which separate in a fan-like fashion (Fig. 1-35).

The cremasteric reflex can be obtained in the male patient by stroking the anterior medial aspect of the upper thigh with a blunt object. The stimulus results in contraction of the cremasteric muscle and elevation of the testis on the same side. This reflex is lost in corticospinal tract lesions and in lesions involving the lower segments of the spinal cord. The anal reflex is produced by gently stroking the skin around the anal margin, which produces contraction of the anal sphincter. The anal reflex is lost in lesions involving the sacral segments of the spinal cord and cauda equina.

Release reflexes are reflex responses present in the newborn infant. These reflexes disappear with maturation of the CNS but can reappear in degenera-

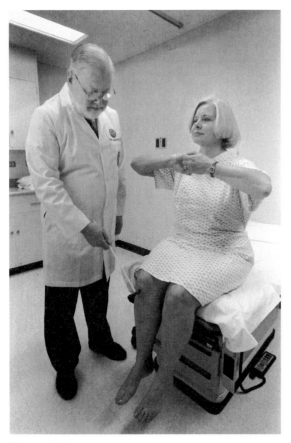

Figure 1-33
The Jendrassik maneuver.

is elicited by tapping the face between the upper lip and the nose gently with the finger. There is a pursing of the lips in response to each stimulus. The sucking reflex can be obtained by gently stroking the upper or lower lip from the midline to the lateral border of the mouth with the finger or with a tongue blade. The lips contract in a sucking movement. This reflex, which is normally present in infants, reappears in diffuse disease of the brain and is usually noted in patients with Alzheimer disease and other dementias. The chewing reflex is an abnormal response obtained by placing a tongue blade in the mouth. The patient begins to make chewing movements, and when the reflex is well developed the jaws may bite down on the tongue blade and make removal difficult. This has been called the bulldog response. The presence of a chewing reflex is indicative of diffuse bilateral lesions involving the cerebral hemispheres.

tive diseases associated with loss of inhibitory activity in the brain. The glabellar reflex is elicited by gently tapping the forehead in the midline just above the bridge of the nose. Under normal circumstances this produces rhythmic contraction of the eyelids, which disappears after a few seconds. The abnormal response consists of persistent closure of the eyes and blepharospasm in response to each stimulus, which is persistent as long as the stimulus is applied. The glabellar reflex is indicative of degenerative disease of the brain and is frequently seen in Parkinson disease, Alzheimer disease, other forms of dementia, frontal lobe infarction, and frontal lobe tumors. The snout reflex cannot be elicited in normal individuals but appears in patients with bilateral cerebral damage, often associated with pseudobulbar palsy. The reflex

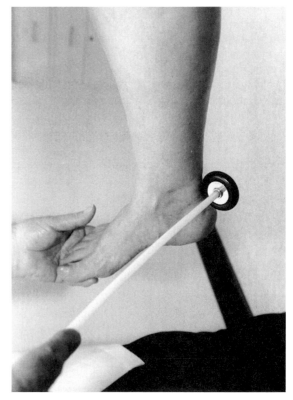

Figure 1-34
The ankle jerk.

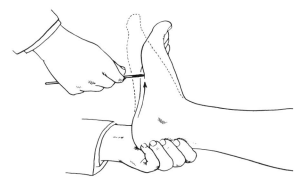

Figure 1-35
The extensor plantar response.

The grasp reflex is a response obtained by stimulation of the palm of the patient's hand. The examiner grasps the patient's hand as if to shake hands and then strokes the palm of the patient with his fingers. The reflex is positive when the patient's fingers flex and grasp the examiner's fingers. In the early stages of this abnormality the patient can release the examiner's fingers on request. Later, release is not accomplished on request and the grasp is sustained (forced grasping). The release can then be accomplished by gently stroking the dorsal surface of the patient's hand. The extreme form of the grasp reflex is the groping reflex, in which the patient actively seeks objects to grasp in the hand and may be frequently found tightly clenching the bed clothes. The grasp reflex is indicative of diffuse bilateral disease involving the cerebral hemispheres. It is commonly seen in the dementias but can occur in many other diseases producing bilateral cerebral damage.

Final Touches of Examination

The examination should be concluded by the performance of several observations that may add to the total picture of the patient's disability.

Examination of Peripheral Pulses The radial pulses should be of equal volume at the wrist and the dorsalis pedis, and posterior tibial pulses should be palpable in the feet. Peripheral vascular disease often accompanies cerebrovascular disease, and the examiner should auscultate for the presence of bruits over the femoral arteries if the peripheral pulses are absent in the feet.

Auscultation for Bruits Auscultation should be carried out over the carotid arteries during the general physical examination for the presence of bruits after the heart has been examined. This will help to localize the bruit to the carotid artery and eliminate the possibility of transmission from the heart. The examiner should also auscultate over the eye for the presence of intracranial bruits. This is accomplished by using the bell of the stethoscope, which is placed over the closed eyelid. The patient is then asked to open the opposite eye, which removes the sound of muscle artifact and permits auscultation into the cranial cavity. Intracranial bruits are usually associated with arteriovenous malformations and are occasionally heard in other conditions such as severe stenosis of the carotid artery or persistent trigeminal artery. As already indicated, auscultation should be carried out over the femoral arteries as they enter the thigh in the inguinal region, particularly when the pedal pulses are absent, since this latter condition is often associated with atherosclerotic narrowing of the iliac or femoral arteries.

Nuchal Rigidity Every patient should be examined for the presence of nuchal rigidity. This can be performed at the end of the cranial nerve examination. The examiner asks the patient to flex the head and place the chin on the chest. The performance of this simple maneuver will lessen the risk of overlooking an early encephalitis, early meningitis, or subarachnoid hemorrhage. The patients who seem to have nuchal rigidity can also be tested for the presence of Brudzinski's sign, which consists of flexion of the knees when the head is flexed on the chest, and of Kernig's sign, which is characterized by back pain and sciatic pain on attempting to straighten the leg when the thigh is flexed at the hip.

Examination of the Peripheral Nerves Palpation of peripheral nerves should be carried out in all cases of suspected peripheral neuropathy. The ulnar nerves are easily palpated in the ulnar groove on the medial aspect of the elbow joint. The common peroneal nerve can be felt as it winds around the head of the fibula. Enlargement of nerves occurs in some cases of chronic peripheral neuropathy.

Examination of the Spine A short cervical spine with low head line may indicate the presence of some congenital abnormality at the base of the skull, such as platybasia or odontoid compression. The cervical spine may show limitation of movement in the presence of cervical spondylosis. Scoliosis is a feature of a number of neurological conditions, including the spinocerebellar degenerations. Scoliosis also occurs in patients who have some degree of paralysis of the paraspinal muscles following poliomyelitis and trauma. There is loss of lumbar lordosis in degenerative disease of the lumbar spine, particularly in herniated lumbar disk. This may be associated with a mild degree of scoliosis and spasm of the erector spinae. There is usually limitation of straight-leg raising (Lasegue's sign) in patients with herniation of lower lumbar disk and sciatic pain.

Pes Cavus The examination of the gait and the Romberg test give the examiner an opportunity to observe the patient's feet for the presence of pes cavus. This condition is found in a number of chronic neurologic conditions including the familial spinocerebellar degenerations and may be observed in patients who have congenital or long-standing lesions involving the corticospinal tracts dating from infancy or early childhood.

REFERENCES

1. LaPointe L (ed): *Aphasia and Related Neurogenic Language Disorders.* New York, Thieme, 1990, pp. 1–52.
2. Marquardt T: *Acquired Neurogenic Disorders.* New York, Prentice-Hall, 1982, pp. 2-65.
3. Rolnick M, Merson R, Roeder K: Communication disorders of neurogenic origin, in GH Kraft, MM Laban, (eds). *Physical Medicine and Rehabilitation Clinics of North America.* Philadelphia, WB Saunders Co, 1996, pp. 619–641.
4. Aronson AE: *Clinical Voice Disorders,* 3rd ed. New York, Thieme, 1992, pp. 79–125.
5. Darley FL, Aronson AE, Brown JR: *Motor Speech Disorders.* Philadelphia, Saunders, 1975, pp. 99–267.
6. Darley FL: *Aphasia.* Philadelphia, Saunders, 1982, pp. 1–85.
7. Basso A, Lecours AR, Moraschini S: Anatomical correlations of the aphasias as defined through computerized tomography: exceptions. *Brain Lung* 26:221, 1985.
8. Broca P: Remarques sur le siege de la faculte du langage articule suivies d'"une observation d'aphemie (perte de la parole). *Bull Soc d'Anat (2nd Series)* 6:330, 1861.

Chapter 2

COMA

DEFINITION

Coma is a state of unresponsiveness in which the patient is unable to sense or respond to the environment.

ETIOLOGY AND PATHOLOGY

Coma occurs in response to:

1. Supratentorial lesions, meningeal infections or subarachnoid hemorrhage producing increased intracranial pressure (ICP), which is transmitted to the brainstem.

2. A lesion in the posterior fossa or brainstem, which produces pressure on the brainstem.

3. A metabolic, endocrine, or anoxic encephalopathy with diffuse involvement of the cerebral hemispheres.

4. Generalized tonic-clonic seizures.

There are many causes of coma, and a systemic approach is required in the examination of comatose patients to avoid overlooking potentially remediable situations. Table 2-1 lists the more common causes of coma.

EXAMINATION OF THE ACUTELY COMATOSE PATIENT

The evaluation of the acutely comatose patient is a common situation encountered in the emergency room. The examination should begin by attempting to obtain information from those who are familiar with or who have had some contact with the patient, including relatives, police, and the emergency services team. A history of hypertension, diabetes, drug abuse, epilepsy, or recent head trauma is invaluable.

Immediate Action

Although the patient may have already been seen by others in the emergency department, the examiner should check to see whether immediate action is necessary. The patient's airway should be clear, and there should be no signs of respiratory obstruction. If there is evidence of respiratory failure, the patient should be intubated and placed on a mechanical ventilator. The comatose patient may be hypotensive or become hypotensive at any time. This complication should be immediately treated with fluid challenge, transfusions, or, if necessary, dopamine infusion. Hypotension is rarely caused by intracranial lesions. If the patient is in cardiac arrest or showing severe cardiac arrhythmias, the cardiopulmonary resuscitation team should be called immediately.

Stabilization

The neurological evaluation begins by ensuring that the patient's condition is stable. Two peripheral intravenous lines, one measuring central venous pressure (CVP) and the other for the administration of intravenous fluids, should be inserted. A Foley catheter is passed into the bladder, and a nasogastric tube passed into the stomach. A cervical collar is applied until a cervical fracture can be ruled out by radiography. A blood sample is obtained and sent for electrolytes, glucose, blood urea nitrogen, serum creatinine, complete blood count, a drug screen, liver function tests, and a blood alcohol level in cases of suspected alcohol intoxication. Arterial blood gases are ordered if hypoxia is suspected. The patient is attached to a cardiac monitor and an electrocardiogram is obtained to rule out a recent myocardial infarct, detect arrhythmias, or discover evidence of electrolyte imbalance. A urine specimen taken from the Foley catheter is tested for the presence of glucose and blood and sent for urinalysis culture and bacterial sensitivity. The nasogastric tube aspirate is sent for analysis if poisoning or intoxication is suspected.

Table 2-1.

Causes of coma

1. Intracranial
   a. Traumatic: penetrating injuries of the brain—closed head injury, concussion, contusion, shearing, epidural hemorrhage, subdural hematoma, intracranial hemorrhage.
   b. Infection: subdural empyema, bacterial or fungal meningitis, chronic meningitis from any cause, brain abscess, viral encephalitis, Reye's syndrome.
   c. Neoplastic: brain tumor, primary or metastatic, meningeal carcinomatosis.
   d. Vascular: infarction, intracerebral hemorrhage, venous-sinus thrombosis, sickle cell disease, isolated angiitis, polyarteritis nodosa.
2. Metabolic
   a. Electrolyte and acid-base disorders: hyper- or hyponatremia, hyper- or hypokalemia, hypercalcemia, hypophosphatemia, hypermagnesemia, hyperammonemia, central pontine myelinosis.
   b. Endocrine disorders: diabetes, nonketotic hyperosmolar coma, hypoglycemia, Cushing's disease, thyrotoxicosis, myxedema, hyper- and hypoparathyroidism, adrenal insufficiency, pituitary apoplexy.
   c. Hepatic coma.
   d. Uremic coma.
   e. Anoxic encephalopathy: airway obstruction, pulmonary dysfunction, cardiac arrest, carbon monoxide, cyanide.
   f. Vitamin deficiencies: thiamine (Wernicke's encephalopathy), niacin, vitamin B_{12}.
   g. Poisons and intoxicants: alcohol, heroin, barbiturates, benzodiazepines, organic solvents, pentachlorophenol.

Once the patient is stabilized, a bedside glucose determination using a reagent strip test should be performed.[1] An intravenous injection of 50 mL of 50% dextrose is given to all patients with a glucose level of less than 80 mg/dL. Dextrose therapy is no longer recommended for all cases of coma because glucose can be detrimental to ischemic brain tissue in patients with elevated blood glucose levels presumably owing to conversion of glucose to lactate in the presence of incomplete ischemia.

However, when an intravenous administration of dextrose is indicated, it should be accompanied by thiamine 100 mg intravenously. This is particularly important to malnourished or alcohol abusing patients, or in those suffering from Wernicke's encephalopathy (ophthalmoplegia, nystagmus, vomiting, ataxia, and mental deterioration). Likewise, patients with hemodialysis, peritoneal dialysis, cancer, postgastric surgery, acquired immunodeficiency syndrome, intractable vomiting, bulimia, hyperemesis gravidarum, eating disorders, fadist diets, and those receiving hyperalimentation are candidates for immediate thiamine therapy.

Patients with suspected opiate overdose (respirations 12 per minute or less, pinpoint pupils, and evidence of opioid abuse such as drug paraphernalia, needle tracks, or bystander corroboration) require intravenous nalaxone 0.1 to 2.0 mg depending on the level of respiratory depression. When intubation is required, a repeated dose of nalaxone 2 mg intravenously every 2 min to a maximum of 10 mg may be required.

Flumazenil 0.2 mg intravenously every 30 seconds up to a maximum of 5 mg is indicated in patients with altered mental status caused by benzodiazepine intoxication. Flumazenil should not be used when benzodiazepines have been used or may be required for seizure control. In addition, flumazenil is not recommended in patients who have taken tricyclic antidepressants where toxicity produces hypertonia, clonus, hyperreflexia, myoclonus, and a tachycardia or multiple premature ventricular contractions. The use of flumazenil in such cases carries an increased risk of inducing seizures.

General Physical Examination

A systematic examination of the patient should be performed. The patient should first be observed. The dress; age; stigmata of chronic illness, such as gingival hypertrophy in the epileptic patient on phenytoin therapy; pattern of respiration; and position of the body and limbs should be noted. The comatosed patient with an acute hemiplegia lies with the affected lower limb externally rotated. The examiner notes the presence of spontaneous movements such as myoclonic jerks or spontaneous decerebration. A general physical examination should be done to identify evidence of organ failure or trauma. The odor of the breath should be noted. The examiner may detect the odor of alcohol, the smell of ketones in diabetic coma, of urine in uremia, and fetor hepaticus in liver failure. The scalp should be palpated by running the fingers of both hands through the hair from the frontal area to the occiput in an effort to detect any depressed fractures or lacerations. The external auditory meatus should be examined for the presence of cerebrospinal fluid (CSF) or hemorrhage indicating fracture of the petrous temporal bone. The mastoid area should be examined for the presence of bruising (Battle's sign), indicating a fracture of the middle cranial fossa. The zygomatic arches should be palpated and the sclera of the eyes examined for hemorrhages. A hemorrhage of the lateral aspect of the eye that is not bordered posteriorly by normal sclera is indicative of a fracture of the anterior cranial fossa. The nose should be examined for fractures of the nasal bones and epistaxis. Persistent drainage of a clear, watery fluid suggests the possibility of a fracture of the cribriform plate with drainage of CSF. The mouth should be examined and any broken or loose teeth removed to prevent aspiration. Lacerations of the tongue are almost always caused by a recent generalized seizure and most commonly occur on the lateral borders of the tongue. The neck should be palpated for the presence of hematomas and abnormalities of the vertebral bodies. The examination continues with palpation of the clavicles and auscultation and observations of the chest to detect absence of breath sounds and paradoxical respirations. The chest should be palpated for rib fractures. The trachea should be in the midline, and the examiner should palpate the left side of the chest for the apex beat and note its position. Auscultation of the heart is carried out and the presence of arrhythmia or murmurs noted. The abdomen is palpated for the presence of muscle rigidity, indicating possible abdominal hemorrhage or infection. The limbs are then examined for the presence of fractures.

Neurological Examination

Given that the comatosed patient is unable to respond, the neurological examination must be modified to obtain responses that are largely reflex and vegetative in nature.

Appreciation of the respiratory pattern and rhythm is important when examining a semicomatose or comatose patient (Table 2-2). Posthyperventilation apnea is present when 3 min of hyperventilation is followed by a period of apnea of more than 30 s. This respiratory response is associated with diffuse metabolic or structural forebrain damage. Cheyne-Stokes respiration is characterized by rhythmic waxing and waning of respiration separated by periods of apnea. This type of respiration is frequently associated with early brainstem compression or bilateral deep cerebral hemisphere damage. Central neurogenic hyperventilation is characterized by regular, rapid, deep, machinery-like breathing and is associated with lesions of the midbrain or pons (or both). Apneustic breathing is characterized by a pause at the completion of inspiration and is associated with pontine lesions. Ataxic breathing is characterized by an irregular rhythm and depth of respiration and is associated with dysfunction of the medullary respiratory centers.

The pupils should be equal in size and briskly reactive to light. Constricted pupils occur when there is paralysis of sympathetic function or stimulation of parasympathetic connections. This occurs in severe bilateral hemorrhage or after ingestion of narcotics. Dilated pupils indicate paralysis of parasympathetic function or stimulation of sympathetic connections, which occurs after overdosage with hallucinogens, central nervous system (CNS) stimulants, or anticholinergic drugs. A unilateral fixed and dilated pupil is indicative of a third nerve paralysis in a comatose patient, providing a mydriatic agent was not applied in an effort to obtain a better view of the fundus, a procedure that should never be performed in an emergency room. Pressure on the third nerve results in pupillary dilatation, which precedes paralysis of extraocular muscles because the fibers subserving the light reflex surround an inner core of fibers that innervate the extraocular muscles. Dilatation of the pupil may indicate herniation of the medial aspect of the temporal lobe over the free edge of the tentorium cerebelli (uncal herniation). This ominous sign indicates the need for immediate treatment of increased ICP. A metabolic abnormality should be suspected when the patient is nonresponsive with absent corneal reflexes and absent extraocular movement, yet the pupils are reactive.

Table 2-2.
Signs of rostral-caudal deterioration and level of dysfunction[a]

Level of dysfunction	Pupil size and pupillary light reflex	Oculocephalic reflexes ("doll's-eye movements") caloric testing	Respiratory pattern	Response to painful stimuli
Normal	Normal Briskly reactive	Calorics; normal nystagmus present	Normal	Appropriate
Hemispheres	Small Reactive	Doll's eyes present Calorics; eyes may be tonically deviated	Cheyne-Stokes or posthyperventilation apnea	Decorticate posturing
Diencephalic	Small 1–3 cm Reacting	Doll's eyes present Calorics; brisk may be tonic deviation	Normal	Decorticate posturing
Midbrain	Midposition 3–5 cm fixed	Doll's eyes present Calorics; poor response, may be internuclear ophthalmoplegia	Central neurogenic hyperventilation	Decerebrate posturing
Pons	Midposition	± present	Central neurogenic hyperventilation or apneustic	Decerebrate posturing or flaccid
Medulla	Midposition and fixed Terminally dilated and fixed	Absent	Ataxic or absent	Flaccid

[a]Plum F, Posner JB: *The Diagnosis of Stupor and Coma.* 3rd ed. Philadelphia, FA Davis, 1980.

The eyes should be examined while at rest. The examiner should note the position of the eyelids and whether they are completely closed. The lids may be gently raised and allowed to close; slow and incomplete closure is associated with deep coma. The corneal reflexes should be tested. There should be a brisk direct and consensual response. If the patient's eyes are open it is possible to evaluate the visual fields by making a threatening gesture with the hands on one side and repeating the procedure on the other side, noting if the patient shows reflex blinking. The position of the eyes at rest should be noted. Complete paralysis of the third nerve produces abduction of the affected eye. Bilateral sixth nerve palsies may occur with increased ICP, and this sign is of no localizing value as an isolated phenomenon and does not necessarily indicate brain stem damage. Fixed conjugate deviation of the eyes indicates an ipsilateral destruc-

tive lesion, a contralateral irritative lesion of the frontal lobe, or a destructive lesion of the contralateral brainstem. Ocular bobbing is associated with an upper brainstem lesion, while skew deviation of the eyes indicates a severe pontine lesion.

The fundus should be examined in all comatose patients. The retina and optic nerves should be carefully evaluated for the presence of papilledema, hemorrhages, hypertensive or diabetic change, or spasm of the retinal arteries. Subarachnoid hemorrhage is often accompanied by a subhyaloid hemorrhage, which appears as a blotlike hemorrhage on the surface of the retina (Fig. 2-1).

Reflex eye movements should be tested in all comatose patients provided there is no evidence of a fracture of the cervical spine. Reflex eye movements are elicited by briskly turning the head to the right followed by turning it to the left and flexing and ex-

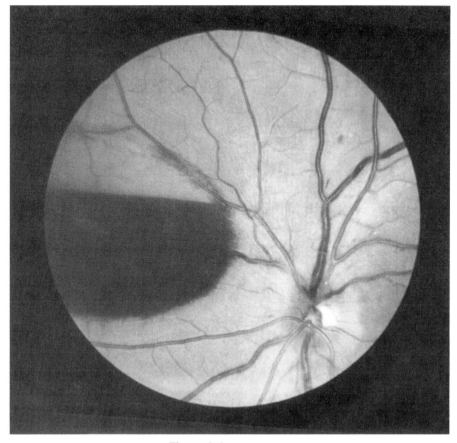

Figure 2-1
Subhyaloid hemorrhage.

tending the head. If the patient's brainstem reflexes are intact, the eyes move in conjugate fashion in the opposite direction to the head movement and the "doll's-eye" movements are said to be present. It is usually not possible to elicit this reflex in the conscious, alert patient because visual fixation overrides the reflex response. Reflex eye movements become increasingly difficult to elicit with progressive brainstem dysfunction. Paralysis of reflex eye movements will be total when the connections between the vestibular nuclei and the sixth nerve are disrupted at the level of the pontomedullary junction. With damage to the paramedian pontine reticular formation, the eyes move in conjugate fashion but fail to cross the midline when the examiner moves the head. With lesions of the medial longitudinal fasciculus there is

abduction of one eye but failure of adduction of the other eye on the side of the medial longitudinal fasciculus lesion.

Caloric testing is used to augment the information obtained when testing reflex eye movements or when the possibility of a cervical spine fracture prohibits movement of the neck. The supine patient should be positioned with the head flexed forward 30°, which places the horizontal semicircular canals in a horizontal position. The external canal should be free of cerumen, and the tympanic membrane should be intact. A slow injection of 50 mL of iced water should be made into the external canal. In the normal situation the eyes will slowly deviate to the ipsilateral side with a quick corrective return to the midline. Under these conditions, nystagmus is named by the fast component: injection of the left ear with iced water produces a right nystagmus. If warm water is injected, the slow phase will be toward the opposite side: warm water injection into the left ear produces a left nystagmus. In patients with dysfunction of the cerebral hemispheres there is an ipsilateral tonic deviation of the eyes following injection of iced water, whereas injection of warm water produces a contralateral tonic deviation. Absence of response to caloric stimulation indicates total disruption of the connections between the vestibular nuclei and sixth nerve nucleus.

Absence of reflex eye movements with preservation of caloric responses indicates the potential for a good outcome in the comatose patient. Absence of both reflex eye movements and caloric responses, however, indicates a poor prognosis. Absence of caloric responses and lack of pupillary light reflexes indicates a fatal outcome in all cases of coma.

In the absence of cervical fracture the head should be flexed forward onto the chest to detect the presence of nuchal rigidity. Tests for the presence of Kernig's and Brudzinski's signs should be performed. Nuchal rigidity suggests the possibility of encephalitis, meningitis, or subarachnoid hemorrhage. A lumbar puncture is indicated in patients who have nuchal rigidity. A magnetic resonance or computed tomography scan should be obtained before a lumbar puncture is performed if equipment is available to rule out the presence of a rapidly expanding supratentorial lesion.

The position of the limbs should be noted and the tone of each compared. In acute hemiplegia the upper limb is flaccid and the lower limb is flaccid and externally rotated. The tendon reflexes should be evaluated for the presence of any asymmetry. It is not unusual to find a bilateral extensor plantar response in a deeply comatose patient. A unilateral response suggests the presence of a contralateral, supratentorial mass lesion. The response of the patient to painful stimuli should be noted. The examiner may press on the supraorbital notch, squeeze the trapezius or any muscle mass, or prick the skin. The patient may either wince in pain and attempt to withdraw from the stimulus, assume a decorticate or decerebrate posture (Fig. 2-2), or remain unresponsive, indicating deep coma.

The neurological status of the patient should be repeatedly evaluated and the responses systematically recorded for later comparison.

Figure 2-2
Decerebrate versus decorticate posturing in the comatose patient.

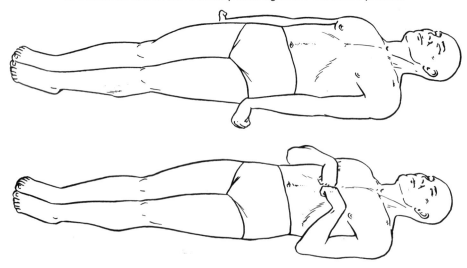

COMPLICATIONS

Deterioration of the neurological status may indicate incipient or ongoing herniation. Five types of herniation are of clinical importance.

1. Rostral-caudal deterioration when there is pressure on the brainstem from above by an expanding mass with progressive loss of brainstem function in a caudal direction (see Table 2-2).

2. (A) Uncal herniation with pressure on the brainstem caused by a herniation of the medial aspect of the temporal lobe over the free edge of the tentorium cerebelli.

Uncal herniation differs from rostral-caudal deterioration in that there is no diencephalic stage in uncal herniation. Coma develops rapidly and is preceded by unilateral dilatation of the pupil on the side of the uncal herniation. This pupil initially shows a poor, then an eventual absence of response to light due to pressure on the third nerve by the herniating mass. This is followed by lateral deviation of the eyes leading to external ophthalmoplegia on the affected side as the oculomotor fibers are paralyzed, then coma, bilateral decerebrate rigidity (see Fig. 2-2), and eventual total flaccidity. Hemiplegia associated with a fixed and dilated pupil is usually contralateral because uncal herniation usually occurs on the same side as an acute supratentorial mass lesion. However, if the mass shifts the brainstem so that the contralateral cerebral peduncle is compressed against the tentorium (Kernohan-Woltman's notch), the hemiplegia will be ipsilateral to the mass lesion. However, this is an unusual situation and the hemiplegia is almost invariably contralateral to the mass lesion in an acute situation. In the more common central diencephalic syndrome of rostral caudal deterioration with central pressure from above on the brainstem, there are no localizing pupillary signs.

Further deterioration in brainstem function is similar to the pontine and medullary stages in Table 2-2 except that the dilated fixed pupil remains larger on the side of the uncal herniation.

3. (B) Cingulate herniation. In cingulate herniation the cingulate gyrus may herniate underneath the falx. This may be associated with compression of the anterior cerebral arteries followed by ischemia and infarction in the region of the paracentral lobules.

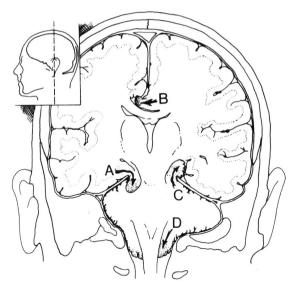

Figure 2-3
Types of brain herniation. Uncal herniation (A); cingulate herniation (B); upward cerebellar herniation (C); and cerebellar tonsillar herniation (D).

4. (C) Upward cerebellar herniation. In posterior fossa lesions cerebellar hemorrhage or infarction may produce coma due to direct pressure on the brainstem or by upward herniation. There may be premonitory headache, vertigo, nausea, and vomiting followed by unreactive or poorly reactive pinpoint pupils, paralysis of upward or conjugate lateral gaze, and bilateral decerebrate rigidity followed by flaccid quadriplegia.

5. (D) Cerebellar tonsillar herniation. Posterior fossa lesions may also produce herniation of the cerebellar tonsils through the foramen magnum. This situation is associated with increasing occipital headache, nuchal rigidity, flexion of the head toward the side of the cerebellar tonsillar herniation, and cardiac and respiratory arrest due to pressure on the medulla (Fig. 2-3).

PROGNOSIS

The outcome in coma is not unpredictable, and a number of general statements can be made.

Except for drug overdose, the presence of coma generally predicts a poor outcome.[2] When a patient in coma is admitted to an intensive care unit (ICU) and coma persists for more than 48 h, the mortality rate is 77 percent. Any patient in shock admitted to an ICU carries a 55 percent mortality rate at 36 h. However, if shock and coma are combined, a 95 percent mortality rate exists at 36 h.

In subarachnoid hemorrhage, only 5 percent of patients recover from coma. Coma and hypoxic encephalopathy carry a 10 percent recovery, coma and hepatic encephalopathy a 27 percent recovery rate.

Any type of coma superimposed with stroke, including intracerebral hemorrhage, cerebral infarction, both ischemic and hemorrhagic type, carries a fatality rate of 65 percent. However, coma with intracerebral hemorrhage carries an 84 percent mortality rate and coma with infarction due to thromboembolism a 60 percent mortality. In contrast, drug overdose carries a mortality rate of 1 percent, even when the patient has been in coma, provided immediate and proper therapy is instituted.

In patients who have received cardiopulmonary resuscitation and are comatose at 72 h, the overwhelming chances are that the patient will recover to a vegetative state and die within 1 year. For those with cardiopulmonary resuscitation, some 13 percent will regain consciousness, and 10 percent will achieve independent functioning. When resuscitation exceeds 30 min, however, there is no survival.

Patients in coma 72 h with a Glasgow Coma Scale score of less than 5 are all dead or in a vegetative state at 1 year. Those who lack signs of brainstem activity (brainstem dead patients) die from cardiac asystole within 3 days in 81 percent and within 7 days in 97 percent of cases.[3]

Trauma (see Chap. 18) carries a considerable mortality if associated with coma. An acute subdural hematoma has a 50 percent mortality rate even if the hemorrhage is drained by craniotomy, traumatic intracerebral hemorrhage a 26 percent mortality whether the hemorrhage is drained or not, an epidural hemorrhage 18 percent mortality after craniotomy. An acute subdural hematoma with a Glasgow Coma Scale score between 3 and 5 carries a 74 percent mortality rate.[5]

Early predictions of poor outcome in coma states can be determined at the time of initial examination in some cases. For instance, if there is absence of pupillary light reflexes at the time of initial examination, less than 20 percent of the patients will regain independent functioning.[4] If pupillary light reflexes are present with conjugate roving eye movements, 40 percent of the patients will make a complete recovery.

In trauma cases at 24 h, if the patient is opening the eyes and responding to pain, there is a 63 percent chance of complete recovery.

PERSISTENT VEGETATIVE STATE

Occasionally, a comatose patient presents with a condition of severe brain damage characterized by preservation of vegetative functions (sleep-wake cycles, autonomic control, and respiratory function) but lacking awareness including all cognitive function and emotion. This vegetative state may be a transient feature during recovery from severe brain damage or a permanent state reflecting failure to recover from brain damage or the end state of a progressive neurodegenerative disease. When awake, patients move the extremities but not in a meaningful way, and there are no purposeful or voluntary responses to visual, auditory, or tactile stimuli. Grunting, moaning, screaming, and smiling may occur, but these are random responses, and there is no comprehension or expression of language. The neuropathological substrate of persistent vegetative state consists of widespread bilateral damage to the cerebral cortex, diffuse axonal injury involving cortical or subcortical and commissural axons in both hemispheres, and bilateral damage to the thalamus or a combination of two or all of these conditions.[5] The essential factor in persistent vegetative state is the preservation of hypothalamic and brainstem function, and brainstem auditory evoked potentials are normal. However, somatosensory evoked potentials show prolonged or absent central conduction time.

Recovery of consciousness from a persistent vegetative state is unlikely after 12 months in adults or children who have traumatic brain injury. Recovery of consciousness is rare after 3 months in adults and children with nontraumatic brain injuries. However, the condition is compatible with survival for months or even years in some cases. The mortality rate for adults with persistent vegetative state after brain injury is 82 percent at 3 years and 95 percent at 5 years.[6] Survival is undoubtedly related to the intensity and skill of nursing care in these cases.

TREATMENT

Increased ICP is defined as a mean CSF pressure of more than 200 mmH$_2$O (15 mmHg). This in itself is not dangerous but when the increased pressure is associated with the presence of a mass lesion, there is distortion and pressure on other structures in the brainstem and the always present risk of sudden decompensation with catastrophic results. Consequently, when a mass lesion is present the mass should be removed whenever possible. In those cases in which surgical decompression is not indicated or is going to be delayed, the treatment is aimed at reducing edema, thus decreasing the likelihood of shifts in pressure and herniation. Vasogenic edema is characterized by increased permeability of brain capillary endothelial cells and major involvement of white matter and is associated with mass lesions such as tumors and abscesses. Corticosteroids and osmotherapy have a beneficial effect in the treatment of this type of edema. Cytoxic edema, which is characterized by cellular swelling, involves both gray and white matter and is a complication of hypoxia following asphyxia or cardiac arrest, hypoosmolality, and severe hypoglycemia. Cytoxic edema responds only to osmotherapy.

Controlled Hyperventilation

Increase of the Pco$_2$ of the arterial system has a potent vasodilatory effect which in turn increases ICP. Controlled hyperventilation, which maintains the Pco$_2$ between 25 and 30, helps to decrease ICP. However, the vasoconstriction may decrease cerebral blood flow to cortical structures resulting in cerebral ischemia or infarction. Consequently, hyperventilation is recommended as a temporary measure only to control ICP until osmotherapy can be instituted.

Head Elevation

Head elevation to 30° will significantly reduce ICP without altering cerebral perfusion pressure in normovolemic patients.

Furosemide

Furosemide 40 mg IV is effective in decreasing ICP without increasing serum osmolality or producing hyponatremia or hypokalemia. Repeated doses can be administered in patients with ICP monitoring. Furosemide decreases edema in intact brain and in areas of pathological change.

Corticosteroid Therapy

Dexamethasone (Decadron) 10 mg IV initially, followed by 6 mg q6h is effective in reducing edema in the treatment of gliomas and metastatic tumors but is not effective in cerebral infarction, cerebral hemorrhage, subarachnoid hemorrhage, or head injury.

Osmotherapy

Osmotherapy has the advantage of acting quickly. However, it decreases the amount of edema only in those areas with intact cellular membranes and vasculature. The effects are short-lived and can be associated with a rebound in ICP. In vasogenic edema, associated with trauma or mass lesions, mannitol is probably the best of the hyperosmolar agents available and should be administered intravenously in doses of 0.25 g/kg q3h or 0.5 to 1.0 g/kg q6h in a 20% solution over 20 min. In the absence of ICP monitoring a serum osmolality ranging from 300 to 320 mOsm/L is recommended. Constant elevation of the serum osmolality to levels greater than 320 mOsm can result in diffusion of osmotically active particles into the brain, which can exacerbate edema. Excessive use of mannitol may also result in reduction of cardiac output and renal perfusion. This must be avoided. Glycerol, another osmotic agent, may be administered orally in a dosage of 1.5 g/kg per day as a 50% or 75% solution in divided doses q6h.

Barbiturate Coma

When all attempts to control increased ICP fail, barbiturate coma may be introduced in patients with traumatic brain injury. High dose Pentobarbital when added to conventional management is useful in aborting elevation of ICP.[7] Consequently, barbiturate coma is used to control ICP in traumatic brain injury and to control seizures and lower ICP in status epilepticus. Pentobarbital and sodium thiopental are the most frequently used barbiturates. If barbiturate coma therapy is to be used, there must be a means of measuring ICP, arterial pressure, electroencephalographic activity, and pulmonary hemodynamics.[8] Consequently, a well equipped, well staffed ICU is a necessity. Details on the use of barbiturate therapy are given in Chap. 4.

Intracranial Pressure Monitoring

It is now possible to monitor the ICP directly and continuously using an intraventricular catheter or a cranial bolt. This method has the advantage of detecting an early rise in ICP, thus avoiding the complications of herniation. As ICP rises there is a point of vascular decompensation with a loss of autoregulation, an increased cerebral blood volume, and a sudden rise in pressure producing the plateau wave that may last for 5 to 20 min, accompanied by signs of neurological deterioration such as pupillary dilatation or decerebrate posturing. This phenomenon indicates an urgent need for the use of measures to decrease ICP. A constant intraventricular pressure of 40 mmHg or more may indicate the need for urgent treatment to avoid impending herniation. Continuous ICP monitoring is also useful in assessing the effectiveness of osmotherapy and in predicting the need for an additional infusion of mannitol. It is often possible to "titrate" the dosage of mannitol to prevent the re-bound of ICP that follows the single infusion of mannitol and to maintain ICP at a safe level.

REFERENCES

1. Doyon S, Roberts JR: Reappraisal of the "coma cocktail." Dextrose, flumazenil, naloxone, and thiamine. *Emerg Med Clin North Am* 12:301, 1994.
2. Snyder JV, Colantonio A: Outcome from central nervous system injury. *Crit Care Clin* 10:217, 1994.
3. Hung TP, Chen ST; Prognosis of deeply comatose patients on ventilators. *J Neurol Neurosurg Psychiatry* 58:75, 1995.
4. Edgren E, Hedstrand U, Kelsey S, et al: Assessment of neurological prognosis in comatose survivors of cardiac arrest. Breti Study Group. Lancet 343:1055, 1994.
5. Kinney HC, Samuels MA: Neuropathology of the persistent vegetative state. A review. *J Neuropath Exp Neurol* 53:548, 1994.
6. The Multi-Society Task Force on PVS: Medical aspects of the persistent vegetative state (second of two parts). *N Engl J Med* 330:1572, 1994.
7. Eisenberg HM, Frankowski RF, Contant CF, et al: High dose barbiturate control of elevated intracranial pressure in patients with severe head injury. *J Neurosurg* 69:15, 1988.
8. Winer JW, Rosenwasser RH, Jimenez F: Electroencephalographic activity and serum and cerebrospinal fluid pentobarbital levels in determining the therapeutic end point during barbiturate coma. *Neurosurgery* 29:739, 1991.

Chapter 3

CONGENITAL DISORDERS

DEVELOPMENTAL DEFECTS OF THE SPINAL CORD

Developmental defects of the spinal cord may be due to failure of closure of the neural tube, abnormalities in development of the spinal cord, or abnormalities in the development of the spinal ganglia and spinal nerves.

The developmental abnormalities occur within the first few weeks of life, and a number of etiological factors have been identified, including genetic predisposition; viral infections, possibly rubella and other viruses; drugs; and irradiation during early pregnancy.

Neural Tube Defects

Definition Neural tube defects are the most common birth defects in the United States and are due to failure of the neural tube to develop normally.

Etiology and Pathology The etiology is uncertain at this time. Neural tube defects occur during early embryonic development at the time of closure of the neural tube. Failure of closure of the cephalic portion of the tube results in anencephaly. Failure of closure at other sites produces variable degrees of cranium bifidum or spina bifida.

Approximately 50 percent of neural tube defects result in anencephaly. Spina bifida occulta, which is the most common defect involving the spinal canal, is characterized by failure of fusion of the vertebral laminae, although the skin and superficial tissues are intact. A spinal meningocele consists of a cyst-like protrusion of meninges through the vertebral defect without involvement of the spinal cord. In myelomeningocele the cyst-like protrusion contains spinal cord or spinal nerves. Complete rachischisis consists of failure of fusion of the posterior spinal cord meninges and severe malformation of the spinal cord.

Dermal cysts are midline structures that develop when the dermis is included during closure of the midline structures. Dermoid cysts often occur in the lower lumbar area and are often connected to the spinal canal by a sinus tract. This is a potential channel for introduction of infection.

Clinical Features Two of every 1000 babies born in the United States have a neural tube defect. Most anencephalic infants are either stillborn or die shortly after birth. In 80 percent of cases of spina bifida, there is an associated defect in the skin. Many of these infants are hydrocephalic and retarded and have no bladder or bowel control and a flaccid paralysis of all limbs. Twenty percent of children with spina bifida have a "closed" lesion in which the defect is covered by skin. These infants are usually of normal intelligence and have few or no physical handicaps.

Diagnostic Procedures Neural tube defects are associated with an increased amount of α-fetoprotein in the maternal circulation and in amniotic fluid. A series of screening tests should be performed to reduce the number of false-positive results. Defects such as anencephaly or hydrocephalus can be recognized by ultrasonography at a relatively early stage of fetal development.

Treatment

Prevention The most effective means of decreasing the incidence of infants born with neural tube defects is by early detection and therapeutic abortion. A woman who has had one child with a neural tube defect has a 5 percent chance of having another.

Surgical Repair Surgical treatment of a myelomeningocele should be carried out within 48 h of birth to reduce the risk of infection. Many of these children will need subsequent treatment for hydrocephalus by ventriculoperitoneal shunting. All children should be followed closely with regular measurement of head circumference to detect the development of hydrocephalus, which can be confirmed by magnetic resonance imaging (MRI) or computed tomography (CT) scanning.

Children who survive but have paraparesis or impairment of bladder/rectal function may need additional surgical treatment later in life, such as orthopedic correction of deformities of the lower limbs, the performance of an ileal loop procedure, or a colostomy. Children with severe cranial deficits are unlikely to survive, and surgery to repair the spinal developmental defect is not recommended.

Diastematomyelia

Definition   Complete duplication of the cord (dystomyelia) is extremely rare; diastematomyelia, in which there is a cleft of the spinal cord, is occasionally encountered.[1]

Etiology and Pathology   The etiology is unknown. The spinal cord is divided in the anteroposterior plane by a fibrous or cartilaginous band, which is attached to a bony septum on the wall of the spinal canal. The spinal cord may show various degrees of reduplication. Diastematomyelia is occasionally associated with a meningocele or congenital dermal cysts.

Clinical Features   The defect is usually associated with a heavily pigmented area of skin in the lumbar area and a growth of dark, coarse, or downy hair. The condition usually produces some degree of atrophy and weakness of the muscles in the lower limb and foot deformity. Sensory impairment may occur, and there may be joint deformities or ulceration of the feet. Sphincter control is impaired and occasionally lost. Examination of the spine reveals the skin abnormality and kyphoscoliosis.

Diagnostic Procedures   Radiographs of the spine reveal widening of the spinal canal and the presence of a bony septum. There may be associated abnormalities of the vertebrae. The cleft of the spinal cord can be demonstrated by MRI scan or CT metrizamide myelography.

Treatment   Removal of the midline septum produces improvement in some cases. Other patients require orthopedic correction of deformities in the lower limbs and urological treatment for sphincter problems.

Klippel-Feil Syndrome

Definition   The Klippel-Feil syndrome is a condition in which there is fusion of one or more vertebrae in the cervical area with shortening of the cervical spine.

Etiology and Pathology   The etiology is unknown. One or more of the cervical vertebrae are fused, and there may be absence of intervertebral discs at several levels. The condition is associated with incomplete closure of the dorsal arch in a number of cases.

Clinical Features   The patient has an abnormally short neck and low hair line, and folds of skin may extend from the ears to the shoulders. Active and passive head movements are reduced. Associated abnormalities such as kyphoscoliosis and Sprengel deformity occur. Patients may present with:

1.   Synkinetic or mirror movements of the limbs, which are said to result from failure of adequate decussation of the corticospinal tracts in the medullary pyramids.

2.   Progressive spastic quadriparesis, which should raise a suspicion of an associated Arnold-Chiari malformation.

3.   Later development of syringomyelia.

4.   Deafness in about 30 percent of cases due to malformation of the middle or inner ear.

5.   Association with a number of systemic congenital abnormalities, including congenital heart disease and renal anomalies such as agenesis of the kidney, horseshoe kidneys, or hydronephrosis.

Treatment   Decompressive surgery is indicated when there is evidence of progressive neurological deficit involving the cervical cord.

Sacrococcygeal Dystrophy

Definition   Sacrococcygeal dystrophy is a defect in the development of the sacrum and coccyx that is often associated with congenital abnormalities of the lumbosacral spinal cord.

Etiology and Pathology   The etiology is unknown. The absence of the sacrum and coccyx produces narrowing of the pelvis and congenital dislocation of the hips.

Clinical Features   There may be flaccid paralysis of the muscles of the pelvic girdle and lower limbs, sensory impairment in the lower limbs, and absence of sphincter control. Marked deformities of the joints of the lower limbs, including arthrogryposis multiplex congenita occur in some cases.

Treatment   Urological treatment is necessary for sphincter problems.

DEVELOPMENTAL DEFECTS OF THE CRANIAL-CERVICAL JUNCTION

Arnold-Chiari Malformation

Definition   The Arnold-Chiari malformation is a condition in which development of the hindbrain, the base of the skull, and the upper cervical canal is abnormal.

Etiology and Pathology   The etiology is unknown, but the Arnold-Chiari malformation probably represents a failure of harmonious development of the brainstem, cerebellum, and upper cervical region. The theory that the malformation is the result of "tethering" of the spinal cord to the sacrum by the filum terminale is unacceptable.

Two types of malformation are recognized: Chiari type I malformation and Arnold-Chiari malformation.

Chiari Type I Malformation   In the Chiari type I malformation there is herniation of the cerebellar tonsils below the foramen magnum. There are no other abnormalities, and the condition is not associated with a spinal myelomeningocele (Fig. 3-1).

Arnold-Chiari Malformation   In the Arnold-Chiari malformation the vermis of the cerebellum extends into the upper cervical canal along with the medulla and the fourth ventricle. The medulla is often folded on itself in an S-shaped fashion. There is an associated meningocele or myelomeningocele in the lumbosacral area, and hydrocephalus is present with dilatation of the entire ventricular system of the brain. Hydrocephalus may be due to an associated aqueductal stenosis or an obstruction of the flow of the cerebrospinal fluid (CSF) at the level of the base of the brain. Other congenital abnormalities of the central nervous system (CNS) are not unusual and include microgyria, fusion of the corpora quadrigemina, cysts of the foramen of Magendie, upward herniation of the cerebellum through an abnormally large tentorial notch, enlargement of the massa intermedia, fusion of the thalami, hydromyelia, and syringomyelia.

Clinical Features   The Chiari type I malformation may be asymptomatic or may cause cerebellar signs and progressive spastic quadriplegia at any time during life. These symptoms may be delayed until adult life. Occasionally, syncope on exertion occurs due to a transient increase of intracranial pressure (ICP).

The Arnold-Chiari malformation usually presents in infancy with progressive enlargement of the head due to hydrocephalus. There is often an associated spinal meningomyelocele. When the diagnosis is delayed, compression of the spinal cord at the cervical medullary junction produces spasticity of the lower limbs with increased tendon reflexes and extensor plantar responses. Cerebellar involvement produces ataxia, which predominantly affects the lower limbs with later involvement of the upper limbs. Compression of the lower brainstem at the cervical medullary junction produces downbeat nystagmus,[2] weakness and atrophy of the muscles of the tongue, the sternocleidomastoid, and the trapezius. There may be periodic venous congestion in the medulla with laryngeal stridor or respiration obstruction, which may be fatal.

Older children and adults may remain asymptomatic for many years and later present with pain in the suboccipital area, neck, and upper extremities, which is aggravated by head movement. There is an associated

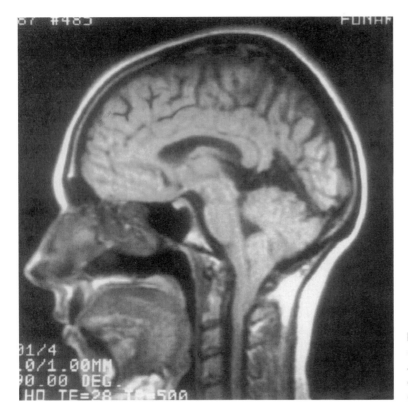

Figure 3-1
Chiari type I malformation. The MRI scan shows significant herniation of cerebellar tonsils shown to the level of the second cervical vertebra.

headache in the suboccipital area, which is increased on exertion. This is followed by weakness and spasticity involving all four limbs, ataxia of gait, and dysphagia. The association of the Arnold-Chiari malformation and syringomyelia in adult life is not unusual.

Diagnostic Procedures

1. MRI scanning. The MRI scan is the study of choice to demonstrate caudal displacement of cerebellar tissue including herniation of the vermis and cerebellar tonsils. Medullary herniation, inferior displacement of the aqueduct and fourth ventricle, and elongation and inferior displacement of the brainstem are usually present.[3,4]

2. CT scanning. CT scanning of the area following injection of contrast material into the subarachnoid space will also reveal the abnormality.

3. Myelography. If MRI or CT scanning is not available, a myelogram may reveal herniation of the cerebellar tonsils below the foramen magnum.

4. Arteriography. A vertebral arteriogram shows abnormal displacement of the posterior inferior cerebellar artery below the foramen magnum. Films taken during the venous phase show the vermian veins, which lie on the surface of the cerebellum, below the foramen magnum.

Treatment The myelomeningocele and hydrocephalus should be promptly treated in the affected infant. When signs of progressive neurological deficit develop later in life, pressure may be reduced by suboccipital decompression and laminectomy.

Platybasia

Definition Platybasia is an upward invagination of the foramen magnum, which causes flattening of the base of the skull and distortion of the contents of the posterior fossa.

Etiology and Pathology The condition occurs as a developmental abnormality but can be acquired later in life as a result of rickets, osteomalacia, or Paget's disease of the bone.

Clinical Features Pressure on the upper cervical spinal cord and medulla produces a progressive spastic quadriparesis occasionally accompanied by wasting of the tongue and dysphagia. Involvement of the cerebellum and cerebellar connections produces ataxia and nystagmus.

Diagnostic Procedures A lateral radiograph of the skull or laminogram of the foramen magnum should be taken. The angle subtended by a line drawn from the glabella to the midpoint of the pituitary fossa and from this point to the anterior margin of the foramen magnum should be constructed. This angle is usually less than 140° under normal circumstances but is increased in platybasia with invagination of the base of the skull.

Treatment Laminectomy, removal of the posterior lip of the foramen magnum, and decompression of the cervical cord and the lower brainstem are advised.

Basilar Impression

Definition Basilar impression or basilar invagination is an upward extension of the odontoid process through the foramen magnum producing compression of the lower brainstem and upper cervical cord.

Etiology and Pathology The etiology is unknown in congenital cases. The condition may occur as an acquired disease in association with the acquired form of platybasia. The effects of compression of the brainstem in platybasia may well be due to impairment of blood supply rather than direct compression by the odontoid process.

Clinical Features See platybasia, above.

Diagnostic Procedures Lateral films of the upper cervical region and the foramen magnum demonstrate projection of the odontoid process into the posterior fossa. This can be confirmed by constructing

McGregor's line—a line drawn from the posterior aspect of the hard palate to the external surface of the most inferior portion of the occipital bone behind the foramen magnum. Under normal circumstances the odontoid process is usually below and not more than 3 mm above McGregor's line. The tip of the odontoid process lies more than 6 mm above McGregor's line in platybasia.[5]

Treatment The treatment is that of platybasia. In addition, some surgeons remove the odontoid process through an anterior approach with fusion of the upper two cervical vertebrae.

DEVELOPMENTAL DEFECTS OF THE BRAINSTEM

Mobius Syndrome

Mobius syndrome is a condition characterized by congenital weakness of the facial muscles associated with bilateral failure of abduction of the eyes. The condition is occasionally familial, but many cases are sporadic. The etiology is unknown. The condition may be due to a congenital abnormality of the neurons of the sixth and seventh cranial nerve nuclei in the brainstem or the result of a primary neuropathy involving the facial and extraocular muscles.

There is bilateral facial weakness and wasting with an inability to abduct the eyes on either side. Some patients show additional features of complete ophthalmoplegia or wasting and paralysis of the pharynx and tongue. Occasionally, wasting of the pectoralis major, syndactyly, club feet, and mental retardation have been described in association with Mobius syndrome.

Cerebellar Dysgenesis

Many forms of congenital abnormality of the cerebellum have been described. These may occur as sole defects or in association with abnormalities involving the brainstem and cerebral hemispheres.[6] Children with cerebellar abnormalities may present with ataxia dating from birth. About 50 percent of these cases have a genetic disorder while others are examples of ataxic cerebral palsy. In some familial cases cerebel-

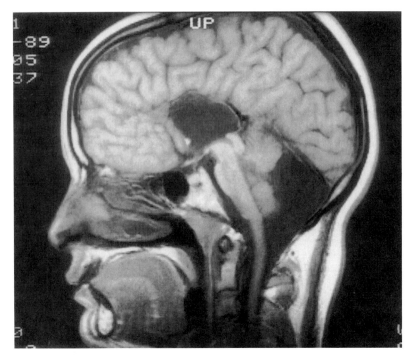

Figure 3-2
Dandy-Walker syndrome. The MRI scan shows a large cyst replacing most of the cerebellum including the vermis and posterior portions of the hemispheres. The scan shows an additional abnormality—agenesis of the corpus callosum.

lar ataxia is associated with mental retardation and additional findings of atrophy of the inferior olives, pons, restiform body, thalamus, and microcephaly.[7] Many cases of congenital cerebellar dysgenesis remain undiagnosed and present as an incidental finding during life or at autopsy.

Dandy-Walker Syndrome

Definition   The Dandy-Walker syndrome is a condition in which maldevelopment of the roof of the fourth ventricle is associated with failure of development of the cerebellar vermis.

Etiology and Pathology   The etiology is unknown. The posterior fossa is enlarged, and the internal occipital protuberance is elevated. The fourth ventricle is dilated and forms a cyst-like protrusion between the cerebellar hemispheres. The brain shows signs of hydrocephalus.

Clinical Features   The condition may present with hydrocephalus in infancy or early childhood. Other cerebral brainstem or cerebellar anomalies are

not unusual and visceral, particularly cardiac abnormalities, occur in a significant number of cases.[8]

Diagnostic Procedures   Either MRI or CT scanning will demonstrate the presence of a midline cystic mass in the posterior fossa, which extends between the cerebellar hemispheres, and diffuse dilation of the ventricular system due to hydrocephalus[9] (Fig. 3-2).

Treatment   The condition responds to a ventricular peritoneal shunting procedure.

Congenital Nystagmus

Definition   Congenital nystagmus is a familial condition, often inherited as a sex-linked recessive or an autosomal dominant trait in which nystagmus is present from birth.

Etiology and Pathology   It is postulated that the nystagmus is due to inequality in the activity of the vestibular reflex mechanisms responsible for saccadic eye movements.

Clinical Features Nystagmus may be either pendular, in which the amplitude and rate of nystagmus is equal in the two directions, or it may be a jerk nystagmus, in which there is a slow and fast component to the nystagmus.

Nystagmus is usually present at rest and always increases in amplitude on lateral gaze. The condition is usually obvious at birth; when it is not, it typically appears in early infancy. In later life there may be associated rhythmic movements of the head. There is more than a chance association of other congenital abnormalities involving the CNS, particularly strabismus.

Diagnostic Procedures The diagnosis is based on the history and physical examination.

Treatment Treatment is usually not required.

Duane Syndrome

Definition Duane syndrome is a congenital disorder of ocular movement inherited as an autosomal dominant trait in a minority of cases.

Etiology and Pathology The etiology is unknown. A number of different pathological changes have been described, including abnormalities in the neurons of the oculomotor nerves and myopathy affecting the lateral rectus muscles.

Clinical Features The syndrome can be detected only on eye movement and is characterized by limitation of abduction, widening of the palpebral fissure and protrusion of the eye on attempted abduction, and narrowing of the palpebral fissure and retraction of the eye into the orbit on adduction. A downward and inward deviation of the eye may accompany adduction. Duane syndrome has been described in association with many other congenital abnormalities.

Spasmus Nutans

Definition Spasmus nutans is an uncommon congenital abnormality characterized by nystagmus and head tilting.

Etiology and Pathology The etiology is unknown. The condition occurs in children who have been kept indoors for an undue period of time in dark or dimly illuminated surroundings. Pathological changes are unknown.

Clinical Features The condition usually begins between 16 and 18 months of age with the development of a horizontal, vertical, rotary, mixed, or monocular nystagmus. The development of nystagmus is accompanied by head nodding, which is usually intermittent and abolishes the nystagmus. Head tilting occurs in 50 percent of patients. No other abnormalities are seen on neurological examination.

Diagnostic Procedures All children with monocular nystagmus should have a CT or MRI scan to rule out a glioma of the optic nerve or optic chiasm.[10]

Treatment Treatment is not necessary because spasmus nutans shows spontaneous resolution 6 months or 1 year after onset.

DEVELOPMENTAL DEFECTS OF THE SKULL

There are several developmental defects of the skull, among them:

1. Cranium bifidum occultum is the mildest developmental defect of the skull. There is a deficiency in the midline fusion of bones of the skull, which usually occurs in the parietal occipital area. The condition is asymptomatic.

2. Meningoceles of the skull usually occur in the parietal occipital area. The bony defect is associated with protrusion of a sac consisting of dura and arachnoid, which contains CSF. This defect occasionally occurs at other sites, including the frontal area, nasal area, and nasopharynx. In a meningoencephalocele the sac also contains neural tissue.

3. Iniencephaly is a rare malformation of the posterior fossa involving the foramen magnum and upper cervical vertebrae. Deformities include retroflexion of the head, malformation of the brain,

and malformation of many other organs of the body. Most patients die shortly after birth.

4. Complete rachischisis occurs when there is failure of fusion of the skull associated with failure of development of the rostral portion of the neural tube resulting in anencephaly. The brain may be represented by a mass of undifferentiated nervous tissue.

5. Dermal sinuses usually occur in the midline parietal occipital area. They may or may not be associated with a dermoid cyst that communicates with the subarachnoid space. This affords a tract between the surface and the subarachnoid space and may be the cause of recurrent meningitis. The dermoid cyst may occasionally discharge highly irritating sebaceous material into the subarachnoid space, which may cause a severe chemical meningitis.

6. Craniosynostosis is a condition characterized by premature fusion of one or more of the cranial sutures. The disorder appears to result from a failure of development of bones at the base of the skull with failure of transmission of forces through the dura to the calvarium. Two forms are recognized: primary craniosynostosis, in which there is failure of one or more of the cranial sutures to remain open, and secondary craniosynostosis, which occurs with diseases such as rickets, vitamin D–resistant rickets, and hypophosphatasia, and following excessive replacement of thyroid hormone in infantile cretinism.

Many syndromes have been associated with craniosynostosis. Some are inherited as autosomal dominant traits, whereas others occur as autosomal recessive traits. There is an association with mental retardation and increased ICP in some cases. The most common condition is Crouzon syndrome. Other forms of craniosynostosis include scaphocephaly, brachycephaly, and trigonocephaly. These conditions are not usually associated with neurological abnormalities.

Treatment is indicated only if the child develops increased ICP and for cosmetic restoration of normal cranial and facial appearance when the deformity is severe. Hydrocephalus should be treated with ventriculoperitoneal shunting.

Craniocleidodysostosis

This condition is due to failure of development of the membranous bones of the face, clavicles, and cranial vault. There is a typical facial appearance with a depressed nasal bridge and high arched palate. The clavicles are rudimentary or only partially developed, and the anterior and posterior fontanelles remain open. There is frequently some abnormality in the underlying brain, particularly involving the frontal lobes and the anterior portion of the corpus callosum. Mental retardation and seizures are common.

Radiography of the skull is characteristic in this condition and shows partial ossification of the frontoparietal and occipital bones with persistence of the fontanelle. The appearance resembles a hot cross bun.

Achondroplasia

Definition Achondroplasia is a condition in which there is abnormal development of cartilaginous bone.

Clinical Features Patients have the typical appearance of an achondroplastic dwarf with a small face, depressed nasal bridge, and short extremities. There is marked lumbar lordosis and anterior flaring of the sacrum. Neurological manifestations include a mild degree of mental retardation, hydrocephalus, and late development of progressive spastic paraparesis due to platybasia or spinal cord compression caused by herniation of one or more intervertebral discs or spondylosis. Sudden death can occur from brainstem compression.[11]

Diagnostic Procedures

1. Hydrocephalus can be diagnosed by MRI scan or radioactive cisternography.

2. The diagnosis of platybasia has already been discussed above.

Treatment

1. Hydrocephalus may be relieved by ventriculoperitoneal shunting.

2. Platybasia, spinal cord, or cauda equina compression from spinal stenosis with progressive neurological deficit will require surgical intervention.[12]

Microcephaly

A small skull is associated with a small brain, but this does not necessarily imply neurological abnormality; approximately 2 percent of people with an unusually small brain or microcephaly have normal intelligence. Microcephaly may be caused by:

1. A primary genetically determined condition that is inherited as an autosomal recessive trait accounts for 20 to 25 percent of cases of microcephaly.

2. A known chromosomal abnormality such as Down's syndrome.

3. Secondary microcephaly resulting from intrauterine infection by known viruses such as rubella or cytomegalovirus.

4. Asphyxia neonatorum.

5. Neonatal trauma.

6. Postpartum meningitis or encephalitis.

Intrauterine diagnosis of microcephaly by ultrasound may not be accurate because some microcephalics have normal head circumference at birth with slowing of head growth after birth.[13]

Macrocrania

An enlarged skull is not necessarily associated with an enlarged brain. The most common cause is hydrocephalus. The condition has also been described in benign intracranial hypertension and in bony abnormalities including osteogenesis imperfecta and craniocleidodysostosis. Asymmetrical enlargement of the skull may develop when subdural hematomas and hygromas occur in infants.

Megencephaly

Megencephaly, or enlargement of the brain, is occasionally seen in conditions affecting the parenchyma of the brain, such as the lipidoses and leukodystrophies.

Hypertelorism

Hypertelorism is a disproportionate enlargement of the lesser wings of the sphenoid bone associated with decrease in size of the greater wings of the sphenoid bone and an excessive distance between the orbits. The condition is seen in many mentally retarded individuals but may occur in perfectly normal individuals.

Fibrous Dysplasia

Definition Fibrous dysplasia is a condition of progressive displacement of normal bone by fibrous-osseous tissue.

Etiology and Pathology The etiology is unknown. Normal bone is progressively replaced by an abnormal proliferation of fibrous connective tissue that contains poorly formed bone trabeculae.

Clinical Features The disease occurs in monostolic and polyostolic forms and can affect any bone in the body. The skull and facial bones are involved in about 25 percent of cases. Extensive involvement of the facial bones gives the characteristic appearance of leontiasis ossea,[14] but the base of the skull shows thickening and sclerosis of bone. The dysplastic process may involve the orbits, paranasal sinuses, nasal fossi, and neurovascular canals. The most common symptom is an asymptomatic cosmetic deformity.[15] Orbital involvement results in pressure on the optic nerve, visual impairment, and eventually total loss of vision in the affected eye.

Malignancies including osteosarcoma, fibrosarcoma, and chondrosarcoma occur in less than 1 percent of cases of fibrous dysplasia. Some cases occur following radiation therapy, which has been recommended for treatment of fibrous dysplasia in the past. The current recommendation is that radiation therapy is ineffective in this disease.[16] Multiple meningiomas have been reported. The rare occurrence of McCune-Albright syndrome of thyrotoxicosis and gigantism/acromegaly has been described in craniofacial fibrous dysplasia.[14]

Diagnostic Procedures

1.   Radiographs of the skull show a pagetoid or ground-glass pattern that consists of a mixture of dense and radiolucent areas, a homogenous sclerotic pattern, or a cystic variety characterized by spherical or ovoid lucency surrounded by a dense rim.[17]

2.   CT scanning is the study of choice in fibrous dysplasia with clear definition of soft tissue and dense bone structures.

Treatment   Surgical removal of tissue compressing the brain or vital structures, such as the optic nerve, and removal of tumors because of pressure effects or potential malignancy are recommended.

DEVELOPMENTAL DEFECTS OF THE FOREBRAIN

Anencephaly is a condition in which there is complete absence of development of the forebrain, which is usually represented by a mass of undifferentiated neural tissue. This condition may or may not be associated with failure of development of the skull. When the skull forms normally, the area which would normally be occupied by the hemispheres contains CSF. This is called hydranencephaly, which can be demonstrated by transillumination of the infant's head.

Severe deformities of the forebrain, or prosencephaly, are often associated with abnormalities involving the basal ganglia, thalamus, spinal cord, and marked deformities of the face, including cyclopia. Most of these conditions are incompatible with life.

Abnormalities of the gyri are usually associated with mental retardation and seizures. These abnormalities include absence of gyri (lissencephaly), numerous small gyri (microgyria), or wide irregular gyri (pachygyria).

A porencephalic cyst is a condition that occurs when there is failure of development of one hemisphere or part of one hemisphere and is often caused by failure of development of a normal blood supply. This condition is often associated with contralateral hemiparesis and some degree of mental retardation. Seizures are not unusual. Less severe defects involving the hemispheres include schizencephaly in which there are clefts communicating with the ventricular system. Inclusions of gray matter in the white matter are not uncommon and may give rise to seizures later in life, particularly when the inclusions occur in the temporal lobes. A number of developmental abnormalities are of no clinical significance, and these include the presence of a central cavity in the septum pellucidum, cavum septum pellucidi, or a more posterior cavity, cavum virgii.

One of the most common malformations of the brain is partial failure of development of the corpus callosum. Agenesis of the corpus callosum is asymptomatic and does not lead to any problems later in life. However, the condition is often associated with other developmental defects, such as the G syndrome, that cause some degree of mental retardation and seizures.[18]

The diagnosis of agenesis of the corpus callosum can be established by MRI or CT scanning demonstrating wide separation of the lateral ventricles, dilatation of the occipital horns of the lateral ventricles, and a high position of the third ventricle.

DEVELOPMENTAL DEFECTS OF THE OPTIC NERVE AND RETINA

The most frequently encountered developmental defect of the optic nerve is of no clinical significance and consists of myelinated fibers that extend out from the edge of the optic nerve onto the retina. The optic nerve and retina have a normal appearance in patients with congenital absence of rods and cones. A midline coloboma or retinal defect occurs when the optic vesicles fail to fuse. This midline cleft may involve the optic disc, as well as the retina, and may extend into the iris.

Pigmentary Degeneration of the Retina

In addition to retinitis pigmentosa a number of conditions are associated with pigmentary degeneration of the retina. The appearance of the retina is not always comparable to that of retinitis pigmentosa. Pigmentary degeneration of the retina may occur in association with spinocerebellar degeneration, hereditary spastic ataxia and spastic paraparesis, the Laurence-

Moon-Biedl syndrome, heredopathia atactica polyneuritiformis (Refsum disease), Kearns-Sayre syndrome, and a rare condition called homocarcinosis, in which spastic paraplegia, progressive mental retardation, and pigmentary degeneration of the retina occur.

CEREBRAL PALSY

Cerebral palsy is a nonprogressive disturbance of brain function due to prenatal factors in the majority of cases and occurs in 0.2 to 0.25 percent of pregnancies.[19] Prenatal factors include genetic abnormalities producing neuronal migration disorders including pachygyria, polygyria, schizencephaly, heteratopia, agenesis of the corpus callosum, and hyperplasia of the cerebellum.[20] Vascular disorders may occur in utero and include focal infarction, symmetrical periventricular ischemia (periventricular leukomalasia), or intraventricular hemorrhage with enlarged ventricles. Intrauterine infection from cytomegalovirus, rubella, herpes simplex, and toxoplasmosis are additional causal factors. Perinatal factors include metabolic disorders and pyridoxine dependency. Encephalopathy following asphyxia and birth trauma occurs in about 3 to 6 per 1000 births.[21] Affected term infants have an Apgar score less than 5 at 1 to 5 min, require resuscitation or ventilator support, and experience convulsions before day 3. Preterm infants who develop cerebral palsy exhibit intracerebral hemorrhage, brain edema, neonatal shock requiring resuscitation, asystole, or evidence of CNS infection. Consequently, cerebral palsy should be regarded as a neurological syndrome of heterogenous background.[22] However, birth asphyxia should only be considered in infants who experience an event or condition during the perinatal period that is likely to severely reduce oxygen delivery and lead to acidosis (e.g., major antenatal hemorrhage or cord prolapse and the failure of function of two organs such as the brain and kidneys consistent with the effect of asphyxia).[19] The risk of cerebral palsy is low in the asymptomatic newborn even after complicated delivery, and the majority of full-term infants who develop cerebral palsy are the products of normal pregnancies and have no perinatal events that may have caused neurological impairment.[23] Five types are now recognized: spastic

diplegia, hemiplegic cerebral palsy, athetotic cerebral palsy, ataxic cerebral palsy, and complex plegia.

Spastic Diplegia

Definition   Spastic diplegia is the most common form of cerebral palsy.[22]

Etiology and Pathology   The most common etiologic factor is low birth weight, suggesting that some prenatal factor is responsible for spastic diplegia. The majority of these children are premature, but some are born full term with normal birth weight. This latter group shows a high proportion of severely retarded infants. Two readily identifiable conditions in low birth weight children are periventricular leukomalacia and intraventricular hemorrhage with ventricular dilatation identified by MRI scan or transcranial ultrasonography. Periventricular leukomalacia has also been demonstrated in full-term children suggesting a silent ischemic hypoxic episode in utero in the third trimester.

Clinical Features   There is usually a history of prematurity, birth weight less than 2000 g, and a delay in reaching such motor milestones as sitting, standing, and walking. Signs of the development of corticospinal tract damage include hypertonia, adductor spasm, increased tendon reflexes, and bilateral extensor plantar responses. Patients have a typical "scissor" gait. There is a high incidence of associated strabismus or squint. Mental retardation, if present, is usually less severe in spastic diplegia than in other forms of cerebral palsy. Twenty-seven percent of patients develop a seizure disorder.

Hemiplegic Cerebral Palsy

Definition   Hemiplegic cerebral palsy is a common form of cerebral palsy and usually results from damage to the sensorimotor cortex that controls one side of the body.

Etiology and Pathology   The cause is multifactorial as already explained, and head trauma at birth, anoxia, and embolism are now believed to be unlikely causes of hemiplegic cerebral palsy.

Clinical Features   The hemiparesis is usually not apparent at birth, and it may not be until much later that the child develops difficulty. Typically, the hemiparesis involves the upper extremity more than the lower, and growth and development are impaired in the affected limbs, the cause of which is unknown and is not related to nutritional nor endocrine factors.[24] In mild cases, the growth asymmetry can be detected by comparing the size of thumbnails on the two sides. Sensory deficits are of a cortical nature. This form of cerebral palsy is associated with the mildest mental retardation of all forms; however, 50 percent of these children develop a seizure disorder.

Athetotic Cerebral Palsy

Athetotic cerebral palsy is characterized by involuntary choreoathetoid movements due to damage to the extrapyramidal system. The factors producing damage to the basal ganglia are unknown, and asphyxia neonatorum with anoxia is no longer considered a factor. Similarly, kernicterus damage to the basal ganglia due to deposition of bilirubin was a leading cause of athetotic cerebral palsy in the past but is unusual now. These children are usually hypotonic at birth and develop generalized choreoathetoid movements after 1 year of age. The speech is severely dysarthric, but 45 percent of patients with athetotic cerebral palsy have an IQ greater than 90.

Ataxic Cerebral Palsy

Ataxic cerebral palsy is a rare form of cerebral palsy characterized by cerebellar ataxia. The condition most commonly occurs in children with cerebellar hemorrhage. Motor development and walking are delayed due to cerebellar ataxia. Speech is dysarthric. In most cases intelligence is normal.

Complex Plegia

Complex plegia is a form of cerebral palsy in which corticospinal, extrapyramidal, or cerebellar function are impaired. Children frequently have unilateral or bilateral motor involvement with spasticity or involuntary movements. Additional difficulties in-

clude mental retardation, limb and truncal ataxia, and seizures.

Diagnostic Procedures

1.   Affected children should be screened for metabolic abnormalities such as hypoglycemia, hypothyroidism, amino acidurias, and pyridoxine dependency.

2.   MRI scanning will demonstrate developmental defects of areas of infarction, leukomalacia, or hemorrhage[20] shortly after birth. Children with spastic diplegia have significant atrophy of the corpus callosum.[25]

3.   Ultrasonography through the anterior fontanel is useful in demonstrating hemorrhage, ventricular enlargement, or periventricular leukomalacia in newborn infants who fail to thrive and in low birth weight infants who are suspected cases of cerebral palsy up to the age of 2 years.

4.   Psychologic testing should be obtained as soon as possible to assess educational potential.

5.   Urodynamic assessment to determine the cause of lower urinary tract dysfunction should lead to more rational treatment of the more than one-third of children with cerebral palsy who have voiding problems.

Treatment

The key to success in the treatment of cerebral palsy is teamwork with a planned approach to the individual child's problem. The child, parents, pediatrician, neurologist, psychologist, physical therapist, and school authorities should be involved. Education programs must be tailored to the needs of the child. Many children with cerebral palsy have normal intelligence and should not be penalized because of dysarthria or involuntary movements. Conversely, many parents develop unrealistic expectations of children who have moderate to severe mental retardation. These cases require tactful handling, and realistic goals should be set.

Seizures should be correctly identified as outlined in Chapter 4 and treated with appropriate anticonvulsant medication as soon as the diagnosis is established.

REFERENCES

1. Simpson RK Jr, Rose JE: Cervical diastematomyelia. Report of a case and review of a rare congenital anomaly. *Arch Neurol* 44:331, 1987.
2. Bronstein AM, Miller DH Rudge P, et al: Down beating nystagmus: magnetic resonance imaging and neuro-otological findings. *J Neurol Sci* 81:173, 1987.
3. el Gammal T, Mark EK: MR imaging of Chiari II malformation. *AJR Am J Roentgenol* 150:163, 1988.
4. Yuh WT, Segall HD, et al: MR imaging of Chiari II malformation associated with dysgenesis of cerebellum and brain stem. *J Comput Tomogr* 11:188, 1987.
5. Adam AM: Skull radiograph measurements of normals and patients with basilar impression; use of Landzert's angle. *Surg Radiol Anat* 9:225, 1987.
6. Young ID, Moore JR: Sex-linked recessive congenital ataxia. *J Neurol Neurosurg Psychiatry* 50:1230, 1987.
7. Robain O, Dulac O: Cerebellar hemispheric agenesis. *Acta Neuropathol (Berl.)* 74:202, 1987.
8. Golden JA, Rorke LB: Dandy Walker syndrome and associated anomalies. *Pediatr Neurosci* 13:38, 1987.
9. Naraganan HS, Gandhi DH: Neurocutaneous melanosis associated with Dandy-Walker syndrome. *Clin Neurol Neurosurg* 89:197, 1987.
10. Hoyt CS: Nystagmus and other abnormal ocular movements in children. *Pediatr Clin North Am* 34:1415, 1987.
11. Hecht JT, Francomano CA, et al: Mortality in achondroplasia. *Am J Hum Genet* 41:454, 1987.
12. Shikata J, Yamamuro T, et al: Surgical treatment of achondroplastic dwarfs with paraplegia. *Surg Neurol* 29:125, 1988.
13. Jaffe M, Terosh E, Oren S: The dilemma in prenatal diagnosis of idiopathic microcephaly. *Dev Med Child Neurol* 29:187, 1987.
14. Daly BD, Chow CC, Cockram CS: Unusual manifestations of craniofacial fibrous dysplasia: clinical, endocrinological and computed tomographic features. *Postgrad Med J* 70:10, 1994.
15. Jan M, Dweik A, Destrieux C, et al: Fronto-orbital sphenoidal fibrous dysplasia. *Neurosurgery* 34:544, 1994.
16. Ruggieri P, Sim FH, Bond JR, et al: Malignancies in fibrous dysplasia. *Cancer* 73:1411, 1994.
17. Brown EW, Megerian CA, McKenna MJ, et al: Fibrous dysplasia of the temporal bone: imaging findings. *AJR Am J Roentgenol* 164:679, 1995.
18. Neri G, Genuardi M, Natoli G, et al: A girl with G syndrome and agenesis of the corpus callosum. *Am J Med Genet* 28:287, 1987.
19. The origins of cerebral palsy—a consensus statement. The Australian and New Zealand Perinatal Societies. *Med J Aust* 162:85, 1995.
20. Sugimoto T, Woo M, Nishida N, et al: When do brain abnormalities in cerebral palsy occur? An MRI study. *Dev Med Child Neurol* 37:285, 1995.
21. Hall DM: Intrapartum events and cerebral palsy. *Br J Obst Gynaecol* 101:745, 1994.
22. Kragelow-Mann I, Hagberg G, Meisner C, et al: Bilateral spastic cerebral palsy—a collaborative study between southwest Germany and western Sweden. III. Aetiology. *Dev Med Child Neurol* 37:191, 1995.
23. Naulty CM, Long LB, Pettett G: Prevalence of prematurity, low birthweight, and asphyxia as perinatal risk factors in a current population of children with cerebral palsy. *Amer J Perinatol* 11:377, 1994.
24. Stevenson RD, Roberts CD, Vogtl L: The effects of non-nutritional factors on growth in cerebral palsy. *Dev Med Child Neurol* 37:124, 1995.
25. Iai M, Tanabe YM, Goto M, et al: A comparative magnetic resonance imaging study of the corpus callosum in neurologically normal children and children with spastic diplegia. *Acta Paediatr* 83:1086, 1994.

Chapter 4

EPILEPSY

Epilepsy is a condition characterized by abnormal recurrent and excessive neuronal discharges precipitated by many different disturbances within the central nervous system (CNS).

Under normal circumstances, neuronal discharge is rhythmic and represents repetitive, excitatory, and inhibitory influences. The summation of neuronal discharges is recorded in the electroencephalogram (EEG).

No single mechanism can explain epileptic activity. Many abnormalities—the results of hereditary disorders, congenital anomalies, trauma, scar formation, infection, hypoxia, hypoglycemia, tumor, cerebral infarction, vasculitis, or a degenerative condition—can lead to an alteration in neuronal function, the result of selective loss of inhibitory neurons in the damaged region of the brain.[1] There may be multiplication in dendritic structure or proliferation of dendrites with increased synaptic contact and synaptic reorganization in a limited area.[2] Epilepsy is the result of dysfunction of a relatively large cell population, which initiates a local paroxysmal discharge, probably the result of excessive glutamate or aspartate release and increased N-methyl-D-aspartate (NMDA) receptor activity. This discharge propagates from the original site through an abnormal dendritic network, lacking inhibitory mechanisms, recruiting neurons at other sites with emergence of a focal seizure. Further propagation leads to a generalized seizure. The excitatory discharge overwhelms inhibitory mechanisms driven by γ-aminobutyric acid (GABA)-ergic neurons. The role of other neurotransmitters in the generation of the epileptic seizure is probably limited. Norepinephrine probably plays an inhibitory role in limiting the spread of seizures. The dopaminergic system has a lesser role as an inhibitory influence in seizure propagation, while the diffuse acetylcholine projections through the brain may enhance the epileptic process. An epileptic discharge spreading to involve all of the brain will result in a generalized seizure. When the discharge does not spread, the seizure will be focal or partial. In partial seizures, the clinical manifestation is determined by the area of the brain involved. All areas of the brain are potentially epileptogenic; consequently, many different seizure patterns are recognized. Epilepsy may be classified according to the clinical presentation of the seizure (Table 4-1).

Table 4-1
Classification of epilepsy

I. Partial seizures
  A. Simple partial seizures
    i. Motor—focal motor; focal motor with march (jacksonian), versive, postural, phonatory
    ii. Sensory—somatosensory, visual, auditory, olfactory, gustatory, vertiginous
    iii. Autonomic
    iv. Psychic—dysphasia, dysmnesia, cognitive, affective, illusions, hallucinations
  B. Complex partial seizures
    i. Simple partial seizures followed by impairment of consciousness
    ii. With impairment of consciousness at onset and in some cases, automatisms
  C. Any partial seizure may evolve to a secondary generalized seizure.

II. Generalized seizures
  A. Absence seizures
    i. Typical absence seizures
      With impairment of consciousness only
      With mild clonic movements
      With tonic components
      With automatisms
      With autonomic components
    ii. Atypical absence
  B. Myoclonic seizures
  C. Tonic seizures
  D. Tonic clonic seizures
  E. Tonic (static) seizures

III. Unclassified seizures that cannot be classified into one of the above categories.

ETIOLOGY AND PATHOLOGY

It is important to emphasize that seizures result only from the electrical discharge of living cells. Necrotic tissue and scar tissue are not the origin of epileptic activity, although sclerosis may produce damage to nearby surviving neurons, altering their metabolism and function with propagation of abnormal discharges to nearby neurons, gradually incorporating them into an abnormal pool of neuronal activity.

CAUSATIVE FACTORS IN SEIZURES

Hereditary Factors in Seizures

Fifty percent of patients with epilepsy have no demonstrable underlying neurological disorder. These "idiopathic" cases have a strong genetic background and patients experience primary generalized seizures. Family studies have shown that the patient and approximately 30 percent of siblings and children of the patient have similar EEG abnormalities. The gene penetrance of this trait is about 14 percent in early childhood, rising to over 50 percent in middle childhood and then decreasing to lower levels in adult life.

Seizures are not an unusual concomitant of some of the rare hereditary diseases, including the leukodystrophies, lipidoses, and aminoacidurias. Tuberous sclerosis and Sturge-Weber disease are frequently accompanied by a seizure disorder. The hypoglycemia that results from several of the glycogen storage diseases and other hereditary hypoglycemias, such as leucine-sensitive hypoglycemia, frequently produce seizures in affected children. Some of the chromosomal abnormalities such as trisomy D are accompanied by intractable seizure activity.

Prenatal and Perinatal Factors in Seizures

A number of infections may be passed transplancentally from mother to fetus, often producing brain damage and seizure activity. These infections include syphilis, toxoplasmosis, rubella, cytomegalovirus, and herpes simplex. The regular maternal use of certain drugs, including alcohol and cocaine, has been implicated in the cause of brain damage in the fetus and subsequent seizure activity. Irradiation in the early months of gestation can also produce brain damage, cerebral maldevelopment, and seizures.

Traumatic insults to the brain during parturition may have a number of effects. There may be direct damage to the brain. Excessive molding of the head as it passes through the birth canal may lead to herniation of the medial aspect of the temporal lobe over the free edge of the tentorium cerebelli. Although this condition resolves as soon as the head is born, the herniation is sufficient to produce damage to the medial aspect of the temporal lobe with subsequent gliosis. There is alteration in metabolism and function in surrounding neurons, with generation of abnormal discharges, which are propagated to nearby neurons, gradually incorporating them into an abnormal pool of neuronal activity. This, coupled with the development of abnormal synaptic connections, draws an increasing number of neurons into an abnormal process and eventually the area becomes epileptogenic later in life.[2] This mechanism is the cause of complex partial seizures (psychomotor or temporal lobe seizures). Perinatal trauma has a number of indirect effects, including cerebral venous thrombosis, which may become associated with later seizure activity.

Perinatal anoxia has many causes. The basic problem lies in failure to establish spontaneous respirations at birth. This can occur in prematurity and in excess maternal sedation during labor. Anoxia is a potent cause of liver damage and kernicterus, which leads to cerebral damage in about 25 percent of surviving infants, with subsequent development of microcephaly, mental retardation, choreoathetosis, and seizures. However, the role of perinatal anoxia in infantile brain damage and subsequent development of seizures has been overemphasized in the past, and it is probable that anoxia is a minor factor in brain damage and subsequent development of seizures.

Toxic, Metabolic, and Nutritional Causes of Seizures

Numerous toxins and drugs are epileptogenic. Commonly encountered toxic causes include alcohol withdrawal; sudden withdrawal of barbiturates or phenytoin in the epileptic; high doses of psychotropic drugs, particularly phenothiazines, butyrophenones, and thioxanthenes; poisoning with carbon monoxide; lead or mercury; the ingestion of antihistamines; and intravenous injection of heroin or cocaine.[3]

Electrolyte disturbances, hyponatremia, hypernatremia, hypocalcemia, and hypomagnesemia produce neuronal irritability and seizures. Seizures frequently accompany hypoglycemia, uremic encephalopathy, and other chronic metabolic encephalopathies.

Pyridoxine deficiencies are a rare but potent cause of neonatal and infantile seizures and should always be considered in an investigation of seizures in this age group. Pyridoxine dependency occurs in infants who receive diets deficient in pyridoxine.

Infectious Causes of Seizures

Seizures are not unusual during the early stage of acute bacterial meningitis and acute encephalitis, particularly in children. Chronic infections such as neurosyphilis, tuberculosis, and fungal and parasitic infestation may also be accompanied by seizures.

Head Trauma, Cerebral Anoxia in Seizures

Severe head trauma is often followed by seizures. The early onset of seizures, within 1 to 7 days after injury, carries a better prognosis than a later onset. Post-traumatic seizures are discussed in Chapter 18. Anoxic encephalopathy can occur at any age and is frequently accompanied by seizures. An increasing number of patients suffering from anoxia or hypoxia are successfully resuscitated following cardiac or respiratory arrest and subsequently present with anoxic encephalopathy, myoclonus, and intermittent seizures.

Vascular and Neoplastic Causes of Seizures

Seizures occur in about 15 percent of patients with chronic cerebrovascular disease. These are usually individuals who have suffered cerebral infarction or cerebral hemorrhage. The rarer arteritides, particu-

larly polyarthritis nodosa, may be associated with the late onset of seizures.

All brain tumors are potentially epileptogenic and the sudden onset of seizures in adult life should always raise the possibility of neoplasia; 40 to 60 percent of tumors produce seizures.

Degenerative and Demyelinating Causes of Seizures

All patients with degenerative diseases of the brain have an increased risk of seizure activity. Seizures are not uncommon during the course of Alzheimer disease. Ten percent of patients with multiple sclerosis will have seizure activity sometime during the course of their disease.

CLINICAL FEATURES

Epidemiology

Epilepsy has a prevalence of 1 to 2 percent, which means that from 2 million to 4 million people suffer from epilepsy in the United States. The condition occurs in all races and has an equal distribution in males and females. Epilepsy occurs in all age groups, but there is a marked difference in incidence in relation to age. Two-thirds of all epileptic patients develop their seizure disorder in childhood or adolescence, with an average incidence of between 46 and 83 per 100,000 in children under 14 years of age[4] (Table 4-2). Fewer than 2 percent of all epileptic patients have their first seizure after the age of 50 years.

Table 4-2
Common causes of seizures in children

1. Febrile seizures
2. Hypertension—nearly all cases are uremic
3. Lead encephalopathy
4. Electrolyte disturbances—particularly hyponatremia
5. Meningitis
6. Encephalitis
7. Cerebral malformations, particularly tuberous sclerosis

SIMPLE PARTIAL SEIZURES

Simple partial seizures occur at any age and are characterized by focal epileptic activity without impairment of consciousness. A partial seizure is the result of focal neuronal seizure activity, which may remain localized or spread to involve nearby neuronal pools or become secondarily generalized. Consequently, a careful history of an event reconstructing clinical presentation of the partial seizure serially in a temporal fashion will illustrate the spread of the disturbance through the brain. Partial seizures usually produce positive symptoms, not negative ones,[5] and the symptoms and signs are stereotyped and paroxysmal.

Although the patient is conscious during a seizure, the history should be obtained from a patient and an observer whenever possible, because experience and observation do not necessarily coincide.

I. Motor Seizures

a. Focal Motor Seizures

There is clonic activity involving a strictly focal area of the body, usually the thumb, fingers, or base. Most simple motor seizures are brief, lasting for a few seconds. However, in some cases, seizures may continue for hours or days (epilepsia partialis continua), which may be followed by a transient weakness of the muscle groups involved in the seizure activity—a condition termed Todd's paralysis. A more serious form of partial motor seizure, occurs in Rasmussen encephalitis, and presents as repeated partial motor seizures or epilepsia partialis continua compounded by the gradual development of hemiparesis. Cognitive impairment can occur in the later stages of this disease.

b. Focal Motor with March (Jacksonian)

There is clonic activity that begins focally and spreads in an orderly fashion to involve other structures on the same side of the body; spread corresponds to the relationship of representative neurons in the motor cortex; for

example, the thumb, finger, wrist, forearm (Fig. 4-1).

c. Versive Seizures

Involuntary movements of the head, eyes, and trunk occur in contraversive fashion (e.g., the head turns toward the involved arm), indicating the presence of a neuroepileptic focus in the contralateral frontal, temporal, or occasionally the occipital lobe.[6] Ipsiversive head movement is an occasional observation in versive seizures. Patients aware of the versive movements usually have frontal lobe foci.

d. Postural Seizures

There is a sudden tonic contraction of the muscles in a limb, with the assumption of an abnormal posture in a hand or foot.

e. Phonatory Seizures

These seizures are characterized by brief involuntary vocalization or, more commonly, brief speech arrest.

f. Atonic Seizures

Focal atonic seizures are partial seizures with ictal paresis or paralysis of one or more parts of the body.[7] The paralysis may precede or occur during the focal motor seizure. There may be a preceding somatosensory sensation affecting the same side of the body, including warmth, a hot sensation, a buzzing, or a nonspecific discomfort. Attacks are brief in duration.

Focal atonic seizures are also the result of negative myoclonus—a lapse of muscle tone or continuous jerking of one or more limbs, interfering with coordination and postural control, associated with a time-linked EEG, sharp wave in the contralateral motor cortex, immediately followed by an electromyographic (EMG) silent period of 20 to 40 msec.[8]

Drop attacks in which the patient experiences diffuse atonia and suddenly drops to the floor have been described in both simple partial and complex partial seizures. The mechanism involves the rapid spread of an ictal discharge to the brainstem through the pontine reticular formation.[9]

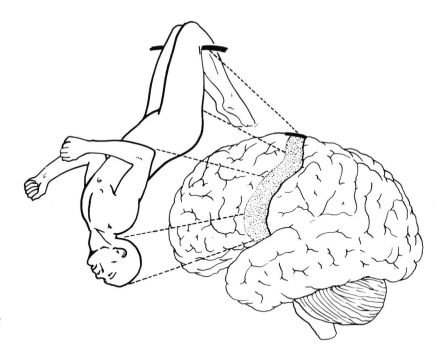

Figure 4-1.
Somatotropic organization of the motor cortex.

II. Sensory Seizures

a. Somatosensory Seizures

There is a sudden sensation of tingling affecting a strictly focal area of the body, or the sensation of a breeze affecting the face or an extremity.

b. Visual Seizures

These seizures usually consist of elementary visual phenomena such as flashes of light or colored balls of light in contrast to the more complex visual symptoms described in some cases of partial complex seizures.

c. Auditory Seizures

A sudden onset of ringing, buzzing, or bell-like sounds can occur as an ictal phenomena. The auditory seizures are usually elementary, but occasionally there are more complex phenomena, including hallucinations of music, singing, or bells.

d. Olfactory Seizures

A sudden, intense hallucination of smell occurs that is usually unpleasant and often described vividly as "burned blood or rotting material." The odor is usually unpleasant but is occasionally a pleasant sensation, often described as the smell of geraniums. Gustatory sensations are often confused with olfactory sensations but occasionally may be hallucinations of taste—sweet, sour, salt, or bitter—and may be described as a "metallic taste."

e. Vertiginous Seizures

Vertiginous seizures consist of a sensation of vertigo of sudden onset, often associated with the sensation of falling. The experience is often quite frightening to the patient.

III. Autonomic Seizures

This seizure type is associated with the sudden onset of anxiety, tachycardia, sweating, piloerection, or borborygmi accompanied by an abnormal sensation rising up through the upper abdomen into the chest. There may be flushing, piloerection, shivering, sweating, and pupillary dilatation accompanying these symptoms.

IV. Psychic Seizures

a. **Aphasic Seizures**

A sudden failure of comprehension and inability to communicate may occur with focal seizure activity confined to discrete areas of the dominant hemisphere.

b. **Dysmnesic Seizures**

This typically consists of déjà vu, which is a sudden intense feeling of familiarity with a place, person, object, or situation. It is often described as having "lived it all before" or "having been there before." Jamais vu is a feeling of unfamiliarity when a familiar visual experience is construed as unfamiliar. The corresponding auditory illusions are termed déjà entendu and jamais entendu.

Other dysmnesic seizures have been described as "a dreamy state" in which there are forced recollections of past memories, often pleasant, reminiscent of a dream. Hallucinatory experiences can occur including autoscopy, a hallucination of out-of-body experience, in which the individual perceives himself in space outside of the body, as though the mind has left the body and is observing events from an outer vantage point.

c. **Cognitive Seizures**

There is an abrupt intrusion of a single thought or train of thoughts into consciousness with exclusion of other thought processes. Hallucinatory experiences can occur, apparently observed from an outer vantage point. Distortion of time can be associated with slowing or acceleration of thought processes. An altered perception of body image can result in the false perception of an increase or a decrease in body size.

d. **Affective Seizures**

An experience of fear, varying from mild discomfort to terror, often associated with an hallucination of a menacing figure located in one visual field has been described. Anger or an intense feeling of hate is probably the result of seizure activity in the amygdala. Other emotions include pleasure, joy, love, or religious ecstasy, but fear is the most common affective experience.

e. **Illusions**

Illusions are false mental images produced by misinterpretation of things that exist, whereas hallucinations are perceptions of an object that has no physical counterpart. Both of these phenomena are occasionally reported during partial seizure activity.

Visual illusions consisting of distortion of size, with an object appearing larger, "macropsia," or smaller, "micropsia," than in reality. Illusions of shape, color, motor, or distance can occur.

f. **Hallucinations**

Visual hallucinations arising from temporal lobe seizure activity tend to be complex (e.g., a rural scene or a human figure) and simple visual hallucinations, such as balls of light and zigzag lines, are characteristic of occipital lobe seizures. Auditory hallucinations are often simple in character, consisting of buzzing, ringing, or clicking. Occasionally, auditory phenomena are more complex, when they tend to be stereotyped, repetitive experiences of voices or music.

Olfactory hallucinations usually indicate seizure activity arising in an anterior temporal focus (uncinate fits). The hallucination is unpleasant in most cases but is occasionally a pleasant experience. Similarly, hallucinations of taste, a bitter, sour, or metallic taste, indicate involvement of the parietal opercular region. Vertiginous components during seizures indicate activity in the insula in most cases.

The interictal neurological examination may be abnormal in cases of partial seizures of recent origin. There is increased tone and increased tendon reflexes on the affected side. The interictal EEG may reveal a focal spike discharge. This tends to increase in frequency and may take on a polyspike configuration at the onset of a partial seizure, or it may even become generalized and paroxysmal in some cases. It is important to rule out the existence of a treatable structural lesion. All partial seizures have the potential to develop into secondary generalized seizures.

Treatment

Partial seizures with onset in adolescence or adulthood are often the result of structural brain lesions and require diagnostic imaging. They are often resistant to antiepileptic drug treatment and may require brain surgery.[10] Carbamazepine, phenytoin, and valproate are of equal efficacy and acceptability for the control of partial seizures, with or without secondary generalized tonic-clonic seizures in adults and children. When the primary antiepileptic drugs produce partial improvement without complete seizure control, the addition of gabapentin or lamotrigine may produce improvement or total control of this form of epilepsy. Evaluation for surgical therapy should be considered when response to anticonvulsant drug therapy is inadequate, with a demonstrable focal or brain lesion or an isolated focus of activity in the EEG, which could be responsible for the partial seizures.[11] Partial seizures with a clear focal lesion in the anterior temporal lobe show the best response to surgical treatment. Rasmussen encephalitis should be treated with hemispherectomy.

COMPLEX PARTIAL SEIZURES (PSYCHOMOTOR EPILEPSY: TEMPORAL LOBE EPILEPSY)

Complex partial seizures present as simple partial seizures associated with or followed by impairment of consciousness. Alternatively, consciousness may be impaired at the onset, when it is the sole manifestation of the seizure, or impairment of consciousness may be followed by automatisms or evolve into a secondary generalized seizure.

I. Temporal Lobe Complex Partial Seizures

It is clear that the designation of temporal lobe seizures is a too-confining alternative term for complex partial seizures. Many complex partial seizures arise from foci outside the temporal lobe, the seizure activity often spreading into temporal lobe structures, while some seizures originating in a temporal lobe focus may spread to extratemporal areas. The association of temporal lobe and frontal lobe activity in complex partial seizures is common and it is not unusual to assume that the focus of epileptic activity is in the temporal lobe in complex partial seizures of frontal lobe origin. This is to be expected when considering the highly interconnected temporal and frontal lobes.[12] Complex partial seizures are, in fact, a set of disorders grouped together under a common rubric.[13]

Complex partial seizures may occur at any age. The essential feature in the recognition of complex partial seizures is the occurrence of impairment or loss of consciousness which may occur at the onset of the seizure or during the seizure. The alteration of consciousness may take the form of a "dreamy state" in which the patient recognizes that something unusual is happening but appreciates the phenomenon in a detached sense, in much the same way as an individual "observes" a dream. However, in some cases the patient has no recollection of events that have occurred during a seizure. The alteration of consciousness may be the onset manifestation of a complex partial seizure, or there may be additional features, which include:

1. Cognitive disturbances

There may be an abrupt onset of a feeling of unreality, such as a sense of detachment or depersonalization accompany the dreamy state. The patient may experience déjà vu or jamais vu. There may be derealization, where reality is perceived as a dream, or autoscopy, a feeling of detachment between mind and body, such that the individual perceives oneself from an outer vantage point.[14] A heightened religious sense can occur during partial complex seizures and persist in the postictal period in a frenzy of religious activity. Time distortion or forced thinking, where a recurrent thought forces itself into a forefront of thinking, is another experience in the cognitive realm. Schizophrenic-like symptoms, both ictal and postictal, can develop in some patients, whereas others show a mental deterioration with the progression of seizure activity.

2. Psychomotor activity

Automatic stereotyped behavior can be observed during the period of altered consciousness. This consists of lip smacking, masticatory movements, picking at clothing, or simple gestures such as scratching or stroking. Unilateral tonic posturing, dystonic posturing of a limb on the opposite side of the seizure discharge, or head and body turning may occur.[15] Occasionally there is continuation of one action already in progress at the onset of the seizure. More complex acts, such as walking, running, disrobing, searching with the hands, or urinating in public, are uncommon. Some patients appear fearful and adopt defensive attitudes to escape or avoid danger. More complex activities, which can appear purposeful, such as rearranging books, ornaments, or furniture in a room, driving a car, or walking several blocks, are occasionally reported. This activity may resemble transient global amnesia.

3. Psychosensory phenomena

Two types of disturbances may occur: hallucinations or perceptual disorders. Visual hallucinations are usually elementary and consist of flashing or balls of light. Occasionally the patient experiences complex stereotyped visual phenomena such as hallucination of a landscape or a human figure. Auditory hallucinations usually take the form of hissing or ringing, but the hallucinations can include voices of persons known or unknown, and the patient may be able or unable to remember the details of the conversations heard during the attack. Hallucinations of smell are usually intense and unpleasant, occasionally being experienced as a pleasant sensation. Hallucinations of movement, particularly vertigo, can be distressing. Perceptual disorders usually take the form of distortion of body size and objects may appear to be larger or smaller during an attack.

4. Speech disturbances

A speech arrest may occur at the beginning of the seizure, or the patient may be dysphasic or dysarthric.

5. Affective disturbances

Intense feeling of fear or dread are not unusual in complex partial seizures associated with appropriate psychomotor activity. This is a stereotyped phenomenon and it recurs during each attack experienced by the patient. Experiences of sadness or happiness, occasionally crying (dacrystic seizures) or laughter (gelastic seizures) or even a feeling of ecstasy have been experienced on rare occasions.

6. Autonomic activity

Many patients experience epigastric sensations such as borborygmi, a feeling of palpitations or abdominal distress at the beginning of partial complex seizures. This is sometimes called "butterflies in the stomach." Abdominal or visceral pain is unusual and has occasionally been reported as the only manifestation of complex partial seizures. Other autonomic symptoms include pallor, flushing, sweating, piloerection, pupillary dilatation or constriction, and excessive salivation. Abdominal sensations may rise up into the chest occasionally accompanied by irregular respirations, tachycardia, and piloerection. Erotic sensations involving the genitalia and including sexual arousal have been described.

7. Secondary generalized seizures

Secondary generalized seizures can develop in patients with complex partial seizures at anytime during an episode of seizure activity.

Patients may experience one or more of the major components of a complex partial seizure. Attacks can vary in one individual from a relatively brief episode with few symptoms to an extremely complex constellation of symptoms. Complex partial seizures are the main cause of accidents in epileptic drivers.[16]

The neurological examination is often normal. Some patients show a slight increase in tendon reflexes on the side opposite the epileptic focus. Patients with complex partial seizures are said to show a marked facial asymmetry that appears on involuntary facial movements such as smiling. The EEG is often abnormal with focal spikes, polyspikes, and episodic high-voltage, slow-wave discharges occurring in one or both midtemporal regions. All cases of complex partial seizures of recent origin in adolescents and adults should be fully investigated. About 50 percent of children and adults experience school difficulties and behavior problems.

The drugs of choice are phenytoin, carbamazepine, or valproic acid. Gabapentin, vigabatrin, lamotrigine, and topiramate are also effective. Clonazepam and clorazepate are useful add-on anticonvulsants in poorly controlled partial complex seizures.

II. Frontal Lobe Seizures

Frontal lobe seizures that present as partial complex seizures are difficult to distinguish from temporal lobe seizures in part because of the several direct projections between the two lobes.

The initial symptoms of frontal lobe seizures often consist of vague sensory, cephalic, or epigastric sensations. More complex symptoms such as forced thinking or forced actions are unusual. Visual or auditory hallucinations are usually elementary, consisting of flashes of irregular-shaped lights or simple sounds such as whistling or humming. Olfactory hallucinations usually arise from seizure activity in the mesio-orbitofrontal cortex, whereas emotional periods of fear, depression, or irritability are indicative of an anterior cingulate or frontal opercular insular focus. Similarly, autonomic phenomena such as thirst, palpitations, belching, defecation, and urination occur in seizures in the medial, frontal, or opercular regions.

Motor cortex involvement is characterized by tonic or clonic movements of the contralateral limb or limbs. Consciousness is often preserved. There may be somatotopic spread (jacksonian march) followed by postictal paralysis (Todd's paralysis), or the activity can spread further, resulting in a second generalized seizure. Persistent unilateral clonic activity is not unusual in the presence of a structural lesion such as a brain tumor presenting with focal motor status epilepticus (epilepsia partialis continua). This can result in permanent neuronal damage with spastic hemiparesis.

Seizures originating in the supplementary sensorimotor cortex are often bizarre in appearance, frequently giving rise to the misdiagnosis of pseudoseizures.[17] The seizures are usually multiple, up to 5 to 20 seizures per day.[18] Each episode is brief with abrupt onset and cessation, lasting 30 s or less, and often occurring during sleep. Postictal confusion is minimal. A seizure consists of tonic posturing of the extremities, abduction of the contralateral upper limb with flexion at the elbow, rotation of the head and eyes to the side of the abnormal limb posture.[19] While consciousness is often preserved, there may be speech arrest, crying, grunting, moaning, and repetition of words, syllables, or laughter.

Both supplementary motor area seizures and frontopolar seizures can present with tonic or dystonic posturing of the contralateral upper and/or lower limbs. However, frontopolar seizures are associated with loss of consciousness, which distinguishes the two conditions.

Ictal speech arrest can occur during seizures arising from a seizure focus in the dominant superior frontal gyrus parasagittal region.[20]

Seizures arising from a dorsolateral frontal focus may resemble supplementary motor area seizures but may begin with forced thinking and progress rapidly to generalized tonic-clonic seizures. Complex partial seizures of cingulate origin are associated with intense fear, complex motor movements, and autonomic phenomena.

Orbitofrontal seizures are often nocturnal and complex. Symptoms include a vocal component with screaming or cursing; an affective component, usually fear; complex motor movements involving axial and limb muscles, with thrashing or pelvic thrusting suggesting a pseudoseizure, but the stereotypical nature of the attack confirms that this is a true epileptic seizure.[21]

Partial complex seizures arising from foci in the frontal lobe are more likely to evolve adversive posturing than seizures of temporal lobe origin.[22]

III. Parietal Lobe Seizures

This seizure type is unusual but can be defined clinically. The most common symptom is a contralateral somatosensory sensation that may present as a sensory jacksonian seizure. The sensation is usually a tingling or numbness, but pain or a thermal sensation can occur. A disturbance of body image results in a sensation of movement of one extremity, the twisting or turning of the body, or a feeling of absence of a limb. Visual illusions present with figures looking larger or smaller, or a perception that objects are in motion. Vertiginous sensations or dysphasia indicate anterior parietal lobe involvement.[23]

IV. Occipital Lobe Seizures

Seizures originating in the occipital lobe are relatively uncommon. Symptoms are usually elementary, consisting of flickering lights or lines, balls, balloons, wheels, fine particles, stars, or light projecting from a central source, resembling the fortification spectra of migraine. Symptoms are usually experienced in the contralateral homonymous visual field. Visual fading, blurring, or loss, with homonymous hemianopia, may proceed to ictal blindness when the seizure activity spreads to the opposite occipital lobe. Contralateral tonic-clonic eye deviation, forced blinking, or eyelid flutter occurs with involvement of the medial occipital cortex.

The subsequent development of more complex visual hallucinations, preceded by elementary visual phenomena, indicates spread of the seizure activity to the ipsilateral temporal lobe.[24]

A benign occipital lobe epilepsy has been described in children and adolescents. Many cases of familial occipital lobe seizures cease in the late teens.

The EEG shows unilateral or bilateral interictal occipital spikes.

The magnetic resonance imaging (MRI) scan is positive in many cases of occipital lobe seizures because the majority of patients have structural lesions in the occipital lobe.

Treatment   As for partial complex seizures.

ABSENCE (PETIT MAL)

Three conditions comprise the syndrome of typical absence: (a) childhood absence, (b) juvenile absence, and (c) juvenile myoclonic epilepsy.

The etiology is unknown, but there is a strong genetic predisposition to absence seizures.[25] It is possible that low-threshold calcium iron currents (T currents), which are partially controlled GABA-b mediated inhibition, alternating with glutamate-mediated excitation, may activate burst firing of thalamic neurons, initiating an absence seizure.[26] Childhood absence occurs in children 2 to 10 years of age. The seizure is sudden in onset and brief; the attacks last from a few seconds to less than 30 s. The child stares

and there may be brief upward movement of the eyes. All activities, including speaking, eating, and gesturing, come to a sudden halt. The attack terminates abruptly. There is no postictal confusion and the patient continues previous activities. Childhood absence attacks can develop in children who have generalized tonic-clonic seizures or tonic-clonic seizures may follow the appearance of absence seizures. In 65 percent, seizures cease, but a significant number of children progress to generalized tonic-clonic seizures or juvenile myoclonic epilepsy.[27] The outcome of absence may be worse than previously stated, with a considerable proportion of patients developing tonic-clonic seizures.[28] Young adults with a history of typical absence seizures, particularly those without remission of their seizures, often have poor psychosocial outcomes.[29] Accidents and injuries are common in absence seizures, particularly bicycle accidents. Injury prevention counseling is indicated and helmet use should be mandatory.[30]

Juvenile myoclonic epilepsy, which is inherited as an autosomal dominant trait, is linked to a genetic defect located on the short arm of chromosome 6. Juvenile myoclonic epilepsy is a common cause of generalized tonic-clonic seizures in teenagers and young adults. The characteristic feature is the occurrence of multiple bilaterally synchronous myoclonic jerks usually occurring in the first few hours after awakening in the morning. Patients also experience occasional generalized tonic-clonic seizures. Absence occurs in up to 30 percent of cases and seizure activity is enhanced by sleep deprivation, fatigue, and alcohol withdrawal. Intelligence is not impaired, and the neurological examination is normal.

The EEG shows burst of frontal irregular spike-wave activity.

ATYPICAL ABSENCE

Progressive Myoclonic Epilepsies

Juvenile myoclonic epilepsy must be differentiated from the rare degenerative conditions associated with myoclonus and epilepsy. These progressive myoclonic epilepsies include Lafora disease, Unverricht-Lunborg disease, late infantile, juvenile and adult neuronal ceroid lipofuscinosis, sialidosis, and mitochondrial encephalopathy with ragged red fibers (MERRF). Unlike juvenile myoclonic epilepsy, these conditions show progressive intellectual and cognitive decline, ataxia, and spasticity.

Treatment   Valproic acid is the drug of choice for the treatment of juvenile myoclonic epilepsy. There is usually poor response to phenytoin and carbamazepine, which may increase seizure activity.

Progressive Myoclonus Epilepsy of Unverricht-Lunborg (Dyssynergia Cerebellaris Myoclonica: Ramsay-Hunt Syndrome)

Unverricht-Lunborg disease is a distinct form of progressive myoclonic epilepsy that is inherited as an autosomal recessive disorder assigned to a genetic defect mapping to the distal region of chromosome 21.[31] There is a high prevalence in the Finnish population.

Symptoms begin between the ages of 6 and 15 years and the course is progressive and characterized by severe stimulus-sensitive myoclonus and tonic-clonic seizures. There is a slow intellectual decline in some cases, and the ataxia is mild. Myoclonus, ataxia, and seizure activity increase for 10 to 20 years, then decline and abate in the fourth decade, leaving many patients only slightly impaired.

The EEG shows progressive slowing of background activity with bursts of generalized spike wave activity. There is a prominent driving response to photic stimulation. High-voltage somatosensory evoked potentials are found in the early stages of the disease.[32]

Mitochondrial Encephalopathy with Ragged Red Fibers (MERRF)

Progressive myoclonus epilepsy is a feature of some cases of MERRF, a condition showing a variable clinical presentation, depending on the affected element in the mitochondrial respiratory chain. The complete clinical presentation of progressive myoclonus epilepsy can occur in MERRF, or there may be only occasional generalized tonic-clonic seizures without myoclonus. The complete picture of MERRF includes a history of migraine, deafness, short stature, myopathy, lactic acidosis, optic atrophy, dementia, dysarthria, neuropathy, and hyperventilation.

The EEG shows slowing of background activity into the 5- to 7-Hz theta range, with intermittent bursts of symmetrical, synchronous 2- to 3-Hz delta activity. Bursts of synchronous spike wave, polyspike, or slow wave discharges in the 2- to 5-Hz range occur intermittently in the recording.

The diagnosis is established by the demonstration of typical ragged red fibers in the muscle biopsy.

Lafora Disease

Lafora disease is a rare inborn error of carbohydrate metabolism characterized by the presence of polyglucan inclusion bodies in the CNS and other tissues. Lafora disease is a form of progressive myoclonus epilepsy inherited as an autosomal recessive trait. The gene responsible has not been identified.[33]

The salient pathological changes consist of the presence of Lafora bodies in many tissues.[34] Lafora bodies are intracytoplasmic basophilic inclusions composed of glucose polymer, with small variable components of phosphate and sulfate groups, which are always present in the brain and often found in cardiac and striated muscle, liver, and skin.

The disease begins in the teens with generalized tonic-clonic and clonic seizures. There are action and resting myoclonus, cerebellar ataxia, visual seizures, and a rapidly progressive dementia. A few cases have been described with occult onset, slow progression, and delayed appearance of seizures and myoclonus.[35]

The diagnosis is established by brain biopsy when Lafora bodies are absent in liver, muscle, and skin biopsies.

The EEG is abnormal. In the early stages of the disease, the background alpha activity is preserved and there are episodes of synchronous spike wave activity. In the second stage, the alpha is interrupted by slower activity and there are bilateral discharges and fast spikes occurring independently and posteriorly over both hemispheres. In the final stage, the background consists of slow activity with superimposed multifocal fast spikes.[36] Divalproex sodium is the drug of choice for control of seizure activity in all stages of Lafora disease but is usually only partially effective for these conditions. Clonazepam should be added slowly to the regimen if necessary for better seizure control. Phenytoin should be avoided because this drug has been reported to increase cerebellar ataxia in Unverricht-Lunborg disease and may have a similar effect in Lafora disease.

There is no effective treatment for Lafora disease. Divalproex sodium and clonazepam may reduce seizure activity in some cases.

Atypical Absence

This type of seizure presents with signs similar to absence seizures, but patients are often retarded and have mixed seizure types, including generalized tonic-clonic seizures, myoclonic seizures, tonic seizures, and atonic seizures. The EEG is more heterogenous, with an irregular spike-wave activity bilaterally, with a frequency of 0.5 to 2.5 Hz and an abnormal background activity of paroxysmal spike or spike-wave complexes.

The condition may respond to ethosuximide, divalproex sodium, or clonazepam, but treatment with standard antiepileptic drugs is often unsatisfactory. Lamotrigine or a ketogenic diet may be beneficial.

Lennox-Gastaut Syndrome

This condition, which begins between the ages of 1 to 2 years, may be regarded as a malignant epilepsy syndrome characterized by multiple seizures types, mental retardation, and slow spike-wave activity in the EEG.[37] About 25 percent of patients give a history of West syndrome. Seizures may be tonic-clonic, tonic-atonic, or atypical absence. Myoclonic seizures are unusual. The EEG is said to be characteristic, with a slow background activity punctuated by bilateral spike wave activity at 2 to 2.5 Hz or paroxysmal fast activity at 10 to 13 Hz. The latter presentation, with multiple seizure types, evolves into a single predominant pattern by the second decade. Intellectual, cognitive, and psychosocial deficits are permanent and status epilepticus is common.

Treatment with standard antiepileptic drugs is usually unsatisfactory; lamotrigine may be beneficial but may cause a life-threatening rash and must be withdrawn at the first signs of skin involvement. Gabapentin has a good safety record and reduces seizure activity at higher doses. Vigabatrin is effective in Lennox-Gastaut syndrome, beginning 25 mg/kg per day and increasing by increments of 25 mg/kg per day up to 200 mg/kg per day if necessary. Topiramate is probably beneficial, but exposure has been limited. Corticosteroids will produce short-term benefit and a ketogenic diet can be useful in some cases. Felbamate can be prescribed as monotherapy for refractory cases of Lennox-Gastaut syndrome. The initial dose of 15 mg/kg per day can be increased slowly to 45 mg/kg per day. Regular hematological and biochemical monitoring should be obtained because of the risk of aplastic anemia or hepatic failure. A signed informed consent before administration of felbamate should be obtained.[38]

Infantile Spasms (West Syndrome)

This syndrome combines the triad of infantile spasms, mental retardation, and EEG findings of hypsarrhythmia.[39]

Infantile spasms occur in childhood during the first year of life, often as early as 3 months of age, with a peak onset after 3 months and before 1 year of age. A typical attack varies from simple head nodding to violent flexion of the head, limbs, and trunk. However, other patterns of extension or flexion/extension may occur. Usually an attack consists of spasms of the flexor muscles of the neck, trunk, and limbs. This results in flexion of the head onto the chest, accompanied by flexion of trunk and limbs. Each episode is brief and is followed by relaxation to a normal posture. Hundreds of seizures may occur in one day. Hemispasms or more complicated movements have been described.

Chronic encephalitis, cerebral malformation, particularly lissencephaly, and degenerative diseases of the brain such as tuberous sclerosis are frequently associated with infantile spasms. Rare conditions that may be remediable include pyridoxine dependency, hypoglycemia, and phenylketonuria. The past history is entirely normal with lack of previous disease, no abnormal neurological signs, normal psychomotor development, and normal computed tomography (CT) and MRI studies.[40] Once the disorder appears, the patient shows rapid deterioration with loss of previously attained developmental levels.

The interictal neurological examination is abnormal. The EEG associated with the spasms has the unique appearance of random high-voltage polyspike and wave activity on a background of mixed delta and theta activity (hypsarrhythmia).

It is important to delineate those patients who can be treated. The injection of 50 mg pyridoxine (vitamin B_6) should be given intravenously during the EEG recording to detect pyridoxine dependency. In such cases, the EEG will improve dramatically. Hypoglycemia and phenylketonuria should be ruled out.

Treatment with standard anticonvulsants such as phenytoin, barbiturates, carbamazepine, and the succinimides has been ineffective.[41] ACTH varying from 20 to 160 IU and prednisone have been the most frequently used therapeutic agents and have achieved control of spasms in 50 to 70 percent of cases. Felbamate (see Lennox-Gastaut syndrome) is recommended in refractory cases. Other antiepileptic drugs such as nitrazepam or vigabatrin, or pyridoxine combined with divalproex sodium, have been recommended. Acetazolamide and a ketogenic diet are occassionally beneficial.[42] No treatment has been shown to improve the long-term intellectual development in infantile spasms.

Tonic Seizures

Tonic seizures occur in children and are characterized by the sudden onset of sustained contraction of axial and limb musculature with loss of consciousness.

The interictal neurological examination is abnormal in mentally retarded children. It is important to differentiate tonic seizures from intermittent decerebate rigidity associated with severe and often acute disease of the cerebral hemispheres.

Tonic-Clonic Seizures (Grand Mal)

Tonic-clonic seizures occur at any age. The seizure is abrupt in onset with no prodromal symptoms. The total neuronal population is involved, with simultaneous loss of consciousness and symmetrical contrac-

tions of all voluntary muscles. If the vocal cords are closing as the diaphragm and intercostal muscles contract, the patient will make an audible sound, often a high-pitched cry. The patient drops to the ground in a decerebrate posture, with all muscles in tonic contraction. During this state, which lasts from a few seconds to 3 minutes, there is absence of respiratory movement and cyanosis. The tonic phase is followed by a clonic phase, which is accompanied by violent expiratory contractions with expulsion of saliva. This stage may be accompanied by tongue-biting on the sides of the tongue, which results in bloodstained saliva. Urinary incontinence is not unusual if the bladder is full. The clonic movements gradually decline in frequency and cease. The patient remains in a coma, with no reaction to painful stimuli, fixed nonreactive pupils, flaccid limbs, and bilateral extensor plantar responses. Arousal is possible after several minutes, but the patient is typically combative, irritable, and extremely confused and usually lapses into sleep. If awakened, some 20 to 30 minutes later the patient complains of severe headache, muscle aches, and extreme fatigue and appears irritable. Full recovery occurs after several hours, but many patients feel mentally dull for several days after the seizure.

An accurate history is particularly important in these patients. One should always try to get a complete and accurate description of the seizure. It is imperative to distinguish patients with focal seizures and secondary generalized seizures from those with primary tonic-clonic seizures. In case of focal onset, the patient may describe an aura or have evidence of Todd's paralysis following the seizure, both of which indicate a focal onset and the possibility of underlying brain damage. Todd's paralysis is a hemiplegia or monoplegia that may persist from days to as long as a week after a seizure.

The interictal neurological examination is usually normal. The interictal EEG is normal in 50 percent of patients. Others show short bursts of generalized spike and wave activity with accentuation by hyperventilation. Isolated spikes or spike and wave activity occur in some cases.

Most tonic-clonic seizures are secondary generalized tonic-clonic seizures rather than primary tonic-clonic seizures, the secondary phenomenon arising on a background of partial seizure activity. Hence, it is important to obtain the history both from the patient and from an observer.

The drugs of choice are carbamazepine, divalproex sodium, or phenytoin. Newer anticonvulsants such as gabapentin may also be effective in controlling primary tonic-clonic seizures.

Atonic Seizures

Atonic seizures have been described as a sudden diminution of muscle tone leading to a slumping to the ground. When these attacks are extremely brief, they are known as drop attacks.[43]

The atonic seizure syndrome consists of focal atonic seizures, negative myoclonus, and drop attacks.

Focal atonic seizures are partial seizures with ictal paralysis of one or more parts of the body. There is a transient ictal hemiplegia, monoplegia, or facial weakness. Attacks are usually brief and precede any convulsive activity anywhere in the body. The atonia can be preceded by an aura such as the aura of a secondary generalized tonic-clonic seizure or the beginning of a partial seizure. However, the aura does not lead to convulsive movements, as might be seen in other seizures, and the weakness without convulsions resembles Todd's paralysis that occurs after a frank convulsive seizure. The cause of focal atonic seizures is probably a negative inhibition of cortical activity by a seizure discharge in an area of the brain known to cause inhibition of movement.

Negative myoclonus consists of a brief lapse of tone in a limb or continuous jerking of the limb with loss of postural tone. More extensive atonia of the limb and axial muscles causes the patient to fall. Diagnosis depends on demonstration of an EMG silent period of 100 to 400 msec time-locked to an EEG sharp wave in the contralateral posterior frontal cortex, the sharp wave preceding the EMG silent period by 20 to 40 msec.

Drop attacks have several identifiable causes, the most common being cardiac or cerebrovascular disease.[44] Other conditions include partial seizures of frontal or temporal lobe origin, seizures induced by cardiac arrest,[45] or dysrhythmias, loss of balance because of dystonic posturing during the seizure, or rapid spread of ictal activity to the pontine reticular formation.[46]

Treatment   Drugs effective against drop attacks include divalproex sodium, benzodiazepines, felbamate, vigabatrin, and lamotrigine.[47]

Seizures in Pregnancy

Most pregnancies in women with epilepsy have a favorable outcome, but stillbirth, perinatal infant death, and malformations occur more often in women with epilepsy than in nonepileptic women. The risk of a major malformation in the fetus is between 3 and 4 percent in nonepileptic women, rising to 6.9 percent in women with epilepsy.[48] Exposure to antiepileptic drugs in the first trimester of pregnancy results in an abnormal fetal outcome in 11.3 percent of cases.[49] All of the marketed antiepileptic drugs can produce teratogenic effects, which include congenital heart problems, neural tube defects, cleft lip and palate, skeletal deformities, and microcephaly.[50] Polytherapy increases the risk of teratogenicity. As the number of antiepileptic drugs used in combination during the first trimester increases, the incidence of fetal malformations rises. Phenytoin and divalproex sodium therapy carries a higher risk than carbamazepine, with the highest risk with polytherapy.[51] Drug-specific malformations consist of neural tube defects associated with divalproex sodium and possibly carbamazepine therapy.[52]

Monotherapy titrated to the lowest effective dose to control seizures is advocated in pregnancy. If one drug fails, another should be substituted and the first drug withdrawn. However, when monotherapy fails to control seizures, polytherapy using drugs with dissimilar pharmacologic properties is advised (e.g., a voltage-dependent sodium channel blocking agent, and gabapentin).[53]

Pregnancy decreases the brain seizure threshold, probably by causing electrolyte imbalance, hormonal alterations, or emotional stress. Pregnancy also results in decreased serum anticonvulsant levels due to decreased intestinal absorption and increased metabolism. Approximately 17 percent of pregnant epileptic patients will experience an increased seizure frequency.[54] This is particularly true in patients who have greater than one seizure per month prior to conception.

In general, isolated seizures do not affect the fetus. However, status epilepticus is a high-risk complication to both mother and fetus and must be treated promptly and aggressively. Free antiepileptic drug levels of carbamazepine, phenytoin, and phenobarbital decrease and valproate level increases during pregnancy;[55] consequently, free drug levels should be monitored carefully, with appropriate adjustments of medication when necessary. Nevertheless, the aim is the achievement of monotherapy at the lowest protective dose.

The treatment of epilepsy during pregnancy should follow certain guidelines:

1. Optimal seizure control should be established in an epileptic woman who is contemplating pregnancy, using antiepileptic drug monotherapy.

2. If the patient is receiving valproate monotherapy with total seizure control, the patient should be informed about the higher risk of spina bifida and also informed about the risk of changing any antiepileptic drugs.

3. Free levels of antiepileptic drug should be obtained every trimester and every week during the last month of pregnancy, and the dose adjusted to maintain a therapeutic drug level.

4. Begin folate supplementation early and continue throughout pregnancy.[56] The role of folate in the prevention of a neural tube defect in pregnancy is not well established.

5. Intrauterine testing with high-resolution ultrasonography should be ordered in patients under 35 years of age and performed at 11 weeks and 19 weeks.

6. Serum α-fetoprotein determination is recommended in all patients over 35 years of age.

7. Amniocentesis is recommended if ultrasonography is abnormal or the α-fetoprotein level is elevated.

8. The newborn infant should be carefully examined for the congenital malformations associated with the anticonvulsant to which it has been exposed. Phytonadione (vitamin K) 1 mg should be administered and clotting factors carefully monitored.

9. The anticonvulsant dosage of the postpartum patient may not drop to preconception levels for several months. The patient should be monitored monthly until a stable plasma level is attained.

SEIZURES IN CHILDREN

The many types of seizures in children are discussed under each category in this chapter. The most common causes of seizures in children are listed in Table 4-2. The key to diagnosis is the history, which must be obtained from the parent and the older child in great detail. The most common mistake is to misdiagnose complex partial seizures (psychomotor seizures), which are common in childhood, as absence (petit mal), a rare form of childhood seizure disorder. Incorrect diagnosis leads to inappropriate therapy and failure of seizure control.

The benign childhood epilepsies are common, comprising about 25 percent of epilepsy in children under 13 years of age. The seizures are usually nocturnal, infrequent, and unilateral and may progress to a secondary tonic-clonic seizure. In many cases, the initial seizure is not repeated, or the child may suffer several seizures over a period of 5 years. The general physical and neurological examinations and laboratory studies and imaging studies are normal.[57] The EEG shows the presence of high-voltage spike or sharp wave and slow wave complexes in the central or midtemporal leads, which are unilateral or occasionally bilateral when they occur independently on the two sides. The condition resolves spontaneously by age 16 years.

Similar benign seizures with frontal, occipital, frontotemporal, and parietotemporal EEG abnormalities have been described. All have an excellent prognosis.

Treatment has been a source of controversy. The recommendation to use anticonvulsant therapy after the second seizure and continue treatment for a 2-year period is widely accepted. Carbamazepine is the drug of choice.

Febrile Seizures

Febrile seizures occur in children between the ages of 6 months and 5 years and constitute 3 to 5 percent of seizures in children. The great majority present with a single generalized tonic-clonic seizure that occurs early in the febrile episode, when there is a sudden elevation in body temperature during a mild systemic infection. The majority of children do not have a recurrence; during the febrile episode the neurological examination and the EEG are normal, the condition is benign, and the prognosis excellent. Benign febrile convulsions of this type are believed to be genetically determined and maternal inheritance is an important factor.

A small group of children who have abnormal neurological findings also develop febrile seizures. These seizures are often prolonged and exhibit focal features; multiple seizures can occur during the febrile episode. The neurological examination and the EEG are abnormal. Consequently, it is possible to identify two distinct groups within the category of febrile seizures—benign febrile seizures and complex febrile seizures, the latter representing epilepsy triggered by fever.

The treatment of febrile seizures is controversial. Prophylactic antiepileptic drugs do not appear to be effective in preventing febrile seizures. Phenobarbital has been recommended in the past but is no more effective than placebo and the drug has detrimental effects on cognitive and intellectual development in children.[58] Rectal diazepam, given at the onset of a febrile episode, has been recommended to prevent febrile seizures in susceptible children.[59]

Reflex Seizures

Epilepsy can be precipitated by a specific stimulus. Generalized tonic-clonic seizures resulting from a light stimulus are probably the most frequently encountered form of reflex seizures. The trigger may be a sudden bright light, sunlight flickering through trees, discotheque lighting, a badly adjusted TV set, or exposure to video games.[60] Many patients have spontaneous seizures in addition to the photosensitive condition.[61] The induction of myoclonic jerks, absence or generalized seizures by viewing patterns, is an unusual phenomenon in this category.

Myoclonus induced by thinking and decision-making may be followed by generalized seizures in some cases. Subjects may experience symptoms while playing chess or cards, performing arithmetical tasks or manipulating spatial information (e.g., Rubic's cube).

Reading epilepsy is rare. This phenomenon consists of myoclonic movements of the jaws while reading, increasing in amplitude and culminating in a generalized seizure.

Seizures induced by music have been termed musicogenic epilepsy. The trigger may be a specific piece of music, exposure to new or unfamiliar musical compositions, hearing music played on a particular instrument, singing, or exposure to unusual sounds such as church bells. Consequently, it is possible that this form of epilepsy may be induced by the affective response to a particular piece of music or by a sound.

Chewing and swallowing can induce seizures, which can also be precipitated by eating a heavy meal or even the odor of food.

Immersion in hot water will induce seizure activity, usually partial complex seizures. The trigger appears to require the use of very hot water (40° to 50° C).

Seizures can be induced by an unexpected auditory, somatosensory, or tactile stimulus. Sudden noise is the most common stimulus in this group. Patients are usually hemiparetic with mental retardation. The condition must be differentiated from hyperekplexia and paroxysmal kinesigenic choreoathetosis.

DRUG-INDUCED SEIZURES

Although the incidence of drug-induced seizures is low, frequent use of drug therapy in modern medical practice makes these seizures a relatively common problem encountered by neurologists. Seizures are more likely to occur in individuals who are epileptic or have a seizure tendency when exposed to drugs with convulsant properties. In addition, high dose and rapid absorption by intravenous administration enhances the likelihood of seizures.

In most cases, the drug-induced episode is a generalized tonic-clonic seizure, but partial seizures and status epilepticus can occur.

Many drugs, which are pharmacologically acceptable substances and recreational drugs, including alcohol or alcohol withdrawal, can induce seizures. The sudden onset of a seizure in an individual newly exposed to a medication or recreational drug should arouse suspicion of a relationship between the substance and the seizure.

EPILEPSY IN THE ELDERLY

The incidence of epilepsy in the elderly is higher than epilepsy in children and young and middle-aged adults. The incidence is 30 per 100,000 at age 40 years, rising to 140 per 100,000 at age 80 years.[62] Seizures are symptomatic in about 50 percent of elderly patients, but the remaining 50 percent must be considered idiopathic. The most common cause is cerebrovascular disease followed by Alzheimer disease, head injury, hepatic and renal failure, other metabolic abnormalities, drug administration or withdrawal, and alcohol use or alcohol withdrawal. The figure for idiopathic seizures should diminish with adequate evaluation of seizures in the elderly population.

Seizures in this age group are usually complex partial seizures often progressing to secondary generalized seizures. Simple partial seizures are not unusual, but primary generalized tonic-clonic seizures are rare.

Status epilepticus is a major complication, in that convulsive status epilepticus carries a high mortality, whereas nonconvulsive status, presenting with an abrupt change in mentation, is often misdiagnosed as stroke, dementia, drug intoxication, or delirium.

The consequences of seizures in the elderly are potentially serious and include injury such as hip fractures or subdural hematoma, prolonged postictal confusion, fixed neurological deficits, and infections, including pneumonia.

Treatment with antiepileptic drugs requires careful monitoring. Adverse effects are not unusual: phenytoin—ataxia; carbamazepine—diplopia; divalproex sodium—tremors; and barbiturates—sedation. Because the standard antiepileptic drugs are protein bound and total serum protein declines with age, determination of drug levels should be in the free or unbound form.[63] Medication should be started at a low dose and gradually increased while antiepileptic drug levels are followed closely, in an effort to avoid adverse reactions. Gabapentin, which is not bound to serum proteins or metabolized in the liver, is a good alternative and effective anticonvulsant and can be used as monotherapy.[64] Lamotrigine[65] and topiramate are also good alternative drugs.

Compliance with therapeutic regimen is often a problem, the result of poor memory, dementia, visual impairment, or low fixed income. Consequently, it is prudent to involve a close family member in management of the medication.

A further complication factor is that elderly patients on antiepileptic drugs often take potentially interacting medications such as benzodiazepines, antidepressants, antipsychotics, antacids, calcium channel blockers, and warfarin, with an increased risk of adverse effects.[66] Consequently, the physician must review all prescribed drugs, because drugs prescribed for concomitant illnesses such as depression, cardiovascular disease, hypertension, and infection may alter the metabolism of antiepileptic drugs. Antiepileptic drugs tend to induce metabolism of other drugs, leading to a decline in intended response.[67]

INTRACTABLE SEIZURES

Failure to respond to antiepileptic drugs occurs in a small number of children and adults and these individuals are said to have intractable epilepsy.

This term can be defined as epilepsy in an individual who has at least one seizure per year who fails to respond to at least three first-line antiepileptic drugs.[68] Nevertheless, at least 40 percent of children with intractable seizures will achieve complete remission and remain seizure free without medication. The introduction of newer antiepileptic drugs such as gabapentin and improved surgical technique should increase this percentage in the next decade.

When seizures persist despite adequate antiepileptic drug therapy, it is prudent to consider:

1. An error in diagnosis
2. An error in classification of seizure type
3. Coexistence of epilepsy and nonepileptic seizures
4. An underlying structural lesion
5. An underlying degenerative disease
6. Antiepileptic drug toxicity

NONEPILEPTIC SEIZURES (PSEUDOSEIZURES)

A pseudoseizure can be considered as a paroxysmal behavioral pattern that mimics epilepsy and is initiated by psychological mechanisms.[69]

Pseudoseizures are sudden paroxysmal experiences that appear epileptic-like but are not caused by abnormal electrical discharges in the brain. These seizures may coexist with true epilepsy or may occur in the absence of epilepsy.

Pseudoseizures are a somatic form of communication involving dissociative mechanisms, are sometimes related to a history of traumatic experiences, particularly child abuse,[70] and commonly exist with other psychiatric disorders.[71]

Clinical Features The diagnosis is established by direct observation and it is essential to watch the patient carefully, sitting or standing at the bedside and avoiding any restraining of movement. Pseudoseizures are more common in women, are of unusually long duration, with side-to-side head movements, back arching, pelvic thrusting, and asynchronous thrashing of all four limbs. Vocalization is not unusual, including verbal abuse or speaking in a child-like voice. Agitated wandering and feelings of depersonalization, with out-of-body experiences or a sensation of rising in the air have been reported. Examination shows a response to painful stimulation and bilateral plantar flexor responses during a pseudoseizure. The EEG, preferably prolonged with video monitoring,[72] fails to show seizure activity during a pseudoseizure. Serum prolactin levels are increased in epilepsy but remain normal in pseudoseizures measured in the immediate postictal period. Arterial oxygen saturation using pulse oximetry falls during an epileptic seizure but remains normal in pseudoseizures. Concomitant organic disease, including a current or prior neurological or neurosurgical disorder, or a systemic disease affecting the brain, is not unusual in pseudoseizures.[73]

The differential diagnosis includes tonic-clonic seizures, complex partial seizures,[74] syncopal attacks, and parasomnias. The most difficult situation is the differentiation from frontal lobe complex partial seizures when asynchronous limb movements and vocalization may closely resemble pseudoseizures. However, frontal lobe complex partial seizures have a shorter ictal course—usually less than 60 s—abrupt onset and cessation, tend to occur in sleep, and exhibit tonic contraction of the upper extremities in abduction.

Treatment Psychotherapy, including family therapy when the patient is a child, should be the primary treatment for pseudoseizures.[75] Antidepressants are indicated when depression is a major factor.

Diagnostic Procedures The history, with an accurate description of the seizure given by the patient and an observer, and the neurological examination, are the most important factors in evaluation of the patient's epilepsy. The patient with a suspected seizure disorder should have:

1. Complete history, general physical examination, and neurological examination. It is important to get an accurate description of the seizure from the patient and an observer and to inquire about the presence or absence of factors discussed under Causative Factors in Seizures (see page 86).

2. EEG. In the majority of cases, the interictal EEG is normal. Characteristic EEG findings are discussed under the particular seizure type. Hyperventilation, photic stimulation, and sleep deprivation are useful measures to unmask a seizure disorder. A 24-h ambulatory EEG with the patient recording activities in a diary is useful in difficult cases. A video-monitored recording with EEG is indicated when the diagnosis of seizure type is in doubt or to differentiate seizures from pseudoseizures.

3. An MRI scan is indicated in simple partial, complex partial, and generalized tonic-clonic seizures to identify or rule out a structural lesion. MRI scanning is particularly sensitive in deducting temporal lobe lesions, including medial temporal sclerosis and gliosis in patients with intractable seizures (Fig. 4-2).

4. The blood should be drawn for electrolytes (Na^+, K^+, CA^{++}, Mg^+), blood urea nitrogen (BUN), creatinine, glucose, liver function, and thyroid function. Further studies (e.g., toxicology screen, alcohol levels) depend on clinical suspicion.

5. Serum amino acids, organic acids, lysosomal enzymes, and ammonia studies are indicated in infantile spasms, Lennox-Gastaut syndrome, and progressive myoclonic seizures.

6. Serum lactate and pyruvate levels are indicated in screening for mitochondrial encephalopathies.

7. When a patient is already taking medication but the diagnosis of a seizure disorder is doubt-

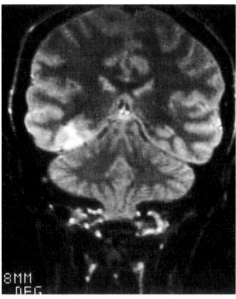

Figure 4-2.
MRI scan showing the presence of a glial scar in the inferomedial aspect of the right midtemporal lobe in a patient with chronic complex partial seizures.

ful, the following evaluations should be performed. If the initial EEG is normal, anticonvulsant medication should be withdrawn slowly and the EEG repeated. If the EEG remains normal and the patient has no seizures, a sleep deprivation EEG should be obtained. If this is normal, a 24-h EEG recording is advised. If this remains normal and the patient has no seizures, it is unlikely that the patient requires treatment.

8. It is important to recognize patients with pseudoseizures. This problem is frequently complicated by the occurrence of pseudoseizures in patients with a genuine seizure disorder. Patients who have pseudoseizures are more likely to bite the tip of the tongue than the side of the tongue, there is no urinary incontinence, the patient responds to deep pain during the seizure, attempts to open the eyes are actively resisted by blepharospasms, the pupils react to light, and there is a bilateral plantar flexor response. The patient is able to recall events that occur during the seizure, the postictal EEG reveals no slowing, and a postictal serum prolactin level is increased in epilepsy but remains normal in pseudoseizures measured in the immediate postictal period.

9. Further diagnostic procedures in epilepsy include lumbar puncture, arteriography, and evaluation for cerebral metastases, all depending on clinical suspicion. The MRI scan is the most sensitive in detecting structural lesions in the temporal lobe, particularly mesiotemporal sclerosis or tumor in patients with intractable seizures (see Fig. 4-3). However, the combination of EEG, ictal single photon emission CT (SPECT) scan and interictal positron emission tomography (PET) scan have the highest sensitivity and specificity for temporal lobe seizures, regardless of the presence of structural abnormalities.[76]

DRUG THERAPY

Because there is no standard dose of any anticonvulsant, the selected drug should be administered in sufficient amounts to achieve a therapeutic plasma concentration. In many cases, it is prudent to begin treatment with small doses of an anticonvulsant to avoid adverse affects, usually drowsiness. This can be accomplished by only increasing the dosage when the patient feels comfortable with the current dose of the medication. Plasma concentrations should be determined when the drug level has reached a steady state, which is generally four half-lives of the drug. Once a steady state has been achieved, the decision to maintain, increase, or decrease the dosage can be determined from the plasma concentration. If seizure control is achieved at levels below the recommended therapeutic plasma levels of the administered drug, it is not necessary to increase the dosage. Similarly, if seizure control is not achieved at the upper level after the recommended therapeutic plasma range, the drug dosage may still be increased until control is achieved or until signs of toxicity occur. Failure to control due to systemic toxicity or neurotoxicity usually occurs early in the treatment.

Determinations of plasma levels of anticonvulsants should be made throughout the course of treatment. To avoid differing recommendations for different drugs, a simple course of action would be as follows:

1. Seven days after beginning treatment
2. Seven days after each change in dosage

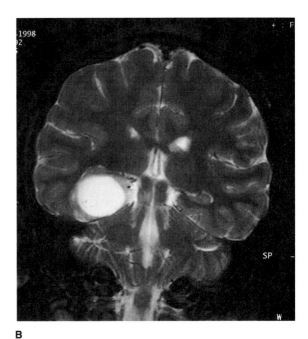

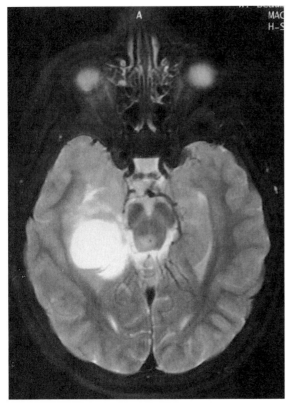

A

B

Figure 4-3.
MRI scan. There is an area of increased signal intensity located in the medial aspect of the right midtemporal lobe. A. Transverse section. B. Coronal section. Oligodendroglioma in a patient with partial complex seizure.

3. Seven days after the addition or withdrawal of a new anticonvulsant
4. If there is a recurrence of or an increase in seizure activity
5. If there is any obvious adverse reaction to the drug, or if signs of toxicity occur
6. At 6-month intervals in controlled patients

Phenytoin (Dilantin)

Action Phenytoin controls the spread of epileptic activity by preventing sodium influx into neurons, thus stabilizing the threshold against hyperexcitability caused by excessive stimulation by exci-

tatory neurotransmitters. Phenytoin is highly bound to serum albumin and has the potential to displace other albumin-bound medications such as valproic acid, warfarin, and nonsteroidal anti-inflammatory drugs (NSAIDs) from binding sites. This results in an increase in activity of phenytoin and the displaced drug. Consequently, careful monitoring of phenytoin and the displaced medication is necessary. Both total and free phenytoin should be measured and valproic levels maintained between 50 to 100 μg/mL.

The displacement of warfarin from binding site can be followed by increased levels of unbound warfarin and an increase in the international normalized ratio (INR). However, phenytoin acts as an inducer of liver enzymes, resulting in increased metabolism of warfarin with decrease in INR in some cases. Consequently, more frequent and careful monitoring of INR and warfarin dosage is advised when one of the two drugs is added in the presence of the other medication.

Phenytoin has a nonlinear metabolic profile owing to saturation of liver enzymes responsible for phenytoin metabolism. Dose increments should not exceed 30 to 50 mg, to avoid sudden elevation in serum levels when enzyme saturation is exceeded.

The half-life of phenytoin within therapeutic range is 20 to 36 h, permitting a single dose daily. However, there may be a precipitous fall in serum concentration and seizure breakthrough should the patient fail to take the one prescribed daily dose. Consequently, a q12h dosage schedule is recommended. If there is omission of one dose, this dose is then taken with the next scheduled dose.

Indications   Generalized tonic-clonic seizures, partial complex seizures

Half-life   20 to 36 h

Steady State   7 to 10 days

Drug Administration   q12h
Available in capsules of 30 mg and 100 mg; tablets 50 mg; suspension 125 mg in 5 mL; ampules for parenteral use; 50 mg/mL supplied in 2-mL and 5-mL ampules. Phenytoin sodium injection must be administered slowly in adults, not exceeding 50 mg/min intravenously. Neonates should be given the drug at rates not to exceed 1 to 3 mg/kg per minute.

Therapeutic Levels   Total phenytoin 10 to 25 μg/mL. Free phenytoin 1 to 3 μg/mL.

Adverse Effects   CNS: ataxia, lethargy, nystagmus, blurred vision, diplopia, memory problems, nausea and vomiting. Peripheral nervous system: peripheral neuropathy. Non-CNS symptoms include hirsutism, gingival hyperplasia, altered facial features, bone mass suppression, decreased sodium, decreased serum folate, and megaloblastic anemia. Phenytoin should be withdrawn if the patient develops a rash.

Phosphenytoin

Action   Phosphenytoin is a water-soluble disodium phosphate ester of phenytoin that is converted in plasma to phenytoin.[77] Phosphenytoin was developed to eliminate the poor aqueous solubility[78] and venous irritation related to intravenous administration of phenytoin.[79] Phosphenytoin is compatible with common intravenous solutions and can be infused rapidly when administered intravenously. The intravenous infusion of phenytoin is limited by the propylene glycol vehicle, which is the cause of hypotension in cardiac arrhythmias reported with intravenous phenytoin.[80] The absence of propylene glycol makes phosphenytoin a safer compound and the treatment of choice for status epilepticus. Once infused intravenously, the phosphate molecule is cleaved from the phosphenytoin biphosphatases, converting the phosphenytoin molecule into active phenytoin.

Indications   Treatment of status epilepticus.

Carbamazepine (Tegretol)

Pharmacokinetics   Carbamazepine acts by blocking voltage-dependent sodium channels in the neuronal membranes.

Carbamazepine has the property of inducing its own metabolism, resulting in increasing dosage requirements during the first several weeks of therapy. This autoinduction is the product of the formation of additional metabolizing enzymes and the process is maximal within the first month of therapy. The drug should be introduced slowly to minimize adverse affects, but the dosage may have to be increased for several weeks to maintain adequate therapeutic serum levels. Withdrawal of carbamazepine is associated with deinduction over a 4-week period. The decrease in metabolic enzyme activity may affect concomitant medication, particularly divalproex sodium, with a rise in serum levels and the occurrence of toxic adverse effects.

Indications   Carbamazepine is effective in the control of generalized tonic-clonic seizures, complex partial seizures, and simple partial seizures.

Half-life   13 to 17 h

Steady State   4 to 6 weeks after initial dose

Metabolism   Carbamazepine is metabolized in the liver to 10,11 epoxide, which is then excreted in the urine.

Initial Dose   200 mg q12

Maximum Daily Dose   200 mg q12h to 800 mg q8h

Availability   100-mg chewable tablets, 200-mg tablets. An extended-release preparation of carbamazepine (Tegretol-XR) is supplied in 100-mg, 200-mg, and 400-mg tablets. Carbamazepine suspension is available 5 mL/100 mg.

Adverse   Effects   CNS: light-headedness, drowsiness, lethargy, memory problems, limb and gait ataxia, dysarthria, blurred vision or diplopia, agitation, restlessness, irritability, insomnia, choreiform movements. Non-CNS: leukopenia, thrombocytopenia, and skin rash.

Therapeutic Blood Levels   8 to 12 μg/mL

Drugs Affecting Serum Levels of Carbamazepine   Increased carbamazepine levels occur in association with propoxyphene, erythromycin, cimetidine, and fluoxetine. Decreased carbamazepine levels occur in association with phenytoin and phenobarbital. Drugs affected by carbamazepine include warfarin, theophylline, doxycycline, oral contraceptives, and lamotrigine.

Oxcarbamazepine

Pharmacokinetics   Oxcarbamazepine has a chemical structure closely related to carbamazepine. Oxcarbamazepine has low protein-binding properties and little induction of liver enzymes.

Adverse Effects   Adverse effects are significantly lower with this medication than with carbamazepine[81] and with a half-life 50 percent higher

than carbamazepine, oxycarbazepine can be administered q12h at higher doses than carbamazepine if necessary.[82]

Indications   Generalized tonic-clonic seizures, complex partial seizures, simple partial seizures

Half-life   < 6 to 7 h

Administration   q12h

Availability   100-mg, 200-mg, 400-mg tablets

Adverse Effects   As for carbamazepine but reduced in severity and frequency. Drowsiness, nausea, diplopia, hyponatremia, a rash, choreoathetosis, thrombocytopenia, and leukopenia can be expected to occur occasionally.

Valproic Acid (Depakene), Divalproex Sodium (Depakote)

Pharmacokinetics   Valproic acid and divalproex sodium have two distinct actions: (1) the blockade of voltage-dependent sodium channels in the neuronal membrane and (2) increased brain levels of the inhibitory neurotransmitter, GABA, which enhances postsynaptic GABA-mediated inhibition. An increased concentration of GABA is the result of competitive inhibition of GABA transaminase, succinic semialdehyde dehydrogenase, and stimulation of enzymes that synthesize GABA, including glutamic acid dehydrogenase.[83]

Valproic acid and divalproex sodium rapidly dissociate to develop the valproate ion in the gastrointestinal tract. Valproate is metabolized in the liver and inhibits the clearance of many hepatically metabolized medications. Inhibition of phenobarbital metabolism can cause a doubling of phenobarbital concentrations while a decrease in plasma protein binding will lower total phenytoin but increase free phenytoin levels.[84]

Indications   Valproate has a broad spectrum of activity, which includes primary and secondary tonic-clonic seizures,[85] myoclonic seizures, complex partial seizures,[86] simple partial seizures, absence and atypical absence seizures.

Half-life   6 to 20 h

Steady State   5 to 10 days

Metabolism   Valproate is metabolized in the liver with production of many metabolites.

Initial Dose   500 mg q12h. Maximal daily dose: 1500 mg q12h to 1500 mg q8h. Valproic acid is available in 250-mg capsules and as a syrup containing 250 mg valproic acid/5 mL. Divalproex sodium is available in single capsules of 125 mg; in 125-mg, 250-mg, and 500-mg tablets; and in 100 mg/mL intravenous solution.

Adverse Effects   CNS: tremor, somnolence, memory problems, ataxia, slurred speech, blurred vision, and neural tube defects in the newborn. Systemic effects include hepatoxicity, particularly in infants and children but rarely in adults. Other adverse effects include significant weight gain, nausea, vomiting, tremor, thrombocytopenia, hepatic dysfunction, and hair loss.

Therapeutic Blood Levels   50 to 100 μg/mL, estimated 2 h after the dose of divalproex sodium.

Drugs Affecting Serum Levels   Increased levels of valproic acid occur with salicylate therapy and cimetidine therapy.
Decreased levels of valproic acid occur with concomitant phenytoin, carbamazepine, phenobarbital, and lamotrigine therapy.
Drugs affected by valproate include increased levels of phenobarbital and lamotrigine.

Phenobarbital

Pharmacokinetics   Phenobarbital acts by blocking voltage-dependent sodium channels in the neuronal membrane and modulates the inhibitory postsynaptic activity of GABA and the action of presynaptic glutamate.
Phenobarbital is metabolized in the liver by the hepatic cytochrome P450 system and competes directly with phenytoin. However, because phenobarbital has a higher binding affinity for the cytochrome P450 system, there may be significant effect on phenytoin metabolism with increased levels of this drug, when the two are administered concomitantly. Chronic administration of phenobarbital induces induction of the P450 enzyme system with a later decrease in phenytoin levels. However, the time-honored combination of phenytoin and phenobarbital has no advantage over phenytoin monotherapy and the practice of combining these two drugs should be abandoned.
Primidone (Mysoline) is metabolized to phenobarbital and has the same actions and side effects as phenobarbital.

Indications   Phenobarbital should be reserved for patients who have not responded to other antiepileptic drugs in the treatment of primary or secondary tonic-clonic seizures, simple partial seizures, and complex partial seizures. Phenobarbital is also useful in the treatment of refractory status epilepticus.

Half-life   72 to 120 h

Steady State   1 to 4 weeks

Metabolism   Phenobarbital is metabolized primarily by hepatic microsomal enzyme systems and the metabolic products are excreted in the urine.

Initial Dose   Phenobarbital 30 to 60 mg q.h.s.; primidone 50 mg q.h.s.

Maximum Daily Dose   Phenobarbital 180 mg per day; primidone 750 to 1000 mg per day.

Availability   Phenobarbital tablets 15 mg, 30 mg, 60 mg, and 100 mg. Elixir 20 mg/5 mL. Parenteral solution for use in status epilepticus. Primidone 50-mg and 250-mg tablets, 250 mg/5 mL suspension.

Adverse Effects   CNS: sedation, cognitive impairment, impaired learning in children, which persists after withdrawal of the drug, depression, restlessness, paradoxical excitement, attention deficit, and impaired attention span.

In addition, barbiturates may be associated with myalgic and arthritic pains, which tend to be maximal in the early morning hours.

Therapeutic Blood Levels   Phenobarbital 10 to 40 μg/mL. Primidone 5 to 12 μg/mL.

Drugs Affecting Serum Levels of Phenobarbital   Valproic acid and divalproex sodium increase phenobarbital serum levels. Consequently, careful monitoring of serum levels should be performed when these drugs are used concomitantly.

Drugs Affected by Phenobarbital   Phenobarbital produces decreased levels of warfarin, chloramphenicol, and phenylbutazone.

Felbamate

Pharmacokinetics   Felbamate acts on both NMDA and GABA cellular receptors. The drug has significant interaction with carbamazepine, phenytoin, and valproate. There is a reduction in carbamazepine levels and an increase in phenytoin and valproate levels following introduction of felbamate therapy.

Indications   Felbamate can be used as monotherapy or as an add-on for partial seizures in children and adults and for treatment of the Lennox-Gastaut syndrome.[87] However, although felbamate is an effective anticonvulsant, this drug has been relegated to the role of a second- or third-line add-on agent because of the risk of aplastic anemia or liver failure.

Half-life   15 to 20 h

Steady State   5 to 7 days

Metabolism   Felbamate is metabolized through the cytochrome P540 isoenzyme system in the liver.

Initial Dose   600 mg twice a day

Maximum Daily Dose   3600 mg

Drug Administration   q8h

Availability   Felbamate is available in tablets of 400 mg or 600 mg, and a suspension of 600 mg/5 mL.

Adverse Effects   Although felbamate is an effective anticonvulsant, the drug has been relegated to the role of a second- or third-line add-on agent because of the risk of aplastic anemia or liver failure.[88] Felbamate should not be used unless the patient has a severe seizure disorder partially controlled by other antiepileptic drugs. Under these circumstances, felbamate requires a complete blood count and platelet count weekly and liver function tests every 2 weeks. Felbamate monotherapy is desirable because the risk of adverse effects increases in patients receiving other antiepileptic drugs. However, if felbamate is required for treatment of refractory seizures, which are usually associated with a Lennox-Gastaut syndrome in children, the product package insert recommendations for monitoring should be followed and the parent or guardian should sign the informed consent included in the package insert.

In addition to the serious side effect of aplastic anemia and hepatic failure, felbamate can cause nausea, vomiting, insomnia, and headaches.

Drugs Affecting Serum Levels of Felbamate   Felbamate concentrations are decreased with concomitant use of phenytoin and carbamazepine, but felbamate levels are increased by divalproex sodium.

Drugs Affected by Felbamate   Felbamate therapy increases phenytoin, divalproex sodium, and carbamazepine levels.

Gabapentin

Pharmacokinetics   The mechanism of action of gabapentin is unknown[89] but gabapentin may enhance the release or actions of GABA.[90]

The drug has no primary metabolic interactions with other antiepileptic drugs and is excreted unchanged through the kidneys and is not metabolized by the liver. This unique property of gabapentin may be a major factor in defining its clinical usefulness.[91]

However, the renal elimination of gabapentin mandates that the drug should be used with caution in patients with renal impairment or in the elderly, who should have regular serum creatinine levels determined during therapy. Unfortunately, initial labeling recommended doses of gabapentin that were only partially effective. Current recommendations suggest higher doses, which can be obtained by 300-mg or 400-mg increments, given at intervals when the patient reports freedom from adverse effects.

Indications Adjunctive therapy of partial seizures with or without secondary generalized therapy. Monotherapy is also effective for partial complex seizures with or without secondary generalization.[92]

Half-life 6 h

Drug Administration q8h orally, beginning with 300 mg q8h, usually effective in doses of 2400 to 2700 mg/day but doses of 3600 mg or 4800 mg/day have been used in some cases.

Availability Available in capsules 100 mg, 300 mg, 400 mg.

Therapeutic Level Not determined

Adverse Effects Somnolence, fatigue, light-headedness, and ataxia

Lamotrigine (Lamictal)

Pharmacokinetics

a. Inhibition of release of the presynaptic excitatory amino acid glutamate
b. Voltage-dependent sodium channel blockade, stabilizing neuronal membrane[93]

Lamotrigine is extensively metabolized to inactive metabolites in the liver, but its half-life can be significantly decreased by hepatic enzyme-inducing antiepileptic drugs. Conversely, the half-life of lamotrigine is increased by valproic acid, which inhibits conjugation of lamotrigine and glucuronic acid.

Indications Simple or partial complex seizures,[94] Lennox-Gastaut syndrome

Half-life 24 h monotherapy, 15 h with phenytoin or carbamazepine, 60 h with divalproex sodium

Drug Administration q12h

Steady State 3 to 15 days

Availability Available in oral tablets 25 mg, 100 mg, 150 mg, 200 mg.

Therapeutic Levels Undefined

Adverse Effects CNS: drowsiness, light-headedness, ataxia, diplopia, headache, nausea, vomiting, and tremor at higher dosage.[95] Systemic rash in 5 percent, which usually occurs in the first 4 to 6 weeks of treatment, with an increased tendency if lamotrigine is combined with divalproex sodium.[96] Serious rashes, including Stevens-Johnson syndrome and toxic epidermal necrolysis, have been reported in less than 1 percent, occurring predominantly in the pediatric population.

Ethosuximide (Zarontin)

Pharmacokinetics Ethosuximide acts by blocking neuronal calcium channels. Ethosuximide is rapidly absorbed and metabolized in the liver. The drug has little reaction with other antiepileptic drugs, but because ethosuximide inhibits hepatic metabolism, valproic acid levels may increase when ethosuximide is combined with divalproex sodium in the treatment of absence plus generalized tonic-clonic seizures or myoclonic seizures.[97]

Indications Treatment of absence (petit mal) seizures

Half-life 30 to 60 h

Drug Administration q.d. or b.i.d.

Availability Available in capsules 250 mg or solution 250 mg/5 mL.

Therapeutic Levels   40 to 80 μg/mL

Adverse Effects   Few; irritability, insomnia, hyperactivity, and nausea have been reported.

Vigabatrin

Pharmacotherapy   Vigabatrin produces irreversible inhibition of gabatransaminase, increasing the amount of GABA available to produce an inhibitory effect on seizure activity.[98] More than 60 percent of vigabatrin dose is absorbed but is not bound to plasma proteins. Vigabatrin is eliminated through the kidneys and does not have any significant drug interactions.

Indications   Vigabatrin is effective in the control of simple and complex partial seizures alone or in partial seizures combined with secondary generalized seizures.[99] The drug is especially effective in infantile spasms.[100] Tests of cognitive function show no detrimental effect, or in some cases, slightly improved function in patients receiving vigabatrin.[101]

Half-life   4 to 8 h

Metabolism   Vigabatrin is readily absorbed, is not protein bound, and is excreted by glomerulofiltration through the kidneys in an unchanged form.

Initial Dose   500 mg increasing by 500-mg increments q12h until seizures are controlled.

Maximum Daily Dose   4000 mg in divided doses q12h

Availability   Vigabatrin is available in tablets of 500 mg.

Therapeutic Levels   Not known

Adverse Effects   The majority of the reported adverse effects of vigabatrin are relatively benign, consisting of drowsiness or fatigue, irritability, nervousness, headache, and confusion occurring during the stage of titration and decreasing on a maintenance dose of the drug. There are occasional reports of psychosis with paranoia, mood swings, auditory hallucinations, and agitation. These symptoms subside following withdrawal of the drug but can be minimized by the use of the minimum dose required to control seizures, beginning with 500 mg per day in adults, 20 mg/kg per day in children.[102] Psychosis has also been attributed to abrupt withdrawal of vigabatrin. Severe persistent visual field constriction has been reported as a rare complication of vigabatrin therapy.[103]

Topiramate (Topamax)

Pharmacokinetics

a. Voltage-dependent sodium channel blockade
b. Inhibition of kainate/AMPA receptors
c. GABA enhancement at some GABA receptors

Topiramate has a 20 to 50 percent hepatic metabolism, depending on concomitant therapy but does not act as an hepatic enzyme inducer. Between 50 and 60 percent of the drug is eliminated unchanged through the kidneys. Topiramate does not affect the metabolism of other antiepileptic drugs, but there is a 50 percent decrease in topiramate serum concentration following addition of phenytoin, carbamazepine, or phenobarbital.[104]

Indications   Monotherapy and add-on for simple partial seizures, complex partial seizures, and secondary generalized tonic-clonic seizures.[105]

Half-life   20 to 30 h monotherapy; 12 to 15 h with concomitant antiepileptic drugs acting as liver enzyme inducers.

Metabolism   Excreted unchanged through the kidneys.

Initial Dose   100 mg q12h

Maximal Daily Dose   300 mg q12h[106]

Drug Administration   q12h

Availability   25-mg, 100-mg, and 200-mg tablets

Therapeutic Drug Level   Unknown

Adverse Effects   Somnolence, mental slowing, fatigue, confusion, light-headedness, ataxia, impaired concentration

Tiagebine (Gabatril)

Pharmacokinetics   Tiagebine acts by inhibiting the uptake of GABA by glial cells and neurons, with enhanced activity of GABA, which is the major inhibitory neurotransmitter in the CNS. There is prolonged hyperpolarization of GABA-ergic receptors, extension of the period of intrasynaptic GABA elevation and a wider diffusion of GABA in the brain.[105] Tiagebine has no effect on the steady-state plasma concentrations of phenytoin, carbamazepine, and divalproex sodium.[106] However, divalproex sodium decreases tiagebine binding and increases free tiagebine concentration, indicating the need for lower doses and slower titration in patients taking divalproex sodium. An increased incidence of malformed fetuses has been reported in laboratory animals receiving tiagebine, but there are no well-controlled studies in women. Consequently, tiagebine should be avoided during pregnancy unless clearly indicated by improved seizure control.

Indications   Tiagebine is indicated in children and adults with refractory, simple, and partial complex seizures.

Half-life   7 to 9 h

Initial Dose   4 mg daily, increasing by 4 mg at weekly intervals.

Maximum Daily Dose   Up to 32 mg per day, at which time the drug should be given in divided doses q8h.

Availability   4-mg, 12-mg, 16-mg, 20-mg tablets

Adverse Effects   Light-headedness, fatigue, somnolence, nausea, irritability, tremor, abdominal pain, depression, poor concentration, and confusion.

Tiagebine does not cause deterioration in cognitive performance during long-term follow-up with higher doses of the drug.[107]

Benzodiazepines

Pharmacokinetics   The benzodiazepines selectively potentiate GABA-ergic inhibitory activity. These drugs, which include diazepam, lorazepam, clonazepam, and clorazepate, have a limited role in control of seizures, and there has been a decline in the use of benzodiazepines in seizure therapy following the introduction of newer antiepileptic drugs in recent years. Intravenous diazepam and lorazepam have an essential role in status epilepticus or severe recurrent seizures, and intravenous diazepam is useful in the control of repeated simple partial seizures when used as a diazepam drip. Rectal diazepam is available for control of repeated seizure activity or prevention of febrile seizures when given at the onset of fever in a susceptible child.

The long-term use of oral benzodiazepines is limited by sedative side effects and the development of tolerance. These complications can be minimized in some cases by increasing the dose at long intervals over several months. Clonazepam (Klonopin) 0.01 to 0.2 mg/kg, is effective in Lennox-Gastaut syndrome and myoclonic or akinetic absence, clorazepate (Tranxene) 15 to 60 mg per day, given in divided doses q6h, is a useful add-on medication in poorly controlled complex partial seizures.

Adverse Effects   CNS depression with sedation, drowsiness and fatigue, ataxia, cognitive impairment, and, occasionally, psychotic behavior. Paradoxical reactions such as personality change, irritability, aggressive behavior, and memory problems can occur.

Acetazolamide

Pharmacokinetics   Acetazolamide acts by inhibition of the enzyme carbonic anhydrase. The anticonvulsant action of acetazolamide is related to inhibition of carbonic anhydrase in the brain, which leads to accumulation of carbon dioxide, resulting in an increase in the concentration of GABA and inhibition of seizure activity.

Indications   As an adjuvant in absence, partial complex seizures, generalized tonic-clonic seizures, and juvenile myoclonic epilepsy.[108]

Half-life   10 to 12 h

Metabolism   Acetazolamide is excreted unchanged in the urine.

Initial Dose   250 mg q12h

Maximum Daily Dose   1000 mg per day q8h or q12h, with extended-release acetazolamide

Availability   Acetazolamide (Diamox) tablets 125 mg and 250 mg. Diamox sustained-release capsules 500 mg.

Adverse Effects   Transient polyuria, hypokalemia, increased risk of kidney stones, muscle weakness, lethargy, diminished appetite, drowsiness, and paresthesias. Metabolic acidosis can occur in the elderly. Blood dyscrasias, including aplastic anemia and thrombocytopenia, have been reported.

Discontinuing Antiepileptic Drugs

The discontinuance of antiepileptic drugs may be considered by the physician and informed patient or parent/guardian if the patient meets the following profile[109]:

1. Seizure-free 2 to 5 years on antiepileptic drugs (mean 3.5 years)
2. Single type of partial seizure (simple partial or complex partial or secondary generalized tonic-clonic seizure) or single type of primary generalized tonic-clonic seizures
3. Normal neurological examination/normal IQ
4. The EEG converts to a normal record with treatment.

It must be emphasized, however, that children meeting the profile can be expected to have a 69 percent chance and adults a 61 percent chance of successful withdrawal. This corresponds to a relapse rate of 31 percent in children and 39 percent in adults.

SURGICAL TREATMENT OF EPILEPSY

The development of epilepsy surgery units, sophisticated EEG techniques, and improved neuroimaging have resulted in an increase in the surgical treatment of epilepsy. Regions of the brain formerly regarded as unapproachable are now open to surgical intervention in patients of all ages with seizures refractory to medical therapy.[110]

The essential factor in modern epilepsy surgery is the input of a multidisciplinary team of highly trained individuals working together in an epilepsy center. A detailed presurgical evaluation is mandatory to identify the offending area of the brain responsible for the seizure activity and to ensure a high rate of success while avoiding new neurological or cognitive deficits. Diagnostic tests include the routine EEG, outpatient long-term EEG monitoring, and video EEG monitoring. These basic studies can be augmented by intraoperative electrocorticography, subdural grid or strip recording, long-term recording, or stereotactic depth electrode recording. Imaging techniques include MRI, MRI spectroscopy, SPECT,[111] and PET.[112] An intracarotid amobarbital injection (Wada test) is indicated in all surgical candidates with frontal, temporal, or parietal lobe seizure foci. The new technique of magnetoelectroencephalography[113] and function MRI will improve the identification of epileptic foci.

Anterior temporal lobe resection[114] for mesiotemporal lobe seizures is the most frequently performed procedure for medication-resistant partial complex seizures. Temporal lobe surgery for partial complex seizures in children produces a significant improvement in seizure control and an improved social/behavioral outcome in the majority of cases.[115] The majority show hippocampal sclerosis or atrophy on high-resolution MRI and temporal lobe hypometabolism on interictal PET scanning. Focal structural lesions such as low-grade astrocytomas, angiomatous malformations, or other congenital defects respond well to surgical treatment.

Frontal lobe partial complex seizures[116] and seizures arising from the insular cortex[117] are characterized by frequent and often disabling seizure activity resistant to pharmacotherapy. Invasive diagnostic procedures, including intracranial monitoring and subdural electrodes,[118] augmented by MRI, PET, and

SPECT scanning, are necessary for the localization of the exact site of epileptic activity, which can be difficult to identify. Surgical results, although impressive, are not as good in frontal lobe partial seizures as in temporal lobe seizures.[119]

Intractable generalized or unilateral seizures resulting from epileptic activity confined to one hemisphere due to Rasmussen encephalitis, multiple porencephalic cysts, Sturge-Weber syndrome, or diffuse cortical dysplasias in children, with an intact contralateral hemisphere, may show dramatic improvement with hemispherectomy.[120]

Sectioning of the corpus callosum is indicated in patients with diffuse brain damage and intractable seizures who have frequent drop attacks resulting in injury.[121] Surgery may abolish the drop attacks without affecting seizure activity occurring independently in either hemisphere.

Mood disorders, particularly depression and anxiety, are common postoperative psychiatric disorders following epileptic surgery. Treatment of depression with selective serotonin uptake inhibitors along with anticonvulsant medication is indicated in patients with postoperative depression.[122]

The incidence of psychosis in uncontrolled epileptic patients ranges from 10 to 25 percent and may persist postoperatively.[123] Appropriate antipsychotic medications such as haloperidol or risperidone are indicated in such cases.

Neuropsychological testing is the best single means of quantifying brain-dependent cognitive abilities before and after surgical treatment of epilepsy and for assessing emotional and social aspects of preoperative and postoperative functioning.[124]

STATUS EPILEPTICUS

Definition   Status epilepticus is a condition in which an individual has two or more seizures or a series of seizures lasting more than 30 min without recovery of consciousness between episodes.

Alternative definitions have been proposed and include:

1. An epileptic seizure that is so frequently repeated or so prolonged as to create a fixed and lasting condition[125]

2. A state of continuing or recurrent seizures in which recovery between attacks is incomplete[126]
3. Continuous seizure activity lasting 30 min or longer[127]

The combination of these definitions covers generalized convulsive status epilepticus, generalized nonconvulsive status epilepticus (absence status), simple partial status epilepticus, and complex partial status epilepticus.

Although generalized convulsive status epilepticus should be considered a medical emergency because of the high risk of neuronal damage beginning approximately 30 min after onset of seizures, other types of status epilepticus should not be neglected but treated promptly to avoid focal neuronal loss. Patients with simple partial status with somatomotor signs— epilepsia partialis continua—have the highest risk in this category.

Etiology and Pathology   Status epilepticus is not an uncommon problem, with an estimated 60,000 to 160,000 cases of generalized tonic-clonic status epilepticus occurring in the United States each year.[128] In one-third, status epilepticus is the presenting symptom in individuals who will develop recurrent epileptic seizures. One-third occur in patients with established epilepsy, usually the result of noncompliance in the use of anticonvulsant medication. The remainder of cases develop in patients without a history of epilepsy.[129] Some common causes of status epilepticus are outlined in Table 4-3. It should be noted that the mortality related to seizure activity is between 1 and 2 percent, but the mortality related to diseases causing status epilepticus, as outlined in Table 4-3, is about 10 percent.[130]

It is possible to recognize five stages clinically and on EEG in status epilepticus. The first stage, lasting some 30 min, consists of intermittent seizure activity, without recovery of consciousness between seizure episodes. This stage is associated with elevated blood pressure, increase in serum lactate, increase in serum glucose, and decrease in serum pH because of lactic acidosis. Neuronal change is reversible during stage one. After 30 min, there is a change to stage two, when the seizure activity waxes and wanes and the blood pressure, serum pH, and

Table 4-3
Some causes of status epilepticus

A. Hereditary and Congenital
   Congenital abnormalities of the brain, including
   lipidosis, leukodystrophies, and aminoacidurias

B. Head Trauma
   Acute head injury, post-traumatic encephalopathy,
   postcraniotomy

C. Infections
   Viral encephalitis, acute purulent meningitis, chronic
   meningitis, particularly tuberculosis, fungal meningitis

D. Metabolic
   Hypocalcemia, hypomagnesemia, hypoglycemia,
   hyponatremia

E. Toxic
   Alcohol withdrawal; drug abuse, particularly cocaine;
   withdrawal of medications, particularly antiepileptic
   drugs and benzodiazepines

F. Vascular
   Cerebrovascular disease, including acute infarction,
   multi-infarct state, cerebral arteritis, cerebral lupus,
   intracerebral hemorrhage, subarachnoid hemorrhage

G. Neoplastic
   Brain tumor, angiomatous malformation

H. Degenerative
   Multiple sclerosis, Alzheimer disease

serum glucose return to normal. Irreversible neuronal damage begins in this stage. In stage three, seizure activity becomes continuous, leading to hyperthermia, respiratory impairment, and increased irreversible neuronal damage. The continuous seizure activity is followed by myoclonus during stage four, when increasing respiratory compromise requires mechanical ventilation. This is followed by cessation of all clinical seizure activity in stage five, but neuronal loss and brain damage continue.[131]

Neuronal damage and death are not uniform in status epilepticus but are maximal in five areas of the brain (layers three, five, and six of the cerebral cortex; the cerebellum; the hippocampus; thalamic nuclei; and the amygdala). The hippocampus is probably the most sensitive to the effects of status epilepticus, with neuronal loss maximal in Sommers' zone. The exact mechanism of neuronal damage or loss is complex but involves reduction of inhibition of neuronal activity through the GABA receptors and increased release of glutamate, which stimulates glutamate receptors, with influx of sodium and calcium ions into the cell and calcium-mediated cell damage.

Clinical Features Repeated seizure activity should always be regarded as a medical emergency. Tonic-clonic status epilepticus requires prompt treatment with the ever-present thought that control must be achieved within 30 minutes if possible and always in under 1 h, to avoid brain damage. This does not mean that one should be sanguine in the presence of partial status epilepticus, which can also lead to focal neuronal damage if not controlled as soon as possible.

1. Generalized tonic-clonic epilepticus. This is the most frequently encountered and potentially the most damaging form of status epilepticus. Activity may begin with a generalized tonic-clonic seizure or as a partial seizure, which changes quickly to a generalized tonic-clonic pattern. In generalized tonic-clonic status, the attack begins with a series of generalized tonic-clonic seizures, without recovery of consciousness between attacks and increasing in frequency. Each seizure lasts 2 to 3 min, with a tonic phase involving the axial muscles and halting respiratory movements. The patient becomes cyanosed during this phase, followed by hyperpnea owing to CO_2 retention. There is tachycardia and elevated blood pressure; hyperpyrexia may develop. Hyperglycemia and increased serum lactate occur, resulting in decreased serum pH and respiratory and metabolic acidosis. Seizure activity is repeated up to five times in the first hour in untreated cases. Eventually, the activity is modified by a progression through stage two to five as outlined above.

2. Clonic-tonic-clonic status epilepticus. Occasionally status epilepticus presents with generalized clonic activity preceding the tonic phase and followed by a second period of clonic activity.

3. Tonic status epilepticus. Tonic status epilepticus occurs in children and adolescents and presents with episodic tonic seizures associated with loss of consciousness but without clonic episodes. This type of activity occurs on a background of chronic encephalopathy and is a feature of Lennox-Gastaut syndrome.

4. Myoclonic status epilepticus is usually seen in patients with an established encephalopathy. Myoclonic jerks are generalized but often asymmetrical and there is impairment of consciousness. This type of status epilepticus is not unusual in severe anoxic encephalopathy when the prognosis is poor but can occur in other toxic, metabolic, infectious, or degenerative conditions.

5. Absence status epilepticus is a rare form of status epilepticus and is usually seen in adolescents or adults. There is an alteration in the level of consciousness and the condition presents as a "dreamy state" with slowed responses, rather like a slow motion movie and may last for a prolonged period of time.[132] There may be a history of primary generalized seizures or absence seizures in childhood. The EEG shows monotonous 3-Hz spike activity in all leads. The response to intravenous benzodiazepine is dramatic.

6. Nonconvulsive status epilepticus. This condition may be difficult to differentiate from absence status or partial complex status epilepticus clinically because the symptoms in the three conditions can be similar. Patients with nonconvulsive status epilepticus present with slower mentation, stupor, or occasionally coma. When conscious, there is a marked change in personality, with paranoia, delusions, irascibility, hallucinations, impulsive behavior, psychomotor retardation, and overt psychosis in some cases. The EEG shows generalized spike wave discharges, unlike the 3-Hz spike wave discharges of absence status.

7. Simple partial status epilepticus
a. Somatomotor status. Seizures begin with myoclonic twitching of corner of the mouth, thumb and fingers on one hand or involve the toes and foot to one side and develop into a jacksonian march on one side of the body. The seizure may remain unilateral and consciousness is not impaired. There is waxing and waning of activity between partial seizures and occasional myoclonus, which is sometimes referred to as epilepsia partialis continua. The EEG often but not invariably shows periodic lateralized epileptiform discharges in the opposite hemi-sphere (PLEDS), which are often associated with an underlying destructive process in the brain. A variant of somatomotor status, which presents with intermittent aphasia or disturbance of language (aphasic status), has been described.

b. Somatosensory status epilepticus is rare but resembles somatomotor status with prolonged unilateral sensory symptoms or a sensory jacksonian march.

8. Complex partial status epilepticus may be regarded as a series of partial complex seizures of sufficient frequency to prevent recovery between episodes. There is waxing and waning of the level of consciousness, automatisms can occur, speech is impaired, and there is a state of prolonged confusion. The EEG may show focal activity in the temporal or frontal lobes on one side, but epileptic discharges are often generalized. The condition can be differentiated from absence status by EEG, but it may be difficult to separate partial complex status epilepticus and nonconvulsive status epilepticus in some cases.

Treatment of Status Epilepticus

Status epilepticus is one of the neurological conditions requiring history, physical examination, diagnostic procedures, and treatment in a continuum of activity as soon as the patient is seen by the emergency ambulance service or in the emergency center. Treatment should be continued in an intensive care unit.

General Measures

1. Establish the airway. If secretions are excessive, the patient will need intubation and oxygen therapy should be instituted.

2. Insert a nasogastric tube, aspirate stomach contents, and send gastric contents for analysis.

3. Insert a venous catheter and obtain blood for complete blood count, electrolytes, including sodium, potassium, calcium, magnesium, blood urea nitrogen, creatinine, glucose, anticonvulsant levels, a drug screen, and an alcohol level.

4. Obtain a blood specimen for arterial blood gases.

5. Have resuscitation equipment available.

6. Start an intravenous infusion of normal saline and give 100 mg thiamine by intravenous push and 50 mL of 50% glucose solution by intravenous push.

7. Examine the patient for signs of head trauma, cardiopulmonary compromise, CNS infection, focal neurological signs, and hyperthermia.

Begin Antiepileptic Drug Therapy

1. Fosphenytoin is currently the drug of choice for seizure control in tonic-clonic status epilepticus. It is water soluble and is converted quickly to phenytoin after administration.[133] Adverse effects include pruritus and headache and are usually transient.[134] The intravenous administration of lorazepam 0.1 mg/kg at 2 mg per minute for immediate seizure control is followed by fosphenytoin in a single loading dose of 20 mg/kg given at 150 mg per minute. The blood pressure, pulse, electrocardiogram, respiratory rate, and EEG should be monitored throughout. If the seizures are controlled, fosphenytoin can be continued intravenously or intramuscularly at 7 mg/kg q12h, with conversion to phenytoin by nasogastric tube or orally when the patient is conscious and able to swallow.

2. If the seizures continue after fosphenytoin infusion, the intravenous administration of lorazepam 0.1 mg/kg (4 to 8 mg) should be repeated at 2 mg per minute.

3. If the seizures persist, give additional intravenous fosphenytoin 7 mg/kg at 150 mg per minute.

4. If the seizures continue, induce pentobarbital coma. The patient should be in an intensive care unit, should be intubated, mechanically ventilated with continuous cardiovascular and respiratory monitoring, and continuous EEG recording.

Pentobarbital should be infused in a dose of 15 mg/kg at 100 mg per minute, followed by intravenous pentobarbital 1 to 2 mg/kg per hour until seizures are controlled or until the EEG achieves burst suppression pattern[135] with interburst intervals of 2 to 30 s.[136] The EEG record should show low-voltage activity during the suppression stage of burst suppression, since induction of a flat EEG recording during suppression is often followed by hypotension, which will compound neuronal damage due to cerebral hypoperfusion. The pentobarbital infusion is then titrated to maintain the burst suppression pattern as described above.

If breakthrough seizures occur, a bolus of 50 mg pentobarbital should be given at 25 mg per minute and the maintenance intravenous infusion increased to 3 mg/kg per hour.

The optimum duration of barbiturate anesthesia remains to be determined. Continuous therapy for as long as 13 days has been reported. One approach is to allow 24 h of seizure control, following which the infusion can be reduced q4 to 6h by 1 mg/kg per hour, if the pentobarbital level is about 50 μg/mL, or reduced by 0.5 mg/kg per hour if the level is below 50 μg/mL. If seizures recur during tapering, a bolus of 50 mg pentobarbital should be infused at the rate of 25 mg per minute and the maintenance infusion increased to the last effective preseizure dose.

Adverse effects of barbiturate anesthesia include hypotension, decreased myocardial contractility, hypothermia, and hypersensitivity reactions. Patients should be repositioned frequently to avoid decubitus ulcers.

Option 2

1. Infuse lorazepam 0.1 mg/kg at 2 mg per minute intravenously or diazepam 0.2 mg/kg at 2 mg per minute intravenously. This is followed with an intravenous infusion of phenytoin 15 to 20 mg/kg at 50 mg per minute. If diazepam has been used, the dose should be repeated 0.2 mg/kg intravenously after 15 min. Blood pressure, pulse, respirations, electrocardiogram, and EEG monitoring are necessary. Phenytoin has been associated with adverse cardiac effects, including dysrhythmias, conduction defects, and hypotension.[137] Soft tissue damage can occur if there is inadvertent venous extravasation of phenytoin.[138] Consequently, blood pressure, pulse, respirations, electrocardiogram, and EEG should always be monitored during phenytoin infusion.

2. If seizures continue after phenytoin infusion, repeat lorazepam or diazepam infusion.

3. If seizures persist, additional phenytoin at 5 mg/kg infused at the rate of 50 mg per minute intravenously should be given to a maximum dose of 13 mg/kg phenytoin.

4. If seizures continue, induce pentobarbital coma (see above).

Absence Status Epilepticus

1. Seizure activity usually responds to intravenous lorazepam 4 mg over 2 min. The dose can be repeated in 10 min if necessary, or intravenous diazepam 10 mg, given at 2 mg per minute and repeated after 10 min if necessary. This should be followed by intravenous or oral divalproex sodium or ethosuximide. Intravenous diazepam 5 mg per hour by drip can be continued until serum valproate levels exceed 50 μg/mL. Ethosuximide therapy requires 10 to 15 mg/kg per day in three divided doses.

Simple Partial Status Epilepticus

Simple partial status epilepticus with continuous motor activity is an indication of continuous electrical discharges arising in the pre-Rolandic motor strip and may be the result of a structural lesion or metabolic abnormality. There is a risk of secondary generalized seizure activity. Treatment consists of correction of any metabolic abnormality and administration of intravenous fosphenytoin or phenytoin (see pages 104–105) followed by oral phenytoin, carbamazepine, or divalproex sodium. Epilepsia partialis continua confined to hand, face, or foot is often refractory to treatment and may persist for a protracted period of time.

Simple partial seizures accompanied by myoclonus are usually associated with focal or generalized encephalopathy, with periodic lateralizing epileptiform discharges on EEG, and are often resistant to treatment. Treatment should be directed to prevention of spread of epileptic activity resulting in generalized seizures. This may entail the use of intravenous fosphenytoin or phenytoin if secondary generalized seizures occur, or use of intravenous phenobarbital 20 mg/kg with a maintenance dose of 90 mg q24h.

Nonconvulsive Status Epilepticus

Elderly patients who have a sudden onset of symptoms without evidence of an acute encephalopathy or structural lesion may show dramatic improvement with intravenous fosphenytoin or phenytoin followed by oral anticonvulsant therapy. Those with a severe generalized encephalopathy such as anoxic encephalopathy or a large cerebral infarction and periodic epileptic discharges in the EEG are highly resistant to anticonvulsant therapy, which may cause further deterioration in some cases that already carry a poor prognosis.

Complex Partial Status Epilepticus

This condition can be associated with progressive neuronal damage and loss in the hippocampus, amygdala, thalamus, intrarhinal, and piriform cortex. The main complication is impaired memory,[139] but serious permanent neurological deficits can occur and prolonged partial or localized seizures are capable of producing neuronal injury or death,[140] which can be prevented by aggressive treatment, as outlined under Clonic-Tonic-Clonic Status Epilepticus. This should be followed by appropriate long-term anticonvulsant therapy and surgery in selected cases.

REFERENCES

1. Sloviter RS: The functional organization of the hippocampal dentate gyrus and its relevance to the pathogenesis of temporal lobe epilepsy. *Ann Neurol* 35:640, 1994.
2. Pringle CE, Blume WT, Munoz DG, et al: Pathogenesis of mesial temporal sclerosis. *Can J Neurol Sci* 20:184, 1993.
3. Choy-Kwong M, Lipton RB: Seizures in hospitalized cocaine users. *Neurology* 39:425, 1989.
4. Hauser WA: Seizure disorders. The changes with age. *Epilepsia* 33 (Suppl 4):S6, 1992.
5. Smith MC, Buelow JM; Epilepsy (review). *Disease A Month* 42:72, 1996.
6. McLachlan RS: The significance of head and eye turning in seizures. *Neurology* 37:1617, 1987.
7. So NK: Atonic phenomena and partial seizures. A reappraisal (review). *Adv Neurol* 67:29, 1995.

8. Guerrini R, Dravet C, Genton P, et al: Epileptic negative myoclonus. *Neurology* 43:1078, 1993.

9. Gambardella A, Reutens DC, Andermann F, et al: Late onset drop attacks in temporal lobe epilepsy: a reevaluation of the concept of temporal lobe syncope. *Neurology* 44:1074, 1994.

10. Grunewald RA, Panayiotopoulos CP: The diagnosis of epilepsies. *J R Coll Physicians London* 30:122, 1996.

11. Kotagal P, Rothner AD: Localization-related epilepsies: simple partial seizures, complex partial seizures, benign focal epilepsy of childhood and epilepsia partialis continua, in Dodson WE, Pellock JM (eds): *Pediatric Epilepsy: Diagnosis and Therapy*. New York, Demos, 1993, p. 183.

12. Luciano D: Partial seizures of frontal and temporal origin. *Neurol Clin* 11:805, 1993.

13. Paradiso S, Hermann BP, Robinson RG: The heterogeneity of temporal lobe epilepsy. Neurology, neuropsychology, and psychiatry. *J Nerv Ment Dis* 183:538, 1995.

14. Devinsky O, Feldmann E, Burrowes K, et al. Autoscopic phenomena with seizures. *Arch Neurol* 46:1080, 1989.

15. Kotagal P, Luders H, Morris HH, et al: Dystonic posturing in complex partial seizures of temporal lobe onset: a new lateralizing sign. *Neurology* 39:196, 1989.

16. Gastaut H, Zifkin BG: The risk of automobile accidents with seizures occurring while driving: relation to seizure type. *Neurology* 37:1613, 1987.

17. Reutens DC, Andermann F, Olivier A, et al: Unusual features of supplementary sensorimotor area epilepsy: cyclic pattern, unusual sensory aura, startle sensitivity, anoxic encephalopathy and spontaneous remission. *Adv Neurol* 70:293, 1996.

18. Bleasel AF, Morris HH, 3rd: Supplementary sensorimotor area epilepsy in adults. *Adv Neurol* 70:271, 1996.

19. King DW, Smith JR: Supplementary sensorimotor area epilepsy in adults. *Adv Neurol* 70:285, 1996.

20. Chee M, So NK, Dinnerd S: Speech and the dominant superior frontal gyrus. correlation of ictal symptoms, EEG and results of surgical resection. *J Clin Neurophysiol* 14:226, 1997.

21. Williamson PD, Spencer DD, Spencer SS, et al: Complex partial seizures of frontal lobe origin. *Ann Neurol* 18:497, 1985.

22. Manford M, Fish DR, Shorvon SD: An analysis of clinical seizure patterns and their localizing value in frontal and temporal lobe epilepsies. *Brain* 119 (Pt 1):17, 1996.

23. Salanova V, Andermann F, Rasmussen T, et al: Parietal lobe epilepsy. Clinical manifestations and outcome in 82 patients treated surgically between 1929 and 1988. *Brain* 118 (Pt 3):607, 1995.

24. Williamson PD, Thadani VM, Darcey TM, et al: Occipital lobe epilepsy: clinical characteristics, seizure spread patterns, and results of surgery. *Ann Neurol* 31:3, 1992.

25. Porter RJ: The absence epilepsies (review). *Epilepsia* 34 (Suppl 3):S42, 1993.

26. Snead OC, 3rd: Basic mechanisms of generalized absence seizures. *Ann Neurol* 37:146, 1995.

27. Wirrell EC, Camfield CS, Camfield PR, et al: Long-term prognosis of typical childhood absence epilepsy: remission or progression to juvenile myoclonic epilepsy. *Neurology* 47:912, 1996.

28. Bouma PA, Westendorp RG, van Dijk JG, et al: The outcome of absence epilepsy: a meta-analysis. *Neurology* 47:802, 1996.

29. Wirrell EC, Camfield CS, Camfield PR, et al: Long-term psychosocial outcome in typical absence epilepsy: Sometimes a wolf in sheeps clothing. *Arch Pediatr Adol Med* 151:152, 1997.

30. Wirrell EC, Camfield PR, Camfield CS, et al: Accidental injury is a serious risk in children with typical absence epilepsy. *Arch Neurol* 53:929, 1996.

31. Lehesjoki AE, Eldridge R, Eldridge J, et al: Progressive myoclonus epilepsy of Unverricht-Lundborg type: a clinical and molecular genetic study of a family from the United States with four affected sibs. *Neurology* 43:2384, 1993.

32. Tassinari CA, Michelucci R, Genton P, et al: Dyssynergia cerebellaris myoclonica (Ramsay-Hunt syndrome): a condition unrelated to mitochondrial encephalomyopathies. *J Neurol Neurosurg Psychiatry* 52:262, 1989.

33. Labauge P, Beck C, Bellet H, et al: Lafora disease is not linked to the Unverricht-Lundborg locus. *Am J Med Genet* 60:80, 1995.

34. Drury I, Blaivas M, Abou-Khalil BW, et al: Biopsy results in a kindred with Lafora disease. *Arch Neurol* 50:102, 1993.

35. Kaufman MA, Dwork AJ, Willson NJ, et al: Late-onset Lafora's disease with typical intraneuronal inclusions. *Neurology* 43:1246, 1993.

36. Ponsford S, Pye IF, Elliot EJ: Posterior paroxysmal discharge, an aid to early diagnosis in Lafora disease. *J R Soc Med* 86:597, 1993.

37. Duchowny M, Harvey AS: Pediatric epilepsy syn-

dromes: an update and critical review. *Epilepsia* 37 (Suppl 1):S26, 1996.

38. Pellock JM: Utilization of new antiepileptic drugs in children. *Epilepsia* 37 (Suppl 1):S66, 1996.

39. Baram TZ: Pathophysiology of massive infantile spasms: perspective on the putative role of the brain adrenal axis. *Ann Neurol* 33:231, 1993.

40. Andermann F, Tenembaum S: Negative motor phenomena in generalized epilepsies: A study of atonic seizures. *Adv Neurol* 67:9, 1995.

41. Haines ST, Casto DT: Treatment of infantile spasms. *Ann Pharmacother* 28:779, 1994.

42. Prasad AN, Stafstrom CF, Holmes GL: Alternative epilepsy therapies: the ketogenic diet, immunoglobulins and steroids. *Epilepsia* 37 (Suppl):S81, 1996.

43. Commission on Classification and Terminology of the International League Against Epilepsy. Proposal for revised clinical and electroencephalographic classification of epileptic seizures. *Epilepsia* 22:489, 1981.

44. Lee MS, Marsden CD: Drop attacks. *Adv Neurol* 67:41, 1995.

45. Liedholm LJ, Gudjonsson O: Cardiac arrest due to partial epileptic seizures. *Neurology* 42:824, 1992.

46. Blume WT: Physiology of atonic seizures. *Adv Neurol* 67:173, 1995.

47. Bourgeois B: Clinical use of drugs useful in the treatment of atonic seizures. *Adv Neurol* 67:361, 1995.

48. Shuster EA: Epilepsy in women. *Mayo Clin Proc* 71:991, 1996.

49. Waters CH, Belai Y, Gott PS, et al: Outcomes of pregnancy associated with antiepileptic drugs. *Arch Neurol* 51:250, 1994.

50. Lindhout D, Omtzigt JGC: Pregnancy and the risk of teratogenicity. *Epilepsia* 33 (Suppl 4):S41, 1992.

51. Kaneko S, Battino D, Andermann E: Multicenter collaborative study groups. Congenital malformations in offspring of mothers with epilepsy (abstract). *Epilepsia* 36 (Suppl 3):S11, 1995.

52. Rosa FW: Spina bifida in infants of women treated with carbamazepine during pregnancy. *N Engl J Med* 324:674, 1991.

53. The U.S. Gabapentin Study Group. No. 5. Gabapentin as add-on therapy in refractory partial epilepsy: a double-blind, placebo-controlled, parallel-group study. *Neurology* 43:2292, 1993.

54. Lopez-Cendes I, Andermann E, Cendes F, et al: Risk factors for changes in seizure frequency during pregnancy of epileptic women: a cohort study (abstract). *Epilepsia* 33 (Suppl 3):57, 1992.

55. Yerby MS, Friel PN, McCormick K: Antiepileptic drug disposition during pregnancy. *Neurology* 42 (Suppl 5):12, 1992.

56. Dansky LV, Rosenblatt DS, Andermann E: Mechanisms of teratogenesis: folic acid and antiepileptic therapy. *Neurology* 42 (Suppl 5):32, 1992.

57. Panayiotopoulos CP: Benign childhood partial epilepsies: benign childhood seizure susceptibility syndromes (editorial). *J Neurol Neurosurg Psychiatry* 56:2, 1993.

58. Farwell JR, Lee YJ, Hirtz DG, et al: Phenobarbital for febrile seizures—effects on intelligence and on seizure recurrence. *N Engl J Med* 322:364, 1990.

59. McKinlay I, Newton R: Intention to treat febrile convulsions with rectal diazepam, valproate, or phenobarbitone. *Dev Med Child Neurol* 31:617, 1989.

60. Ferrie CD, De Marco P, Grunewald RA, et al: Video game induced seizures. *J Neurol Neurosurg Psychiatry* 57:925, 1994.

61. Ritaccio AL: Reflex seizures. *Neurol Clin* 12:57, 1994.

62. Hauser WA: Seizure disorders: the changes with age. *Epilepsia* 33 (Suppl 4):56, 1992.

63. Willmore LJ: Management of epilepsy in the elderly (review). *Epilepsia* 37 (Suppl 6):S23, 1996.

64. Goa KL, Sorkin EM: Gabapentin: A review of its pharmacological properties and clinical potential in epilepsy. *Drugs* 46:409, 1993.

65. Goa KL, Ross SR, Chrisp P: Lamotrigine: A review of its pharmacological properties and clinical efficacy in epilepsy. *Drugs* 46:152, 1993.

66. Cloyd JC, Lackner TE, Leppik IE: Antiepileptics in the elderly. Pharmacoepidemiology and pharmacokinetics. *Arch Fam Med* 3:589, 1994.

67. Thomas RJ: Seizures and epilepsy in the elderly. *Arch Intern Med* 157:605, 1997.

68. Camfield PR, Camfield CS: Antiepileptic drug therapy: when is epilepsy truly intractable? *Epilepsia* 37 (Suppl 1):S60, 1996.

69. Kuyk J, Van Dyck R, Spinhoven P: The case for a dissociative interpretation of pseudoepileptic seizures. *J Nerv Ment Dis* 184:468, 1996.

70. Bowman ES: Etiology and clinical course of pseudoseizures. Relationship to trauma, depression, and dissociation. *Psychosomatics* 34:333, 1993.

71. Nash JL: Pseudoseizures: an update. *Comp Therapy* 21:486, 1995.

72. Devinsky D, Sanchez-Villasenor F, Vazquez B, et al: Clinical profile of patients with epileptic and nonepileptic seizures. *Neurology* 46:1530, 1996.

73. Krahn LE, Rummans TA, Sharbrough FW, et al:

Pseudoseizures after epilepsy surgery. *Psychosomatics* 36:487, 1995.

74. Iancu I, Kotler M, Lauffer N, et al: Seizures and the Dandy-Walker syndrome: a case of suspected pseudoseizures. *Psychother Psychosom* 65:109, 1996.

75. Ramchandani D, Schindler B: Evaluation of pseudoseizures. A psychiatric perspective. *Psychosomatics* 34:70, 1993.

76. Spencer SS: The relative contributions of MRI, SPECT, and PET imaging in epilepsy. *Epilepsia* 35 (Suppl 6):S72, 1994.

77. Ramsay RE, De Toledo J: Intravenous administration of fosphenytoin: options for the management of seizures. *Neurology* 46 (Suppl 1):S17, 1996.

78. Bebin M, Bleck TP: New anticonvulsant drugs. Focus on flunarizine, fosphenytoin, midazolam and stiripentol. *Drugs* 48:153, 1994.

79. Jamerson BD, Dukes GE, Brouwer KL, et al: Venous irritation related to intravenous administration of phenytoin versus fosphenytoin. *Pharmacotherapy* 14:47, 1994.

80. Eldon MA, Loewen GR, Voigtman RE, et al: Safety, tolerance, and pharmacokinetics of intravenous fosphenytoin. *Clin Pharmaco Ther* 53:212, 1993.

81. Thomas RJ: Seizures and epilepsy in the elderly. *Arch Intern Med* 157:605, 1997.

82. Schwabe S: Oxcarbamazepine: clinical development program. *Epilepsia* 35 (Suppl 5):S51, 1994.

83. Marks WA, Morris MP, Badensteiner JB, et al: Gastritis with valproate therapy. *Arch Neurol* 45:903, 1988.

84. Leppik IE, Wolff DL: Antiepileptic medication interactions. *Neurol Clin* 11:905, 1993.

85. Richens A, Davidson DL, Cartlidge NE, et al: A multicenter comparative trial of sodium valproate and carbamazepine in adult epilepsy. Adult EPITEG Collaborative Study *J Neurol Neurosurg Psychiatry* 57:682, 1994.

86. Beydoun A, Sackellares JC, Shu V: Safety and efficacy of divalproex sodium monotherapy in partial epilepsy: a double-blind concentration-response design clinical trial. *Neurology* 48:182, 1997.

87. Ritter FJ, Leppik IE, Dreifuss FE, et al: Efficacy of felbamate in childhood epileptic encephalopathy (Lennox-Gastaut syndrome). The felbamate study group in Lennox-Gastaut syndrome. *N Engl J Med* 328:29, 1993.

88. O'Neil MG, Perdun CS, Wilson MB, et al: Felbamate-associated fatal acute hepatic necrosis. *Neurology* 46:1457, 1996.

89. Pranzatelli MR, Nadi NS: Mechanism of action of antiepileptic and antimyoclonic drugs. *Adv Neurol* 67:329, 1995.

90. Dichter MA: Integrated use of old and new antiepileptic drugs. *Curr Opin Neurol* 8:95, 1995.

91. McLean MJ: Gabapentin. *Epilepsia* 36 (Suppl 2):S73, 1995.

92. Bergey GK, Morris HH, Rosenfeld W, et al: Gabapentin monotherapy: 1. An 8-day, double-blind, dose-controlled, multicenter study in hospitalized patients with refractory complex partial or secondarily generalized seizures. The US gabapentin study group 88/89. *Neurology* 49:739, 1997.

93. Cheung H, Kamp D, Harris E: An in vitro investigation of the action of lamotrigine on neuronal voltage-activated sodium channels. *Epilepsy Res* 13:107, 1992.

94. Matsuo F, Bergen D, Faught E, et al: Placebo-controlled study of the efficacy and safety of lamotrigine in patients with partial seizures. US lamotrigine protocol 0.5 clinical trial group. *Neurology* 43:2284, 1993.

95. Brodie MJ: Lamotrigine. *Lancet* 339:1397, 1992.

96. Gilman JT: Lamotrigine: an antiepileptic agent for the treatment of partial seizures. *Ann Pharmacother* 29:144, 1995.

97. Pellock JM: Efficacy and adverse effects of antiepileptic drugs. *Pediatr Clin North Am* 36:435, 1989.

98. Guberman A: Vigabatrin. *Can J Neurol Sci* 23:S13, 1996.

99. French JA, Mosier M, Walker S, et al: Vigabatrin Protocol 024 Investigative Cohort. A double-blind placebo-controlled study of vigabatrin three g/day in patients with uncontrolled complex partial seizures. *Neurology* 46:54, 1996.

100. Fisher R, Kalviainen R, Tanganelli P, et al: Newer antiepileptic drugs as monotherapy: data on vigabatrin. *Neurology* 47 (Suppl 1):S2, 1996.

101. Monaco F: Cognitive effects of vigabatrin: a review. *Neurology* 47 (Suppl 1):S6, 1996.

102. Ferrie CD, Robinson RO, Panayiotopoulos CP: Psychotic and severe behavioural reactions with vigabatrin: a review. *Acta Neurol Scand* 93:1, 1996.

103. Backstrom JT, Hinkle RL, Flicker MR: Severe persistent visual field constriction associated with vigabatrin. Manufacturers have started several studies. *BMJ* 314:1694, 1997.

104. Bourgeois BF: Drug interaction profile of topiramate. *Epilepsia* 37 (Suppl 2):S14, 1996.

105. Meldrum BS: Update on the mechanism of action of antiepileptic drugs. *Epilepsia* 37 (Suppl 6):S4, 1996.

106. Gustavson LE, Cato A, Guenther HJ, et al: Lack of clinically important drug interactions between tiagabine and carbamazepine, phenytoin or valproate. *Epilepsia* 35 (Suppl 3):S159, 1995.

107. Kalviainen R, Aikia M, Mervaala E, et al: Long-term cognitive effects of tiagabine. *Epilepsia* 36 (Suppl 3):S149, 1995.

108. Reiss WG, Oles KS: Acetazolamide in the treatment of seizures. *Ann Pharmacother* 30:514, 1996.

109. Practice parameter: a guideline for discontinuing antiepileptic drugs in seizure-free patients—summary statement. Report of the Quality Standards Subcommittee of the American Academy of Neurology. *Neurology* 47:600, 1996.

110. Engel J Jr: Surgery for seizures. *N Engl J Med* 334:647, 1996.

111. Newton MR, Berkovic SF, Austin MC, et al: SPECT in the localisation of extratemporal and temporal seizure foci. *J Neurol Neurosurg Psychiatry* 59:26, 1995.

112. Chugani HT, Shewmon DA, Shields WD, et al: Surgery for intractable infantile spasms: neuroimaging perspectives. *Epilepsia* 34:764, 1993.

113. Ebersole JS, Squires KC, Eliashiv SD, et al: Application of magnetic source imaging in evaluation of candidates for epilepsy surgery. *Neuroimaging Clin N Am* 5:267, 1995.

114. Blume WT: Temporal lobe epilepsy surgery in childhood: rationale for greater use. *Can J Neurol Sci* 24:95, 1997.

115. Duchowny M, Levin B, Jayakar P, et al: Temporal lobectomy in early childhood. *Epilepsia* 33:298, 1992.

116. Wieser H, Hajek M: Frontal lobe epilepsy. Compartmentalization, presurgical evaluation and operative results. *Adv Neurol* 66:297, 1995.

117. Roper SN, Levesque MF, Sutherling WW, et al: Surgical treatment of partial epilepsy arising from the insular cortex: Report of two cases. *J Neurosurg* 79:266, 1993.

118. Spencer SS, Spencer DD, Williamson PD, et al: Combined depth and subdural electrode investigation in uncontrolled epilepsy. *Neurology* 40:74, 1990.

119. Liajek M, Wieser HG: Extratemporal, mainly frontal epilepsies: surgical results. *J Epilepsy* 1:103, 1988.

120. Carson BS, Javedan SP, Freeman JM, et al: Hemispherectomy: a hemidecortication approach and review of 52 cases. *J Neurosurg* 84:903, 1996.

121. Spencer SS, Spencer DD, Saas K, et al: Anterior total and two-stage corpus callosum section: differential and incremental. *Epilepsia* 34:561, 1993.

122. Krahn LE, Rummans TA, Peterson GC: Psychiatric implications of surgical treatment of epilepsy. *Mayo Clin Proc* 71:1201, 1996.

123. Spencer SS: Long-term outcome after epilepsy surgery. *Epilepsia* 37:807, 1996.

124. Trenerry MR: Neuropsychologic assessment in surgical treatment of epilepsy. *Mayo Clin Proc* 71:1196, 1996.

125. Commission on Classification and Terminology of the International League Against Epilepsy. Proposal for revised clinical and electroencephalographic classification of epileptic seizures. *Epilepsia* 22:489, 1981.

126. Watson C: Status epilepticus. Clinical features, pathophysiology and treatment. *West J Med* 155:626, 1991.

127. Treatment of convulsive status epilepticus. Recommendations of the Epilepsy Foundation of America's Working group on status epilepticus. *JAMA* 270:854, 1993.

128. Leppik IE: Status epilepticus. *Neurol Clin* 4:633, 1986.

129. Hauser WA: Status epilepticus: epidemiologic considerations. *Neurology* 40 (Suppl 2):9, 1990.

130. Leppik IE: Status epilepticus: the next decade. *Neurology* 40 (Suppl 2):4, 1990.

131. Lothman E: The biochemical basis and pathophysiology of status epilepticus. *Neurology* 40 (Suppl 2):13, 1990.

132. Fagan KJ, Lee SI: Prolonged confusion following convulsions due to generalized nonconvulsive status epilepticus. *Neurology* 40:1689, 1990.

133. Baron B, Hankin S, Knapp L: Advantages of intravenous fosphenytoin (Cerebyx) compared with IV phenytoin (Dilantin) (absts). *Neurology* 45 (Suppl 4):A202, 1995.

134. Sloan EP: Emergency department seizure treatment with fosphenytoin. *Emerg Med* April Suppl 17, 1996.

135. Van Ness PC: Pentobarbital and EEG burst suppression in treatment of status epilepticus refractory to benzodiazepines and phenytoin. *Epilepsia* 31:61, 1990.

136. Shorvon S: Tonic clonic status epilepticus. *J Neurol Neurosurg Psychiatry* 56:125, 1993.

137. Donovan PJ, Cline D: Phenytoin administration by constant intravenous infusion: selective rates of administration. *Ann Emerg Med* 20:139, 1991.

138. Weinstein M: Severe soft tissue injury following intravenous infusion of phenytoin. *Arch Intern Med* 149:1905, 1989.

139. Treiman DM, Delgado-Escueta AV, Clark MA: Impairment of memory following prolonged complex partial status epilepticus. *Neurology* 31:109, 1981.

140. Krumholz A, Sung GY, Fisher RS, et al: Complex partial status epilepticus accompanied by serious morbidity and mortality. *Neurology* 45:1499, 1995.

Chapter 5

HEADACHE

A headache is a pain or discomfort that occurs over the superior aspect of the head and occasionally spreads to the face, teeth, jaws, and neck. Pain-sensitive structures in the cranial cavity include the venous sinuses and their cortical tributaries, the large arteries of the base of the brain, the dural lining of the floor of the anterior and posterior fossae, the 5th, 9th, and 10th cranial nerves, and the first three cervical nerves. These structures contain pain-sensitive nerve endings that may be stimulated by traction, inflammation, pressure, neoplastic infiltration, and biochemical substances that are liberated in certain types of headaches. Stimulation of pain-sensitive structures above the tentorium cerebelli tends to produce headaches in the frontotemporal or parietal area. Stimulation of pain-sensitive structures in the posterior fossa produces pain in the occipital and suboccipital areas. All of the tissues of the scalp, face, and neck are sensitive to painful stimulation. Headaches can occur in diseases of the eye and orbital contents, the nasal cavity and paranasal sinuses, the teeth, and external and middle ears.

In summary, headache may be caused by:

1. Traction or thrombosis of or displacement of venous sinuses or their cortical tributaries
2. Traction, dilatation, or inflammation involving the dura of the anterior and posterior fossae or the intracranial or extracranial arteries
3. Traction, displacement, or disease of the 5th, 9th, and 10th cranial nerves and the first three cervical nerves
4. Changes in intracranial pressure
5. Diseases of the tissues of the scalp, face, eye, nose, ear, and neck

MIGRAINE

Definition Migraine is a condition of paroxysmal or occasionally constant headaches that are the product of a primary brain dysfunction resulting in a neurovascular reaction in genetically predisposed individuals.[1]

Epidemiology Migraine affects about 18 percent of women and 6 percent of men across their life span.[2] Prevalence peaks between the ages of 25 and 55—the most productive years—and is an important cause of lost work time.[3] Probably 11 percent of persons in the United States suffer from migraine[4]—a total of at least 28 million people. Migraine is more prevalent in boys than girls before the age of 12 years[5] but becomes increasingly common in women after puberty, and migraine is more prevalent in the age group 25 to 44 years. However, onset of migraine after age 40 years is recognized.[6] There is a significant difference in prevalence among races, with migraine in females occurring in 20.4 percent of Caucasians compared to 16.2 percent in African-Americans and 4.8 percent in Asians.[7] The widespread belief that migraine is associated with a high socioeconomic status is erroneous because migraine is more common in persons from low family income sources.[8] Women have a decreasing prevalence of migraine with increasing levels of education, but a positive family history of Raynaud disease and coffee consumption of more than six cups per day are associated with increased likelihood of migraine.[9] Loss of productivity in the United States has been estimated to be $1.4 billion a year by those of the work force who suffer from migraine.

Etiology and Pathology Research into the causes and mechanisms of migraine is in an active phase, and a number of attractive hypotheses have been proposed in recent years. An attempt to reconcile apparently divergent views leads to the following conclusions.

1. Every migraineur has a migraine threshold that can be exceeded and migraine can be triggered by a number of factors acting on the brain. These

factors include ingestion of certain foods—eggs, alcohol, caffeine,[10] chocolate, red wine,[11] shellfish, for example—and both emotional and physical stress[12] or relaxation. Stress is significant if the individual has experienced a particularly stressful day 1 to 3 days before or on the day of onset of the migraine.[13] Alterations in the level of circulating hormones during the menstrual cycle,[14] exposure to certain medications such as nitroglycerin, reserpine, and contraceptives, minor head trauma,[15] exposure to bright lights, excessive noise or odors, or changes in meteorologic pressure can initiate an attack of migraine.

2.   These factors and other unidentified factors that may act through the cerebral cortex, thalamus, or hypothalamus produce a series of changes in brain function. In some cases premonitory symptoms occur hours or days before the onset of headache.[16] Photophobia, phonophobia, and osmophobia are most common,[17] and migraineurs are significantly more photophobic and phonophobic between attacks.[18] Changes in mood, usually depression or anger, or occasionally a feeling of well-being, are not unusual. Other changes consist of fatigue, excessive yawning, and feeling chilled, with muscle and neck stiffness. There may be fluid retention or increased urinary frequency and other contrasting symptoms such as increased appetite or anorexia and constipation or diarrhea. In general, migraine patients experience poorer subjective well-being/quality of life even between attacks.[19] Premonitory symptoms suggest early hypothalamic involvement, although abnormal response to stress, menstruation, flickering lights, loud noise, or strong odors suggest that other areas of the brain may be involved primarily.

3.   In migraine with aura, a process of excitation and inhibition of cortical neurones is triggered in the brain, spreading through the cortex as a wave of neuronal activity followed by inhibition at a rate of 2 to 3 mm per minute. The spreading depression first described by Leao in animal models in 1944[20] corresponds to the rate of propagation of the migraine aura calculated by Lashley in 1941,[21] who made drawings of his own developing visual aura preceding a migraine attack. Spreading depression may be related to low extracellular magnesium since the magnesium ion gates the N-methyl-D-aspartate receptor. A low extracellular magnesium level might increase receptor sensitivity to glutamate and result in the intracellular changes of spreading depression. Alternatively, the condition may be a transient inhibition of neuronal activity in the brain accompanied by a flux of sodium, calcium, and chloride ions into the neuron. Whatever mechanism, the result is a brief burst of electrical activity followed by electrical silence, which progresses as an expanding concentric wave propagated through the brain at the same rate as a developing migraine aura.

4.   In migraine with or without aura, projections from the brain probably through the hypothalamus stimulate neurons in the locus ceruleus and dorsal raphe nuclei in the brainstem.

5.   The locus ceruleus connections to the thoracic sympathetic outflow release norepinephrine from the adrenal medulla and other sites. Increased levels of norepinephrine then trigger the release of 5-hydroxytryptamine (5-HT) from platelets, which is metabolized rapidly, leading to a phase of 5-HT depletion.

6.   Lower 5-HT levels depress the function of the serotonergic endogenous pain control system arising from the dorsal raphe nuclei and remove an inhibitory effect on transmission of pain impulses through the spinal tract of the trigeminal nerve.

7.   Projections from the locus ceruleus and dorsal raphe nuclei to the trigeminal nerve produce antidromic stimulation of sensory fibers projecting to bipolar neurons in the trigeminal ganglion. These neurons contain substance P and calcitonin gene-related peptide (CGRP), which is released when the neuron is stimulated.[22] These neurons innervate large cerebral arteries and the dura through the ophthalmic division of the trigeminal nerve. The release of vasoactive neuropeptides including substance P and CGRP results in neurogenic inflammation, vasodilatation, and vascular permeability. The local tissue responds by the release of potassium, histamine, and serotonin from local cells and by the synthesis of prostaglandin, leukotrienes, and bradykinin. These changes initiate depolarization of pain receptors and long-lasting enhancement of receptor activity.

8.   The majority of C fibers in the trigeminal nerve, which are depolarized by stimulation of pain

receptors, are concentrated in the pia and dura. In migraine, increased input through the depolarized C fibers is projected through the ophthalmic division of the trigeminal nerve, with a second projection in the spinal tract extending caudally to the C2–3 level. The intense input then recruits sensory neurons from the C2–3 sensory pool, resulting in a posterior spread of head pain to the occipital area. The input then crosses the midline from the spinal tract of the trigeminal nerve and the C2–3 neuron projections, ascending in the quintothalamic tract to the posteroventral medial nucleus and intralamina nuclei of the thalamus, and thence to the cerebral cortex.

9. The intense depolarization of C fibers in the trigeminal nerve probably leads to further antidromic stimulation of fibers in that nerve, establishing a trigeminal vascular reflex through the trigeminal nerve, which is uninhibited and perpetuates the migraine headache.

10. Projections from the locus ceruleus and trigeminal nuclei in the brainstem may synapse in the superior salivary nucleus of the seventh cranial nerve. Efferent fibers from the superior salivary nucleus pass through the greater superficial petrosal nerve to the sphenopalatine ganglion, which projects to the carotid plexus, producing vasodilatation in the internal and external carotid artery territories. This results in further stimulation of pain receptors already affected by neurogenic inflammation. Thus, a second trigeminal vascular reflex would be established.

11. The system remains uninhibited because of the lack of activity of 5-HT receptors on the pial and dural blood vessels. These receptors are nonfunctional because of lowered circulating 5-HT and fail to block noxious neurotransmission from pain receptors on affected blood vessels, which project through C fibers contained in the trigeminal nerve.

Clinical Features A careful and detailed history with a temporal description of all events is the most important factor in the diagnosis of migraine. This requires the investment of time and patience by the physician, who must guide the patient through a series of developments that culminate in a complete description of an unmistakable event—the migraine headache.[23] This approach is essential because migraine is much more than a headache and the history often unfolds as a series of incidents occurring over several hours, but the end product is obvious. Furthermore, the general physical and neurological examinations are likely to be normal, thus adding nothing to the interview. Similarly, there are no useful diagnostic procedures in migraine. The diagnosis depends on the history obtained by an examiner who listens to the patient.

However, the diagnosis, though the first objective, is a preliminary step in developing a treatment plan. The patient should be given an explanation of the nature of migraine in lay terms, coupled with reassurance that the condition is essentially benign. Trigger factors should be identified and a treatment regimen proposed for control of the acute attack and long-term prevention. Patient cooperation in treatment is essential, and regular follow-up appointments with the physician should be scheduled. Finally, the physician should be available to answer questions and give further advice, usually by telephone, when the patient needs reassurance and change in therapy in what is often a crisis situation to the patient.

The following are the more common types of migraine headaches.

Migraine with Aura The headache is usually preceded by visual symptoms known as an aura. The attack begins with an aura in which the patient may experience scintillating scotomata, sparks or flashes of light, or scotomata with irregular projections in reverse angle resembling the ground defenses of a medieval fortified city—sometimes termed fortification spectra. Occasionally, large paracentral or central field defects, homonymous hemianopia, or cortical blindness can occur.[24] Photophobia is not uncommon, but distortion of shape or size of objects or alteration of body perception are unusual experiences.[25] Prodromal olfactory hallucinations are less frequent. Unilateral paresthesias are a common phenomenon readily forgotten by the patient unless questioned about this symptom. Others experience impaired sensation or unpleasant hypersensitivity to touch or contact with clothing. Hemiparesis can occur before the headache but is more likely to develop during the headache. Similarly, dysphasia may develop early or later in the course of the migraine attack. Diplopia, tinnitus, hearing impairment,[26] vertigo, and ataxia indicate early brainstem involvement. Dysarthria, drowsiness, and impaired level of consciousness are rare early manifestations of migraine aura.

Five to 20 min after the aura begins, the patient develops a headache. The headache is unilateral or bilateral and usually frontal or frontotemporal, but it may occur in any part of the cranial cavity. In about 40 percent of cases the headache is bilateral. The pain may be pulsating or a constant ache that increases in severity and is often but not invariably intense. The patient may feel that the entire head is involved, and the pain can spread down into the neck and face. There is photophobia, visual blurring, phonophobia, and, in some cases, osmophobia. Marked gastrointestinal upset with anorexia, nausea, and diarrhea is common, and though most migraineurs experience vomiting[27] over the many years of suffering headaches, vomiting is only an occasional event in most cases. There is a feeling of fatigue with depression and irritability or anger if the patient is disturbed, and the victim prefers to lie quietly in a darkened room. The condition gradually subsides over a period of hours but occasionally lasts all day and is terminated by sleep. Many patients recognize that sleep will relieve the headache and try to go to sleep in quiet and darkened surroundings as soon as possible. In a few cases, however, the headache may persist for 2 or 3 days or more and occasionally for more than a week—a condition that has been called migraine status. This is associated with considerable prostration, and the inability to eat or drink coupled with vomiting can result in dehydration. When the headache resolves, the patient is left with a feeling of fatigue, heaviness, and aching in the head. The scalp may be tender, and there may be listlessness and poor concentration for several days. The termination of an attack is often accompanied by diuresis.

Migraine without Aura   Migraine without aura begins with a headache. This has all the characteristics of migraine headache in development, form, and subsequent spread. All the symptoms described above in migraine with aura can be present, and migraine without aura is analogous to migraine with aura except for the initial presentation.

Hemiplegic Migraine   Familial hemiplegic migraine is an autosomal dominant condition that is genetically heterogenous, with 50 percent of families linked to chromosome 19p.[28] Twenty percent of family members with familial hemiplegic migraine also have progressive cerebellar ataxia, and all of the patients in this group with ataxia are linked to chromosome 19p.[29] A mutation in the gene results in dysfunction in calcium-mediated channels in the neurons. These channels mediate 5-HT release, and impairment may predispose individuals to migraine attack.[30]

Another locus for familiar hemiplegic migraine has been identified and mapped to chromosome 1q31.[31]

Nonfamilial Hemiplegic Migraine   In this condition the affected individuals have occasional attacks of migraine with or without aura and without hemiplegic symptoms. However, hemiparesis can occur in some attacks and is of longer duration than in the familial forms of hemiplegic migraine. Cerebral infarction can occur. There is also considerable risk of repeated cerebral infarction.

Basilar Migraine   Patients with basilar migraines have a history of motion sensitivity and motion sickness in 33 percent of cases and episodic vertigo in 25 percent. They are phonophobic and complain of fluctuations in their hearing.[32] The headache is usually bilateral and occipital and may be preceded or accompanied by visual field defect, diplopia, vertigo, ataxia, tinnitus, impaired hearing, dysarthria, bilateral paresis or hemiparesis, and bilateral paresthesias. Consciousness may be impaired. The patient appears to be confused, restless, and sometimes incoherent or dysphasic. This stage is occasionally followed by a period of stupor. Symptoms of neurological deficit may persist for several hours following the onset of headache. The electroencephalogram (EEG) may be normal or show paroxysmal activity including spike wave complexes, increased beta activity, or frontal intermittent rhythmic delta activity. In the absence of clinical seizures, these patients respond to antimigraine therapy. Seizure activity requires the addition of an anticonvulsant.

Basilar migraine has been described following hyperextension–flexion (whiplash) injury to the neck. The condition will respond to antimigraine therapy and physical therapy.

Ophthalmoplegic Migraine Ophthalmoplegic mi-graine is a form of migraine in which the patient develops ipsilateral ophthalmoplegia at the height of the migraine attack. Ophthalmoplegia is believed to be the result of compression of the third nerve and occasionally compression of the fourth and sixth nerves and the ophthalmic division of the fifth nerve in the lateral wall of the cavernous sinus by a dilated internal carotid artery. Patients with ophthalmoplegic migraine typically give a history of migraine with or without aura and without oculomotor involvement many years before the development of an ophthalmoplegic migraine attack. The ophthalmoplegia and headache are usually unilateral and occur on the same side. It is rare for the patient to experience attacks that move from one side to the other. It is a feature of ophthalmoplegic migraine that the headache always precedes the oculomotor deficit by several hours or even days in protracted cases. Paresis always outlasts the pain, and there have been occasional reports of permanent oculomotor deficits.

Migrainous Psychosis Personality changes are not unusual in migraine, but severe emotional cognitive and intellectual change can occur in rare cases. The patient may appear to be confused and may exhibit abnormal behavior, anxiety, fear, anger, or hallucinations. There may be loss of contact with surroundings and an occasional lapse into coma. The condition can be familial. When conditions occur without headache (see Acephalgic Migraine) or when the patient is dysphasic and unable to indicate the presence of headache, migrainous psychosis may mimic an acute encephalopathy.

Complex Migraine Migraine is usually regarded as a benign condition, but the oligemia associated with spreading depression is occasionally sufficient to cause ischemia and cerebral infarction[33] with permanent neurological deficits including hemiplegia and hemisensory loss.[34] Although more common in migraine with aura, migrainous infarction can also accompany migraine without aura.[35] Angina pectoris associated with coronary artery spasm has been reported to occur spontaneously in migraine.[36] Cardiac arrhythmias and cardiac or respiratory arrest are also rare complications of basilar migraine.

Acephalgic Migraine Prodromal symptoms of migraine can occur without subsequent development of headache. The most common symptom is the scintillating scotoma, and it is not unusual for these visual symptoms to occur as an isolated phenomenon in a migraineur. Other neurological symptoms include paroxysmal vertigo,[37] transient hemiparesis, or hemisensory symptoms, which can cause alarm to patient or physician when the expected headache fails to develop. However, the patient will usually admit to the presence of a dull or slight headache and give an unmistakable history of migraine.

Familial acephalgic migraine has been described in which the aura is similar in affected family members with migraine.[38]

Migraine can also present as recurrent unilateral neck pain associated with tenderness of the ipsilateral carotid artery.[39]

Migraine in Children Migraine is not unusual in children. It has been estimated that 5 percent of children aged 11 have migraine, which is more common in boys in the prepuberty years. Many of these children have an antecedent history of periodic cyclic vomiting and episodic vertigo, recurrent abdominal pain, or transient neurological deficits such as hemiparesis, ptosis, diplopia, or ataxia without headache. Migraine is often precipitated by fatigue, exertion, anxiety, exercise, and illness and aggravated by routine physical activity. Minor head trauma is a potent cause of migraine in children. Complex migraine with visual aura and transient neurological deficit is not uncommon. However, approximately 50 percent of children with migraine have migraine without aura.[40] There is a positive family history of migraine in many cases.

Migraine often presents as a bilateral pulsating headache in children with the development of the characteristic unilateral headache, photophobia, and phonophobia later in life. Some children develop migraine in the late afternoon after-school hours. These attacks are probably precipitated by fatigue. Prostration is prominent in childhood migraine, with rapid recovery after an attack. Sumatriptan is both effective and safe in childhood migraine in doses of 0.06 mg/kg.[41] Propanolol is most effective in prophylaxis. Calcium channel blockers or cypropheptadine can be used in propanolol-resistant cases.

Migraine in Epilepsy   There is more than a chance relationship between migraine and epilepsy, and the coexistence of the two conditions can be regarded as:

1. A chance association of two common conditions without either condition influencing the other

2. A pathological change in the brain, giving rise to both migraine and epilepsy[42]
    —Arteriovenous malformation[43]
    —Lupus erythematosus
    —Mitochondrial encephalopathy lactic acidosis and stroke (MELAS)

3. Migraine occurring as an ictal headache during seizure activity
    —Benign occipital epilepsy
    —Partial complex seizures[44]
    —Benign rolandic epilepsy[45]

4. Seizures occurring during or shortly after the aura of migraine as a feature of basilar migraine[46]

The association is confined to patients suffering from migraine with aura. Most likely a mechanism of migraine-induced seizures is spreading depression that is associated with lower intraneuronal magnesium and increased potassium and glutamate release resulting in neuronal instability and seizure activity. Combined treatment with antimigraine and anticonvulsant drugs is recommended.

Migraine in Pregnancy   Approximately 60 to 70 percent of women with migraine report improvement during pregnancy. However, migraine may occur for the first time during pregnancy, preexisting migraine may worsen, particularly during the first trimester, or the patient may become headache free later in pregnancy.[47] The majority of women who continue to

have migraine attacks during pregnancy experience significant improvement in the number and severity of attacks.[48] However, migraine recurrence is a frequent experience in the postpartum period. The role of oral contraceptives is controversial because there are several reports of increases in migraine in women taking oral contraceptives while other studies have reported improvement. There is little doubt, however, that there is a relationship between menstruation and migraine headaches.

Migraine in Menstruation   The term "menstrual migraine" should be reserved to migraine attacks occurring on day 1, ± 2 days of the menstrual cycle.[49] Migraine without aura is the most frequently encountered type of migraine in this classification.[50] The migraine attack is believed to be the result of a fall in estrogen levels during the late phase of the menstrual cycle.[51] However, prostaglandin release, which is maximal during the first 48 h of menstruation, is another possible mechanism.[52] Migraine attacks should be treated as outlined under Treatment of Migraine. Prophylactic treatment using nonsteroidal anti-inflammatory drugs (NSAIDs) such as naproxen 500 mg, 1 q8h for 5 days, beginning the day prior to the expected onset of headache, is often effective. Alternatively, 100-μg estradiol patches can be used, beginning 3 days before menstruation, replacing the patch the day before menstruation and further replacement on the second day of menstruation.

Retinal Migraine   Migraine is occasionally accompanied by a monocular scotoma or blindness during or after an attack of migraine.[53] The condition is usually benign, but there are occasional reports of permanent visual impairment in one eye with branch occlusion of the retinal artery.[54]

Migraine and Intracranial Vascular Malformations   Although the majority of cases of migraine occurring in patients with vascular malformations (AVM) are no more than a coincidence, some evidence indicates that there is a higher prevalence of migraine in patients with AVM and a positive correlation between the site of headache and location of the AVM.

Differential Diagnosis The differential diagnosis of the more common types of headache is given in Table 5-1.

Diagnostic Procedures In most cases, a diagnosis of migraine can be established by history alone. The neurological examination is normal, and further diagnostic procedures are not necessary and may occasionally lead to confusion. For example, an EEG is usually normal between attacks of migraine but may show a focal slowing if taken during or shortly after an attack of migraine. The abnormality may suggest the presence of a space-occupying lesion or infarction and culminate in further procedures unless the EEG changes in migraine are appreciated. However, the EEG is not effective in screening for structural causes of migraine,[55] and magnetic resonance imaging (MRI) or computed tomography (CT) scanning should be reserved for those who have an abnormal neurological examination, sudden onset of headache without prior migraine, and persistent migraine not responding to therapy. Repeated neuroimaging in migraine with normal neurologic examination does not appear to be valuable. However, in older patients with headache or when headache occurs with neurological abnormalities, particularly motor symptoms, seizures, or galactorrhea, the likelihood of clinically relevant abnormal neuroimaging is significant.[56]

Treatment

1. Mild migraine headaches often respond to simple analgesics[57] such as aspirin or aspirin with codeine; aspirin, acetaminophen, and caffeine; ibuprofen; ketoprofen;[58] or propoxyphene. However, because there is some delay in absorption of oral medications from the stomach in the migraine attack, simple analgesics may not be effective except in mild cases. The combination of acetaminophen 500 mg, aspirin 500 mg, and caffeine 130 mg is reported to be as effective as sumatriptan 25 mg orally in alleviating the pain of acute migraine.[59] An analgesic with butabarbital is effective in some patients, probably because the addition of the barbiturate induces sleep, which usually relieves migraine. A combination of lysine acetylsalicylate and metoclopramide 10 mg orally[60] with a second dose 2 h later if necessary[61] will relieve mild migraine headaches in most cases. Capsules containing isometheptine mucate dichloralphenazone and acetaminophen (Midrin) are effective in some cases, particularly if taken at the onset of headache. The adult dose is 2 capsules initially followed by 1 capsule every hour until the headache is relieved, with a maximum of 5 capsules in 12 h.

2. Moderately severe migraine headache. When the migraine headache is of sufficient intensity to preclude working, the patient often prefers to retire to a quiet, darkened room and lie with a cold compress applied to the head. The attack will usually subside if the migraineur manages to sleep for a few hours, and sleep may be induced by the use of a barbiturate preparation or a benzodiazepine that has been effective in the past.

When attacks are of sufficient frequency to interfere with employment or similar functions, oral ergotamine tartrate 1 mg combined with caffeine 100 mg is useful if taken during the aura or early in the attack. The usual dose of 2 tablets can be repeated in 30 min if the headache increases in severity. Sublingual tablets of ergotamine tartrate 2 mg are probably more effective than oral preparations and can be repeated in 30 min but often induce vomiting. Ergotamine suppositories are more effective in such cases. Migraine-associated nausea and vomiting responds to ondansetron 8 mg orally in most cases. The drug is well tolerated and is a good option for those who need to function throughout the day because it does not induce fatigue.

Naproxen sodium 500 mg taken at the first sign of migraine headache is an effective alternative to ergotamine preparations. There is some delay in absorption of naproxen, but this does not affect peak plasma concentrations. When symptoms persist, a further 500 mg naproxen may be taken after 30 min, with a final 500 mg 1 h after the initial dose of the medication, should that be necessary. Naproxen sodium is as effective as ergotamine tartrate and may have less adverse effects and is therefore a preferred alternative therapy for some patients.[62]

The trend at this time is toward the use of sumatriptan for treatment of moderately severe and severe migraine. Sumatriptan is a specific serotonin (5-HT1D) receptor agonist that enhances receptor

Table 5-1

Differential diagnosis and treatment of headache

Headache type	Epidemiology	Location	Signs and symptoms	Treatment	Prevention
Migraine	Family history Children, M > F Adults, F > M	Unilateral, but may be bifrontal	Nausea, photophobia, phonophobia, osmophobia, desire to lie in a darkened room. There may be neurological deficits.	aspirin, acetominophen, caffeine aspirin, acetominophen, butabarbital Bellergal ibuprofen acetominophen, isometheptine mucate, dichloralphenazone (Midrin) Moderate: Sumatriptan, ergotamines, naproxen sodium, indomethicin Severe: Sumatriptan, ergotamine tartrate, dihydroergotamine Status: Sumatriptan dihydroergotamine metoclopramide prochlorperazine chlorpromazine flunarazine dromperidal	beta blockers calcium channel blockers tricyclics methysergide cyproheptadine naproxen sodium divalproex sodium
Cluster	Adolescents and adults, M > F	Unilateral orbitofrontal	Lacrimation, unilateral nasal congestion, occasionally ptosis and miosis	ergotamines sumatriptan corticosteroids beta blockers calcium channel blockers lithium carbonate divalproex sodium methysergide indomethicin intransasal capsaicin or Lidocaine	

Table 5-1 *(continued)*
Differential diagnosis and treatment of headache

Headache type	Epidemiology	Location	Signs and symptoms	Treatment	Prevention
Tension	F > M	Bilateral, generalized, or occipital	Long duration, associated anxiety and depression	anxiolytics, antidepressants	
Hypertensive	Family history	Bilateral, occipital or frontal	Hypertension retinopathy, may be papilledema with hypertensive encephalopathy	Treatment of hypertension	
Increased intracranial pressure		Varies	Nausea, vomiting, papilledema	Treatment of elevated intracranial, pressure, steroids, mannitol, furosemide, head elevated 35 degrees, surgery	
Temporal arteritis	Adults	Unilateral, Temporal, can be in other areas of scalp	Tender temporal arteries, impairment of vision, elevated sedimentation rate	corticosteroids	
Subarachnoid hemorrhage, encephalitis, meningitis		Bilateral, occipital	Sudden onset with subarachnoid hemorrhage and encephalitis. Meningitis may also be sudden in onset or somewhat more protracted. Examination shows nuchal rigidity and fever in meningitis and encephalitis.	Treatment of meningitis or subarachnoid hemorrhage	

activity promoting vasoconstriction, reduces the neurogenic inflammatory response, and inhibits pain transmission through the trigeminal nerve and its central connections. The drug is equally effective in migraine with aura and migraine without aura[63] and is useful in treatment of cluster headaches. Sumatriptan is contraindicated in hemiplegic migraine and basilar migraine and should not be used in patients with known cerebrovascular disease, subarachnoid hemorrhage, and ischemic heart disease, myocardial infarction, or angina pectoris given that there is a potential to induce coronary artery spasm. The use of sumatriptan is also precluded in Prinzmetal angina and uncontrolled hypertension. Sumatriptan cannot be used within 24 h of administration of an ergotamine preparation[64] or 2 weeks following withdrawal of a monoamine oxidase inhibitor.

Sumatriptan subcutaneously relieves migraine headache and its accompanying symptoms in almost 80 percent of patients within 2 h of administration. The drug is superior to other acute treatments for migraine[65] and is effective whether given early or late in the course of the headache. The expense of the medication is offset by the rapidity of its action, the rapid control of symptoms, the reduced need for emergency treatment, the ability to remain at work or to return to work in many cases,[66] and improved quality of life.[67] There is improved work productivity and a net benefit for the employer.[68] Nonresponders have more severe vomiting and photophobia with initial worsening of headache after sumatriptan administration and tend to treat attacks too early.[69]

Oral sumatriptan is effective in moderate to severe migraine with mild nausea, photophobia, and phonophobia. The drug is supplied in 25-mg and 50-mg tablets (United States and Europe) and 100-mg tablets (Europe). The 50-mg tablet is usually effective and should be used as a starting dose which provides relief from headache within 2 h in 73 percent of cases and 78 percent within 4 h after administration. Alternative therapy includes the nasal spray of 5 or 20 mg sumatriptan[70] or the subcutaneous injection of 6 mg. Although self-injection using an autoinjection device is the most rapid and effective therapy, there is a growing preference for the 20-mg nasal spray, which is associated with complete pain relief or mild residual headache in 65 percent of cases 2 h postadminis-

tration. An additional dose of sumatriptan can be given 2 h after the initial dose for persistent headache and again for recurrence, which is featured in 30 to 40 percent of cases within 24 h.

Adverse effects of sumatriptan are usually mild and consist of local bleeding and pain at the site of injection when the drug is administered subcutaneously. Muscle tension, pain in the extremities, paresthesias, flushing, nausea, and vomiting can occur following subcutaneous or oral administration.[71] Chest pain following administration of sumatriptan is not thought to be of cardiac origin in most cases, although isolated examples of myocardial infarction have been described shortly after using sumatriptan.[72] One case of cardiac arrest occurred in a 35-year-old woman with occult coronary artery disease shortly after receiving a first-time dose of sumatriptan subcutaneously. The patient was resuscitated and shown to have had a myocardial infarction. Patients with risk factors for coronary artery disease should be evaluated carefully for cardiovascular disease prior to the use of sumatriptan.[73]

Additional 5-HT1D agonists available for the treatment of migraine include zolmitriptan, which acts both peripherally and centrally in the brainstem on the trigeminal vascular system. The drug is well tolerated[74] and is a highly and consistently effective[75] treatment for migraine[76] in doses of 2.5 mg[77] or 5.0 mg, with similar adverse effects to sumatriptan.

Three other orally active 5-HT1D receptor agonists (rizatriptan, electriptan, and naratriptan) improve on the bioavailability and extended duration of action of this family of drugs.[78] Naratriptan has a longer half-life than sumatriptan and this is expected to have additional benefit in reducing recurrence of migraine headache. Naratriptan has similar adverse effects when compared to sumatriptan. A dose of a 1.0 mg or 2.5 mg tablet of naratriptan is effective and well tolerated in controlling migraine headache.[79]

When migraine and the accompanying symptoms of photophobia, phonophobia, nausea, vomiting, prostration, weakness, and incapacity are severe, the patient will usually seek treatment in a hospital emergency center. The first premise in treatment is to realize the migraineurs are ill with severe pain and discomfort. They are not seeking narcotics; the one thought is to obtain relief from intense suffering, which may have been present for anywhere from several hours to 2 or 3 days. Consequently, there may be dehydration from repeated vomiting, and intravenous fluids should be given urgently in such cases.

The physician has a choice:

1.   Give sumatriptan 6 mg subcutaneously if ergotamines have not been used in the last 24 hours. This will usually produce relief from headache in 1 to 2 h.[80] If symptoms persist, sumatriptan can be repeated in 2 h.

2.   Dihydroergotamine mesylate (DHE) is an effective alternative to sumatriptan for moderate and severe attacks of migraine[81] as well as intractable migraine (status migrainous).[82] Dihydroergotamine is a 5-HT1D, 5-HT1A, 5-HT1B receptor agonist and has significant effect on 5-HT2, 5-HT3 norepinephrine and dopamine receptors.[83] The drug can be given by intramuscular injection or subcutaneously, 1 mg by self-injection[84] for moderately severe migraine preceded by 10 mg metoclopramide orally to reduce nausea. A nasal spray is also available as an alternative method of administration of DHE. Intravenous DHE is usually effective in the treatment of severe migraine or intractable migraine. A combination of dihydroergotamine plus metoclopramide hydrochloride (Reglan) injected intravenously is as effective as sumatriptan in the treatment of migraine. Metoclopramide (10 mg) should be injected intravenously into the tubing because the intravenous fluids are already running. This is followed by 1.0 mg of dihydroergotamine given intravenously by slow injection over a 3-minute period. The combination reduces adverse effects, particularly the nausea associated with DHE, and produces relief in about 80 percent of cases. If there is a history of angina pectoris, myocardial ischemia, or myocardial infarction, the DHE should be injected intramuscularly to avoid potential vasoconstriction.

Adverse effects include nausea, vomiting, chest pain, muscle aching, and transient rise in blood pressure. DHE should not be given to individuals age 55 years or older, should be avoided in pregnancy and lactation, is contraindicated in bradycardia, valvular heart disease, coronary heart disease, hypertension, and in collagen vascular disease or vasculitis. Reports of peripheral vascular spasm are rare, but DHE should not be used in peripheral vascular disease and excessive use avoided because ergotamine can cause limb-vascular spasm.[85]

3.   Prochlorperazine edisylate (Compazine), a D2 dopamine receptor antagonist given in a dose of 10 mg intravenously, is very effective in migraine.[86] The medication should be administered by slow intravenous infusion at the rate of 2 mg per minute.

4.   Chlorpromazine (Thorazine) 12.5 mg intravenously given at the rate of 1 mg every 2 min and repeated in 12.5 mg doses every 20 min to a total of 37.5 mg intravenously is also effective.[87]

5.   Flunarizine, a calcium channel blocker with significant dopamine antagonist action and affinity for dopamine D2 receptors, is effective particularly in the treatment of severe migraine with aura. Intravenous flunarizine 20 mg should be given by slow infusion.[88]

6.   Metoclopramide, another dopamine D2 receptor antagonist given 10 mg intravenously, is effective and has fewer adverse effects.[89]

7.   Haloperidol, a potent dopamine receptor antagonist given in a 6-mg dose intravenously, has a reportedly high efficacy in controlling severe migraine headache.[90]

8.   Droperidol, another dopamine receptor antagonist, can be given in an intravenous dose of 2.5 mg every 30 min until the patient is headache free or to a maximum of three doses.[91]

Other medications reported to be of benefit include butorphanol tartrate (Stadol) 2 mg intramuscularly or 1 mg by nasal spray into one nostril. An additional 1-mg dose may be given an hour later if the headache has not been relieved by that time. Intranasal lidocaine in a 1% solution applied to the nostril on the same side as the headache is temporarily effective in abolishing the headache in most cases.[92]

Migraine Status (Status Migrainosis)   When migraine persists for more than 72 h, the patient should be classified as migraine status. Dehydration, electrolyte imbalance, or repeated vomiting can occur, and intravenous fluids are required. Treatment with 0.5 to 1 mg dihydroergotamine combined with 10 mg metoclopramide given over a 3-min period q6h intravenously is usually effective in such cases but may require 2 or 3 days of therapy before symptoms are controlled. A combination of DHE and prochlorperazine or chlorpromazine is equally effective. Adverse effects following repeated DHE dosing include nausea, vomiting, diarrhea, muscle cramps, and abdominal discomfort. Nausea and vomiting usually respond to metoclopramide or prochlorperazine, and diphenoxylate is effective in controlling diarrhea. Sumatriptan 6 mg subcutaneously is also effective in controlling migraine status when given q6h but cannot be used within 24 h of administration of DHE.

There is a tendency to underdose patients suffering from migraine status, and the interval between administration of medications should be flexible in an attempt to achieve a pain-free state. Once this is accomplished, the time between doses of medication can be increased gradually until the migraine attack is controlled.

Prevention of Migraine There are five main classes of prophylactic agents—beta blockers, calcium channel blockers, serotonin modulators, antiinflammatory drugs, and ergot alkaloids.

1. Beta-adrenergic blocking agents are effective in the prevention of migraine. Propranolol (Inderal) is effective in some patients, beginning with 20 mg t.i.d. and increasing by 20-mg increments to as high as 240 mg if necessary. Converting to a long-acting preparation of propranolol can be made at the appropriate times during the buildup of the dosage. The drug should not be used in patients who are suffering from chronic bronchitis, chronic obstructive pulmonary disease, or asthma. There are few adverse effects, but patients should be monitored for bradycardia and hypotension. Other beta-blocking agents such as timolol 5 mg p.o. daily, atenolol 25 mg daily,[93] bisoprolol 5 mg daily,[94] and labetalol are also effective in the prophylaxis of migraine.

2. Calcium channel-blocking agents have been disappointing in most cases, but nicardipine slow-release 30 mg increasing to 45 mg or 60 mg a day can produce significant reduction in frequency of migraine attacks. Nimodipine, a cerebral-selective calcium channel blocking agent, 60 mg q6h, has few adverse effects. Flunarizine, another cerebral-selective calcium channel antagonist, 10 mg daily, is reported to be the most effective of the calcium channel blocking agents.[95]

3. Serotonin modulators include the tricyclic antidepressants and the serotonin uptake inhibitors. Amitriptyline 10 mg q.h.s. may be slowly increased until effective or to a maximum of 150 mg in divided doses in 24 h. It is important to increase the dose of this medication slowly to avoid adverse effects, which include drowsiness, dryness of the mouth, blurring of vision, and excessive perspiration, which can be quite troublesome. Other antidepressants that block serotonin reuptake include doxepin, trazodone, fluoxetine, sertraline, and paroxetine.

4. Cyproheptadine (Periactin), a histamine and serotonin receptor antagonist, is occasionally effective if given in the dose of 4 mg q.i.d. The most prominent adverse effect is drowsiness and increased appetite with weight gain. Methysergide, another serotonin receptor antagonist, is given in doses of 2 mg daily, increasing slowly to a total of 3 or 5 tablets in divided doses daily (maximum 8 mg). The dosage should be increased only when the patient is free from adverse effects, including drowsiness, ataxia, and nausea. Methysergide should not be used for more than 6 months because of the risk of retroperitoneal fibrosis. Pleural, pulmonary, and cardiac fibrosis following long-term use of methysergide have also been reported on occasions.

5. The NSAIDs are most effective if taken regularly for short periods of time (e.g., naproxen in the treatment of menstrual migraine). Long-term use carries a significant risk of gastritis and peptic ulceration. Naproxen is effective in doses of 375 to 500 mg q12h.

6. Anticonvulsant drugs. Divalproex sodium is an effective prophylactic drug in the treatment of migraine.[96] The drug is thought to act by elevating levels of the inhibitory amino acid γ-aminobutyric acid (GABA) and reducing levels of the excitatory amino acid glutamate in the central nervous system (CNS).[97] An initial dose of 500 mg q.d. may be effective in some cases but should be increased to 500 mg q12h if required. Further increments can be added if necessary, increasing the dose to 1250 mg q12h.[98] These high doses require determination of serum val-

proate levels, and serum levels should be maintained between 50 and 100 µg/mL, taken 2 h after dose of divalproex sodium. Adverse effects include weight gain, tremors, and hair loss.[99] Hepatic toxicity is a rare occurrence. Liver function tests and platelet counts should be obtained in the early months of therapy.

Unusual Presentations of Migraine Migraine headaches preceded by severe abdominal pain, nausea, and vomiting are a feature of migraine in children rather than adults.[100] It is probable that some cases of cyclic vomiting in younger children are examples of migraine. A significant number of these children develop migraine later in life. Recurrent abdominal pain in older children can be an early expression of migraine when the cause of the pain is obscure.[101]

The association of migraine and stroke is rare,[102] but migraine is one of the causes of stroke in children and adolescents.[103] Stroke can occur in migraine with or without aura[104] and as a complication of hemiplegic migraine. A report that propanolol may potentiate cerebral vasospasm indicates that this drug should be avoided in patients who experience hemiparesis during migraine attacks.[105]

There have been reports of migraine associated with cerebrospinal fluid pleocytosis. These cases are probably examples of recurrent low-grade viral aseptic meningitis.[106]

The headache in migraine usually occurs in the frontotemporal area, but migraine may occasionally present in the face, occipital area,[107] or as recurrent neck pain.

Persistent aura in the absence of MRI evidence of infarction is a rare complication of migraine and responds to divalproex sodium.[108]

CLUSTER HEADACHES

Definition Cluster headaches are severe unilateral headaches of relatively short duration that occur daily or several times a day. Episodic cluster headaches occur in periods lasting 7 days to 1 year, separated by pain-free periods lasting 14 days or more. When attacks occur for more than 1 year without remission or with remission lasting less than 14 days, the condition is termed chronic cluster headaches. Chronic cluster headaches have usually evolved to the condition of unremitting headaches, which began as classical episodic cluster headaches.

Etiology and Pathology Cluster headaches are associated with vasodilatation that occurs in the distribution of one internal and external carotid artery, but this may be a secondary phenomenon rather than a primary cause of headache. The most likely cause of cluster headaches is an intermittent dysfunction of the peripheral[109] or central sympathetic nervous system.[110] An alternative hypothesis suggests that there is a periodic intense antidromic discharge though the trigeminal nerve resulting in a neurogenic inflammatory response and the release of substance P CGRP and other vasoactive polypeptides producing stimulation of pain receptors in the affected area and vasodilatation. The cause of the periodic discharges through the trigeminal system is unknown. There is a constriction of the internal carotid and its branches at the height of a cluster headache as a prelude to the rapid termination of the pain with persistence of vasoconstriction for several hours, indicating a refractory state until the next cluster headache attacks.

Clinical Features There is a male-to-female ratio of between 4:1 to 20:1, but the male preponderance decreases with age.[111] The epidsodic form is more frequent than the chronic form of the disease, the latter occurring in about 10 percent of cases. Cluster headaches have been reported in children beginning as early as 10 years of age. There is a positive family history in 7 percent of families of patients with cluster headaches.[112] This suggests an autosomal dominant inheritance in these families.[113]

The onset is usually abrupt, occurring in a healthy individual without any precipitating events. Headaches occur daily for 6 to 12 weeks, then cease abruptly. Remission may last for periods varying from 14 days to years before a further period of cluster headaches develops. There may be a seasonal pattern initially, but this does not persist in most cases. Cluster periods may lengthen and remissions become shorter in about 10 percent of patients who ultimately develop a chronic, nonremitting form of the disease with daily attacks for an indefinite period of time. Rarely, chronic cluster headaches revert to the episodic form of the disease. The least frequently encountered pattern is a chronic form of cluster headaches without a preceding episodic pattern.

An attack begins without warning with an abrupt rise to maximum intensity within a few minutes, the pain continuing at that intensity for the remainder of the episode. It is strictly unilateral, involving the orbit and the adjacent temporal area, and consists of a steady, excruciating pain lasting 30 to 120 minutes untreated. Relief is rapid, with the pain declining and resolving in no more than a few minutes. Frequency varies from several episodes a day to one every several days. Nocturnal attacks are frequent and occur with the onset of the rapid movement (REM) stage of sleep.

Attacks are always unilateral but can occur on either side in a few cases. Autonomic symptoms are prominent, with ipsilateral conjunctival injection, tearing, nasal congestion, and occlusion rhinorrhea. Ipsilateral ptosis and myosis, Horner syndrome, which is a permanent sign in 5 percent of cases, and, rarely, eyelid edema and ipsilateral facial flushing with sweating are occasional features. The patient with cluster headaches is extremely distressed, restless, vocal, often pacing in agony, unable to sit or lie down. Nausea and vomiting are rare. Rarer examples of cluster headaches occurring in the face, head, or neck outside the trigeminal nerve territory have been reported.[114] Cluster headache suffers are said to be type A individuals with above-average alcohol and tobacco consumption.

Differential Diagnosis

1. *Acute glaucoma.* This condition can be differentiated by the presence of visual loss, "steamy" appearance of the cornea, and the presence of raised intraocular pressure in glaucoma.

2. *Temporal arteritis.* Temporal arteritis tends to occur in older patients, but the headache can be paroxysmal and mimic cluster headaches. The sedimentation rate is elevated in temporal arteritis, and a temporal artery biopsy establishes the diagnosis.

3. *Ophthalmoplegic migraine (see page 127).*

4. *Tolosa-Hunt syndrome (see page 137).*

Treatment

THE ATTACK

1. Oxygen inhalation at 6 to 8 L/min through a loose face mask to avoid rebreathing is effective in 60 to 80 percent of cases.[115]

2. Oral preparations are not effective in treating cluster headaches because of poor absorption of the medication. However, ergotamine tartrate by rectal suppository 1 to 2 mg may be helpful.

3. Dihydroergotamine 1 mg intramuscularly or subcutaneously by self-administration or by nasal spray is an effective treatment that can be repeated after 1 h.

4. Sumatriptan 6 mg subcutaneously is the treatment of choice[116] but cannot be given in a patient who has taken ergotamines in the previous 24 h. An injection of sumatriptan 6 mg subcutaneously should be given at the onset of each headache.[117] Alternatively, sumatriptan nasal spray 20 mg can be used in the same manner.

5. Corticosteroids. Methylprednisolone, beginning 80 mg orally in a single dose at breakfast time and tapering by 8 mg a day has been recommended. Recurrence of headache is likely to occur as the dose is tapered, but it may be possible to continue at the lowest effective dose on alternate days for several weeks to prevent adverse effects from the corticosteroid.

6. Verapamil 80 mg orally three times a day may take up to 3 weeks to control headache. This drug can be started along with corticosteroids.

7. Lithium carbonate 300 mg orally three times a day is most effective in the chronic form of the disease. Several weeks of treatment may be necessary before the headaches are controlled. Serum levels of lithium should be checked every week and the level kept between 0.8 to 1 mEq/L.

8. Divalproex sodium. This slow-release form of valproic acid, beginning 250 mg q8h orally and increasing as necessary to produce a blood level greater than 50 mg/mL at the trough level, is an effective form of therapy (see page 106).

9. Methysergide. The use of this drug is limited by adverse effects and the development of fibrosis. The beginning dose of 2 mg a day is increased every 5 days, up to 2 mg four times a day. If attacks cease, the drug should be continued at the lowest effective dose for 3 to 6 months. Patients should be warned about retroperitoneal, pulmonary, or heart valve fibrosis. If methysergide therapy is continued, a chest x-ray should be obtained every 6 months and a CT scan or MRI scan of the abdomen every 12 months.

10. When single therapies fail, combined therapy such as corticosteroids and verapamil or methysergide and verapamil can be tried.

11. Other preparations that may control cluster headaches include indomethacin, mexiletine, and nimodipine or the intranasal application of capsaicin[118] in those who have failed to show response to measures outlined above.

12. When all other therapies have been tried and failed, admission to hospital with regular infusion of dihydroergotamine can be tried (see Migraine Status, page 133).

13. Surgical treatment. Refractory cases of cluster headache are occasionally treated surgically. Various techniques have been described in an attempt to interrupt the afferent pain pathway and the parasympathetic outflow, often with limited success. Percutaneous radio frequency gangliorhizolysis of the fifth cranial nerve is probably the most successful of several procedures. Nervous intermedius section combined with microvascular decompression of the trigeminal nerve may be helpful.

CHRONIC PAROXYSMAL HEMICRANIA AND HEMICRANIA CONTINUA

This disorder resembles cluster headaches but is distinguished by headaches of shorter duration and by greater frequency of daily attacks. The pain is strictly unilateral and is associated with ipsilateral ptosis, conjunctival injection, lacrimation, and nasal congestion. Chronic paroxysmal hemicrania, like cluster headaches, can occur in episodic chronic or episodic evolving into chronic forms.

Hemicrania continua is a rare unilateral nonparoxysmal headache of moderate intensity that may be associated with transient stabbing pains in the affected area. An episode may last from a few days to many weeks while the headache may become chronic and persistent.

Both conditions show a rapid and complete response to indomethacin 25 mg to 150 mg a day, with absolute relief within 48 h and within 24 h in most patients.[119] When indomethacin is not tolerated, verapamil 240 mg to 320 mg per day or aspirin 1000 mg per day or naproxen 500 mg per day may be effective.[120]

SHORT-LASTING UNILATERAL NEURALGIFORM HEADACHE WITH CONJUNCTIVAL INJECTION AND TEARING (SUNCT)

This rare condition presents with unilateral brief episodes of orbital and periorbital pain of 5 to 250 s in duration. The headache may be accompanied by conjunctival injection, tearing, rhinorrhea, and unilateral sweating.[121] Attacks tend to occur in the morning and evening, and night attacks are unusual. Occasionally there are bouts of pain of longer duration.[122] The symptoms are of shorter duration than cluster headaches or chronic paroxysmal hemicrania, and there is a waxing and waning in frequency and severity of symptoms. SUNCT status has been described where the patient experiences recurrent pain for most of the day.[123] The condition is benign and responds to indomethacin.

TOLOSA-HUNT SYNDROME

Definition The Tolosa-Hunt syndrome is a unilateral headache involving one orbit associated with ophthalmoplegia, which develops several days later.

Etiology and Pathology The syndrome results from an idiopathic inflammation of the wall of the anterior cavernous sinus, or the superior orbital fissure, or orbital apex.[124]

Clinical Features   There is severe headache involving the orbit on the affected side associated with ophthalmoplegia that develops several days after the onset of the headache. The ophthalmoplegia usually presents with a third nerve paralysis followed by involvement of the fourth, sixth, and ophthalmic division of the fifth cranial nerve. Horner syndrome due to involvement of the carotid sympathetic plexus is not unusual. Optic neuritis has been described in some cases. The condition typically persists for several days but eventually remits spontaneously in most cases.

Treatment   The Tolosa-Hunt syndrome shows a good response to corticosteroids. Methylprednisolone 80 mg daily produces rapid resolution of symptoms, and the dose can be progressively reduced as response occurs.

TENSION HEADACHES

Definition   *Tension headache* is a syndromic condition of headaches that occur in those subjected to stress, anxiety, or depression.

Etiology and Pathology   The majority of tension headaches are examples of prolonged or fluctuating episodes of migraine. Sustained contraction of the muscles of the scalp, face, neck, and shoulders is probably a secondary phenomenon. Tension headaches are probably benign recurrent headaches caused by abnormal central cortical hypothalamic or brainstem discharges similar to the mechanisms responsible for migraine. The depression seen in tension headaches may be the result of chronic decrease in central serotonin levels.

Clinical Features   The diagnosis of tension headaches depends on the history obtained by the examiner who must reconstruct the complaint moment by moment and will often find that the patient-labeled "tension headache" has a history of episodes where the description is clearly that of migraine. The majority of headaches, however, will be milder with a steady bilateral, often band-like, pressure in the head, suboccipital area, or neck lasting for a few hours and recurring two or three times a week. They are not associated with vomiting, rarely associated with nausea, but anorexia is not uncommon. There may be some mild degree of photophobia. The general physical and neurological examinations are normal.

Diagnostic Procedures   The patient should be subjected to a minimum of diagnostic procedures because the diagnosis is established by a detailed history and normal physical examination.

Treatment   The physician should attempt to identify the stress or emotional problem underlying the headache. The cause should be explained to the patient. The patient should then be reassured that the condition does not indicate an underlying disease based on the adequate general physical and neurological examinations that have already been performed. Anxiety may be controlled by regular use of a mild tranquilizer such as alprazolam 0.25 to 0.5 mg q.h.s., which has the added benefit of inducing sleep. Depressed patients may also benefit from the use of an antidepressant such as the serotonin reuptake inhibitor fluoxetine or from a tricyclic antidepressant such as amitriptyline or nortriptyline, given 10 mg q.h.s. and increasing slowly to 75 to 100 mg daily to minimize side effects.

When the tension-type headache is associated with a severe emotional problem, the patient requires referral for psychotherapy. Physical therapy with ice packs or hot packs, ultrasound, and an exercise program may be of benefit in some cases.

CHRONIC DAILY HEADACHE

Definition   Chronic daily headaches previously categorized as chronic tension headaches are usually cases of transformed migraine.[125] In some cases there is evidence of medication overuse.

Clinical Features   There is a history of migraine beginning at an early age in which attacks become more frequent and ultimately occur on a daily basis.[126] The term "chronic migraine" has been suggested for this condition.[127] Many are depressed individuals with hypochondriacal traits. Most are using excessive amounts of analgesics or ergotamine-containing medications. A history of insomnia in early morning, wakening with severe headache is not unusual.

Treatment   The overused analgesic or ergotamine must be withdrawn slowly, then discontinued, and an effective preventive agent substituted. When withdrawal results in severe headaches, regular use of intramuscular or intravenous dihydroergotamine or subcutaneous or oral sumatriptan is often effective in controlling severe bouts of headache pain. Patients need counseling and support during the withdrawal period and long-term continuity of care to prevent relapse.

HEADACHES AND CEREBROVASCULAR DISEASE

Cerebral Infarction   Headaches occur in about 30 percent of patients with stroke. Of those patients with headache, 50 percent have intracerebral hemorrhage; 26 percent cerebral infarction; and 15 percent lacunar infarction by CT scan. Headache is a more frequent feature of stroke in the vertebral basilar circulation (46 percent) than in the carotid distribution (23 percent). Unilateral headache is usually ipsilateral to an infarct or hemorrhage, and severity is not related to the size of an ischemic infarct.[128]

Hypertensive Encephalopathy   Generalized headache is a prominent feature of hypertensive encephalopathy and usually precedes the onset of seizures. Patients have a sustained high blood pressure and hypertensive retinopathy. Papilledema, which indicates the presence of cerebral edema, is present in most cases. Hypertensive encephalopathy is a medical emergency and should be treated with intravenous antihypertensive agents to lower blood pressure to acceptable levels as quickly and safely as possible.

Subarachnoid Hemorrhage   The headache in subarachnoid hemorrhage is one of the most severe pains experienced by man. Conscious patients complain of sudden onset of generalized headache that is often maximal in the occipital area and radiating into the neck. There is marked nuchal rigidity. The headache of subarachnoid hemorrhage requires a regular dose of narcotics such as morphine sulfate 15 mg q4h or meperidine hydrochloride (Demerol) 100 mg q4h.

Unruptured Cerebral Aneurysm   Large aneurysms of the terminal internal carotid artery or the circle of Willis may produce a chronic, dull unilateral headache when there is pressure on the parasellar structures. A sentinel headache is an occasional antecedent of a subarachnoid hemorrhage. In about 30 percent of the cases, the headache (thunderclap headache) is sudden in onset, severe, and unlike any headache experienced previously. It is usually focal in the fronto-occipital or retro-orbital areas and may be accompanied by vomiting, neck pain, syncope, visual symptoms, or focal motor or sensory symptoms. The headache subsides after several hours to days. The sentinel headache is usually a retrospective complaint for which few seek medical advice because it resolves completely. In some cases it may be the result of leakage of a minute amount of blood through a small tear in the wall of an aneurysm, which is rapidly corrected by clotting (see Thunderclap Headache, page 143).

Arteriovenous Malformation   Unilateral headache indistinguishable from migraine with or without aura is the most frequently presenting symptom in unruptured arteriovenous malformation (AVM) followed in frequency by seizures and focal motor deficits. The migraine headache is usually but not invariably on the side of the AVM. Features such as recent onset, a short duration of less than 4 h, a prolonged aura, or focal neurological signs suggest the presence of an AVM.

Cerebrovascular Insufficiency   Patients with cerebrovascular insufficiency often complain of chronic headache. This occurs in the frontotemporal area in cases of internal carotid insufficiency and is probably due to development of collateral circulation through the external carotid system. Dull occipital headache is not unusual in vertebral basilar insufficiency and is often exacerbated following a transient ischemic episode. This suggests that the headache is caused by vasodilatation and is possibly related to the development of collateral circulation. However, a number of patients with vertebral basilar insufficiency and occipital headache are probably experiencing discomfort from an associated cervical spondylosis.

Cerebral Arteritis Inflammation of the branches of the superior temporal artery causing temporal arteritis (giant cell arteritis) produces severe unilateral headache. The inflamed vessels are usually but not always tender on palpation. Temporal arteritis should be considered in every elderly individual who has recent onset of unilateral headache. Pain may occur in the temporal, frontal, vertex, or occipital areas and may be unilateral, bilateral, or generalized. The sedimentation rate is elevated. The condition shows a dramatic response to corticosteroid therapy (see page 265).

Headaches in Anemia and Polycythemia The occurrence of headaches and anemia may be related to increased cerebral blood flow and decreased cerebrovascular resistance. There is marked reduction of cerebral blood flow in polycythemia. The headaches that occur in this condition may be the result of chronic cerebral ischemia.

Headaches Due to Meningeal Inflammation The headache of bacterial meningitis or viral encephalitis is the result of inflammation of the meninges at the base of the brain and in the posterior fossa. The inflammatory process also involves nerve roots in the cervical area producing reflex contraction of the neck muscles. The headache often begins in the occipital area but becomes generalized in most cases of meningitis and encephalitis and is accompanied by pain and stiffness of the neck, which is increased when the head is flexed. All patients with recent onset of headache should be tested for the presence of nuchal rigidity, which should be a routine procedure in all neurological examinations.

Headaches Due to Decreased Intracranial Pressure A postlumbar puncture headache should be an unusual experience, and most cases can be avoided by reassuring the patient before the examination is performed. A few patients will experience headaches several hours after lumbar puncture, which is presumed to be due to leakage of cerebrospinal fluid (CSF) at the site of the needle puncture. This results in depletion of CSF volume and dilatation of cerebral veins in an attempt to maintain a constant intracranial volume. Because the veins are pain sensitive, dilatation results in headache. In most, the headache is localized to the occipital or frontal regions and is accompanied by nausea in 50 percent of cases. Neck stiffness may be experienced in about 30 percent, and visual blurring, diplopia, or photophobia occurs in about 10 percent of patients.[129] In most cases the headache will resolve if the patient is placed in the prone position in bed and given extra oral or intravenous fluids if nauseated and adequate analgesic. However, the headache is exacerbated on assuming the erect position in the early stages. The duration of postpuncture recumbency has not been shown to be related to the development of headaches and is no longer regarded as a prophylactic measure. The development of postlumbar puncture headache is, however, related to needle size, needle tap design, and technique of insertion. Consequently, prevention of headache should be directed toward a meticulous technique, proper positioning of the patient, ensuring that antiseptics are allowed to dry or are removed by sterile swab to prevent transmission into the puncture site, and the use of a 25-gauge Whitacre needle. The needle bevel should be oriented so that it is parallel to the longitudinal dural fibers during insertion.

If postlumbar puncture headache ensues, ensure that the diagnosis is correct and initiate therapy with bed rest and adequate oral analgesics. When conservative measures fail, an intravenous bolus of 500 mg caffeine sodium benzoate is usually effective. This should be repeated if the headache is not relieved in 2 to 4 h. An epidural block patch should be avoided unless all other measures fail.[130]

Headaches Due to Increased Intracranial Pressure Increased intracranial pressure from any cause will produce stretching of the nerve endings in the meninges and pressure on the blood vessels at the base of the brain. This often results in generalized headache that increases in severity with increasing intracranial pressure. Reduction of increased intracranial pressure to normal levels produces prompt resolution of the headache.

Headaches and Brain Tumor   The most common site for headache in brain tumor is bifrontal in patients who have a supratentorial tumor or increased intracranial pressure. The value of headache in localizing a brain tumor is limited to the unilateral headaches without raised intracranial pressure when the tumor is always ipsilateral to the headache. Factors associated with headache in brain tumor include increased intracranial pressure, tumor size, and the amount of midline shift as demonstrated by MRI scan. The presence of these factors supports the concept that headache is the result of traction on intracranial pressure-sensitive structures, including large blood vessels, the dura, and certain cranial nerves. Increasing headache, nausea and vomiting, and resistance to common analgesics are indicative of increased intracranial pressure, but papilledema will only be present in about 50 percent of cases. Infratentorial tumors tend to produce bifrontal headaches but only after the development of increased intracranial pressure.

POST-TRAUMATIC HEADACHES

There are at least three types of headache occurring in the posttraumatic period:

1.   Unilateral or bilateral headaches similar to migraine with or without aura may be provoked by trivial head injury in susceptible individuals who frequently give a history of pretrauma migraine. This is the most common form of post-traumatic headache, and the diagnosis is obvious to an examiner who obtains a detailed step-by-step history from the patient.

2.   Dysautonomic headache following injury to the neck and damage to the sympathetic outflow either in the spinal cord or lower cervical nerve roots. This condition is characterized by unilateral frontotemporal headaches, facial hypohidrosis, ptosis, and myosis. There is a good response to propranolol 20 mg three times a day with increasing dosage to as

high as 240 mg daily in the slow-release form or in divided doses.

3.   Headaches arising in the occipital area and projecting to the frontotemporal area are usually unilateral and aggravated by neck movements. Many are related to damage or bruising to the greater occipital nerves on one or both sides.

HEADACHES IN SYSTEMIC DISEASE

Headaches frequently accompany an infectious process. In many cases this is probably due to an increase in cerebral blood flow associated with an elevated temperature. Other certain infectious diseases such as influenza, malaria, typhus, and typhoid are associated with severe headaches, probably caused by circulating toxins that produce further dilatation of the extra and intracerebral arteries. It is not unusual to find some degree of neck stiffness in children with fever and headaches. This condition of meningismus is often mistaken for early meningitis, and the diagnosis must be clarified by lumbar puncture. This procedure should be performed in any patient with a febrile illness who has a severe headache and who develops abnormal neurological signs suggesting an early encephalitis or meningitis.

Episodic headaches of rapid onset with severe bilateral throbbing are a feature of pheochromocytoma due to release of adrenaline and noradrenaline into the circulation. The blood pressure is very high at the onset of the headache, and the urine contains excessive 5-hydroxyindoleacetic acid.

HEADACHES IN OBSTRUCTIVE PULMONARY DISEASE

Impaired respiratory exchange with retention of carbon dioxide causes cerebral vasodilatation and chronic headache. Headache is a feature of chronic emphysema and may also occur in patients who suffer from hypoventilation due to extreme obesity (pickwickian syndrome).

Headaches due to carbon dioxide retention can be relieved by improving pulmonary function.

HEADACHES IN HYPOGLYCEMIA

Although headaches are a feature of hypoglycemia, this condition is all too frequently erroneously cited as a cause of headaches in patients with other forms of headache. The demonstration of hypoglycemia should not depend on a single casual blood glucose determination but rather on adequate study of the problem. Patients with headache due to hypoglycemia respond to appropriate treatment.

HEADACHES IN HEAT EXHAUSTION

Headache is a feature of heat stroke and heat exhaustion and probably results from increased cerebral blood flow secondary to temperature elevation. Additional factors may be dehydration and lowered CSF pressure that produces increased traction on pain-sensitive structures within the cranial cavity. This complication and the headache respond to appropriate correction of fluid and electrolyte imbalance.

TOXIC CAUSES OF HEADACHE

1. Hangover headache. The hangover headache, which is a throbbing, generalized headache resembling migraine, appears to be the result of vasodilatation. However, ingestion of alcohol may precipitate migraine in certain individuals. In most cases hangover headache is the result of ingestion of small quantities of aromatic substances that are contained in alcoholic beverages rather than the alcohol itself. Treatment consists of rest, fluid replacement, and the use of simple analgesics, but in many cases relief is obtained only after a period of sleep.

2. Carbon monoxide poisoning. Carbon monoxide poisoning results in the reduction of arterial oxygen saturation and cerebral vasodilatation. Although acute carbon monoxide poisoning causes loss of consciousness, chronic poisoning produces severe paroxysmal headaches. These headaches resolve when the source of carbon monoxide is removed.

3. Headaches following ingestion of medication. A number of medications produce vasodilatation and headache. Thus, headache is often seen after ingestion of nitrates such as amyl nitrate or nitroglycerin. Sudden headache may occur in patients receiving monoamine oxidase inhibitors who eat cheese or drink red wine, both of which have a high tyramine content.

4. Chinese restaurant and hot dog headache. Ingestion of foods containing monosodium glutamate, which is used abundantly in Chinese food, or foods containing nitrates such as cured meats and hot dogs may cause throbbing headaches in susceptible individuals.

5. Headaches in diseases of the eye. It is a common assumption that headaches are caused by refractory errors, but this is a rather uncommon event. Occasionally hypermetropic children complain of headache toward the end of the school day. This can be corrected by a prescription of suitable glasses.

Infections involving the superficial structure of the eye or the tissue surrounding the eye frequently produce periorbital headache. This includes conjunctivitis, dacryocystitis, and keratitis. Pain is particularly severe in herpes zoster ophthalmicus. Orbital cellulitis will also produce pain and discomfort in the orbital and frontotemporal areas. Headache also accompanies inflammation within the eye such as uveitis, iritis, and endo- or panophthalmitis. Acute optic neuritis often presents with acute onset of pain in and around the eye and a frontal headache. The pain is exacerbated by eye movement and is associated with sudden dimness or loss of vision.

Acute glaucoma produces severe unilateral headache, vomiting, and prostration, and the condition resembles an acute and severe attack of migraine. However, the cornea is steamy, the pupil is dilated, and a diagnosis can be quickly established by ophthalmological examination. Chronic glaucoma is a cause of intermittent frontal headache. Visual symptoms are often minimal, but the diagnosis can be established by determination of intraocular pressure.

6. Headaches in disease of the nose and paranasal sinuses. Acute sinusitis may produce frontal headache, particularly if the ethmoidal or

sphenoidal sinuses are involved. Patients are febrile and toxic and have an elevated white cell count. The condition responds to antibiotics and analgesics.

Chronic sinusitis is a rare cause of headache. Patients with chronic sinus infection may experience headache when there are problems in changes of atmospheric pressure, which occurs during flying. There may be a failure to equalize pressure in a congested sinus during the descent of an aircraft with the sudden occurrence of severe pain over the affected sinus. The condition is relieved by nasal decongestants.

7. Tumors of the paranasal sinuses produce chronic headache or facial pain that tends to be referred to the site of the involved sinus. Tumors of the maxillary sinus produce pain over the cheek and upper teeth, often associated with epistaxis and followed by the later development of headache on the same side. Ethmoidal sinus tumors cause pain over the bridge of the nose. Frontal sinus tumors produce unilateral frontal headache. Nasopharyngeal tumors can cause unilateral nasal obstruction with headache, epistaxis, pain in the throat on the affected side, which is often referred to the ipsilateral ear, and some decrease in hearing on that side. Tumors in the nasopharyngeal area can also involve the maxillary and mandibular divisions of the fifth cranial nerve, producing constant pain in the maxillary and mandibular areas of the face. Early nasopharyngeal tumors can be difficult to diagnose, and the nasopharynx should always be examined when the patient complains of unilateral facial pain, pharyngeal pain, or pain in the ear.

MISCELLANEOUS CAUSES OF HEADACHE

Cervical Spondylosis and Cervical Osteoarthritis Patients with degenerative disease in the cervical spine often complain of headache in the occipital region. This may be caused by: (1) compression of the cervical nerves and involvement of the greater occipital nerves; (2) prolonged contraction of skeletal muscles in the neck and posterior scalp; (3) referred pain from diseased joints in the cervical spine and cervical disk disease or cervical spondylosis; (4) compression of the vertebral arteries by osteo-

phytes in the neck, producing vertebral basilar insufficiency and occipital headache.

Headaches during the Menopause The menopause is not a cause of headache. Although it is possible that headache could develop because of hormonal changes, this cause is unlikely and most cases can be related to tension and depression.

Headaches during Sexual Activity The occurrence of headache during or immediately following orgasm is probably due to contraction of muscles in the neck, jaw, and scalp during sexual intercourse. In the majority of cases headache is infrequent and unpredictable, but in some individuals the headache may occur regularly. Men are affected more than women, and there is a history of migraine, which is often undiagnosed in many who experience this form of headache. The patient should be reassured that this is a benign condition. Treatment with an oral over-the-counter agent such as a compound of aspirin 250 mg and acetaminophen 250 mg and caffeine 65 mg, 2 tablets prior to intercourse, is often effective.

Cough Headache Recurrence of severe generalized headache following a bout of coughing is probably due to sudden rise in intracranial pressure. Some of these patients have herniation of the cerebellar tonsils into the spinal canal (Chiari type I malformation), and a minority require surgical decompression to relieve the symptom.

Lancinating Ocular Headaches Patients occasionally complain of sudden intense pain passing through the eye, which is often described dramatically as the passage of a needle through the eye. The condition is benign, and the cause is unknown, but most patients give a history of migraine or cluster headaches. There is no effective treatment.

Thunderclap Headaches The abrupt onset of intense headache that usually lasts for several hours has been termed a thunderclap headache. The concept of such a headache indicates an impending rupture of a saccular aneurysm (a sentinel headache) owing to leaking of blood prior to rupture was supported by anecdotal reports of thunderclap headaches in survivors of subarachnoid hemorrhage. However, respective studies have shown that there are many examples of repeated thunderclap headaches occurring in individuals who do not have a saccular aneurysm.[131] In addition, studies of patients with unruptured aneurysms have revealed that thunderclap headaches can occur in a minority without evidence of hemorrhage or subsequent rupture.[132] Consequently, thunderclap headaches are usually benign and probably represent abrupt onset of migraine. If there is doubt in an individual who has prolonged or repeated thunderclap headaches or onset following unusual exertion, a lumbar puncture should be performed and magnetic resonance angiography obtained to rule out aneurysm.[133]

Ice Cream Headaches This condition is also benign and consists of the sudden development of intense unilateral headaches affecting the orbit and frontal areas following the ingestion of substances of low temperature. The condition resolves very rapidly as soon as the patient ceases to swallow the frozen substance. Ice cream headaches tend to recur under similar conditions, and the affected individual should learn to avoid rapid ingestion of extremely cold substances.

Ice Pick Headaches Sudden intense painful stabbing pains lasting no more than a second and located in the scalp are occasionally experienced by individuals who are known to suffer from migraine. Ice pick headaches are unusual in nonmigraineurs. The pain occurs at irregular intervals without warning and in some cases is associated with a migraine attack or scintillating scotomata, sudden change in posture, or physical exertion.[134] An identical phenomenon has been described in patients with cluster headaches, or giant cell (temporal) arteritis, the latter condition presenting with intense unilateral headache and superimposed lancinating pains.

Hypnic Headaches This rare condition occurs in elderly individuals who suddenly awaken from a dream at a particular time of night with a headache that is usually diffuse but occasionally unilateral.[135] Symptoms persist for 30 to 60 min, often accompanied by nausea, and abate. The headache responds to lithium 300 to 600 mg at bedtime.

REFERENCES

1. Goadsby PJ: Current concepts of the pathophysiology of migraine. *Neurol Clin* 15:27, 1997.
2. Stewart WF, Lipton RB, Celentano DD, et al. Prevalence of migraine headaches in the United States. Relation to age, income, race, and other sociodemographic factors. *JAMA* 267:64, 1992.
3. Lipton RB, Stewart WF, von Korff M: Burden of migraine: societal costs and therapeutic opportunities. *Neurology* 48 (Suppl 3):S4, 1997.
4. Stewart WF, Lipton RB: Work-related disability: results from the American migraine study. *Cephalalgia* 16:231, 1996.
5. Abu-Arefeh I, Russell G: Prevalence of headache and migraine in schoolchildren. *BMJ* 309:765, 1994.
6. Cull RE: Investigation of late onset migraine. *Scot Med J* 40:50, 1995.
7. Stewart WF, Lipton RB, Liberman J: Variation in migraine prevalence by race. *Neurology* 47:52, 1996.
8. Stewart WF, Simon D, Shechter A, et al: Population variation in migraine prevalence a meta-analysis. *J Clin Epidemiol* 48:269, 1995.
9. Stang P, Sternfeld B, Sidney S: Migraine headache in a prepaid health plan: ascertainment, demographics, physiological and behavioral factors. *Headache* 36:69, 1996.
10. Mannix LK, Frame JR, Solomon GD: Alcohol, smoking and caffeine use among headache patients. *Headache* 37:572, 1997.
11. Sandler M, Li NY, Jarrett N, et al: Dietary migraine: recent progress in the red (and white) wine story. *Cephalalgia* 15:101, 1995.
12. Holm JE, Lokken C, Myers TC: Migraine and stress. A daily examination of temporal relationships in women migraineurs. *Headache* 37:553, 1997.
13. Mosley TH Jr, Penzien DB, Johnson CA: Time series analysis of stress and headache. *Cephalalgia* 11 (Suppl 1):306, 1991.
14. Johannes CB, Linet MS, Stewart WF, et al: Relationship of headache to phase of the menstrual cycle among young women. a daily diary study. *Neurology* 45:1076, 1995.
15. Packard RC, Ham LP: Pathogenesis of posttraumatic headache and migraine. a common headache pathway? *Headache* 37:142, 1997.

16. Silberstein SD, Lipton RB: Overview of diagnosis and treatment of migraine. *Neurology* 44 (Suppl 7):S6, 1994.

17. Saper JR: Diagnosis and symptomatic treatment of migraine. *Headache* 37 (Suppl 1):S1, 1997.

18. Main A, Dowson A, Gross M: Photophobia and phonophobia in migraineurs between attacks. *Headache* 37:492, 1997.

19. Dahlof CG, Dimenas E: Migraine patients experience poorer subjective well-being/quality of life even between attacks. *Cephalalgia* 15:31, 1995.

20. Leao APP: Spreading depression of activity in the cerebral cortex. *J Neurophysiol* 7:259, 1944.

21. Lashley KS: Patterns of cerebral integration indicated by the scotomas of migraine. *Arch Neurol Psychiatry* 46:331, 1941.

22. Goadsby PJ, Edvinsson L: Joint 1994 Wolfe award presentation. Peripheral and central trigeminovascular activation in cat is blocked by the serotonin (5HT)— D receptor agonist 311C90. *Headache* 34:394, 1994.

23. MacGregor EA: The doctor and the migraine patient. improving compliance. *Neurology* 48 (Suppl 8):S16, 1997.

24. Liu GT, Schatz NJ, Galetta SL, et al: Persistent positive visual phenomena in migraine. *Neurology* 45:664, 1995.

25. Rolak LA: Literary neurologic syndromes. Alice in Wonderland. *Arch Neurol* 48:649, 1991.

26. Viirre ES, Baloh RW: Migraine as a cause of sudden hearing loss. *Headache* 36:24, 1996.

27. Lipton RB, Solomon S, Newman LC, et al: Gastrointestinal symptoms in migraine: results from the AASH-Gallup survey. *Headache* 35:563, 1995.

28. Joutel A, Tournier-Lusserve E, Bousser MG, et al: Hemiplegic migraine. *Presse Med* 24:411, 1995.

29. Terwindt GM, Ophoff RA, Haan J, et al: Familial hemiplegic migraine: a clinical comparison of families linked and unlinked to chromosome 19 OMGRG. *Cephalalgia* 16:158, 1996.

30. Ophoff RA, Terwindt GM, Vergouwe MN, et al: Wolff award 1997. Involvement of the Ca^{2+} channel gene in familial hemiplegic migraine and migraine with and without aura. Dutch migraine genetics research group *Headache* 37:479, 1997.

31. Gardner K, Barmada MM, Ptacek LJ, et al: A new locus for hemiplegic migraine maps to chromosome 1q31. *Neurology* 49:1231, 1997.

32. Baloh RW: Neurotology of migraine. *Headache* 37:615, 1997.

33 Mendizabal JE, Greiner F, Hamilton WJ, et al: Migrainous stroke causing thalamic infarction and amne-

34. Narbone MC, La Spina P, et al: Migraine stroke: a possible complication of both migraine with and without aura. *Headache* 36:481, 1996.

35. Welch KM, Levine SR: Migraine-related stroke in the context of the International Headache Society classification of head pain. *Arch Neurol* 47:458, 1990.

36. Lafitte C, Even C, Henry-Lebras F, et al: Migraine and angina pectoris by coronary artery spasm. *Headache* 36:332, 1996.

37. Abu-Arafeh I, Russel G: Paroxysmal vertigo as a migraine equivalent in children: a population-based study. *Cephalalgia* 15:22, 1995.

38. Shevell MI: Familial acephalgic migraine. *Neurology* 48:776, 1997.

39. De Marinis M, Accornero N: Recurrent neck pain as a variant of migraine: description of four cases. *J Neurol Neurosurg Psychiatry* 62:669, 1997.

40. Maytal J, Young M, Shechter A, et al: Pediatric migraine and the International Headache Society (IHS) criteria. *Neurology* 48:602, 1997.

41. Linder SL: Subcutaneous sumatriptan in the clinical setting: the first 50 consecutive patients with acute migraine in a pediatric neurology office practice. *Headache* 36:419, 1996.

42. Verma A, Rosenfeld V, Forteza A, et al: Occipital lobe tumor presenting as migraine with typical aura. *Headache* 36:49, 1996.

43. Monteiro JM, Rosas MJ, Correia AP, et al: Migraine and intracranial vascular malformations. *Headache* 33:563, 1993.

44. Welch KM, Lewis D: Migraine and epilepsy. *Neurol Clin* 15:107, 1997.

45. Bazil CW: Migraine and epilepsy. *Neurol Clin* 12:115, 1994.

46. De Romanis F, Buzzi MG, Assenza S, et al: Basilar migraine with electroencephalographic findings of occipital spike-wave complexes: a long-term study in seven children. *Cephalalgia* 13:192, 1993.

47. Silberstein SD: Migraine and pregnancy. *Neurol Clin* 15:209, 1997.

48. Granella F, Sances G, Zanferrari C, et al. Migraine without aura and reproductive life events: a clinical epidemiological study of 1300 women. *Headache* 33:385, 1993.

49. MacGregor EA: Menstruation, sex hormones and migraine. *Neurol Clin* 15:125, 1997.

50. Fettes I: Menstrual migraine. Methods of prevention and control. *Postgrade Med* 101:67, 1997.

51. Cupini LM, Matteis M, Troisi E, et al: Sex-hormone-

related events in migrainous females. A clinical comparative study between migraine with aura and migraine without aura. *Cephalalgia* 15:140, 1995.

52. Nattero G, Allais G, De Lorenzo C, et al: Biological and clinical effects of naproxen sodium in patients with menstrual migraine. *Cephalagia* 11 (Suppl 11):201, 1991.

53. Lee AG, Brazis PW, Miller NR: Posterior ischemic optic neuropathy associated with migraine. *Headache* 36:506, 1996.

54. Beversdorf D, Stommel E, Allen C, et al: Recurrent branch retinal infarcts in association with migraine. *Headache* 37:396, 1997.

55. Gronseth GS, Greenberg MK: The utility of the electroencephalogram in the evaluation of patients presenting with headache: a review of the literature. *Neurology* 45:1263, 1995.

56. Wheeler SD: Value of repeat neuroimaging in headache when first study normal. Presented at the 39th Annual Scientific Meeting of the American Association for the Study of Headache. June 19–22 1977, New York.

57. Sheftell FD: Role and impact of over-the-counter medications in the management of headache. *Neurol Clin* 15:187, 1997.

58. Karabetsos A, Karachalios G, Bourlinou P, et al: Ketoprofen versus paracetamol in the treatment of acute migraine. *Headache* 37:12, 1997.

59. Lipton RB, Stewart WF, Ryan RE, et al: Efficacy and safety of acetaminophen, aspirin and caffeine in alleviating migraine headache pain: three double-blend randomized placebo conrolled trials. *Arch Neurol* 55:210, 1998.

60. Tfelt-Hansen P, Henry P, Mulder LJ, et al: The effectiveness of combined oral lysine acetylsalicylate and metoclopramide compared with oral sumatriptan for migraine. *Lancet* 346:923, 1995.

61. Hugues FC, Lacoste JP, Danchot J, et al: Repeated doses of combined oral lysine acetylsalicylate and metoclopramide in the acute treatment of migraine. *Headache* 37:452, 1997.

62. Welch KM: Drug therapy of migraine. *N Engl J Med* 329:1476, 1993.

63. Moschiano F, D'Amico D, Grazzi L, et al: Sumatriptan in the acute treatment of migraine without aura: efficacy of 50-mg dose. *Headache* 37:421, 1997.

64. Wilkinson M, Pfaffenrath V, Schoenen J, et al: Migraine and cluster headache. Their management with sumatriptan. a cortical review of the current clinical experience. *Cephalalgia* 15:337, 1995.

65. Boureau F, Chazot G, Emile J, et al: Comparison of subcutaneous sumatriptan with usual acute treatments for migraine. French sumatriptan study group *Eur Neurol* 35:264, 1995.

66. Stewart WF, Lipton RB: Work-related disability: results from the American migraine study. *Cephalalgia* 16:231, 1996.

67. Mushet GR, Miller D, Clements B, et al: Impact of sumatriptan on workplace productivity, non work activities, and health-related quality of life among hospital employees with migraine. *Headache* 36:137, 1996.

68. Legg RF, Sclar DA, Neme NL, et al: Cost benefit of sumatriptan to an employer. *J Occup Environ Med* 39:652, 1997.

69. Visser WH, de Vriend RH, Jaspers NH, et al: Sumatriptan nonresponders: a survey in 366 migraine patients. *Headache* 36:471, 1996.

70. Ryan R, Elkind A, Baker CC et al: Sumatriptan nasal spray for the acute treatment of migraine. Results of two clinical studies *Neurology* 49:1225, 1997.

71. Ottervanger JP, van Witsen TB, Valkenburg HA, et al: Adverse reactions attributed to sumatriptan. A postmarketing study in general practice. *Eur J Clin Pharmacol* 47:305, 1994.

72. Mueller L, Gallagher RM, Ciervo CA: Vasospasm-induced myocardial infarction with sumatriptan. *Headache* 36:329, 1996.

73. Kelly KM: Cardiac arrest following use of sumatriptan. *Neurology* 45:1211, 1995.

74. Zagami AS: 311C90: long-term efficacy and tolerability profile for the acute treatment of migraine. International 311C90 long-term study group. *Neurology* 48 (Suppl 3):S25, 1997.

75. Dowson AJ: 311C90: patient profiles and typical case histories of migraine management. *Neurology* 48 (Suppl 3):S29, 1997.

76. Rapoport AM, Ramadan NM, Adelman JU, et al: Optimizing the dose of sumatriptan (Zomig, 311C90) for the acute treatment of migraine. A multicenter double-blind, placebo controlled, dose range-finding study. The O17 clinical trial study group. *Neurology* 49:1210, 1997.

77. Solomon GD, Cady RK, Klapper JA, et al: Clinical efficacy and tolerability of 2.5 mg zolmitriptan for the acute treatment of migraine. The O42 clinical trial study group. *Neurology* 49:1219, 1997.

78. Mathew NT, Asgharnejad M, Peykamian M, et al: Naratriptan is effective and well tolerated in the acute treatment of migraine. Results of a double-blind placebo-controlled, crossover study. The naratruptan S2WA3003 study group. *Neurology* 49:1485, 1997.

79. Moskowitz MA, Cutrer FM: Attacking migraine headache from beginning to end. *Neurology* 49:1193, 1997.

80. Akpunonu BE, Mutgi AB, Federman DJ, et al: Subcutaneous sumatriptan for treatment of acute migraine in patients admitted to the emergency department: a multicenter study. *Ann Emerg Med* 25:464, 1993.

81. Saper JR: Diagnosis and symptomatic treatment of migraine. *Headache* 37 (Suppl 1):S1, 1997.

82. Silberstein SD, Young WB: Safety and efficacy of ergotamine tartrate and dihydroergotamine in the treatment of migraine and status migrainosus. Working panel of the Headache and facial pain section of the American Academy of Neurology. *Neurology* 45:577, 1995.

83. Peroutka SJ: The pharmacology of current antimigraine drugs. *Headache* 30 (Suppl 1):5, 1990.

84. Becker WJ, Riess CM, Hoag J: Effectiveness of subcutaneous dihydroergotamine by home injection for migraine. *Headache* 36:144, 1996.

85. Paraskevopoulos JA, Teasdale DE, Cuschieri RJ: Severe reversible arterial spasm with ergotamines. *Br J Clin Pract* 49:214, 1995.

86. Coppola M, Yealy DM, Leibold RA: Randomized placebo controlled evaluation of prochlorperazine versus metoclopramide for emergency department treatment of migraine headache. *Ann Emerg Med* 26:541, 1995.

87. Bell R, Montoya D, Shuaib A, et al: A comparative trial of three agents in the treatment of acute migraine headache. *Ann Emerg Med* 19:1079, 1990.

88. Peroutka SJ, Wilhout T, Jones K: Clinical susceptibility to migraine with aura is modified by dopamine D2 receptor (DRD2) alleles. *Neurology* 49:201, 1997.

89. Tek DS, McClellan DS, Olshaker JS, et al: A prospective, double-blind study of metoclopramide hydrochloride for the control of migraine in the emergency department. *Ann Emerg Med* 19:1083, 1990.

90. Fisher H: A new approach to emergency department therapy of migraine headache with intravenous haloperidol: a case series. *J Emerg Med* 13:119, 1995.

91. Wang SJ, Silberstein SD, Young WB: Droperidol treatment of status migrainosus and refractory migraine. *Headache* 37:377, 1997.

92. Maizels M, Scott B, Cohen W, et al: Intranasal lidocaine for treatment of migraine. A randomized, double-blind controlled trial. *JAMA* 276:319, 1996.

93. Kowacs PA, Werneck LC: Atenolol prophylaxis in migraine secondary to an arteriovenous malformation. *Headache* 36:625, 1996.

94. Van de Ven LL, Franke CL, Koehler PJ: Prophylactic treatment of migraine with bisoprolol a placebo-controlled study. *Cephalalgia* 17:596, 1997.

95. Leone M, Bussone G: Current approaches to the prophylaxis of migraine. *CNS Drugs* 3:163, 1995.

96. Mathew NT, Saper JR, Silberstein SD, et al: Migraine prophylaxis with divalproex. *Arch Neurol* 52:281, 1995.

97. Silberstein SD, Wilmore LJ: Divalproex sodium: migraine treatment and monitoring. *Headache* 36:239, 1996.

98. Taylor K, Goldstein J: High-dose versus low-dose valproic acid as a prophylactic medication. *Headache* 36:514, 1996.

99. Silberstein SD: Divalproex sodium in headache. Literature review and clinical guidelines. *Headache* 36:547, 1996.

100. Abu-Arafeh I, Russell G: Prevalence and clinical features of abdominal migraine compared with those of migraine headache. *Arch Dis Child* 72:413, 1995.

101. Mavromichalis I, Zaramboukas T, Giala MM: Migraine of gastrointestinal origin. *Eur J Pediatr* 154:406, 1995.

102. Wober-Bingol C, Wober C, Karwautz A, et al: Migraine and stroke in childhood and adolescence. *Cephalalgia* 15:26, 1995.

103. Rothrock J, North J, Madden K, et al: Migraine and migrainous stroke: risk factors and prognosis. *Neurology* 43:2473, 1993.

104. Narbone MC, Leggiadro N, La Spina P, et al: Migraine stroke: a possible complication of both migraine with and without aura. *Headache* 36:481, 1996.

105. Mendizabal JE, Greiner F, Hamilton WJ, et al: Migrainous stroke causing thalamic infarction and amnesia during treatment with propranolol. *Headache* 37:594, 1997.

106. Caminero AB, Pareja JA, Arpa J, et al: Migrainous syndrome with CSF pleocytosis: SPECT findings. *Headache* 37:511, 1997.

107. Caputi CA, Firetto V: Therapeutic blockade of greater occipital and supraorbital nerves in migraine patients. *Headache* 37:174, 1997.

108. Rothrock JF: Successful treatment of persistent migraine aura with divalproex sodium. *Neurology* 48:261, 1997.

109. Drummond PD: The site of sympathetic deficit in cluster headache. *Headache* 36:3, 1996.

110. Havelius U, Heuck M, Milos P, et al: Ciliospinal reflex response in cluster headache. *Headache* 36:568, 1996.

111. Manzoni GC: Male preponderance of cluster

headache is progressively decreasing over the years. *Headache* 37:588, 1997.

112. Russell MB, Andersson PG, Thomsen LL: Familial occurrence of cluster headache. *J Neurol Neurosurg Psychiatry* 58:341, 1995.

113. Russell MB, Andersson PG, Iselius L: Cluster headache is an inherited disorder in some families. *Headache* 36:608, 1996.

114. Solomon S, Lipton RB, Newman LC: Nuchal features of cluster headache. *Headache* 30:347, 1990.

115. Gallagher RM, Mueller L, Ciervo CA: Analgesic use in cluster headache. *Headache* 36:105, 1996.

116. Ekbom K, Krabbe A, Micieli G, et al: Cluster headache attacks treated for up to three months with subcutaneous sumatriptan (6 mg) sumatriptan cluster headache long-term study group. *Cephalalgia* 15:230, 1995.

117. Centonze V, Polito BM, Attolini E, at al: Use of high sumatriptan dosages during episodic cluster headache. three clinical cases. *Headache* 36:389, 1996.

118. Fusco BM, Marabini S, Maggi CA, et al: Preventative effect of repeated nasal applications of capsaicin in cluster headaches. *Pain* 59:321, 1994.

119. Pareja J, Sjaastad O: Chronic paroxysmal hemicrania and hemicrania continua. Interval between indomethacin administration and response. *Headache* 36:20, 1996.

120. Evers S, Husstedt IW: Alternatives in drug treatment of chronic paroxysmal hemicrania. *Headache* 36:429, 1996.

121. Pareja JA, Shen JM, Kruszewski P, et al: SUNCT syndrome: duration, frequency, and temporal distribution of attacks. *Headache* 36:161, 1996.

122. Kruszewski P, Zhao JM, Shen JM, et al: SUNCT syndrome: forehead sweating pattern. *Cephalalgia* 13:108, 1993.

123. Pareja JA, Caballero V, Sjaastad O: SUNCT syndrome. Statuslike pattern. *Headache* 36:622, 1996.

124. Zournas C, Trakadas S, Kapaki E, et al: Gadopentetate dimeglumine-enhanced MR in the diagnosis of Tolosa-Hunt syndrome. *Am J Neuroradiol* 16 (4 Suppl):942, 1995.

125. Mongini F, Defilippi N, Negro C.: Chronic daily headache. A clinical and psychological profile before and after treatment. *Headache* 37:83, 1997.

126. Solomon S, Lipton RB, Newman LC: Clinical features of chronic daily headache. *Headache* 32:325, 1992.

127. Manzoni GC, Granella F, Sandrini G, et al: Classification of chronic daily headache by International Headache Society criteria: limits and new proposals. *Cephalalgia* 15:37, 1995.

128. Vestergaard K, Andersen G, Nielsen MI, et al: Headache in stroke. *Stroke* 24:1621, 1993.

129. Leibold RA, Yealy DM, Coppola M, et al: Post-dural-puncture headache: characteristics, management and prevention. *Ann Emerg Med* 22:1863, 1993.

130. Morewood GH: A rational approach to the cause, prevention and treatment of postdural puncture headache. *Can Med Assoc J* 149:1087, 1993.

131. Linn FH, Wijdicks EF, van der Graaf Y, et al: Prospective study of sentinal headache in aneurysmal subarachnoid haemorrhage. *Lancet* 344:590, 1994.

132. Raps EC, Rogers JD, Galetta SL, et al: The clinical spectrum of unruptured intracranial aneurysms. *Arch Neurol* 50:265, 1993.

133. Hughes RL: Identification and treatment of cerebral aneurysms after sentinel headache. *Neurology* 42:1118, 1992.

134. Raskin NH: Short-lived head pains. *Neurol Clin* 15:143, 1997.

135. Gould JD, Silberstein SD: Unilateral hypnic headache: a case study. *Neurology* 49:1749, 1997.

Chapter 6

MOVEMENT DISORDERS

A number of neurological disorders are characterized by the presence of conspicuous involuntary movements. Although these movements occur in many different unrelated pathological conditions, their appearance permits convenient clinical classification. Involuntary movements have certain common properties.

1. In most cases, the type of movement is recognized by observation.
2. Involuntary movements are often accentuated by stress.
3. Involuntary movements disappear during sleep.

The following terms are used in describing involuntary movements:

Chorea: abrupt spasmodic, irregular movements of short duration involving the fingers, hands, arms, face, tongue, or head.

Athetosis: irregular slow, sinuous movements usually involving the hands and fingers.

Choreoathetosis: a combination of choreiform and athetotic movements.

Dystonia: an abnormal sustained movement or posture due to a disturbance of muscle tone in agonists and antagonists.

Myoclonus: sudden shocklike contractions of muscle or a group of muscles.

Palatal myoclonus (synonym: palatal nystagmus): rapid rhythmic contractions of one side of the palate, producing a rhythmic movement of the uvula, which is usually accompanied by synchronous movements of the pharynx. The condition often spreads to involve the face, tongue, platysma, shoulders, and diaphragm.

Myokymia: persistent irregular twitching of muscles producing a quivering, "bag of worms" appearance, often seen in the periorbital region (facial myokymia).

Fasciculations: irregular contractions and relaxations of muscle fascicles innervated by the same motor unit, which are visible through the skin.

Tic: repetitive, spasmodic movements that occur in an irregular fashion and resemble volitional movements.

Habit spasm: a tic of long duration.

Clonus: a rhythmic movement produced by rapid contraction and relaxation of muscle, usually seen in increased muscle tone.

Tremor: a rhythmic movement of short amplitude.

CHOREA

Sydenham (Rheumatic) Chorea

Definition Sydenham chorea is a neurological manifestation of rheumatic fever in which antistreptococcal antibodies are believed to cross-react with neuronal tissue, particularly in the basal ganglia.[1]

Etiology and Pathology Sydenham chorea probably represents the cerebral form of rheumatic fever, which is a systemic disease characterized by inflammation, degeneration, and fibrosis of collagen. The heart and arterial system are particularly susceptible to rheumatic involvement. The exact etiology of rheumatic fever is still unclear, but the condition is believed to be an abnormal immune response involving group A streptococci.

Rheumatic chorea is associated with vasculitis and occasionally an exudate surrounding or necrosis of the smaller cerebral arteries. There is a perivascular cellular infiltration around the affected arteries and neurons in the cerebral cortex, basal ganglia, and cerebellum.

Clinical Features   Girls are affected twice as frequently as boys.[2] The incidence of rheumatic fever has decreased dramatically in the United States and other developed countries[3] following the introduction of antibiotic therapy. However, the disease is not uncommon in children living in developing countries, where it is a significant cause of morbidity. The interval between the attack of rheumatic fever and the detection of chorea varies from 2 to 9 months. Many children exhibit concomitant psychological dysfunction, including behavioral problems of obsessive-compulsive nature, associated with hyperactivity, irritability, emotional lability, distractibility, and age-regressed behavior.[4] These symptoms often fluctuate and can precede the appearance of chorea by several weeks. Choreiform movements involve the fingers and hands initially, followed by gradual involvement of the upper limbs and spread to the face and tongue. Examination may reveal a mild fever and tachycardia, and the patient presents with choreiform movements that are increased by excitement or stress. When the tongue is protruded, it suddenly jerks back into the mouth. The hands show a typical posture when the arms are outstretched, with flexion at the wrist, extension of the metacarpal phalangeal and interphalangeal joints, and extension and abduction of the thumb. The wrist is pronated when the arms are held above the head. In severe cases, there may be continuous movements with flinging of the limbs. The speech is dysarthric, with an irregular explosive quality due to contraction of the respiratory muscles. Constant movements of the head may lead to loss of hair over the occipital area. Involvement of the pharyngeal muscles produces dysphagia and increases the risk of aspiration pneumonia.

There is generalized hypotonia and muscle weakness, and coordination is slowed and impaired, with irregular overflinging during rapid alternating movements. The tendon reflexes are normal, but the knee jerks are pendular. There is a bilateral plantar flexor response. Sensation is normal. Evidence of systemic rheumatic involvement (e.g., fever, carditis, polyarteritis, erythema marginatum) may be present. Chorea usually lasts for about 4 to 6 weeks, but prolonged episodes, up to 3 years, have been observed.[5] Persistence is rare. Recurrence occurs in 20 percent of cases.

Diagnostic Procedures

1.   The sedimentation rate or C-reactive protein is elevated.

2.   The antistreptolysin O (ASO) test is the most reliable serological test. However, by the time chorea appears, the antibody titers may have declined.

3.   Increased expression of rheumatic B-cell alloantigen D8/17[6] helps to differentiate rheumatic chorea from other forms of chorea.

4.   Other serological tests that may be helpful in documenting rheumatic chorea include antistreptokinase and antineuronal antibodies.[7]

5.   Magnetic resonance imaging (MRI) demonstrates increased volume of the caudate nucleus putamen and globus pallidus in rheumatic chorea,[8] compatible with swelling due to inflammation.

6.   Positron emission tomography (PET) demonstrates increased glucose metabolism in the basal ganglia in rheumatic chorea.[9]

7.   Lumbar puncture. The cerebrospinal fluid (CSF) is normal.

Differential Diagnosis

1. Infections
   a. A viral encephalitis presents with headache followed by alteration in the level of consciousness. Cortical spinal tract involvement and extensor plantar responses are usually present. The CSF is abnormal.
   b. Postinfectious encephalomyelitis. Brain, spinal cord, and cortical spinal tracts are involved, with extensor plantar responses and sensory deficits. The MRI scan is abnormal with areas of increased signal intensity in the white matter of the brain and spinal cord.
   c. Chronic meningoencephalitis. Tuberculosis, sarcoidosis, or partially treated bacterial meningitis can present with signs of diffuse brain involvement as well as chorea, and the CSF examination is abnormal.
   d. Neurosyphilis may present as a syphilitic arteritis or general paresis. In both cases, the

serologic test for syphilis is positive, and the CSF examination is abnormal.[10]

e. Human immunodeficiency virus (HIV) enters the central nervous system (CNS) at an early stage of infection and may produce chorea as one of the manifestations of an HIV encephalitis. Appropriate antibody testing will be positive.

f. In Mycoplasma pneumoniae encephalitis[11] the CSF examination and antibody testing will be abnormal.

2. Anoxic encephalopathy

a. Cardiopulmonary arrest usually follows myocardial infarction and requires emergency resuscitation. The resulting anoxic encephalopathy may be associated with choreiform movements.

b. Respiratory arrest or distress with prolonged anoxia can result in anoxic encephalopathy in which chorea may be a prominent symptom.

c. Cardiopulmonary bypass with hypothermia[12] or postpump chorea[13] may be the result of anoxic encephalopathy occurring during the bypass procedures and the chorea may be a feature of this complication.

3. Collagen vascular diseases

a. Lupus erythematosus may be responsible for many cases masquerading as rheumatic chorea in children or adolescents in developed countries. Appropriate antibody testing should be considered in all cases of chorea in these age groups.[14]

b. Antiphospholipid antibody syndrome, which is associated with cerebral infarction, migraine, recurrent abortion, and venous thrombosis, is another disease in which chorea may be a prominent feature. Antiphospholipid antibodies are present in the serum and there is a false-positive VDRL.[15]

c. Acute glomerulonephritis.[16] Chorea has been described in association with this autoimmune condition.

4. Metabolic encephalopathy. Both nonketotic hyperglycemia[17] and hypoglycemia[18] can be associated with chorea.

5. Drug-induced chorea. Many drugs have been associated with choreiform movements. The list includes phenothiazines, carbamazepine, gabapentin,[19] valproic acid,[20] cocaine,[21] cyclosporine,[22] and theophylline.[23]

6. Infarction.[24] Infarction due to vasculitis or embolism affecting the basal ganglia may result in choreiform movements. Although this is likely to occur in older individuals, infarction in such conditions as the antiphospholipid antibody syndrome can occur in adolescents.

Treatment

1. Bed rest. In acute chorea the affected individual is weak and fatigued, and the institution of bed rest is helpful.

2. The head and limbs should be protected from trauma when there are severe involuntary movements.

3. Most cases show an early resolution and medication is not necessary. However, when the movements are prolonged, chlorpromazine beginning with 10 mg q8h gradually increasing until the choreiform movements are controlled, is very effective in many cases.

4. A short course of corticosteroids produces dramatic improvement in others. Prednisone 60 mg daily for 7 to 14 days is usually effective.

5. Severe cases will respond to haloperidol (Haldol) beginning 1 mg q12h and increasing slowly until adequate response occurs.

6. Carbamazepine can be used as an alternative in difficult cases.

7. Prophylaxis. About 50 percent of patients with rheumatic chorea develop overt signs of rheumatic carditis. This may be prevented with prophylactic penicillin, given as benzathine penicillin G, 1.2 million units intramuscularly every month, or oral penicillin A, 250,000 units q12h until 21 years of age.

Prognosis The prognosis is good. Neurological complications of rheumatic chorea are now rare, because of institution of early and more effective treatment. A few children show minor intellectual impairment or emotional lability, which requires special attention on returning to school. This usually resolves. Recurrence is rare, particularly in patients treated with prophylactic penicillin.

Chorea Gravidarum

Chorea gravidarum is a rare condition related to rheumatic fever since many patients report attacks of chorea when not pregnant. One-third give a history of rheumatic heart disease and one-third show clinical evidence of heart disease. However, with the decline of rheumatic fever, most cases seen today are secondary to systemic lupus erythematosus (SLE) or may herald the onset of SLE. Chorea may also occur during estrogen therapy or with the use of oral contraceptives, suggesting that chorea may be induced by hormonal changes in some cases.[25]

Acute psychosis with anxiety, delirium, or mania is the most important complication of chorea gravidarum. Speech disturbances, which may be dysphasic or dysarthric, have been reported. Chorea gravidarum may recur during subsequent pregnancies.

Senile Chorea

Chorea is occasionally seen in elderly patients and occurs with or without dementia. Senile chorea with dementia is probably due to neuronal degeneration of the basal ganglia in patients with Alzheimer disease. A few cases may be related to the late onset of Huntington disease. However, measurements of CAG trinucleotide repeats in the Huntington gene have shown normal repeat lengths, indicating that senile chorea is a distinct disease.[26] Cases without dementia are rare and are probably due to degenerative changes or multiple lacunar infarcts confined to the basal ganglia.

Hemichorea

Choreiform movements involving one limb are occasionally seen following a mild stroke. These patients usually exhibit pronounced sensory change in the affected limb, suggesting the presence of a lesion in the posterior ventrolateral nucleus of the thalamus. Other cases show the presence of infarction in the ipsilateral subthalamic nucleus.[27]

Symptomatic Chorea

Chorea is occasionally seen during acute encephalitis and is a feature of some chronic diseases, including SLE, multiple sclerosis, and the leukodystrophies. Chorea has been observed in a number of metabolic conditions including hyperthyroidism, hypocalcemia, and hypernatremia. Choreiform movements have been described during treatment with phenothiazines, phenytoin (Dilantin), carbamazepine (Tegretol), anticholinergic drugs, amphetamine-like drugs, digoxin, cimetidine, methylphenidate, and cyclizine. The presence of chorea has also been recorded in blood dyscrasias, including polycythemia vera and sickle cell disease. Chorea and dystonia can occur as a remote effect of carcinoma. Pimozide or tetrabenazine may be effective in senile chorea, hemichorea, or symptomatic chorea.

Benign Hereditary Chorea

This is a rare condition in which the symptoms of chorea appear in late infancy or early childhood. The chorea affects the upper limbs more than the lower limbs. There is associated generalized hypotonia and the condition remains unchanged, without significant progression into adult life. There is no mental deterioration. Benign hereditary chorea is a distinct genetic entity that is not linked to Huntington disease.[28] Improvement has been reported with corticosteroids, but the relatively benign nature of the chorea hardly warrants long-term steroid therapy.

Familial Calcification of the Basal Ganglion

This condition is occasionally associated with the presence of chorea, which is nonprogressive. Diagnosis is established by the demonstration of calcification of the basal ganglia by computed tomography (CT) or MRI scanning.

Chorea in Systemic Lupus Erythematosus

Systemic lupus erythematosus is probably the most common cause of chorea in children and adolescents in North America. The condition usually presents in females and may recur intermittently for many years. Occasionally chorea precedes the development of other manifestations of SLE, suggesting that all cases of chorea in young persons should be screened for SLE. This is particularly important because neurological complications of SLE include cerebral infarction, migraine, seizures, and a disabling psychosis often followed by dementia. Treatment with corticosteroids may be effective for isolated chorea due to SLE, but immunosuppression is often required for patients who have established neurological symptoms of psychosis and dementia.

Chorea in Primary Antiphospholipid Antibody Syndrome

Circulating antibodies to phospholipids—antiphospholipid antibodies—detected as lupus anticoagulant or anticardiolipin antibodies, have been associated with multiple cerebral infarction, amaurosis fugax, seizures, migraine, dementia, multiple spontaneous abortions, and chorea.[29] These antibodies may occur in SLE and other autoimmune diseases but also occur as primary antibodies in individuals who do not fulfill the criteria for SLE or other associated diseases. Chorea may present as an isolated symptom or as one of the several complications of the antiphospholipid syndrome.[30] MRI scans show the presence of discrete areas of increased signal intensity in the white matter of the brain.[31] Treatment should include anticoagulation or aspirin in symptomatic patients to prevent thrombotic stroke. Hydroxychloroquine is effective in preventing complications in the antiphospholipid syndrome.[32] Corticosteroid therapy will alleviate chorea and dementia.

Neuroacanthocytosis

This rare condition is characterized by the onset in adult life of a progressive neurological deficit consisting of choreiform movements, seizures, buccolingual dyskinesia, orofacial tics, neurogenic muscular atrophy with areflexia, dementia, and acanthocytosis. Psychiatric symptoms, including personality change, impulsive behavior, apathy, depression, anxiety, obsessive-compulsive behavior, and paranoia are features of this disease.

The condition resembles Huntington disease, which can be excluded by the presence of acanthocytosis.[33] CT or MRI scanning shows atrophy of the caudate nucleus and lentiform nucleus. Serum creatinine kinase levels are elevated, but β-lipoprotein levels are normal, excluding a β-lipoproteinemia.

ATHETHOSIS

The common athetotic syndromes are discussed under cerebral palsy (see Chapter 3). Athetosis is occasionally encountered in a number of genetically determined conditions with metabolic defects, including the aminoacidurias, in particular, phenylketonurias; disorders of lipid metabolism, including the lipidoses and leukodystrophies; the Lesch-Nyhan syndrome, a genetically determined disorder of purine metabolism; and Wilson disease (hepatolenticular degeneration). a genetically determined disorder of copper metabolism. Athetosis is not unusual in degenerative diseases of the brain, including tuberous sclerosis, Hallervorden-Spatz disease, ataxia telangiectasia, and the dementias, in particular, Alzheimer disease.

Dentatorubropallidoluysian Atrophy

This rare disorder is inherited as an autosomal dominant trait and is the result of an unstable CAG trinucleotide repeat expansion on the short arm of chromosome 12.[34] Pathological changes consist of neuronal loss and gliosis in the dentate nuclei, red nucleus, globus pallidus, and subthalamic nucleus. Age of onset is clearly related to the degree of repeat expansion. The larger the expansion, the younger the age of onset. The symptoms consist of myoclonus epilepsy, choreoathetosis, ataxia, psychiatric symptoms, and dementia. Younger patients present with myoclonus and epilepsy; older patients present with a constellation of choreoathetosis, ataxia, psychiatric symptoms, and dementia resembling Huntington disease. Seizures may be controlled with anticonvulsant therapy, but there is no treatment that slows the progression of the disease or reduces the choreoathetosis. The diagnosis can be established by the demonstration of mutant protein in cultured lymphoblastic cells.[35]

Paroxysmal Choreoathetosis

Definition Paroxysmal choreoathetosis is a condition characterized by sudden paroxysms of choreoathetosis. Two distinct types have been recognized. In paroxysmal kinesiogenic choreoathetosis (PKC), the choreoathetosis is precipitated by sudden movement and is of short duration. In paroxysmal dystonic choreoathetosis, the choreoathetosis occurs spontaneously and may last for several hours.

Etiology and Pathology PKC is related to the epilepsies, whereas paroxysmal dystonic choreoathetosis is an autosomal dominant condition resulting from a genetic defect located on distal chromosome 2q.[36] The cause of paroxysmal choreoathetosis is unknown, but PKC has been described in progressive supranuclear palsy, following head injury,[37] after thalamic infarction,[38] and in hypoglycemia. Paroxysmal dystonic choreoathetosis can occur following caffeine or alcohol consumption and also occurs in hypothyroidism and hypoglycemia[39] and in obsessive-compulsive disorder.[40]

Clinical Features PKC begins in childhood with the development of sudden paroxysms of choreoathetoid movements, which may occur several times a day. The attacks are precipitated by sudden voluntary movement or by movement after a prolonged period of immobility. The paroxysms begin in the distal limbs and spread rapidly to involve the proximal muscles, the trunk, and the neck. This produces a bizarre contortion, coupled with writhing movements, and the patient may collapse to the floor. There is no loss of consciousness. The paroxysms may be confined to one side of the body. Careful observation often reveals brief choreiform movements of the fingers and feet between attacks. Some patients can abort attacks by voluntary acts such as clenching the fist or flexing the toes and arching the feet. The relationship to epilepsy is established by the precipitation of attacks by hyperventilation and the beneficial effect of anticonvulsant medication. The neurological examination, including mentation, is normal between attacks, and there is no effect on intellect.

Paroxysmal dystonic choreoathetosis is rare. The symptoms are similar to the kinesiogenic form of

Table 6-1
Choreoathetosis

Hereditary

1. Huntington disease
2. Familial paroxysmal choreoathetosis
3. Wilson disease (hepatolenticular degeneration)
4. Lesch-Nyhan syndrome
5. Hallervorden-Spatz disease
6. Familial calcification of the basal ganglia

Acquired

1. Infarction of caudate nucleus of putamen
2. Drug induced—lithium, phenytoin, carbamazepine, amphetamines

the disease, but the movements occur spontaneously, without warning, may last several hours, and are not precipitated by sudden movement.

Diagnostic Procedures Results of MRI and CT scanning are usually normal. High-voltage paroxysmal discharges have been reported in the electroencephalogram (EEG) during hyperventilation in PKC.

Differential Diagnosis Conditions characterized by choreoathetosis are listed in Table 6-1.

Treatment Phenytoin (Dilantin) in therapeutic doses, usually controls attacks of PKC. Carbamazepine (Tegretol) is also effective.

Paroxysmal dystonic choreoathetosis usually responds to clonazepam.[41] Acetazolamide and low-dose haloperidol are also effective.

Hallervorden-Spatz Disease

Definition Hallervorden-Spatz disease is a rare familial condition inherited as an autosomal recessive trait, although rare sporadic cases have been reported. The disease usually begins in infancy or childhood, but onset in adults has been described.

Etiology and Pathology An accumulation of cysteine in the globus pallidus and a deficiency of cysteine dioxygenase have been described,[42] but this has not been confirmed in most cases.

The brain shows rust-colored pigmentation in the globus pallidus and pars reticulata of the substantia nigra. There is a loss of neurons with iron deposits in surviving neurons, which are surrounded by astrocytes and extracellular deposits of iron.[43] Axons show distal swellings presenting as spheroid bodies.

Clinical Features The condition usually begins in infancy or childhood, and children present with progressive difficulties with gait due to corticospinal tract involvement. This is followed by rigidity, dystonia, dysarthria, and choreoathetotic movements of the limbs. There is progressive cognitive decline. About 50 percent of patients show pigmentary degeneration of the retina and optic atrophy.

Diagnostic Procedures

1. Acanthocytosis occurs in some cases.

2. The MRI reveals marked hypointensity of the globus pallidus and, usually, the substantia nigra, consistent with iron deposits in these structures. A small area of hyperintensity in the T2-weighted spin echo sequence, located in the anteromedial or central aspect of the hyperintense area—the eye of the tiger sign—is usually present.[44]

Treatment The condition is refractory to oral medications, but continuous intrathecal baclofen infusions through a baclofen pump are beneficial in some patients with generalized dystonia.[45]

Huntington Disease (Huntington Chorea)

Definition Huntington disease is an hereditary degenerative disease of the CNS characterized by emotional disorders of depression, irritability, and apathy; cognitive disturbances with a slowly progressive dementia; and the presence of motor symptoms with choreoathetosis, rigidity, and bradykinesis.

Etiology and Pathology The disease is inherited as an autosomal dominant trait. The Huntington's allele is located on the short arm of chromosome 4 and consists of an extended CAG trinucleotide repeat.[46] The number of trinucleotide repeats necessary to cause phenotypical Huntington disease appears to exceed 40.[47] However, the length of the trinucleotide expansion does not seem to correlate with the rate of disease progression.[48]

The brain shows cortical atrophy most prominent in the frontal lobes, and ventricular dilatation that is more marked in the frontal horns of the lateral ventricles, resulting from atrophy of the caudate nucleus. Microscopic examination shows a profound loss of medium-sized spiny neurons, which make up 80 percent of the neurons in the caudate nucleus and putamen, with sparing of the larger neurons. There is a reactive gliosis in the basal ganglia with the presence of prominent characteristic astrocytes. It should be realized, however, that Huntington disease is a generalized neuronal atrophy, and there is neuronal loss of lesser extent in most of the gray matter of the cerebral hemispheres and cerebellum. The striatum, which is particularly vulnerable to the disease process, has decreased levels of neurotransmitters, including substance P γ-aminobutyric acid, metenkephalin, and dynorphin.[49] The cause of the neuronal loss and subsequent neurotransmitter decline remains elusive, but an imbalance between the production and removal of free radicals caused by the gene mutation in Huntington disease could lead to neuronal death.[50] Alternatively, neuronal death may be the result of a gene defect producing a failure of energy metabolism at the mitochondrial level in Huntington disease.[51]

Clinical Features Huntington disease is seen in all races and has a prevalence of approximately 6.5 cases per 100,000 population.

The mean age of onset ranges from 35 to 42 years, but 6 percent develop symptoms before 21 years and 2 percent before 15 years of age. In some cases, choreiform movements begin as late as the sixth to eighth decade when the progression of the disease is slow. The earliest manifestation of the disease consists of depression or irritability coupled with a slowing of cognition and difficulty in problem-solving. There are subtle changes in coordination and the appearance of minor choreiform movements, particularly in the fingers. The symptoms then progress to irregular choreoathetoid movements of fingers and wrists, with later involvement of more proximal muscle groups in the upper limbs. The gait is ataxic in the fully developed state and has a bouncing quality due to irregular choreoathetoid movements. Choreoathetoid movements of the face and tongue result in nonrepetitive facial and mouth movements, and the patient is dysarthric and dysphagic. A slowly progressive dementia presents as a loss of memory coupled with impairment of judgment and insight. Many patients develop depression and suicidal thoughts. However, there is a lack of correlation between psychiatric symptoms and cognitive decline, motor symptoms, or CAG repeat length in Huntington disease. This may be the result of differential degeneration of striatocortical circuits or the tendency for psychiatric disturbances to be more prevalent in certain families with the disease.[52] Ultimately, cognitive deficits increase, the disease progresses relentlessly, and the patient eventually becomes bedridden.

There are two variants of Huntington disease:

1. Variant 1 (Westphal). This more rapid form of Huntington disease consists of the development of rigidity beginning with the trunk and proximal limb musculature and gradually involving all muscle groups. There is rapid dementia and death occurs within a few years of disease onset. Examination shows masklike facies, generalized rigidity, and evidence of corticospinal tract involvement, with increased reflexes and bilateral extensor plantar responses.

2. Juvenile. This variant occurs in children and adolescents. Progressive rigidity, ataxia, and dementia with seizures are followed by death within a few years of onset.

Diagnostic Procedures

1. The MRI or CT scans demonstrate reduced basal ganglia volume in early Huntington disease (Fig. 6-1).[53] This is primarily a reduction in putamen volume rather than volume reduction of the caudate nucleus.[54] Late cases show basal ganglia atrophy and signs of diffuse brain atrophy.
2. Glucose tolerance testing is abnormal in some cases.[55]
3. Position-emission tomography shows lowered D_1 and D_2 dopamine receptor binding in Huntington disease.[56]

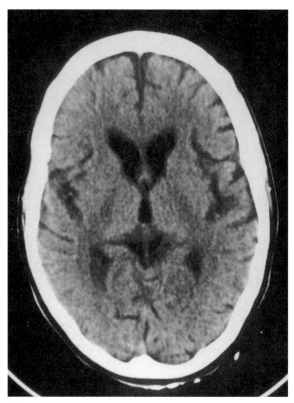

Figure 6-1
CT scan. Axial study of brain showing atrophy of the caudate nucleus bilaterally, a characteristic change in Huntington disease.

4. Single photon emission CT (SPECT) scan regional cerebral blood flow (rCBF) measurements show a reduction in rCBF in the caudate nucleus greater than in the putamen.
5. Direct gene testing by polymerase chain reaction will identify Huntington disease and asymptomatic carriers. However, identification of a carrier does not necessarily imply the inevitable development of Huntingon disease in the future.[57]

Treatment

A. CHOREOATHETOSIS   There is little evidence that treatment of choreoathetosis is effective in Huntington disease, although most physicians feel compelled to place patients on medication in an attempt to reduce involuntary movements.

In the early stages of the disease, some benefit may occur with the use of benzodiazepines, particularly clonazepam, which can be started in a dose of 0.5 mg q.h.s., increasing as high as 9 mg in a divided dosage over a period of several months. The use of dopamine receptor antagonists including phenothiazines, butyrophenones, or thioxanthenes is popular, but it is probably better to use a mild alternative because it is inevitable that adverse effects will develop from these medications in the long term. Thioridazine beginning 10 mg q.h.s. and increasing by 10-mg increments as high as 100 mg/day is usually well tolerated and may have some benefit in reducing involuntary movements. It is unusual to see adverse effects with this drug. However, the use of the more potent dopamine receptor blocking agents such as haloperidol inevitably leads to the development of adverse effects, including acute dystonic reactions, tardive dyskinesia, akathisia, increased rigidity, and parkinsonian symptoms. Nevertheless, haloperidol has been widely used in treatment of choreoathetosis in Huntington disease. This drug should be started at 0.5 mg/day with gradual increase until the patient shows some signs of decrease in involuntary movements. However, treatment in doses greater than 10 mg haloperidol per day yields little increased benefit over low doses of this drug. In addition, higher doses increase the early development of adverse effects. Fluphenazine in similar dosage to haloperidol is also effective in some cases and is an acceptable alternative medication.

Dopamine-depleting agents, which include reserpine and tetrabenazine, are also used in the treatment of Huntington disease. Reserpine is given in an initial dose of 0.1 mg/day and can be increased at 7- to 10-day intervals to doses as high as 3 mg/day. The main problem with reserpine is its known tendency to cause depression in patients who are already susceptible to this problem. Frequent inquiries should be made about depression when treating patients and any signs of this complication should lead to tapering off reserpine and discontinuing this drug. Hypotension is not usually a problem but can occur. Tetrabenazine is less likely to cause depression, but signs of increased rigidity, parkinsonism, or akathisia are not uncommon. Tetrabenazine is usually given in doses of 12.5 mg, increasing by 12.5 mg every 7 days, to a maximum of 25 mg q.i.d.

B. RIGIDITY Rigidity is usually seen in advanced Huntington disease, and in the juvenile form of the disorder. The condition is difficult to treat and response to medication is unpredictable.

Baclofen, beginning 10 mg/day and increasing slowly to as high as 120 mg/day in divided doses, combined with a benzodiazepine such as clonazepam 0.5 mg/day, increasing slowly to as high as 9 mg in divided doses, may be helpful in some cases.

Antiparkinsonian medications have been of temporary benefit in Huntington disease, with reduction of bradykinesias and rigidity. Amantadine 100 mg q12h can be tried initially and may be helpful for a period of a few months. The medication can then be changed to carbidopa/levodopa 25/100 twice or three times a day and gradually increasing the dose to effect. If bromocriptine, which is a dopamine receptor agonist, is used, the dose should be as low as 1.25 mg daily, increasing by 1.25 mg weekly to effect. High doses can be achieved in such a scheme, and 30 to 50 mg/day may be of benefit. Prominent dystonia with torticollis can be treated with the injection of the appropriate muscles with botulinum toxin.

C. MYOCLONUS Myoclonus is an unusual complication of Huntington disease but can be prominent in some cases. There is usually a good response to clonazepam beginning at 0.5 mg/day and increasing as high as 9 mg/day in divided doses, if necessary. Divalproex sodium, beginning at 250 mg/day and increasing by 250-mg increments to as high as 3000 mg/day, may also be effective.

There is an increased incidence of epilepsy in Huntington disease, although fortunately, it is not a prominent symptom. Treatment of epilepsy is outlined in Chapter 4.

D. DYSPHAGIA Impaired coordination of the complex coordinated movements involving swallowing is a feature of Huntington disease. Consequently, dysphagia leading to aspiration, aspiration pneumonia, or actual suffocation is a common cause of death. Dysphagia does not respond to medication, and patients and caregivers must be instructed in those maneuvers that will facilitate swallowing and avoid aspiration. The patient should be fed in an upright position, whether sitting or in bed and instructed to eat slowly. The caregiver selects manageable pieces of easily chewable food when feeding the patient. The oral cavity should be cleared before the next bite and the patient should avoid breathing when swallowing.

As the disease progresses, the patient eventually develops dysphagia at every meal and alternative methods of feeding must be considered. The nasogastric tube may be a temporary stopgap method to supply nutrition. However, the question of performing a gastrostomy and inserting a gastrostomy tube has to be considered in patients with profound impairment of swallowing.

This method of feeding is relatively complication free, but the patient should be given some sustenance by mouth, using substances known to produce little risk of aspiration. Finally, of course, the nutrition will be entirely dependent on the gastrostomy route.

E. DYSARTHRIA   The progressive dysarthria of Huntington disease rarely responds to medication and there is a relentless decline in articulation with the passage of time. In the initial stages, the patient should be asked to repeat sentences slowly so that the observer can understand what is being said, and in some cases, it may be necessary to resort to a communication board containing the alphabet, where the patient will laboriously spell out words during efforts to communicate. Very often, the caregiver will be able to understand the patient much better than the physician during interviews in the office setting. Referral to a speech pathologist may be of help. The patient's failure to communicate should not be taken as an indication of dementia, and it should always be assumed that the patient can understand exchanges between caregivers and the physician when the patient is within hearing range. Inability to communicate does not mean a hearing deficit nor lack of comprehension and careless exchanges between caregiver and physician, discussing a disability or prognosis, can be catastrophic to the listening patient.

F. COGNITIVE DECLINE   Huntington disease is usually associated with a slow cognitive decline, be-

ginning with impairment of attention and ability to learn new material. Judgment, insight, and memory deficits make their appearance somewhat later in the disease.

The early cognitive difficulties may present with problems in the workplace and at home. There may be impairment of emotional response and angry outbursts, in some cases accomplished by combative behavior. As cognition declines, the patient has decreasing ability to function both in the workplace and at home and often has to assume a subsidiary role in the family, which can lead to further irritation and compound depression.

Family members, for their part, must be aware of the growing difficulties in cognition that the patient is experiencing and make allowances for these problems, providing more time for completion of tasks, curbing a tendency to criticize, and using tact when observing difficulties that the patient may have in daily functioning.

G. DEMENTIA   The dementia in Huntington disease is usually mild but, as already indicated, it tends to be overestimated because of communication difficulties secondary to dysarthria. Ultimately, however, the patient does have progressive deficits in retention, recall, judgment, insight, and recent memory, which can be documented by testing at 6-month intervals, using the Mini Mental Status Examination.

H. DEPRESSION   Depression is a prominent symptom of Huntington disease and the suicide rate is significantly higher in patients with this disorder. Families should be fully aware of this risk and should convey their impressions to the physician when it is apparent that the patient is becoming depressed. Antidepressant medication can be started at an early stage and the medication given in low dose with slow increments to a standard level of therapy. This reduces the risk of adverse effects, which are not unusual with the available antidepressants.

The serotonin uptake inhibitor fluoxetine, beginning with 10 mg and increasing by 10-mg increments as high as 60 mg/day, is probably the most effective antidepressant. Similar serotonin uptake inhibitors, including paroxetine and sertraline, are of equal efficacy. Tricyclic antidepressants such as nortriptyline, amitriptyline, and imipramine can be used but do not have the success of the serotonin uptake inhibitors. In addition, the tricyclic antidepressants can cause dry mouth, blurred vision, constipation, and urine retention at higher dosage. However, if one of these medications is selected, then the dosage should be low initially, that is, 10 mg of any of the chosen tricyclics, gradually increasing by 10-mg increments as high as 150 mg/day. It is possible to control these medications by measuring blood levels. Physicians are advised to ask the patient about suicidal ideation at each visit to the office, and it is recommended that the caretaker take charge of all medications that could be used in a suicide attempt and that these pills are not available to the patient at any time. In protracted cases of depression, monoamine oxidase (MAO) inhibitors have been recommended but require following a low-tyramine diet, which is often not practical. Electroconvulsive therapy has been used in refractory cases.

I. MANIC-DEPRESSIVE PSYCHOSIS Patients with manic-depressive illness may well respond to carbamazepine, valproic acid, or fluphenazine in appropriate dosage.

J. OBSESSIVE-COMPULSIVE DISORDER Some patients with Huntington disease do show signs of obsessive-compulsive disorder, particularly in the early stages; this may well respond to fluoxetine or clomipramine.

K. PSYCHOSIS Overt psychosis requires the use of stronger neuroleptic medications, including fluphenazine, haloperidol, or higher doses of thioridazine. In some cases, clozapine is an effective antipsychotic or lithium carbonate has a calming effect in therapeutic doses.

L. IRRITABILITY Many patients show lack of emotional control and become quite irritable when they are aware that memory is failing and that they are in need of increasing help from caregivers. Irritability can be treated with fluoxetine or a benzodiazepine such as clonazepam or oxazepam. A combination of the serotonin uptake inhibitor and a benzodiazepine is often effective.

M. APATHY Apathy should always suggest depression. Patients will usually respond positively to questions about depression and are readily forthright in their responses. Depression requires appropriate treatment, particularly because of the risk of suicide.

N. ANXIETY Many patients show anxiety, particularly in the early stages of the disease when it becomes an established fact that the diagnosis is one of Huntington disease and the individual is aware of the long-term outlook in this condition. Consequently, anxiety tends to occur before the responses are dulled by cognitive decline. Anxiety can be treated with alprazolam or buspirone. The latter can be given in 5 mg twice a day, increasing by 5-mg increments to as high as 15 mg three times a day.

O. SLEEP DISTURBANCES Sleep disturbances are not unusual in Huntington disease and may represent primary insomnia or may occur in patients with major depression or anxiety. One of the most common problems is napping during the day. Every effort should be made to avoid this problem, which usually occurs in the afternoon and is almost irresistible in established cases. The caregiver should see that the patient is kept occupied during the afternoon, particularly in the summer months, when the patient can be taken outside and involved in simple tasks until the evening meal. However, the use of a mild sleeping preparation may be necessary, and the antidepressants amitriptyline or trazodone have the added benefit of sedative properties. Amitriptyline should be given as 10 mg at night and can be increased to 25 to 50 mg at night. The beginning dose of trazodone is 25 mg increasing to 50 mg at night. Other effective medications include Benadryl 50 mg q.h.s. or a benzodiazepine such as clonazepam or oxazepam.

P. SMOKING The presence of choreiform movements makes smoking an unsafe pursuit in patients with Huntington disease. However, the patient who finds smoking a relief or who becomes somewhat obsessed by the need for cigarettes can have problems as the disease progresses. Nicotine patches or bupropion 150 mg q/2h p.o. may be helpful in some cases. When smoking persists, then general safety measures should be instituted, limiting smoking to a safe part of the house and making sure that the patient does not smoke in bed.

Q. FALLING Ambulatory patients develop an increasing tendency to fall because of the combination of choreiform movements, spasticity, and rigidity. The problem may be of considerable concern while the patient is still walking independently and advice given to the patient to avoid accidents is often ignored. Similarly, offers to accompany a patient when the patient is walking up or down stairs often evoke resentment. The risk of fractures or head injury with subdural hematoma should be repeatedly stressed to the patient, and hopefully, this will eventually lead to some curtailing of independent walking.

When the patient is unable to walk and resorts to the use of a wheelchair, risks of falling still exist because of the involuntary movements, which can overturn a wheelchair. The fitting of rear or side wheels to the wheelchair may be useful in such cases.

R. SEXUAL DISORDERS Increased libido can occur in men, who may begin to make increasing sexual demands on the spousal partner, even to the extent of becoming aggressive or angry if their requests are denied. Inappropriate sexual advances to strangers may occur. Treatment with Provera 6 to 80 mg p.o. q.d. or Depo-Provera 500 mg IM every week may be effective in some cases.

S. INCONTINENCE Incontinence tends to occur in advanced stages of Huntington disease and is often the result of detrusor hyperreflexia. Consequently, anticholinergic agents such as oxybutynin 5 mg b.i.d. or t.i.d. or hyoscyamine timed release 0.375 mg b.i.d., combined with regular toileting, is usually effective. If incontinence should continue, then appropriate urological investigation with cystometrography should be performed.

Prognosis The disease is fatal. The interval between diagnosis and death is about 15 years and few survive beyond 20 years. Death is the result of aspiration pneumonia in most cases and length of survival is related to quality of care.

Wilson Disease (Hepatolenticular Degeneration)

Definition Wilson disease is a disorder of copper metabolism inherited as an autosomal recessive trait and is the result of a defect in a gene that encodes a copper-transporting P-type adenosine triphosphatase.[58]

Etiology and Pathology The defective gene in Wilson disease is located on chromosome 13.[59] The genetic defect results in faulty transport and impaired elimination of copper. In the healthy state, copper is absorbed through the intestinal mucosa and transported by ceruloplasmin, a globulin that binds copper molecules. Copper is then secreted in saliva, gastric juice, and bile and is eliminated through the gastrointestinal tract. Wilson disease is characterized by impaired biliary excretion of copper with accumulation of copper in hepatocytes in the liver, causing copper toxicity. Ultimately, copper that cannot be stored is passed into other tissues in the body. This results in an increase in urinary excretion of copper, but the mechanism is insufficient to maintain a copper balance, and copper is deposited in many tissues, including the brain. Free copper is toxic to cells, resulting in cell death.

Ceruloplasmin levels are usually low in Wilson disease, suggesting an impairment in copper transport, but this is no longer regarded as the primary cause of Wilson disease, which is clearly the result of faulty biliary excretion of copper.[60]

Pathological changes consist of deposition of copper in liver cells, which eventually produces cirrhosis of the liver. Deposition of copper in kidney cells produces damage to the renal tubules and consequent aminoaciduria, alkaline urine, low serum uric acid, and low serum phosphate level in chronic cases. Copper is deposited in Descemet's membrane of the cornea, which produces a characteristic Kayser-Fleischer ring. Deposition of copper in the brain produces damage in the caudate nucleus and putamen, which may show cavitation. The globus pallidus is shrunken but rarely cavitated. Lesions are also seen in the subthalamic nucleus, thalamus, red nucleus claustrum, blood vessels, and myelinated fiber bundles, and there are minor cortical changes. Microscopic examination reveals neuronal loss. Surviving neurons are pyknotic. Vascular changes consist of capillary swelling and proliferation, swelling of arterial endothelium, and perivascular thickening occurring in the basal ganglia.

Clinical Features Wilson disease occurs in childhood, adolescence, and adult life up to the age of 40 years. The condition affects both sexes and there is often a marked similarity in the presentation of the illness in members of an affected family. First symptoms may be psychiatric, neurological, or hepatic. Psychiatric and behavioral abnormalities consisting of personality changes, including irritability, anger, depression, suicidal ideation and attempted suicide. Deteriorating academic and work performance, sexual preoccupation, and reduced sexual inhibition[61] are the initial presentation in about 30 percent of cases. Consequently, many patients in the group receive psychiatric treatment before the diagnosis of Wilson disease is established.[62]

There are three types of neurological presentation.

1. The classical dystonic form. This most common form of Wilson disease is characterized by the appearance of choreoathetotic movements of the fingers and hands, which spreads to involve the more proximal muscles of the upper limbs, followed by involvement of the lower limbs, head, and trunk. Tremor, which is a prominent feature and may be present at rest or as an intention tremor, can be associated with head titubation. A proximal component produces the characteristic wing-beating tremor when the upper limbs are extended. Speech is dysarthric and gradually becomes unintelligible in the later stages of the disease and finally aphonic. Dysphagia and drooling occur. Constant choreoathetotic movements give the gait a peculiar, dancing quality. As the disease progresses the patient can no longer walk and finally becomes bedridden with the limbs fixed by contractures. Death occurs from intercurrent infection.

2. The pseudosclerotic form presents with prominent cerebellar dysfunction, including intention tremor and scanning speech. The condition has a superficial resemblance to multiple sclerosis, hence the prefix pseudosclerotic.

3. The pseudoparkinsonian form is rare and is characterized by generalized muscle rigidity and bradykinesis. The gait has a festinant quality resembling that seen in parkinsonism. The patient is severely dysarthric and may have some absence of facial expression.

Liver disease occurs in about 50 percent of cases with onset usually in the early teens. Cirrhosis is often mild, but episodes of acute hepatitis can occur and a fulminating, often fatal hepatitis has been described.[63] Chronic active hepatitis or chronic progressive cirrhosis are the most common forms of hepatic involvement in Wilson disease, with progression to eventual hepatic failure, ascites, esophageal varices, splenomegaly, and hepatic encephalopathy.

Kayser-Fleischer rings, though not pathognomonic, are the hallmark of Wilson disease.[64] Initially, Kayser-Fleischer rings appear as crescents in the superior and inferior aspects of the cornea at the corneal-scleral junction. The crescents gradually extend and eventually join to form a complete ring. The color is usually brownish red or brownish green and should not be confused with arcus senilis, a much more common condition. A definitive diagnosis can be made by slit lamp examination.

About 20 percent of patients with Wilson disease develop sunflower cataracts, which do not interfere with vision but can be seen by slit lamp examination.

Diagnostic Procedures

1. Ceruloplasmin levels are reduced below 20 mg/dL.
2. Serum copper levels are usually elevated in Wilson disease, about 80 to 150 mg/dL.
3. Urinary copper excretion is increased to more than 100 mg/24 h. Urine must be collected in copper-free containers.
4. The presence of Kayser-Fleischer rings can be confirmed by slit lamp examination in early cases. Alternatively, the copper content of the cornea can be measured by x-ray excitation spectrometry.
5. Patients with chronic Wilson disease show the presence of aminoaciduria, glycosuria, and alkaline urine.

6. Cirrhosis of the liver is usually mild in Wilson disease. Excess copper concentrations can be demonstrated on liver biopsy.
7. In very early cases, the diagnosis of Wilson disease can be established with a radioactive copper kinetic study, using the stable copper isotope Cu^{65} and demonstrating significantly increased biological half-time for removal of copper from the plasma pool.[65]
8. Results of MRI scanning are usually abnormal, with increased signal intensity in the thalamus, basal ganglia, brainstem, especially the midbrain and pons,[66] and cerebellar nuclei (Fig. 6-2). White matter involvement can be demonstrated in the frontotemporal and occipital lobes and in the cen-

trum semiovale. Generalized atrophy and ventricular dilatation may be present. Basal ganglia lesions are usually symmetrical, white matter lesions multiple and asymmetrical. Dystonia correlates with lesions of the putamen, dysarthria with lesions of the putamen and caudate nucleus.
9. Diagnosis of Wilson disease can be established in asymptomatic siblings by DNA linkage analysis using the polymerase chain reaction.[67]

Treatment The objective of treatment is to decrease the absorption of copper from the intestinal tract and promote excretion of copper from the tissues into the urine. This can be accomplished by:

1. Reduction of dietary copper to below 1 mg/day.
2. Patients presenting with neurological disease should be treated with tetrathiomolybdate, which produces rapid and safe control of copper by blocking copper absorption from the intestine and rendering blood copper nontoxic.[68]
3. Those presenting with mild liver failure require trientine hydrochloride and zinc therapy. Trientine, a chelating agent, increases urinary output of copper; zinc delays absorption of copper from the intestinal tract.[69]
4. Presymptomatic patients should be treated with zinc and all patients can eventually be placed on maintenance therapy with zinc.
5. D-Penicillamine is an effective chelating agent that is given in doses of 1 to 4 g/day in divided doses on an empty stomach. Supplementary vitamin B_6 should be given during the administration of D-penicillamine to minimize the risk of optic neuritis. Adverse effects include fever, morbilliform rashes, bone marrow suppression, and SLE. When necessary, these reactions can be minimized by concomitant administration of oral corticosteroids and penicillamine therapy can be continued. The use of penicillamine is decreasing as new, less toxic agents become available.

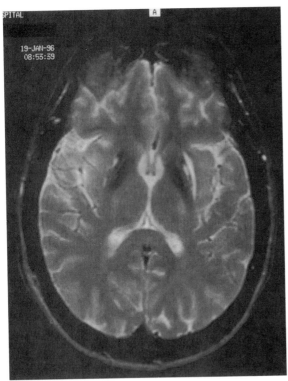

Figure 6-2
MRI scan. T2-weighted image showing symmetrical dark areas in the globus pallidus bilaterally, indicating the presence of copper deposits in a case of hepatolenticular degeneration (Wilson disease).

Prognosis Untreated patients usually die within 4 years of the appearance of symptoms. However, survival for 10 years or more has been described in some cases. The prognosis is improved significantly with the appropriate use of chelating agents and zinc. A normal life span can be expected following treatment in asymptomatic patients with Wilson disease.[70]

Spasmodic Torticollis

Definition Spasmodic torticollis is a form of dystonia characterized by intermittent and recurrent involuntary movements of the head due to contraction of the neck muscles.

Etiology and Pathology The condition may be inherited as an autosomal dominant or autosomal recessive trait. Other causes include congenital abnormalities in the sternocleidomastoid muscle, congenital abnormalities of the cervical spine, hemiatlas or hypoplasia of the atlas, neurovascular compression of the 11th nerve by the vertebral artery,[71] or posterior inferior cerebellar artery, unilateral lesions over the mesencephalon or diencephalon following viral encephalitis, and a bilateral breakdown of the normal metabolic relationship between the thalamus and the basal ganglia. The most likely cause, however, is a functional disturbance of motor control mechanisms believed to reflect a bilateral disturbance within the basal ganglia or the outflow from these structures.[72]

Clinical Features Spasmodic torticollis may begin in adolescence or adult life. There is often a history of preceding trauma to the neck. The onset is usually gradual with intermittent rotation and flexion of the head to one side. This gradually increases in severity and in severe cases, there may be prolonged periods of dystonic deviation of the head. In most cases, the head movement is intermittent and is associated with periodic irregular contractions of the neck musculature. Bilateral involvement is rare but has been described with extension of the head (retrocollis). The movements can often be decreased by counterpressure on the side of the head using the hand, or resting the head against a wall. Some patients experience increased cervical pain due to progressive cervical arthritic changes, with nerve root compression secondary to the involuntary head movement. Spasmodic torticollis is occasionally complicated by blepharospasm or a mandibular dystonia and writer's cramp.[73]

Diagnostic Procedures

1. Electromyography (EMG) shows persistent muscle contraction in the affected neck muscles, including the sternocleidomastoid, splenius capitus, and trapezius muscles.
2. Thyroid function tests should be obtained because there may be more than a chance association between hyperthyroidism and spasmodic torticollis. Some improvement may occur if the patient is restored to the euthyroid state.
3. An MRI or CT scan of the cervical spine should be obtained when there is severe neck pain.

Treatment

1. Mild cases may respond to benzodiazepines such as diazepam 10 to 40 mg q.d. or lorazepam 3 to 6 mg q.d. in b.i.d. or t.i.d. dosage. In either case, treatment should begin with a low dose of the medication followed by gradual addition of increments, thus avoiding drowsiness.
2. High doses of trihexyphenidyl (Artane) 20 to 40 mg/day are usually effective in patients with chronic rather than phasic head turning.[74]
3. Haloperidol (Haldol) 0.5 mg b.i.d., increasing to as high as 5 mg q.d. may be effective.
4. Baclofen (Lioresal) up to 120 mg/day has produced improvement in some cases.
5. Sensory feedback methods have produced some benefit in a few cases.
6. Injection of two or more involved neck muscles using botulinum toxin under EMG control is the most effective available treatment, with resolution of symptoms lasting several weeks or months.[75] The most frequent adverse side effect is dysphagia. Repeated injections are required if symptoms recur.
7. Surgical treatment with intradural selective rhizotomies[76] or selective peripheral denervation[77] should be reserved for patients in whom treatment with botulinum toxin injections fails.

8. Selective sensory stimulation applied to specific anatomic sites identified by repeated trials is beneficial for some patients.[78]

Dystonia Musculorum Deformans

Definition Dystonia musculorum deformans is a condition characterized by progressive dystonic involvement of limbs in the childhood-onset disease and a more restricted cervical cranial or brachial muscle involvement in focal adult-onset disease, with rare involvement of the trunk and lower limbs.

Etiology and Pathology The etiology is unknown. Metabolic studies indicate relative metabolic overactivity in the lentiform nucleus and premotor cortex, but not in the thalamus, suggesting that hyperkinetic movements may arise through excessive activity of the direct putamenopallidal inhibitory pathway,[79] resulting in abnormal input to the motor areas of the cortex.[80] Some cases of childhood-onset limb disease are inherited as an autosomal dominant trait, with a genetic abnormality located in the EYTI gene on chromosome 9q34.[81]

Clinical Features The childhood-onset limb disease usually begins with difficulty in gait due to intermittent dystonic posturing of the feet. If the patient is carefully observed, there will also be intermittent dystonic posturing of the hand at the wrist at this stage. The dystonic movements gradually become more frequent and involve the whole of the lower limb. The patient tends to present with a moment-to-moment variation in the position of the limbs and trunk, due to the unpredictable occurrence of dystonia.

In the fully developed cases, limb and axial muscles on both sides are involved, and the patient is no longer able to walk. The body is in constant dystonic motion, producing unpredictable contortions of the trunk, limbs, and head with involvement of the neck muscles. The head may be moved in any direction and the speech becomes dysarthric.

Examination of the patient reveals normal mentation and dystonic movements of muscle groups with absence of other neurological abnormalities.

In the focal adult-onset disease, dystonia is restricted to the cervical, cranial, brachial, and hand muscles and rarely involves the trunk and lower limbs.

Diagnostic Procedures The diagnosis presents no difficulty in advanced cases. Early cases are missed unless the patient is observed carefully, particularly during walking.

The EEG is said to show diffuse slowing in advanced cases. There are no focal features.

Treatment

1. Repeated injections of botulinum toxin into affected muscles will frequently relieve symptoms of dystonia musculorum deformans. Treatment is necessary for an indefinite period of time.[82]
2. Intrathecal baclofen delivered through an implanted pump mechanism has had beneficial results.[83]
3. Surgical treatment using bilateral pallidoansotomy[84] or thalamotomy[85] produces improvement or slight improvement in about 80 percent of cases.
4. Trihexyphenidyl (Artane) is often effective but requires a high dosage. Treatment should commence with 2 mg daily, gradually increasing by 2-mg increments until the dystonia is controlled or adverse effects prevent further increase in dosage.[86]

Prognosis Spontaneous remissions often occur. If childhood-onset limb disease does not respond to therapy, the patient may be permanently disabled by this condition and either confined to the wheelchair or bedridden. Such patients, with complete dystonia musculorum deformans, often die from intercurrent infection. In focal adult-onset disease, the condition does not affect the life span.

Writer's Cramp

Definition This is a form of focal dystonia involving the hand, wrist, and forearm, with occasional involvement of upper arm and shoulder.

Clinical Features The pen is picked up and gripped in an abnormal fashion. The wrist is hyperextended or flexed, and the writing is slow, laborious, and accompanied by sudden jerking; there is a feeling of tension, with aching or pain in the forearm. The contralateral hand may be used to support the writing hand. Ultimately, the individual ceases to write and the pen may perforate the paper as the dystonia increases.

Similar focal dystonias have been reported in musicians and athletes.

Treatment Injection of botulinum toxin into the affected forearm muscles, with EMG control, is the most effective treatment for writer's cramp.[87]

Spasmodic Dysphonia

Spasmodic dysphonia, usually considered to be a psychogenic disorder in the past, is the result of adductor dystonia of the vocal cords. The speech is staccato and strained, with irregular, abrupt pauses. An abductor dystonia has been described, resulting in reduction of speech to a whisper. Treatment with botulinum toxin injections into the vocal cords (adductor dystonia) or into the tricoarytenoid muscles (abductor dystonia) is effective but must be repeated, usually at 6-month intervals.

Oromandibular Dystonia

Dystonia of the masticatory muscles results in dystonic movements of the jaw and mouth. There may be dystonia on jaw opening or closing, trismus, pressing of the lips, lateral displacement of the lower jaw, bruxism, jaw pain, dysarthria, and difficulty chewing. Movements are often triggered by speaking or chewing.

Limb Dystonia

Limb dystonia involving the upper limb is usually writer's cramp or a similar dystonia occurring in an individual who experiences prolonged stress to the upper limb muscles (e.g., a violin or guitar player). Lower limb dystonia is not uncommon in tardive dyskinesia and tardive dystonia; it can occur in re-

sponse to therapy in Parkinson disease but can also occur spontaneously in Parkinson disease in younger patients. The foot is usually inverted and drawn into plantar flexion, with the toes plantar flexed and the sole of the foot arched. Spontaneous dystonia of the foot can also occur after prolonged running or other forms of exercise involving repetitive stimulation to the feet.

Blepharospasm

Involuntary spasm producing closure of the eyelids in middle-aged or elderly individuals is syndromic. Blepharospasm probably results from abnormalities in the brainstem and basal ganglia[88] producing prolonged contraction of the orbicularis oculi, combined in some cases with involuntary inhibition of the levator palpebrae,[89] an abnormal blink reflex in many — but not all — cases,[90] and abnormal eye movements or oculogyric crises in others.[91] Consequently, blepharospasm is not a homogeneous disease entity but rather the product of different pathophysiological mechanisms.[92]

Periodic injections of botulinum toxin into multiple sites in the orbicularis oculi and into the pretarsal portion of the orbicularis oculi muscle of the upper lid relieves blepharospasm in most cases.

Meige Syndrome

This condition, occurring in middle-aged or elderly individuals, is the result of dystonic stimulation mediated through the facial nerve. The signs of orofacial mandibular dystonia and blepharospasm are characteristic. The changes, which resemble tardive dyskinesia, are not induced by neuroleptic drugs and are unlike the open mouth dystonia of Bruegel syndrome. Lower pontine lesions can be identified in some cases.[93] There may be temporary improvement with haloperidol, tetrabenazine, or intravenous Cogentin. Botulinum toxin injection into the affected facial muscles is the treatment of choice.

Bruegel Syndrome

This dystonia is characterized by a wide open mouth and reflects a dystonic abnormality affecting the trigeminal nerve, producing jaw opening. There is no blepharospasm, the eyes remain open, and there is no focal myokymia, features that distinguish Bruegel syndrome from Meige syndrome.[94] Medication is ineffective. Treatment consists of injection of botulinum toxin into the submental muscle complex.

Ballism

Definition Ballism is an unusual condition characterized by the abrupt onset of violent flinging movements affecting the limbs, neck, and trunk, often on one side of the body (hemiballism) or involving a single limb (monoballism).

Etiology and Pathology The majority of cases are due to a lesion involving the contralateral subthalamic nucleus or afferent and efferent subthalamopallidal connections. There have been rare examples of ballism in which lesions were confined to the contralateral globus pallidus, putamen, caudate nucleus, or thalamus. Most cases are associated with occlusion of a small artery producing a well circumscribed infarct. Other rare causes include focal hemorrhage from an arteriovenous malformation, embolism, metastatic tumor, abscess, tuberculoma, encephalitis, multiple sclerosis, phenytoin intoxication, stereotaxic thalamotomy, and hypoglycemia.

Clinical Features The onset is usually abrupt and the patient presents with almost continuous violent flinging movements affecting the proximal muscles of the shoulders, arms, pelvis, and thighs. There may be contraction of the neck muscles producing violent movements of the head and associated facial grimacing. The movements of the limbs are essentially nonrepetitive and represent completely uncoordinated contractions of agonists and antagonist muscles.

The movements cease during sleep but are extremely exhausting, and many elderly patients succumb from progressive exhaustion and intercurrent infection, particularly pneumonia. In some cases, spontaneous remission occurs approximately 6 weeks following onset of the movements.

Diagnostic Procedures Once the ballistic movements are controlled, every effort should be made to determine and treat causative lesions.

1. Protective measures should be taken to prevent damage to the limbs by placing the patient in a bed with heavily padded head board, foot board, and side rails. The affected limbs can be restrained until there is a response to treatment.
2. In the majority of cases, good control can be maintained by oral diazepam.
3. Clozapine is very effective, and possibly the treatment of choice, because it has few adverse effects.[95]
4. Neuroleptics such as haloperidol should be reserved for intractable cases because adverse effects such as parkinsonism and tardive dyskinesia are more likely to occur in elderly patients.

Prognosis Because most cases of ballism can now be controlled, the prognosis becomes that of the underlying disease.

Myoclonus

Definition Myoclonus may be defined as sudden, brief muscle jerks, simple in character, occurring at irregular or regular intervals, in focal, multifocal, or generalized fashion.

Etiology and Pathology Myoclonus may be physiological as in hypnagogic myoclonus, essential when there is no underlying abnormality, epileptic, or symptomatic. The phenomenon occurs in response to neuronal discharges in either the brain, brainstem, or spinal cord, or may represent a sudden loss of antigravity muscle activity (negative myoclonus).

Clinical Features

1. Physiological myoclonus occurs in normal individuals with nocturnal myoclonus.
2. Essential myoclonus occurs as an isolated symptom and is often familial and nonprogressive. However, essential myoclonus can occur in association with dystonia, a condition inherited as an

autosomal dominant trait, showing a dramatic improvement with ingestion of alcohol.[96]

3. Epileptic myoclonus. Myoclonic jerks are a feature of epilepsy occurring in generalized tonic-clonic seizures with or without progressive encephalopathy, benign myoclonus of infancy, absence seizures, juvenile myoclonic epilepsy, and photosensitive epileptic myoclonus.

4. Symptomatic myoclonus.
   a. Hereditary. Lipidoses and leukodystrophies, Lafora disease, MERRF syndrome (myoclonus epilepsy with ragged red fibers).
   b. Trauma. Myoclonus can follow closed head injury, penetrating wounds injuring the brain, heat stroke, or decompression sickness.
   c. Infection. Myoclonus may be a feature of acute viral encephalitis, particularly herpes simplex encephalitis, acute purulent meningitis, subacute sclerosing panencephalitis, chronic encephalitis, and Creutzfeldt-Jakob disease.
   d. Metabolic. The phenomenon is a feature of anoxic encephalopathy, hepatic encephalopathy, uremic encephalopathy, hyponatremia, hypocalcemia, and hypokalemia.
   e. Neoplastic. Tumors of the brain, brainstem, or spinal cord or angiomatous malformations can be associated with myoclonus.
   f. A number of toxic conditions can be associated with myoclonus, including bismuth intoxication, exposure to heavy metals, methyl bromide poisoning, lithium therapy particularly in high dosage, and use of opioids and tricyclic antidepressants.
   g. Degenerative. Myoclonus occurs in Unverricht-Lundberg disease, the spinocerebellar degenerations, multisystem disease, Alzheimer disease, and corticobasal degeneration.
   h. Basal ganglion disease. Movement disorders, including Huntington disease, Wilson disease, Parkinson disease, Hallervorden-Spatz disease, and progressive supranuclear palsy are occasionally associated with myoclonus.
   i. Lesions of the brainstem. The characteristic feature of brainstem disease is palatal myoclonus, which follows brainstem infarction and is occasionally seen in slowly progressive brainstem gliomas.
   j. Lesions of the spinal cord. Spinal cord tumors and angiomatous malformations may cause myoclonus.

Diagnostic Procedures   The diagnosis of myoclonus is usually apparent by history and observation. EMG can be helpful in differentiating type and location.

Differential Diagnosis   Myoclonus must be differentiated from tics, complex tics, chorea, tremor, fasciculations, myokymia and hemifacial spasm.

Treatment   Essential myoclonus responds to alcohol, but this is an impractical form of therapy. Benztropine, propranolol, 5-hydroxytryptophan, and clonazepam are effective therapeutic agents. Epileptic myoclonus persisting after adequate control of seizures requires the addition of clonazepam, primidone, 5-hydroxytryptophan, or acetazolamide.

Myoclonus Following Anoxic Encephalopathy

Generalized myoclonus may be associated with anoxic encephalopathy. The condition may be transient or permanent when it is associated with severe brain damage. Myoclonus or seizures can be expected to occur in approximately 50 percent of adult survivors of cardiopulmonary resuscitation. Myoclonic jerks are frequently induced by voluntary motor activity (action myoclonus) following recovery of consciousness.

Treatment

1. L-5-Hydroxytryptophan. This drug is a precursor of 5-hydroxytryptamine (serotonin), which is depleted in some conditions associated with myoclonus. Patients should be treated with 100 to 300 mg q.d. of α-methyldopahydrazine (carbidopa) beginning 2 days before the administration of L-5-hydroxytryptophan and continuing during the treatment with this drug. This will reduce the peripheral effects of 5-hydroxytryptamine. L-5-Hydroxytryptophan is administered in capsules with meals, beginning with 10 mg/kg body weight q.d. and increasing slowly un-

til the myoclonus is controlled, or until adverse effects including nausea, vomiting, anorexia, and toxic psychosis make further administration unacceptable.

2. Clonazepam, divalproex sodium, carbamazepine, and levodopa are also effective in postanoxic myoclonus.

TICS

Definition Tics are brief, intermittent, repetitive stereotyped movements resulting from contraction of one muscle or several muscle groups.

Etiology and Pathology Tics often occur in families, suggesting a genetic factor in some cases. It is possible that a disturbance producing increased activity in ascending dopaminergic pathways from the brain to the basal ganglia[97] or to the limbic system with projections to the cerebral cortex may be the substrate for tics. Alternatively, the biochemical abnormality may be a hyperfunction of cerebral cholinergic pathways.[98]

Clinical Features

1. Sensory tics. There is a brief, uncomfortable sensory experience relieved by a motor tic or vocalization.
2. Motor tics. This type of tic consists of a rapid clonic movement that may be focal or generalized. Occasionally motor tics can present as a dystonia with a brief change in posture involving the affected area of the body.
3. Vocal tics consist of simple sounds such as barking, coughing, growling, grunting, or sniffing. Occasionally, utterances can be complex in nature or coprolaliac, causing embarrassment.

Treatment

1. Clonazepam 0.5 mg qhs increasing to 6 mg daily or clonidine 0.05 mg q.h.s. increasing slowly to 0.1 mg q8h with the last dose at bedtime is often sufficient to suppress simple tics.
2. If clonazepam or clonidine fails to suppress tics, a

neuroleptic such as haloperidol may be added to the medication regimen or substituted for clonidine. Haloperidol can be introduced at bedtime using 0.25 mg, increasing slowly, to effect, by no more than 2 mg/day. Adverse effects are not infrequent.
3. If haloperidol is not effective, pimozide[99] or fluphenazine may be of benefit. Risperidone and tetrabenazine, which deplete CNS dopamine will also control tics.
4. Injections of botulinum toxin into the affected muscles is a possible alternative in refractory cases.

Tourette Syndrome

Definition Tourette syndrome is a polygenic disorder, part of a spectrum of related disorders that include tics, attention deficit hyperactive disorder (ADHD), motor hyperactivity, obsessive-compulsive disorder (OCD), conduct disorder (CD), oppositional defiant disorder (ODD), and poor impulse control.

Etiology and Pathology The syndrome is believed to be associated with increased D_2 dopamine receptors[100] and dopamine transporters in the basal ganglia,[101] resulting in dysfunction of projection systems that mediate activity in the cingulate and orbitofrontal cortex.[102]

Clinical Features The onset is in the prepuberty years—mean age of onset, 7 years—with a male preponderance of 5:1.[103] The disease often presents as ADHD followed by eye, face, and head tics, with later neck, shoulder, and upper limb tics. Respiration and phonation become involved, and the patient develops a vocal component consisting of grunting or barking. The expulsion of air imparts an explosive quality to the speech with occasional associated hissing sounds. Some patients develop repetitive verbal expressions, occasionally of obscene sexual character (coprolalia). The patient is unable to control this unfortunate symptom, which may be uttered in a loud voice, causing considerable embarrassment. In addition to coprolalia, patients may show echolalia in which there is repetition of words, and echopraxia in which there is repetition of acts. School-related difficulties occur in 36 percent of patients with Tourette syndrome and are strongly associated with comorbid ADHD[104] and, to a lesser extent, with learning disabilities and OCD. Tics are in themselves related to increased risk of academic difficulties.

Examination of patients with Tourette syndrome often reveals only minor neurological abnormalities. Many patients are left-handed or ambidextrous.

Diagnostic Procedures

1. The EEG is abnormal in many cases, although there is no definite pattern to the abnormality.
2. MRI studies have shown that there is a reduction in volume of the lenticular nucleus in the left hemisphere of patients with Tourette syndrome, compared to normal controls, and reduction in volume and attenuation of the left-sided prominence of the lenticular nucleus, compared to the right side, observed in control groups.[105]

Treatment

1. Treatment of tics is discussed on page 168.
2. Patients with ADHD may respond to methylphenidate (Ritalin) 10 mg in the morning and at noon, increasing to 20 mg in the morning and noon if necessary. Dextroamphetamine 10 mg morning and noon is an effective alternative. Pemoline (Cylert) 37.5 mg morning and noon has less stimulant properties but is also effective in ADHD. Selegiline (Eldepryl) 5 mg q12h has been reported to improve ADHD and tics in children with Tourette syndrome.
3. Patients with OCD respond to serotonin uptake inhibitors such as fluoxetine or clomipramine. Serotonin uptake inhibitors should not be taken in conjunction with MAO inhibitors such as selegiline.
4. ODD should be treated with carbamazepine, divalproex sodium, or lithium carbonate.

Prognosis Some 40 percent of patients show a complete remission in adolescence; 30 percent have a marked reduction in severity, and the remainder show a persistence of symptoms throughout life but often lose the vocal component of the disease.

Exaggerated Startle Reaction

Hyperexplexia, or exaggerated startle reaction, is not unusual in conditions where there is inhibition of brainstem or spinal cord interneurons, removing their normal inhibitory effect on motor neurons. Hyperexplexias may be seen in toxic, metabolic, and degenerative disorders; delirium tremens; withdrawal from long-term drug therapy, including barbiturates, benzodiazepines, and analeptic drugs; high-dose steroid therapy; and in the lipidoses and leukodystrophies.

Hereditary hyperexplexia has also been described in families, where the condition is inherited as an autosomal dominant trait with a genetic deficit localized to chromosome 5.[106] This mutation is the result of a single amino acid substitution that alters glycine binding to the inhibitory glycine receptor.[107]

Clinical Features There may be increased muscle tone and an exaggerated startle response in infancy. The muscle tone improves in childhood, but startle responses increase in response to noise, unexpected touch, or movement, and there is nocturnal myoclonus. The responses continue in the adult with sudden loss of muscle tone, frequent falling, and injuries. The startle response cannot be suppressed and is not accompanied by vocalization. Familial hyperexplexia has been titled "jumping Frenchmen of Maine" in North America and latah in Malaysia and Indonesia.

Treatment Clonazepam is usually effective in treating this condition.

Restless Legs Syndrome

This disturbance syndrome usually occurs in middle-aged or elderly individuals but has been described in adolescents. It may be associated with diabetic or uremic neuropathies, but the cause cannot be determined in most cases. Symptoms consist of a sensation of creeping, crawling, prickling, or burning dysesthesias in the lower extremities, which is worse in the evening and relieved by movement. There is an inner feeling of tension and distress and the symptoms often interfere with ability to fall asleep. Restless legs syndrome is frequently associated with periodic leg movements during sleep.

Treatment The affected individual should avoid caffeine and alcohol in the evening. Antidepressants, particularly serotonin uptake inhibitors, should be avoided or used only in the morning. There is a good response to carbidopa/levodopa (Sinemet 25/100) 1 tablet 30 min before bedtime, increasing to 2 tablets if necessary, or bromocriptine 2.5 to 5 mg in the evening, which is equally effective. Clonazepam 0.5 to 2 mg q.h.s., taken 1 h before bedtime or an opioid such as codeine 30 mg can be used in refractory cases. Divalproex sodium[108], pramipexole, or gabapentin[109] may be beneficial in refractory cases.

TREMOR

Benign Familial (Essential) Tremor

Definition Benign familial tremors are the most common movement disorders[110] in which the prefix benign is questionable because there is often significant disability. The condition is characterized by bilateral symmetrical postural tremor that presents in the fingers and hands, is absent at rest, and is not associated with extrapyramidal signs.

Etiology and Pathology The disorder is inherited as an autosomal dominant trait and a positive family history has been observed in 96 percent of patients, indicating that a negative family history is often inaccurate, and that the term "essential tremor," indicating an isolated case, is redundant.[111] The genetic abnormality is unknown,[112] but penetrance is virtually complete by age 65 years.[113] Autopsy studies have not revealed any abnormality.[114] However, studies of regional cerebral blood flow indicate that benign familial tremors are associated with abnormal bilateral cerebellar, red nuclear, and thalamic activation, indicating overactivity of cerebellar connections.[115]

Clinical Features The tremor typically appears in young adults and increases with age[116] and there is a prevalence of approximately 300 to 400/100,000.[117] The first symptoms consist of tremor less than 7 Hz[118] involving the fingers and hands, and about 50 percent of cases are alcohol responsive. The tremor presents in a mild form in the hands, often with a slight asymmetry in amplitude. Writing may be affected in the early stage. Using eating utensils becomes difficult later. Lifting a glass or cup markedly accentuates a tremor, and the patient develops a characteristic method of grasping the object with two hands, in an often futile effort to prevent spillage. Tremor of the head, facial muscles, jaw, voice, tongue, trunk, and lower extremities occurs in some cases after several years and can be exacerbated by stress, anger, or excitement. The typical rhythmic dysphonia of benign familial tremor, with a typical rhythmic quavering when speaking, is characteristic.[119] Other associated symptoms consist of migraine, which occurs in 20 percent of cases of benign familial tremor,[120] and episodic vertigo. The lower limbs and trunk are usually spared, but the hand tremor may become so intense on intention that it is a major disability.

Benign familial tremor is frequently misdiagnosed as Parkinson disease[121] and there is a high frequency of familial tremor among relatives of patients with Parkinson disease, suggesting some pathophysiological relationship between these two distinct conditions.[122] However, this may be no more than a chance relationship (Table 6-2).

The neurological examination is characterized by the presence of the tremor, which is accentuated by intention and demonstrated dramatically by lifting a cup or glass of water.

Diagnostic Procedures

1. The diagnosis depends on the history and the presence of typical tremor.
2. The workup should be minimal.[123]
3. Ballistic movements are associated with the triphasic pattern of agonist-antagonist-agonist muscle activity seen in normal subjects, measured by EMG with a significant delay in the second agonist activity.[124]

Table 6-2
Differential diagnosis of tremor

Tremor	Symptoms	Signs	Treatment
Benign (essential) also physiological	Occurs at rest or with movement Exacerbated by emotion	6 to 12 cps[a]—involves UE[b] and head	propranolol (Inderal) or metoprolol (Lopressor) diazepam (Valium) primidone (Mysoline) methazolamine (Neptazane)
Intention (action)	Increases with movement	3 to 5 cps—involves UE	propranolol (Inderal) diazepam (Valium)
Resting (Parkinson)	Present at rest Exacerbated by emotion	3 to 7 cps (typically 6)—involves extremities and head in characteristic "pill-rolling"	dopamine agonist (e.g., L-dopa, bromocriptine) anticholinergics
Metabolic	Symptoms of basic disorder	10 to 20 cps—involves UE[b] and head, signs of metabolic disorder (hyperthyroidism, liver disease, etc.)	Correct disturbed metabolic state
Alcohol withdrawal	Appears 8–12 h after last ingestion of alcohol	6 to 10 cps—involves extremities and head	chlordiazepoxide (Librium) diazepam (Valium) oxazepam (Serax)

[a] cps, cycles per second

[b] UE, upper extremities

Treatment

1. β-Adrenergic blockers. Propranolol (Inderal) 80 mg LA 1 every morning or 1 q12h is an effective treatment in many cases. Other β-adrenergic blockers are also effective, but this class of drug should not be used in asthmatics.

2. Primidone (Mysoline). Primidone 125 mg daily increasing to 250 mg q8h, if necessary, is almost as effective as propranolol and should be used in patients who cannot take β blockers.

3. Carbonic anhydrase inhibitors, including acetazolamide 25 to 50 mg, 1 q8h, are moderately effective in some cases.[125] Methazolamide is less effective.[126]

4. Benzodiazepines, including clonazepam or lorazepam, will reduce tremor but must be adminis-tered in a single small dose initially (0.5 mg p.o.) and gradually increased to avoid drowsiness.

5. Nimodipine 30 mg 1 q8h is effective in some, but not all, cases.[127]

6. Chronic electrical stimulation of the nucleus ventralis intermedius of the thalamus is well tolerated and effective but shows deterioration with time in about 20 percent of cases.[128]

7. Thalamotomy using a stereotactic technique can be performed with a high degree of safety and is of significant benefit in patients with benign familial tremor who have disabling tremor and who are refractory to medical treatment.[129]

8. Intermittent electrical stimulation of the medial caudate nucleus, using stereotactic placement of stimulating electrodes, is a most promising technique for control of this disorder.[130]

Involuntary Movements Complicating Neuroleptic Therapy

The neuroleptics (phenothiazines, butyrophenones and thioxanthenes, clozapine, and risperidone) are major tranquilizers that decrease muscle tone and diminish motor activity. Neuroleptics possess antipsychotic properties and the ability to produce adverse effects, probably due to blocking of some dopamine receptors in the CNS, increased sensitivity of nigrostriatal dopamine neurons, and the induction of glutaminergic activity, resulting in neurotoxic effects. One of these effects could be impairment of mitochondrial energy metabolism by inhibition of complex 1 of the electron transport chain.[131]

Several involuntary movement disorders can complicate neuroleptic therapy.

1.   Acute dystonic reaction. This is characterized by the sudden onset of dystonic movements of the face, torticollis, and tonic deviation of the eyes or opisthotonus after ingestion or injection of a neuroleptic such as prochlorperazine, a common practice in an emergency room setting to control vomiting. The condition is frequently misdiagnosed as a conversion (hysterical) reaction. Parenteral injection of benztropine (Cogentin) 2 mg or diphenhydramine (Benadryl) 25 mg produces dramatic response. However, the patient should be kept under observation for several hours because there is a risk of recurrence when the treatment can be repeated. The availability of nonneuroleptic agents for the treatment of vomiting (ondansetron-Zofran) obviates the need for injection of neuroleptics in such cases.[132]

In prospective long-term neuroleptic therapy, the concomitant use of benztropine orally significantly reduces the risk of an acute dystonic reaction.

2.   Parkinsonism. A gradual development of rigidity, tremor, and bradykinesis can occur beginning about 3 weeks following the introduction of neuroleptic therapy. Drug-induced parkinsonism occurs in 15 to 60 percent of neuroleptic-treated individuals, is common in elderly patients in whom there is a clear-cut, dose-induced response, and may persist when the neuroleptic is discontinued. This suggests that drug-induced parkinsonism occurs in individuals with a pre-existing nigrostriatal dopamine deficiency

(a preclinical Parkinson disease).[133] Nevertheless, it seems prudent to use the minimal effective dose of neuroleptic drugs, coupled with daily benztropine therapy to avoid or delay the onset of drug-induced parkinsonism when long-term neuroleptic therapy is contemplated.

3.   Akathisia. The patient with akathisia is usually under treatment for schizophrenia, is often young, and is receiving high doses of antipsychotic medication, often in the form of a deponeuroleptic. Akathisia presents with a characteristic inner restlessness associated with a compulsion to move, with an inability to sit still for more than a short period of time. This is associated with symptoms of dysphoria, including tension, panic, irritability, and impatience.[134] The presence of akathisia may be as high as 40 percent in patients treated with neuroleptics.[135]

Treatment should be directed toward lowering the dose of neuroleptic drugs. When symptoms persist, propranolol 40 to 120 mg/day is most likely to be effective. Anticholinergic drugs and benzodiazepines, singly or in combination, are a second choice.

Tardive Dyskinesia

Definition   Tardive dyskinesia consists of repetitive, involuntary movements of the mouth, lips, and tongue, occasionally accompanied by dystonic posturing or choreoathetotic movements of trunk and limbs.

Etiology   The etiology is not clear. As already discussed, the changes following introduction of neuroleptic therapy are complex and adverse effects may be solely the consequence of the antipsychotic drug therapy or may reflect an intrinsic predisposition to these events.[136]

Tardive dyskinesia is a syndrome. Most cases begin during the administration of neuroleptics and may become more evident when the medication is stopped. The syndrome is also seen following administration of metoclopramide, antihistamines, and tricyclic antidepressants and in chronic alcohol abuse. The risk of tardive dyskinesia is increased in neuroleptic-treated patients with diabetes mellitus and may be a feature of a degenerative brain disease, including Alzheimer disease and cerebrovascular disease.

Clinical Features Tardive dyskinesia is a late complication of neuroleptic therapy. Risk of persistent tardive dyskinesia is 4.8 percent after 1 year, 7.2 percent after 2 years, and 15.6 percent after 4 years. Poor response to treatment, high dose of neuroleptics, duration of therapy, advanced age, and female sex appear to increase the risk of developing tardive dyskinesia.[138]

The first indication is the appearance of brief repetitive movements of the lips and eyes. The fully developed syndrome consists of sucking movements, lip smacking, or sudden withdrawal of lips, exposing the teeth. The jaw may be retracted or moved laterally. The tongue is often thrust forward or rolled into the mouth. Each patient develops a stereotyped pattern sometimes accompanied by a grunting expiratory sound. The extremities and trunk are held in the dystonic posture or exhibit choreoathetoid movements. About one-third of the patients have features of parkinsonism. The onset may be accompanied by a depressive episode and some patients have a pseudodementia that resolves on withdrawal of neuroleptics. The course of tardive dyskinesia is variable but the condition is often not progressive.[139] Complications of tardive dyskinesia include:

1. The patient loses weight and becomes dehydrated because of inability to sustain nutrition.

2. Parkinsonism may restrict movements and the patient may become bedridden, with increased susceptibility to infection.

3. There is substantial impairment of speech with abnormalities of phonation, intelligibility, and rate of speech production.[140]

4. Jaw movements may become extremely painful. Dislocation has been reported.

5. Anticholinergic agents, alcohol, oxazepam, diazepam, and levodopa increase the movements of tardive dyskinesia.

6. A Tourette-like syndrome has been reported to occur concurrently with tardive dyskinesia, and the term tardive–Tourette-like syndrome has been used to describe this condition. The syndrome is treated as tardive dyskinesia.

7. Chronic oral or genital pain of sufficient magnitude to cause profound distress has been reported.[141]

Differential Diagnosis

1. Parkinson disease. Patients with Parkinson disease may have a head and neck tremor, and other signs of parkionsism are present. The dyskinesias accompanying Parkinson disease respond to changes in the dose of dopaminergic agents.

2. Essential tremor. A positive family history and improvement of the movements with alcohol or propranolol are typical.

3. Orofacial dyskinesia (Miege disease) is characterized by blepharospasm, photophobia, otomandibular dystonia, and exacerbation with physostigmine.

4. In palatal myoclonus, there are rhythmic movements of the palate and occasionally of the eyes and head, which respond to serotonergic agents and clonazepam.

5. Choreiform movements of the face can occur in Huntington disease, Sydenham chorea, Wilson disease, and with the use of carbamazepine (Tegretol), phenytoin (Dilantin), ethosuximide (Zarontin), dopaminergic drugs, and imipramine (Tofranil).

6. Dyskinesias of the head may occur with cerebellar or labyrinthine disease.

7. In hemifacial spasm, only one-half of the face is involved.

8. Facial tics are essentially repetitive and stereotyped movements.

Treatment

1. Agents that block dopamine receptors (dopamine antagonists) are effective in some cases. Haloperidol (Haldol) 1 mg daily, increasing to 2 mg q8h, may be effective, although the effect is often temporary.

2. Catecholamine-depleting agents (reserpine, tetrabenazine) are also temporarily effective. Reserpine may cause severe depression.

3. Baclofen 20 to 80 mg/day. This gaba-mimetic has been used with success in the treatment of tardive dyskinesia.

4. Calcium channel blocking agents, including verapamil 80 mg q6h or 240 mg SR, or nifedipine are potentially useful in the treatment of tardive dyskinesia[142] because they influence the release of dopamine in the basal ganglia.

5. Antiserotonergic agents such as cyproheptadine and some of the tricyclic antidepressants have been reported to be effective.

6. Other drugs, including α-methyldopa (Aldomet), α-methyl-para-tyrosine, oxiperomide, sulpiride, divalproex sodium (Depakote), and apomorphine may produce some improvement in particularly difficult cases.

7. Vitamin E significantly reduces the dystonic movements of tardive dyskinesia.[143]

8. Chronic pain responds to the catecholamine-depleting agents, reserpine, or tetrabenazine.

Prognosis Many drugs are temporarily effective in tardive dyskinesia. Improved control may be obtained by regularly changing medication known to produce temporary benefits in a particular patient. Some cases show resolution after withdrawal of neuroleptic drugs. In others, symptoms increase or remain unchanged for many months and then subside, indicating that tardive dyskinesia is often reversible.[144] However, a few patients show indefinite continuation of involuntary movements.

Tardive Dystonia

Definition Tardive dystonia is a late-onset complication of neuroleptic treatment, occurring in approximately 2 percent of patients in the course of treatment with neuroleptic medication, and is characterized by sustained muscle contraction, producing abnormal posture.

Etiology and Pathology Etiology is unknown. Tardive dystonia is believed to be the result of bilateral pathological changes in the basal ganglia which,

together with neuroleptics, represent predisposing factors for the development of tardive dystonia.[145] The fundamental abnormality appears to be the repetitive stimulation of D_1 dopamine receptors by endogenous dopamine, resulting in increased sensitivity of D_1 dopamine receptor-mediated output in the presence of D_2 receptor blockage by neuroleptics, which have a high affinity for D_2 receptors.

Clinical Features Tardive dystonia may be focal, segmental or, rarely, generalized and consists of prolonged, often painful contraction of muscles. The condition usually starts by affecting the face and neck muscles and then progresses to other muscle groups. The limbs are held in prolonged dystonic posture or the trunk displaced in an abnormal dystonic fashion. Inequality in dystonic contraction of the neck muscles produces a condition resembling spasmodic torticollis,[146] whereas oculofacial muscle involvement results in blepharospasm or oculogyric crises.[147] A combination of tardive dystonia and tardive dyskinesia is encountered occasionally and tardive dystonia-tardive dyskinesia can be accompanied by akathisia, tremor, chorea, or myoclonus.[148]

Treatment

1. Neuroleptic medication should be stopped, if possible, or changed to a less potent D_2 receptor-blocking agent.
2. Clozapine alone[149] or in combination with clonazepam is effective in many cases.[150]
3. Verapamil beginning with 240 SR can be effective, particularly in myoclonic tardive dystonia when other medications fail.[151]
4. Baclofen 40 to 180 mg q.d. will occasionally result in improvement of dystonia.[152]
5. Injections of botulinum toxin can produce improvement in focal tardive dystonia, particularly where there are spasmodic torticollis-like changes or hemifacial spasm and blepharospasm.[153]

Prognosis Many drugs are temporarily effective. The combination of clozapine and clonazepam appears to give more persistent results in this disorder.[154]

Neuroleptic Malignant Syndrome

Definition This syndrome is an acute idiosyncratic reaction to neuroleptic medication, owing to a central dopamine receptor blockade.[155]

Etiology and Pathology Neuroleptic malignant syndrome follows a diffuse dopamine receptor blockade in the CNS, producing an acute reduction in brain dopamine activity.[156]

Clinical Features Neuroleptic malignant syndrome is usually associated with the use of haloperidol but may follow introduction of any neuroleptic drug, including long-acting preparations such as fluphenazine. Most cases develop within 10 days of starting therapy, but the syndrome can occur at any time during a course of treatment, particularly following an increase in drug dosage. Although usually described as a complication of neuroleptic therapy, neuroleptic malignant syndrome is related to non-neuroleptic drugs including metoclopramide,[157] domperidone,[158] amphetamines, reserpine, tetrabenazine, tricyclic antidepressants with lithium or with an MAO inhibitor, and withdrawal of antiparkinsonian medication. Neuroleptic malignant syndrome has also been associated with the use of cocaine[159] and 3.4 methylene dioxymethamphetamine (MDMA), known as "Ecstasy."[160] Symptoms are usually abrupt in onset and consist of fever, encephalopathy with fluctuating confusion and agitation progressing to coma, a labile blood pressure, tachycardia, diaphoresis in association with dystonia, and generalized tremor. Examination shows severe generalized muscle rigidity that can produce pain in some cases, with sufficient muscle damage to produce rhabdomyolysis, myoglobinuria, and renal failure. Occasionally, the onset begins with dystonia, tremor, gaze palsy, or forced deviation of the eyes preceding fever. The course is often rapid in untreated cases, with deterioration leading to cardiac failure, pulmonary congestion, pneumonia, renal failure, and death.

Diagnostic Procedures

1. There is no specific test for neuroleptic malignant syndrome.

2. Creatinine kinase often shows marked elevation.
3. The complete blood count shows an elevated white cell count.
4. Decreased serum iron levels have been reported.

Differential Diagnosis

1. Other causes of fever should be considered.
2. Hypothalamic tumors or viral encephalitis can disturb temperature regulation.
3. Catatonia usually presents with psychotic behavior preceding the catatonic state.
4. Malignant hyperthermia, a genetically determined condition, occurs shortly after the use of general anesthesia. The condition is not associated with encephalopathy and autonomic disturbance.

Treatment

1. Discontinue the neuroleptic drug. Long-acting depo-injectible neuroleptics can be a problem.
2. Reduce body temperature using cooling blankets and ice water enemas.
3. Monitor the blood pressure, urinary output, electrolytes, and temperature change.
4. Administer bromocriptine 75 to 100 mg/day by nasogastric tube.
5. Give dantrolene sodium intravenously 0.25 mg/kg q12h and convert to oral dantrolene as improvement occurs.[161]

Prognosis The outlook is good, provided that the condition is recognized and treated promptly. The outcome is usually successful with awareness of the syndrome, prompt diagnosis, and treatment in an intensive care setting.

The Rabbit Syndrome

This late and uncommon complication of neuroleptic therapy consists of orofacial movements producing a regular, rhythmic pouting of the lips, accentuated by finger tapping just above the upper limb. The tongue is not involved.[162] The condition can be associated with drug-induced parkinsonism due to the use of neuroleptics and has been reported following treatment with tricyclic antidepressants[163] or occasionally occur spontaneously.[164]

Treatment Anticholinergic medication such as trihexyphenidyl relieves the symptoms of the rabbit syndrome in most cases.[165]

Parkinsonism

Definition Parkinsonism is a syndromic neurodegenerative disorder characterized by rigidity, tremors, bradykinesis, and impaired postural reflexes. The most common form of parkinsonism is Parkinson disease (paralysis agitans), but parkinsonism is seen in a variety of disorders.

1. Parkinson disease (paralysis agitans).
2. Postencephalitic parkinsonism.
3. Arteriosclerotic parkinsonism.
4. Drug-induced parkinsonism.
5. Parkinsonism secondary to infectious diseases.
6. Toxic parkinsonism following exposure to manganese, carbon monoxide, or carbon disulfide.
7. Parkinsonism following anoxic encephalopathy.
8. Post-traumatic parkinsonism following closed head injury.
9. Parkinsonian features in Alzheimer disease and other chronic neurological degenerative disorders.

The signs and symptoms of parkinsonism are related to a reduction in the activity of the neurotransmitter dopamine in the basal ganglion. There may be a failure of production of dopamine in the pars compacta of the substantia nigra, a failure of axonal transmission along the axons of the nigrostriatal pathway, a failure to release dopamine at the axonal terminals, or a failure of uptake of dopamine by dopamine receptors in the basal ganglia. The failure of the dopaminergic nigrostriatal system results in a relative overactivity of other receptor-dependent systems in the basal ganglia. This imbalance influences other portions of the brain via the thalamus and thalamic connections. The ultimate effect is felt at the level of the final common pathway of the motor system, the anterior horn cell, where there are two basic defects:

1. Increased inhibition of the gamma motor neuron.
2. Increased alpha motor neuron activity.

The cardinal symptoms of parkinsonism (i.e., tremor, rigidity, bradykinesis, and impaired postural reflexes) may be experienced as follows:

1. Tremor is the result of inhibition of gamma motor neuron activity. This inhibition leads to loss of gamma circuit sensitivity resulting in a decrease in the fine control of motor movement. This lack of control permits the appearance of involuntary movements generated at other levels in the CNS. The tremor of parkinsonism is probably initiated by rhythmic discharges of the alpha motor neurons under the influence of impulses generated in the ventrolateral nucleus of the thalamus. This activity is normally suppressed by action of the gamma motor neuron circuit but can appear as tremor when the circuit is inhibited.

2. Rigidity is due to increased tone in both antagonists and protagonists, and there appears to be a failure of inhibition of motor neuron activity in both protagonists and antagonists during movement. The increased alpha motor neuron activity in both protagonists and antagonists results in rigidity, which is present throughout the full range of movement in the affected limb.

3. Bradykinesis is the end result of a disorder of integration of optic labyrinthine proprioceptive and other sensory impulses in the basal ganglia. This results in an alteration in reflex activity influencing the gamma and alpha motor neurons.

4. Impaired postural reflexes are the result of a failure of integration of proprioceptive, labyrinthine and, to a lesser extent, optic impulses at the level of the thalamus and basal ganglia, which disturbs the awareness of body position in space.

Parkinson Disease (Paralysis Agitans)

Etiology and Pathology The etiology is unknown. A number of possible factors must be considered.[166]

1. The evidence for genetic risk factors in Parkinson disease is weak. Familial Parkinson disease is rare and monozygotic and dizygotic twin studies do not indicate a genetic component in the nonfamilial form of this disease.[167]

2. Toxic changes to nigrostriatal neurons is a possible factor in Parkinson disease, given the established development of parkinsonism following exposure to exogenous toxins such as 1-methyl-4-phenyl-1236-tetrahydropyridine (MPTP),[168] manganese,[169] tetrahydroisoquinolone (TIQ),[170] and carbon monoxide. Toxic exposure to unknown toxins possibly occurs in rural living, drinking well water, farming and herbicide or pesticide exposure,[171] and industrial chemical exposure.[172]

3. A number of infections have been associated with parkinsonism. The list includes encephalitis lethargica, a putative viral infection, which was recognized in the second decade of this century and disappeared in the late 1920s. The main interest in this disease was the long latent period from acute infection to the appearance of symptoms of parkinsonism, in some cases years or decades later. Several other putative infections include influenza, syphilis, nocardia asteroides, herpes simplex, eastern equine and Japanese B encephalitis. In all cases, the resulting parkinsonism differs from Parkinson disease, but the long latent period in encephalitis lethargica suggests that infection leading to premature death of neurons in the substantia nigra, coupled with natural attrition of these cells, could impose a limit on production of dopamine and ultimately the appearance of clinical parkinsonism. A similar mechanism could occur in Parkinson disease.

4. Closed head injury is occasionally followed by signs of parkinsonism. This association is well documented in boxers who suffer repeated trauma to the head, with the signs of parkinsonism developing many years later.[173] A similar course has been described after anoxic encephalopathy.[174] This delayed appearance of parkinsonism probably has the same explanation as the delayed appearance in encephalitis lethargica.

5. There is a normal age-related loss of dopaminergic neurons in all individuals, which amounts to about 35 percent over a typical human life span.[175] This loss is presumably insufficient to reduce synthesis of dopamine below the critical level, which results in symptoms of Parkinson disease. However, there may be a genetic predisposition to accelerate neuronal loss in the substantia nigra or the process could be accelerated by factors such as infection, trauma, or toxins or the production of free radicals. The latter is currently the preferred hypothesis regarding the pathogenesis of Parkinson disease at this time.

6. Free radicals in neuronal degeneration. A free radical is an atom or molecule with an unpaired orbiting electron, making it unstable and extremely reactive. Free radicals are a normal product of all cells, which are protected by oxyradical scavenger enzymes. The production of free radicals is accelerated in the dopamine-containing cells of the substantia nigra, which contain high concentrations of neuromelanin[176] and iron. The iron is buffered by increased levels of the iron-binding protein, ferritin.[177] A failure to buffer iron by ferritin allows neuromelanin, which has the capacity to bind free iron, to provide an electron to convert the iron to its ferrous state. At the same time, the metabolism of dopamine results in the production of hydrogen peroxide, which is normally cleared by oxyradical scavenger enzymes. However, excessive production of hydrogen peroxide may exceed clearance mechanisms and react with ferrous iron to form the hydroxyl radical, which is cytotoxic.

Although a definite etiology has not been established in Parkinson disease, the most likely explanation is that the disease results from a combination of accelerated aging, genetic predisposition, exposure to toxins, and an abnormality in oxidative mechanisms.[178]

Pathological changes are stereotyped. Sections of the midbrain show marked diminution or absence of melanin in the area of the substantia nigra. Microscopic examination reveals a loss of neurons in the zona compacta; the surviving neurons are abnormal and contain intracytoplasmic hyalin inclusions (Lewy bodies). Pathological changes are not confined to the substantia nigra. There is a diffuse neuronal loss involving the whole of the brain and brainstem, with particular involvement of the cerebral cortex, basal ganglia, thalamus, oculomotor nuclei, locus coeruleus, and dorsal motor nucleus of the vagus.

Clinical Features Parkinson disease usually occurs in middle-aged or elderly individuals, although 5 percent report an onset of symptoms before age 40 years.[179]

1. The tremor of Parkinson's disease often appears unilaterally and may be confined to one upper limb for months or even years. The tremor of 4 to 5 Hz is first seen in the fingers and thumb, and there may be a characteristic apposition of forefinger and thumb producing the so-called pill-rolling tremor. The tremor eventually spreads to involve the entire affected limb and appears in the opposite limb. In severe cases, the tremor involves all four limbs, the head and neck producing titubation, and the facial musculature, tongue, and jaw. The tremor is markedly increased by tension or exertion and disappears during sleep.

2. Rigidity is an increased response to muscle stretch that appears in both antagonists and agonists. Both muscle groups contract and their tendons may be visible during movement. The muscles contract without recruitment during passive movement so that the activation of one motor unit is associated with the deactivation of another, maintaining uniform tension in the muscle. Rigidity usually appears unilaterally and proximally in an upper limb, spreading later to involve all of the muscles of that limb and eventually the opposite side and muscles of the neck and trunk. One of the earliest signs of rigidity is loss of associated movements of an arm when walking. More advanced cases show extension of the wrist, flexion of the metacarpal phalangeal joints, and hyperextension of the interphalangeal joints.

3. The bradykinesis of Parkinson disease is not related to rigidity and is probably the result of biochemical dysfunction of the basal ganglia. There is a decrease in inhibitory dopaminergic stimulation of neurons in the globus pallidus, which results in increased inhibitions of neurons in the ventrolateral nucleus of the thalamus. This, in turn, results in loss of stimulation of the neurons of the motor cortex, leading to bradykinesis. The patient shows loss of facial expression, slowing of lip and tongue movements during talking, loss of fine movements in writing and handling small objects, and difficulty in rising from a chair and initiating gait.

4. Most patients with Parkinson disease experience weakness and easy fatigue once the disease becomes generalized. This compounds bradykinesis and increases immobility. Fatigue correlates with depression but not with disease severity, and many nondepressed patients have significant complaints of fatigue.[180]

5. Although dystonia is frequently encountered as a complication of therapy (end-of-dose dystonia) and reflects a reduction in dopaminergic stimulation by decreasing circulating drug levels,[181] dystonic postures may be seen in hands and feet in the early cases of Parkinson disease, before the diagnosis is established.[182] Dystonia does not negate the diagnosis of Parkinson disease.[183]

6. The typical facial appearance of patients with idiopathic parkinsonism is caused by bradykinesis. The face is "masklike" with infrequent blinking and lack of expression. In addition, there is a somewhat "greasy" appearance to the skin of the face and occasional drooling due to loss of the swallowing movements that normally dispose of saliva.

7. Micrographia, or the gradual development of the small, cramped writing, is characteristic of Parkinson disease when the dominant hand is involved. This is the first symptom in some cases.

8. Festinant gait. Bradykinesis results in the typical small steps seen in Parkinson disease. In the fully developed state, the patient has a flexed posture with the head flexed on the chest, the shoulders bent forward, the back arched forward, and the arms held immobile at the sides when walking. Muscle rigidity prevents rapid compensation for loss of balance, and many patients show propulsion, an "inability to catch up with their center of gravity," and quicken their pace if propelled forward. This may result in a fall. Similarly, if suddenly unbalanced, the patient may display lateropulsion or retropulsion and eventually fall. Serious injury can occur in these falls.

9. Freezing is seen in more advanced cases of Parkinson disease when the patient will suddenly stop and have trouble resuming walking. This is particularly troublesome when walking through a confined space such as a doorway or in turning.

10. Rigidity and bradykinesis of the respiratory muscles, vocal cords, pharyngeal muscles, tongue, and lips results in the slow, monotonous speech of poor volume so characteristic of patients with Parkinson disease. In some cases, the voice is reduced to a slowed whisper.

11. The established parkinsonian patient shows infrequent blinking, impaired upward gaze, poor convergence, and defective voluntary and following eye movements, which are saccadic in quality. An exaggerated blink reflex (glabellar reflex) can be obtained by rhythmic percussion of the forehead just above the root of the nose.

12. Many patients with Parkinson disease experience discomfort or actual pain, which is usually poorly localized but may be cramplike and situated in either the axial muscles or the limbs. Some patients experience paresthesias in the extremities.

13. Autonomic nervous system disorders occur frequently in Parkinson disease, the result of progressive loss of neurons in central and peripheral autonomic centers involved in sympathetic and parasympathetic activity. This basic problem may be compounded by other factors, including the effect of aging, medication, and the presence of other chronic diseases such as diabetes mellitus and diabetic peripheral neuropathy. The most disabling autonomic disturbance is orthostatic hypotension, which tends to be a problem in advanced cases. Urinary tract dysfunction, with urgency, frequency, nocturia, and incontinence, is present in a significant number of elderly patients. Retention can occur, usually the result of a concomitant bladder outlet obstruction.

Constipation is a common complaint, secondary to autonomic dysfunction and impaired intestinal motility. This may be compounded by medication used in the treatment of Parkinson disease.

Sexual dysfunction, manifested by erectile difficulties and ejaculatory disturbances in the male and vaginismus and anorgasmia in the female, occur in more than 50 percent of patients with mild to moderate Parkinson disease. Other problems include lack of desire and arousal, leading to a decrease in sexual frequency. Many factors are involved in addition to autonomic dysfunction, including bradykinesis, rigidity, dyskinesias, drooling, anxiety, and depression. Antiparkinsonian drugs may cause hypo- and occasionally hypersexuality. Concomitant use of propranolol, clonidine, the thiazides, benzodiazepines, digoxin, and serotonin uptake inhibitors, can alter sexual functioning adversely.[184]

Thermal regulation abnormalities are a feature of advanced Parkinson disease and are enhanced by medication. The most common complaint is periodic hyperhidrosis, often associated with hypertension, tachycardia, and flushing. Hypothermia has been observed in some patients.

Seborrhea of the scalp, face, nasolabial folds, eyebrows, the external auditory meatus, retroauricular areas, and presternal regions is a problem in longstanding generalized Parkinson disease, often associated with seborrheic dermatitis of the axillae and inguinal areas.

14. Many patients develop an impairment of involuntary swallowing mechanisms. Salivary secretions accumulate in the mouth and pharynx, resulting in troublesome drooling in some cases.

15. Orthostatic hypotension is often a feature of advanced Parkinson disease and may be enhanced by drug therapy.

16. Depression may further impede the restricted activities of the patient with Parkinson disease. Significant depression occurs in at least 40 percent of cases and should be recognized and treated.[185] Referral to a psychiatrist or psychologist is appropriate for patients with severe depression. Tricyclic antidepressants may enhance the effect of levodopa. Serotonin uptake inhibitors are effective in alleviating depression in most cases. Tricyclic antidepressants and serotonin uptake inhibitors should not be used in conjunction with selegiline.

17. Dysphagia (nonfluent swallowing movement) is common in patients with Parkinson disease. There is abnormal bolus formation, delayed swallowing reflex, vallecular stasis, and piriform sinus residue.[186] Some patients have tracheal aspiration, but there is little evidence of pulmonary aspiration, despite frequent choking.

18. Although visual acuity is not affected in Parkinson disease, contrast sensitivity, the minimal amount of contrast (light/dark) necessary to distinguish the presence of two objects, is impaired in advanced disease. This has practical implications in that a patient may not be able to identify two objects of similar color in juxtaposition to each other or may fail to identify an object in dim lighting. The impairment improves with levodopa or dopamine receptor agonist therapy.[187]

19. There is generalized neuronal loss in Parkinson disease and 50 percent of patients show a progressive dementia. This may be associated with delusions and visual or auditory hallucinations. Dementia may antedate Parkinson disease by months or years in some cases. There are similarities in cognitive dysfunction in patients with frontal lobe lesions and Parkinson disease. Both have a disturbance in the frontal regulation of attentional processes. A degeneration of the dopaminergic mesocortical innervation of the frontal cortex in Parkinson disease is a possible neurochemical substrate of frontal attention disturbances.[188]

Diagnostic Procedures The history and physical examination are diagnostic and few tests are needed after the full initial clinical evaluation. At each office visit, the patient should have:

1. Blood pressure recorded lying and standing to detect orthostatic hypotension, which may be aggravated by medication.
2. Assessment of response to stress because patients may appear to respond well to treatment until they are subjected to mild stress. The patient should be given a simple task such as standing with the arms extended, asked to open and close the fingers rapidly on one side and at the same time, count back from 100. This stress is usually sufficient to produce increased tremor or rigidity in the other limb when the patient is not fully responding to medication.
3. Measurement of functional activity. The patient should be asked to write his or her name and the date on the top of a large sheet of paper. This should be followed by writing a simple sentence

and drawing concentric circles with both the right and left hand. This record should be attached to the patient's clinical notes and is a graphic measurement of functional activity, which can be compared at each visit.

4. Optional studies:
   a. EEG may show progressive slowing of background activity in serial recordings.
   b. MRI or CT scanning will show diffuse cortical atrophy with widening of the sulci and hydrocephalus ex vacuo in advanced cases.
   c. Serial neuropsychological testing will indicate a progressive loss of cognitive and intellectual functioning over a period of several years.

Treatment See page 182.

Prognosis Although there has been marked improvement in the survival of patients with Parkinson disease following the introduction of levodopa, the disease does significantly reduce life span in most patients who have developed the generalized form of the disease in their fifties or sixties. Because there is a progressive neuronal loss, the condition continues to progress, despite response to medication. Ultimately the effect of medication decreases and the patient deteriorates, becomes bedridden, and dies from intercurrent infection.

Postencephalitic Parkinsonism

Definition Postencephalitic parkinsonism was first described during the epidemic of encephalitis lethargica from 1917 to 1928. Encephalitis lethargica (Von Economo) was a putative viral encephalitis of worldwide distribution. Some cases of parkinsonism were parainfectious. The majority were postinfectious with an interval of many years or decades between infection and overt symptoms. The population with postencephalitic parkinsonism related to encephalitis lethargica has largely disappeared because of the passage of time. However, sporadic cases of postencephalitic parkinsonism still occur, owing mainly to the effects of viral encephalitis, such as herpes simplex encephalitis, eastern equine encephalitis, or Japanese B encephalitis.

Etiology and Pathology There is marked pallor of the substantia nigra and locus ceruleus corresponding to the severe loss of neurons in these structures. Surviving neurons show Alzheimer neurofibrillary tangles. Neuronal loss and the fibrillary changes are also seen in the basal ganglia and hypothalamus.

Clinical Features Patients show the tremor, rigidity, and bradykinesis of parkinsonism with additional features that include:

1. Changes in mentation, including hallucinations, psychoses, and dementia.
2. Oculogyric crises—tonic deviation of the eyes, usually in a vertical plane, lasting from several minutes to an hour or more.
3. Smooth conjugate eye movements are replaced by coarse saccadic eye movements.
4. Blepharospasm or lid retraction.
5. Nystagmus.
6. Cranial nerve palsy.
7. Irregular respiratory movements.
8. Autonomic disturbances, including excessive perspiration, excessive salivation with drooling, disturbances of bladder function, and postural hypotension.

Diagnostic Procedures

1. On EEG, there is a reduction of background alpha activity and gradual replacement with slower frequencies recorded symmetrically from both hemispheres.
2. The MRI or CT scans show ventricular dilatation and diffuse brain atrophy in advanced cases.
3. Serial neuropsychological testing indicates a progressive loss of intellectual functioning over a period of several years.

Treatment See page 182.

Prognosis Postencephalitic parkinsonism is a slowly progressive condition that results in total disability and considerable reduction of life span in many cases. Death usually occurs from intercurrent infection.

Arteriosclerotic Parkinsonism

Etiology and Pathology Arteriosclerotic parkinsonism is due to infarction of the brain, which damages the substantia nigra, the nigrostriatal pathways, or the basal ganglia, producing disruption of dopaminergic systems in the brain.

The brain shows gross evidence of atrophy and numerous lacunar infarcts in the brainstem and basal ganglia. Large areas of infarction may be present in one or both hemispheres.

Clinical Features Patients show the tremor, rigidity, and bradykinesis of parkinsonism with additional features including:

1. History of repeated transient ischemic attacks or minor strokes.
2. History and physical findings compatible with one or more episodes of infarction.
3. Dementia.
4. Pseudobulbar emotional response, usually pseudobulbar crying, indicating bilateral involvement of the brain.

Diagnostic Procedures The metabolic, cardiac, and cerebral abnormalities of ischemic cerebrovascular disease can be demonstrated (see page 182).

Treatment The treatment is a combination of treatment for Parkinson disease and ischemic cerebrovascular disease.

Prognosis Prognosis is poor because there is a high risk of further episodes of cerebral infarction and a high risk of myocardial infarction.

Drug-Induced Parkinsonism

The blocking of dopamine receptors by drugs—predominantly phenothiazines, butyrophenones, or thioxanthenes, or by metoclopramide—results in rigidity, masklike facies, bradykinesis and, less frequently, parkinsonian tremor. Dopaminergic drugs and dopamine agonists are not effective treatments because the receptor sites are blocked. Anticholinergic drugs alleviate some symptoms by suppression of the uninhibited central cholinergic system. Symptoms of parkinsonism may completely disappear when the causative drug is withdrawn.

Parkinsonism Secondary to Infectious Diseases

Parkinsonian symptoms occasionally occur in patients recovering from viral encephalitis. Parkinsonian features have been described and treated in neurosyphilis, arrested tuberculosis, meningitis, sarcoidosis, and chronic meningoencephalitis due to fungi and yeasts.

Toxic Parkinsonism

Signs of parkinsonism, with rigidity and bradykinesis rather than tremor, can occur in susceptible individuals engaged in the mining, crushing, or smelting of manganese ores or exposed to manganese-containing fungicides.[189] Parkinsonian symptoms have occurred following recovery from carbon monoxide poisoning,[190] hypoxia, exposure to toxic solvents such as carbon disulfide,[191] ingestion or inhalation of cyanide,[192] ingestion of methanol,[193] and the injection of MTPT, a toxic by-product of the illicit synthesis of meperidine. The latter preparation is in itself nontoxic, but upon crossing the blood–brain barrier, it is converted into MPP^+, which accumulates in mitochondria, interfering with mitochondrial metabolism and ultimately producing cell death.[194]

Parkinsonian Features in Chronic Neurological Conditions

Parkinsonism can occur in any degenerative condition that is associated with neuronal loss in the substantia nigra and impairment of nigrostriatal function. Parkinsonian features are not unusual in Alzheimer disease, which is often misdiagnosed as Parkinson disease. Other conditions that often show the rigidity and bradykinesis of parkinsonism during the course of the disease include Huntington disease, Wilson disease, multisystem atrophy, particularly olivopontocerebellar degeneration, progressive supranuclear

palsy, Creutzfeldt-Jakob disease, and the parkinsonian-dementia complex.

Treatment of Parkinson Disease and Parkinsonism Parkinsonism may be regarded as a condition in which there is a relative insufficiency of dopamine in the CNS. The five dopamine receptors are grouped into type 1-like receptors (D_1 and D_5) and type 2-like receptors (D_2, D_3, and D_4). Dopamine produces inhibition of the D_1 receptor neurons and stimulation of the D_2 receptor neurons. Under normal conditions, there is a balance of activity in D_1 and D_2 pathways in the striatum, with the inhibitory D_1 pathway projecting to the globus pallidus and inhibiting the efferent projection from the globus pallidus to the thalamus. The D_2 pathway, however, stimulates the inhibitory efferent projections from the globus pallidus to the thalamus. This pallidothalamic pathway has an inhibitory effect on thalamocortical drive, which is reduced when the D_1 pathway drive is decreased and D_2 pathway activity is increased.

Restoration of dopamine levels in the striatum in Parkinson disease should adjust the balance of D_1 and D_2 receptor activity and restore normal thalamocortical activity. Consequently, treatment of Parkinson disease by increasing dopamine levels in the basal ganglia has been the mainstay of modern therapy. However, dopamine is rapidly metabolized and does not cross the blood–brain barrier, but L-dopa has the property of entering the CNS where it is converted to dopamine, thus restoring function in the basal ganglia.

L-Dopa was introduced in the 1960s and was the first effective treatment for Parkinson disease. The drug was destroyed by peripherally acting dopadecarboxylase and less than 10 percent crossed the blood–brain barrier to enter the CNS, where it was converted to dopamine. Consequently, large oral doses were required to overcome the peripheral destruction of the drug and adverse effects, particularly vomiting, were frequent and distressing to patients with Parkinson disease. This effect was overcome with the introduction of carbidopa/levodopa (Sinemet).

The therapeutic effect of Sinemet is exactly the same as levodopa. However, carbidopa inhibits peripheral decarboxylation of levodopa to dopamine. Dopamine and carbidopa do not cross the blood–brain barrier. Therefore, more levodopa is available to cross the blood–brain barrier for conversion to dopamine in the brain.

1. Sinemet is available in a standard preparation of three strengths: 10/100, 25/100, 25/250, where the first number indicates carbidopa content and the second, levodopa content. This preparation is considered the most effective in the treatment of Parkinson disease.[195] A controlled-release preparation, Sinemet CR, is available as Sinemet CR 50/200 or 25/100. The use of sustained-release Sinemet is predicated on the hypothesis that continuous dopamine stimulation is superior to intermittent stimulation of receptors in the basal ganglia. However, starting L-dopa therapy with controlled-release medication does not appear to have any advantage over standard Sinemet therapy.[196]

   The initial dose of Sinemet 25/100 can be as low as 1 tablet q4h for three doses each day.[197] This is often effective in early cases of Parkinson disease because there is an uptake of exogenous dopamine into presynaptic dopamine storage sites, prolonging the effect of the last dose for several hours. The dose can be adjusted as the need for dopamine increases, by adding 1 tablet of Sinemet 10/100 at each dose. A similar increase can be made 7 days later if necessary. Ideally, the aim should be to achieve a state where there is minimal evidence of rigidity in the neck muscles, elicited by passive extension or flexion of the neck. The dose of Sinemet should be increased at 7-day intervals, with monitoring of the blood pressure sitting and standing, to avoid induction of orthostatic hypotension. When the dose is adjusted after the second increase, it is better to begin with the first dose of the day, with additional increments progressively throughout the day. This method allows early saturation of the peripheral dopa-decarboxylase and increases the effect of smaller doses of Sinemet later in the day. The effect of Sinemet can be prolonged by the use of a low-protein diet at breakfast and lunch.

If a decision is made to replace the standard Sinemet with the sustained-release preparation, it should be remembered that the bioavailability of the drug is diminished to 70 percent on replacing Sinemet with Sinemet CR.[198] Consequently, the calculated dose should be increased by 20 percent to achieve a similar therapeutic result.

Many patients will experience adverse effects during Sinemet therapy:

a. Nausea and vomiting tend to occur in the early stages of therapy and require lowering of the dose of Sinemet or prolonging the interval between an increase in dosage or both. Vomiting can be controlled by ondansetron (Zofran) 4 to 8 mg p.o., q12h or trimethobenzamide (Tigan) 250 mg p.o. with each dose of Sinemet.

b. Orthostatic hypotension is common. The blood pressure should be recorded supine and standing at each office visit.

c. Cardiac arrhythmias may occur. This complication is due to the β-adrenergic effect of dopamine on the conduction system of the heart and can be treated with β-adrenergic blocking agents such as propranolol.

d. Involuntary movements. About 80 percent of patients develop choreoathetosis after months or, in some cases, years of treatment. The patient may not notice mild movements, which are usually tolerated by the family. Severe movements can be reduced by lowering the dose of Sinemet and accepting some return of parkinsonian symptoms or by changing to a controlled-release preparation that maintains a less fluctuating level of serum L-dopa for a longer period of time. A combination of a lower dose of Sinemet CR and a receptor agonist[199] (bromocriptine, pergolide, or pramipexole) is a good alternative. Changing to small doses of Sinemet at frequent intervals, with the addition of selegiline, is also beneficial.[200]

e. "On-off" phenomenon. Some patients experience sudden changes from immobility to normal function or severe dyskinetic movements. This "on-off" phenomenon is often disabling and can be controlled by a low-protein diet at breakfast and lunch and a change to smaller, more frequent doses of Sinemet. The addition of selegiline or pramipexole monotherapy may be effective in some patients who are experiencing this unfortunate complication of therapy, and the drug may relieve the "on-off" phenomenon for a protracted period of time.

f. Psychoses and abnormal behavior. Mild symptoms of anxiety and agitation can occur during the induction period. The dose of Sinemet should be reduced to the minimum and increased slowly, that is, once a week in small increments. At the same time, the physician should encourage the patient to persist with the medication because rejection is rarely followed by acceptance in the future.

Hallucinations are quite common and are often more acceptable to the patient, who finds them pleasant, while the patient's family often finds the patient's hallucinations objectionable, if not humiliating. Mild, benign hallucinations should be accepted, however, rather than lowering the dose of Sinemet, which will result in an increase in parkinsonian symptoms.

More serious symptoms of psychoses, with paranoid delusions, loss of insight, poor judgment, and confusion about medication schedules or use are more likely to occur in patients who show dementia before starting treatment but are not necessarily restricted to Parkinson disease with dementia.

g. Sinemet may induce drowsiness or insomnia. A reversal of the sleep cycle can occur, with excessive sleeping during the day and insomnia at night. The urge to sleep after lunch is almost irresistible in many patients with advanced Parkinson disease.

h. The tendency for depression may be enhanced by Sinemet. The condition can be treated with antidepressant medications, however, it should be remembered that serotonin uptake inhibitors are effective but should not be used with selegiline or any MAO inhibitor.

i. Disturbances in walking. Hesitancy in initiation of walking or sudden immobility in a confined space such as a doorway (freezing) usually develops after prolonged Sinemet therapy. There is no response to changes in medication, and the patient must be told to initiate a step by counting when walking, marching (left-right-left-right), or stepping over an object or an imaginary object.

2. Bromocriptine is a dopamine D_2 receptor agonist and a D_1 receptor antagonist. It is indicated as adjunct therapy[201] when there is a poor or incomplete response to Sinemet therapy, unacceptable adverse effects, or severe dyskinesia or when there is a persistent "on-off" phenomenon on Sinemet therapy. It is preferred by some physicians to initiate therapy in early cases of mild Parkinson disease.[202] The initial dose is 1.25 mg daily, increasing by 1.25 mg every week until the patient experiences maximum benefit or unacceptable adverse effects. A low dose initially, followed by low-dose increments every week, reduces the risk of adverse effects and increases patient acceptance. There is usually a good response when the dosage exceeds 25 mg daily, but it may not be achieved until doses of 45 to 50 mg daily are administered. The adverse effects are the same as those for levodopa. When bromocriptine is added with the intention of replacing Sinemet, the Sinemet should be reduced as the bromocriptine is increased. It can be used with other antiparkinsonian drugs, including anticholinergics, selegiline, and amantadine. Bromocriptine should not be given to patients with severe dementia because of the risk of increasing confusion and agitation. Bromocriptine will increase orthostatic hypotension and may cause peripheral edema.

3. Pergolide mesylate is a potent dopamine receptor agonist, acting by stimulating both D_1 and D_2 receptor sites. Pergolide is used as an adjuvant to levodopa therapy after patients begin to develop dyskinesia and "on-off" fluctuations. Some centers advocate combination therapy at an early stage in the treatment of Parkinson disease, before the development of dyskinetic movements. Under these conditions, pergolide has distinct advantages over bromocriptine in that pergolide has a longer half life and fewer adverse effects than bromocriptine. The recommended treatment plan for patients receiving levodopa is as follows:

a. Change Sinemet CR 50/200 to 1 tablet at 0600, 1 tablet at 1100, ½ tablet at 1600, and ½ tablet at 2200 hours.

b. Begin pergolide 0.05 mg tablet, ½ at breakfast and ½ at lunch for 1 week.

c. During the second week, give 0.05-mg tablets, 1 at breakfast, lunch, and dinner.

d. During the third week, 0.05-mg tablets, 2 at breakfast, 2 at lunch, and 2 at dinner.

e. The fourth week, give 0.25-mg tablets, ½ at breakfast, ½ at lunch, and ½ at dinner.

f. In the fifth week, 0.25-mg tablets, 1 at breakfast, 1 at lunch, and 1 at dinner. Continue this dosage.

When changing from bromocriptine to pergolide a dosage ratio of 10:1 bromocriptine to pergolide, is recommended, and the change should be gradual. If the patient is also receiving Sinemet, the dose of Sinemet should be reduced during the change from bromocriptine to pergolide, then advanced to optimal control of symptoms.

Adverse effects of pergolide are not uncommon and include dyskinesia, dizziness, hallucinations, confusion, somnolence, insomnia, nausea, constipation, diarrhea, dyspepsia, and rhinitis. Some evidence indicates that dopamine agonists such as pergolide, although less effective than Sinemet, might have an important role in slowing the progression of Parkinson disease.[203]

4. Anticholinergic drugs act by inhibiting the cholinergic system in the basal ganglia. The cholinergic system is normally inhibited by the nigrostriatal dopaminergic system, but the lack of inhibitory input results in overactivity of the excitatory cholinergic system. Anticholinergic drugs are more effective in the treatment of parkinsonian tremor than rigidity or bradykinesis and may have an additive effect when taken concurrently with dopamine or dopamine agonists. Trihexyphenidyl (Artane) and benztropine (Cogentin) are used for the control of tremor and are the only drugs that are effective in drug-induced parkinsonism, which is the result of neuroleptics such as the phenothiazines or butyrophenones. The anticholinergic drugs do not usually show additional benefit when given more than three times a day.

Dry mouth, constipation, and urinary retention are the most common complications of the anticholinergic drugs. Impairment of memory, judgment, and insight can occur. Hallucinations may be troublesome, particularly in demented patients.

5. Amantadine increases dopamine release from presynaptic storage sites, blocks dopamine reuptake, and stimulates dopamine receptors. However, its therapeutic effect is weak, but it is a useful adjuvant and may produce additional improvement in patients who cannot tolerate high doses of Sinemet or dopamine receptor agonist medications.

Amantadine is available in capsules of 100 mg and the initial dose is 1 capsule q12h. Higher doses do not produce additional benefit. The adverse effects include livido reticularis and edema involving the lower extremities. Insomnia and vivid dreams or nightmares are occasionally troublesome. Severe psychiatric symptoms are unusual. Orthostatic hypotension, heart failure, and urinary retention are rare.

6. Selegiline (Eldepryl) (deprenyl) is an MAO type B inhibitor. MAO type B is mainly concentrated as an intracellular enzyme on the outer membrane of the mitochondria, where it functions in the catabolism of catecholamines, including dopamine. The blocking of this action by selegiline increases the concentration of dopamine and should be beneficial in decreasing the symptoms of Parkinson disease. However, the effect of selegiline is marginal therapeutically and at best, the drug serves an adjuvant role. The initial impression that selegiline was neuroprotective and delayed the progression of Parkinson disease is no longer universally accepted. Nevertheless, selegiline is believed to increase dopamine in the basal ganglia[204] and may have an antioxidant effect in the neurons of the striatum. The early use of selegiline 5 mg q12h delays the use of the levodopa and possibly slows progression of the disease.[205] Adverse effects are few, but there are occasional complaints of nausea, light-headedness, abdominal pain, and hallucinations, which require discontinuing selegiline therapy.

7. Pramipexole is a dopamine agonist acting as a full agonist of the D_2 receptor group with preferential affinity for the D_3 receptor. In addition, the drug

may have antioxidant properties, suggesting that pramipexole could be cytoprotective to dopamine neurons.[206] The drug has been safe and well tolerated when used as monotherapy in early Parkinson disease.[207] Pramipexole is also effective as adjuvant therapy, when combined with Sinemet in advanced Parkinson disease, when the dose of Sinemet can be reduced, resulting in delayed development of adverse effects. The titration schedule for pramipexole begins with 0.125 mg t.i.d., followed by an increase to 0.25 mg t.i.d. after 7 days. The dose is increased by 0.25 t.i.d. every 7 days to 1.5 mg t.i.d.—a total of 4.5 mg/day. Adverse effects of pramipexole therapy include somnolence, dizziness, nausea, musculoskeletal pains, dystonic movements, headache, constipation, insomnia, and fatigue. Most of these effects will resolve, given time. Consequently, the dose should not be increased until the patient is free from any of these symptoms.

8. The use of miscellaneous drugs in the treatment of Parkinson disease:
   a. Apomorphine has a limited role in the treatment of Parkinson disease. This drug, which is a mixed D_1 and D_2 type dopamine receptor agonist, needs to be administered by subcutaneous injection or through sublingual, intranasal, or rectal routes. The use of apomorphine should be restricted to patients who have unpredictable "on-off" periods during therapy with other antiparkinsonism medications. Continuous apomorphine infusions through portable minipumps have been used in a limited fashion. Vomiting is a problem and can be controlled by domperidone 20 mg q8h. Inflammatory responses may develop at subcutaneous injection sites.
   b. Peripheral L-dopa metabolism is through two pathways: the first, dopa-decarboxylase, is inhibited by the dopa-decarboxylase inhibitor in Sinemet. The alternative route for metabolism of L-dopa is via catechol-0-methyltransferase, COMT. Consequently, inhibitors of COMT have a potential role in the therapy of Parkinson disease, in that they should increase availability of levodopa to the brain and reduce the need for L-dopa-containing medication. Tol-

capone 100 to 200 mg q8h is a COMT inhibitor with significant effect in inhibiting the peripheral breakdown of L-dopa and increasing the concentration of L-dopa, which crosses the blood–brain barrier resulting in higher concentrations of dopamine in the brain. A reduction in carbidopa/levodopa dosage may be necessary to prevent the development of involuntary dystonic movements.

Complications of Parkinson Disease and Therapy

1. Autonomic dysfunction
   a. Orthostatic hypotension. Autonomic nervous system disorders occur frequently in Parkinson disease, the result of progressive loss of neurons in central and peripheral autonomic centers involved in sympathetic and parasympathetic activity. This basic problem may be compounded by other factors, including the effect of aging, medication, and the presence of other chronic diseases such as diabetes mellitus and diabetic peripheral neuropathy. The most disabling autonomic disturbance is orthostatic hypotension, which tends to be a problem in advanced cases. Sinemet and dopamine receptor agonists exacerbate orthostatic hypotension in Parkinson disease. The first step in such cases is to withdraw any antihypertensive drugs that may have been taken for many years and are no longer necessary. Salt intake should be increased and the patient instructed to use thigh high elastic stockings or wear a leotard. Fludrocortisone 0.1 mg every morning, increasing to q8h if necessary, increases circulating blood volume, but patients should be monitored for supine hypertension and congestive heart failure. Indomethacin 25 mg q8h p.o., which inhibits vasodilating prostaglandins, is also effective. Sympathomimetics, including ephedrine or phenylpropanolamine or clonidine, may also be of benefit in countering orthostatic hypotension.
   b. Urinary tract dysfunction. Urgency, frequency, nocturia, and incontinence are present in a sig-

nificant number of elderly patients and may respond to medications such as oxybutynin (Ditropan) 5 mg q.h.s., tolterodine tartrate (Detrol) 2mg q12h, or dicyclomine (Bentyl) 10 mg q8h. Persistence of symptoms, retention, or suspicion of bladder outlet obstruction warrant a full urologic evaluation.

c. Constipation is a common complaint secondary to autonomic dysfunction and impaired intestinal mobility. This may be compounded by medication used in Parkinson disease. Constipation should be treated with a program of regular bowel movement each morning after breakfast. A high-fiber diet and exercise are recommended. Stool softeners such as sodium docusate 100 mg q12h or Milk of Magnesia 30 mL q.h.s. are often effective. Enemas may be necessary twice a week. Delayed gastric emptying often responds to cisapride 20 mg t.i.d. before meals.

d. Sexual dysfunction, manifested by erectile difficulties and ejaculatory disturbances in the male and vaginismus and anorgasmia in the female, occur in more than 50 percent of patients with mild to moderate Parkinson disease. Other problems include lack of desire and arousal, leading to a decrease in sexual frequency. Many factors are involved in addition to autonomic dysfunction, including bradykinesia, rigidity, dyskinesias, drooling, anxiety, and depression. Antiparkinsonian drugs may cause hypo- and occasionally hypersexuality. Concomitant use of propranolol, clonidine, thiazides, benzodiazepines, digoxin, and serotonin uptake inhibitors can alter sexual functioning adversely.[208]

Treatment of sexual dysfunction requires identification of the cause. Depression may respond to a serotonin uptake inhibitor (not to be given with selegiline) or other antidepressant medication. Referral to a sex therapist or a urologist specializing in male sexual dysfunction may be necessary.

2. Thermoregulation abnormalities are a feature of advanced Parkinson disease and are enhanced by medication. The most common complaint is periodic hyperhidrosis, often associated with hypertension, tachycardia, and flushing. Hypothermia has been observed in some patients.

Profound sweating may accompany end-of-dose "off" phenomenon, due to excessive sympathetic stimulation of sweat glands. There is usually a good response to β-adrenergic blocking agents such as propranolol. Reduction of Sinemet dosage and substitution of a dopamine receptor agonist is beneficial.

3. Dysphagia. Nonfluent swallowing movements are common in Parkinson disease. There is abnormal bolus formation, a delayed swallowing reflex, follicular stasis, and piriform sinus residue.[209] Some patients have tracheal aspiration, but there is little evidence of pulmonary aspiration, despite frequent choking. The use of a soft diet is advised because this allows easier movement of food from the mouth to the esophagus. Liquids are often the cause of aspiration and can be thickened, which may take care of this problem. Meals should always be taken when the patient is receiving benefit from medication, rather than during "off" times.

4. Sialorrhea. Drooling of saliva is a frequent accompaniment of advanced Parkinson disease and distressing both to patient and family. The addition of anticholinergic drugs may lead to a smaller volume of saliva and is helpful under such circumstances.

5. Although visual acuity is not affected in Parkinson disease, contrast sensitivity—the minimal amount of contrast (light/dark) necessary to distinguish the presence of two objects—is impaired in advanced cases. This has practical implications, in that a patient may not be able to identify two objects of similar color in juxtaposition to each other or may fail to identify an object in dim lighting. The impairment improves with levodopa or dopamine agonist therapy.[210]

6. Parkinson disease is not a painless condition. Many patients experience severe pain with dystonia. Others have truncal and limb pain, including pseudoradicular pain, paraspinal pain, aching in limb muscles, and burning dysesthesias. Painful radicular pains, arthritic pains, and dysesthesias

of neuropathy require appropriate investigation and treatment. Dystonic pains often respond to increasing doses of Sinemet or addition of a dopamine agonist such as pergolide or pramipexole.

7. The tendency to depression may be enhanced by Sinemet or other antiparkinsonian medication, particularly the dopamine receptor agonists. Mild cases of depression can be treated with small doses of amitriptyline, beginning with 10 to 25 mg/day and increasing by 10-mg increments every 2 weeks until the symptoms are relieved or adverse effects are unacceptable. Amitriptyline should be given at night because it is effective in inducing sleep, which is often disturbed in patients with depression. If adverse effects of amitriptyline are unacceptable, nortriptyline may be effective in equal dosage.

    Serotonin uptake inhibitors such as fluoxetine are also effective in alleviating depression in most cases. Tricyclic antidepressants and serotonin uptake inhibitors should not be used in conjunction with selegiline.

8. Approximately 25 to 40 percent of patients with Parkinson disease have dementia.[211] Although there is no definitive treatment for dementia in Parkinson disease, it is important to make sure that the patient is not suffering from a concomitant dementia including Alzheimer disease, Pick disease, corticobasal degeneration, diffuse Lewy body disease, progressive supranuclear palsy, or multisystem atrophy. Treatable causes of dementia should be excluded and all patients should receive thyroid function tests, determination of vitamin B_{12} and serum folate, a serologic test of syphilis, and an MRI or CT scan of the head to rule out a space-occupying lesion. Depression is a potent cause of dementia in patients with Parkinson disease and once recognized, can be treated, as outlined above.

9. Cognitive impairment may complicate treatment of patients with Parkinson disease. Lack of insight is often followed by rejection of suggested medication schedules. Similarly, a patient with cognitive impairment may not follow instructions regarding dosage and timing of medication ad-

ministration and may resent interference by a family member who attempts to assume responsibility for the correct administration of medication. There are similarities in cognitive dysfunction in patients with frontal lobe lesions and Parkinson disease. Both have a disturbance in the frontal regulation of attention or processing. A degeneration of the dopaminergic mesocortical innervation of the frontal cortex in Parkinson disease is a possible neurochemical substrate of frontal intentional disturbances.[212]

10. Psychosis, including symptoms of confusion, paranoid delusions, and hallucinations, particularly at night, often respond to clozapine or risperidone, but adverse effects of these drugs, including leukopenia and extrapyramidal symptoms, are a problem. The use of olanzapine, which does not precipitate leukopenia nor worsen symptoms of Parkinson disease, is an effective alternative. Treatment should begin with 1 mg/day increasing slowly to as high as 15 mg/day, if necessary.[213]

11. Freezing is seen in more advanced cases of Parkinson disease, when the patient will suddenly stop and have trouble resuming walking. Freezing can indicate an excessive dopamine effect or inadequate dopamine dosage. If there are prominent signs of parkinsonism, with rigidity at the time of freezing, then the patient is underdosed and should respond to larger doses of Sinemet. Those patients who develop freezing despite an adequate therapeutic effect of Sinemet in terms of reduced rigidity and bradykinesis may respond to the addition of a dopamine receptor agonist with appropriate reduction in Sinemet therapy or the introduction of pramipexole into the therapeutic regimen, again with reduction of Sinemet. When there is no response to change in medication, then the patient must be taught to initiate a step by counting when walking, marching (left-right-left-right), or stepping over an object or an imaginary object.

Dyskinesias Choreoathetoid movements almost invariably occur in patients with Parkinson disease after the passage of time.[214] The most common form occurs at peak dose effect and has been termed "peak-dose dyskinesia" or improvement-dyskinesia-improvement (I-D-I). There may be response to a slow reduction of Sinemet therapy, but this may precipitate the patient into a bradykinetic state. Under these circumstances, a dopamine receptor agonist such as pramipexole, bromocriptine, or pergolide can be added and slowly titrated to effect. The second dyskinetic response is a persistent dystonia, which occurs at the beginning and the end of a levodopa cycle. The term dyskinesia-improvement-dyskinesia (D-I-D) response has been given to this complication. The condition may respond to increasing the frequency of Sinemet dosage, the use of a sustained-release preparation of Sinemet, or the addition of a dopamine receptor agonist such as bromocriptine, pergolide, or pramipexole. This problem becomes urgent when the patient experiences severe pain associated with a dystonia, which usually affects the foot. Dramatic improvement can occur with the introduction of pergolide in such cases.

Sleep Disturbance A number of sleep disturbances are identified in patients with Parkinson disease.

1. Many patients experience insomnia. The common cause of this phenomenon is afternoon sleeping with reversal of the sleep cycle. It is difficult to break this habit, which usually occurs immediately after lunch, and the family must be encouraged to keep the patient active during the early afternoon. If the patient is depressed, appropriate therapy with an antidepressant (see above) is indicated and preparations such as benzodiazepines, which induce sleepiness, should be withdrawn. Depression should be treated with appropriate antidepressants (see above). The use of a bedtime dose of amitriptyline or nortriptyline may be particularly effective in these cases.

Nighttime insomnia is usually the result of daytime sleeping but at other times is the result of an associated sleep disorder such as sleep apnea or narcolepsy. Treatment with methylphenidate 5 to 10 mg, 1 in the morning and 1 at noon, or selegiline 5 mg morning and noon may be of benefit.

Some patients experience nightmares, often related to the introduction of an antiparkinsonian medication, which should then be withdrawn and an appropriate substitution given. Nightmares that are an increased complication of parkinsonism associated with dementia may respond to low-dose clozapine. Polysomnography may be necessary in some cases, particularly when the bed partner reports behavior such as aggression or wandering in the middle of the night. This condition usually responds to clonazepam 0.25 to 1 mg q.h.s. When the patient appears to be restless at night without wandering or aggressive behavior, the possibility of discomfort should be considered because many Parkinson patients are unable to change their position in bed and experience increasing difficulties during the night as the effect of medication decreases. The substitution of a long-acting Sinemet preparation at bedtime may alleviate this situation, or the introduction of dopamine receptor agonists such as pramipexole, pergolide, or bromocriptine with their longer half-life may be advantageous. Both selegiline and amantadine can produce insomnia and when there is interruption of nighttime sleeping, these drugs should either be withdrawn or given in two doses, one in the morning and one no later than noon. Other conditions consist of restless legs syndrome and periodic limb movements of sleep.

2. Restless legs syndrome, a condition consisting of an irresistible urge to move the extremities, is increased when the individual attempts to sleep at bedtime. Some cases are due to akathisia. Others are idiopathic. The substitution of a slow-release form of Sinemet may be helpful, or substitution of Sinemet by pergolide or pramipexole may be effective. In some patients with restless legs syndrome, low-dose clonazepam or the use of a small dose of an opiate such as codeine 30 to 60 mg at bedtime is often very effective. Periodic limb movements with sleep (nocturnal myoclonus) usually respond to an increase in Sinemet, particularly when the controlled-release preparation is given at bedtime.

General Measures There seems little doubt that patients with Parkinson disease show some slowing of progression of disease and benefit from a regular program of exercise. Patients should be encouraged to develop a program of exercise at least three times a week and to continue this indefinitely. Physical therapy and occupational therapy are also useful in the treatment of Parkinson disease in that both can benefit patients who are taught to walk in an improved fashion and to use their hands and upper limbs appropriately, considering their disability. An exercise program should be coupled with adequate nutrition. Patients with Parkinson disease tend to eat slowly and may have inadequate food intake because of this problem. Many patients lose weight, which is only partially due to inadequate food intake, but this should always be considered when it is obvious that weight loss is a problem.

Frequent falls may be the result of bradykinesis, rigidity, or the presence of impaired postural reflexes. Falling may also occur in patients with orthostatic hypotension, particularly if the individual needs to empty the bladder during the night and suffers a syncopal episode going to or coming back from the bathroom. When falling is a problem, the use of a wheeled walker, particularly the more modern type with caliper brakes, is of great benefit to patients with Parkinson disease. Finally, however, some patients have to resort to the use of a wheelchair. Despite frequent falls, subdural hematomas are rather unusual but should always be considered if there is a change in mentation in a patient with advanced Parkinson disease, where falling has been recorded.

Surgical Management of Parkinson Disease
Surgical management of Parkinson disease has a long history and was well established prior to the introduction of levodopa therapy in the 1960s. The number of surgical procedures then declined dramatically, until it became apparent that complications of medical treatment occurring in a population with increasing life expectancy presented a further opportunity for surgical treatment.

Thalamotomy with ablation of the nucleus ventrolateralis or nucleus ventrointermedius of the thalamus effectively relieves tremor in Parkinson disease and is about 90 percent effective in patients who have failed to respond to medical treatment. Stereotactic techniques have minimized complications such as contralateral hemiparesis. Bradykinesis, rigidity, and levodopa-induced dyskinesias can be relieved by stereotactic pallidotomy.

Thalamic stimulation through chronically implanted electrodes results in reduction of tremor in Parkinson disease. Pallidal stimulation is indicated for tremor, bradykinesis, rigidity, and persistent dyskinesias.[215] Subthalamic stimulation may reduce medication-induced dyskinesia.

The efficacy of human fetal ventral mesencephalic tissue implantation in refractory cases of Parkinson disease, with rapid fluctuation in symptoms, is under review in several countries at this time.[216] Genetically engineered autologous cell transplantation is under review in primate animal models.

Hemiparkinson-Hemiatrophy Syndrome

This rare condition presents with hemiatrophy of one side or part of one side of the body, followed by symptoms of parkinsonism, most marked on the side of the hemiatrophy. Signs of hemiatrophy can occur in children or adolescents with the onset of parkinsonian symptoms in the fourth or fifth decade. MRI or CT scans show brain asymmetry. The course is slowly progressive and the parkinsonism responds to levodopa therapy.

REFERENCES

1. Swedo SE, Leonard HL: Childhood movement disorders and obsessive-compulsive disorder. *J Clin Psychiatry* 55(Suppl 32):7, 1994.
2. Schipper HM: Sex hormones in stroke chorea and anticonvulsant therapy. *Semin Neurol* 8:181, 1988.
3. Eshel G, Lahat C, Azizi E, et al: Chorea as a manifestation of rheumatic fever—a 30 year survey (1960–1990). *Eur J Pediatr* 152:645, 1993.
4. Swedo SE: Sydenham's chorea: a model of childhood autoimmune disorders [clinical conference]. *JAMA* 272:1788, 1994.
5. Al-Eissa A: Syndenham's chorea: a new look at an old disease. *Br J Clin Pract* 47:14, 1993.
6. Feldman BM, Zabriskie JB, Silverman ED, et al: Diagnostic use of B-cell alloantigen D8/17 in rheumatic chorea. *J Pediatr* 123:84, 1993.
7. Swedo SE, Leonard HL, Schapiro MB, et al: Syndenham's chorea: physical and psychological symptoms of St. Vitus dance. *Pediatrics* 91:706, 1993.

8. Giedd JN, Rapoport JL, Kruesi MJ, et al: Syndenham's chorea: magnetic resonance imaging of the basal ganglia. *Neurology* 45:2199, 1995.

9. Goldman S, Amrom D, Szliwowski HB, et al: Reversible striatal hypermetabolism in a case of Syndenham's chorea. *Mov Disord* 8:355, 1993.

10. Jones AL, Bouchier IA: A patient with neurosyphilis presenting as chorea. *Scot MJ* 38:82, 1993.

11. Beskind DL, Keim SM: Choreoathetotic movement disorder in a boy with *Mycoplasma pneumoniae* encephalitis. *Ann Emerg Med* 23:1375, 1994.

12. Kupsky WJ, Drozd MA, Barlow CF: Selective injury of the globus pallidus in children with post-cardiac surgery choreic syndrome. *Dev Med Child Neurol* 37:135, 1995.

13. Medlock MD, Cruse RS, Winek SJ, et al: A 10-year experience with postpump chorea. *Ann Neurol* 34:820, 1993.

14. Besbas N, Damargue I, Ozen S, et al: Association of antiphospholipid antibodies with systemic lupus erythematosus in a child presenting with chorea: a case report. *Eur J Pediatr* 153:891, 1994.

15. Furie R, Ishikawa J, Dhawan V, et al: Alternating hemichorea in primary antiphospholipid syndrome: evidence for contralateral striatal hypermetabolism. *Neurology* 44:2197, 1994.

16. Springate J, Vetrano A, Cachero S, et al: Chorea following acute glomerulonephritis. *Clin Pediatr* 31:632, 1992.

17. Chang MH, Li JY, Lee SR, et al: Non-ketotic hyperglycaemic chorea: a SPECT study. *J Neurol Neurosurg Psychiatry* 60:428, 1996.

18. Hefter H, Mayer P, Benecke R: Persistent chorea after recurrent hypoglycemica. A case report. *Eur Neurol* 33:244, 1993.

19. Buetefisch CM, Gutierrez A, Gutmann L: Choreoathetotic movements: a possible side effect of gabapentin. *Neurology* 46:851, 1996.

20. Lancman ME, Asconape JJ, Penry JK: Choreiform movements associated with the use of valproate. *Arch Neurol* 51:702, 1994.

21. Daras M, Koppel BS, Atos-Radzion E: Cocaine-induced choreoathetoid movements (crack dancing). *Neurology* 44:751, 1994.

22. Combarros O, Fabrega E, Polo JM, et al: Cyclosporine-induced chorea after liver transplantation for Wilson's disease. *Ann Neurol* 33:108, 1993.

23. Stuart AM, Worley LM, Spillane J: Choreiform movements observed in an 8-year-old child following use of an oral theophylline preparation. *Clin Pediatr* 31:692, 1992.

24. Kirk A, Harding SR: Cardioembolic caudate infarction as a cause of hemichorea in lupus anticoagulant syndrome. *Can J Neurol Sci* 20:162, 1993.

25. Omdal R, Roalso S: Chorea gravidarum and chorea associated with oral contraceptives—diseases due to antiphospholipid antibodies. *Acta Neurol Scand* 86:219, 1992.

26. Shinotoh H, Calne DB, Snow B, et al: Normal CAG repeat length in the Huntington's disease gene in senile chorea. *Neurology* 44:2183, 1994.

27. Crozier S, Lehericy S, Verstichel P, et al: Transient hemiballism/hemichorea due to an ipsilateral subthalamic nucleus infarction. *Neurology* 46:267, 1996.

28. Yapijakis C, Kapaki E, Zournas C, et al: Exclusion mapping of the benign hereditary chorea gene from the Huntington's disease locus: report of a family. *Clin Genet* 47:133, 1995.

29. Milstone A, Fan A, F, Fuchs H: Antiphospholipid syndrome associated with seizures. *South Med J* 89:738, 1996.

30. Mackworth-Young CG: The Michael Mason Prize Essay 1994. Antiphospholipid antibodies and disease. *Br J Rheumatol* 34:1009, 1995.

31. Toubi E, Khamashta MA, Panarra A, et al: Association of antiphospholipid antibodies with central nervous system disease in systemic lupus erythematosus. *Am J Med* 99:397, 1995.

32. Finazzi G, Brancaccio V, Moia M, et al: Natural history and risk factors for thrombosis in 360 patients with antiphospholipid antibodies: a four-year prospective study from the Italian registry. *Am J Med* 100:530, 1996.

33. Rinne JO, Daniel SE, Scaravilli F, et al: The neuropathological features of neuroacanthocytosis. *Mov Disord* 9:297, 1994.

34. Ikeuchi T, Koide R, Tanaka H, et al: Dentatorubral-pallidoluysian atrophy: clinical features are closely related to unstable expansions of trinucleotide (CAG) repeat. *Ann Neurol* 37:769, 1995.

35. Yazawa I, Nukina N, Ichikawa Y, et al: Dentatorubropallidoluysian atrophy proteins in lymphoblastic cells. *Neurology* 47:586, 1996.

36. Fink JK, Rainer S, Wilkowski J, et al: Paroxysmal dystonic choreoathetosis: tight linkage to chromosome 2q. *Am J Hum Genet* 59:140, 1996.

37. Richardson JC, Howes JL, Celinski MJ, et al: Kinesiogenic choreoathetosis due to brain injury. *Can J Neurol Sci* 14:626, 1987.

38. Drake ME: Paroxysmal kinesiogenic choreoathetosis in hyperthyroidism. *Postgrad Med J* 63:1089, 1987.

39. Shaw C, Haas L, Miller D, et al: A case report of

paroxysmal dystonic choreoathetosis due to hypoglycemia induced by an insulinoma. *J Neurol Neurosurg Psychiatry* 61:194, 1996.

40. Jan JE, Freeman RD, Good WV: Familial paroxysmal kinesiogenic choreoathetosis in a child with visual hallucinations and obsessive-compulsive behavior. *Dev Med Child Neurol* 37:366, 1995.

41. Marsden CD: Paroxysmal choreoathetosis. *Adv Neurol* 70:467, 1996.

42. Perry TL, Norman MG, Young V, et al: Hallervorden Spatz disease. Cysteine accumulation and cysteine dioxygenase deficiency in the globus pallidus. *Ann Neurol* 18:482, 1985.

43. Halliday W: The nosology of Hallervorden Spatz disease. *J Neurol Sci* 134(Suppl 84), 1995.

44. Boyacigil S, Tokoglu F, Pasaoglu E, et al: Hallervorden Spatz disease. *Australias Radiol* 40:351, 1996.

45. Albright AL, Barry MJ, Fasich P, et al: Continuous intrathecal baclofen for symptomatic generalized dystonia. *Neurosurgery* 38:934, 1996.

46. Huntington's Disease Collaborative Research Group: A novel gene containing a trinucleotide repeat that is expanded and unstable on Huntington's disease chromosomes. *Cell* 72:971, 1993.

47. Siemers E, Foroud T, Bill DS, et al: Motor changes in presymptomatic Huntington disease carriers. *Arch Neurol* 53:487, 1996.

48. Kieburtz K, MacDonald M, Shih C, et al: Trinucleotide repeat length and progression of illness in Huntington's disease. *J Med Genet* 31:872, 1994.

49. Furtado S, Suchowersky O: Huntington's disease: recent advances in diagnosis and management. *Can J Neurol Sci* 22:5, 1995.

50. Borlongan CV, Kanning K, Poulos SG, et al: Free radical damage and oxidative stress in Huntington's disease. *J Fla Med Assoc* 83:335, 1996.

51. Gu M, Gash MT, Mann VM, et al: Mitochondrial defect in Huntington's disease caudate nucleus. *Ann Neurol* 39:385, 1996.

52. Zappacosta B, Monza D, Meoni C, et al: Psychiatric symptoms do not correlate with cognitive decline, motor symptoms or CAG repeat length in Huntington's disease. *Arch Neurol* 53:493, 1996.

53. Aylward EH, Brandt J, Codori AM, et al: Reduced basal ganglia volume associated with the gene for Huntington's disease in asymptomatic at-risk persons. *Neurology* 44:823, 1994.

54. Harris GJ, Aylward EH, Peyser CE, et al: Single photon emission computed tomographic blood flow and magnetic resonance volume imaging of basal ganglia in Huntington's disease. *Arch Neurol* 53:316, 1996.

55. Grafton ST, Mazziotta JC, Pahl JJ, et al: A comparision of neurological, metabolic, structural and genetic evaluations in persons at risk for Huntington's disease. *Ann Neurol* 28:614, 1990.

56. Weeks RA, Harding AE, Brooks DS, et al: PET demonstrates a parallel loss of D^1 and D^2 dopamine receptors in asymptomatic gene carriers of Huntington's disease. *Neurology* 45(Suppl 4):A220, 1995 [abstract].

57. Giordani B, Berent S, Bolvin MJ, et al: Longitudinal neuropsychological and genetic linkage analysis of persons at risk for Huntington's disease. *Arch Neurol* 50:59, 1995.

58. Schilsky ML: Wilson's disease: genetic basis of copper toxicity and natural history. *Semin Liver Dis* 16:83, 1996.

59. Frydman M, Bonné-Tamir B, Farrer LA, et al: Assignment of the gene for Wilson disease to chromosome 13. *Proc Natl Acad Sci USA* 82:1819, 1985.

60. Chowrimootoo GF, Ahmed HA, Seymour CA: New insights into the pathogenesis of copper toxicosis in Wilson's disease: evidence for copper incorporation and defective canalicular transport of caeruloplasmin. *Biochem J* 315(Pt 3):851, 1996.

61. Akil M, Brewer GJ: Psychiatric and behavioral abnormalities in Wilson's disease. *Adv Neurol* 65:171, 1995.

62. Jackson GH, Meyer A, Lippman S: Wilson's disease. Psychiatric manifestations may be the clinical presentation (Review). *Postgrad Med* 95:135, 1994.

63. O'Donnell JG, Watson ID, Fell GS, et al: Wilson's disease presenting as acute fulminating hepatic failure. *Scot Med J* 35:118, 1990.

64. Finelli PF, Kayser-Fleischer ring. Hepatolenticular degeneration (Wilson's disease). *Neurology* 45:1261, 1995.

65. Lyon TD, Fell GS, Gaffney D, et al: Use of a stable copper isotope (65 Cu) in the differential diagnosis of Wilson's disease. *Clin Sci* 88:727, 1995.

66. Huang CC, Chu NS: Wilson's disease: resolution of MRI lesions following long-term otal zinc therapy. *Acta Neurol Scand* 93:215, 1996.

67. Maier-Doberberger T, Mannhalter C, Rack S, et al: Diagnosis of Wilson's disease in an asymptomatic sibling by DNA linkage analysis. *Gastroenterology* 109:2015, 1995.

68. Brewer GJ: Practical recommendatioins and new therapies for Wilson's disease (Review). *Drugs* 50:240, 1995.

69. Dahlman T, Hartvig P, Lofholm M, et al: Long-term treatment of Wilson's disease with triethylene

tetramine dihydrochloride (Trientine). *QJM* 88:609, 1995.

70. Kumar A, Riely CA: Inherited liver diseases in adults. *West J Med* 163:382, 1995.

71. Kikuchi K, Kowada M, Kojima H: Hypoplasia of the internal carotid artery associated with spasmodic torticollis: the possible role of altered vertebral basilar haemodynamics. *Neuroradiology* 37:362, 1995.

72. Deuschl G, Seifert C, Heinen F, et al: Reciprocal inhibition of forearm flexor muscles in spasmodic torticollis. *J Neurol Sci* 113:85, 1992.

73. Lowenstein DH, Aminoff MJ: The clinical course of spasmodic torticollis. *Neurology* 38:530, 1988.

74. Gauthier S: Idiopathic spasmodic torticollis: pathophysiology and treatment. *Can J Neurol Sci* 13:88, 1986.

75. Anderson TJ, Rivest J, Stell R, et al: Botulinum toxin treatment of spasmodic torticollis. *J R Soc Med* 85:524, 1992.

76. Friedman AH, Nashold BSJ, Sharp R, et al: Treatment of spasmodic torticollis with intradural selective rhizotomies. *J Neurosurg* 78:46, 1993.

77. Braun V, Richter HP: Selective peripheral denervation for the treatment of spasmodic torticollis. *Neurosurgery* 35:58, 1994.

78. Leis AA, Dimitrijevic MR, Delapass JS, et al: Modification of cervical dystonia by selective sensory stimulation. J Neurol Sci 110:79, 1992.

79. Eidelberg D, Moeller JR, Ishikawa T, et al: The metabolic topography of idiopathic torsion dystonia. *Brain* 118(Pt 6):1473, 1995.

80. Van der Kamp W, Rothwell JC, Thompson PD, et al: The movement-related cortical potential is abnormal in patients with idiopathic torsion dystonia. *Mov Disord* 10:630, 1995.

81. Bressman SB, Heiman GA, Nygaard TG, et al: A study of idiopathic torsion dystonia in a non-Jewish family: evidence for genetic heterogeneity. *Neurology* 44:283, 1994.

82. Mezaki T, Kaji R, Hamano T, et al: Optimisation of botulinum treatment for cervical and axial dystonias: experience with a Japanese type A toxin. *J Neurol Neurosurg Psychiatry* 57:1535, 1994.

83. Paret G, Tirosh R, Ben Zeev B, et al: Intrathecal baclofen for severe torsion dystonia in a child. *Acta Paediatr* 85:635, 1996.

84. Iacano RP, Kuniyoshi SM, Lonser RR, et al: Simultaneous bilateral pallidoansotomy for idiopathic dystonia musculorum deformans. *Pediatr Neurol* 14:145; 1996.

85. Yamashiro K, Tasker RR: Stereotactic thalamotomy for dystonia patients. *Stereotact Funct Neurosurg* 60:81, 1993.

86. Lang AE: High dose anticholinergic therapy in adult dystonia. *Can J Neurol Sci* 13:42, 1986.

87. Cole R, Halett M, Cohen LG: Double-blind trial of botulinum toxin for treatment of focal hand dystonia. *Mov Disord* 10:466, 1995.

88. Behari M, Raju GH: Electrophysiological studies in patients with blepharospasm before and after botulinum toxin A therapy. *J Neurol Sci* 135:74, 1996.

89. Aramideh M, Ongerboer de Visser BW, Brans JW, et al: Pretarsal application of botulinum toxin for treatment of blepharospasm. *J Neurol Neurosurg Psychiatry* 59:309, 1995.

90. Eekhof JL, Aramideh M, Bour LJ, et al: Blink reflex recovery curves in blepharospasm torticollis spasmodica and hemifacial spasm. *Muscle Nerve* 19:10, 1996.

91. Aramideh M, Bour LJ, Koelman JH, et al: Abnormal eye movements in blepharospasm and involuntary levator palpebrae inhibition. Clinical and pathophysiological considerations. *Brain* 117(Pt 6):1457, 1994.

92. Aramideh M, Ongerboer de Visser BW, Devriese PP, et al: Electromyographic features of levator palpebrae superioris and orbicularis oculi muscles in blepharospasm. *Brain* 117(Pt 1):27, 1994.

93. Aramideh M, Ongerboer de Visser BW, Holstege G, et al: Blepharospasm in association with a lower pontine lesion. *Neurology* 46:476, 1996.

94. Gilbert GJ: Bruegel syndrome: its distinction from Miege syndrome. *Neurology* 46:1767, 1996.

95. Beshir K, Manyam BV: Clozapine for the control of hemiballismus. *Clin Neuropharmacol* 17:477, 1994.

96. Quinn NP: Essential myoclonus and myoclonic dystonia—a review. *Mov Disord* 11:119, 1996.

97. Singer HS: Neurobiological issues in Tourette's syndrome. *Brain Dev* 16:353, 1994.

98. Sandyk R: Cholinergic mechanisms in Tourette's syndrome. *Int J Neurosci* 81:95, 1995.

99. Regeur L: Clinical evaluation and pharmacological treatment of Gille de la Tourette syndrome and other hyperkinesias. *Acta Neurologic Scand* (Suppl) 137:48, 1992.

100. Singer HS, Hahn I-H, Moran TH: Abnormal dopamine uptake sites in postmortem striatum from patients with Tourette's syndrome. *Ann Neurol* 30:558, 1991.

101. Peterson BS: Considerations of natural history and pathophysiology in the psychopharmacology of Tourette syndrome. *J Clin Psychiatry* 57(Suppl 9):24, 1996.

102. Weeks RA, Turjanski N, Brooks DJ: Tourette's syndrome: a disorder of cingulate and orbitofrontal function? *QJM* 89:401, 1996.

103. Witelson SF: Clinical neurology as data for basic neuroscience: Tourette's syndrome and the human motor system. *Neurology* 43:859, 1993.

104. Abwender DA, Como PG, Kurlan R, et al: School problems in Tourette's syndrome. *Arch Neurol* 53:509, 1996.

105. Peterson B, Riddle MA, Cohen DJ, et al: Reduced basal ganglia volumes in Tourette's syndrome using three-dimensional reconstruction techniques from magnetic resonance images. *Neurology* 43:941, 1993.

106. Floeter MK, Andermann F, Andermann E, et al: Physiological studies of spinal inhibitory pathways in patients with hereditary hyperexplexia. *Neurology* 46:766, 1996.

107. Rajendra S, Lynch JW, Pierce KD, et al: Startle disease mutations reduce the agonist sensitivity of the human inhibitory glycine receptor. *J Biol Chem* 269:18739, 1994.

108. Ehrenberg B, Eisensehr I, Walters A: Influence of valproate on sleep and periodic limb movement disorder. *Sleep Res* 24:227, 1995.

109. Mellick GA, Mellick LB: Successful treatment of restless leg syndrome with gabapentin. *Sleep Res* 24:290, 1995.

110. Britton TC: Essential tremor and its variants. *Curr Opin Neurol* 8:314, 1995.

111. Busenbark K, Barnes P, Lyons K, et al: Accuracy of reporting family histories of essential tremor. *Neurology* 47:264, 1996.

112. Louis ED, Ottman R: How familial is familial tremor? The genetic epidemiology of essential tremor. *Neurology* 46:1200, 1996.

113. Bain PG, Findley LJ, Thompson PD, et al: A study of hereditary essential tremor. *Brain* 117(Pt 4):805, 1994.

114. Elble RJ: The role of aging in the clinical expression of essential tremor. *Exp Gerontol* 30:337, 1995.

115. Wills AJ, Jenkins IH, Thompson PD, et al: A positron emission tomography study of cerebral activation associated with essential and writing tremor. *Arch Neurol* 52:299, 1995.

116. Louis ED, Marder K, Cote L, et al: Differences in the prevalence of essential tremor among elderly African Americans, whites and Hispanics in Northern Manhattan, N.Y. *Arch Neurol* 52:1201, 1995.

117. Metzer WS: Essential tremor: an overview. *J Ark Med Soc* 90:587, 1994.

118. Koller WC, Busenbark K, Gray C, et al: Classification

119. Woo P, Casper J, Colton R, et al: Dysphonia in the aging: physiology versus disease. *Laryngoscope* 102:139, 1992.

120. Baloh RW, Foster CA, Yue Q, et al: Familial migraine with vertigo and essential tremor. *Neurology* 46:458, 1996.

121. Metzer WS: Severe essential tremor compared with Parkinson disease in male veterans: diagnostic characteristics, treatment and psychosocial complications. *South Med J* 85:825, 1992.

122. Jankovic J, Beach J, Schwartz K, et al: Tremor and longevity in relatives of patients with Parkinson's disease, essential tremor and control subjects. *Neurology* 45:645, 1995.

123. Anouti A, Koller WC: Diagnostic testing in movement disorders. *Neurol Clin* 14:169, 1996.

124. Britton TC, Thompson PD, Day BL, et al: Rapid wrist movements in patients with essential tremor. The critical role of the second agonist burst. *Brain* 117 (Pt 1):39, 1994.

125. Busenbark K, Pahwa R, Hubble J, et al: The effect of acetazolamide on essential tremor. An open-label trial. *Neurology* 42:1394, 1992.

126. Busenbark K, Pahwa R, Hubble J, et al: Double-blind controlled study of methazolamide in the treatment of essential tremor. *Neurology* 43:1045, 1993.

127. Biary N, Bahou Y, Sofi MA, et al: The effect of nimodipine on essential tremor. *Neurology* 45:1523, 1995.

128. Benabid AL, Pollak P, Gao D, et al: Chronic electrical stimulation of the ventralis intermedius nucleus of the thalamus as a treatment of movement disorders. *J Neurosurg* 84:203, 1996.

129. Burchiel KJ: Thalamotomy for movement disorders. *Neurosurg Clin N Am* 6:55, 1995.

130. Pahwa R, Wilkinson S, Smith D, et al: High-frequency stimulation of the globus pallidus for the treatment of Parkinson's disease. *Neurology* 49:249, 1997.

131. Goff DC, Tsai G, Beal MF, et al: Tardive dyskinesia and substrates of energy metabolism in C.S.F. *Am J Psychiatry* 152:1730, 1995.

132. Alberts VA, Catalano G, Poole MA: Tardive dyskinesia as a result of long-term prochlorperazine use. *South Med J* 89:989, 1996.

133. Koller WC, Langston JW, Hubble JP, et al: Does a long preclinical period occur in Parkinson's disease? *Neurology* 41(Suppl 2):8, 1991.

134. Halstead SM, Barnes TR, Speller JC: Akathesia,

prevalence and associated dysphoria in an in-patient population with chronic schizophrenia. *Br J Psychiatry* 164:177, 1994.

135. Sachdev P: The epidemiology of drug-induced akathesia. Part II chronic tardive and withdrawal akathesias. *Schizophr Bull* 21:451, 1995.

136. Chakos MH, Alvir JM, Woerner MG, et al: Incidence and correlates of tardive dyskinesia in the first episode of schizophrenia. *Arch Gen Psychiatry* 53:313, 1996.

137. Jeste DV, Caligiuri MP, Paulsen JS, et al: Risk of tardive dyskinesia in older patients. A prospective longitudinal study of 266 outpatients. *Arch Gen Psychiatry* 52:756, 1995.

138. Sweet RA, Mulsant BH, Gupta B, et al: Duration of neuroleptic treatment and prevalence of tardive dyskinesia in late life. *Arch Gen Psychiatry* 52:478, 1995.

139. Jeste DV, Caligiuri MP: Tardive dyskinesia. *Schizophr Bull* 19:303, 1993.

140. Khan R, Jampala VC, Dong K, et al: Speech abnormalities in tardive dyskinesia. *Am J Psychiatry* 151:760, 1994.

141. Ford B, Greene P, Fahn S: Oral and genital tardive pain syndromes. *Neurology* 44:2115, 1994.

142. Cates M, Lusk K, Wells BG: Are calcium-channel blockers effective in the treatment of tardive dyskinesia? *Ann Pharmacother* 27:191, 1993.

143. Dabiri LM, Pasta D, Darby JK, et al: Effectiveness of vitamin E for treatment of long-term tardive dyskinesia. *Am J Psychiatry* 151:925, 1994.

144. Latimer PR: Tardive dyskinesia: a review. *Can J Psychiatry* 40(7 suppl 2):S49, 1995.

145. Assion HJ, Heinemann F: Tardive dystonia. A rare neuroleptic-induced disease picture. *Nervenartz* 65:795, 1994.

146. Kaufman DM: Use of botulinum toxin injections for spasmodic torticollis of tardive dyskinesia. *J Neuropsychiatry Clin Neurosci* 6:50, 1994.

147. Sachdev P: Tardive and chronically recurrent oculogyric crisis. *Mov Disord* 8:93, 1993.

148. Stacy M, Cardoso F, Jankovic J: Tardive stereotype and other movement disorders in tardive dyskinesias. *Neurology* 43:937, 1993.

149. Trugman JM, Leadbetter R, Zalis ME, et al: Treatment of severe axial tardive dystonia with clozapine: case report and hypothesis. *Mov Disord* 9:441, 1994.

150. Shapleske J, Mickay AP, McKenna PJ: Successful treatment of tardive dystonia with clozapine and clonazepam. *Br J Psychiatry* 168:516, 1996.

151. Abad V, Ovsiew F: Treatment of persistent myoclonic tardive dystonia with verapamil. *Br J Psychiatry* 162:554, 1993.

152. Greene P: Baclofen in the treatment of dystonia. *Clin Neuropharmacol* 15:276, 1992.

153. Shulman LM, Singer C, Weiner WJ: Improvement of both tardive dystonia and akathisia after botulinum toxin injection. *Neurology* 46:844, 1996.

154. Gerlach J, Peacock L: Motor and mental side effects of clozapine. *J Clin Psychiatry* 55(Suppl B):107, 1994.

155. Bristow MF, Kohen D: Neuroleptic malignant syndrome. *Hosp Med* 55:517, 1996.

156. Caroff SN, Mann SC: Neuroleptic malignant syndrome. *Med Clin N Am* 77:185, 1993.

157. Shaw A, Matthews EE: Postoperative neuroleptic malignant syndrome. *Anaesthesia* 50:246, 1995.

158. Spirt MJ, Chan W, Thieberg M, et al: Neuroleptic malignant syndrome induced by domperidone. *Dig Dis Sci* 37:946, 1992.

159. Wetli CV, Mash D, Karch SB: Cocaine-associated agitated delirium and neuroleptic malignant syndrome. *Am J Emerg Med* 14:425, 1996.

160. Demirkiran M, Jankovic J, Dean JM: Ecstacy intoxication: an overlap between serotonin syndrome and neuroleptic malignant syndrome. *Clin Neuropharmacol* 19:157, 1996.

161. Burke C, Fulda GJ, Castellano J: Neuroleptic malignant syndrome in a trauma patient. *J Trauma* 39:796, 1995.

162. Todd R, Lippman S, Manshad M, et al: Recognition and treatment of rabbit syndrome, an uncommon complication of neuroleptic therapies. *Am J Psychiatry* 140:1519, 1993.

163. Fornazzari L, Ichise M, Remington G, et al: Rabbit syndrome, antidepressant use and cerebral perfusion SPECT scan findings. *J Psychiatry Neurosci* 16:227, 1991.

164. Yassa R, Lal S: Prevalence of the rabbit syndrome. *Am J Psychiatry* 143:656, 1986.

165. Wada Y, Yamaguchi N: The rabbit syndrome and antiparkinsonian medication in schizophrenic patients. *Neuropsychobiology* 25:149, 1992.

166. Calne DB: Is idiopathic parkinsonism the consequence of an event or a process? *Neurology* 44:5, 1994.

167. Marttila RJ, Kaprio J, Koskenvuo M, et al: Parkinson's disease in a nationwide twin cohort. *Neurology* 38:1217, 1988.

168. Calne DB, Langston JW, Martin WR, et al: Positron emission tomography after MPTP: observations relating to the cause of Parkinson's disease. *Nature* 317:246, 1985.

169. Calne DB, Chu NS, Huang CC, et al: Manganism and idiopathic parkinsonism: similarities and differences. *Neurology* 44:1583, 1994.

170. Yoshida M, Ogawa M, Suzuki K, et al: Parkinsonism produced by tetrahydroisoquinoline (TIQ) or the analogues, in Narabayoshi H, Nagatsu T, Yanagisawa N, Mizuno Y (eds): *Advances in Neurology,* vol 60: *Parkinson's Disease from Basic Research to Treatment.* New York, Raven Press 1993, p 207.

171. Butterfield PG, Valanis BG, Spenser PS: Environmental antecedants of young-onset Parkinson's disease. *Neurology* 43:1150, 1993.

172. Koller WC: When does Parkinson's disease begin? *Neurology* 42(Suppl 4):27, 1993.

173. Semchuk KM, Love EJ, Lee RG: Parkinson's disease: a test of the multifactorial etiologic hypothesis. *Neurology* 43:1173, 1993.

174. Bhatt MH, Obeso JA, Marsden CD: Time course of postanoxic akinetic-rigid and dystonic syndromes. *Neurology* 43:314, 1993.

175. Fearnley JM, Lees AJ: Aging and Parkinson's disease: substantia nigra regional selectivity. *Brain* 114:2283, 1991.

176. Ahlskog JE: Treatment of Parkinson's disease. From theory to practice. *Postgrad Med* 95:52, 1994.

177. Schapira AH: Advances in the understanding of the cause of Parkinson's disease. *J R Soc Med* 87:373, 1994.

178. Jankovic J: Theories on the etiology and pathogenesis of Parkinson's disease. *Neurology* 43(Suppl 1):21, 1993.

179. Quinn N, Critchley P, Marsden CD: Young onset Parkinson's disease. *Mov Disord* 2:73, 1987.

180. Friedman J, Friedman H: Fatigue in Parkinson's disease. *Neurology* 43:2016, 1993.

181. Bravi D, Mouradian MM, Roberts JW, et al: End-of-dose dystonia in Parkinson's disease. *Neurology* 43:2130, 1993.

182. LeWitt PA, Burns RS, Newman RP: Dystonia in untreated parkinsonism. *Clin Neuropharmacol* 9:293, 1986.

183. Poewe WH, Lees A, Stern GM: Dystonia in Parkinson's disease: clinical and pharmacological features. *Ann Neurol* 23:73, 1988.

184. Koller WC, Silver DE, Lieberman A: An algorithm for the management of Parkinson's disease. *Neurology* 44(Suppl 10):S1, 1994.

185. Cummings JL: Depression and Parkinson's disease: a review. *Am J Psychiatry* 149:443, 1992.

186. Edwards LL, Quigley EM, Harned RK, et al: Characterization of swallowing and defecation in Parkinson's disease. *Am J Gastroenterol* 89:15, 1994.

187. Hutton JT, Morris JL, Elias JW, et al: Spatial contrast sensitivity is reduced in bilateral Parkinson's disease. *Neurology* 41:1200, 1991.

188. Brown RG, Marsden CD: Cognitive function in Parkinson's disease: from description to theory. *Trends Neurosci* 13:21, 1990.

189. Lu LS, Huang CC, Chu NS, et al: Levodopa failure in chronic manganism. *Neurology* 44:1600, 1994.

190. Lee MS, Marsden CD: Neurological sequelae following carbon monoxide poisoning: clinical course and outcome according to clinical types and brain computed tomography scan findings. *Mov Disord* 9:550, 1994.

191. Peters HA, Levine RL, Matthews CG, et al: Extrapyramidal and other neurological manifestations associated with carbon disulfide fumigant exposure. *Arch Neurol* 45:537, 1988.

192. Rosenberg NL, Myers JA, Martin WR: Cyanide-induced parkinsonism. Clinical MRI and 6-fluorodopa PET studies. *Neurology* 39:142, 1989.

193. McLean DR, Jacobs H, Mielke BW: Methanol poisoning. A clinical and pathological study. *Ann Neurol* 8:161, 1980.

194. DiMonte DA: Mitochondrial DNA and Parkinson's disease. Neurology 41(Suppl 2):38, 1991.

195. Stacy M, Brownlee HJ: Treatment options for early Parkinson's disease. *Am Fam Physician* 53:1281, 1996.

196. Ahlskog JE: Treatment early of Parkinson's disease: are complicated strategies justified? *Mayo Clin Proc* 71:659, 1996.

197. Silverstein PM: Moderate Parkinson's disease. Strategies for maximizing treatment. *Postgrad Med* 99:52, 1996.

198. Tolosa E, Valldeorida F: Mid stage parkinsonism with mild motor fluctuations. *Clin Neuropharmacol* 17(Suppl 2):S19, 1994.

199. Olanow CW, Fahn S, Muenter M, et al: A multicenter double-blind placebo controlled trial of pergolide as an adjunct to Sinemet in Parkinson's disease. *Mov Disord* 9:40, 1994.

200. Quinn N: Drug treatment of Parkinson's disease. *BMJ* 310:575, 1995.

201. Paulson GW: Management of the patient with newly diagnosed Parkinson's disease. *Geriatrics* 48:30, 1993.

202. Calne DB: Initiating treatment for idiopathic parkinsonism. *Neurology* 44(7 Suppl 6):S19, 1994.

203. Wolters EC, Tissingh G, Bergmans PL, et al: Dopamine agonists in Parkinson's disease. *Neurology* 45(3 Suppl 3):S28, 1995.

204. Gerlach M, Youdim MB, Riederer P: Pharmacology of selegiline. *Neurology* 47(6 Suppl 3):S137, 1996.

205. Olanow CW: Selegiline. Current perspectives related to neuroprotection and mortality. *Neurology* 47 (6 Suppl 3):S210, 1996.

206. Carvey PM, Pieri S, Ling ZD: Attenuation of levodopa-induced toxicity in mesencephalic cultures by pramipexole. *J Neurol Trans* 104:209, 1997.

207. Parkinson Study Group: Safety and efficacy of pramipexole in early Parkinson disease. *JAMA* 278: 125, 1997.

208. Brown RG, Jahanshahi M, Quinn N, et al: Sexual dysfunction in patients with Parkinson's disease and their partners. *J Neurol Neurosurg Psychiatry* 53:480, 1990.

209. Wintzen AR, Badrising UA, Roos RA, et al: Dysphagia in ambulant patients with Parkinson's disease. Common, not dangerous. *Can J Neurol Sci* 21:53, 1994.

210. Hutton JT, Morris JL, Elias JW: Levodopa improves spatial contrast sensitivity in Parkinson's disease. *Arch Neurol* 50:721, 1993.

211. Koller WC, Montgomery EB: Issues in the early diagnosis of Parkinson's disease. *Neurology* 49(Suppl 1): S10, 1997.

212. Stam CJ, Visser SL, Op de Coul AW: Disturbed frontal regulation of attention in Parkinson's disease. *Brain* 116:1139, 1993.

213. Wolters EC; Jansen EN, Tuynman-Qua HG, et al: Olanzapine in the treatment of dopaminomimetic psychosis in patients with Parkinson's disease. *Neurology* 47:1085, 1996.

214. Waters CH: Managing the late complications of Parkinson's disease. *Neurology* 49(Suppl 1):S49, 1997.

215. Davis KD, Wolters EC, Taub E, Houle S, et al: Globus pallidus stimulation activates the cortical motor system during alleviation of parkinsonian symptoms. *Nature Med* 3:671, 1997.

216. Kordower JH, Freeman TB, Snow BJ, et al: Neuropathological evidence of graft survival and striatal re-innervation after the transplantation of fetal mesencephalic tissue in a patient with Parkinson's disease. *N Engl J Med* 332:1118, 1995.

Chapter 7

MULTIPLE SCLEROSIS

Multiple sclerosis is a demyelinating disease of the central nervous system (CNS) caused by an autoimmune reaction that is the result of a complex interaction of genetic and environmental factors.

Epidemiology

Multiple sclerosis is more common in women, with a female:male ratio of 2.1:1. The disease is rare in children and has a peak incidence at 30 to 33 years of age, with a decline in the late forties. The upper limit of age at onset has usually been accepted as 59 years, but late onset of multiple sclerosis after the age of 60 years is reported.[1] However, these cases probably represent late occurrence of overt symptoms in individuals who have had the disease in a subclinical or unrecognized fashion for many years.

The natural history of multiple sclerosis has been studied extensively and it is clearly a disease of temperate zones, with an increase in the prevalence gradient south to north in the northern hemisphere, and north to south in the southern hemisphere. Three zones of high, medium, and low prevalence rates can be recognized. High-frequency prevalence rates of more than 30 per 100,000 population occur in areas lying between latitudes 45° and 65° north or south. This includes northern Europe, southern Canada, the northern United States, New Zealand,[2] and southern Australia.[3] These areas of high frequency are bounded by areas of medium frequency with prevalence rates of 5 to 25 per 100,000 and include southern Europe, the southern United States, and most of Australia. Tropical areas of Asia, Africa, and South America have low prevalence rates of less than 5 per 100,000. Anomalies do occur, however, with levels as high as 170 per 100,000 reported in Switzerland,[4] 53 per 100,000 in southern Spain,[5] 59 per 100,000 in Sardinia, and 32 to 58 per 100,000 in Italy and Sicily.[6]

These figures cannot be attributed to climate alone, however, because there are well-documented ethnic differences. Multiple sclerosis predominantly affects people of northern European extraction.[7] In the United States, African-American men are less likely to develop multiple sclerosis when compared to white men in the same geographic area. Studies in Japan, Korea, and Hong Kong indicate a very low prevalence in populations in these countries. Similarly, persons of Asian extraction who have lived for several generations in the United States have a low prevalence rate for multiple sclerosis.

Such findings suggest a genetic factor in multiple sclerosis, and family studies have demonstrated that the risk of multiple sclerosis is increased for relatives of patients with the disease. Studies in Vancouver, British Columbia indicate a family rate for multiple sclerosis approaching 20 percent, with a lifetime age-correlated risk for the sibling of a patient of more than 25 times the lifetime risk in the general population.[8] Twin studies indicate a concordance of 26 percent for monozygotic pairs compared to 2.4 percent in like-sex dizygotic twins—a figure similar to that for nontwin siblings of multiple sclerosis patients. This supports the view that differences in monozygotic and dizygotic twins have a genetic basis.[9]

At the present time, evidence suggests that multiple sclerosis is influenced by several genes, the major histocompatibility (MHC) complex class 2, HLA-DRII allele having the strongest association with the disease in northern European populations. However, the association of different class 1 and class 2 alleles has been reported in other populations. Consequently, the current impression is that multiple sclerosis is probably polygenic,[10] the result of complex genetic factors involving the interaction of genes and coding within and outside of the MHC complex. However, epidemiologic studies in Israel[11] and the Faroe Islands[12] point to involvement of environmental factors in multiple sclerosis. The ongoing study of the disease in the inhabitants of the Faroe Islands—now experiencing a fourth epidemic of multiple sclerosis—suggests that multiple sclerosis is the result of an unidentified infection transmitted person to person and requiring a prolonged exposure of at least 2 years.[13] Susceptibility is limited to ages 11 years to 45 years at the start of exposure and a further 6 years to onset in those who develop clinical signs of multiple sclerosis. However, these figures are the results of a study in one isolated community, and although they express findings in that community, they should not be extrapolated to multiple sclerosis on a global scale, because multiple sclerosis has been clearly demonstrated in children as young as 5 years.

At the present time, it is considered probable that both genetic and environmental factors are involved in multiple sclerosis,[14] with infection as the major environmental agent, in that both viral[15,16] and bacterial[17] infections can initiate or precipitate attacks of multiple sclerosis. Evidence for a direct involvement of a viral agent such as human T-cell lymphotropic virus (HTLV)-1,[18] herpes simplex virus (HSV)-1, HSV-6, scrapie, parainfluenza virus 1, measles virus, coronavirus, simian virus, chimpanzee cytomegalovirus, and LM7 retrovirus in multiple sclerosis is less compelling.[19] The role of environmental factors other than infection has been studied, including the relationship of trauma and multiple sclerosis, indicating that patients are at no greater risk to experience an exacerbation of multiple sclerosis after trauma than at other times,[20] nor is it likely that trauma is ever a causal factor in initiating the disease process.[21] The role of emotional stress in multiple sclerosis is more controversial because stress is difficult to define and quantitate.[22]

Etiology, Pathology, and Pathogenesis

The etiology is unknown. The pathological changes in multiple sclerosis show variation, depending on the age of focal demyelination (the plaque). In the acute state, there is active demyelination with accumulation of sudanophilic myelin breakdown products. The area is edematous and there is marked perivascular cuffing around veins and venules by lymphocytes and macrophages. Plaques are frequently located in the periventricular distribution, particularly in the cerebral hemispheres, but plaques can occur at any site in the white matter and often penetrate into the gray matter of the cortex and deeper gray matter structures

in the cerebrum and cerebellum. Because multiple sclerosis is a disease of the CNS, plaque formation is not uncommon in the brainstem, cerebellum, spinal cord, and the optic nerves, which are structurally part of the CNS, in which the oligodendrocytes are antigenically similar to the oligodendrocytes in the spinal cord.

All multiple sclerosis lesions show a variable degree of axonal loss, ranging from 10 to 20 percent in milder forms of the disease, to 80 percent in severe, acute multiple sclerosis.[23]

Epidemiologic studies support the concept that multiple sclerosis results from an aberrant immune reactivity[24] occurring in a genetically susceptible host who has acquired a specific, or one or more nonspecific, neurotropic infections at a critical age.[25] Genetic susceptibility is thought to be associated with genes within or close to the HLA-DR DQ subregion, located in the short arm of chromosome 6.[26] This primary infection results in a self-sustaining, organ-specific autoimmune disorder that remains latent until activated by a subsequent infection years after the primary event. An alternative explanation suggests that the mechanism is one of persistent systemic viral infection, which contributes to the changes in the CNS periodically, or to a persistent CNS viral infection that is targeted by T cells unpredictably, resulting in an inflammatory response producing myelin damage (bystander response). The common factor in any one of these theoretical situations is the activation of an autoimmune event within the CNS, directed against myelin antigen-specific T cells,[27] but no specific antigen has as yet been identified. Antibodies to myelin basic protein appear to be the most frequent finding in multiple sclerosis,[28] but reactivity to other myelin antigens is a possibility. Candidates include proteolipid protein, the most abundant myelin protein in humans,[29] myelin oligodendrocyte glycoprotein, myelin-associated protein, minor myelin proteins, or heat shock proteins.[30]

The autoimmune reaction probably begins with a systemic infection that is associated with liberation of γ-interferon, resulting in activation of CD4 T lymphocytes. The lymphocytes attach to adhesion molecules on the surface endothelium of postcapillary venules, roll along the surface of the endothelium, producing endothelial cell activation,[31] followed by passage of the CD4 T lymphocytes into the CNS—in effect, disrupting the blood–brain barrier. Once within the CNS, the T-lymphocyte receptors respond to antigen presented by MHC class 2 molecules on macrophages and astrocytes, but oligodendrocytes are usually preserved at this stage.[32] The antigen T-cell receptor interaction is followed by stimulation of helper T cells, T-cell proliferation, and B-cell and macrophage activation, with release of cytokines such as γ-interferon, tissue necrosis factor, interleukin-12, and proteases.[34] The cytokines induce a local inflammatory reaction with further disruption of the blood–brain barrier, followed by a major influx of CD4 lymphocytes and monocytes into the lesion.[35] Myelin damage results from the combined effect of cytotoxic cytokines, particularly tissue necrosis factor[36] and cytotoxic cells.

Oligodendrocytes appear to survive and proliferate in the presence of acute demyelination and interact with hypertrophied astrocytes, an association that may represent a short-term protective mechanism.[37] Consequently, active demyelination and remyelination can occur in acute lesions. Oligodendrocyte depletion in chronic multiple sclerosis lesions may be a slow, insidious process, spanning a protracted period during which there is gradual cell dropout.

Classification of Multiple Sclerosis

Although multiple sclerosis can affect any site in the CNS, it is possible to recognize eight types of the disease (Table 7-1):

1. Relapsing-remitting multiple sclerosis. This is the classical form of multiple sclerosis that often begins in the late teens or twenties with a severe attack followed by complete or incomplete recovery. Approximately 70 percent of patients with multiple sclerosis experience a relapsing-remitting course initially.[38] Further attacks occur at unpredictable intervals, each followed by increasing disability. The relapsing-remitting pattern tends to change into the secondary progressive form of the disease in the late thirties.

2. Primary progressive multiple sclerosis. The disease runs a steady deteriorating course that may be interrupted by periods of quiescence without im-

Table 7-1
Eight Types of Multiple Sclerosis

1. Relapsing-remitting
2. Primary progressive
3. Secondary progressive
4. Relapsing progressive
5. Benign
6. Spinal form
7. Neuromyelitis optica (Devic disease)
8. Marburg variant

provement. The rate of progression is variable; at its most severe, this form of multiple sclerosis can terminate in death within a few years. In contrast, the more chronic form of progressive multiple sclerosis is similar to the benign form of the disease.

3. Secondary progressive multiple sclerosis. The relapsing-remitting form of the disease frequently develops into secondary progressive multiple sclerosis after a variable period of time but usually in the late thirties.

4. Relapsing progressive multiple sclerosis. Occasional cases are encountered where patients with a progressive form of multiple sclerosis have superimposed relapses with no significant recovery.

5. Benign multiple sclerosis. About 20 percent of cases have the benign form of multiple sclerosis. This may be defined as multiple sclerosis in which the patient is able to function at the level of full employment or provide care of home and family independently 10 years after the appearance of the first symptoms. It is extremely unlikely that these patients will ever be incapacitated by the disease and they should continue to live a full life span with only occasional minor symptoms.

The existence of a benign form of multiple sclerosis increases the importance of recording the date of the first symptoms in patients who appear to have few residual abnormal signs several years after the onset of the disease. These patients may be informed that they have a benign form of multiple sclerosis 10 years following their first recorded symptom and that the benign course will continue in the years ahead.

6. Spinal form of multiple sclerosis. This form of multiple sclerosis presents with symptoms and signs of predominantly spinal cord involvement from the beginning and maintains this pattern. There may be a clear-cut pattern of relapse and remission initially, followed by the secondary progressive form of the disease after several years, or the presentation may be one of steady deterioration from the onset.

7. Neuromyelitis optica (Devic syndrome). Most cases of this syndrome are believed to be examples of multiple sclerosis presenting with acute transverse myelitis followed by optic neuritis. Many patients follow a relapsing-remitting course indistinguishable from multiple sclerosis.

8. Marburg variant. This rare and malignant form of multiple sclerosis is associated with a fulminating course of progressive impairment of consciousness, severe visual loss, dysarthria, dysphagia, respiratory insufficiency, and rapid deterioration. It is indistinguishable from acute disseminated encephalomyelitis. The Marburg variant may result from the autoimmune process of multiple sclerosis occurring in an individual with developmentally immature myelin basic protein.[39]

Clinical Features

The diagnosis of multiple sclerosis is based on the clinical demonstration of multiple levels of involvement of the CNS. Symptoms may be grouped under several headings.

Sensory Symptoms   Sensory symptoms are the most common symptoms experienced by patients with multiple sclerosis. These symptoms are often forgotten or ignored by both patient and physician. Even prolonged sensory symptoms fail to evoke concern, in contrast to the almost immediate response that occurs with weakness or paralysis. Consequently, many patients date the onset of multiple sclerosis from the first appearance of weakness, visual loss, or other symptoms of dramatic onset rather than forgotten or poorly recorded sensory symptoms.

Sensory symptoms include impairment of sensation (hypesthesia), tingling (paresthesias), and un-comfortable sensations (dysesthesias) often referred to as "burning," which may be present for days, weeks, or months[40] without objective abnormalities. All patients with suspected multiple sclerosis should be carefully questioned about the occurrence of previous sensory symptoms.

Motor Symptoms   Paralysis or paresis of upper or lower limbs is the most common presenting symptom in patients with multiple sclerosis. Paraparesis is a common early complaint when the patient gives a history of increasing weakness and stiffness of the lower extremities, associated with progressive impairment of gait. Examination shows signs of upper motor neuron involvement with spasticity, increased tendon reflexes, and extensor plantar responses. These findings may be quite subtle in the early states of the disease.

Visual Symptoms   Optic neuritis presents with sudden visual loss and pain on eye movement and a unilateral headache. The condition may be followed by a rapid progression to total loss of vision in the affected eye (Fig. 7-1) When vision is preserved, there is monocular blurring; a central, paracentral, or centrocecal scotoma; and impairment of color vision. In optic neuritis, there may be edema of the optic discs, but the appearance can be normal in retrobulbar neuritis, when the inflammatory response is localized and located proximally in the optic nerve. Temporal pallor is a later development because of demyelination of the maculopapular bundle. However, subclinical involvement of the optic nerve can occur and may be present without symptoms, when the patient first presents with signs of multiple sclerosis or may be identified when the patient presents with the first symptoms of optic neuritis, indicating prior subclinical involvement of the optic nerve.

Recovery from optic neuritis is unpredictable. Many patients experience no further problems for several years and then develop symptoms of brain or spinal cord involvement, indicating multiple sclerosis. However, not all optic neuritis is multiple sclerosis, and only 50 percent of adolescents and young adults who present with the sudden onset of optic neuritis subsequently develop multiple sclerosis.

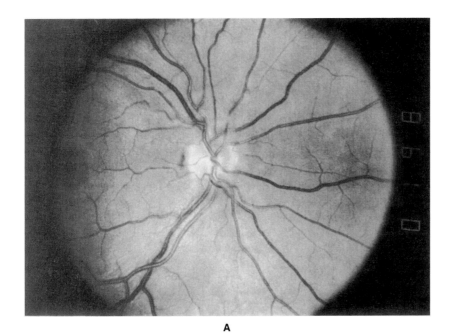

A

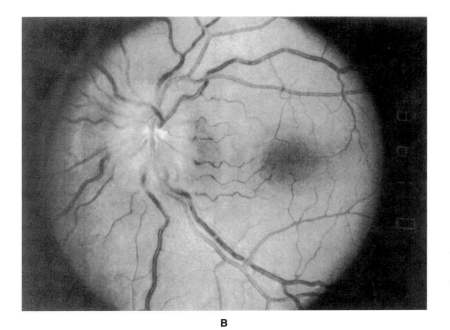

B

Figure 7-1

Acute optic neuritis in a patient with multiple sclerosis. **A.** *Unaffected right eye shows a distinct disc margin.* **B.** *Swollen left optic head of acute optic neuritis.*

Those with a large time interval between the optic neuritis and the development of additional symptoms have a better prognosis. The clinician should always inquire about the possibility of preceding symptoms in any patient who presents with optic neuritis because the presence of symptoms some years before the more dramatic visual symptoms might indicate a more benign prognosis.

Diplopia is indicative of third or sixth nerve involvement in the brainstem. The fourth nerve is rarely involved in isolation. Internuclear ophthalmoplegia is pathognomonic of multiple sclerosis (see page 31) and rarely has another etiology. Unilateral or bilateral Marcus Gunn pupil (page 26) is often present in optic or retrobulbar neuritis.

Bladder Involvement The early symptoms of bladder dysfunction consist of occasional urgency of micturition followed by mild nocturia occurring once a night. The events gradually increase in number, disturbing the sleep of the patient and the bed partner. There is a concomitant increase in urinary frequency and urgency during the day, ultimately resulting in incontinence. Impaired bladder control is usually the result of spinal cord involvement in multiple sclerosis and decreasing bladder control usually parallels increasing paraparesis. However, this is not an inevitable relationship and some patients retain adequate bladder function even when paraplegic.

The anatomical center for bladder control lies in the tegmentum of the pons. The center is under the influence of a higher level of control located in the medial aspect of the frontal lobes. Thus, the frontal lobes can signal the pontine bladder control center to inhibit bladder function or to initiate bladder emptying at will or when convenient. The pontine center then inhibits or permits bladder contraction through connections that traverse the spinal cord and exit through the parasympathetic outflow in the S2–S4 sacral nerves supplying the bladder.

A number of abnormal responses are associated with interruption of bulbar or spinal cord connections in multiple sclerosis.

1. Detrusor hyperreflexia. The interruption of the afferent impulses from the detrusor muscle of the bladder to the pontine micturition center by spinal cord disease results in an uninhibited reflex at the sacral cord level. The detrusor muscle is no longer inhibited as bladder volume increases and detrusor contraction is initiated in response to smaller volumes of urine, resulting in increasing frequency.
2. Detrusor sphincter dyssynergia. The normal pattern of voiding is disturbed. The normal relaxation of the external sphincter is impaired and detrusor contraction is poorly coordinated and accompanied by contraction rather than relaxation of the external sphincter. The result is poor flow of urine and incomplete emptying of the bladder.[41]
3. Detrusor hypocontractility is a failure to empty the bladder secondary to insufficient detrusor pressure or a fading contraction on voiding.[42]

Cerebellar Symptoms Tremor, dysarthria, truncal ataxia, and limb ataxia are frequent symptoms of multiple sclerosis. Occasionally, cerebellar dysfunction is the dominant feature in multiple sclerosis, when a patient presents with adequate vision and muscle strength shows serious disability from the cumulative effects of the several forms of cerebellar ataxia.

Brainstem Symptoms Many patients with multiple sclerosis develop signs of brainstem involvement. Involvement of the oculomotor and sixth cranial nerves as they traverse the substance of the brainstem results in diplopia. Internuclear ophthalmoplegia due to involvement of the interaxial fibers connecting the third, fourth, and sixth nerve nuclei is not uncommon. Sensory loss over the face indicates involvement of the afferent fibers entering the pons from the trigeminal nucleus. Facial weakness may be due to involvement of the seventh nerve in the pons. Episodic dysarthria and dysphagia indicate involvement of the vagus nerve in the medulla, and dysarthria may be due to involvement of the vagus nerve, the glossopharyngeal nerve, and the hypoglossal nerve as they course through the medulla. Involvement of the corticospinal tracts in the brainstem can produce a progressive spastic quadriparesis; involvement of the cerebellar connections results in limb and truncal ataxia.

Spinal Cord Symptoms Most patients with established multiple sclerosis have signs of spinal cord involvement. These signs include some degree of spastic paraparesis with increased tone in both lower limbs, bilateral ankle clonus, increased tendon reflexes, and bilateral extensor plantar responses. It is not unusual to see a progression of paraparesis with increasing disability. This does not necessarily indicate progression of the disease but may be due to progressive gliosis of plaques in the spinal cord. This scarring produces increasing traction on and destruction of axons descending from higher centers in the CNS and results in increasing spasticity and paraparesis.

Abnormal Bowel Function Constipation may be a major problem in advanced multiple sclerosis. Bowel incontinence can be a devastating experience to a patient with multiple sclerosis, particularly if the loss of control occurs in a social situation or in a crowded area such as a shopping center. Many patients react to the incident with reluctance to leave home and are extremely apprehensive if they do so.

Memory Deficits and Dementia Impaired cognitive processing is not unusual in multiple sclerosis when patients often display a verbal working memory deficit owing to a central processing problem.[43] This has a significant impact on reading or other tasks that require the maintenance of verbal information over a short period of time. Dementia occurs in approximately 50 percent of cases, with less cognitive impairment in patients with relapsing-remitting disease than in those with the progressive form.[44] The disease can, however, remain predominantly spinobulbar in form, with little involvement of the white matter in the cerebral hemispheres and preservation of intellect. Patients with demyelination in the periventricular white matter of the brain often show an explosive emotional response with inappropriate laughter or occasional crying during conversation. This condition results from the interruption of an inhibitory dopaminergic pathway connecting the thalamus and the frontal lobe. Despite the laughter, which has been incorrectly termed euphoria, many patients are depressed and are embarrassed by the inability to control this often incongruous response.

Depression Depression, or bipolar affective disorder, is clearly associated with multiple sclerosis and may precede the onset of symptoms of multiple sclerosis in some cases.[45] Character or personality changes with impulsiveness or less inhibition in social interactions[46] may present problems or embarrassment to family members.

Sexual Dysfunction Sexual dysfunction is not uncommon in both men and women with multiple sclerosis. Men experience difficulty in achieving an erection because of diminished penile sensation or difficulty maintaining an erection. Others report failure of orgasm. Sexual dysfunction in women with multiple sclerosis includes lower limb spasticity, lack of vaginal lubrication, and diminished vaginal sensation, any of which can interfere with sexual functioning.

Seizures Epilepsy occurs in 1 to 5 percent of patients with multiple sclerosis, a higher frequency than in the normal population.[47] Seizures are associated with lesions in the cortical or subcortical area and the onset is usually associated with the presence of new lesions in the cortical gray matter or in subcortical regions. When seizures are associated with clinical relapse, the seizures rarely recur. Seizures not related to clinical relapse tend to recur occasionally but control is usually straightforward. Patients with multiple sclerosis, seizures, and progressive cognitive decline have a poor prognosis and are susceptible to status epilepticus.[48]

Tonic Spasms Tonic spasms are paroxysmal, unilateral stereotypical spasms of short duration precipitated by movement or hyperventilation, lasting 30 to 90 s and involving part or the whole of one side of the body. The attacks may be heralded by brief clonic movements. During an attack, the affected limb or limbs are usually extended, but the hands, fingers, feet, and toes may be drawn into a pseudodystonic posture. There may be a spread to the face on the same side with head turning. Speech may be affected by the distortion of the face. The patient is fully alert and usually experiences minimal pain or discomfort. The affected limbs may have a slight degree of weakness after an attack. The condition is believed to be the result of acute demyelination involving the corticospinal tracts in the brainstem or spinal cord.[49]

Lhermitte's sign   Flexion of the head may result in an electric-like shock passing down the spine and into the limbs. This phenomenon, known as Lhermitte's sign, while not pathognomonic, is highly suggestive of multiple sclerosis and may also precede the development of other symptoms by months or years in some cases.

Spasticity   The majority of patients with multiple sclerosis will show some evidence of spasticity, which may vary from a slight increase in tone to severe spastic paraplegia in flexion with limbs held in a permanent flexed posture at the knees and hips. In the mildest of cases, spasticity may present with no more than a slight increase in tendon reflexes and extensor plantar responses. In the most severe cases, spasticity may dominate the clinical picture and be responsible for severe disability.

Psychiatric Symptoms   Psychosis can occur in both chronic, progressive and relapsing-remitting forms of multiple sclerosis when it heralds increasing activity of the disease process.[50] Paranoia or hallucinations are unusual and are occasionally prominent symptoms when there is extensive involvement of both frontal and temporal lobes.

Fatigue   The majority of patients experience fatigue.[51] The onset may be sudden and debilitating, with inability to continue even the simplest of tasks. Fatigue tends to be provoked by a high atmospheric temperature and many patients relate difficulties in functioning in the summer. Some are extremely sensitive to heat and report profound weakness after a hot bath or shower. A febrile illness has the same effect, with the appearance of symptoms suggesting a relapse of the disease. However, there is rapid return to the prefebrile state once the fever subsides.

Pain   Multiple sclerosis is not a painless disease and pain is occasionally a prominent feature. As many as 80 percent of patients experience painful muscle spasms, intermittent or constant limb pain, or spinal pain. Primary pain is usually dysesthetic, occurring most commonly in the lower limbs. However, truncal and upper limb dysesthesias can occur. The dysesthesias may be augmented by tic-like pains, tonic seizures are occasionally painful, and in some cases, Lhermitte's sign is experienced as pain rather than paresthesias. Chronic pain can occur as a dysesthesia in the extremities, in girdle-like fashion around the waist or abdomen, as low back pain or pain in the shoulders due to disuse with capsular adhesions.

Trigeminal neuralgia or atypical facial pain can occur at any stage of the disease. The occurrence of trigeminal neuralgia in a young person should always arouse the suspicion of multiple sclerosis.

Debilitated patients who use a wheelchair often develop joint pains from abnormal posture or from propelling the wheelchair manually. Spasticity and muscle cramps can cause severe pain.

Headache   Migraine headaches are not unusual in multiple sclerosis. Retro-orbital pain presenting as a dull ache, and increasing on eye movement, occurs in optic and retrobulbar neuritis.

Respiratory Impairment   The incidence of respiratory failure in multiple sclerosis is low[52] and usually occurs in the presence of extensive spinal cord or brainstem involvement.[53] Clinical indications of impending respiratory failure include orthopnea, paradoxical movements of the chest wall and abdominal muscles during respiration, and use of accessory muscles of respiration. Patients with suspected impairment of pulmonary function should be monitored carefully with a number of pulmonary function tests, including force vital capacity (FVC), maximal voluntary ventilation (MVV), and maximal expiratory pressure (MEP), coupled with the index score for pulmonary function,[54] which provides a clinical tool for the rapid assessment of significant respiratory dysfunction in multiple sclerosis.

Pregnancy   Multiple sclerosis does not reduce fertility.[55] An apparent reduction in fertility may be secondary to physical disability and to counseling against pregnancy by physicians. Other factors include a decision by women with multiple sclerosis to forego marriage, to have fewer children, or to undergo sterilization. Multiple sclerosis does not affect the course of pregnancy and there is no difference in the duration of labor or frequency of difficult delivery, premature labor or stillbirth.

Relapse rates of multiple sclerosis during pregnancy are significantly reduced, particularly in the third trimester,[56] but there is a significant increase in relapse rates during the first 3 months postpartum.[57] Consequently, these facts should be discussed with a woman seeking advice prior to pregnancy and to her partner, explaining the present knowledge concerning pregnancy and multiple sclerosis. It is important that the partner realize that he will have to assume more responsibility for child care and reduce the burden of responsibility on the mother.[58]

There is an apparent beneficial effect of pregnancy in autoimmune diseases such as rheumatoid arthritis, suggesting that the beneficial effects of pregnancy could be the result of immunomodulation or immunosuppression. However, the explanation for the alteration in the immune system remains illusive.[59]

Diagnostic Procedures

1. The diagnosis of multiple sclerosis is established by careful interpretation of clinical signs and symptoms. These indicate multiple levels of CNS involvement. The diagnosis may be strengthened by interpretation of other findings discussed below, but diagnosis remains a matter of clinical judgment.

2. All patients should be fully investigated for the presence of infection. This includes aerobic and anaerobic blood cultures, urinalysis, culture and sensitivity, and chest x-ray to rule out pneumonia. Many patients have infections that are latent or occult. This dramatically affects response to treatment unless infection is eradicated. Patients with decubitus ulcers, which are chronic and deep, should receive bone scans to rule out the presence of osteomyelitis.

3. Magnetic resonance imaging (MRI). An MRI scan of the brain is abnormal in 95 percent of definite cases of multiple sclerosis, but abnormal MRI findings alone are not sufficient to confirm a diagnosis of multiple sclerosis without compatible clin-

ical abnormalities.[60] MRI scans are abnormal in only 70 percent of patients with probable multiple sclerosis and 30 to 50 percent of patients with possible multiple sclerosis, and some patients with multiple sclerosis may have normal MRI findings.

When patients have a diagnosis of probable multiple sclerosis, a positive MRI scan will raise the category to definite in about 50 percent of cases. The results of positive MRI scanning in those categorized as possibly having multiple sclerosis are less impressive, with only 5 percent changing category from possible to definite. Nevertheless, progression to definite multiple sclerosis is more likely in those with disseminated MRI lesions at presentation and less likely in those without disseminated lesions.[61] Other characteristic features are immediate proximity to the ventricles, lesions greater than 6 mm in diameter, and the presence of infratentorial lesions.[62] Lesions present as multiple areas of increased signal intensity on proton density or T2-weighted image and as hypointense images using T1-weighted images.[63] These lesions are situated predominantly in a periventricular distribution around the lateral ventricles and in the white matter of the brainstem, cerebellum, and spinal cord (Figs. 7-2, 7-3). Lesions in the corpus callosum, which may show atrophy on sagittal images, are more specific for multiple sclerosis. However, the diagnosis of multiple sclerosis requires a history of two attacks with clinical evidence of two separate lesions. An MRI abnormality can now substitute for one of these lesions when it is clearly not related to the other clinically defined lesion. However, an individual who has had a single attack with a single lesion on MRI scan cannot be said to have definite multiple sclerosis and may have a monophasic acute disseminated encephalomyelitis. A repeat MRI scan taken 6 weeks later and demonstrating new lesions would justify a diagnosis of probable multiple sclerosis and lead to additional studies, including evoked potentials and examination for IgG and oligoclonal bands in the cerebrospinal fluid[64] beyond 3 months.

Frequent interval MRI scans have shown that newly encountered lesions found on T2-weighted images have a transient enhancement following administration of gadolinium. In about two-thirds of the cases, these enhancing lesions will continue to show

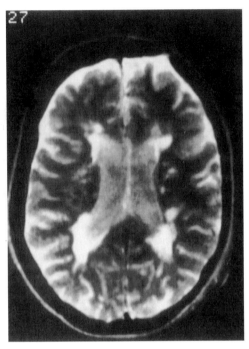

Figure 7-2
MRI scan in chronic multiple sclerosis. Note the confluent periventricular plaques and the moderate ventricular dilatation.

4. Examination of the cerebrospinal fluid (CSF). Acute exacerbations of multiple sclerosis may be accompanied by a lymphocytic or polymorphonuclear pleocytosis in the CSF. This is short-lived and does not usually exceed 200 cells per cubic millimeter. The CSF protein is elevated, particularly in early cases and during acute exacerbations. The level rarely exceeds 100 mg/dL. Gamma globulin elevation is seen in many cases and exceeds 13 percent of the total protein content. About 70 percent of patients have evidence of abnormal intrathecal IgG synthesis, as demonstrated by the IgG index.[70]

$$\frac{\text{IgG CSF/IgG serum}}{\text{albumin CSF/albumin serum}}$$

An index greater than 0.7 indicates synthesis of IgG within the CNS. The presence of IgG oligoclonal bands is a more sensitive measure of local IgG production. However, this finding is nonspecific and

faded enhancement for 4 to 6 weeks with less than 2 percent showing enhancement beyond 3 months.[65] Enhanced lesions tend to appear in clusters over time and lesions seen in T2-weighted MRI scans can regress in size but are unlikely to disappear. Serial studies have shown that the MRI attack rate greatly exceeds the clinical attack rate. There is a much lower rate of new lesions defined by MRI in primary progressive multiple sclerosis than in secondary progressive multiple sclerosis[66] and in the relapsing-remitting form of the disease.

Serial studies have also shown a considerable amount of clinically silent disease activity in relapsing-remitting and secondary progressive multiple sclerosis,[67] but there is a lack of correlation between MRI and clinical disability.[68] Nevertheless, MRI as a measure of multiple sclerosis activity is now widely accepted as a surrogate marker of disease in treatment trials of evolving therapies.[69]

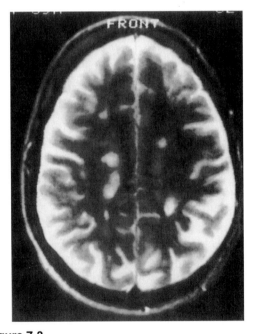

Figure 7-3
T2-weighted MRI shows multiple discrete areas of increased signal in the centrum semiovale. This patient had severe disabling multiple sclerosis. MRI scans with equivalent signal changes may be seen in patients with minimal clinical signs.

oligoclonal bands in the CSF have been seen in patients suffering from cerebral infarction, brain tumors, paraneoplastic syndromes, diabetes mellitus, borreliosis, neurosyphilis, human immunodeficiency virus (HIV) infection, various connective tissue diseases, and hypothyroidism. Consequently, testing must include both serum and CSF. Detection in CSF alone or primarily in the CSF is an indication of local IgG synthesis, which is usually associated with multiple sclerosis. Oligoclonal bands (Table 7-2) are detected in 90 percent of the patients with clinically definite multiple sclerosis. This figure drops to 50 percent in optic neuritis and isolated brainstem and spinal cord disease. Elevation of myelin basic protein is present in approximately 80 percent of cases of acute multiple sclerosis or multiple sclerosis in exacerbation. Antibodies to myelin, myelin basic protein (MBP), myelin oligodendrocyte glycoprotein (MOG), myelin-associated glycoprotein (MAG), and proteolipid protein (PLP) are present in cells in the CSF[71] but are not specific for multiple sclerosis.

5. Visual evoked potentials are positive in about 80 percent of patients with multiple sclerosis. Many of these patients have not had any visual symptoms. Similarly, auditory evoked potentials are positive in about 70 percent of patients with multiple sclerosis and a number of these cases do not show clinical signs of brainstem involvement. Somatosensory evoked potentials are positive in about 60 percent of cases of multiple sclerosis. The presence of abnormal evoked potentials provide additional objective evidence of a heterogenous involvement of the CNS.

Table 7-2
Oligoclonal Bands

Not specific for multiple sclerosis. Can occur in any disease with demyelination.
Multiple sclerosis
Neurosyphilis
Viral encephalitis
Bacterial meningitis
Cerebral lupus erythematosus
Lyme disease
Neurosarcoidosis

6. Neuropsychological testing is useful, particularly in the early stages of apparent intellectual and cognitive failure, when it is necessary to distinguish between early dementia and depression.

7. Urological evaluation. Patients with established symptoms of urgency and frequency of micturition sufficient to cause inconvenience should have a limited urological evaluation with measurement of postvoid residual urine and a cystometrogram.[72]

8. Ophthalmology evaluation. An opinion from an ophthalmologist should be obtained in the event of visual problems. Baseline evaluations of visual acuity, visual fields, color vision and the presence of scotomata are determined accurately and can be used for a comparison should visual deterioration continue.

Differential Diagnosis

Multiple sclerosis can mimic almost any chronic disease affecting the CNS. The diagnosis is usually not difficult in well established cases, with evidence of multiple areas of involvement in the CNS, but early cases often present a problem in diagnosis. Various conditions (Table 7-3) can be confused with multiple sclerosis.

1. The leukodystrophies. The adult forms of metachromatic leukodystrophy, Fabry disease, X-linked adrenaleukodystrophy, globoid leukodystrophy, and leukodystrophy with diffuse Rosenthal fiber formation can present with progressive deterioration and evidence of multiple areas of involvement in the CNS. There is a peripheral neuropathy with slowing of nerve conduction velocities in metachromatic leukodystrophy, which is not present in multiple sclerosis. The demonstration of metachromatic material, low levels of arylsulfatase, and very long-chain fatty acids will establish the diagnosis. The diagnosis of leukodystrophy with diffuse Rosenthal fiber formation can be made only by brain biopsy.

2. Spinocerebellar degenerations. Autosomal dominant spinocerebellar degenerations, sporadic late-onset olivopontocerebellar atrophies (multisystem disease), and Friedrich's ataxia are occasionally misdiagnosed as multiple sclerosis. Diagnostic procedures in late-onset ataxias include MRI scanning of

Table 7-3

*MRI-Detected Abnormalities in White Matter
Resembling Changes in Multiple Sclerosis*

Acute disseminated encephalomyelitis
Adult-onset leukodystrophies
Multisystem disease
Spinocerebellar degeneration
Closed head injury
HIV encephalitis
HTLV-1 myelitis
Progressive multifocal leukoencephalopathy
Neurobrucellosis
Chronic granulomas
Behçet disease
Sjögren syndrome
Brain tumors
Lymphoma
Cerebrovascular disease
Migraine ischemia
Cerebral vasculitis
B_{12} deficiency
Moyamoya
Aging
Drug-induced encephalopathy
Cerebral lupus erythematosus
Neurosarcoidosis
Effects of radiation therapy

the brain and spinal cord and nerve conduction studies. Metabolic evaluation consists of peripheral blood smears for acanthocytosis; determination of plasma amino acids, vitamin E, lactate and pyruvate levels; lipid and lipoprotein determination; and urinary organic acid to identify abetalipoproteinemia, hypobetalipoproteinemia, vitamin E dysmetabolism, mitochondrial cytopathies, and organic acidemias.

3. Syphilis. Both meningeal and vascular syphilis may mimic multiple sclerosis. The diagnosis is established by abnormalities in the CSF and a positive serologic test for syphilis.

4. Wilson disease (hepatolenticular degeneration) usually presents with symptoms and signs of hepatic involvement and neurological dysfunction. However, a number of patients have minimal hepatic involvement with a broad range of neurological signs, including dysarthria, involuntary movements, and deteriorating coordination, followed by progressive dementia and behavioral abnormalities. A misdiagnosis of multiple sclerosis, particularly in those with marked cerebellar ataxia or psychiatric disorder, is not uncommon. Diagnosis is established by a positive slit lamp examination for Kayser-Fleischer rings, cataracts, and determination of serum, copper and ceruloplasmin, and of 24-hour urinary excretion of copper.[73]

5. The antiphospholipid syndrome, which usually presents with deep venous thrombosis or stroke, can mimic multiple sclerosis when repeated minor strokes produce focal deficits and optic neuritis in a young adult.[74] Moreover, some patients will show the presence of areas of increased signal intensity in the periventricular area on a T2-weighted MRI. The diagnosis of the antiphospholipid syndrome is established by a positive anticardiolipin and lupus anticoagulant in the serum.

6. Lyme disease is of major concern in the eastern United States and appears to be spreading south and west. The disease is the cause of intermittent neurological symptoms. In the mildest form, it causes Bell's palsy, but there is a chronic encephalomyelitis with intermittent signs of CNS involvement.

There may be a history of tick bite followed by a migratory rash and arthralgias. Lyme titers or Lyme polymerase chain reaction in the blood or spinal fluid will be positive in these patients.[75]

7. Behçet disease. The presence of cranial neuropathies, cerebellar ataxia, hemiparesis, quadriparesis, pseudobulbar palsy, and peripheral neuropathy in an individual with oral ulcers, genital ulcers, and uveitis suggests Behçet disease. An MRI may reveal findings resembling those seen in multiple sclerosis.

8. HTLV-1 infection. This retrovirus produces a myelopathy and spastic paraparesis and is an occasional cause of more widespread white matter disease. Under these circumstances, it may be difficult to distinguish HTLV-1 infection from multiple sclerosis and appropriate antibody detection in both blood and CSF is necessary.

9. Subacute combined degeneration of the

spinal cord may resemble multiple sclerosis, particularly if there is an associated dementia and optic atrophy. Serum B_{12} levels are low in this condition. Although most cases of serum B_{12} deficiency are acquired, inherited defects have been described in infants and children. Late-onset adult cases mimicking multiple sclerosis have occurred, suggesting that patients diagnosed with multiple sclerosis should be screened for B_{12} deficiency. Similarly, folate dysmetabolism in the rare hereditary adult presentation may resemble multiple sclerosis.

10.   Brain tumor. The presence of a fixed single neurologic deficit in a young adult should always suggest the possibility of a brain tumor rather than multiple sclerosis. The diagnosis is established by MRI or computed tomography (CT) scanning.

11.   The arteritides. Both polyarteritis nodosa and systemic lupus erythematosus can produce multiple lesions in the CNS. However, other organs are often involved and there is evidence of peripheral neuropathy with an elevated sedimentation rate, abnormal nerve conduction velocities, and a positive nerve biopsy. Abnormal antibodies in lupus erythematosus should reveal the presence of this condition, but abnormal antibodies are not always present in isolated cerebral lupus erythematosus. Similarly, isolated cranial arteritis can mimic multiple sclerosis and is often accompanied by a normal sedimentation rate and a lack of any abnormal serum antibody levels. Diagnosis of this condition is established by angiography, which reveals beading and irregularity in the lumen of the intracranial arteries.

12.   Transverse myelitis. Multiple sclerosis is a relatively rare cause of transverse myelitis. Unless there is definite evidence of multiple areas of involvement of the CNS, other conditions causing transverse myelitis should be considered.

13.   Mitochondrial disorders. The association of optic atrophy, ataxia, spasticity, and hyperreflexia, usually associated with multiple sclerosis, can occur in Leber's optic atrophy, now believed to be the result of mitochondrial DNA mutations. An electrocardiogram and molecular diagnostic tests are suggested in suspected cases of Leber disease.

Other mitochondrial metabolic disorders can mimic multiple sclerosis, including MELAS syndrome (mitochondrial encephalomyopathy, lactic acidosis, and stroke-like episodes), chronic milder forms of the MEERF syndrome (myoclonus epilepsy and ragged red fibers), and the adult form of Leigh syndrome.

14.   Sjögren syndrome. There is a marked similarity in the clinical presentation of multiple sclerosis and Sjögren syndrome with CNS involvement. Both conditions may have optic neuritis, spinal cord involvement, psychiatric manifestations, abnormal evoked potentials, similar CSF profiles, and indistinguishable abnormalities on MRI and CT scans. Features that may distinguish Sjögren syndrome include the sicca complex, xerophthalmia, xerostomia, or recurrent salivary gland enlargement, peripheral neuropathy, vasculitis in skin or muscle, elevated sedimentation rate, abnormal antinuclear antibody, positive rheumatoid factor, anti-RO(SSA) or anti-LA(SSB) antibodies and decreased complement.

15.   Hereditary spastic paraparesis with progressive lower limb weakness and spasticity, hyperreflexia, and urinary incontinence can mimic multiple sclerosis, particularly when there is an associated optic atrophy. A positive family history suggesting an autosomal dominant trait and the slow progression of the disease should lead to the exclusion of multiple sclerosis.

Treatment

1.   Infection. Because there is strong evidence that the first attack or exacerbation of multiple sclerosis may be caused by viral or bacterial[77] infection, all infections should be treated promptly.

2.   Bed rest. Patients with acute multiple sclerosis or an acute exacerbation of multiple sclerosis benefit from complete bed rest. Patients who are removed from the necessity of self-care and added worries of the home environment improve with rest. However, the period of rest should not be protracted and no more than a few days in the great majority of patients. Once the patient shows improvement, the institution of a graded program of physical therapy becomes paramount.

3.   Corticosteroids. Evidence suggests that high doses of intravenous corticosteroids (glucocorticoids) may arrest the progress of multiple sclerosis.

Corticosteroids have several beneficial effects, including inhibition of secretion by antigen-presenting cells and T cells of the cytokines, tumor necrosis factor α, and interleukin-6. An additional effect may be inhibition of secretion of γ-interferon and interleukin-12 by T cells.[78,79]

About 85 percent of patients with relapsing-remitting multiple sclerosis shows objective signs of neurological improvement during treatment with intravenous corticosteroids.[80] Fifty percent of patients with progressive multiple sclerosis are improved by intravenous corticosteroids, although for many, the response is limited to a reduction in spasticity.[81] This figure may improve if attention is paid to prevention of infection in the posttreatment period.

The short-term use of intravenous corticosteroids is attended by few side effects. Some patients experience insomnia during treatment, a few show signs of euphoria; gastric upset with epigastric pain responds to ranitidine 150 mg q12h. Hypomania or depression are unusual events. The daily dose and duration of therapy have not been determined, but an intravenous dose of 1000 mg methylprednisolone over 3 h daily for 7 days, followed by alternate-day oral methylprednisolone, beginning with 96 mg (16 mg tablets × 6) at breakfast, and reducing by 8 mg q.o.d., will allow the hypothalamic-pituitary-adrenal axis to recover by the end of therapy.[82] In the majority, this regimen will result in at least 6 months' remission and several months or even years in many cases. The treatment can be repeated if relapse occurs.

As indicated under Diagnostic Procedures, all patients will have received full investigation for infection, including blood cultures, urinalysis, culture and sensitivity, and chest x-ray to rule out pneumonia before receiving corticosteroid therapy. Infections should be treated before and during treatment with corticosteroids. One of the major causes of failure or poor response to corticosteroids is the presence of a concomitant, untreated infection.

4. Immunosuppressive therapy. Long-term treatment with immunosuppressants may reduce the frequency of relapses in patients with multiple sclerosis. Azathioprine is probably the safest drug in this category and has reduced relapse to 70 percent in 3 years, compared to 80 percent in the placebo group.[83]

Azathioprine has few adverse effects and has not been shown to carry an increased risk of inducing neoplasia,[84] unlike the more powerful immunosuppressive therapies used to prevent transplant rejection.[85]

Methotrexate, a drug used widely in the treatment of chronic autoimmune diseases such as rheumatoid arthritis and psoriasis, will reduce progression of disability in chronic progressive multiple sclerosis.[86] Low-dose therapy using 7.5 mg per week orally is effective, and adverse effects are few, but regular monitoring with complete blood counts and liver function tests is advised. Currently, low-dose oral methotrexate appears to be the best therapy for slowing deterioration in chronic progressive multiple sclerosis.[87]

Cladribine, a specific antilymphocytic agent that is incorporated into DNA and induces lymphocyte apoptosis, is reported to produce improvement in patients with chronic progressive multiple sclerosis.[88] The drug, which is administered intravenously, has been reported to induce lymphopenia and severe but reversible aplastic anemia; the safety of cladribine has yet to be determined.

Results of studies of cyclosporine in multiple sclerosis have been equivocal. The drug may be beneficial in patients with frequently recurring or nearly continuous disease activity but unacceptable toxicity[89] and marginal benefit[90] have limited the use of cyclosporine in multiple sclerosis.

5. Total lymphoid irradiation, originally introduced for the treatment of Hodgkin disease, has theoretical benefits in multiple sclerosis, in that treatment produces a significant reduction in CD4 and CD8 lymphocytes. Potential risks of therapy, such as malignancy, have limited the use of this modality, and the results of some studies have been equivocal.[91]

6. Plasmapheresis has marginal benefit in multiple sclerosis[92] and has not been accepted as an established therapy for this disease.

7. Interferon β. Interferon β-1b (Betaseron) is reportedly effective in reducing clinical attacks of multiple sclerosis by approximately 30 percent over 24 months, when compared to placebo.[93] Treatment reduces frequency of major attacks by 50 percent and

produces immediate and significant reduction in contrast-enhanced MRI lesions[94] and fewer new lesions in patients receiving interferon B.[95] The dose is 8 million units subcutaneously every other day.

Interferon β-1a (Avonex) is also an available alternative therapeutic agent. It also lowers multiple sclerosis attack frequency by 30 percent and decreases disease activity, measured by gadolinium-enhanced MRI.[97] The dose is 6 million units intramuscularly, once weekly.

Adverse effects of interferons include fever, chills, headache, and myalgia. These "flu-like" symptoms begin 4 to 6 h after injection and last for a few hours. The response tends to resolve after a few weeks of therapy but can persist for several months in a minority of cases. Acetaminophen or ibuprofen, given 1 h before injection, reduces the flu-like response. The dose of acetominophen or ibuprofen can be repeated, should the flu-like symptoms still occur. The persistence of adverse effects requires reduction of the dose by 50 percent, that is, 4 million units of Betaseron and gradually increasing the dose to 8 million units over a period of 4 weeks. Prednisone 20 mg given 2 h before the injection of interferon β is also effective in reducing adverse effects.

Other adverse effects include redness at injection sites, which occurs in many patients receiving Betaseron. The local reaction lasts for many weeks before resolution. Necrosis at the injection site is rare, but persistence of painful skin reactions requires the cessation of treatment.

Interferon β has been associated with depression, which usually responds to a serotonin uptake inhibitor such as fluoxetine. Inquiry should be made regarding thoughts of suicide, which, if present, are an indication to stop treatment with interferon β.

The development of virus-neutralizing antibodies has been reported in 35 percent of multiple sclerosis patients receiving interferon β-1b. The appearance of antibodies has minimal effect on clinical response and does not appear to be a reason for discontinuing therapy. The action of interferon β in multiple sclerosis appears to be multifactorial, including sequestration of T lymphocytes into lymphoid tissue and impaired migration of T lymphocytes through the blood–brain barrier by inhibition of adhesion molecules on endothelial cells; decreased release of cytokines, including γ-interferon, from T lymphocytes; decreased tissue necrosis factor production by macrophages; and paradoxically, increased interleukin-6 production.[98]

8. Copolymer 1. The development of copolymer 1 was based on the premise that myelin basic protein is encephalitogenic and can cause experimental allergic encephalomyelitis (EAE) in animals. However, although some regions of the protein are encephalitogenic, other regions will suppress the development of EAE. This led to the synthesis and testing of several copolymers of amino acids, based on the amino acid composition of myelin basic protein. One such copolymer, designated copolymer 1, suppressed EAE in guinea pigs and other animals. The mechanism of suppression is not certain, but copolymer 1 seems to inhibit human T-cell lines specific for myelin basic protein.[99] Consequently, the application of copolymer 1 to multiple sclerosis was a natural development in therapy. A double-blind placebo-controlled trial of copolymer 1 in patients with relapsing-remitting multiple sclerosis over a 24-month period indicated a statistically significant reduction in the copolymer treated group, compared to the placebo group.[100] The dose is 30 mg copolymer 1 daily by subcutaneous injection. Side effects are mild, consisting of a local reaction at the site of injection and rare transient palpitations, flushing, sweating, or a feeling of chest tightness and anxiety.

9. Immunoglobulin therapy. Treatment with intravenous immunoglobulin has received some attention in recent years and there is some indication that IVIG may be safe and effective in reducing the frequency of exacerbations in relapsing-remitting multiple sclerosis.[101]

10. Physical therapy. All patients with multiple sclerosis should be evaluated by a physiatrist and should be placed in a graded program of physical therapy. This program should be under constant review so it can be modified, depending on the results of corticosteroid and other therapies, as well as the benefit of the physical therapy itself.

11. Spasticity. Increased muscle tone, exaggerated tendon reflexes, clonus, and spontaneous

muscle spasms are often present in patients with advanced multiple sclerosis. An acute increase in spasticity can occur during an exacerbation of multiple sclerosis, or spasticity may present as an insidious deterioration over a period of months, when the deterioration is often not apparent to patient or therapist. Baclofen (Lioresal) is effective in reducing spasticity and can be given in doses up to 120 mg daily. The tendency is to underdose. The medication should be given in an initial dose of 20 mg q12h orally, with gradual increments over several weeks to an effective level. High doses, although reducing spasticity, may increase weakness in some cases. Diazepam (Valium) or clonazepam (Klonopin) are potent spasmolytic agents. The tendency to drowsiness can be mitigated by beginning with a low dose and only increasing when the patient is comfortable, that is, not drowsy.

Dantrolene sodium (Dantrium) is effective in reducing spasticity but has limited applications because it almost invariably causes weakness. However, it can be useful for treatment of spasticity in nonambulatory patients with severe prolonged muscle contractions, who will not be adversely affected by the decrease in voluntary muscle power associated with the use of this drug. Adverse effects include damage to the liver, drowsiness, and light-headedness. An initial dose of 25 mg/day may be increased by 25 mg increments every week, to a maximum dose of 100 mg/day.

Tizanidine is an effective antispastic agent[102] with an antispasticity effect comparable to baclofen.[103] Tizanidine dosage should be titrated beginning with 2 mg at night and gradually increasing by 2 mg every 4 days in divided doses, until therapeutic goals have been achieved without adverse effects. The larger dose should be given at bedtime to minimize adverse effects. The average daily dose is 18 to 24 mg, and the total daily dose should not exceed 36 mg.[104] Adverse effects include dry mouth, drowsiness, hypotension, light-headedness, abnormal liver function tests, and the rare occurrence of hallucinations. These adverse effects tend to decrease in intensity as the duration of therapy increases.

Sudden muscle spasms (charley horses), whether nocturnal or diurnal, often respond to clonazepam, which is particularly useful for nocturnal spasms, in that clonazepam not only reduces spasm but also induces sleep without contributing to fatigue the next day.[105]

When patients fail to respond to oral medication, intrathecal baclofen delivered through a programmed pump placed in the abdominal wall, with an intrathecal catheter in the spinal canal, produces remarkable reduction of spasticity and spasms in patients with severe spastic paraparesis. Potentially ambulatory patients have returned to walking in some cases.

Botulinum toxin is effective in reducing spasticity when injected into selected muscles but has had limited application to date.

12. Visual difficulties. Patients should be encouraged to report visual deterioration at the onset of the problem. Because optic neuritis can develop rapidly, further deterioration should be treated promptly, with intravenous or oral corticosteroids in a high dose. In many cases, this produces rapid improvement in symptoms or stabilizes the condition, with subsequent slower but steady improvement in visual acuity.

13. Weakness. It is very difficult to strengthen a muscle weakened by central denervation. The potassium channel blocking agents 4-aminopyridine and 3-4-diaminopyridine may improve action potential provocation in demyelinated axons and improve neurological function.[106] Body cooling, using cooling vests or repeated cold showers in the summer months, are effective in those who are heat sensitive.

14. Fatigue may strike without warning. Families should be informed about the fatigue factor and the unpredictable development of this symptom. This prevents resentment when the patient is suddenly unable to attend a long-planned social function and when there is a need for extra rest periods during the day. The intense fatigue associated with a febrile illness will respond once the body core temperature returns to normal. Every patient with recent onset of fatigue should be evaluated for depression, medication effect, or intercurrent illness.

A number of drugs may help eliminate fatigue, including amantadine 100 mg twice a day, pemoline (Cylert) 37.5 mg morning and noon, methylphenidate (Ritalin) 10 mg morning and noon, fluoxetine

(Prozac) 20 mg every morning, or selegiline 5 mg q12h orally.

15. Pain is a common feature of multiple sclerosis. The treatment consists of physical therapy, when appropriate, and medication. Mild chronic pain may respond to acetaminophen or propoxyphene and acetaminophen (Darvocet-N). Nonsteroidal anti-inflammatory drugs should be used with caution to avoid gastric ulceration. Ibuprofen 600 mg, given with meals, is an effective analgesic. Tramadol (Ultram) 50 mg with misoprostol (Cytotec) 100 μg, to limit the risk of gastric ulceration, will control moderately severe pain. Gabapentin beginning 300 mg 12h and increasing, as tolerated, to as high as 2700 mg in divided doses, or amitriptyline 10 mg q.h.s., increasing slowly by 10-mg increments to 80 to 100 mg daily, are both useful in pain control. Trigeminal neuralgia usually responds to carbamazepine but the response is less predictable in atypical facial pain. A painful Lhermitte's sign often shows response to carbamazepine or clonazepam as do tic-like extremity pains. If opioids are prescribed, the medication should be prescribed by one practitioner. The risk of addiction with oral opioids is low, but dependency can occur. Neurolytic nerve blocks are required occasionally, including epidural blocks for chronic sciatic pain.

Migraine headaches respond to sumatriptan or other therapies outlined in Chapter 5.

16. Ankle edema. Swelling of the ankles in patients with limited walking or in those who are nonambulatory and confined to a wheelchair is a gravity effect with fluid accumulating in the dependent tissues of the feet and ankles. Consequently, the use of diuretics is of little value. The patient should lie supine for several hours a day, with the ankles elevated above the level of the heart. This can be accomplished by having the patient lie supine with the feet elevated on a firm cushion or over the armrest of a sofa, thus permitting gravity-driven drainage over the lower limbs. The use of leotards or elastic stockings may also be helpful.

17. Restricted mobility. Many patients with limited mobility resist the use of a wheelchair and require a great deal of persuasion to use an electric cart. The idea that this will lead to further weakening is frequently expressed and is, of course, not true. The severe paraparetic with good upper limb function should be encouraged to use an electric cart. The increased mobility and broadening of the patient's social contacts is truly remarkable, once this is accepted, and the electric cart is an essential therapeutic tool in many cases.

18. Decubitus ulcers. Skin care is one of the paramount needs in the wheelchair-bound paraplegic patient or in those who are bedridden. With few exceptions, skin breakdown and the development of decubitus ulcers is the result of neglect by caregivers. Treatment requires removal of pressure in the affected area and bacterial culture, followed by the use of appropriate antibiotics when the ulcer is infected. When the ulcer fails to heal or when the patient appears to be deteriorating, the suspicion of an underlying osteomyelitis indicates the need for a radioactive bone scan to confirm this diagnosis. A protracted course of intravenous antibiotics is indicated in such cases. Deep (third degree) decubitus ulcers usually require debridement and plastic surgery with surgical reconstruction.

19. Urinary tract infection. Cystitis is common in female patients with multiple sclerosis and has an increased frequency in male patients using self-catheterization. Although pyelonephritis is uncommon, it can occur in severely debilitated patients and is a potent factor in chronic illness, with anemia, weight loss, and fatigue. Urinary tract infections require urinary culture and sensitivity testing, with the use of appropriate antibiotic therapy. Attention to the symptoms of infection and immediate treatment facilitates the use of a Foley catheter or suprapubic catheter and increases the safety of self-catheterization.

20. Management of bladder dysfunction.

A. Detrusor hyperreflexia. The early symptoms of bladder dysfunction are usually caused by detrusor hyperreflexia, with urgency, frequency, and occasional nocturia. Most patients can be managed with an anticholinergic such as oxybutynin chloride 5 mg q12h and increasing to 5 mg q8h if necessary. Tolterodine (Detrol) 2 mg q12h is equally effective and has fewer adverse effects. Imipramine PM 75 to 100 mg q.h.s. is a useful alternative, particularly when nocturia is a problem. Pro-Banthine 15 mg with meals and at bedtime is an effective alternative. Hyoscyamine time release 0.375 mg at night is also effective in reducing nocturia.

B. Sphincter detrusor dyssynergia with poor flow, interrupted stream, and increased postvoid residual responds to prazosin 0.5 mg/day, increasing by 0.5-mg increments to an effective dose, if there are no hypotensive effects.[107] Doxazosin mesylate tablets 1 mg q.h.s., increasing by increments to effect, are also helpful.

C. Incomplete emptying with a post-micturition residual volume greater than 150 mL requires intermittent self-catheterization. This technique has revolutionized the management of bladder dysfunction in multiple sclerosis[108] but requires instruction and is a clean rather than sterile procedure. Repeated bladder infections are not unusual during the first few months of self-catheterization but are reduced as the bladder begins to tolerate the presence of bacteria and clean technique improves. Anticholinergic drugs can be continued in patients performing intermittent self-catheterization.

D. Surgical procedures. Severe or total incontinence requires the use of an indwelling catheter or suprapubic catheter.[109] There seems to be little difference in the development of infection in these two techniques, but some patients find a suprapubic catheter with continuous drainage into a catheter bag more convenient than the transurethral catheter, and the choice should be offered, when appropriate.

Augmentation cystoplasty to increase the storage volume in a severely contracted hyperreflexic bladder is of occasional benefit for patients who can perform self-catheterization.

21. Intention tremor is a common sign in multiple sclerosis and many patients develop resting tremor enhanced by action in the later stages of the disease. These are difficult symptoms to control. Devices to dampen tremor, such as weights applied to the wrists, are of limited benefit. Medication is unpredictable. Propranolol (Inderal) beginning 20 mg tid and increasing to as high as 240 mg/day when the long-acting preparation can be used, may be effective in some cases. Other drugs of occasional benefit include clonazepam, primidone, and hydroxyzine. Carbonic anhydrase inhibitors such as acetazolamide and Neptazane may help in some cases, and isoniazid in high doses has been reported to decrease tremor, but adverse effects are not uncommon. In many cases, a combination of drugs is the most effective approach to this problem.

22. Unsteadiness (ataxia). No medications are available to modify ataxia. The physician must persuade the patient who is at risk from falling to take reasonable precautions to reduce the effects of ataxia. Light-weight wheeled vehicles with hand brakes are useful, rather than the standard walker, which is slow and cumbersome. Severe ataxia is an indication for the use of an electric cart, even though the patient has little or no weakness, and this should be encouraged at an early stage, because improvement in ataxia is unusual.

23. Contractures. Paraplegia and flexion with knee and hip contractures are common manifestations of neglect and should not happen in a well planned treatment program. Contractures can be prevented by physical therapy, appropriate splinting, and the use of antispasticity agents such as baclofen or tizanidine. If contractures are established, early surgical intervention is necessary to release joints and restore normal limb posture. The baclofen pump has major benefit when contractures are the result of severe flexor spasticity.

24. Diplopia is often temporary during an exacerbation of multiple sclerosis and should be treated by patching one eye. The patch should be alternated over each eye daily. When diplopia is an established symptom, the use of prisms in eyeglasses may help. Surgical correction by an ophthalmologist is needed occasionally.

25. Impairment of bowel control. Bowel incontinence can be a devastating event in patients with multiple sclerosis, sufficient in some cases to convert an outgoing, gregarious patient into a recluse. The problem can be solved by development of the innate but dormant gastrocolic reflex. The patient is instructed to attempt bowel movements immediately after breakfast each day. The reflex may not function for several weeks, but eventually, it will return and bowel evacuation becomes an automatic function in the morning. The patient is then free of worry about incontinence for the rest of the day.

Constipation is a common complaint. A stool softener such as docosate sodium 100 mg b.i.d. or bulk agents such as Metamucil may suffice in mild cases. When constipation is established, the patient should take 30 mL Milk of Magnesia, plus 2 senna tablets (Senokot) at night, if there has been no bowel movement for 2 days. This should result in a bowel movement after breakfast the next morning. An alternative method is to use lactulose syrup 1 to 2 tablespoons daily. In refractory cases, bisacodyl suppository (Dulcolax) 10 mg can be used in the morning. Failure of bowel movement after these measures requires the periodic use of an enema.

Fecal impaction is a problem in bedridden or immobile patients. Manual removal of fecal material followed by enemas may be necessary. The venerable but extremely effective milk and molasses enema is recommended as a last resort.

26. Sexual dysfunction. Sexual dysfunction is not uncommon in both men and women with multiple sclerosis, occurring in almost 80 percent of men with advanced multiple sclerosis and in approximately 50 percent of women with similar disability.

In men, failure to achieve erection rarely responds to oral therapy with yohimbine or hormonal replacement, with parenteral testosterone which, in reality, should only be used for hypogonadal disorders. Penile prostheses are cumbersome and subject to infection. Intercavernous injection of alprostadil (prostaglandin E)[110] or propiverine combined with phentolamine increases arterial inflow into the penis, while decreasing venous outflow. Both methods are effective, with restoration of ability to achieve satisfactory intercourse in the majority of cases. Adverse effects include mild pain and dizziness. The dose of alprostadil or propiverine should be titrated to achieve a satisfactory but not prolonged erection. Adverse effects are infrequent and include prolonged erection, priapism, hematoma, hypotension, and fibrosis.

Another method using transurethral suppositories of alprostadil is an equally successful alternative therapy, with fewer adverse effects.[111] It is probable that sildenafil citrate tablets will supersede most methods for improving erectile function in males. The use of this drug is effective in most cases of erectile dysfunction with few serious adverse effects, the most common of which are headache in 16% of patients, flushing in 10%, and dyspepsia in 7%.

Female sexual problems include loss of vaginal sensation or lubrication. The latter can be treated with vaginal lubricant. Loss of vaginal sensation requires empathy and understanding by a concerned partner who is prepared to assist in the development of satisfactory sexual foreplay.

Loss of vaginal sensation can be treated in some cases with a vibrator, which enhances sensation in the vaginal area.

27. Cognitive dysfunction. About 40 percent of patients have cognitive difficulties,[112] which are usually mild. The main deficits relate to retention and recall, short-term memory, attention, and delayed processing of information. When these difficulties interfere with the ability to function, neuropsychological testing should be performed to measure the extent of deterioration and to exclude depression, which is a major cause of impaired memory in multiple sclerosis. A small percentage of patients do show significant disability with cognitive impairment, sufficient to interfere with daily activities. These situations can be treated with a cognitive rehabilitation program, allowing the patient to circumvent or minimize these difficulties. Dementia, if sufficient to produce declining ability to function independently, is rare[113] and often associated with atrophy of the corpus callosum.

28. Respiratory impairment treatment should be directed to the control of infection followed by intravenous corticosteroid therapy. The dictum—if in doubt, don't wait, intubate and place the patient on a ventilator—is applicable in these cases.

29. Bulbar dysfunction. Dysarthria is not unusual in multiple sclerosis but is rarely of sufficient magnitude to interfere with communication. Should this happen, the services of a speech pathologist are indicated.

Dysphagia is, however, common and often undetected in patients with multiple sclerosis. This involves a disturbance of both the oral and pharyngeal phase of swallowing, and evaluation by a speech therapist, including radiological investigations with a barium swallow and visual fluoroscopy, is indicated. The speech pathologist can then suggest changes in diet and the use of various maneuvers to facilitate swallowing. In advanced cases, when dysphagia is a major problem, the patient should be fed through a percutaneous gastrostomy tube.[114]

30. Community services. Patients with severe multiple sclerosis who are unable to continue their employment, or who become increasingly dependent on others, face the prospect of growing problems at home and in the community. Most are not equipped to cope with the stress of chronic illness and should receive social service assessment and advice whenever possible. This results in a smoother transition from hospital to home and better adjustment to home conditions, with improved support for the patient and the family. To this end, identification and referral to community resources available to multiple sclerosis patients should be implemented in all cases with more than a minor degree of disability.

31. Simple prophylactic measures.

A. Combat infection. In many cases, a relapse occurs after an infection. It is prudent, therefore, to treat all infections in multiple sclerosis patients seriously and to resort to the early use of antibiotics. This will not have any effect on viral infections but antibiotic therapy will reduce the risk of secondary bacterial infections such as sinusitis, bronchitis and pneumonia.

B. Avoid fatigue. Some patients note relapse following periods of unexpected exercise. Ambulatory patients with multiple sclerosis should avoid sudden unexpected athletic activities or prolonged exertion. Those who wish to exercise should develop an incremental program of activity and stop whenever they experience fatigue.

C. Emotional stress. As a group, multiple sclerosis patients experience more emotional stress than those who are well. There are increased rates of divorce, more financial problems, and fewer opportunities for gainful employment. Substandard care for the chronically disabled and limitations on mobility because of a lack of transportation or lack of proper building access adds to the emotional distress of multiple sclerosis sufferers. Whether such stress leads to exacerbation is debatable, but every effort should be made to reduce emotional distress by appropriate treatment or referral to community agencies.

Patients with depression will often benefit from the use of appropriate antidepressants such as fluoxetine (Prozac), sertraline (Zoloft), or paroxetine (Paxil), which can be combined with psychotherapy in appropriate cases.

D. Avoid excessive, prolonged exposure to sunlight. Patients with multiple sclerosis experience considerable weakness with the reappearance of previous symptoms if exposed to a hot environment, in particular, after prolonged exposure to sunlight. The patient should be warned about this possibility and reassured that the symptoms will resolve once the body core temperature decreases.

Prognosis

The prognosis in multiple sclerosis has improved in the last two decades.[115] The mean survival is now 20 to 25 years. This can be attributed to better treatment and control of infection in debilitated patients. The physician should be frank with the patient and relatives in discussing the prognosis. Multiple sclerosis resembles a chronic infectious disease in presentation and prognosis. Consequently, multiple sclerosis may be benign, relapsing and remitting, primary or secondary progressive, severely disabling, or fatal. In general, patients who present with mild symptoms and who have several mild relapses tend to remain in the mild category and do not become severely disabled. Approximately 20 percent of patients remain fully active and fully employed 10 years after the diagnosis of multiple sclerosis and should be informed that they have a benign form of the disease and will not be disabled by multiple sclerosis. However, these patients must also be informed that mild exacerbations of multiple sclerosis will continue at unpredictable times well past the fiftieth year. More than 50 percent of patients continue to work full-time,[116] whereas 33 percent are paraparetic, paraplegic, or quadriplegic, and 25 percent require intermittent or constant catheterization for bladder dysfunction.[117]

The prognosis of multiple sclerosis can be improved by avoiding any precipitating factors. The patients should be advised to identify and treat infections promptly, to avoid unusual physical or emotional stress, and to avoid prolonged exposure to sunlight. All infections should be treated with the early use of antibiotics. Patients with chronic multiple sclerosis who are bedridden or confined to a wheelchair often experience slow deterioration, which is not appreciated by patients or by relatives. The prognosis can be improved in these cases by regular reevaluation at 6-month intervals, followed by prompt attention to obvious areas of deterioration. Patients with urinary tract problems should be reevaluated frequently. Loss of function in the limbs calls for prompt reinstitution of physical therapy and treatment with intravenous corticosteroids. Paraparesis should not render a patient bedridden. Prescription of the correct type of wheelchair and instruction in the proper transfer from bed to chair permit broader contact with friends and relatives, improve morale, and improve the long-term outlook for the patient. Pregnancy is associated with clinical stability in most cases, but the postpartum period carries a risk of exacerbation of multiple sclerosis by two or three times the expected relapse rate. Patients should be told that there is some increased risk of multiple sclerosis in the offspring if one parent has the disease, but the actual risk is small.

REFERENCES

1. Azzimondi G, Stracciari A, Rinaldi R, et al: Multiple sclerosis with very late onset: report of six cases and review of the literature. *Eur Neurol* 34:332, 1994.
2. Kurland LT: The evolution of multiple sclerosis epidemiology. *Ann Neurol* 36(Suppl 1): S2, 1994.
3. McLeod JG, Hammond SR, Hallpike JF: Epidemiology of multiple sclerosis in Australia. With NSW and SA survey results. *Med J Australia* 160:117, 1994.
4. Beer S, Kesselring J: High prevalence of multiple sclerosis in Switzerland. *Neuroepidemiology* 13:14, 1994.
5. Fernandez O, Luque G, San Román C, et al: The prevalence of multiple sclerosis in the Sanitary District of Veléz-Málaga, southern Spain. *Neurology* 44:425, 1994.
6. Rosati G: Descriptive epidemiology of multiple sclerosis in Europe in the 1980s: a critical overview. *Ann Neurol* 36(Suppl 2): S164, 1994.
7. Weinshenker BG: Epidemiology of multiple sclerosis. *Neurol Clin* 14:291, 1996.
8. Sadovnick AD, Ebers GC: Genetics of multiple sclerosis. *Neurol Clin* 13:99, 1995.
9. Mumford CJ, Wood NW, Kellar-Wood H, et al: The British Isles survey of multiple sclerosis in twins. *Neurology* 44:11, 1994.
10. Compston A: The epidemiology of multiple sclerosis: principles, achievements and recommendations. *Ann Neurol* 36(Suppl 2): S211, 1994.
11. Kahana E, Zilber N, Abramson JH, et al: Multiple sclerosis: genetic versus environmental aetiology: epidemiology in Israel updated. *J Neurol* 241:341, 1994.
12. Sadovnick AD, Ebers GC: Epidemiology of multiple sclerosis: a critical overview. *Can J Neurol Sci* 20:17, 1993.
13. Kurtzke JF, Hyllested K, Heltberg A, et al: Multiple sclerosis in the Faroe Islands. 5. The occurrence of the fourth epidemic as validation of transmission. *Acta Neurol Scand* 88:161, 1993.
14. Sadovnick AD: Genetic epidemiology of multiple sclerosis: a survey. *Ann Neurol* 36(Suppl 2): S194, 1994.
15. Sibley WA, Bamford CR, Clark K: Clinical viral infections and multiple sclerosis. Lancet 1:1313, 1985.
16. Johnson RT: The virology of demyelinating disease. *Ann Neurol* 36(Suppl): S54, 1994.
17. Fujimoto T, Duda RB, Szilvasi A, et al: Streptococcal preparation OK-432 is a potent inducer of IL-12 and a T helper cell 1 dominant state. *J Immunol* 158:5619, 1997.

18. Myhr KM, Frost P, Gronning M, et al: Absence of HTLV-1 related sequences in MS from high prevalence areas in western Norway. *Acta Neurol Scand* 89:65, 1994.

19. Kennedy PG, Steiner I: On the possible viral aetiology of multiple sclerosis. *QJM* 87:523, 1994.

20. Sibley WA, Bamford CR, Clark K, et al: A prospective study of physical trauma and multiple sclerosis. *J Neurol Neurosurg Psychiatry* 54:584, 1991.

21. Siva A, Radhakrishnan K, Kurland LT, et al: Trauma and multiple sclerosis: a population-based cohort study from Olmsted County, Minnesota. *Neurology* 43:1878, 1993.

22. Chelmicka-Schorr E, Arnason BG: Nervous system-immune system interactions and their role in multiple sclerosis. *Ann Neurol* 36(Suppl 1): S29, 1994.

23. Lassmann H, Suchanek G, Ozawa K: Histopathology and the blood–cerebrospinal fluid barrier in multiple sclerosis. *Ann Neurol* 36(Suppl 1): S42, 1994.

24. Oksenberg JR, Begovich AB, Erlich HA, et al: Genetic factors in multiple sclerosis. *JAMA* 270:2362, 1993.

25. Ebers GC, Sadovnick AD: The role of genetic factors in multiple sclerosis susceptibility. *J Neuroimmunol* 54:1, 1994.

26. Warren KG, Catz I, Johnson E, et al: Anti-myelin basic protein and anti-proteolipid protein specific forms of multiple sclerosis. *Ann Neurol* 35:280, 1994.

27. Olsson T: Critical influences of the cytokine orchestration on the outcome of myelin antigen-specific T-cell autoimmunity in experimental autoimmune encephalomyelitis and multiple sclerosis. *Immunol Rev* 144:245, 1995.

28. Warren KG, Catz I: Relative frequency of autoantibodies to myelin basic protein and proteolipid protein in optic neuritis and multiple sclerosis cerebrospinal fluid. *J Neurol Sci* 121:166, 1994.

29. Hafler DA, Weiner HL: Immunologic mechanisms and therapy in multiple sclerosis. *Immunol Rev* 144:75, 1995.

30. van Oosten BW, Truyen L, Barkhof F, et al: Multiple sclerosis therapy. A practical guide. *Drugs* 49:200, 1995.

31. Wakefield AJ, More LJ, Difford J, et al: Immunohistochemical study of vascular injury in acute multiple sclerosis. *J Clin Pathol* 47:129, 1994.

32. Brück W, Schmied M, Suchanek G, et al: Oligodendrocytes in the early course of multiple sclerosis. *Ann Neurol* 35:65, 1994.

33. Ffrench-Constant C: Pathogenesis of multiple sclerosis. *Lancet* 343:271, 1994.

34. Burger D, Dayer JM: Inhibitory cytokines and cytokine inhibitors. *Neurology* 45(Suppl 6): S39, 1995.

35. Hohlfeld R, Meinl E, Weber F, et al: The role of autoimmune T lymphocytes in the pathogenesis of multiple sclerosis. *Neurology* 45(Suppl 6): S33, 1995.

36. Hartung H-P, Archelos JJ, Zielasek J, et al: Circulating adhesion molecules and inflammatory mediators in demyelination. a review. *Neurology* 45(Suppl 6): S22, 1995.

37. Raine CS: The Dale E. McFarlin Memorial Lecture: the immunology of the multiple sclerosis lesion. *Ann Neurol* 36:S61, 1994.

38. Weinshenker BG, Bass B, Rice GP, et al: The natural history of multiple sclerosis: a geographically based study. I. Clinical course and disability. *Brain* 112:133, 1989.

39. Wood DD, Bilbao JM, O'Connors P, et al: Acute multiple sclerosis (Marburg type) is associated with developmentally immature myelin basic protein. *Ann Neurol* 40:18, 1996.

40. Lynch SG, Rose JW: Multiple sclerosis. *Disease-a-Month* 42:1, 1996.

41. Betts CD, D'Mellow MT, Fowler CJ: Urinary symptoms and the neurological features of bladder dysfunction in multiple sclerosis. *J Neurol Neurosurg Psychiatry* 56:245, 1993.

42. Hinson JL, Boone TB: Urodynamics and multiple sclerosis. *Urol Clin North Am* 23:475, 1996.

43. Ruchkin DS, Grafman J, Krauss GL, et al: Event-related brain potential evidence for a verbal working memory deficit in multiple sclerosis. *Brain* 117:289, 1994.

44. Murray TJ: The psychosocial aspects of multiple sclerosis. *Neurol Clin* 13:197, 1995.

45. Hutchinson M, Stack J, Buckley P: Bipolar affective disorder prior to the onset of multiple sclerosis. *Acta Neurol Scand* 88:388, 1993.

46. Rodgers J, Bland R: Psychiatric manifestations of multiple sclerosis: a review. *Can J Psychiatry* 41:441, 1996.

47. Thompson AJ, Kermode AG, Moseley IF, et al: Seizures due to multiple sclerosis: seven patients with MRI correlations. *J Neurol Neurosurg Psychiatry* 56:1317, 1993.

48. Matthews WB: Symptoms and signs, in Matthews WB (ed): *McAlpine's Multiple Sclerosis,* 2nd ed. Edinburgh Churchill-Livingstone, 1991, pp. 61–63.

49. Rose MR, Ball JA, Thompson PD: Magnetic resonance imaging in tonic spasms of multiple sclerosis. *J Neurol* 241:115, 1993.

50. Feinstein A, du Boulay G, Ron MA: Psychotic illness in multiple sclerosis. A clinical and magnetic resonance imaging study. *Br J Psychiatry* 161:680, 1992.

51. Sandroni P, Walker C, Starr A: "Fatigue" in patients with multiple sclerosis. Motor pathway conduction and event-related potentials. *Arch Neurol* 49:517, 1992.

52. Carter JL, Noseworthy JH: Ventilatory dysfunction in multiple sclerosis. *Clin Chest Med* 15:693, 1994.

53. Howard RS, Wiles CM, Hirsch NP, et al: Respiratory involvement in multiple sclerosis. *Brain* 115:479, 1992.

54. Smeltzer SC, Skurnick JH, Troiano R, et al: Respiratory function in multiple sclerosis. Utility of clinical assessment of respiratory muscle function. *Chest* 101:479, 1992.

55. Weinreb HJ: Demyelinating and neoplastic diseases in pregnancy. *Neurol Clin* 12:509, 1994.

56. Abramsky O: Pregnancy and multiple sclerosis. *Ann Neurol* 36(Suppl 1): S38, 1994.

57. Cook SD, Troiano R, Bansil S, et al: Multiple sclerosis and pregnancy. *Adv Neurol* 64:83, 1994.

58. Stenager E, Stenager EN, Jensen K: Effect of pregnancy on the prognosis for multiple sclerosis. A 5-year follow up investigation. *Acta Neurol Scand* 90:305, 1994.

59. Hutchinson M: Pregnancy in multiple sclerosis (editorial). *J Neurol Neurosurg Psychiatry* 56:1043, 1993.

60. Brod SA, Lindsey JW, Wolinsky JS: Multiple sclerosis: clinical presentation, diagnosis and treatment. *Am Fam Physician* 54:1301, 1996.

61. Filippini G, Comi GC, Cosi V, et al: Sensitivities and predictive values of paraclinical tests for diagnosing multiple sclerosis. *J Neurol* 241:132, 1994.

62. Rolak LA: The diagnosis of multiple sclerosis. *Neurol Clin* 14:27, 1996.

63. Francis GS, Evans AC, Arnold DL: Neuroimaging in multiple sclerosis. *Neurol Clin* 13:147, 1995.

64. Olsson T: Cerebrospinal fluid. *Ann Neurol* 36(Suppl 1): S100, 1994.

65. McFarland HF, Franke JA, Albert PS, et al: Using gadolinium-enhanced MRI lesions to monitor disease activity in MS. *Ann Neurol* 32:758, 1992.

66. Thompson AJ, Kermode AG, Wicks D, et al: Major differences in the dynamics of primary and secondary progressive multiple sclerosis. *Ann Neurol* 29:53, 1991.

67. Thompson AJ, Miller D, Youl B, et al: Serial gadolinium enhanced MRI in relapsing/remitting multiple sclerosis of varying disease duration. *Neurology* 42:60, 1992.

68. McDonald WI, Miller DH, Thompson AJ: Are magnetic resonance findings predictive of clinical outcome in therapeutic trials in multiple sclerosis. The dilemma of interferon beta. *Ann Neurol* 36:14, 1994.

69. Paty DW: The interferon-beta 1b clinical trial and its implications for other trials. *Ann Neurol* 36(Suppl 1): S113, 1994.

70. Andersson M, Alvarez-Cermeno J, Bernardi G, et al: Cerebrospinal fluid in the diagnosis of multiple sclerosis: a consensus report. *J Neurol Neurosurg Psychiatry* 57:897, 1994.

71. Link H, Sun JB, Wang Z, et al: Virus-reactive and autoreactive T cells are accumulated in cerebrospinal fluid in multiple sclerosis. *J Neuroimmunol* 38:63, 1992.

72. Sirls LT, Zimmern PE, Leach GE: Role of limited evaluation and aggressive medical management in multiple sclerosis: a review of 113 patients. *J Urol* 151:946, 1994.

73. Natowicz MR, Bejjani B: Genetic disorders that masquerade as multiple sclerosis. *Am J Med Genet* 49:149, 1994.

74. Scott TF, Hess D, Brillman J: Antiphospholipid antibody syndrome mimicking multiple sclerosis clinically and by magnetic resonance imaging. *Arch Intern Med* 154:917, 1994.

75. Rahn DW, Malawista SE: Lyme disease: recommendations for diagnosis and treatment. *Ann Intern Med* 114:472, 1991.

76. Miller DH, Kendall BE, Barter S, et al: Magnetic resonance imaging in central nervous system sarcoidosis. *Neurology* 38:378, 1988.

77. Rapp NS, Gilroy J, Lerner AM: Bacterial infection in exacerbation of multiple sclerosis. *Arch Phys Med Rehabil* 76:1061, 1995.

78. Whitaker JN: Rationale for immunotherapy in multiple sclerosis. *Ann Neurol* 36(Suppl 1): S103, 1994.

79. Travis J: Microbial trigger for autoimmunity? *Science News* 151:380, 1995.

80. Durelli L, Cocito D, Riccio A, et al: High dose intravenous methylprednisolone in the treatment of multiple sclerosis: clinical-immunologic correlations. *Neurology* 36:238, 1986.

81. Milligan NM, Newcombe R, Compston DA: A double-blind controlled trial of high dose methylprednisolone in patients with multiple sclerosis: 1. clinical effects. *J Neurol Neurosurg Psychiatry* 50:511, 1987.

82. Wenning GK, Wietholter H, Schnauder G, et al: Recovery of the hypothalamic-pituitary-adrenal axis from suppression by short-term, high-dose intra-

venous prednisolone therapy in patients with MS. *Acta Neurol Scand* 89:270, 1994.

83. Yudkin PL, Ellison GW, Ghezzi A, et al: Overview of azathioprine treatment in multiple sclerosis. *Lancet* 338:1051, 1991.

84. Amato MP, Siracusa G, Fratiglioni L, et al: azathioprine therapy and cancer risk in multiple sclerosis: a prospective long-term study. *Ann Neurol* 28:282, 1990.

85. Hughes RAC: Immunotherapy for multiple sclerosis (editorial). *J Neurol Neurosurg Psychiatry* 57:3, 1994.

86. Goodkin DE, Rudick RA, Vanderbrug Medendorp S, et al: Low-dose (7.5 mg) oral methotrexate reduces the rate of progression in chronic progressive multiple sclerosis. *Ann Neurol* 37:30, 1995.

87. Pender MP: Recent advances in the understanding, diagnosis and management of multiple sclerosis (review). *Aust N Z J Med* 26:157, 1996.

88. Sipe JC, Romine JS, Koziol JA, et al: Cladribine in treatment of chronic progressive multiple sclerosis. *Lancet* 344:9, 1994.

89. Kappos L, Patzold U, Dommasch D, et al: Cyclosporine versus azathioprine in the long-term treatment of multiple sclerosis results of the German multicenter study. *Ann Neurol* 23:56, 1988.

90. Zhao GJ, Li DK, Wolinsky JS, et al: Clinical and magnetic resonance imaging changes correlate in a clinical trial monitoring cyclosporine therapy for multiple sclerosis. The MS Study Group. *J Neuroimaging* 7:1, 1997.

91. Buffoli A, Micheletti E, Capra R, et al: Progressive multiple sclerosis. Evaluation of the effectiveness of total lymph node irradiation. *Radiol Med (Torino)* 81:899, 1991.

92. Sorensen PS, Wanscher B, Szpirt W, et al: Plasma exchange combined with azathioprine in multiple sclerosis using serial gadolinium-enhanced MRI to monitor disease activity: a randomized single-masked cross-over pilot study. *Neurology* 46:1620, 1996.

93. The IFNB Multiple Sclerosis Study Group. Interferon beta-1b is effective in relapsing-remitting multiple sclerosis. 1. Clinical results of a multicenter randomized double-blind, placebo-controlled trial. Comments. *Neurology* 43:655, 1993.

94. Arnason BG: Interferon beta in multiple sclerosis. *Clin Immunol Immunopathol* 81:1, 1996.

95. Calabresi PA, Stone LA, Bash CN, et al: Interferon beta results in immediate reduction of contrast-enhanced MRI lesions in multiple sclerosis patients followed by weekly MRI. *Neurology* 48:1446, 1997.

96. Paty DW, Li DK: The UBC MC/MRI Study Group and the IFNB Multiple Sclerosis Study Group. Interferon beta-1b is effective in relapsing-remitting multiple sclerosis. II. MRI analysis results of a multicenter, randomized, double-blind, placebo-controlled trial. *Neurology* 43:662, 1993.

97. Jacobs L, Cookfair D, Rudick R, et al: Results of a phase III trial of intramuscular recombinant beta interferon as treatment for multiple sclerosis (abstract). *Ann Neurol* 36:259, 1994.

98. Brod SA, Marshall GD Jr, Henninger EM, et al: Interferon beta 1b treatment decreases tumor necrosis factor alpha and increases interleukin-6 production in multiple sclerosis. *Neurology* 46:1633, 1996.

99. Arnon R, Sela M, Teitelbaum D: New insights into the mechanism of action of copolymer 1 in experimental allergic encephalomyelitis and multiple sclerosis. *J Neurol* 243(4 Suppl 1): S8, 1996.

100. Johnson KP: A review of the clinical efficacy profile of copolymer 1: new U.S. phase III trial data. *J Neurol* 243(4 Suppl 1): S3, 1996.

101. Achiron A, Gabbay U, Gilad R, et al: Intravenous immunoglobulin treatment in multiple sclerosis. Effect on relapses. *Neurology* 50:398, 1998.

102. United Kingdom Tizanidine Trial Group. A double-blind, placebo-controlled trial of tizanidine in the treatment of spasticity caused by multiple sclerosis. *Neurology* 44 (Suppl 4): 60, 1994.

103. Young RR: Role of tizanidine in the treatment of spasticity. *Neurology* 44(Suppl 9): S1, 1994.

104. Nance PW: Tizanidine: an alpha$_2$-agonist imidazoline with antispacticity effects. *Today's Therapy Trends* 15:11, 1997.

105. Schapiro RT: Symptom management in multiple sclerosis. *Ann Neurol* 36(Suppl 1): S123, 1994.

106. Bever CT: The current status of studies of aminopyridines in patients with multiple sclerosis. *Ann Neurol* 36(Suppl 1): S118, 1994.

107. Fowler CJ, van Kerrebroeck PE, Nordenbo A, et al: Treatment of lower urinary tract dysfunction in patients with multiple sclerosis. Committee of the European study group of sudims. *J Neurol Neurosurg Psychiatry* 55:986, 1992.

108. Webb RJ, Lawson AL, Neal DE: Clean intermittent self-catheterisation in 172 adults. *Br J Neurol* 65:20, 1990.

109. Barnes DG, Shaw PJR, Timoney AG, et al: Management of the neuropathic bladder by suprapubic catheterisation. *Br J Urol* 72:169, 1993.

110. Linet OI, Ogrinc FG: Efficacy and safety of intracavernous alprostadil in men with erectile dysfunction. The Aprostadil Study Group. *N Engl J Med* 334:873, 1996.

111. Padma-Nathan H, Hellstrom WJ, Kaiser FE, et al: Treatment of men with erectile dysfunction with transurethral alprostadil. Medicated urethral system for erection (MUSE) study. *N Engl J Med* 336:1, 1997.

112. Rao SM, Leo GJ, Bernarden L: Cognitive dysfunction in multiple sclerosis. 1. Frequency, patterns, and prediction. *Neurology* 41:685, 1991.

113. Fontaine B, Seilhean D, Tourbah A, et al: Dementia in two histologically confirmed cases of multiple sclerosis: one case with isolated dementia and one case associated with psychiatric symptoms. *J Neurol Neurosurg Psychiatry* 57:353, 1994.

114. Thompson AJ: Multiple sclerosis: symptomatic treatment. *J Neurol* 243:559, 1996.

115. Bronnum-Hansen H, Koch-Henriksen N, Hyllested K: Survival of patients with multiple sclerosis in Denmark: a nationwide long-term epidemiologic survey. *Neurology* 44:1901, 1994.

116. Grønning M, Hannisdal E, Mellgren SI: Multivariate analyses of factors associated with unemployment in people with multiple sclerosis. *J Neurol Neurosurg Psychiatry* 53:388, 1990.

117. Rodriguez M, Siva A, Ward J, et al: Impairment, disability and handicap in multiple sclerosis: a population-based study in Olmsted County, Minnesota. *Neurology* 44:28, 1994.

Chapter 8

CEREBROVASCULAR DISEASE

Cerebrovascular disease is one of the major causes of morbidity and death in the United States. Stroke has an increased incidence and prevalence with increasing age but is not a disease confined to the elderly. The incidence appears to be 0.5 per 1000 at age 40 years, rising to approximately 70 per 1000 at age 70 years, with an annual incidence varying from 1.5 to 4 per 1000 population and a prevalence from 5 to 20 per 1000 population. More than 700,000 individuals suffer stroke each year in the United States[1] and stroke is the third leading cause of death in adults.[2] There is a 20 percent mortality rate in the first 3 days[3] and a 25 percent mortality rate in the first year.[4]

Although the lifetime risk of stroke is higher in men, the risk of dying of stroke is highest in women. This is the result of women being older than men at the onset of stroke and the longer life expectancy in women, who account for a larger proportion of elderly stroke victims.[5]

For each 100 survivors, 10 are able to return to work without impairment, 30 have mild residual disability, 50 have more severe disability requiring special services in a home care situation, and 10 need permanent institutional care.

ANATOMY OF THE BLOOD SUPPLY OF THE BRAIN

The brain is supplied by two paired arteries, the internal carotid arteries anteriorly and the vertebral arteries posteriorly. The vertebral arteries unite to form the basilar artery. These two arterial systems form the circle of Willis at the base of the brain, a unique anastomotic system that gives rise to all of the vessels supplying the cerebral hemispheres (Fig. 8-1).

Internal Carotid Artery

The internal carotid artery rises in the neck as one of two branches of the common carotid artery. It ascends in the neck and enters the carotid canal in the petrous temporal bone where it ascends, loops forward and medially, and ascends again to enter the cranial cavity. The artery enters the cavernous sinus and passes forward, closely related to sella and hypophysis medially, and the third, fourth, sixth, and ophthalmic and maxillary divisions of the fifth cranial nerves laterally. The terminal portion of the internal carotid artery ascends and pierces the dura medial to the anterior clinoid process, where the artery is closely related to the optic nerve. The cavernous and terminal portions of the internal carotid artery are frequently referred to as the carotid siphon.

The branches of the internal carotid artery include:

1. Petrous portion
   A. Caroticotympanic artery—supplies the anterior and part of the medial wall of the middle ear.
2. Cavernous portion
   A. Cavernous arteries—small vessels supplying the hypophysis and the wall of the cavernous sinus.
   B. Hypophyseal arteries—supply the hypophysis.
   C. Semilunar artery—supplies the trigeminal (gasserian: semilunar) ganglion.
   D. Anterior meningeal arteries—supply the dura of the anterior cranial fossa.
3. Supraclinoid portion
   A. Ophthalmic artery
   B. Anterior choroidal artery
   C. Posterior communicating artery
4. Terminal portion
   A. Anterior cerebral artery
   B. Middle cerebral artery

Ophthalmic Artery

The ophthalmic artery rises from the supraclinoid portion of the internal carotid artery, pierces the dura,

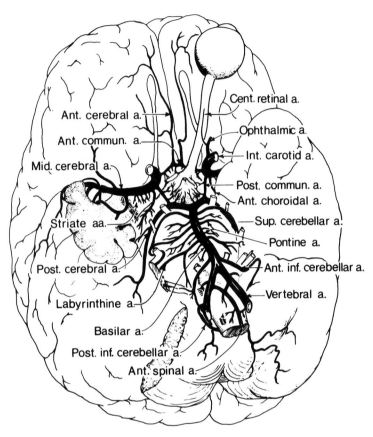

Figure 8-1
Circle of Willis.

and accompanies the optic nerve through the optic foramen and into the orbit. The artery passes medially, superior to the optic nerve, to the roof of the orbit, where it divides into the supratrochlear and dorsal nasal arteries. Branches of the ophthalmic artery anastomose with branches of the external carotid system. This anastomosis may supply blood to intracranial structures by reversal of flow following insufficiency or occlusion of the internal carotid artery.

The branches of the ophthalmic artery include:

1. Central retinal artery—arises from the ophthalmic artery and enters the optic nerve close to the eye. The artery emerges from the center of the optic disc in the optic cup and divides into several branches supplying the optic disc and retina.

2. Ciliary arteries—several in number, which supply the sclera, choroid, lens and conjunctiva of the eye.

3. Lacrimal artery—arises from the ophthalmic artery near the optic foramen and runs laterally along the upper border of the lateral rectus muscle to supply the lacrimal gland.

4. Supraorbital artery—arises from the ophthalmic artery and passes above the eye to accompany the supraorbital nerve. The artery supplies the skin, muscle, and other structures over the forehead and anastomoses with branches of the superficial temporal artery.

5. Ethmoidal arteries—supply the ethmoidal sinuses, the nasal cavity, and the dura of the anterior fossa.

6. Dorsal nasal artery—distributed to the outer sur-

face of the nose and anastomoses with the angular artery.

7. Frontal artery—supplies the medial aspect of the forehead.

8. Superior and inferior palpebral arteries—encircle the eyelids near the facial margins.

9. Muscular branches—supply the extraocular muscles.

10. Anterior choroidal artery—arises from the terminal portion of the internal carotid artery and passes posteriorly along the optic tract to reach the lateral geniculate body. The artery then enters the choroidal fissure and supplies the choroid plexus in the inferior horn of the lateral ventricle. In its course, the artery supplies the optic tract, the cerebral peduncle, the lateral portion of the lateral geniculate body, the posterior two-thirds of the posterior limb of the internal capsule, the retrolenticular and infralenticular portions of the internal capsule, the optic radiation, the hippocampus, the choroid plexus, the tail of the caudate nucleus, and the amygdala.

Posterior Communicating Artery

The posterior communicating artery arises from the terminal portion of the internal carotid artery and passes posteriorly, immediately above the oculomotor nerve, to anastomose with the posterior cerebral artery. Branches of the posterior communicating artery supply the thalamus, subthalamus, internal capsule, mamillary bodies, optic chiasm, and optic tract.

Anterior Cerebral Artery

The anterior cerebral artery arises from the terminal portion of the internal carotid artery and passes anteromedially above the optic nerve to come into contact with the opposite anterior cerebral artery. The two arteries are connected by a short anterior communicating artery, then pass around the genu and body of the corpus callosum to anastomose with branches of the posterior cerebral artery at the level of the parietooccipital fissure.

The branches of the anterior cerebral artery include:

1. Anterior communicating artery—supplies the optic chiasm and hypothalamus.

2. Perforating branches—penetrate the anterior perforating substance and lamina terminalis to supply the rostrum of the corpus callosum and the septum pellucidum.

3. Recurrent branch (medial striate artery, recurrent artery of Heubner)—is distributed to the head of the caudate nucleus and the anterior limb of the internal capsule.

4. Cortical branches
   A. Orbital branches—supply the orbital and medial surfaces of the frontal lobe.
   B. Frontopolar branch—supplies the anterior portion of the medial aspect of the superior frontal gyrus and extends about 1 inch onto the superior lateral surface.
   C. Pericallosal branch—supplies the cingulate gyrus and corpus callosum.
   D. Callosal marginal branch—supplies the cingulate gyrus, the medial aspect of the superior frontal gyrus, and the paracentral lobule.

Middle Cerebral Artery

The middle cerebral artery should be regarded as the intracranial extension of the internal carotid artery. Emboli entering the internal carotid artery invariably enter the middle cerebral artery. The middle cerebral artery runs laterally in the lateral fissure between frontal and temporal lobes (Fig. 8-2) to reach the surface of the insula, where it divides into several branches.

1. Lenticulostriate arteries — perforating branches that arise close to the origin of the middle cerebral artery and penetrate the substance of the brain to supply the head of the caudate nucleus, putamen, globus pallidus, and internal capsule.

2. Cortical branches—radiate outward from the middle cerebral artery as it lies on the insula. Cortical branches that can be recognized by arteriography are the orbitofrontal, frontal, pre-Rolandic, post-Rolandic, anterior parietal, posterior parietal, an angular branch following the line of the lateral fissure, and the anterior, middle, and posterior temporal branches extending over the surface of the temporal lobe.

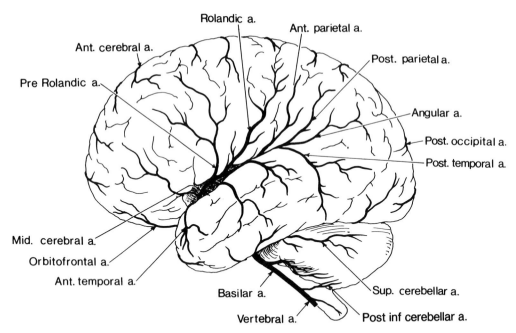

Figure 8-2
The middle cerebral artery and its branches.

Vertebral Artery

The vertebral artery arises from the first portion of the subclavian artery in the neck. The anatomical course can be considered in four parts.

First part—ascends posteromedially and enters the foramen of the transverse process of the sixth cervical vertebra.

Second part—ascends through the foramina of the transverse processes of the upper sixth cervical vertebra.

Third part—curls backward in a groove behind the superior articular process of the atlas and passes through the foramen magnum.

Fourth part—pierces the dura to lie on the ventral surface of the medulla, where it ascends to the lower border of the pons to unite with the vertebral artery from the opposite side, forming the basilar artery.

The branches of the vertebral artery include:

1. Spinal branches accompany the nerve roots into the spinal canal. Only one or two of these branches anastomoses with the anterior spinal artery.

2. Muscular branches—supply the deep muscles of the neck.

3. Meningeal branches—arise from the vertebral arteries at the level of foramen magnum and supply the dura of the posterior fossa and the falx cerebri.

4. Anterior spinal artery—arises from the vertebral artery near its termination and descends over the surface of the medulla to unite with the artery from the opposite site and form one anterior spinal artery. This artery lies on the ventral surface of the spinal cord and terminates as a fine vessel in the cauda equina. The anterior spinal artery supplies the medial and inferior portions of the medulla, including the medullary pyramids, and all of the spinal cord, except the posterior columns and posterior horns of the gray matter.

5. Posterior inferior cerebellar artery—arises from the fourth portion of the vertebral artery and passes around the medulla, onto the inferior surface of the cerebellum, where it divides into two branches. The posterior inferior cerebellar artery supplies the lateral portion of the medulla and the inferior cerebellar peduncle. The medial branch supplies the inferior vermis, the medial aspect of the cerebellar hemisphere, and the choroid plexus of the fourth ventricle. The lateral branch supplies the inferior surface of the cerebellar hemisphere. There is a well-developed anastomosis with the anterior inferior cerebellar and superior cerebellar arteries.

Basilar Artery

The basilar artery (Fig. 8-3) takes origin at the inferior border of the pons from the junction of the two vertebral arteries and ascends in the median groove of the pons to terminate at the upper border of the pons by dividing into the two posterior cerebral arteries.

The branches of the basilar artery include:

1. Pontine branches—supply the pons.
2. Internal auditory artery—accompanies the seventh and eighth cranial nerves into the internal auditory meatus and supplies the inner ear.
3. Anterior inferior cerebellar artery—arises just above the lower border of the pons and passes around the pons onto the inferior surfaces of the cerebellar hemisphere and anastomosis with the posterior inferior cerebellar artery.
4. Superior cerebellar artery—arises just below the termination of the basilar artery and passes around the pons, separated from the posterior cerebral artery by the oculomotor nerve. The superior cerebellar artery supplies the superior and middle

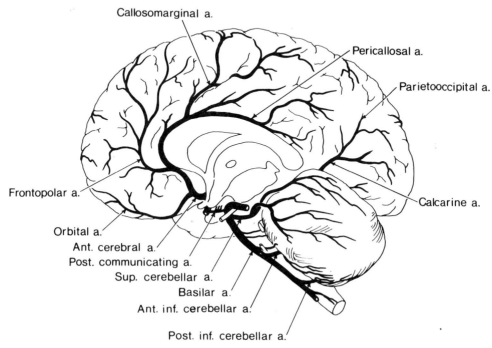

Figure 8-3
The basilar artery and its branches.

cerebellar peduncles, the pineal gland, the choroid plexus of the third ventricle, and the superior surface of the cerebellum.

Posterior Cerebral Artery

The posterior cerebral artery arises at the termination of the basilar artery, where it is separated from the superior cerebellar artery by the oculomotor nerve. The posterior communicating artery, a branch of the internal carotid artery, joins the posterior cerebral artery, which winds around the cerebral peduncle onto the tentorial surface of the occipital lobe.

The branches of the posterior cerebral artery include:

1. Posteromedial arteries—enter the posterior perforated substances to supply the medial surface of the thalamus and the wall of the third ventricle.
2. Posterior choroidal artery—runs beneath the splenium of the corpus callosum to supply the choroid plexus of the third ventricle.
3. Posterolateral arteries—supply the lateral thalamus and the midbrain.
4. Anterior temporal branches—supply the uncus and the fusiform gyrus of the temporal lobe.
5. Posterior temporal branches—supply the inferior temporal gyrus.
6. Calcarine branches—supply the medial surface of the occipital lobe with a short extension onto the superior lateral surface of the hemisphere and the occipital pole. The posterior cerebral artery anastomoses with the anterior cerebral artery at the level of the parietooccipital fissure on the medial surface of the hemisphere.

Arterial Circle of Willis

This unique anastomosis, which lies at the base of the brain, is derived from the internal carotid and vertebral arterial systems (see Fig. 8-1). The anterior portion of the circle is formed by the two anterior cerebral arteries derived from the internal carotid arteries and connected by the anterior communicating artery. The posterior portion of the circle consists of the two posterior cerebral arteries, which are the terminal branches of the basilar artery. The posterior cerebral

arteries are connected to the internal carotid artery on each side by the posterior communicating arteries. The circle of Willis encloses the optic chiasm, the infundibulum, the tuber cinereum, and the mamillary bodies.

ANATOMY OF THE VENOUS DRAINAGE OF THE BRAIN

The cerebrovenous system can be divided into two subdivisions, the superficial external venous drainage and the deep internal venous drainage. Both systems eventually drain into the venous sinuses.

The upper lateral surface of the cerebral hemisphere is drained by the superficial cerebral veins, which enter the superior longitudinal sinus. The superficial middle cerebral vein also drains the lateral surface of the cerebral hemispheres and passes forward in the lateral fissure to enter the cavernous sinus. The superficial middle cerebral vein communicates with the superior longitudinal sinus through the superior anastomotic vein of Trolard and with the transverse sinus through the inferior anastomotic vein of Labbé. The inferior cerebral veins drain the orbital surface of the frontal lobe, the lateral aspect of the temporal lobe, and the lateral aspect of the occipital lobe to empty into the cavernous sinus and transverse sinuses. The veins over the insula unite to form the deep middle cerebral vein, which passes anteriorly deep to the lateral fissure and joins the basal vein of Rosenthal. This latter structure arises in the anterior perforating substance by the union of the anterior cerebral vein and the veins of the corpus callosum. The basal vein is joined by the deep middle cerebral vein as it passes posteriorly in close relationship to the uncus and hippocampus. The basal vein then winds around the midbrain to unite with the basal vein from the opposite side, at the origin of the great cerebral vein.

The deep internal group of cerebral veins drain the central structures of the cerebral hemisphere and are closely related to the ventricular system.

The terminal (thalamostriate) vein arises from the inferior horn of the lateral ventricle and follows the tail of the caudate nucleus into the body of the lateral ventricle, lying between the caudate nucleus and the thalamus. The terminal vein runs forward to the intraventricular foramen and is joined by the anterior caudate vein, the septal vein, which drains the septum pellucidum, and the choroidal vein, which drains the choroid plexus of the lateral ventricle to form the internal cerebral vein. This structure turns at its origin, forming the venous angle, and then passes along the roof of the third ventricle and through the velum interpositum to join with the opposite internal cerebral vein. The great vein of Galen is formed by the union of the internal cerebral veins and the junction of the basal veins of Rosenthal. After a short course, the great cerebral vein is joined by the inferior sagittal sinus to form the straight sinus.

The intracranial venous sinuses are thin-walled endothelial-lined structures lying within the dura. The superior longitudinal sinus takes origin at the foramen cecum anteriorly and passes in the superior surface of the falx cerebri to the internal occipital protuberance, then turns to the right to form the right transverse sinus. The superior longitudinal sinus receives the superior cerebral veins. The walls of the sinus contain granulations that are responsible for the absorption of cerebrospinal fluid (CSF) into the venous system. The inferior longitudinal sinus arises in the free margin of the falx cerebri by the union of a number of small veins and runs posteriorly to terminate in the straight sinus at the junction of the falx cerebri and the tentorium cerebelli. The straight sinus is formed by the union of the great vein of Galen and the inferior longitudinal sinus and passes posteriorly in the junction of the falx cerebri and tentorium cerebelli. The straight sinus terminates at the internal occipital protuberance by becoming the left transverse sinus. The transverse sinuses arise at the internal occipital protuberance and run along the edge of the tentorium cerebelli to end at the base of the petrous temporal bone, where they become the sigmoid sinuses. The transverse sinuses receives most of the venous drainage from the cerebellum. The sigmoid sinuses are a direct continuation of the transverse sinuses, beginning at the base of the petrous temporal bone and terminating at the jugular foramen as the internal jugular vein.

The cavernous sinus arises anteriorly from the superior ophthalmic vein at the superior orbital fissure and passes posteriorly, close to the sella turcica

and terminates by dividing into the superior and inferior petrosal sinuses. The cavernous sinuses communicate with each other through the intercavernous sinuses, which lie anteriorly and posteriorly to the sella turcica. The lateral walls of the cavernous sinuses contain the third, fourth, and sixth nerves and the ophthalmic and maxillary divisions of the trigeminal nerve. The intracavernous portion of the internal carotid artery is contained within the cavernous sinus. The superior petrosal sinus arises from the cavernous sinus at the apex of the petrous temporal bone and passes along the edge of the tentorium cerebelli to terminate in the transverse sinus. The inferior petrosal sinus also rises at the apex of the petrous temporal bone and enters a groove lying in the junction of the petrous temporal and occipital bones to terminate in the jugular bulb of the internal jugular vein.

STROKE (BRAIN ATTACK)

Although the incidence and mortality from stroke declined in the last three decades, this trend has been reversed as the population ages, indicating the need for a dedicated program to educate physicians, patients, and care providers about the early stages of stroke and to increase programs for stroke prevention. One can start by emphasizing that whatever is accomplished in reducing the risk of stroke also reduces the risk of myocardial infarction, a condition that still obtains immediate attention in the public arena. Perhaps the substitution of the term "brain attack" for stroke might strike a more responsive chord, the term signifying a more immediate and ominous threat to the victim. Indeed, early diagnosis is now essential, following the introduction of new therapeutic measures that require prompt intervention and treatment to prevent permanent neurological deficits.[6]

Stroke—The Background

Most, but not all, risk factors for stroke are related to accelerated atherosclerosis, but all risk factors can be considered under five headings:

1. Diseases of blood vessels
2. Concomitant heart disease

3. Abnormalities of blood constituents
4. Reduced cerebral perfusion
5. Infection

These five factors may act individually or in combination, but the end result is the same: a focal reduction in cerebral blood flow that is of sufficient magnitude to produce a spectrum of events varying from temporary interference with cerebral activity to death of tissue or infarction.

Diseases of Blood Vessels

Atherosclerotic Plaques Most transient ischemic attacks (TIAs) and strokes occur in patients who have cerebral atherosclerosis. The process begins with endothelial injury of unknown cause and proliferation of collagen to produce fibrointimal thickening. This is followed by proliferation of muscle cells giving rise to the fibrous plaque. There is a progressive encroachment on the lumen, with development of intraplaque hemorrhages. The breakdown of blood within the plaque leads to the presence of cholesterol, which may form a cholesterol abscess. The cholesterol abscess within the plaque contains neutrophils and monocytes that may remain dormant

unless activated by circulating cytokines, including interleukin-1 (IL-1) and tissue necrosis factor (TNF). The production of cytokines is enhanced by an inflammatory response associated with infection and studies have shown an increase in infection by both bacteria and viruses in the weeks preceding the onset of cerebral infarction in adults and children. Circulating cytokines may then activate the vascular endothelium, stimulating procoagulant activity.[7] Fissure formation in the surface of the plaque, followed by extrusion of lipid material containing activated leukocytes into the lumen of the artery can present a surface that might precipitate intraluminal thrombosis or embolism.[8] In many cases, this is asymptomatic, but embolization can cause TIAs or more serious neurological deficits. Emboli occasionally make a transient appearance in the retinal circulation (Fig. 8-4). The atheromatous ulcer formed by the discharge of cholesterol presents an ideal surface for platelet adherence and luminal thrombosis, and is the main source of cerebral microembolism in patients with high-grade internal carotid artery stenosis.[9] In some cases, the ulcer will heal or calcify. However, the material released from an atheromatous plaque is a powerful procoagulant and can lead to local thrombosis with partial or complete obstruction of the lumen.

Figure 8-4
Carotid atherosclerotic embolism. Boxcar appearance of interrupted blood flow from presumed cholesterol emboli.

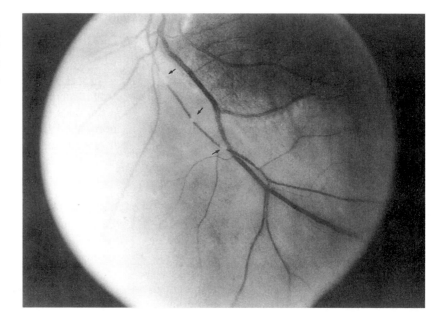

The demonstration of neutrophil activation within the first few hours after thromboembolic stroke has been established.[10] Activation of neutrophils by infection prior to cerebral infarction is an important risk factor in stroke in children[11] and adults under the age of 50 years.[12] Recent bacterial and viral infection and, in particular, respiratory tract infection, is an important risk factor for ischemic stroke.[13] A systemic infection,[14] remote inflammatory process, or local trauma could influence previously prepared endothelium to promote the development of a thrombus and lead to subsequent embolism. Thus, intraluminal thrombosis with or without embolism is the product of many factors.

Common sites of plaque formation are the bifurcation of the common carotid artery, the origin and terminal portions of the vertebral arteries, the basilar artery, and the origin of the middle cerebral arteries.

There has been a somewhat belated recognition that ascending aortic atherosclerosis with plaque formation can be a source of cerebral embolism and stroke.[15,16] It is illogical to recognize heart disease or plaque formation in the carotid or vertebral arteries as a potent course of embolism and ignore the proximal feeding vessel in this process. The use of transesophageal echocardiography (TEE) to visualize the ascending aorta should be a routine procedure in suspected embolic cerebral infarction. Surgical treatment of symptomatic aortic atherosclerotic disease by aortectomy and graft replacement is feasible in carefully selected patients.[17]

Factors that contribute to accelerated development of atherosclerosis include:

A. Hypertension. Chronic hypertension is a primary risk factor for stroke and appears to accelerate the atherosclerotic process. The risk of stroke increases proportionally with increased levels of systolic or diastolic blood pressure,[18] and treatment of isolated hypertension in the elderly may be associated with a 36 percent reduction in the incidence of stroke.[19] Up to 75 percent of people with elevated blood pressure in a community may be unidentified or inadequately treated and physicians can still further reduce the incidence of stroke by identification and improved treatment of hypertension.[20] Many patients with chronic cerebrovascular disease have labile hypertension and casual measurements of blood pressure may give an erroneous impression of normotensive levels. Such patients are nearly all susceptible to a considerable rise in blood pressure in response to stress and may have sustained periods of hypertension during the day, leading to accelerated atherosclerosis. Therefore, intermittent hypertension should be treated when identified. However, caution should be exercised in treating hypertension, because some patients show excessive response to even small doses of antihypertensive agents. Although autoregulation is preserved in atherosclerosis and perfusion is stable over a wide range of perfusion pressures, between 50 and 150 mmHg, both lower diastolic and upper systolic limits are raised in chronic hypertension and precipitous lowering of blood pressure may produce systolic pressure readings that are so low in a hypertensive individual that autoregulation fails and there is a precipitous fall in cerebral blood flow. Optimum blood pressure control for persons with hypertension, using antihypertensive agents, is an important component of stroke prevention. This should be coupled with nonpharmacologic treatment, including weight reduction, reduced alcohol intake in those with high intake, cessation of cigarette smoking, and exercise.[21]

B. Diabetes mellitus. Diabetes mellitus is a risk factor for ischemic stroke in large vessel disease but is of questionable import in small vessel disease.[22] Approximately 30 percent of patients with cerebral atherosclerosis have evidence of diabetes mellitus and the incidence of stroke is twice as high in diabetics as in nondiabetics, with equivalent atherosclerotic disease. The prevalence of high-grade carotid artery stenosis is also significantly higher in diabetics.[23] Men with diabetes or with increased glucose levels who are not considered diabetic have an increased risk of stroke.[24] The risk of stroke is further increased when diabetes is associated with hypertension, hypercholesterolemia, and smoking. This combination appears to greatly accelerate atherosclerosis, although there is no evidence to show that accelerated atherosclerosis is more common in the patient with severe rather than mild diabetes, or that strict control of diabetes mellitus reduces the risk of developing stroke. Nevertheless, the coexistence of hypertension and poorly controlled diabetes is significant in the early occurrence of stroke,[25] but diabetes does appear to have an independent role as a risk factor for stroke in subjects who do not have hypertension. In addition, diabetes mellitus is an independent predictor of recurrent stroke.[26]

C. Abnormal serum lipid levels. Patients in their late thirties, forties, and early fifties who have TIAs or acute stroke often show evidence of hyperlipidemia. This condition is considered an important cause of generalized atherosclerosis and when detected should be treated appropriately. Hypercholesterolemia may be a significant factor in 20 percent of Caucasians with cholesterol levels exceeding 220 mg. Lowering of serum triglycerides in elderly patients with symptoms of cerebrovascular disease and hypertriglyceridemia is effective in improving cerebral profusion and cognition.

D. Hypothyroidism. Some of the stroke population have shown a significant prevalence of hypothyroidism. Because this condition can contribute to atherosclerosis, all patients with cerebrovascular disease should be investigated for hypothyroidism.

E. Hyperuricemia. Several studies have shown a relationship between hyperuricemia and chronic cerebrovascular disease. Hyperuricemia is usually asymptomatic and patients rarely have symptoms of gout, but there is some evidence of increased predisposition to stenosis of extracranial vessels in the neck of patients with cerebrovascular disease and hyperuricemia. Consequently, hyperuricemia, whether symptomatic or asymptomatic, should be treated if detected.

F. An increase in serum homocysteine levels is a recognized factor in stroke in childhood and may contribute to stroke in young adults.[27]

G. Obesity. Both hypertension and overt diabetes mellitus are common in obese patients. In addition, obesity has been shown to be an independent factor contributing to accelerated atherosclerosis. An obese patient should have a strict program of weight reduction.

H. Cigarette smoking. The relationship between cigarette smoking and increased risk of cerebrovascular disease is well established. The combination of smoking, hypertension, and diabetes mellitus is particularly hazardous.[25] Cigarette smoking is a more important risk factor for stroke than excessive alcohol consumption.[28]

I. Lack of exercise. Some evidence suggests that regular exercise reduces the development of atherosclerosis and decreases the risk of stroke.

J. Heavy alcohol consumption is associated with accelerated atherosclerosis and drinking for intoxication may trigger the onset of brain infarction in young adults.[29]

K. Recent infection, primarily bacterial infection, may be a significant factor increasing morbidity in patients admitted to the hospital for treatment of recent stroke. Increased body temperature has a significant association with stroke severity, infarct, size mortality, and functional outcome.[30]

L. Dementia after stroke is a significant independent risk for long-term stroke recurrence after adjusting for other risk factors.[31]

Other Disorders of Cranial or Extracranial Blood Vessels

1. Arteriosclerosis. Hypertrophic arteriosclerosis in chronic hypertension is not uncommon in the cerebral vessels. Reduplication of the elastic lamina and hyalinization of vessel walls produces narrowing of the lumen, which may reduce cerebral blood flow.

2. Arteritis. Inflammation of the vessel wall from any cause (e.g., syphilis, sarcoidosis, polyarteritis nodosa) leads to a narrowing of the lumina with a reduction in cerebral blood flow. About 5 percent of patients with TIAs or cerebral infarction have syphilitic arteritis, which can cause a severe stroke in younger patients.

3. Fibromuscular dysplasia, a rare condition, may produce significant stenosis of the carotid arteries.[32]

4. Cervicocranial artery dissection is one of the commoner causes of stroke in young patients.

5. Cerebral infarction and TIAs are common complications of organ transplantation. Recipients older than 40 years of age and those with diabetes mellitus are at greater risk for this condition.

Heart Disease The association of heart disease and stroke has received much attention in the last decade. Cardiac disease and stroke are highly correlated and prevention and treatment of cardiac disease may shift the balance of stroke risk.[33] Embolism of cardiac origin is a major cause of cerebral infarction and there has been a steady increase in identification of cerebral embolism as the cause of stroke in at least 30 percent of cases in some series. Furthermore, myocardial infarction is the leading cause of death following stroke, and the increasing survival of persons with heart disease increases the number at risk for stroke.

After one embolic event, nonvalvular atrial fibrillation carries a risk of recurrence between 2 and 15 percent in the first year and 5 percent yearly thereafter.[34] Silent brain infarction of the lacunar type, situated in a deep white matter, is not unusual in nonvalvular atrial fibrillation.[35] Atrial fibrillation associated with mitral stenosis or other forms of valvular heart disease increases the risk of stroke 17-fold.

Other recognized cardiac causes of embolism include recent myocardial infarction with mural thrombosis, coronary artery disease, coronary artery bypass grafting,[36] left ventricular hypertrophy, calcified aortic stenosis, mitral annular calcification, hypertensive myocardial hypertrophy, patent foramen ovale with interatrial septum aneurysm, bacterial endocarditis, and nonbacterial thromboendocarditis.

During the last decade, there has been a progressive emphasis on the role of patent foramen ovale and interatrial septal aneurysm in the genesis of stroke.[37] Paradoxical embolism from a venous source through a right-to-left shunt is usually incriminated but difficult to prove.[38] The presenting stroke is often severe, but recurrence is uncommon.[39]

The role of mitral valve prolapse is less compelling and uncomplicated mitral valve prolapse is not associated with increased risk of stroke.[40]

Abnormalities of Blood Constituents

1. Hypercoagulability. This is fully discussed in Chapter 11.
2. Embolism. Although embolism of cardiac origin is the most common cause of cerebral embolism, other sites in the arterial system are recognized sources of emboli.
   A. Platelet emboli may originate on atherosclerotic plaques in the ascending aorta, carotid, or vertebral circulation and occlude small vessels in the brain, producing local transient ischemia.
   B. Cholesterol discharged from cholesterol abscesses in atherosclerotic plaques can also occlude small vessels in the brain.
   C. Thromboemboli may arise from thrombi that form over atherosclerotic plaques in any arteries supplying blood to the brain. This includes emboli arising from ulcerative plaques in the ascending aorta, innominate artery, left subclavian artery, the carotid arteries, and the vertebral arteries. Plaque ulceration and lumen thrombosis are the main source of cerebral microemboli in high-grade internal carotid artery stenosis.

Reduced Cerebral Perfusion

1. Diminished cardiac output. Diminished cardiac output may be a significant factor in the production of focal ischemia of the brain when there is significant narrowing of the extracranial, internal carotid, or vertebral arteries (70 percent or more reduction in lumen) or narrowing of the intracranial arteries owing to cerebrovascular disease. Diminished cardiac output occurs in orthostatic hypotension, aortic valve stenosis or insufficiency, from a subaortic stenosis, cardiac dysrhythmias, arteriosclerotic heart disease, and certain primary cardiomyopathies.

2. Steal syndromes. Steal syndromes may be extracranial or intracranial. The best-known extracranial steal syndrome is the subclavian steal syndrome in which blood flows normally up one vertebral artery toward the basilar artery then flows down the opposite vertebral artery into the subclavian artery. The subclavian steal is caused by diminished pressure in the subclavian artery due to severe proximal stenosis of the vessel. Intracranial steal syndromes are not uncommon and depend on the development of a collateral circulation from one area of the brain to another area of diminished perfusion pressure. This may lead to diversion of blood from part of the brain sufficient to produce symptoms of transient ischemia.

3. Kinking and compression of intracranial vessels. Internal, carotid and vertebral arteries occasionally undergo kinking or compression in the neck

with head turning. This results in the reduction or cessation of flow through the affected vessel. Atherosclerotic vessels frequently lose elasticity, resulting in the formation of redundant coils or kinks, even when the head is in a normal position. The internal carotid artery can be narrowed or occluded by the lateral mass of the atlas when the head is turned to the opposite side. This may result in the production of carotid insufficiency. The vertebral arteries are sometimes compressed by osteophytes arising from the margins of the cervical vertebrae and interpeduncular joints when the head is turned to one side. This osteophyte compression of the vertebral arteries as they pass through the intervertebral foramina produces vertebrobasilar insufficiency. These abnormalities can be detected by ultrasonography or arteriography and in many cases can be corrected by appropriate surgical treatment.

TRANSIENT ISCHEMIC ATTACKS

Transient ischemic attacks are episodes of transient focal ischemia involving the brain or brainstem. They are commonly 2 to 30 min in duration and, by definition, last less than 24 h. The onset is sudden and symptoms usually reach maximum intensity within 2 min. The episodes usually resolve rapidly with a 50 percent recovery in 1 h and a 90 percent recovery in 4 h. The frequency varies. Some patients experience a single attack, whereas others experience multiple attacks at different intervals.

Although the concept of the TIA is firmly established in medical parlance, it should be recognized that most TIAs are the result of a small cerebral or brainstem infarct. Careful examination will reveal unilateral increase in tone, persistent but slight asymmetry of reflexes, or mild intention tremor in many cases. Some but not all will have abnormalities on magnetic resonance imaging (MRI). The subsequent development of a major infarct in patients who have had TIAs or in those who have suffered an acute attack with an obvious persistent neurological deficit is the same—a cumulative risk of 25 percent in 3 years.

The symptoms of TIA depend on the site of focal ischemia of the brain. There are two categories of TIA: those that occur in response to ischemia in the carotid arterial system and those resulting from disturbed blood flow in the vertebrobasilar system.

Clinical Features

Carotid Artery Insufficiency

1. Visual symptoms. Dimness of vision or loss of vision affecting the eye on the side of the carotid insufficiency (amaurosis fugax) may occur due to involvement of the ophthalmic arterial system. Homonymous hemianopia can occur when there is a cerebral hemisphere ischemia.

2. Language dysfunction. Dysphasia or aphasia is the result of ischemia of the dominant hemisphere.

3. Motor symptoms. Contralateral hemiparesis or hemiplegia occurs with hemispheric ischemia.

4. Sensory symptoms. Contralateral numbness, coldness, or parethesias involving the hand, upper limb, and lower limb is the result of ischemia of the parietal lobe.

Vertebrobasilar Insufficiency

1. Visual symptoms. Dimness of vision, hemianopia, alexia without agraphia, color anomia, simple or complex visual hallucinations, visual perseveration, and prosopagnosia are products of occipital lobe ischemia.

2. Eye movement disorders. These include Parinaud syndrome, vertical gaze paresis, paralysis of downward gaze, bilateral ptosis, blepharospasm, pupillary abnormalities, nystagmus, decreased blinking, and internuclear ophthalmoplegia.

3. Cranial nerve deficits. Diplopia, facial numbness, facial weakness, tinnitus, vertigo, dysarthria, or dysphagia are the result of brainstem ischemia. Isolated vertigo occurring in episodic fashion in an elderly patient is often the result of a TIA.

4. Motor symptoms. Paresis or paralysis of one or more limbs. A partial Horner syndrome with pupil asymmetry and a mild ptosis occurs in most cases.

5. Coordination deficits. Ataxia or clumsiness of upper or lower limbs, or both, on one side or both

sides, rubral tremor, hemiballismus, or choreoathetosis may result from cerebellar ischemia or ischemic involvement of cerebellar connections in the brainstem.

6. Sensory symptoms. Paresthesias on one or both sides of the face and upper or lower limbs, or thalamic pain, can occur with ischemia in the territory supplied by the posterior cerebral arteries.

7. Drop attacks. Sudden loss of tone in the lower limbs may result from ischemia of the medullary pyramids.

8. Altered consciousness. This includes brief episodes of impairment or loss of consciousness, abulia, drowsiness, confusion, agitation, and altered sleep-wake cycle.

9. A combination of any or all of the above. Numbers 6 and 7 are unlikely to be caused by vertebrobasilar insufficiency unless they are accompanied by one or more of the other manifestations of transient ischemia.

Diagnostic Procedures

TIA and Cerebral Infarction

1. Complete blood count and sedimentation rate may reveal anemia, which contributes to ischemia by reducing oxygen transport to the brain, polycythemia, which reduces blood flow and oxygen availability, an elevated white cell count, which may indicate an unsuspected infection, or an elevated sedimentation rate, which suggests a vasculitis (arteritis) (Table 8-1).

2. Urinalysis may show signs of infection or renal damage, which is not unusual in the chronic atherosclerotic patient. Glycosuria, suggests the presence of diabetes mellitus and urinalysis culture and sensitivity is abnormal in urinary tract infection.

3. Blood urea nitrogen and serum creatinine are elevated in prerenal problems such as dehydration and in renal disease.

4. A fasting blood glucose and a 2-h postprandial blood glucose determination should be obtained to reveal the presence of diabetes mellitus. An elevated glycosylated hemoglobin level also suggests the presence of diabetes mellitus.

5. Cardiac evaluation. The relationship between cerebrovascular disease and cardiac disease is twofold: (a) atherosclerosis of the cervical cranial vessels is usually associated with coronary artery disease, and (b) the heart is a frequent and often unsuspected source of emboli in patients with TIAs or stroke. Consequently, all patients with a TIA or stroke should receive a full cardiac evaluation. This would include a 24-h cardiac monitor and transthoracic and transesophageal echocardiography. TEE is safe and provides superior resolution of the left atrium, left atrial appendage, aortic arch, and other cardiac basal structures.[41] Further tests such as cardiac catheterization would be conducted at the discretion of the consulting cardiologist. There is a significant increase in detection of cardiac abnormalities with TEE in patients with stroke who have embolism of cardiac origin.[42] Although atrial myxoma is rare, cerebral embolism is a common complication of this tumor.

6. Duplex ultrasound. Ultrasonography using both real-time and Doppler methods provides an opportunity to detect abnormalities in the carotid and vertebral arteries. The reliability of ultrasonography has increased remarkably but ultrasonography is not a substitute for arteriography. The development of transcranial Doppler ultrasonography allows identification of the circle of Willis with its main intracranial branches. Consequently, this permits demonstration of intracranial artery stenosis with a high degree of reliability.

7. A chest x-ray may reveal an unexpected tumor as a source of cerebral metastases, which may mimic TIA. The heart is enlarged in chronic hypertension and heart disease. An unsuspected pneumonia may be a significant factor in the onset of stroke.

8. Serum lipids. Fasting cholesterol and triglycerides are elevated in a significant number of patients with TIA or stroke.

9. Serum uric acid. Hyperuricemia occurs in about 30 percent of patients with cerebrovascular disease.

10. Thyroid function tests. Hypothyroidism is associated with accelerated atherosclerosis.

11. Patients who may have a collagen vascular disease often show an elevated sedimentation rate

Table 8-1

Evaluation of the patient with acute stroke due to thromboembolism

---

1. Complete blood count and sedimentation rate to reveal anemia, polycythemia, and elevated white cell count, which might indicate unsuspected infection or elevated sedimentation rate, suggesting a vasculitis (arteritis).

2. Urinalysis culture and sensitivity to detect signs of renal damage, glycosuria, or urinary tract infection.

3. Blood urea nitrogen and serum creatinine: often elevated in dehydration or indicating the presence of renal disease.

4. Fasting blood glucose levels: 2-h postprandial blood glucose determination or elevated glycosylated hemoglobin level, suggesting the presence of diabetes mellitus.

5. Full cardiac evaluation, including 24-h cardiac monitoring, echocardiogram, and transesophageal echocardiogram, to detect source of emboli and to reduce risk of myocardial infarction, the leading cause of death in stroke, due to thromboembolism. TEE provides adequate visualization of the ascending aorta by a transesophageal approach to exclude ulcerative plaques as a source of embolism.

6. Duplex ultrasonography (real-time and Doppler ultrasonography) of carotid arteries and vertebral arteries and trans-cranial Doppler sonography to study intracranial extensions of the vessels, including the circle of Willis, middle cerebral arteries, basal artery, and posterior cerebral arteries.

7. Chest x-ray to exclude aspiration pneumonia or an unexpected tumor or cerebral mestastasis, which may mimic TIA. A chest x-ray may also show enlargement of the heart and chronic hypertension or heart disease and reveal unsuspected pneumonia, which may be a significant factor in the onset of stroke.

8. Metabolic screen for cholesterol and triglycerides, which are elevated in a significant number of patients with TIA or stroke.

9. Serum uric acid. Uric acid acts as a lipid transport and is elevated in about 30 percent of patients with cerebrovascular disease.

10. Thyroid function tests. Hypothyroidism is associated with accelerated atherosclerosis.

11. Determination of antinuclear factor, anticardiolipin, antithrombin-III, Sjögren, SSA and SSB, complement C3, C4, CH50 in cases of suspected collagen vascular disease.

12. Platelet count and coagulation profile in young patients with stroke who may have a coagulation deficit, particularly in the presence of intracranial hemorrhage or hemorrhagic infarction.

13. MRI and CT scans. A CT scan is usually obtained in the emergency center to differentiate between ischemic and hemorrhagic infarction, or intracerebral hemorrhage. MRI is usually an interval study to delineate the extent of cerebral infarction, or hemorrhage and clearly delineate the extent of infarction when the CT scan is normal.

14. Electrolyte determination every 48-h for sodium, potassium, calcium, magnesium, and phosphate. Electrolyte abnormalities contribute to further neuronal damage in the penumbra.

15. Lumbar puncture in cases with nuchal rigidity suggesting subarachnoid hemorrhage, encephalitis, or meningitis, where MRI and CT scans are equivocal.

16. Ophthalmic consultation is indicated in patients with neurovascular glaucoma or ischemic optic neuropathy who may have significant stenosis of the carotid artery and its branches.

17. Four-vessel conventional arteriography is indicated in all cases where there is demonstrable significant stenosis of the carotid or vertebral arteries, demonstrated by duplex ultrasonography or magnetic resonance angiography, and where there is a question of surgical intervention.

18. Serological test for syphilis.

19. Evaluation of swallowing should be conducted within 24 h of admission in conscious patients to avoid aspiration when feeding. Serial swallowing tests are indicated in patients who have impaired swallowing mechanisms.

20. Evaluation for possible hypercoagulable state should be conducted in all young patients with stroke.

and other symptoms suggesting this diagnosis. Such cases require determination of antinuclear factor, anticardiolipin, antithrombin III, Sjögren, SSA and SSB, complement C3, C4, and CH50.

12. Platelet count and anticoagulation profile. A coagulation disorder may predispose to the development of a hemorrhagic infarction in an area of ischemic infarction.

13. The MRI and computed tomography (CT) scans may reveal the presence of an unexpected cerebral infarction, subdural hematoma, or tumor. A CT scan is usually obtained in the emergency center before admission to differentiate between an ischemic and hemorrhagic infarction or intracerebral hemorrhage. The clinical neurological examination and the noncontrast CT scan is 95 percent accurate in establishing the diagnosis.[43] However, CT scanning may not be abnormal for 3 to 5 days after ischemic cerebral infarction. The MRI is superior to CT and high-signal intensity regions in the MRI scan with contrast enhancement indicating cerebral infarction or ischemia are consistently seen on T2-weighted images within the first few hours following onset of a stroke.[44] The superiority of MRI is most striking in brainstem infarction; however, MRI is occasionally negative in patients with symptoms and signs of cortical, lacunar, or brainstem strokes.[45] The role of MRI in detecting lesion size, using diffusion-weighted and perfusion-weighted images to detect the extent of the ischemic area is a promising extension of MRI in stroke.[46]

14. Electrolyte determination every 48 h for sodium, potassium, calcium, magnesium, and phosphate. Electrolyte abnormalities contribute to further neuronal damage in the penumbra.

15. Lumbar puncture. The need for lumbar puncture has decreased considerably following the introduction of MRI and CT scanning, but there are indications for lumbar puncture when scans are negative but the patient has a focal neurological deficit and nuchal rigidity, suggesting subarachnoid hemorrhage, encephalitis, or meningitis.

16. Ophthalmic consultation. Patients with neurovascular glaucoma without a precipitating fundus condition may have severe carotid artery stenosis leading to retinal ischemia and glaucoma. Ischemic

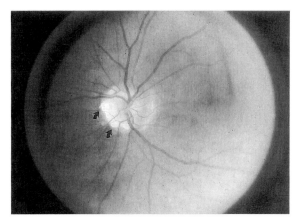

Figure 8-5

Disc drüsen: glistening lumps (arrows) in the nerve head, blurring the disc margin, sometimes confused with papilledema. Condition may be associated with ischemic optic neuropathy.

optic neuropathy and disc drüsen (Fig. 8-5) is generally associated with stenosis and occlusion of the ophthalmic artery rather than stenosis of the internal carotid artery. Retinal artery occlusion is associated with retinal edema and infarction (Fig. 8-6).

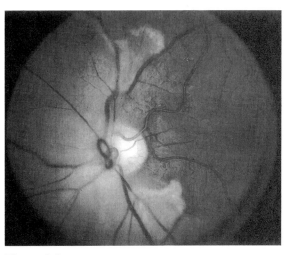

Figure 8-6

Retinal edema and infarction. There is sharp delineation between the healthy retina and the poorly perfused (pale) retina, resulting from a recent branch retinal artery occlusion.

17. Arteriography. Four-vessel conventional arteriography remains the standard procedure for the evaluation of cervical and intracarotid vessels before the decision to recommend carotid endarterectomy or other surgical procedures on the carotid or vertebral arteries.[47] There is, however, an increasing reliance on a combination of duplex ultrasonography and magnetic resonance angiography (MRA) for evaluation of the internal carotid arteries in patients with carotid stenosis who may be candidates for endarterectomy.[48]

18. Serological test for syphilis. Syphilitic arteritis is still an occasional cause of TIA and stroke.

Differential Diagnosis of TIAs

1. Epilepsy. The recent onset of partial seizures in a middle-aged or elderly person may suggest TIAs. This is particularly common in partial complex seizures when the patient complains of transient loss of consciousness, or transient clouding or loss of consciousness has been noted by family members. A tonic seizure is unlikely to be mistaken for a TIA, but the subsequent hemiparesis (Todd's paralysis) in some patients may be misdiagnosed as a stroke if the history is not obtained in detail.

2. Cardiac disorders. The majority of patients with cerebrovascular disease have some degree of cardiovascular disease and are therefore subject to sudden changes in cardiac rhythm such as paroxysmal fibrillation, paroxysmal tachycardia, and heart block. These disorders may be associated with temporary neurological deficits. Myocardial infarction may produce precipitous reduction in cardiac output with impairment of cerebral circulation and transient neurological deficits due to reversible anoxia.

3. Postural (orthostatic) hypotension. The role of postural hypotension in the production of TIAs has been overemphasized in the past. Nevertheless, the postural hypotension of Parkinson disease, other neurodegenerative diseases, syringomyelia, peripheral neuropathy, and idiopathic orthostatic hypotension may produce syncope resembling TIAs.

4. Hypoglycemia may be associated with transient neurological deficits. The condition is not usually difficult to diagnose when the onset is sudden because of the prominence of autonomic symptoms. However, gradual development of hypoglycemia following an overdose of a slow-release insulin preparation may produce clouding of consciousness and focal or neurological signs causing considerable difficulty in diagnosis.

5. Syncope. Fainting spells are not usually difficult to diagnose because they are frequently precipitated by sudden stress. They may, however, occur with or without obvious precipitating factors, in the presence of anemia, or in debilitated persons and may mimic a TIA.

6. Renal and hepatic failure. Transient clouding of consciousness is not unusual in established uremia and hepatic encephalopathy. The diagnosis is established by history and appropriate tests.

7. Electrolyte imbalance. Hyponatremia and hypocalcemia may produce sudden neurological deficits with clouding of consciousness and focal neurological signs. Severe electrolyte abnormalities are usually detected in such cases.

8. Medication and drugs. Alcohol, barbiturates, nonbarbiturate sleeping preparations, anticonvulsants, and tranquilizers may produce nystagmus and slurring of speech and clouding of consciousness of a temporary nature.

9. Migraine. The neurological deficits accompanying certain migraine attacks (i.e., ophthalmoplegia, hemiplegia, aphasia, unilateral sensory loss, hemianopia, vertigo, dysarthria, and clouding of consciousness) may closely mimic TIAs. A history of migraine and the accompanying headache usually clarify the diagnosis. Migraine attacks occasionally occur with neurological deficits, but without subsequent headache. This condition, called a migraine equivalent, may produce considerable difficulty in diagnosis.

10. Labyrinthine disorders. Middle-aged and elderly patients with acute onset of vertigo should receive a careful neurological examination because many of them show additional signs of brainstem involvement, indicating a TIA, and are erroneously diagnosed as having labyrinthitis or Meniere disease.

11. Ocular disturbances. Glaucoma, retinal vascular disease, and sudden changes in refraction in

diabetic patients receiving insulin therapy may produce symptoms of transient blurring or dimness of vision and suggest vascular insufficiency.

12. Intracranial mass lesion. It is not unusual for intracranial mass lesions such as tumors, subdural hematomas, and cerebral abscesses to cause transient neurological deficits suggesting TIAs. The situation will be clarified as the patient is fully evaluated for either cerebrovascular disease or suspected tumor.

13. Psychiatric disorders. Transient impairment or loss of consciousness occurring in an emotionally disturbed individual with a conversion reaction may be mistaken for a TIA. The light-headedness and occasional syncope associated with hyperventilation and anxiety neurosis may also suggest a transient impairment of cerebral circulation. In both cases, a careful history will usually clarify the situation and establish the diagnosis.

Treatment

Patients with TIAs are high-risk candidates for both cerebral infarction and myocardial infarction. Consequently the treatment should include the following:

1. Hypertension should be appropriately managed, but hypotensive episodes must be avoided.

In view of the association of chronic hypertension and atherosclerosis, it is better to maintain the blood pressure in the lower hypertensive range in patients who have had either TIA or a stroke (see below for the management of hypertension).

2. Any cardiac abnormalities identified in the evaluation process should be treated.

3. Any hematological or metabolic abnormality identified in the evaluation process should be adequately treated. Reduction of elevated cholesterol levels using an HMG-CoA reductase inhibitor protects against nonfatal or fatal strokes.[49]

4. Anticoagulants. There is no conclusive evidence that anticoagulants prevent the development of stroke in patients with TIA.[50] The effectiveness of heparin or low molecular weight heparinoid has not been established as a therapeutic measure in TIA or stroke.[51] Nevertheless, when the TIAs are frequent and are associated with atrial fibrillation, the patient

should receive anticoagulants.[52] Similarly, other cardiac abnormalities that could give rise to embolism, identified in the cardiac evaluation, are an additional reason for anticoagulant therapy. A TIA occurring in an individual known to have a greater than 90 percent stenosis of the appropriate internal carotid artery[53] or those with an intraluminal thrombus or carotid or vertebral dissection should receive anticoagulants.[54] An MRI or CT scan should be obtained to rule out intracranial bleeding, followed by activated clotting time (ACT) or a partial thromboplastin time (PTT) and platelet count. If the results of the ACT or PTT or platelet count are within normal limits, 5000 units heparin should be given as an intravenous bolus, followed by a slow mechanical infusion of 1000 units heparin each hour. The ACT or PTT should be repeated 4 h after the beginning of IV heparin infusion and every 4 h during treatment. The dose of heparin should be adjusted according to the results of testing, with the aim of obtaining a PTT time of 55 to 85, or an ACT of 190. If bleeding occurs at any site, the infusion should be terminated. Effects of heparin can be reversed with protamine sulfate if necessary, but this would be an unusual situation. In all cases, the hemoglobin and hematocrit should be checked every 48 h to detect occult bleeding. Once the patient stabilizes, he or she should be converted to warfarin sodium (Coumadin). An initial dose of 10 mg daily should be given orally and the dose regulated according to daily prothrombin time (PT) and International Normalized Ratio (INR). When the PT is one and a half times normal, or preferably the INR is between 2.5 and 3, the heparin should be discontinued and the Coumadin continued. Bleeding during Coumadin therapy can be controlled with vitamin K (phytonadione). The use of aspirin, phenylbutazone, and chloramphenicol should be avoided during Coumadin therapy. Cholesterol embolization is occasionally enhanced by anticoagulation with warfarin, when the drug interferes with plaque healing and shards of cholesterol emboli enter the circulation. Patients present with evidence of involvement of multiple cerebral arteries, and there is a purple color on the plantar surfaces of the feet several weeks after the beginning of treatment. Other features include livido reticularis, cyanosis, infarction of the digits, fever, elevated sedimentation rate, evidence of visceral ischemia, and a rising creatinine level. Diagnosis can be confirmed by the presence of retinal emboli, by transcranial Doppler ultrasonography, or by skin biopsy. The syndrome has been seen following cardiac and aortic surgery and cardiopulmonary bypass surgery as well as anticoagulation.

5.   Antiplatelet agents. Chronic use of acetyl salicylic acid (aspirin), 81 to 325 mg daily, reduces the incidence of stroke. Patients with nonvalvular atrial fibrillation who have absence of risk factors, including recent congestive heart failure, left ventricular fractional shortening of 25 percent or less, previous thromboembolism, systolic blood pressure greater than 160 mmHg, or female sex older than 75 years, are considered to carry a low risk of stroke. Treatment with aspirin, 325 mg daily, rather than anticoagulation is recommended in such cases.[55] The combination of aspirin and dipyridamole has a highly significant effect for the prevention of stroke and the combined therapy is more effective than either agent prescribed singly.[56] Ticlopidine 250 mg bid or clopidogrel bisulphate 75mg bid are alternative agents that may be more effective in stroke prevention than aspirin during the first year of treatment.[57]

6.   Surgical treatment has proved to be of definite benefit in patients with TIA when the carotid plaque is producing greater than 50 percent narrowing of the lumen of the artery.

Prognosis

Many patients have suffered single or multiple episodes of transient ischemia before a stroke but have failed to seek medical advice. Prospective studies of the natural history of TIA show differing figures for subsequent cerebral thrombosis, depending on the age group, vocation, and race of the population studied.

The risk of stroke appears to be greatest in the first year following the TIA and stroke tends to occur after a small number of TIAs, with a decreasing risk as the attacks continue. Between 10 and 25 percent of patients with TIA develop cerebral infarction within a year following the first TIA, and about 5 percent of patients per year develop stroke each subsequent year. Consequently, a TIA is a sign indicating a major

risk of cerebral or brainstem infarction. Because vascular disease is not confined to one system, a TIA is also a sign indicating a major risk of myocardial infarction.

CEREBRAL INFARCTION

Definition   A cerebral infarction occurs when there are ischemia and necrosis of an area of the brain following a reduction of blood supply below the critical level necessary for cell survival.

Etiology   There are two major causes of cerebral infarction: thrombosis and embolism.

Thrombosis

The term "cerebral thrombosis" is only partially correct because infarction may result from thrombosis of the internal carotid or vertebral arteries as well as the cerebral arteries and their branches.

The majority of cases of cerebral infarction follow thrombosis and occlusion of an atherosclerotic vessel. Consequently, cerebral thrombosis occurs in an individual who has one or more risk factors, producing accelerated atherosclerosis. Cerebral thrombosis also occurs as a complication of other diseases, for example, arteritis affecting the cerebral (or cervical) arteries or abnormalities of coagulation and possibly following a critical fall in perfusion of the brain.

Cerebral Embolism

The most common location of cerebral embolism is a thrombotic embolus involving the middle cerebral artery. Emboli originating in or passing through the heart have a much greater chance of entering the common carotid arteries than the vertebral arteries. An embolism in a common carotid artery tends to enter the internal carotid artery and pass into the middle cerebral artery, which is the largest branch and the anatomic continuation of the internal carotid artery. About 15 percent of all ischemic strokes and 30 percent of strokes in the elderly are associated with atrial fibrillation. In patients with atrial fibrillation, embolism is more likely to occur at the onset of paroxysmal atrial fibrillation and within a year of the transition to chronic atrial fibrillation. The increased use of TEE has identified atheromatous disease of the ascending aorta and proximal aortic arch as a source of embolism in stroke.[58] The several risk factors of cerebral embolism are listed in Table 8-2.

Cerebral infarction will occur only when there is a critical reduction of blood flow to an area of the brain. The brain has a well-developed anastomotic system that affords considerable protection against reduction in blood flow and there are no end arterial systems in the brain. The anastomotic potential begins with the circle of Willis. In addition, the anterior, middle, and posterior cerebral arteries communicate with each other through numerous anastomotic con-

Table 8-2

Major risk factors in
thromboembolic cerebral infarction

1. Heart disease
2. Hypertension
3. Diabetes mellitus
4. Abnormal serum lipids
5. Hypothyroidism
6. Hyperuricemia
7. Obesity
8. Cigarette smoking
9. Alcohol
10. Age
11. Lack of exercise
12. Arteriolosclerosis
13. Arteritis
14. Fibromuscular dysplasia
15. Organ transplant recipients
16. Sickle cell disease
17. Hypercoagulable states

A. Primary: Protein C deficiency, protein S deficiency, antithrombin III deficiency, presence of factor V Leiden

B. Secondary: Positive anticardiolipin; antithrombin III; arteritis with reduced complement C3, C4, and CH50; circulating lupus anticoagulant and homocystinemia

C. Platelet hyperaggregability

nections, but there is variability of the territorial distribution of the major cerebral vessels.[59] This is one factor that influences the site and size of infarction following major vessel occlusion. Consequently, infarction will occur when (a) there is a failure of blood flow through a major vessel and (b) there is a failure of blood flow through the anastomotic vessels supplying the ischemic area of the brain.

The site of infarction depends on the effectiveness of anastomotic connections. For example, if there is a gradual stenosis at the origin of an atherosclerotic middle cerebral artery with the development of adequate blood flow through the anastomotic channels from the posterior and anterior cerebral circulations at the time of the thrombosis of the middle cerebral artery, (a) infarction will not occur at all or, (b) if infarction occurs, the infarct will be located close to the origin of the middle cerebral artery, which is the edge of the area supplied by the anastomotic vessels. On the other hand, the sudden occlusion of a healthy middle cerebral artery might be followed by a large infarction in the middle cerebral artery territory, because there has been no prior stimulus to encourage the development of an effective collateral circulation. Similarly, thrombosis of an atherosclerotic middle cerebral artery will be followed by a major infarction with edema producing hemispheric swelling, shift of the midline structures, and hydrocephalus with increased intracranial pressure (Fig. 8-7) when the anterior and posterior cerebral arteries are also atherosclerotic and incapable of supporting an adequate collateral circulation.

Pathology One of the earliest changes following ischemia is the production of proinflammatory interleukins by microglia and astrocytes, including interleukins IL-1, IL-2, and IL-6 and tissue necrosis factor-alpha (TNF-α). These cytokines activate receptor sites on the surface endothelium of the microvasculature and on leukocytes flowing freely through these vessels. The leukocytes are then tethered to the surface of the endothelium by adhesion molecules termed selectins present on the surface of the leukocytes and endothelium.[60] The leukocytes then roll along the endothelium to a site close to where the leukocyte will ultimately migrate through the vessel wall. The rolling ceases and the second stage begins,

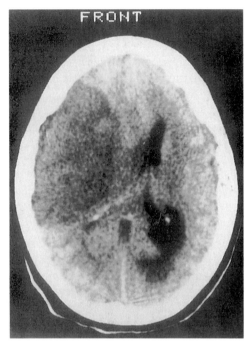

Figure 8-7
CT scan, large infarction the result of occlusion right middle cerebral artery in the presence of poor collateral circulation. There is edema, hemisphere swelling, shift of the midline structure, and hydrocephalus involving the left lateral ventricle.

marked by a flattening out of the leukocyte on the endothelium, mediated by CD18 adhesion molecules expressed on leukocytes binding to intercellular adhesion molecules (ICAM 1 and ICAM 2) on the endothelial surface.[61] In the final stage of leukocyte migration, a leukocyte begins to extravasate between endothelial cells, leaving the bloodstream and entering the parenchyma. Adhesion of leukocytes to the endothelium, followed by leukocyte migration, results in a number of responses. The leukocytes may block smaller arterioles, resulting in further ischemia in the affected area. There is a further release of the proinflammatory cytokines IL-1, IL-2, IL-6, and TNF-α, resulting in activation of other leukocytes, promoting additional adhesion to the vascular endothelium, and extending the damage to arteries and arterioles. In addition, cytokines can promote thrombosis by binding circulating anticoagulants, including protein C, protein S, and antithrombin III and by inhibiting tissue plasminogen activator release.[62]

Transient endothelial migration of leukocytes into the parenchyma of the central nervous system (CNS) is associated with further release of cytokines from microglia, astrocytes, and infiltrating leukocytes, producing neuronal cytotoxic injury.[63] Thus, neuronal injury and death are not solely the results of anoxia but also include the effect of cytokines liberated from several sources.

In the first 24 h after infarction, leukocytes that have migrated into the perivascular spaces occasionally reach the subarachnoid space, producing a transient polymorphonuclear pleocytosis in the CSF. The leukocytes in the microvasculature are gradually replaced by mononuclear cells that migrate through the endothelium into the necrotic area of the infarct. Active phagocytosis of dead material proceeds over a period of several months. There is proliferation of astrocytes in the surrounding area and partial replacement of dead tissue by glia, but the center of the infarct often remains as a glial cyst.

In the early period following infarction, the area immediately surrounding the infarct (the penumbra) contains neurons and glial cells receiving a marginal blood supply. These cells are damaged but potentially viable for a few hours after the onset of stroke, in that electrical failure has occurred while structural integrity is maintained and energy metabolism is preserved.[64] There is a gradual expansion of the infarct during this period, until the penumbra is obliterated.[54] Spontaneous reperfusion after cerebral infarction occurs in 42 percent of cases within the first week after infarction but does not occur early enough to preserve tissue function and clinical improvement following reperfusion occurs in only 2 percent of cases. Consequently, reperfusion must occur in the early stages of stroke if the neurons in the penumbra are to be preserved. Later reperfusion is of no benefit to the penumbra and may, in some cases, be associated with hemorrhagic transformation.

The result of the ischemic state is the change from aerobic to anaerobic glycolysis, the development of lactic acidosis, a rapid decline in high-energy phosphate production, and the inhibition of protein synthesis, all of which may contribute to neuronal damage. Adenosine triphosphate is depleted and there is release of the neurotransmitters, glutamate and aspartate; progressive disturbance of energy metabolism; and finally, anoxic depolarization.[65] This is followed by influx of calcium and sodium ions and efflux of potassium ions because of pump failure in the neuronal membrane. The excessive influx of calcium reacts with intracellular phospholipids with the formation of free radicals known to cause further intracellular damage and neuronal death.[66] Calcium influx into the neuron also stimulates production of nitric oxide; release of cytokines in the ischemic area is followed by release of large amounts of nitric oxide by microglia. Both mechanisms contribute to neuronal damage or death by excessive accumulation of nitric oxide,[67] which damages the mitochondrial electron transport chain and mitochondrial DNA. The penumbra then can be regarded as an area of restricted blood supply in which energy metabolism is preserved but progressively depleted, with expansion of the core of the infarct until the penumbra is obliterated. This process occurs over a period of approximately 3 to 4 h.[68] Consequently, the therapeutic window for successful reperfusion is short, if successful tissue salvage is to be achieved. A similar constraint applies to the use of neuroprotective agents in the treatment of acute cerebral or brainstem infarction.

The cascade that eventually leads to neuronal death might be blocked by a number of interventions, including (a) restoration of blood supply, (b) prevention of early edema in the penumbra, (c) control of hyperglycemia or systemic acidosis, (d) prevention of propagation of the thrombus, impeding collateral circulation, (e) preventing glutamate release from the axon by inhibiting presynaptic voltage-sensitive ion channels controlling exocytosis, (f) using N-methyl-D-aspartate (NMDA) and other receptor antagonists to block receptor activity, (g) enhancing glutamate and other excitatory amino acid reuptake by glial cells, (h) blocking resynthesis of glutamine and reuptake by axon terminals, (i) blocking calcium channels in NMDA and non-NMDA receptors, (j) inhibiting the production of nitric oxide, and (k) inhibiting the production of free radicals.

NMDA receptor antagonists are the most advanced agents in clinical development for treatment of stroke. A blockade of NMDA receptors consistently reduces infarct volume in vivo in focal ischemia models. Neuropsychological symptoms and cardiovascular side effects are a problem.[69]

Clinical Features Infarction of the brain in an area supplied by a cerebral artery tends to produce a clearly recognizable clinical syndrome. Each syndrome is discussed separately.

Occlusion of the Internal Carotid Artery

1. Occlusion is preceded by TIAs in about 50 percent of cases.

2. Infarction usually occurs in the region of the brain supplied by the middle cerebral artery, producing contralateral signs, including homonymous hemianopia, a central type of facial paralysis, hemiparesis or hemiplegia, and hemisensory loss. Involvement of the dominant hemisphere produces dysphasia or aphasia, whereas involvement of frontal lobe produces deviation of the head and eyes toward the side of the infarction. Onset is usually followed by some impairment of consciousness, which varies from drowsiness to coma, depending on the development of cerebral edema. Infarcts are likely to be cortical or large subcortical infarcts.[70]

3. Occlusion of an internal carotid artery can be asymptomatic when the collateral circulation in the middle cerebral territory is adequate.

4. When the involved internal carotid artery supplies both anterior cerebral arteries, the ipsilateral middle cerebral artery and the posterior cerebral artery through the posterior communicating artery, occlusion of the internal carotid artery may produce ischemia and infarction involving both frontal lobes and all of the hemisphere on the affected side. This usually results in severe cerebral edema, uncal herniation, brainstem compression, and death within a few days.

Occlusion of the Middle Cerebral Artery

1. Symptoms of occlusion of the middle cerebral artery are often indistinguishable from

those of occlusion of the internal carotid artery (Fig. 8-8).

2. The most common symptoms consist of the sudden onset of contralateral signs, including homonymous hemianopia, central type of facial weakness, flaccid hemiparesis or hemiplegia, and hemisensory loss. The patient is dysphasic or aphasic if the dominant hemisphere is involved and the head and eyes are often deviated toward the side of the infarction and away from the side of weakness (Fig. 8-9). The head and eye deviation usually resolves within a few days, and there is gradual improvement in strength, which is much more apparent in the lower limb than the upper limb. This improvement is associated with progressive spasticity, increased tendon reflexes, and an extensor plantar response on the affected side. Persistence of a homonymous hemianopia indicates a poor prognosis for recovery. Early

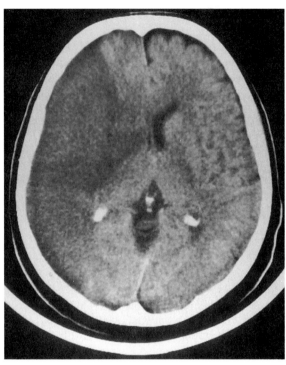

Figure 8-9
CT scan with contrast enhancement. Large infarction in the right middle cerebral artery territory. There is edema producing effacement of the right lateral ventricle and right to left shift of the midline structures.

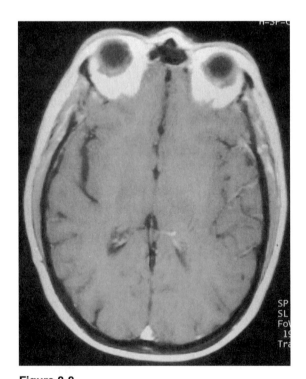

Figure 8-8
MRI scan. T1 axial image with contrast showing effacement of the left sylvian fissure in early left middle cerebral artery occlusion with infarction.

seizures also indicate a poorer prognosis, particularly in elderly patients with large hemorrhagic infarction of a parietal lobe.[71]

Occlusion of the Anterior Cerebral Artery

1. Occlusion of the recurrent branch (Huebner's artery) produces ischemia and infarction involving the anterior limb of the internal capsule and anterior portion of the caudate nucleus and putamen. Involvement of these structures results in contralateral paralysis or paresis of the face and upper limb. There may be some rigidity or dystonia due to basal ganglia involvement.

2. Occlusion of the distal cortical branches causes infarction of the paracentral lobule producing paralysis and sensory loss in the contralateral lower limb.

3. Complete occlusion of the anterior cerebral artery results in a combination of numbers 1 and 2 (i.e., contralateral hemiparesis and hemisensory loss). In addition, right-handed persons show dyspraxia of the left hand because of ischemia or infarction involving the corpus callosum.

4. Bilateral occlusion of the anterior cerebral arteries produces bilateral frontal lobe ischemia. Survivors may have minimal limb weakness, but patients who are fully conscious show a remarkable apathy. There is an apparent indifference to surrounding activity and no interest in food, but the affected individual will chew and swallow if fed. This state is associated with lack of discrimination in acceptance of any material as food, if it is fed to the patient. Language is intact, but it is extremely difficult to hold a conversation because of lack of motivation. Speech is monotonous and slowed. Patients with this condition are incontinent of bowel and bladder due to bilateral involvement of sphincter control centers lying on the medial aspects of the frontal lobes. This incontinence is a "neglect" situation and the patient shows a complete indifference to bladder emptying or bowel movement.

Occlusion of the Anterior Choroidal Artery Infarction in the distribution of the anterior choroidal artery is usually combined with massive infarction in the territory of the internal carotid artery. Infarcts restricted to anterior choroidal artery occlusion alone are rare.[72] However, occlusion of the anterior choroidal artery can cause infarction of the posterior limb of the internal capsule, thalamus, midbrain, temporal lobe, or lateral geniculate body, depending on the territory supplied by this vessel. The following features may be seen:

1. The most common sign is hemiplegia.
2. Hemisensory loss is usually transient.
3. Visual field defects, including homonymous upper quadrantanopia, hemianopia, or upper and lower quadrantanopia, sparing the horizontal median, can occur. The latter indicates involvement of the lateral geniculate body.
4. Bilateral anterior choroidal artery infarcts are associated with pseudobulbar symptoms and paralysis of vertical gaze.

Occlusion of the Posterior Cerebral Artery

1. Occlusion of the penetrating branches to the midbrain results in ischemia or infarction involving the cerebral peduncle, the third nerve, and the red nucleus. This produces contralateral hemiparesis, ipsilateral or contralateral cerebellar ataxia, and tremor due to ischemia of the red nucleus or involving the fibers passing from the cerebellum to the ipsilateral or contralateral red nucleus and ipsilateral third nerve paralysis.

2. Occlusion of penetrating branches supplying the subthalamic nucleus or its efferent or afferent connections results in a contralateral or occasionally ipsilateral ballism (hemiballismus) with involuntary flinging movements of the affected limb and severe hemiataxia.[73]

3. Occlusion of the thalamostriate branches produces infarction of the posterolateral ventral nucleus of the thalamus (Fig. 8-10). This results in

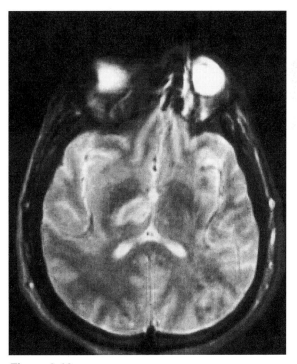

Figure 8-10
Right thalamic infarct. MRI scan showing a well-circumscribed area of increased signal intensity in the region of the right thalamus.

severe contralateral hemisensory loss. The symptoms vary from sensory loss affecting the hand (useless hand syndrome) to complete hemisensory involvement (hemisensory stroke). The hemisensory loss is sometimes accompanied by a mild hemiparesis owing to involvement of the internal capsule. This usually results in some residual spasticity and increased reflexes. After a period varying from 1 week to several months, the affected limb and trunk show some return of sensory function. This is occasionally accompanied by a severe burning pain that is accentuated by mild painful stimuli (hyperalgesia) or non-noxious stimulation such as contact with clothing in extreme cases (allodynia).[74] This condition of central poststroke pain (or thalamic pain) is extremely distressing and debilitating and is often misdiagnosed.

4.   Bilateral occlusion of the thalamostriate arteries can occasionally arise from occlusion of a single trunk of one posterior cerebral artery or from a basilar artery that supplies all of the thalamostriate arteries and results in bilateral paramedian thalamic infarction. The onset is sudden, with somnolence or loss of consciousness followed by apathy, persistent amnesia resembling Korsakoff syndrome, dementia, lack of spontaneity, slowing of thought, poor insight, confabulation, perseveration, dysgraphia, and impairment of downward gaze.

5.   Occlusion of the distal branches that supply the occipital lobe results in a contralateral homonymous hemianopia (Fig. 8-11). A cortical blindness results if both posterior cerebral arteries are involved. Right-handed individuals with left occipital lobe infarction may show alexia without agraphia (inability to read with preservation of writing). This syndrome is the result of ischemia to the posterior portion of the corpus callosum, preventing the transfer of information from the surviving right occipital lobe for interpretation in the left hemisphere. Depression and obsessive thinking, anomia, and color anomia are features of dominant hemisphere infarction and visual perseveration and metamorphosis may occur. Headache is not uncommon in posterior cerebral artery occlusion. Visual hallucinations, including complex hallucinations, are well recognized in posterior cerebral artery infarction.

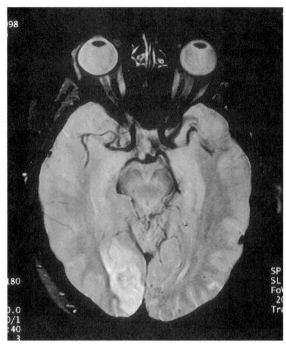

Figure 8-11
MRI scan. Area of increased signal intensity indicating a right occipital infarction owing to an occlusion of the calcarine branch of the right posterior cerebral artery.

6.   Occlusion of the main trunk of the posterior cerebral artery (Fig. 8-12) is often sudden, suggesting an embolic cause. Signs consist of a homonymous hemianopia associated with one or more of the following: hemisensory loss, hemiparesis, dyslexia, unsteady gait, poor hand coordination, confusion, and poor memory when the hippocampal area of the dominant hemisphere is involved. It is not unusual to find a contralateral homonymous hemianopia without any other sign of neurological deficit despite complete occlusion of the posterior cerebral artery.

Occlusion of the Vertebral Artery   The following are characteristics of occlusion of the vertebral artery:

1.   Occlusion of one vertebral artery may be asymptomatic because of adequate collateral circula-

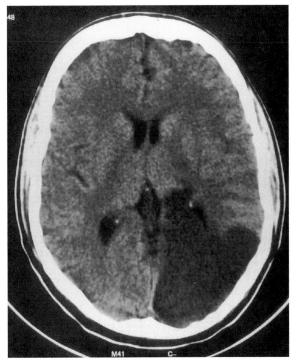

Figure 8-12
CT scan. Large infarct involving the occipital lobe and medial temporal lobe following occlusion of the left posterior cerebral artery.

tion unless the opposite vertebral artery is small or severely atherosclerotic.

2. Vertebral artery occlusion may result in a small infarction in the medulla or pons when the contralateral circulation is poor and when there is marked atherosclerosis of the basilar artery or its penetrating branches. This type of stroke is sudden in onset, with development of a number of possible symptoms, including ataxia, diplopia, facial weakness, vomiting, vertigo, dysarthria, dysphonia, and dysphagia. Vomiting may be severe in some cases, with minor vertigo or dizziness.[75] Many patients make a good recovery over a period of weeks or months.

3. Thrombosis of the fourth portion of the vertebral artery may present with symptoms of posterior inferior cerebellar artery thrombosis (see below).

4. Occlusion of the vertebral artery is occa-

sionally followed by symptoms suggesting basilar artery thrombosis (see below).

Occlusion of the Posterior Inferior Cerebellar Artery (Lateral Medullary Syndrome) This artery supplies the lateral portion of the medulla and the inferior surface of the cerebellum and arterial occlusion may be followed by infarction in any portion or all of this region (Figs. 8-13 and 8-14).

The onset is sudden, with intense vertigo due to involvement of the inferior vestibular nucleus and vomiting, pallor, and diaphoresis because of stimulation of the vomiting center and vestibular vagal and descending sympathetic pathways. At the same time, there may be complaints of unilateral facial pain or paresthesias due to irritation of the spinal tract of the fifth cranial nerve. These early symptoms tend to subside, but the patient is left with severe deficits, including:

a. Involvement of the nucleus ambiguous or 10th nerve traversing the medulla, resulting in ipsilateral paralysis of the palate, larynx, and pharynx, producing dysarthria, dysphonia, and dysphagia. Unilateral involvement of one nucleus ambiguous can result in bilateral pharyngeal paralysis with acute onset of dysphagia as the sole or predominant symptom.[76]

b. Infarction of the inferior cerebellar peduncle and/or cerebellum results in nystagmus, which is maximal in looking toward the side of the lesion, and an ipsilateral cerebellar ataxia.

c. Involvement of the descending sympathetic fibers in the medullary reticular formation usually causes a partial rather than a complete Horner syndrome, with meiosis and ptosis on the side of the lesion.

d. Infarction of the lateral spinothalamic tract produces a contralateral loss of pain and temperature sensation involving the limbs and trunk.

e. Involvement of the spinal tract of the fifth nerve results in an ipsilateral loss of pain and temperature sensation over the face.

f. Inconsistent signs, including mild ipsilateral facial weakness and mild contralateral hemiparesis, are occasionally seen when the ischemia spreads beyond the usual boundaries of the lateral medullary infarct.

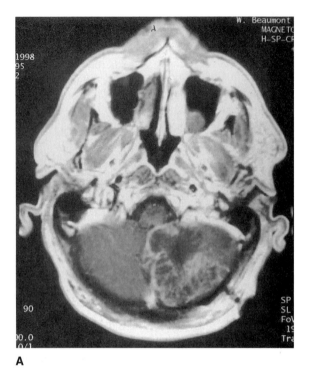

A

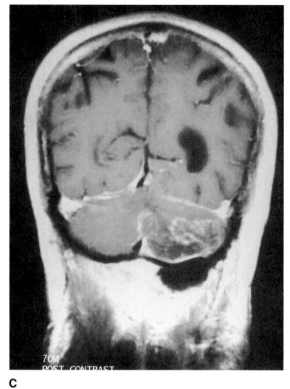

C

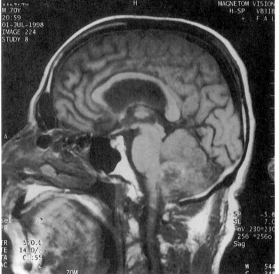

B

Figure 8-13
*MRI scan. Axial (**A**), saggital (**B**), and coronal (**C**) views showing a large left cerebellar infarct with gyral enhancement.*

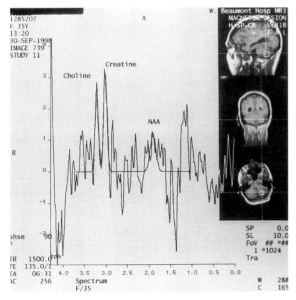

Figure 8-14
MRI spectroscopy. Left cerebellar infarction. Spectroscopy indicates reduced choline, creatine, and NAA with marked elevation in lactate, which presents as an enlarged biphasic wave form.

Occlusion of the Anterior Inferior Cerebellar Artery   The anterior inferior cerebellar artery is one of the long circumferential branches arising from the lower portion of the basilar artery supplying the anterior and inferior surface of the cerebellum, the cerebellar vermis, and the lower pons.

Infarction following occlusion of the anterior inferior cerebellar artery shows marked variation, depending on the efficiency of the collateral circulation in the pons and cerebellum. The presentation may include vertigo, nausea, vomiting, nystagmus, dysarthria and dysphagia, and ipsilateral signs including partial Horner syndrome, depressed corneal reflex, impaired sensation of the face, ipsilateral facial weakness, and ipsilateral hearing loss when the internal auditory artery rises from the anterior inferior cerebellar artery. There may be mild contralateral hemiparesis and hemisensory impairment with increased tendon reflexes and an extensor plantar response on the contralateral side. Recovery is usually partial but often includes resolution of the majority of functional loss.

Occlusion of the Basilar Artery and its Branches

1.   Emboli arising from atheromatous plaques in the basilar artery (or vertebral artery) and the distal branches of the basilar artery may give rise to single or multiple small strokes in the midbrain, thalamus or occipital lobes (Fig. 8-15) (see Occlusion of the Posterior Cerebral Artery).

2.   Thrombosis of a small penetrating artery entering the pons produces a ventromedial infarct in the brachium pontis with involvement of the corticobulbar and corticospinal tracts, pontine nuclei, descending sympathetic fibers, and the fibers passing to the middle cerebellar peduncle. This results in contralateral hemiparesis, ipsilateral cerebellar signs, and a partial Horner syndrome. Repeated thrombosis involving penetrating arteries on both sides of midline result in accumulating neurological deficits and eventually a severe dysarthria, dysphagia, and quadriparesis.

3.   Thrombosis of the short circumferential arteries arising from the basilar artery results in infarction of the lateral or tegmental area of the pons.

a.   Infarcts in the ventrolateral portion of the pons involve the root of the fifth cranial nerve, the sixth cranial nerve, the medial lemniscus, and the medial cerebellar peduncle, with involvement of the fibers in the corticospinal tract subserving the lower extremity. This results in vertigo, diplopia, ipsilateral sensory loss over the face, ipsilateral cerebellar signs with lateropulsion, dysarthria, Horner syndrome, and contralateral hemiparesis with greater weakness and loss of vibration and position sense in the lower extremity.

b.   Infarcts of the tegmental area of the pons are usually lacunar infarcts with involvement of the fifth, sixth, and seventh cranial nerves resulting in ipsilateral loss of sensation over the face, facial weakness, diplopia, and vertigo. There may be some involvement of the medial lemniscus, medial longitudinal fasciculus, and the superior cerebellar peduncle. This will result in an internuclear ophthalmoplegia, contralateral hemisensory loss, ipsilateral cerebellar signs, dysarthria, and a mild contralateral hemiparesis.[77] Bilateral ventrotegmental pontine infarcts present with acute pseudobulbar palsy, bilateral

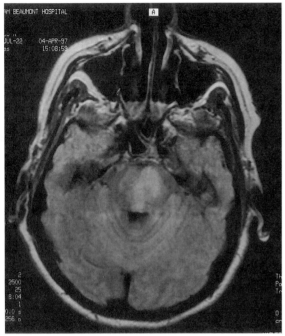

A

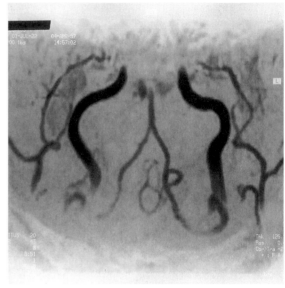

B

Figure 8-15
A. *MRI scan in pontine infarction. **B**. MRA scan showing occlusion of the terminal portion of the basilar artery.*

corticospinal tract involvement and tegmental signs of cranial nerve palsies.

4.   Occlusion of the superior cerebellar artery. This artery supplies the midbrain, the superior cerebellar peduncle, and the superior surface of the cerebellum. Infarction produces signs of ipsilateral or contralateral rubral tremor or myoclonus. There is a Horner syndrome on the side of the lesion and involvement of the corticospinal tract and spinothalamic tract results in contralateral hemiparesis and loss of pain and temperature sensation.

5.   Complete thrombosis of the basilar artery. This condition is usually a catastrophic affair with rapid onset of coma and a high mortality rate. Survivors show signs of brainstem involvement, including quadriplegia, which may persist with the return of consciousness. The condition is aptly termed the locked-in syndrome. This may be coupled with signs of occipital lobe infarction producing severe impairment of vision or permanent cortical blindness. Re-

covery may occur over a period of several months and is quite good in some survivors, whereas others show severe neurological deficits, including multiple bilateral cranial nerve involvement, impairment of ocular movements, and nystagmus, loss of sensation over the face, facial paralysis, dysarthria, and dysphagia. Bilateral corticospinal tract involvement results in spastic quadriparesis. Involvement of the lateral spinothalamic tracts or the medial lemnisci results in severe bilateral sensory loss. Pulmonary complications are the leading cause of death.

6.   Occlusion of the terminal portion of the basilar artery. This condition usually results from embolism and has been termed "saddle embolism." The embolus usually arises from a mural thrombus following a myocardial infarction. Subtle embolism can occur in any cardiac condition associated with thrombosis, including rheumatic heart disease, subacute bacterial endocarditis, prolapsed mitral valve, patent foramen ovale, calcified aortic valves, and atrial fib-

rillation. Emboli occasionally arise more distally at the origin of the vertebral arteries in atherosclerotic individuals. Saddle embolus produces occlusion of both posterior cerebral arteries and if extensive, will also produce occlusion of both superior cerebellar arteries.

Symptoms include cortical blindness due to involvement and infarction of both occipital lobes. It is not infrequent to find some sparing of a small area in the occipital lobe with visual field constriction and an unusual field pattern such as altitudinal hemianopia. Occasionally there is extensive damage to the visual association areas associated with anosognosia or denial of blindness (Anton syndrome). These patients, although totally blind, will describe situations visually and supply answers to questions that require vision.

Diagnostic Procedures All patients with cerebral infarction due to thrombosis or embolism should receive full evaluation for diseases of the blood vessels, abnormalities of blood constituents, and reduced cerebral perfusion. These investigations have been outlined in the diagnostic procedures for TIAs.

Treatment (Table 8-3) Stroke is an emergency. Ischemic stroke is similar to myocardial infarction in that the pathogenesis is loss of blood supply to tissue, which can result in irreversible damage if blood flow is not restored quickly.[78]

Treatment of the Comatose Patient

1. Respiratory care. The airway should be established and maintained. Comatose patients require

Table 8-3
Treatment of acute stroke due to thromboembolism

1. Maintain blood pressure at high normal or low hypertensive range.
2. Heparinize patients with suspected cerebral embolism.
3. Control diabetes mellitus.
4. Treat any infection with antibiotics following chest x-ray demonstrating aspiration pneumonia or results of urinary culture and sensitivity.
5. Treat hypothyroidism.
6. Treat hyperuricemia.
7. Foley catheter in bladder in obtunded stuporous, semicomatose, or comatose patients. Urinalysis, culture, and culture every 2 days to detect urinary tract infection. If present, treat with appropriate antibiotics.
8. Assess swallowing mechanisms daily. Insert nasogastric tube if aspiration is detected and withhold all fluids or food. Elevate head of bed to 35 degrees to prevent regurgitation and maintain a head elevation throughout treatment.
9. Intravenous fluids to maintain fluid and electrolyte balance.
10. If conscious and swallowing without aspiration, begin light diet.
11. If swallowing impaired, begin feeding by nasogastric tube after 24 h.
12. Physical therapy with passive limb movement beginning on the first day, modifying the program to a more active one as the patient improves.
13. Treat any cardiac abnormalities as recommended by a cardiac consultant.
14. Consider use of rt-PA or prourokinase by intra-arterial infusion or by intravenous infusion if less than 6 h since onset of stroke.
15. Examine chest early to detect early respiratory infection or pneumonia.
16. Treat hypercoagulable abnormalities in young patients with stroke.
17. Dietitian to see patient to prescribe appropriate diet for obese patients.
18. Stop smoking.

insertion of a short airway. There should be no hesitation in passing a low-pressure cuffed endotracheal tube if pharyngeal secretions are excessive and impede respiratory exchange.[79] Maintenance of normal oxygenation of the blood and near-normal P_{CO_2} levels is the immediate goal.[80] All patients should be suctioned frequently to clear the airway. This may be aided by turning the patient 2 h from right lateral to supine to the left lateral position. The drainage of pulmonary secretions into the pharynx where secretions can be removed by suctioning is facilitated by elevation of the foot of the bed. The chest should be examined frequently by auscultation and suspected atelectasis or pneumonia confirmed by x-ray. Any infection should be treated promptly with antibiotics and cultures of secretions should be obtained for identification of organisms and sensitivity to antibiotics. The importance of respiratory care cannot be overemphasized, particularly in those who are immobilized for long periods of time, such as patients with prolonged coma and those with a "locked-in" syndrome.

   2.   Management of hypertension. Many patients are hypertensive on admission to the hospital, but the hypertension resolves during the first few days. Consequently, there should be some restraint exercised in prescribing antihypertensive medication for patients who are moderately hypertensive at the time of admission. Catheterization of a distended bladder and removal of a large volume of urine that has accumulated in a comatose state may lead to a rapid decline from hypertensive to a normotensive state. Similarly, reduction in blood pressure may occur with the removal of any impediment to respiratory exchange. Treatment of hypertension is recommended for systolic pressure greater than 220 mmHg or diastolic pressure more than 120 mmHg.[81]

   Patients who show sustained severe hypertension with diastolic pressure above 140 mmHg require urgent treatment using intravenous nitroprusside (Nipride) 10 μg/kg per min. Nitroprusside should be given with the patient lying flat in bed and any hypotension can be immediately controlled by elevating the foot of the bed. It should be emphasized that such drastic measures are rarely necessary in patients with cerebral infarction. When control of hypertension is less urgent, that is, systolic pressure below 230 mmHg and diastolic pressure below 140 mmHg, an

intravenous injection of labetalol 20 mg over 2 min should be given. This can be repeated every 20 min until a satisfactory reduction of blood pressure occurs. Labetalol, which is a selective α_1-adrenergic blocking agent and nonselective β-adrenergic blocking agent can reduce arterial blood pressure with little effect on intracranial pressure.[82] Calcium channel antagonists and angiotensin-converting enzyme inhibitors can cause cerebral vasodilatation and increased intracranial pressure. They should be reserved for treatment of moderate hypertension. Hypertension of 220 mmHg systolic may be controlled by the use of nifedipine 20 mg sublingually or orally, which can be repeated in 6 to 12 h if necessary. Alternatives include furosemide (Lasix) 40 to 80 mg intravenously or intramuscularly or oral labetalol beginning with 100 mg bid and increasing to 400 mg bid. In a comatose patient, high-normal or low hypertensive levels may be maintained by intravenous labetalol.

   Comatose patients occasionally become hypotensive because of excessive use of antihypertensive agents or other drugs. The blood pressure is often unstable in such patients and caution is required in the use of antihypertensive agents. However, should hypotension occur, there is usually a prompt response to a fluid challenge. Vasoactivation such as dopamine (isotropine) or isoproterenol may be required in some cases. When the response is poor, the failure to respond may be due to adrenal insufficiency. Therefore, all patients who have failed to respond to pressure agents should receive intravenous corticosteroids such as hydrocortisone 100 mg q8h.

   3.   Care of the heart. An electrocardiogram should be obtained in the emergency center at the time of admission, and a consultation requested from a cardiologist or internist if there is any electrocardiographic abnormality, congestive heart failure, or persistent arrhythmia. Such patients should receive cardiac monitoring for at least 24 h following admission to the hospital, and the procedure should be continued at the discretion of the cardiologist or internist. Acute myocardial infarction is not unusual in patients with acute cerebral infarction and many others suffer from arteriosclerotic heart disease or other intracardiac abnormalities.

4. Care of the bladder. The comatose patient frequently fails to empty the bladder, which may become distended, and this situation may contribute to an excessive rise in blood pressure. All comatose patients should be catheterized and an indwelling catheter inserted through the urethra into the bladder. The risk of infection is high and the catheter should be removed as soon as possible, as the patient regains consciousness, and trials of voluntary bladder control should be instituted in the conscious patient in an early phase of treatment.

Some comatose patients require prolonged catheterization. Under such circumstances, the risk of a bladder infection which can ascend through the ureters to the kidney, must be kept in mind. Any rise in temperature should automatically suggest a urinary tract infection and appropriate studies should be carried out. It should be realized that prolonged dependency on a bladder catheter after the patient becomes conscious will increase difficulties in ultimately regaining sphincter control. The bladder catheter should be changed every month in those patients who require prolonged bladder control by a catheter.

5. Care of skin and joints. The comatose patient has a tendency to develop decubiti over the pressure points. This can be minimized by turning the patient every 2 h as indicated in respiratory care. Pressure areas should be protected with suitable lambskin or soft plastic appliances and the patient nursed on an air pressure mattress. Decubiti tend to form over the heels and the sacral areas. Any reddening of skin in those areas should be treated promptly with removal of all pressure and application of tincture of benzoin. Patients with hemiparesis or quadriparesis develop ankylosis of joints in a few days unless these joints are moved through a full range of motion passively, several times a day. This can be accomplished by the physician on rounds, those nursing the patient, as well as physical therapists and occupational therapists. The tendency to ankylosis is most apparent in the shoulder joints but can involve other joints, particularly when the limb is totally paralyzed. Thus, paralyzed or severely paretic limbs should be supported in a position of function. In the lower limbs, this entails maintaining the limb in a neutral position and prevention of external rotation by the use of sandbags against the thigh. The foot should be placed in a function position at right angles to the ankle and maintained in that position with a suitable splint if necessary. This splint should be padded to protect the heel from pressure. As spasticity develops, the knees should be slightly flexed over a pillow, and the knees should be separated by another pillow to prevent contact due to adductor spasticity. The upper limbs should be placed in a position of function with the arm slightly abducted and the pillow placed in the axilla to prevent adduction. The forearm and elbow should be placed on a pillow with the hand elevated over the pillow and the elbow elevated higher than the shoulder. This prevents the development of edema. The hand is then slightly extended at the wrist and the fingers placed around a hand, roll in a position of function. These positions are maintained until the patient regains consciousness and begins to move the affected limbs, at which time a graded program of physical and occupational therapy should be instituted.

6. Deep venous thrombosis and the accompanying risk of pulmonary thromboembolism warrants the use of subcutaneous heparin 5000 units q8h. Should edema develop, ultrasonography is required to detect any thrombosis of lower limb and pelvic veins. Full intravenous heparinization should be instituted if venous thrombosis is established.

7. Water and electrolyte balance. Comatose patients require intravenous fluids for at least 24 h. Every effort should be made to correct water deficits, and if intravenous fluids are continued, the average adult usually requires 3000 mL/day. If electrolytes are normal, this should be given as a 5% solution of glucose with 0.5 normal saline; and 20 mEq potassium added to each 1000 mL of intravenous fluid once satisfactory urinary output is established. Adequate intake and output records must be kept, and electrolytes should be measured every 24 h. A nasogastric tube should be passed during the first 2 or 3 days and fluids should then be given through the tube for at least a 24-h period. Once the nasogastric tube has been passed, the patient should be nursed with the head elevated at 35°. This minimizes the risk of aspiration. After 24 h, a liquid diet can be given through the nasogastric tube. This is usually given in divided amounts to a total of 2000 mL over 24 h with

addition of 1000 mL water, again in divided doses every 2 h. However, tube feeding may be carried out using a pump mechanism with continuous delivery of the dietary substance in similar amounts. Nasogastric feedings can be slowly discontinued as the patient recovers consciousness and begins to swallow. At this stage, swallowing mechanisms should be tested frequently, because the risk of aspiration is high and although many patients appear to have normal swallowing mechanisms, they are at high risk for aspiration pneumonia. Under such circumstances, it is better to err on the side of caution and to maintain tube feeding until it is established that there is little risk of aspiration. Suitable diets are available for those who have difficulty in taking thin liquids when oral feeding is resumed. However, as the patient improves and the nasogastric tube has been removed, the patient should take sufficient nourishment and fluids by mouth. This may require a calorie count by a nutritionist. At that time, attention should also be given to supplementing the bulk of the diet to prevent development of fecal impaction.

Acute Cerebral Infarction in Conscious Patients During the first few days following a stroke, conscious patients are often seriously ill and require care similar to that for a comatose patient. Equal stress should be placed on a prevention of pulmonary or bladder infection, and adequate attention toward an electrolyte imbalance. Headaches occur in 25 percent of patients with stroke and unilateral headache is usually ipsilateral to the infarction.[83] Conscious patients should be screened for swallowing problems in the first 24 h and dysphagia management instituted if it is necessary to reduce the risk of aspiration pneumonia.[84] This risk can be further reduced by spending an increasing time seated out of the bed each day and by ambulating the patient as soon as possible. A program of physical therapy can be instituted on day one. Certain drugs should be avoided if possible during the acute phase of treatment, including benzodiazepines, dopamine receptor antagonists, phenytoin, and phenobarbital, all of which appear to have a detrimental effect on recovery.[85]

Treatment of Cerebral Edema in Acute Cerebral Infarction Patients with acute infarction de-

velop some level of cerebral edema. This may be minor when the infarct is small but may be of considerable magnitude in the presence of larger infarction. Under such circumstances, the edema may lead to an increase in intracranial pressure. This will result in a decrease in the level of consciousness in a conscious patient and an increase in the level of stupor or coma in the unconscious patient, with the development of signs of brainstem compression (see Chap. 2). Every effort should be made to reduce cerebral edema in this situation, and the patient can be treated with intravenous hyperosmolar solutions such as mannitol intravenously.

In cases where there is rapid deterioration because of increased intracranial pressure secondary to cerebral edema, intravenous mannitol, maintaining the serum osmolality between 300 and 320 is often effective. Intracranial pressure monitoring has marginal value in large hemispheric infarctions.[86]

Cerebral Embolism with Infarction This condition should be treated with anticoagulation beginning with intravenous heparin. This may be followed by long-term anticoagulation if indicated, using warfarin sodium and maintaining prothrombin time at 1.5 times normal and an INR between 2.5 and 3.0, unless there is atrial fibrillation with valvular heart disease, in which case the INR should be maintained between 3.0 and 3.5. Chronic anticoagulation is particularly important in rheumatic or nonrheumatic atrial fibrillation. The risk of converting an ischemic infarct into a hemorrhagic infarct is small and is outweighed by the risk of further cerebral embolism, which is reduced significantly through anticoagulation.

It should be realized that anticoagulants do not appear to be of benefit in the treatment of cerebral infarct of nonembolic origin. Anticoagulants should be restricted to patients with chronic atrial fibrillation and those other conditions outlined under TIAs.[87] Chronic anticoagulation increases the risk of secondary stroke from a brain hemorrhage or death in the absence of atrial fibrillation.

Poststroke Depression Poststroke depression of a significant degree occurs in about 50 percent of patients following acute infarction. Lesions in the region of the left basal ganglia tend to play a crucial role in the development of a major depression following the acute phase of a stroke.[22] This debilitating problem may hinder physical therapy, rehabilitation, and patient recovery. Appropriate antidepressant therapy and referral for psychotherapy should be obtained at an early stage once this problem is recognized.

Thrombolytic Therapy for Acute Stroke Clot lysis and restoration of circulation may limit the extent of brain injury in acute ischemic stroke and improve outcome after stroke.[88] Available thrombolytic agents are recombinant tissue plasminogen activator, urokinase, and prourokinase. Local intra-arterial fibrinolytic therapy using an intra-arterial infusion of urokinase, tissue plasminogen activator, or prourokinase delivered through an intra-arterial catheter may lead to recannulation of an occluded artery and have some benefit if the technique is used at an early stage following occlusion and infarction.[89] The window of opportunity for such treatment is less than 6 h following infarction. Intravenous thrombolysis using recombinant tissue plasminogen activator, given in a dose of 0.9 mg/kg up to a maximum of 90 mg with 10 percent of the dose given as a bolus and the remainder infused over 1 h, improves outcome in ischemic stroke if the infusion is given within 3 h of the onset of the stroke.[90]

Intravenous streptokinase is not recommended for the management of acute ischemic stroke.[91] Oral nimodipine 30 to 60 mg q6h may be effective in reducing mortality, morbidity, and acute ischemic infarction if begun within 12 h of onset of symptoms.[92] Other calcium channel blocking agents are currently under review and may be available in the near future. The use of neuronal protective agents blocking NMDA receptors or drugs acting as scavengers for free radicals or inhibiting nitric oxide synthetase are currently under investigation.[93]

The role of angioplasty in the treatment of carotid stenosis, whether simple angioplasty, double balloon angioplasty, or angioplasty with stenting, has not been established at this time and requires more experience and further studies to define safety and identification of suitable candidates for these procedures.

Surgical Treatment Approximately 25 percent of elderly persons have internal carotid artery stenosis.[94] Many are asymptomatic and blood flow through the stenosed vessel remains constant and does not decrease until the stenosis exceeds 90 percent. Beyond that, the flow decreases progressively and precipitously. Nevertheless, complete occlusion can occur without symptoms because of the development of an effective collateral circulation, mainly through the circle of Willis. On the other hand, the stenosis can become symptomatic at an early stage of development if the plaque presents an active procoagulant surface with microembolism.

Symptoms of carotid stenosis are similar to those of middle cerebral artery stenosis (middle cerebral arteries should be regarded as a direct anatomical continuation of the internal carotid artery) and include TIAs and minor or major cerebral infarction. The advantage of carotid endarterectomy in patients with 70 percent or greater stenosis of the internal carotid artery, and who have suffered a minor stroke or TIA, are now firmly established,[95–97] and the benefit of carotid endarterectomy in symptomatic patients with 50 to 70 percent stenosis has now been substantiated.[98] Further development of carotid endarterectomy requires identification of active plaque at an early stage of plaque development because microembolism increases the risk of cerebral infarction. Long-term transcranial Doppler ultrasonography of intracranial arterial blood flow can reveal clinically silent abnormal high-pitched intensity signals, indicating thromboembolism.[99] Carotid stenosis greater than 50 percent, is a proven indication for carotid endarterectomy, which reduces the risk of stroke significantly.[100] Stenotic plaque with less than 50 percent stenosis should also be removed by endarterectomy if clinically symptomatic.[101] Similarly, a patient with an asymptomatic stenotic plaque with cerebral microemboli detected by transcranial Doppler ultrasonography should be considered a candidate for carotid endarterectomy.[102] The presence of angiographically defined ulceration, regardless of the degree of carotid stenosis, is also an indication for carotid endarterectomy.[103] However, carotid surgery is only beneficial in reducing stroke morbidity and mortality in selected patients who were operated on by selected surgeons and cared for by selected physicians at selected hospitals within therapeutic trials.[104] Mortality is higher in hospitals that have a low volume of carotid surgeries and lower in high volume hospitals.

Prognosis   Survivors of cerebral infarction run a high risk of a second stroke or myocardial infarction and approximately 50 percent of patients who have had cerebral infarction die from subsequent myocardial infarction. In addition to age, the major risk factors include hypertension, diabetes mellitus, smoking, and pre-existing cardiovascular disease with atrial fibrillation, which are singly or collectively related to increased mortality in stroke. However, there is only a weak association of ischemic stroke with elevated cholesterol levels and an inverse relationship between total fat intake and stroke.[105]

CERVICOCRANIAL ARTERIAL DISSECTION

Dissection of the internal carotid artery is recognized as a cause of stroke in younger patients with an annual incidence of 2.6 per 100,000.[106] The extracranial internal carotid artery is involved in most cases. Isolated intracranial dissection is rare, and isolated dissection of the middle cerebral artery is exceptionally unusual.[107] Dissection of the vertebral artery is uncommon and is usually the result of trauma.

Etiology and Pathology   Trauma to the cervicocranial vessels is often documented in dissection in both carotid and vertebral systems,[108] but trauma may be trivial in some cases. Spontaneous dissection has been associated with cystic medial necrosis, fibromuscular dysplasia, moyamoya disease, atherosclerosis, arteritis (Fig. 8-16), homocystinuria, and collagen abnormalities, including Ehlers-Danlos syndrome and pseudoxanthoma elastica.

Clinical Features   Internal carotid dissection often presents with sudden ipsilateral headache, ipsilateral Horner syndrome, and pain and tenderness over the carotid artery, which is exacerbated by head flexion followed hours or even days later by symptoms of cerebral infarction. Additional features include neck pain, amaurosis fugax, dysgeusia, and cranial nerve

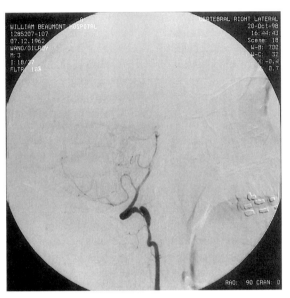

Figure 8-16
Cerebral arteriogram showing dissection of the terminal portion of the right vertebral artery in a patient with arteritis.

palsies.[109] The latter consists of oculomotor palsies[110] or low cranial nerve palsies.[111] Vertebral artery dissection, either intracranial or extracranial, can also occur spontaneously but also follows traumatic injury to the neck in automobile accidents or chiropractic manipulation.[112] Symptoms are those of occipital headache, unbearable lateral neck pain,[113] followed by lateral medullary infarction, brainstem infarction, upper cervical spinal cord infarction,[114] or subarachnoid hemorrhage. Intracranial dissections have a poorer prognosis than extracranial dissections, with a much higher permanent disability in those with intracranial involvement.[115]

Diagnostic Procedures

1. A combination of extracranial Doppler sonography and transcranial Doppler sonography and duplex sonography will detect carotid dissection in 95 percent of cases.[116]
2. An MRI scan shows a typical narrowed, eccentric signal void surrounded by a semilunar signal hyperintensity on T1- and T2-weighted images in

about 80 percent of patients with cervicocranial dissection.[117]

3. Four-vessel angiography of carotid and vertebral arteries should be performed when results of ultrasonography and MRI and MRA scanning are equivocal.

Treatment

1. Anticoagulation with heparin with later conversion to warfarin sodium has been recommended to restrict further propagation of clot in the affected blood vessel.
2. Surgical treatment with carotid endarterectomy, evacuation of clot, and repair of damaged endothelial tears has been attempted in some cases.

Prognosis   Most patients experience some degree of permanent neurological deficit following arterial dissection of either carotid or vertebral arteries. Recurrences are unusual.

CENTRAL POSTSTROKE PAIN (THALAMIC PAIN)

Central pain occurring within a week to 6 months after a stroke is often called thalamic pain but can occur with infarction involving the spinothalamic system anywhere in its course and sparing of the lemniscal pathway.[118] The pain has been described with infarcts involving the ventral posterolateral thalamus with right diencephalic predominance[74] but has also been associated with subcortical parietal lobe,[119] capsular, and lower brainstem infarcts including the lateral medullary syndrome[120] and spinal cord disease.

The pain is described as a burning pain that may be associated with intermittent sharp components (electrical pain). It is usually constant but can be intermittent and is aggravated by noxious stimuli (hyperalgesia) or non-noxious stimuli (allodynia), when pain can be induced by a cold stimulus or by touch.

Treatment   There is usually a good response to amitriptyline beginning 10 mg qhs and increasing slowly to avoid adverse effects, to 75 to 100 mg qhs.[121] Carbamazepine and gabapentin produce some

relief but are less effective than amitriptyline. A combination of these medications may be necessary in some cases.

DEMENTIA IN CEREBROVASCULAR DISEASE

There are several causes of dementia in cerebrovascular disease:

1. Dementia is common after cerebral infarction.[114] The incidence of dementia within the first year, in persons who survived the first cerebral infarct, is nearly nine times greater than would have been expected had the individual remained healthy (Fig. 8-17).

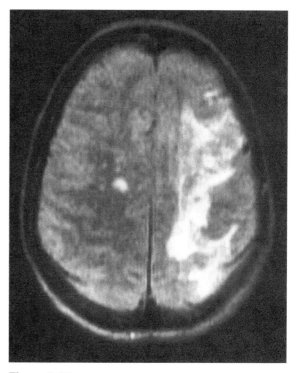

Figure 8-17
MRI scan showing increased signal within the left hemisphere compatible with gliosis secondary to previous infarction. There is a white matter infarct present in the right hemisphere.

2. Cerebral infarction may predispose to an increase in Alzheimer disease. The reason for this observation is not clear[122]; however, patients with a clinically diagnosed vascular disease often have concomitant Alzheimer disease at autopsy.[123]

3. A second stroke is a highly significant event in the development of dementia. Dementia is more common in patients with left hemisphere lesions, exclusive of dysphasia, particularly infarction involving the left medial frontal and left temporal regions.[124]

4. Dementia is a feature of Binswanger disease and cadasil. Binswanger disease may be an extreme example of leukoaraiosis and lesser degrees of the condition may explain some of the intellectual impairment in the elderly.[125]

5. The presence of multiple lacunar infarcts secondary to atherosclerotic or amyloid angiopathy,[126] involving the deeper penetrating arteries, is associated with dementia (multi-infarct dementia).

6. Dementia has been associated with embolism owing to chronic atrial fibrillation and multiple cerebral infarction. Chronic nonrheumatic atrial fibrillation increases the risk of stroke and some patients with neurologically asymptomatic nonrheumatic atrial fibrillation have impaired cognition, with significant impairment in attention and memory.[127]

7. Microvascular disease and severe microinfarction involving the cerebral white matter and deep gray matter are potent causes of vascular dementia.[128]

Clinical Features The most common causes of dementia in middle-aged and elderly persons are Alzheimer and dementia in cerebrovascular disease. However, many patients with Alzheimer disease have cerebrovascular disease, which may be an incidental and noncontributing factor in the progressive dementia. Consequently, the diagnosis of dementia owing to cerebrovascular disease should only be made when the individual exhibits certain well-defined criteria: an abrupt onset, stepwise deterioration, history of stroke, focal neurological symptoms, and focal neurological signs. Factors of lesser weight include chronic hypertension, cardiovascular disease, the presence of other risk factors for cerebrovascular

disease, the presence of hemiparesis, increased tendon reflexes, extensor plantar responses, blepharospasm, impersistence of gaze, sucking and rooting reflexes, and grasp reflexes—all occurring in a stepwise fashion, with emotional lability manifested by pathological laughing or crying (pseudobulbar crying).

Diagnostic Procedures Diagnostic procedures should be performed to identify those factors that contribute to accelerated atherosclerosis. Patients should be fully investigated (as outlined in TIA discussion). CT and MRI scans may be particularly helpful. Other imaging studies, including single photon emission CT (SPECT) and positron emission tomography (PET) scanning, may be of additional benefit in arriving at the correct diagnosis.

Treatment Hypertension, diabetes mellitus, and smoking should be rigidly controlled and any metabolic and cardiac abnormalities corrected. Improvement in cerebral blood flow may be associated with improvement in cognition in dementia in cerebrovascular disease, and there may be some benefit from the regular use of aspirin and dipyridamole, ticlopidine, or clopidogrel.

Prognosis Many patients die from myocardial infarction, whereas others die from a massive cerebral or brainstem infarction. The survivors show a progression of dementia or progression of neurological deficits, and die from intercurrent infection once they are reduced to a bedridden state.

THE OVERLAP SYNDROME

Because Alzheimer disease and vascular dementia are the two most common causes of dementia, it is not unusual to encounter strokes in patients with Alzheimer disease. Consequently, the presence of a stroke followed by progressive dementia should not be assumed to be dementia caused by cerebrovascular disease. Most patients who have suffered a stroke are not demented and certainly do not experience progressive dementia. Dementia in cerebrovascular disease occurs in the presence of repeated strokes with stepwise deterioration in intellectual and cognitive functioning, focal neurological symptoms, and focal neurological signs.

THE LACUNAR SYNDROME

This condition is associated with small areas of infarction deep in the cerebral white matter of the cerebral hemispheres or in the pons, resulting from:

1. Small vessel disease with lipohyalinosis and fibrinoid degeneration
2. Decreased perfusion of penetrating arteries from proximal narrowing of larger vessels
3. Branch artery atheromatous occlusion
4. Embolism[129]

However, the widespread use of MRI and CT scanning has shown that the lacunar state is not uncommon in asymptomatic individuals. Consequently, the diagnosis of lacunar syndrome should be approached with caution.

The lacunar stroke may be defined as a unilateral motor or sensory deficit without visual field deficit or disturbance of consciousness or language. The CT scan may show a small, sharply marginated hypodense lesion in the subcortical area, with the diameter smaller than 20 mm.[130] Multiple lacunes are strongly related to hypertension and diabetes mellitus.[131]

Lacunar infarction is an acute onset of focal neurological deficits lasting more than 24 h. There are six recognized lacunar syndromes:

1. Pure motor, hemiplegia or hemiparesis
2. Dysarthria, clumsy hand syndrome
3. Ataxic hemiparesis
4. Sensorimotor stroke
5. Pure sensory stroke
6. Unilateral dystonia and involuntary movements such as choreoathetosis following lacunar infarction of the putamen or globus pallidus[132] or hemiballismus owing to subthalamic infarction

Risk factors include hypertension, diabetes mellitus,[133] heart disease, heavy alcohol consumption, cig-

arette smoking, and lack of physical exercise.[134] Lacunar infarcts are the most common finding in cerebral infarction in young adults.

Diagnostic Procedures All patients should receive full evaluation for diseases of the blood vessels, atherosclerosis, arteriosclerosis heart disease abnormalities of blood constituents, and reduced cerebral perfusion. These investigations have been outlined under diagnostic procedures for TIAs. Future developments of MRI with diffusion and perfusion studies, PET, and SPECT will define the location and extent of damage to cerebral tissue, and may permit earlier identification of blood vessel involvement in the lacunar state.

Treatment Control of risk factors (smoking, hypertension, diabetes mellitus) and treatment with antiplatelet agents or anticoagulants are of limited value, suggesting that the process of lacunar infarction has advanced to a point where treatment of risk factors is ineffective.

BINSWANGER DISEASE

Binswanger disease is a progressive dementia of presumed vascular etiology, characterized by the thinning and hyalinization of the walls of small penetrating arteries or occasionally amyloid angiopathy[135] in the basal ganglia and periventricular regions. There is diffuse white matter loss, often in a patchy and multifocal fashion, with sparing of the U fibers and cortical gray matter. Loss of white matter volume leads to hydrocephalus and ischemia of the deep gray matter results in lacunar infarcts in the basal ganglia, thalamus, and pons.[136]

The disease occurs equally in both sexes with onset between 55 and 75 years. The clinical picture is characterized by acute strokes with symptoms and signs compatible with lacunar infarction. Subacute onset of focal neurological deficits and seizures may develop over a period of several days, and there is a stepwise progression of motor, cognitive, intellectual, and behavioral deficits during a 5- to 10-year period. Periods of stability and occasional periods of improvement can occur. Examination shows dementia with apathy, abulia, poor judgment, lack of insight, altered effective responses, impaired memory, dysphasia, and dyspraxia. Corticospinal and extrapyramidal signs, abnormal often dyspraxic gait, and pseudobulbar signs with emotional lability and presence of release reflexes—grasp, snout, sucking, rooting, reflexes—occur in advanced cases.

The majority of patients with Binswanger disease have chronic hypertension that could cause degenerative changes in the penetrating arteries in the white matter. Other putative factors include diabetes mellitus, polycythemia, thrombocytosis, hyperlipidemia, hyperglobulinemia, and pseudoxanthoma elasticum,[137] increased fibrinogen levels that increase serum viscosity, and the antiphospholipid antibody syndrome.

The MRI and CT scans show hydrocephalus, patchy, irregular white matter abnormalities extending into the centrum semiovale and corona radiata, and multiple lacunar infarcts in the basal ganglia, thalamus, and pons. The advent of MRI scanning was followed by a surge of interest in Binswanger disease because of the presence of multiple areas of increased signal intensity in the white matter was a frequent finding in elderly persons. It should be emphasized that these areas of signal abnormality are not unusual in asymptomatic elderly patients and do not establish the diagnosis of Binswanger disease. The diagnosis is established by clinical findings in association with MRI abnormalities.

The evaluation of patients with Binswanger disease should include hematocrit, fibrinogen levels, hemoglobin A_1C, serum lipid profile, antiphospholipid antibody determination, and serological tests for syphilis.

Treatment should be directed to the control of hypertension, diabetes mellitus, and any of the factors predisposing to increased serum viscosity, such as reduction of serum fibrinogen by plasmapheresis.[138] Because some of these factors are now reversible or respond to therapy, treatment may prevent or delay the late stages of severe dementia in this disease.

CADASIL

Definition   Cerebral autosomal dominant arteriopathy with subcortical infarcts and leukoencephalopathy (CADASIL) is an inherited arterial disease of the brain mapped to chromosome 19.[139]

Etiology and Pathology   The etiology is unknown. There is a widespread vasculopathy affecting the arterioles, with deposition of eosinophilic-congophilic material in vessel walls.[140]

Clinical Features   There is a positive family history of attacks of migraine beginning between ages 20 to 40 years, followed by symptoms of cerebral infarction occurring after age 40 years. Progressive subcortical infarction produces dementia, pseudobulbar palsy, and mood disorders, with severe episodes of depression. The clinical presentation and course of the disease bear a striking resemblance to Binswanger disease. Death occurs in the sixth or seventh decade.

Diagnostic Procedures   The MRI scan reveals hydrocephalus and prominent signal abnormalities in the subcortical white matter and basal ganglia.

HYPERTENSIVE ENCEPHALOPATHY

Hypertensive encephalopathy is a syndrome characterized by marked elevation of blood pressure and evidence of increased intracranial pressure.

Etiology and Pathology   Most patients with hypertensive encephalopathy have a long history of essential hypertension. In other cases, the elevation of blood pressure is secondary to another disease process such as acute glomerulonephritis, chronic nephritis, pheochromocytoma, Cushing disease, or acute toxemia of pregnancy.

There is diffuse cerebral edema and cerebral vasospasm. Microscopic examination reveals petechial hemorrhages and fibrinoid necrosis of the arteries.

The patient complains of severe headache with nausea and vomiting. Visual disturbances, including blurring of vision and scotomata, are frequent. Confusion, with progression to stupor, convulsions, and coma are seen in untreated cases. Examination of the fundi reveals papilledema and hypertensive retinal changes. Focal neurological signs are not characteristic but may be seen as a postictal phenomenon or when intracranial hemorrhage occurs.

Diagnostic Procedures   The MRI and CT scans reveal diffuse cerebral edema.

Treatment   Hypertensive encephalopathy is a medical emergency and the blood pressure should be reduced as rapidly and safely as possible.

Prognosis   Untreated hypertensive encephalopathy is fatal. Follow-up care and appropriate long-term medication allow patients to survive for many years.

CEREBRAL ARTERITIS

A number of rare conditions are associated with inflammation of the cerebral arteries, which may lead to thrombosis and infarction. The arteritides include syphilitic arteritis (see Chap. 16), polyarteritis nodosa, systemic lupus erythematosus (SLE), giant cell arteritis, and thrombotic thrombocytopenic purpura. Both heroin and cocaine abuse may result in cerebral infarction, caused by vasculitis in some cases.[141]

Polyarteritis Nodosa

Definition   Polyarteritis nodosa is an inflammatory arteritis of small or medium-sized arteries in multiple organs, including the kidney, liver, muscles, peripheral nerves, bowel, skin, and the central nervous system.

Etiology and Pathology   The etiology is unknown. Pathological changes consist of inflammation of all layers of the arterial wall with areas of necrosis and occasional aneurysm formation. Developing and healing lesions may coexist in the affected vessels, and thrombosis is not unusual.

Clinical Features   Polyarteritis nodosa is more common in males, with a male to female ratio of 3:1. The condition can present in many ways. Systemic signs and symptoms include fever, weakness, weight loss, arthralgia, myalgia, and muscle cramps. Abdominal pain is not unusual and may indicate mesenteric thrombosis or pancreatic involvement. Peptic ulceration with hematemesis or melena are occasional complications. Testicular pain is a common complaint. Liver involvement is indicated by hepatic enlargement and jaundice. Skin lesions include erythema purpura and ulcers; lividoreticularis is quite common. Coronary artery involvement predisposes to myocardial infarction. Pleuritic pain and pneumonia may be recurrent complaints.

Neurological complications include a symmetrical peripheral neuropathy in about 25 percent of cases, due to involvement of the vasa nervorum. Mononeuropathies and mononeuritis multiplex may occur. Cerebral symptoms are rare and include cerebral infarction with hemiparesis and aphasia, intracerebral hemorrhage, seizures, cranial nerve palsies, particularly involving the eighth nerve, with hearing loss and subarachnoid hemorrhage. Spinal cord involvement may produce a transverse myelitis or an anterior spinal artery occlusion (see Chap. 12).

Diagnostic Procedures

1. Complete blood count. The white blood count is usually elevated between 10,000 to 20,000 cells per cubic millimeter and eosinophilia may be present.
2. The sedimentation rate is elevated.
3. A high proportion of cases shows the presence of aneurysms in the renal and hepatic vasculature, which can be demonstrated by arteriography.
4. Hepatic B surface antigen or antibody titer is positive in 30 to 50 percent of cases.
5. The diagnosis can be established by a muscle biopsy and/or sural nerve biopsy and by cerebral arteriography.

Treatment   The disorder can be suppressed by corticosteroids beginning with methylprednisolone 96 mg daily and converting to alternate day therapy when symptoms subside. The treatment may have to be continued for many months or years on an alternate-day basis, using the minimal amount of steroids to keep the patient symptom free and the sedimentation rate normal.

Prognosis Approximately 50 percent of patients are alive after 5 years of steroid therapy.

Systemic Lupus Erythematosus

Systemic lupus erythematosus is a multisystem, autoimmune disease in which antibodies against many cellular constituents, including DNA, nuclear protein, and mitochondria are formed.

Etiology and Pathology The cause is unknown. There appears to be hereditary susceptibility to SLE. There is more than a chance association between SLE and human leukocyte antigens (HLA). There has been recent interest in a viral etiology followed by the isolation of certain viruses in patients with SLE. The development of numerous autoimmune antibodies in this disease suggests that there is a basic defect in the autoimmune system, probably in the T-lymphocyte population. The disease has been related to the use of certain drugs, including hydralazine, procainamide, phenytoin, reserpine, and isoniazid. It is probable that these drugs produce some change in the immune system.

The essential pathological changes consist of a vasculitis with necrosis and the deposition of fibrinoid material within the vessel walls. The fibrinoid deposits contain immunoglobulins, DNA, fibrinogen, and the third component of complement (C3). The deposition of this material in the subendothelial tissues produces narrowing of the vessel lumen and thrombosis in some cases. The affected vessels show a perivascular lymphocytic infiltration.

Clinical Features The disease is more common in women than in men, with a ratio of 9:1 and it occurs predominantly in the 20- to 40-year-old age group. Patients with SLE usually have a number of the following signs: facial erythema, discoid lupus rash, Raynaud phenomenon, alopecia, photosensitivity, oral or nasopharyngeal ulceration, recurrent arthritis without deformity, chronic false-positive serologic tests for syphilis, proteinuria of more than 3.5 g/day, cellular casts in the urine, recurrent pleuritis or pericarditis, recurrent psychosis and convulsions, and the presence of leukopenia, hemolytic anemia, or thrombocytopenia.

Neurological manifestations of SLE include mood disorders, delirium, dementia, and psychotic symptoms, suggesting schizophrenia with delusions, hallucinations, and paranoia. Episodic clouding of consciousness may occur, or there may be focal neurological signs, including hemiparesis or aphasia with cerebral infarction, suggesting a stroke. Intracerebral hemorrhage and subarachnoid hemorrhage have been reported. Seizures occur in about one-third of patients with cerebral involvement. Brainstem lesions produce nystagmus, vertigo, cerebellar ataxia, and cranial nerve palsies. A visual loss can occur from involvement of the optic nerve, producing central scotoma or homonymous hemianopia when there is involvement of the optic pathways. Some patients show cortical blindness. Spinal cord involvement produces transverse myelitis. Peripheral neuropathies or mononeuropathies are a feature of SLE and myopathy has been described. The multisystem involvement of the central nervous system and the relapsing and remitting course frequently leads to a consideration of multiple sclerosis.

Diagnostic Procedures

1. Lumbar puncture. There is a pleocytosis with elevated protein content in patients with aseptic meningitis secondary to SLE. Red blood cells are present in subarachnoid hemorrhage and intracranial hemorrhage.
2. A complete blood count may show the presence of anemia, leukopenia, and thrombocytopenia.
3. The diagnosis is suggested by an intranuclear antibody titer greater than 1 in 64 and a false-positive VDRL may be present.
4. Confirmatory tests include decreased levels of complement fractions C3, C4, and CH50. Testing for the presence of antibodies Sjögren SSA and Sjögren SSB and the presence of anticardiolipin antibodies should be performed.
5. There may be evidence of a hypercoagulable state, with decreased fibrinolysis, decreased plasminogen activation, and decreased tissue plasminogen activation.
6. The electroencephalogram will be abnormal in patients with cerebral involvement. Abnormalities include seizure discharges or focal slowing in the

presence of infarction.

7. The CT scan reveals cerebral infarction, cerebral hemorrhage, or gradual development of cerebral atrophy and hydrocephalus on serial studies. The MRI may show white matter lesions that resemble findings in multiple sclerosis.

Treatment The use of high doses of cortico-steroids has been equivocal in the treatment of SLE. The occurrence of psychosis and myopathy has been attributed to the use of steroids rather than the disease in some cases. Purine antagonists, for example, aza-thioprine (Imuran) and alkylating agents, for example, cyclophosphamide (Cytoxan), chlorambucil (Leukeran), or cyclosporine may be effective in re-fractory cases with life-threatening disease. Anticoagulants have been advised in patients with cerebral infarction and a hypercoagulable state.

Prognosis Approximately 70 percent of patients with SLE are alive at 5 years and 60 percent at 10 years after the onset of disease. Death is usually due to renal failure.

Giant Cell Arteritis

Definition Giant cell arteritis is an inflammatory disease of blood vessels, characterized by the presence of an inflammatory exudate, including giant cells, involving all layers of the vessel wall.

Etiology and Pathology The etiology is unknown. Pathological changes consist of intimal proliferation with obliteration of the vascular lumen and inflammation of all layers of the vessel wall and the presence of typical giant cells. Inflammatory exudate contains lymphocytes, eosinophils, and polymorphonuclear cells. In chronic cases, the larger vessels may show the presence of concentric fibrosis.

Clinical Features Three distinct entities constitute the syndrome of giant cell arteritis: polymyalgia rheumatica, temporal arteritis, and the aortic arch syndrome (Takayasu disease, pulseless disease).

Polymyalgia rheumatica may precede the development of other forms of giant cell arteritis by many years. The condition consists of fluctuating episodes of muscle and joint pain associated with proximal muscle weakness, malaise, nausea, low-grade fever, and weight loss of many years' duration. The condition often disappears 4 to 8 years after onset, even if untreated, and only 10 to 15 percent of patients with polymyalgia rheumatica develop temporal arteritis.

Temporal arteritis occurs in elderly patients with a marked preponderance of cases in patients of Scandinavian origin and is associated with HLA markers, HLA-DR4, HLA-DR7, and HLA-B12. Headache is the presenting symptom in 60 percent of cases and usually presents as a unilateral headache in the supraorbital region, associated with tenderness in the distribution of the superficial temporal artery. However, the headache of temporal arteritis may be generalized or occur in any part of the head. Independent claudication of the jaw muscles when chewing is virtually pathognomonic. Temporal arteritis should be considered in every elderly individual who begins to complain of headache. Sudden visual loss proceeding to blindness may occur in 36 percent of cases[142] (Fig. 8-18). Alopecia and blanching of the tongue are frequent concomitants. Necrosis of the tongue is an occasional complication.[143] Patients show signs of systemic disease with fever, arthralgia, and weight loss.

The *aortic arch syndrome* is a chronic form of giant cell arteritis in which there is progressive narrowing and occlusion of major branches of the aorta. This may present with TIA, subclavian steal syndrome, angina, or aortic insufficiency. Hypertension may be secondary to stenosis of the renal arteries.

Diagnostic Procedures

1. The complete blood count shows elevation of the white cell count.
2. The sedimentation rate is usually elevated to 70 to 100 mm/h but may be normal in 5 percent of cases.
3. Serum IL-6 concentration is elevated and decreases within 24 h of prednisone therapy.
4. The diagnosis is established by biopsy of the superficial temporal artery in case of temporal arteritis.

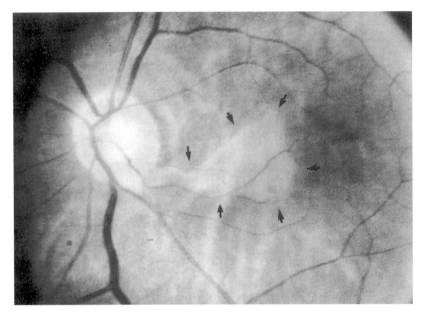

A

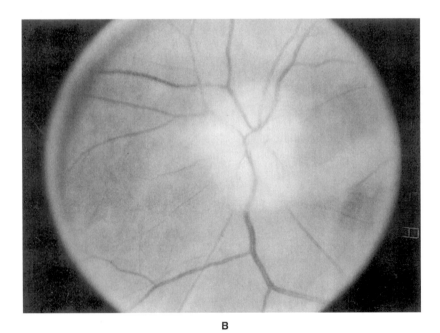

B

Figure 8-18

*Temporal (giant cell) arteritis. **A**. Retinal vessel occlusion showing infarcted area of the retina (arrows). **B**. Complete infarction of the optic nerve 3 days later. This 66-year-old patient had experienced amaurosis fugax in the opposite eye, then visual loss in the ipsilateral eye, followed by complete loss of vision in that eye 3 days later. The classical pale swollen appearance of the optic nerve is the signal for temporal artery biopsy.*

Treatment Giant cell arteritis responds well to corticosteroids. However, there are rare reports of steroid resistance with persistence of giant cells in biopsied material, despite prompt chemical response to corticosteroid therapy. The patient should be started on 96 mg methylprednisolone in a single dose orally and continued at 96 mg daily until there is a satisfactory response. This therapy usually produces rapid relief of symptoms of temporal arteritis and the dose can be continued and gradually decreased when the sedimentation rate is normal. Some visual improvement may persist in about one-third of patients with visual loss. A maintenance dose may be required and may be continued for several years, if necessary. Treatment should be given prior to biopsy of the superficial temporal artery because pathological abnormalities do not change for several days after the beginning of corticosteroid therapy, thus giving ample time for biopsy.

The aortic arch syndrome will respond to corticosteroids in uncomplicated cases. Therapy should be continued until the sedimentation rate is below 20 mm/h and the sedimentation rate monitored regularly to detect recurrence. Major complications of grade 2 retinopathy, persistent hypertension above 200/110, grade 3 or grade 4 aortic regurgitation, and angiographic demonstration of aortic or arterial aneurysm associated with a progressive course have a mortality rate of greater than 50 percent in 15 years. Selected cases benefit from aortic or cervical artery reconstructive surgery. Death is usually the result of congestive heart failure, myocardial infarction, or cerebral infarction.

Idiopathic Thrombocytopenic Purpura

This is a relatively benign condition characterized by bleeding into the skin and other tissues. It may follow a viral infection or occur in patients with SLE, lymphoma, or human immunodeficiency virus infection. Hemorrhages in the brain usually consist of multiple capillary petechiae and rarely present as large areas of hemorrhage into the parenchyma of the brain or spinal cord. The platelet count is reduced, the tourniquet test is positive, and the bleeding time is prolonged and the clotting time normal. Treatment consists of platelet

transfusions, intravenous corticosteroids, intravenous γ-globulin, and splenectomy.

Thrombotic Thrombocytopenic Purpura

This disorder is usually acute in onset, with purpura, hemolytic anemia, and neurological symptoms. The essential lesion is the occlusion of small arteries by thrombi composed of aggregated platelets and fibrin.

Symptoms include fever, headaches, altered levels of consciousness, focal or generalized seizures, arthralgias, abdominal pain, and vomiting. Focal signs of dysphasia, hemiplegia, cranial nerve involvement, and papilledema indicate brain involvement. The disease carries a high mortality rate, but prognosis has improved with plasmapheresis and intravenous γ-globulin therapy.

Scleroderma

Involvement of the cerebral arteries with disseminated cerebral angiitis in scleroderma is an unusual event. Scleroderma can cause cranial and peripheral neuropathies and myopathy in addition to the more common systemic involvement.

Sjögren's Syndrome

Sjögren's syndrome is occasionally associated with arteritis, which can cause a chronic myositis, peripheral neuropathy, and cranial neuropathies of the third, fifth, seventh and twelfth nerves. Trigeminal neuropathy, with loss of sensation in all three divisions of the nerve and depressed corneal reflexes, is the most common form of cranial nerve involvement. Cranial arteritis is rare.

Granulomatous Angiitis

Definition Granulomatous angiitis, or isolated angiitis, is a rare condition characterized by vasculitis restricted to the nervous system.

Etiology and Pathology The etiology is unknown. There is angiitis with a mononuclear infiltration and granuloma formation in about 50 percent of cases involving the arteries and occasionally the veins of the CNS. The angiitis is focal and segmental, with involvement of the small and medium-sized arteries and veins of the leptomeninges and parenchyma.

Clinical Features This rare form of subacute vasculitis is confined to the CNS. Although the etiology is unknown, a number of cases have been reported in association with Hodgkin disease, lymphoma, cerebral amyloid angiopathy, neurosarcoidosis, or following herpes zoster ophthalmicus.

The vasculitis presents with symptoms of severe headache resembling migraine, followed by changes in mental status, including memory failure and intellectual deterioration, with focal deficits such as hemiparesis, dysphasia, alexia, and partial seizures. Isolated angiitis of the spinal cord has been described with progressive paraparesis, radicular pain, and bladder dysfunction. The course of granulomatous angiitis is one of progressive deterioration and death within 3 years. Few survive.

Diagnostic Procedures

1. The routine laboratory tests such as complete blood count, sedimentation rate, standard testing for collagen vascular disease, cryoglobulins, and circulating immune complex determinations are usually normal.

2. Cerebral angiography shows narrowing or beading of intermediate or small arteries at multiple sites (Fig. 8-19).[144] Other causes of cerebral arteritis, including herpes zoster, bacterial meningitis, syphilis, tuberculosis, fungal infections, Hodgkin disease, SLE, rheumatoid arthritis, scleroderma, systemic necrotizing vasculitis, Wegener granulomatosis, lymphomatoid granulomatosis, vasculitis due to heroin, methylamphetamine, cocaine, allopurinol, or radiation vasculitis must be excluded.

3. The angiogram may be normal in some cases.

4. The MRI findings include multiple bilateral infarcts in both gray and white matter. Because abnormalities tend to be more prominent in white matter, T2-weighted images may suggest demyelinating disease.[145]

5. Lumbar puncture. The CSF may show a slight-to-moderate elevation in protein content.

6. Tissue biopsy is needed to establish the diagnosis when there is spinal cord involvement, and in those with normal arteriography when leptomeningeal biopsy is recommended.[146]

Treatment The response to corticosteroids is unpredictable, but this form of therapy should be tried initially. If relapse occurs, immunosuppressive therapy with cyclophosphamide and high-dose intravenous methylprednisolone for 7 days, followed by 100 mg on alternate days, may induce a sustained clinical remission. Treatment may be necessary intermittently or continuously for many years.

Prognosis The prognosis has been poor and the condition was invariably fatal until the introduction of a combination of prednisone and cyclophosphamide therapy. The use of plasmapheresis and intravenous immunoglobulin (IVIG) has yet to be established.

Neurological Complications of other Arteritides

Neurological complications have rarely been described in other forms of arteritis, including Wegener granulomatosis with a diffuse symmetrical peripheral neuropathy, Schonlein-Henoch purpura with hemiplegia, seizures, chorea, subarachnoid hemorrhage, particularly in children, and the arteritis associated with rheumatoid arthritis, showing peripheral neuropathy and focal neurological signs, including hemiparesis. Scleroderma occasionally involves the CNS and may produce secondary neurological symptoms due to hypertension or uremia following sclerodermic involvement of the heart, lungs, or kidneys. Involvement of the small intestine may produce malabsorption, vitamin B deficiency, and subacute degeneration of the cord in scleroderma, Crohn's disease, and ulcerative colitis.

TRANSIENT GLOBAL AMNESIA

Definition Transient global amnesia is a syndrome characterized by sudden total amnesia lasting several hours without other signs of neurological involvement, followed by complete recovery.

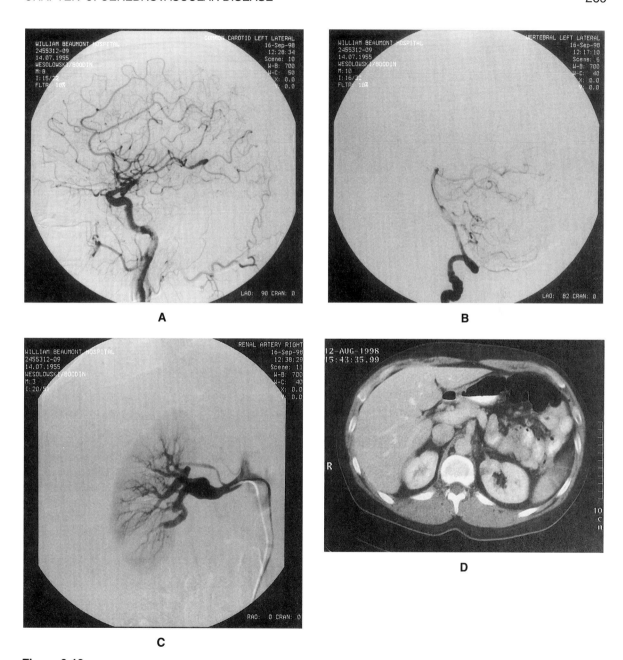

Figure 8-19

A. Cerebral arteriogram. There are multiple areas of altered caliber of the cerebral vessels compatible with cerebral arteritis. *B*. Cerebral arteritis. Arteriogram showing many areas of alteration in caliber of arteries in the posterior fossa. *C*. Renal arteriogram. There are several areas of aneurysmal dilatation of the renal artery. *D*. CT scan. Axial view, abdomen, showing multiple infarcts involving kidney, spleen, and liver.

Etiology and Pathology   The etiology is unknown. Although it is not unusual to obtain a history of migraine,[147] the relationship to migraine is not established but spreading depression involving the medial aspect of both temporal lobes is a plausible explanation for transient global amnesia.[148]

The onset is sudden and follows exertion such as manual labor, athletic activity, sexual intercourse, or an intense emotional experience in many cases.

Clinical Features   Transient global amnesia occurs in middle-aged or elderly individuals who are apparently healthy. The onset is sudden and there is a period of total amnesia lasting several hours. During the time, the individual behaves in a normal or near-normal fashion but cannot recall verbal or nonverbal material presented only minutes before and often repeats the same question many times.[149] Individuals who are acquainted with the patient can detect subtle changes in behavior. The attack usually terminates slowly, with the patient showing gradual improvement in identification of those around him. The rate of recurrent attacks, subsequent stroke, and development of dementia is low.

Diagnostic Procedures   When signs of cerebral atherosclerosis are present, the attack should be investigated as a TIA.

Treatment   Any underlying disease (e.g., hypertension) should be treated. The patient should be informed that further attacks of transient global amnesia are unusual but have been reported.

LOCKED-IN SYNDROME

Definition   The locked-in syndrome is characterized by quadriparesis and lower bulbar palsy due to bilateral infarction of the ventral pons.

Etiology and Pathology   Most cases of this syndrome are due to basilar artery thrombosis with bilateral infarction of the ventral pons. The condition can occur following head and neck trauma, with vertebral artery damage and occlusion. The syndrome occasionally occurs in multiple sclerosis and pontine gliomas that involve the ventral pons bilaterally.

Clinical Features   In the majority of cases with thrombosis of the basilar artery, the onset is sudden, with the development of acute hemiparesis and rapid progression to quadriparesis. Initially there may be severe dysarthria and dysphonia, with rapid progression to a state of mutism. The patient is unable to handle oral and pharyngeal secretions and aspiration pneumonia occurs at an early stage.

Examination shows complete quadriplegia with mutism and paralysis of all functions supplied by the cranial nerves bilaterally from the fifth to the twelfth cranial nerves. Horizontal eye movement is impaired, but vertical eye movement and blinking are preserved. This preservation of oculomotor function gives the patient an opportunity to communicate by eye blinking.

These patients give the superficial impression of coma because of quadriplegia and mutism. However, they are fully conscious and alert and can communicate, as indicated, by vertical eye movements or blinking.

Diagnostic Procedures   Cerebral angiography is the definitive procedure in identifying basilar artery thrombosis and should be performed urgently at the time of admission. An MRI or CT scan will exclude a pontine hemorrhage. The MRI scan or MRA may indicate basilar artery occlusion.

Treatment   Patients with locked-in syndrome should receive full supportive treatment, as many recover from this seemingly hopeless condition (see treatment of cerebral infarction). Reversal of locked-in state by treatment with intra-arterial thrombolytic agents within 12 h of basilar artery thrombosis has had a good clinical outcome, indicating the need for an aggressive approach to diagnosis and therapy in locked-in syndrome.[150]

CEREBRAL INFARCTION DUE TO CEREBRAL VENOUS OR DURAL SINUS THROMBOSIS

Definition   This is a thrombosis of the cerebral venous system, followed by cerebral infarction.

Etiology and Pathology   Cerebral venous thrombosis and dural sinus thrombosis may be caused by infection following otitis media, mastoiditis, acute sinusitis, or furunculosis of the face. Noninfectious thrombosis may be associated with head trauma, sickle cell disease, neoplasia, homocysteinemia, the immediate postpartum period, and the presence of lupus anticoagulant.

Clinical Features

1. Superior sagittal sinus thrombosis (Fig. 8-20). The condition usually presents with generalized headache followed by seizures and progressive weakness of one or both lower extremities. The patient becomes obtunded or stuporous and there are signs of increased intracranial pressure with papilledema and distention of scalp veins. Young children show bulging of the anterior fontanelle. Thrombosis of the posterior half of the superior sagittal sinus may result in benign intracranial hypertension.

2. Cerebral venous thrombosis. The condition is usually seen in the immediate postpartum period. The patient may present with seizures,[151] which can be followed by the development of headache and hemiparesis.

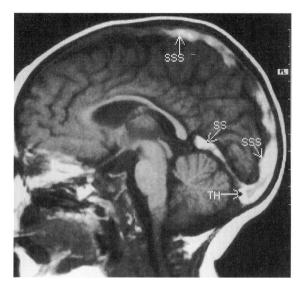

Figure 8-20
Dural sinus thrombosis. MRA scan showing thrombosis of the superior sagittal sinus and straight sinus.

3. Transverse sinus thrombosis and cavernous sinus thrombosis. These conditions are usually caused by infection. Transverse sinus thrombosis may be asymptomatic or associated with papilledema, headache, neck pain, nausea, vomiting, and ataxia. Cavernous sinus thrombosis is usually characterized by edema of the orbit and eyelids with ptosis, chemosis, and orbital edema. The third, fourth, and ophthalmic division of the fifth and the sixth cranial nerves which traverse the lateral wall of the cavernous sinus are usually involved.

Diagnostic Procedures

1. The MRI and CT scans show abnormalities in one or both cerebral hemispheres in patients with hemorrhagic infarction.

2. An MRA scan may indicate the absence of blood flow in the affected sinus.

3. Patients with benign intracranial hypertension (pseudotumor cerebri) should undergo venous transcranial Doppler ultrasonography, angiography, or brain MRI studies before assuming that the condition is idiopathic.[152]

4. Venous transcranial Doppler ultrasound is a reliable, noninvasive and rapid technique for intracranial venous sinus examination.[153]

5. Angiography. The venous stage of angiography demonstrates lack of filling of the affected vessel.

6. Lupus anticoagulant can be demonstrated in some cases.

7. The electroencephalogram shows focal slowing, often associated with intermittent spike wave activity on this side of ischemia or infarction.

Treatment

1. Seizures should be controlled with an adequate dose of anticonvulsants.
2. Patients with increased intracranial pressure of sufficient magnitude to produce papilledema should receive intracranial pressure monitoring and appropriate treatment with hyperosmolar agents such as mannitol.
3. Patients with lupus anticoagulant responded to anticoagulants and prednisone therapy.

Prognosis In most cases, residual neurological deficits cannot be predicted, but a good recovery is not unusual. Seizures may require long-term anticonvulsant therapy.

NEUROLOGICAL COMPLICATIONS OF DRUG ABUSE

The repeated intravenous injection of illicit drugs may produce a number of cerebrovascular complications:

1. Chronic heroin and cocaine users can develop arterial vasospasm or a cerebral arteritis, with cerebral infarction or subarachnoid hemorrhage.[154] Recent illicit drug use occurs in 12 percent of young adult stroke patients.[155]

2. Repeated intravenous injection without sterile precautions is associated with a significant risk of subacute bacterial endocarditis and the subsequent development of embolism and mycotic aneurysms. The presence of mycotic aneurysm may be complicated by subarachnoid hemorrhage or cerebral infarction.

3. Ingestion of amphetamines or phenylpropanolamine, often found in dietary medications, has resulted in intracerebral hemorrhage. The recent increase in IV amphetamine use is a particularly dangerous and disturbing trend in illicit drug administration.

CEREBROVASCULAR COMPLICATIONS OF MIGRAINE

Migraine is usually a benign condition but occasionally patients with more complex forms of migraine will develop cerebral infarction. The infarctions are usually in the distribution of the posterior cerebral artery but can also involve the territory of the middle cerebral artery.

REFERENCES

1. Broderick J, Brott T, Kothari R, et al: The Greater Cincinnati/Northern Kentucky Stroke Study: preliminary first-ever and total incidence rates of stroke among blacks. *Stroke* 29:415, 1998.

2. Goldstein LB, Matchar DB: Clinical assessment of stroke. *JAMA* 271:1114, 1994.

3. Petersen P, Boysen G: Ischaemic stroke—prevention and treatment. *J Intern Med* 231:103, 1992.

4. Sacco RL, Benjamin EJ, Broderick JP, et al: American Heart Association Prevention Conference, IV. Prevention and rehabilitation of stroke. Risk factors. *Stroke* 28:1507, 1997.

5. Bonita R: Epidemiology of stroke. *Lancet* 339:342, 1992.

6. Borsan WG, Brott TG, Broderick JP, et al: Urgent therapy for acute stroke. Effects of a stroke trial on untreated patients. *Stroke* 25:2132, 1994.

7. DiGraba TJ: Expression of inflammatory mediators and adhesion molecules in human atherosclerotic plaque. *Neurology* 49(Suppl 4):S15, 1997.

8. Buja LM, Willerson JT: Role of inflammation in coronary plaque disruption. *Circulation* 89:503, 1994.

9. Sitzer M, Muller W, Siebler M, et al: Plaque ulceration and lumen thrombus are the main source of cerebral microemboli in high-grade internal carotid artery stenosis. *Stroke* 26:1231, 1995.

10. Bednar MM, Gross CE, Balazy M, et al: Antineutrophil strategies. *Neurology* 49(Suppl 4):S20, 1997.

11. Riikonen R, Santavuori P: Hereditary and acquired risk factors for childhood stroke. *Neuropediatrics* 25:227, 1994.

12. Syrjanen J, Valtonen VV, Iivanainen M, et al: Preceding infection as an important risk factor for ischaemic brain infarction in young and middle aged patients. *BMJ Clin Res Ed* 296:1156, 1988.

13. Grau AJ, Buggle F, Becher H, et al: Recent bacterial and viral infection is a risk factor for cerebrovascular Ischaemia: clinical and biochemical studies. *Neurology* 50:196, 1998.

14. Grau AJ, Banerjee T, Stieehen-Weihn C, et al: Preceding infection as a risk factor in cerebral ischemia. *Stroke* 24:182, 1993.

15. Amarenco P, Cohen A, Tzourio C, et al: Atherosclerotic disease of the aortic arch and the risk of ischemic stroke. *N Engl J Med* 331:1474, 1994.

16. Jones EF, Kalman JM, Calafiore P, et al: Proximal aortic atheroma. An independent risk factor for cerebral ischemia. *Stroke* 26:218, 1995.

17. Belden JR, Caplan LR, Bojar RM, et al: Treatment of multiple cerebral emboli from an ulcerated thrombogenic ascending aorta with aortectomy and graft replacement. *Neurology* 49:621, 1997.

18. Wolf PA, Belanger AJ, D'Agostino RB: Management of risk factors. *Neurol Clin* 10:177, 1992.

19. SHEP Cooperative Research Group. Prevention of

stroke by antihypertensive drug treatment in older persons with isolated systolic hypertension. Final results of the Systolic Hypertension in the Elderly Program (SHEP). *JAMA* 265:3255, 1991.

20. Dunbabin DW, Sandercock PA: Preventing stroke by the modification of risk factors. *Stroke* 21(Suppl IV): IV-36, 1990.

21. Whisnant JP. Effectiveness versus efficacy of treatment of hypertension for stroke prevention. *Neurology* 46:301, 1996.

22. WHO Stroke-1989. Recommendations on stroke prevention, diagnosis, and therapy. Report of the WHO task force on stroke and other cerebrovascular disorders. *Stroke* 20:1407, 1989.

23. Yasaka M, Yamaguchi T, Svhichiri M: Distribution of atherosclerosis and risk factors in atherothrombotic occlusion. *Stroke* 24:206, 1993.

24. Burchfiel CM, Curb JD, Rodriguez BL, et al: Glucose intolerance and 22-year stroke incidence. The Honolulu Heart Program. *Stroke* 25:951, 1994.

25. Rohr J, Kittner S, Feeser B, et al: Traditional risk factors and ischemic stroke in young adults: the Baltimore-Washington Cooperative Young Stroke Study. *Arch Neurol* 53:603, 1996.

26. Petty GW, Brown RD Jr, Whisnant JP, et al: Survival and recurrence after first cerebral infarction. a population-based study in Rochester, Minnesota, 1975–1989. *Neurology* 50:208, 1998.

27. van den Berg M, van der Knaap MS, Boers GH, et al: Hyperhomocysteinaemia; with reference to its neuroradiological aspects. *Neuroradiology* 37:403, 1995.

28. Lee TK, Huang ZS, Ng SK, et al: Impact of alcohol consumption and cigarette smoking on stroke among the elderly in Taiwan. *Stroke* 26:790, 1995.

29. Hillbom M, Haapaniemi H, Juvela S, et al: Recent alcohol consumption, cigarette smoking, and cerebral infarction in young adults. *Stroke* 26:40, 1995.

30. Reith J, Jorgensen HS, Pedersen PM, et al: Body temperature in acute stroke: relation to stroke severity, infarct size, mortality and outcome. *Lancet* 347:422, 1996.

31. Moroney JT, Bagiella E, Tatemichi TK, et al: Dementia after stroke increases the risk of long-term stroke recurrence. *Neurology* 48:1317, 1997.

32. Naradzay JF, Gaasch WR: Acute stroke. *Emerg Med Clin N Amer* 14:197, 1996.

33. Gorelick PB: Stroke prevention. *Arch Neurol* 52:347, 1995.

34. van Latum JC, Koudstaal PJ, Venables GS, et al: Predictors of major vascular events in patients with a transient ischemic attack or minor ischemic stroke

and with nonrheumatic atrial fibrillation: European Atrial Fibrillation Trial (EAFT) study group. *Stroke* 16:801, 1995.

35. EAFT Study Group. Silent brain infarction in nonrheumatic atrial fibrillation. *Neurology* 46:159, 1996.

36. Vanninen R, Aikia M, Kononen M, et al: Subclinical cerebral complications after coronary artery bypass grafting: prospective analysis with magnetic resonance imaging, quantitative electroencephalography, and neuropsychological assessment. *Arch Neurol* 55:618, 1998.

37. Di Tullio M, Sacco RL, Gopal A, et al: Patent foramen ovale as a risk factor for cryptogenic stroke. *Ann Inter Med* 117:461, 1992.

38. Cabanes L, Mas JL, Cohen A, et al: Atrial septal aneurysm and patent foramen ovale as risk factors for cryptogenic stroke in patients less than 55 years of age. A study using transesophageal echocardiography. *Stroke* 24:1865, 1993.

39. Bogousslavsky J, Garazi S, Jeanrenaud X, et al: Stroke recurrence in patients with patent foramen ovale: the Lausanne Study. Lausanne Stroke with Paradoxical embolism study group. *Neurology* 46:1301, 1996.

40. Orencia AJ, Petty GW, Khandheria BK, et al: Risk of stroke with mitral valve prolapse in population-based cohort study. *Stroke* 26:7, 1995.

41. Brown RD Jr, Evans BA, Wiebers DO, et al: Transient ischemic attack and minor ischemic stroke: an algorithm for evaluation and treatment. Mayo Clinic Division of Cerebrovascular Diseases. *Mayo Clin Proc* 69:1027, 1994.

42. Klotzsch C, Janssen G, Berlit P: Transesophageal echocardiography and contrast-TCD in the detection of a patent foramen ovale: experiences with III patients. *Neurology* 44:1603, 1994.

43. Kothari RU, Brott T, Broderick JP, et al: Emergency physicians. Accuracy in the diagnosis of stroke. *Stroke* 26:2238, 1995.

44. Elster AD, Moody DM: Early cerebral infarction: gadopentetate dimeglumine enhancement. *Radiology* 177:627, 1990.

45. Alberts MJ, Faulstich ME, Gray L: Stroke with negative brain magnetic resonance imaging. *Stroke* 23:663, 1992.

46. Tong DC, Yenari MA, Albers GW, et al: Correlation of perfusion- and diffusion-weighted MRI with NIHSS score in acute (<6.5 hour) ischemic stroke. *Neurology* 50:864, 1998.

47. Atlas SW: MR angiography in neurologic disease. *Radiology* 193:1, 1994.

48. Polak JF, Kalina P, Donaldson MC, et al: Carotid endarterectomy. preoperative evaluation of candidates with combined Doppler sonography and MR angiography. Work in progress. *Neuroradiology* 186:333, 1993.

49. Bucher HC, Griffith LE, Guyatt GH: Effect of HMG-coA reductase inhibitors on stroke. A meta-analysis of randomized controlled trials. *Ann Intern Med* 128:89, 1998.

50. Camarata PJ, Heros RC, Latchaw RE: "Brain attack": the rationale for treating stroke as a medical emergency. *Neurosurgery* 34:144, 1994.

51. The Publications Committee for the Trial of ORG 10172 in Acute Stroke Treatment (TOAST) Investigators. Low molecular weight heparinoid, ORG 10172 (Danaparoid), and outcome after ischemic stroke: a randomized controlled trial. *JAMA* 279:1265, 1998.

52. Chaturvedi S, Hachinski V: Transient ischemic attacks. Rethinking concepts in management. *Postgrad Med* 96:42, 1994.

53. Sherman DG, Dyken ML Jr, Fisher M, et al: Antithrombotic therapy for cerebrovascular disorders. *Chest* (Suppl 4):529S, 1992.

54. Ojemann RG, Heros RC, Cromwell RM: Dissection of internal carotid, vertebral and intracranial arteries. *Surgical Management of Cerebrovascular Disease,* Baltimore: Williams and Wilkens ed. 2, pp. 125–136, 1988.

55. The SPAF III Writing Committee for the Stroke Prevention in Atrial Fibrillation Investigators. Patients with nonvalvular atrial fibrillation at low risk of stroke during treatment with aspirin: Stroke prevention in atrial fibrillation III Study. *JAMA* 279:1273, 1998.

56. Diener HC, Cunha L, Forbes C, et al: European Stroke Prevention Study 2. Dipyridamole and acetylsalicylic acid in the secondary prevention of stroke. *J Neurol Sci* 143:1, 1996.

57. Hass WK, Easton JD, Adams HP Jr, et al: A randomized trial comparing ticlopidine hydrochloride with aspirin for the prevention of stroke in high-risk patients. Ticlopidine aspirin stroke study group. *N Engl J Med* 321:501, 1989.

58. Horowitz DR, Tuhrim S, Budd J, et al: Aortic plaque in patients with brain ischemia: diagnosis by transesophageal echocardiography. *Neurology* 42:1602, 1992.

59. van der Zwan A, Hillen B, Tulleken CA, et al: A quantitative investigation of the variability of the major cerebral arterial territories. *Stroke* 24:1951, 1993.

60. Kishimoto TK, Rothlein R: Integrins, ICAMs, and selectins: role and regulation of adhesion molecules in neutrophil recruitment to inflammatory sites. *Adv Pharmacol* 25:117, 1994.

61. Rothlein R. Overview of leukocyte adhesion. *Neurology* 49(Suppl 4):S3, 1997.

62. Sherman DG: Advances in stroke management. *Neurology* 49(Suppl 4):S1, 1997.

63. Clark WM: Cytokines and reperfusion injury. *Neurology* 49(Suppl 4):S10, 1997.

64. Hossmann KA: Viability thresholds and the penumbra of focal ischemia. *Ann Neurol* 36:557, 1994.

65. Pulsinelli W: Pathophysiology of acute ischaemic stroke. *Lancet* 339:533, 1992.

66. Fisher M, Garcia JH: Evolving stroke and the ischemic penumbra. *Neurology* 47:884, 1996.

67. Paakkari I, Lindsberg P: Nitric oxide in the central nervous system. *Ann Med* 27:369, 1995.

68. Ginsberg MD, Pulsinelli WA: The ischemic penumbra, injury thresholds, and the therapeutic window for acute stroke. *Ann Neurol* 36:553, 1994.

69. Muir KW, Lees KR: Clinical experience with excitatory amino acid antagonist drugs. *Stroke* 26:503, 1995.

70. Mounier-Vehier F, Leys D, Pruvo JP: Stroke patterns in unilateral atherothrombotic occlusion of the internal carotid artery. *Stroke* 26:422, 1995.

71. Arboix A, Comes E, Massons J, et al: Relevance of early seizures for in-hospital mortality in acute cerebrovascular disease. *Neurology* 47:1429, 1996.

72. Levy R, Duyckaerts C, Hauw JJ: Massive infarcts involving the territory of the anterior choroidal artery and cardioembolism. *Stroke* 26:609, 1995.

73. Crozier S, Lehericy S, Verstichel P, et al: Transient hemiballism/hemichorea due to an ipsilateral subthalamic nucleus infarction. *Neurology* 46:267, 1996.

74. Nasreddine ZS, Saver JL: Pain after thalamic stroke. right diencephalic predominance and clinical features in 180 patients. *Neurology* 48:1196, 1997.

75. Fisher CM: Vomiting out of proportion to dizziness in ischemic brainstem strokes. *Neurology* 46:267, 1996.

76. Buchholz DW: Clinically probable brainstem stroke presenting primarily as dysphagia and nonvisualized by MRI. *Dysphagia* 8:235, 1993.

77. Bassetti C, Bogousslavsky J, Barth A, et al: Isolated infarcts of the pons. *Neurology* 46:165, 1996.

78. Futrell N, Millikan CH: Stroke is an emergency. *Disease-A-Month* 42:199, 1996.

79. Naradzay JF, Gaasch WR: Acute stroke. *Emerg Med Clin N Amer* 14:197, 1996.

80. Pryse-Phillips W, Yegappan MC: Management of acute stroke. Ways to minimize damage and maximize recovery. *Postgrad Med* 96:75, 1994.

81. Brainin M: Antihypertensive therapy in stroke; acute therapy, primary and secondary prevention. *Acta Med Austriaca* 22:54, 1995.

82. Tietjen CS, Hurn PD, Ulatowski JA, et al: Treatment modalities for hypertensive patients with intracranial pathology: options and risks. *Crit Care Med* 24:311, 1996.

83. Veskergaard K, Andersen G, Nielsen MI, et al: Headache in stroke. *Stroke* 24:1621, 1993.

84. Odderson IR, Keaton JC, McKenna BS: Swallow management in patients on an acute stroke pathway: quality is cost effective. *Arch Phys Med Rehabil* 76:1130, 1995.

85. Goldstein LB and the Sygen in Acute Stroke Study Investigators. Common drugs may influence motor recovery after stroke. *Neurology* 45:865, 1995.

86. Schwab S, Aschoff A, Spranger M, et al: The value of intracranial pressure monitoring in acute hemispheric stroke. *Neurology* 47:393, 1996.

87. The Stroke Prevention in Reversible Ischemic Trial (SPIRIT) Study Group. A randomized trial of anticoagulants versus aspirin after cerebral ischemia of presumed arterial origin. *Ann Neurol* 42:857, 1997.

88. Adams HP Jr, Brott TG, Furlan AJ, et al: Guidelines for thrombolytic therapy for acute stroke: a supplement to the guidelines for the management of patients with acute ischemic stroke. A statement for healthcare professionals from a Special Writing Group of the Stroke Council, American Heart Association. *Circulation* 94:1167, 1996.

89. Hund E, Grau A, Hacke W: Neurocritical care for acute ischemic stroke. *Neurol Clin* 13:511, 1995.

90. The National Institute of Neurological Disorders and Stroke rt-PA Stroke Study Group. Tissue plasminogen activator for acute ischemic stroke. *N Engl J Med* 333:1581, 1995.

91. Donnan GA, Davis SM, Chambers BR, et al: Trials of streptokinase in severe acute ischaemic stroke. *Lancet* 345:578, 1995.

92. Mohr JP, Orgogozo JM, Harrison MJG, et al: Meta-analysis of oral nimodepine trials in acute ischemic stroke. *Cerebrovascular Dis* 4:197, 1994.

93. Jonas S: Prophylactic pharmacologic neuroprotection against focal cerebral ischemia. *Ann NY Acad Sci* 765:21, 1995.

94. Pujia A, Rubba P, Spencer MP: Prevalence of extracranial carotid artery disease detectable by echo-Doppler in an elderly population. *Stroke* 23:818, 1992.

95. The European Carotid Surgery Trialists Collaborative Group. Risk of stroke in the distribution of an asymptomatic carotid artery. *Lancet* 345:209, 1995.

96. Hobson RW 2nd, Weiss DG, Fields WS, et al: Efficacy of carotid endarterectomy for asymptomatic carotid stenosis. The Veterans Affairs Cooperative study group. *N Engl J Med* 328:221, 1993.

97. Mayberg MR, Winn HR. Endarterectomy for asymptomatic carotid artery stenosis. Resolving the controversy (editorial). *JAMA* 273:1459, 1995.

98. Biller J, Feinberg WM, Castaldo JE, et al: Guidelines for carotid endarterectomy, a statement for healthcare professionals from a special writing group of the Stroke Council, American Heart Association. *Stroke* 29:554, 1998.

99. Siebler M, Kleinschmidt A, Sitzer M, et al: Cerebral microembolism in symptomatic and asymptomatic high-grade internal carotid artery stenosis. *Neurology* 44:615, 1994.

100. North American Symptomatic Carotid Endarterectomy Trial Collaborators. Beneficial effect of carotid endarterectomy in symptomatic patients with high-grade carotid stenosis. *N Engl J Med* 325:445, 1991.

101. Valton L, Larrue V, Pavy Le Traon A, et al: Cerebral microembolism in patients with stroke or transient ischaemic attack as a risk factor for early recurrence. *J Neurol Neurosurg Psychiatry* 63:784, 1997.

102. Barnett HJ, Haines SJ: Carotid endarterectomy for asymptomatic carotid stenosis. *N Engl J Med* 328:276, 1993.

103. Eliasziw M, Streifler JY, Fox AJ, et al: Significance of plaque ulceration in symptomatic patients with high-grade carotid stenosis. *Stroke* 25:304, 1994.

104. Caplan LR: Stroke Treatment: promising but still struggling. JAMA 279:1304, 1998.

105. Gillman MW, Cupples LA, Millen BE, et al: Inverse association of dietary fat with development of ischemic stroke in men. *JAMA* 278:2145, 1997.

106. Schievink WI, Mokri B, Whisnant JP: Internal carotid artery dissection in a community. Rochester, Minnesota, 1987-1992. *Stroke* 24:1678, 1993.

107. Sharif AA, Remley KB, Clark HB. Middle cerebral artery dissection: a clinicopathologic study. *Neurology* 45:1929, 1995.

108. Peters M, Bohl J, Thomke F, et al: Dissection of the internal carotid artery after chiropractic manipulation of the neck. *Neurology* 45:2284, 1995.

109. Mokri B, Silbert PL, Schievink WI, et al: Cranial nerve palsy in spontaneous dissections of the extracranial internal carotid artery. *Neurology* 46:356, 1996.

110. Schievink WI, Mokri B, Garrity JA, et al. Ocular motor nerve palsies in spontaneous dissections of the cervical internal carotid artery. *Neurology* 43:1938, 1993.

111. Mokri B, Schievink WI, Olsen KD, et al: Spontaneous dissection of the cervical internal carotid artery. Presentation with lower cranial nerve palsies. *Arch Otolaryngol Head Neck Surg* 118:431, 1992.

112. Lee KP, Carlini WG, McCormick GF, et al: Neurologic complications following chiropractic manipulation: a survey of California neurologists. *Neurology* 45:1213, 1995.

113. Silbert PL, Mokri B, Schievink WI: Headache and neck pain in spontaneous internal carotid and vertebral artery dissections. *Neurology* 45:1517, 1995.

114. Sturzenegger M, Mattle HP, Rivoir A, et al: Ultrasound findings in spontaneous extracranial vertebral artery dissection. *Stroke* 24:1910, 1993.

115. de Bray JM, Penisson-Besnier I, Dubas F, et al: Extracranial and intracranial vertebrobasilar dissections: diagnosis and prognosis. *J Neurol Neurosurg Psychiatry* 63:46, 1997.

116. Sturzenegger M, Mattle HP, Rivoir A, et al. Ultrasound findings in carotid artery dissection: analysis of 43 patients. *Neurology* 45:691, 1995.

117. Zuber M, Meary E, Meder JF, et al: Magnetic resonance imaging and dynamic CT scan in cervical artery dissections. *Stroke* 25:576, 1994.

118. Holmgren H, Leijon G, Borvie J, et al: Central poststroke pain—somatosensory evoked potentials in relation to location of the lesion and sensory signs. *Pain* 40:43, 1990.

119. Schmahmann JD, Leifer D: Parietal pseudothalamic pain syndrome. Clinical features and anatomic correlates. *Arch Neurol* 49:1032, 1992.

120. MacGowan DJ, Janal MN, Clark WC, et al: Central poststroke pain and Wallenberg's lateral medullary infarction: frequency, character, and determinants in 63 patients. *Neurology* 49:120, 1997.

121. Leijon G, Boivie J: Central post-stroke pain—a controlled trial of amitriptyline and carbamazepine. *Pain* 36:27, 1989.

122. Kokmen E, Whisnant JP, O'Fallon WM, et al: Dementia after ischemic stroke: a population-based study in Rochester, Minnesota (1960-1984). *Neurology* 46:154, 1996.

123. Hulette C, Nochlin D, McKeel D, et al: Clinical-neuropathologic findings in multi-infarct dementia: a report of six autopsied cases. *Neurology* 48:66B, 1997.

124. Tatemichi TK, Desmond DW, Paik M, et al: Clinical determinants of dementia related to stroke. *Ann Neurol* 33:568, 1993.

125. Ylikoski R, Ylikoski A, Erkinjuntti T, et al: White matter changes in healthy elderly persons correlate with attention and speed of mental processing. *Arch Neurol* 50:818, 1993.

126. Greenberg SM, Vonsattel JP, Stakes JW, et al: The clinical spectrum of cerebral amyloid angiopathy: presentations without lobar hemorrhage. *Neurology* 43:2073, 1993.

127. Farina E, Magni E, Ambrosini F, et al: Neuropsychological deficits in a symptomatic atrial fibrillation. *Acta Neurol Scand* 96:310, 1997.

128. Esiri MM, Wilcock GK, Morris JH: Neuropathological assessment of the lesions of significance in vascular dementia. *J Neurol Neurosurg Psychiatry* 63:749, 1997.

129. Gan R, Sacco RL, Kargman DE, et al: Testing the validity of the lacunar hypothesis: the Northern Manhattan Stroke Study experience. *Neurology* 48:1204, 1997.

130. van Zagten M, Boiten J, Kessels F, et al: Significant progression of white matter lesions and small deep (lacunar) infarcts in patients with stroke. *Arch Neurol* 53:650, 1996.

131. Mast H, Thompson JL, Lee SH, et al: Hypertension and diabetes mellitus as determinants of multiple lacunar infarcts. *Stroke* 26:30, 1995.

132. Giroud M, Lemesle M, Madinier G, et al: Unilateral lenticular infarcts: radiological and clinical syndromes, aetiology and prognosis. *J Neurol Neurosurg Psychiatry* 63:611, 1997.

133. Gandolfo C, Caponnetto C, Del Sette M, et al: Risk factors in lacunar syndromes: a case-control study. *Acta Neurol Scand* 77:22, 1988.

134. You R, McNeil JJ, O'Malley HM, et al: Risk factors for lacunar infarction syndromes. *Neurology* 45:1483, 1995.

135. Bogucki A, Papierz W, Szymanska R, et al: Cerebral amyloid angiopathy with attenuation of the white matter on CT scans: subcortical arteriosclerotic encephalopathy (Binswanger) in a normotensive patient. *J Neurol* 235:435, 1988.

136. Caplan LR: Binswanger's disease—revisited. *Neurology* 45:626, 1995.

137. Mayer S, Tatemichi TK, Spitz J, et al: Recurrent ischemic events and diffuse white matter disease in patients with pseudoxanthoma elasticum. *Cerebrovasc Disord* 4:294, 1994.

138. Walzl M, Lechner H, Walzl B, et al: Improved neurological recovery of cerebral infarctions after plasmapheretic reduction of lipids and fibrinogen. *Stroke* 24:1447, 1993.

139. Verin M, Rolland Y, Landgraf F, et al: New phenotype

of the cerebral autosomal dominant arteriopathy mapped to chromosome 19: migraine as a prominent clinical feature. *J Neurol Neurosurg Psychiatry* 59:579, 1995.

140. Chabriat H, Vahedi K, Iba-Zizen MT, et al: Clinical spectrum of CADASIL: a study of 7 families. Cerebral autosomal dominant arteriopathy with subcortical infarcts and leukoencephalopathy. *Lancet* 346:934, 1995.

141. Daras M, Tuchman AJ, Koppel BS, et al: Neurovascular complications of cocaine. *Acta Neurol Scand* 90:124, 1994.

142. Liu GT, Glaser JS, Schatz NJ, et al: Visual morbidity in giant cell arteritis. Clinical characteristics and prognosis for vision. *Ophthalmology* 101:1779, 1994.

143. Liorente Pendass S, De Vicente Rodriguez JC, Gonzalez Garcia M, et al: Tongue necrosis as a complication of temporal arteritis. *Oral Surg Oral Med Oral Pathol* 78:448, 1994.

144. Harris KG, Tran DD, Sickels WJ, et al: Diagnosing intracranial vasculitis: the roles of MR and angiography. *AJNR* 15:317, 1994.

145. Alhalabi M, Moore PM: Serial angiography in isolated angiitis of the central nervous system. *Neurology* 44:1221, 1994.

146. Ehsan T, Hasan S, Powers JM, et al: Serial magnetic resonance imaging in isolated angiitis of the central nervous system. *Neurology* 45:1462, 1995.

147. Melo TP, Ferro JM, Ferro H: Transient global amnesia. A case control study. *Brain* 115:261, 1992.

148. Olesen J, Jorgensen MB: Leao's spreading depression in the hippocampus explains transient global amnesia. A hypothesis. *Acta Neurol Scand* 73:219, 1986.

149. Sakashita Y, Kanai M, Sugimoto T, et al: Changes in cerebral blood flow and vasoreactivity in response to acetazolamide in patients with transient global amnesia. *J Neurol Neurosurg Psychiatry* 63:605, 1997.

150. Wigdicks EF, Nichols DA, Thielen KR, et al: Intra-arterial thrombolysis in acute basilar artery thromboembolism: the initial Mayo Clinic experience. *Mayo Clin Proc* 72:1005, 1997.

151. Chang YJ, Huang CC, Wai YY: Isolated cortical venous thrombosis—discrepancy between clinical features and neuroradiologic findings. A case report. *Angiology* 46:1133, 1995.

152. Daif A, Awada A, al-Rajeh S, et al: Cerebral venous thrombosis in adults. A study of 40 cases from Saudi Arabia. *Stroke* 26:1193, 1995.

153. Valdueza JM, Schultz M, Harms L, et al: Venous transcranial Doppler ultrasound monitoring in acute dural sinus thrombosis. Report of two cases. *Stroke* 26:1196, 1995.

154. Qureshi AI, Akbar MS, Czander E, et al: Crack cocaine use and stroke in young patients. *Neurology* 48:341, 1997.

155. Sloan MA, Kittner SJ, Feeser BR, et al: Illicit drug-associated ischemic stroke in the Baltimore-Washington Young Stroke Study. *Neurology* 50:1688, 1998.

Chapter 9

SUBARACHNOID HEMORRHAGE

Subarachnoid hemorrhage (SAH) is a syndrome in which there is bleeding into the subarachnoid space. It may be spontaneous or secondary to trauma. Spontaneous SAH may result from an intracerebral hemorrhage that ruptures into the ventricular system and subsequently gains access to the subarachnoid space. Less frequently, spontaneous SAH may result from an intracerebral hemorrhage that ruptures directly into the subarachnoid space; or it may follow primary SAH. In primary SAH, spontaneous rupture of a blood vessel lying in the subarachnoid space results in bleeding into the subarachnoid space. Primary SAH accounts for approximately 9 percent of acute cerebrovascular episodes. Rupture of an aneurysm or bleeding from an arteriovenous malformation (AVM) is, by far, the most common cause of primary SAH. Table 9-1 lists less common etiologies of SAH.

ANEURYSMS

Aneurysms have been described in 1 to 18 percent of autopsied cases of SAH, depending on the pathologist's definition of an aneurysm. Aneurysms are usually single, but multiple aneurysms occur in about 15 percent of cases. Ninety percent of aneurysms occur

Table 9-1
Subarachnoid hemorrhage

A. Common causes
  1. Traumatic subarachnoid hemorrhage
  2. Spontaneous subarachnoid hemorrhage
     a. Intracerebral hemorrhage with rupture into the subarachnoid space
     b. Primary subarachnoid hemorrhage
        1. Ruptured saccular aneurysm
        2. Bleeding AVM
        3. Ruptured mycotic aneurysm
B. Rare causes
  1. Developmental defects, including pseudoxanthoma elasticum, Ehlers-Danlos syndrome, Marfan's syndrome,[84] Sturge-Weber disease, hereditary hemorrhagic telangiectasia, telangiectasia pontis, autosomal dominant polycystic kidney disease[85]
  2. Herpes simplex encephalitis, acute hemorrhagic leukoencephalitis, brain abscess, tuberculous meningitis, syphilitic vasculitis
  3. Neoplasm, primary or metastatic brain tumor, hemangioblastoma of the cerebellum or brainstem[86]
  4. Blood dyscrasias. Leukemia, Hodgkin disease, thrombocytopenia, sickle cell anemia,[87] hemophilia, aplastic anemia, pernicious anemia, anticoagulant therapy, congenital deficiency of factor VII
  5. Hypertension
  6. Vasculitis. Polyarteritis nodosa, anaphylactic purpura, Wegener's granulomatosis,[88] primary angiitis of the CNS[89]
  7. Arteriosclerosis with rupture of an arteriosclerotic vessel
  8. Rupture of a dissecting aneurysm of the carotid or vertebral/posterior cerebral arteries
  9. Subdural hematoma with rupture into the subarachnoid space
  10. Endometriosis of the spinal canal

in the anterior portion of the circle of Willis and 10 percent occur in the vertebrobasilar system. The most common sites for aneurysm formation are at the terminal portion of the internal carotid artery, the junction of the anterior cerebral and anterior communicating arteries, or at the origin of the middle cerebral artery (Fig. 9-1). The reported incidence of SAH has shown considerable variability in different countries, but death from SAH has been reported to be 15 to 16 per 100,000 per year in the United States.[1] The condition is more common in men under the age of 40 and has a higher incidence in women after the age of 50, but the overall incidence is equal in the two sexes. However, SAH occurs predominantly between ages 40 and 60, with a peak frequency between ages 55 and 65.[2] The rupture of a cerebral aneurysm is the most common cause of primary SAH, occurring in 70 to 90 percent of cases.[3] This figure has increased steadily in the last 30 years, as methods of detection have improved. Familial SAH, owing to a ruptured aneurysm, occurs in 5 to 10 percent of cases and is inherited as an autosomal dominant or autosomal recessive trait.[4] Hemorrhage tends to occur at a younger age in familial cases with a predilection for bleeding from aneurysms of the middle cerebral artery; furthermore the outcome tends to be worse in familial SAH when compared to sporadic SAH. Other conditions include bleeding from an AVM in 6 percent and "SAH of unknown cause" in 15 percent.[5]

Pathology

Two current theories address the development and rupture of cerebral aneurysms (excluding mycotic aneurysms)—an inherited or congenital weakness of the arterial wall or arteriosclerosis. An inherited abnormality of type III collagen was first suggested more than 20 years ago,[6] but recent studies have not provided support for this concept.[7] Nevertheless, the occurrence of familial cases of SAH caused by ruptured aneurysm and the occasional occurrence of a ruptured aneurysm in a child or adolescent tend to support the proposed relationship between congenital or inherited weakness of the vessel wall and aneurysm formation. In most cases, however, aneurysms are the result of a degenerative process in the arterial

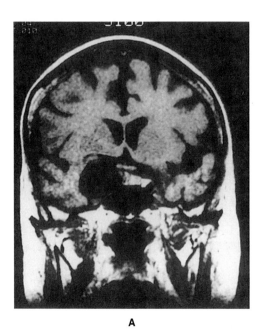
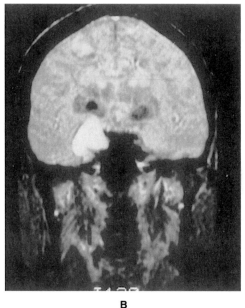

A   B

Figure 9-1
MRI scan coronal sections T1 (A) and T2 (B) weighted images showing a large aneurysm of the terminal portion of the right internal carotid artery.

wall and are classified as saccular aneurysms. Futhermore, atherosclerosis is postulated as the most important factor in the development and subsequent rupture of saccular aneurysms. The evidence is indirect, however, with a demonstration that a history of smoking,[8] elevated serum cholesterol levels, high apolipoprotein B concentrations, and hypertension[9] are risk factors in the rupture of cerebral aneurysms.[10-12] Recent heavy alcohol consumption carries a significant risk for aneurysm rupture and SAH, but alcohol drinking does not appear to be a risk factor for the process of aneurysm development.[13] The increased identification of risk factors for atherosclerosis suggests that atherosclerosis is an important factor in the development of saccular aneurysms before rupture. The predilection for saccular aneurysms to form at the bifurcation of major cerebral arteries strengthens the atherosclerotic hypothesis because atherosclerotic changes tend to develop primarily at these same sites (Fig. 9-2).

Pathological changes following SAH consist of staining of the subarachnoid space due to the presence of blood. The high-pressure jet of blood from a ruptured aneurysm frequently penetrates the brain parenchyma, forming an intracerebral hematoma. Occasionally the blood tears through the dura into the subdural space, creating a subdural hematoma. The brain may show evidence of edema and ischemic infarction secondary to interruption of blood supply due to arterial spasm or compression of the circle of Willis by a hematoma.

Microscopic examination of the site of a saccular aneurysm reveals that the internal elastic lamina terminates on either side, close to the aneurysm. The aneurysm has a very thin wall of fibrous tissue and is often lined by laminated blood clot. Areas of calcification may occur in long-standing aneurysms.

Clinical Features

The signs and symptoms of SAH caused by rupture of an aneurysm depend on the site of the aneurysm (Table 9-2).

Some patients have prodromal symptoms several days or weeks preceding aneurysm rupture. At least one-third experience the sudden onset of a severe headache lasting a few hours to several days and then subsiding. This symptom has been termed the "sentinel headache." However, sentinel headaches are rarely associated with cerebral aneurysm or SAH.[14] Intracavernous internal carotid aneurysms, or aneurysms arising at the junction of the internal carotid and posterior communicating arteries, may compress the third nerve in the lateral wall of the cavernous sinus, producing third nerve palsy with ptosis and involvement of the pupil. Similarly, pressure on the ophthalmic or maxillary division of the fifth cranial nerve in the lateral wall of the cavernous sinus produces orbital or facial pain. Focal motor seizures or partial complex partial seizures are a rare complication of large aneurysms that irritate the cortical gray matter.

Rupture of an aneurysm usually occurs when a patient is active and alert. Many patients give a history of onset while working or engaged in other activities such as athletics or sports.[15] Rupture of an aneurysm has been recorded during sexual intercourse, defecation, and immediately following micturition. Nevertheless, rupture can occur when the patient is asleep or quietly sitting and resting.

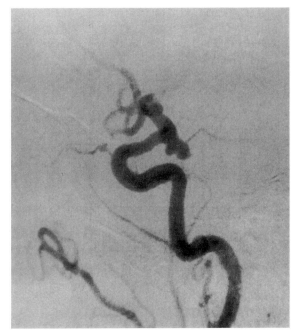

Figure 9-2
Cerebral arteriogram demonstrating a lobulated aneurysm arising at the origin of the posterior communicating artery from the internal carotid artery.

Table 9-2

Signs and symptoms of aneurysms according to site of origin

Origin of aneurysm	Structure involved	Signs and symptoms
Internal carotid, cavernous portion	Compression of cranial nerves III, IV, VI; compression of ophthalmic division of cranial nerve V; compression of pituitary; rupture into cavernous sinus producing an AV fistula	Mydriasis, diplopia, ptosis, trigeminal neuralgia, atypical facial pain, hypopituitarism, noise in the head
Internal carotid, supraclinoid portion	Compression of optic nerve, compression of optic chiasm, compression of cranial nerve III	Visual failure, optic atrophy, visual field defects, mydriasis, diplopia, ptosis
Ophthalmic artery	Compression of optic nerve, compression of pituitary	Visual failure, optic atrophy, hypopituitarism
Middle cerebral artery	Irritation of the cortex	Usually causes few signs and symptoms before rupture, partial seizures
Anterior cerebral artery	Compression of optic chiasm, compression of olfactory tract	Visual field defects, unilateral anosmia
Posterior communicating artery	Compression of cranial nerve III, compression of cranial nerve VI	Mydriasis, diplopia, ptosis
Posterior cerebral artery	Compression of the midbrain	Usually causes few signs and symptoms before rupture, hydrocephalus, stupor, akinetic mutism
Basilar artery	Compression of cranial nerve V, compression of cranial nerve VII, compression of midbrain	Trigeminal neuralgia, atypical facial pain, facial paralysis, hydrocephalus
Vertebral artery	Compression of cranial nerves IX, X, compression of brainstem	Paralysis of the palate, pharynx, dysphonia, dysphagia, vertigo, ataxia, vomiting

The onset of SAH from a ruptured aneurysm is sudden in about 90 percent of cases, and there is rapid loss of consciousness in 20 percent. The majority of patients complain of severe generalized headache with pain extending into the occipital and cervical region, with nuchal rigidity, photophobia, lethargy, altered mentation, nausea, and vomiting. Other symptoms include transient vertigo and a feeling of faintness or confusion. Seizures occurring within 12 h after bleeding are not uncommon. Pa-

tients occasionally report hearing loss, visual impairment, and diplopia. Many patients experience a brief loss of consciousness with gradual improvement, but a small number remain comatose from the onset of the illness. Onset with hemiparesis may mimic infarction. When first examined, most patients show some impairment of consciousness, lack of abnormal neurological signs or seizures, and the presence of nuchal rigidity, which should alert the examiner to the probability of subarachnoid hemorrhage.[16] Funduscopic examination may reveal the presence of a subhyaloid hemorrhage and papilledema may develop within 6 h of the onset of SAH.

About 10 percent of patients with SAH due to ruptured aneurysm have a more gradual onset, with evolution of symptoms over a period ranging from several hours to several days. Although severe headache is a major complaint in the great majority of conscious patients, not all patients report headache, and approximately 2 percent of patients are headache free.

Complications

1. Arterial vasospasm occurs in approximately 30 percent of cases of SAH and has a peak incidence 6 to 8 days postbleed. However, it can occur from 4 to 12 days after aneurysm rupture.[17] Once vasospasm develops, it can persist for several days to several weeks.

Patients with a large volume of blood in the basal cisterns carry the highest risk of spasm.[18] Blood in the sylvian fissure indicates intermediate risk.[19] About 12 percent of patients with extensive vasospasm will develop permanent neurological deficits or die.

The pathogenesis of vasospasm is obscure. It probably related to the presence of oxyhemoglobin in the subarachnoid blood clot,[20] leading to the release of cytokines that stimulate release of endothelin, an agent known to cause vasospasm. Increased concentrations of endothelin have been demonstrated in plasma and cerebrospinal fluid (CSF) after SAH.[21]

An alternative hypothesis proposes that the presence of blood in the subarachnoid space leads to inflammation and the release of platelet activating factor from inflammatory cells, platelets, and vascular endothelium, resulting in contraction of the muscle in cerebral arterial walls and vasospasm.[22]

2. Rebleeding following ruptured aneurysm is maximum in the first 24 h with a cumulative risk of about 20 percent in the next 14 days. Rebleeding results in death in about 60 percent of affected cases.

3. Intracerebral hematoma can produce a contralateral homonymous hemianopia and hemiparesis.

4. A subdural hematoma may result from rupture of an aneurysm into the subdural space.[23]

5. Acute hydrocephalus is the result of occlusion of the subarachnoid space by breakdown products of red blood cell disintegration and the ensuing inflammatory response. Hydrocephalus occurs in more than 50 percent of cases of SAH within 30 days of the hemorrhage but can occur quickly within a period of several hours following SAH. Ventricular peritoneal shunting may be required in those who show delayed neurological deterioration and persistent ventricular enlargement.[24]

6. Cardiac arrhythmias and in some cases cardiac injury[25] with pulmonary edema presumably the result of cerebral or brainstem injury are recognized complications of SAH.[26]

7. Inappropriate secretion of antidiuretic hormone may occur in severe SAH or as a postoperative complication. Some patients develop hyponatremia due to inhibition of renal tubular sodium absorption rather than inappropriate secretion of antidiuretic hormone.

8. Pulmonary and urinary tract infections, dehydration, electrolyte disturbances, and the development of decubiti are not unusual in comatosed patients.

9. Epilepsy develops in 9 percent of patients who survive SAH, occurring within 4 weeks after the hemorrhage in the majority of cases.[27]

Diagnostic Procedures

1. Computed tomography (CT) scanning is the procedure of choice in the diagnosis of SAH and will confirm the diagnosis in 85 percent of cases, if this study is performed within 48 h of bleeding. A CT scan will reveal blood in the basal cisterns in most patients with SAH (Fig. 9-3), and the extent of an intracerebral hematoma, cerebral infarction, cerebral edema, and acute hydrocephalus are readily demonstrated. Intraventricular and intracerebral bleeding and hydrocephalus have adverse effects on survival. Localized thick or diffuse collections of subarachnoid blood in the basal cisterns are associated with a high risk of vasospasm and a poorer prognosis.[28] Aneurysms are occasionally seen in an enhanced CT scan (Fig. 9-4).

2. Magnetic resonance imaging (MRI) scanning has no advantage in the diagnosis in the early

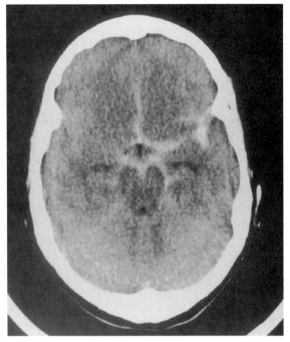

Figure 9-3
CT scan with contrast enhancement taken in the emergency center in a patient with subarachnoid hemorrhage. The basal cisterns, interhemispheric fissure, and the left sylvian fissure are displayed prominently by accumulating blood.

stages of SAH. However, MRI may detect the site of blood clot when it is no longer detectable by CT and is useful in detecting the probable source of hemorrhage in cases with multiple aneurysms.[29] Magnetic resonance angiography should always be performed in cases of SAH when cerebral angiography fails to demonstrate an aneurysm and is regarded as the superior technique when compared to digital subtraction angiography in some centers.[30]

3.   Lumbar puncture reveals a bloody CSF under increased pressure. The supernatant fluid is xanthochromic within 6 h of SAH. There is a polymorphonuclear pleocytosis within 24 h, and later, appearance of mononuclear cells. Red blood cells usually disappear from the CSF by 5 days; their persistence indicates that further hemorrhage has occurred. Xanthochromia usually lasts for about 28 days. An estimate of the date of onset of SAH can be

made by measuring the presence of oxyhemoglobin and bilirubin in the xanthochromic fluid by CSF spectrophotometry. Oxyhemoglobin appears at the onset of SAH and gradually disappears. Bilirubin appears after 2 or 3 days and increases in amount as oxyhemoglobin decreases. Recurrent hemorrhage is associated with a late rise in the presence of oxyhemoglobin. Lumbar puncture continues to have an important role in the diagnosis of SAH.[31]

4.   Skull x-rays occasionally show the presence of calcification in the wall of an aneurysm. Erosion of the lateral wall of the sella or anterior clinoid processes may occur. Pineal shift occurs in the presence of a large hematoma. An ophthalmic aneurysm can cause enlargement of the optic foramen.

5.   Four-vessel arteriography with multiple views to demonstrate the origin of each of the major intracranial arteries should be performed as early as possible in all cases of SAH (Fig. 9-5). The objective of this study is the demonstration of the origin of the aneurysm to define the neck of the aneurysm, and to detect the presence of multiple aneurysms (Fig. 9-6),

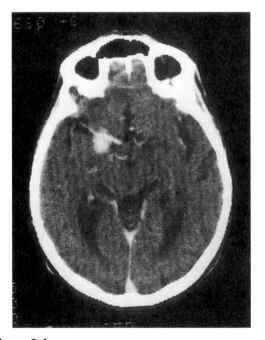

Figure 9-4
CT scan with contrast enhancement showing a saccular aneurysm of the right middle cerebral artery.

or demonstrate the presence or absence of vasospasm. The complication rate of arteriography performed by an experienced neuroradiologist, using modern techniques, is less than 1 percent. Rebleeding from a ruptured aneurysm during arteriography is rare, occurring in less than 3 percent of cases. The risk of

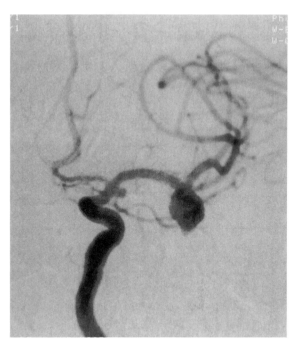

Figure 9-6
Cerebral arteriogram. There is a large aneurysm located at the junction of the M1 and M2 segments of the left middle cerebral artery and a small aneurysm rising at the terminal portion of the left internal carotid artery.

rebleeding is significantly higher during the first 6 h after the initial event.[32] Consequently, it is prudent to delay arteriography for at least 6 h after the initial hemorrhage.

6. CT angiography. High-quality CT angiography provides adequate depiction of aneurysms in 90 percent of cases allowing surgery to be performed on the basis of CT angiography alone.[33]

7. Transcranial Doppler ultrasound monitoring is a useful procedure in the detection of vasospasm leading to delayed ischemic neurological deficits complicating SAH.[34]

Differential Diagnosis

1. Migraine headache. The first "migraine headache" in a young individual may be confused with a SAH. An MRI or CT scan and a lumbar

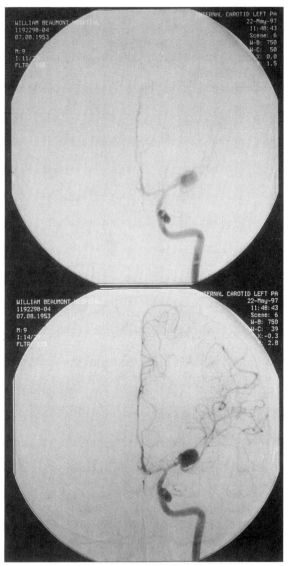

Figure 9-5
Serial arteriograms of an aneurysm located at the junction of the M1 and M2 segments of the left middle cerebral artery.

puncture should be performed if the diagnosis is in doubt. A CT scan is sufficient to exclude 97.5 percent of SAH in patients presenting to the emergency center with a "worst ever" headache.[35]

2.   Systemic infection. Some systemic infections such as influenza can be associated with severe headache. Lumbar puncture will reveal a normal CSF in such cases, and this procedure should always be performed if there is any doubt about the diagnosis.

3.   Acute meningitis or encephalitis. The acute onset of severe headache and nuchal rigidity occurs in these acute inflammatory conditions and also occurs in SAH. Lumbar puncture should be performed because of the presence of nuchal rigidity and will establish the correct diagnosis.

4.   Hypertensive encephalopathy. Patients with severe hypertension may present with severe headache. Systemic evidence of hypertension, such as hypertensive retinopathy, cardiac enlargement, and proteinuria are usually present. There is no nuchal rigidity.

5.   Cervical arthritis. This condition may be present in patients who develop acute headache from other causes such as migraine. The neck stiffness is present in all directions of head movement and is not of recent onset.

6.   Intracerebral hemorrhage. The acute onset of hemiparesis may occasionally occur following forceful rupture of an aneurysm into the brain parenchyma or result from the development of vasospasm. Most cases with SAH will have severe headache and nuchal rigidity. Magnetic resonance imaging or CT scan and lumbar puncture will establish the correct diagnosis in most cases, but arteriography may be necessary to differentiate between spontaneous intracerebral hemorrhage and ruptured aneurysm.

Treatment

Surgical Treatment   The majority of neurosurgeons believe that patients with ruptured cerebral aneurysm and SAH who have a normal neurological examination, or who show mild impairment of consciousness or mild focal neurological deficits (Hunt-

Hess classification grades 1–3),[36,37] should undergo surgery to obliterate the ruptured aneurysm, prevent rebleeding, and remove subarachnoid clot, thus minimizing the development of vasospasm.

The belief that early surgery precipitates vasospasm and cerebral infarction has not been substantiated and at least 30 percent of patients develop vasospasm as a result of the initial hemorrhage.[38] The operative mortality rate in poorer grade patients (grades 4 and 5) is high, approaching 75 percent. Early surgical treatment is precluded in such cases[39] and there is a mandatory delay until clinical improvement occurs. However, there is recognition that early surgery can produce quality survival in a higher percentage of patients with poor grade SAH when associated with immediate measures to relieve intracranial pressure (ICP), to evacuate an intracerebral or subdural hematoma, and to relieve acute hydrocephalus.[40] In addition, early surgery prevents rebleeding, which is often catastrophic,[41] with the highest incidence of 4 percent within the first 48 h after the initial hemorrhage and a mortality rate of 70 percent. Although early surgery only marginally improves survival, the quality of life of the survivors is significantly better.[42]

The preoperative management of patients with ruptured cerebral aneurysm is an important factor in achieving good surgical results and includes the use of antihypertensive agents, cerebral selective calcium channel blocking drugs such as nimodipine,[43] and adequate analgesia, as described in "Medical Management." Postoperative management, including treatment of vasospasm, is covered in the same section.

Medical Management   A number of circumstances may delay or contraindicate immediate surgical intervention for, and treatment of, an aneurysm following SAH. About 20 percent of cases are the result of a nonaneurysmal SAH from various other causes (see Table 9-1), which require appropriate treatment, depending on the diagnosis and basic medical management. Other reasons for medical management include impaired levels of consciousness, ranging from stupor to coma, plus moderate- to -severe neurological deficits (Hunt-Hess classification grades

4 and 5); delay in diagnosis for several days with concomitant illness, including pneumonia, heart disease, or renal insufficiency; demonstrable arterial spasm on arteriography; and patients or next of kin who refuse to give permission for surgery. Under these circumstances, medical management is recommended as follows:

1. At least 3 weeks of strict bed rest with adequate nursing care is a necessity.
2. Adequate use of narcotics in the conscious patient. Most patients will require morphine 15 mg intramuscularly q4h p.r.n. for control of severe headache. Lesser doses are inadequate. Subarachnoid hemorrhage produces one of the most severe and distressing headaches known, and it is unfortunate that headaches are often inadequately treated.
3. In addition to narcotics, patients may require the regular administration of phenothiazine or barbiturate to allay restlessness.
4. Hypertension should be controlled unless there are signs of increasing cerebral vasospasm.
5. Cerebral edema should be controlled by ICP monitoring and mannitol 1 g/kg in a 20% solution over 20 min. The mannitol should be repeated as necessary to maintain an ICP reading below 20 mmHg measured at the level of the foramen of Monro (midhead) in a supine patient. Sustained rise in ICP suggests acute hydrocephalus, which will require surgical intervention and ventricular drainage. Because early detection of hydrocephalus, or rebleeding, is essential, serial CT scans are performed on a daily basis until the patient shows signs of improvement. Mortality is significantly higher in patients with acute hydrocephalus and early detection is imperative.[44] Consequently, when hydrocephalus is causing clinical deterioration, external ventricular drainage is indicated. This can be discontinued gradually once the CSF is clear. In a few cases, the procedure fails and a temporary ventricular peritoneal shunt is required.
6. Interarterial embolization using Gugliemi detractable coils is now a well-established method of treatment for surgically inaccessible aneurysms or in cases with vasospasm and poor-grade clinical status.[45]
7. Progressive neurological deficits due to cerebral vasospasm occur in 30 percent of patients with SAH from a ruptured cerebral aneurysm, and this complication carries significant morbidity and mortality. The calcium channel blocking agent nimodipine has been reported to prevent vasospasm and to improve neurological outcome in patients with neurological deficits associated with vasospasm. A dose of 60 mg nimodipine q4h for 21 days, beginning immediately after admission to the hospital, is recommended. Treatment with hypervolemic therapy is recommended, requiring the use of an indwelling arterial catheter for blood pressure monitoring, a Swan-Ganz catheter to measure pulmonary capillary wedge pressure, transcutaneous pulse oximetry to detect signs of early pulmonary decompensation from hypervolemic therapy, hourly assessment of fluid balance, and daily chest films to detect incipient congestive heart failure or pulmonary edema. Treatment begins with infusion of plasma protein fractionate to create positive fluid balance of 1 to 2 L, at the same time, maintaining the pulmonary artery wedge pressure between 18 to 20 mmHg and central venous pressure at 10 mmHg. If volume expansion fails to produce clinical improvement, arterial blood pressure is elevated to a systolic pressure of 180 to 220 mmHg, using intravenous dopamine. This should be combined with monitoring of cerebral blood flow to assess increased blood flow in ischemic areas of the brain, and occasionally paradoxical decrease in cerebral blood flow in nonischemic areas in some cases, which could have a deleterious effect.[46] However, blood pressure elevation should be restricted to cases of postoperative vasospasm with successful surgical obliteration of the ruptured aneurysm.

Other methods of treating vasospasm include selective intraarterial infusion of 300 mg papaverine hydrochloride over 1 h into the vessels exhibiting vasospasm but results have been equivocal in some studies[47] and repeated papaverine infusion may be necessary to prevent recurrence of vasospasm.[48] Papaverine infusion is not as effective as balloon angiography in the treatment of vasospasm.[49] Transluminal balloon angioplasty has also been used with some success,[50] but the rate of delayed ischemic infarction is higher in endovascular treatment than in early surgical treatment probably the result of the presence of unremoved blood in endovascular cases.[51] Intrathecal thrombolytic therapy with urokinase or tissue plasminogen activator, infused into the basal cisterns immediately after surgery, with continuous irrigation and drainage of the subarachnoid space for 7 days, accelerates blood clot lysis and reduces the incidence of cerebral vasospasm and cerebral infarction.[52]

8. Endovascular treatment with Guglielmi coils should be considered in patients with giant aneurysms, fusiform aneurysms,[53] and in those with a Hess-Hunt grade 3 to 5, or when surgery is contraindicated because of other complications.[54] Patients with moderate deficits after SAH have similar outcomes following open surgery or embolization of unruptured or ruptured aneurysms.[55] There is a risk of further SAH during embolization, but the incidence is low.[56]

9. Continuous cardiac monitoring should be performed, irrespective of early or delayed surgical treatment, because 90 percent of patients develop cardiac arrhythmias, of which 50 percent are serious and require prompt treatment.[57,58] A neurogenically mediated cardiac injury, possibly due to massive sympathetic discharge, can give rise to left ventricular decompensation and sudden onset of pulmonary edema after SAH.[59]

10. Seizures occur in 10 to 20 percent of cases, shortly after SAH, and should be controlled by anticonvulsant medication.[60] Early seizures rarely persist or recur and bear no relationship to the subsequent development of epilepsy.

11. Hyponatremia secondary to inappropriate secretion of antidiuretic hormone is not unusual in patients who have more than minor neurological deficits. Treatment with fluid restriction should be instituted if possible, unless hypervolemic therapy is needed for cerebral vasospasm, when intravenous fluids with high sodium content can be infused.

Care After Recovery

All patients who have suffered a ruptured aneurysm and SAH require close follow-up after discharge from the hospital. Symptoms of increasing headache, lethargy, decreasing mentation, or increasing neurological deficits should alert the physician to the possibility of hydrocephalus. Seizures can occur, with onset days to months after the hemorrhage, and require appropriate anticonvulsant therapy.

Prognosis

The outcome of SAH following rupture of an aneurysm varies from center to center but the fatality rate has decreased in the last three decades due to improved management of patients with SAH.[61] This may be related to the fact that at least 12 percent of patients die before they receive medical attention.[62] In addition, elevated glucose levels on admission predict a higher risk of death and a poorer outcome.[63] In general, it can be said that 30 percent of patients die within 24 h and 40 percent die within 7 days. Of the survivors, 50 percent will have a second SAH, which carries a 40 percent mortality rate; 60 percent of patients with SAH caused by ruptured aneurysm die within 6 months of the initial bleed. The risk of rebleeding in survivors is low after 6 months and approximately 1 percent of survivors eventually rebleed each year.[64] However, patients with aneurysm or SAH have significant neurological complications in 50 percent of cases and those with a good neurological outcome often have neuropsychological deficits when examined with a battery of cognitive tests.[61] Short-term memory impairment occurs in more than 50 percent, and 21 percent have reduced long-term memory. Other problems include disability in complex choice reaction and concentration; 10 percent have dysphasic language disturbances.[65] Less than half of surviving patients who were fully employed at the time of the SAH return to full-time employment 12 months after the hemorrhage.[66] Cognitive dysfunction is significantly worse in older patients than in younger patients examined 3 to 4 years after aneurysmal SAH.[67] Given the poor prognosis for ruptured saccular aneurysms, the use of preventative surgery should be considered in those with unruptured aneurysms. Clipping of these aneurysms has a mortality of 2.6 percent and morbidity of 10.5 percent.[68]

ARTERIOVENOUS MALFORMATION

Definition

An AVM is a congenital nonneoplastic mass composed of tortuous blood vessels that apparently results from agenesis of an interposing capillary system. The condition is occasionally inherited as an autosomal dominant trait.[69]

Etiology and Pathology

The absence of an intervening capillary bed permits a greatly decreased vascular resistance, and the abnormal vessels undergo progressive dilatation. Most AVMs (90 percent) are supratentorial and are located in the parietal cortex (Figs. 9-7 and 9-8). However, AVMs can occur anywhere in the brain or spinal cord. They consist of thin-walled dilated communications between arterial and venous systems. The surrounding brain shows staining, numerous small hemorrhages, and gliosis with the disruption of surrounding neurons.

Clinical Features

Partial or generalized seizures occur in 18 percent of cases.[70] Other patients report migraine-like headaches on the side of the malformation. The neurological examination may reveal the presence of focal deficits, including homonymous hemianopia, dysphasia, and hemiparesis. Often a bruit can be heard on auscultation over the orbit or skull.

The risk of bleeding from an AVM is 3 to 4 percent per year, or 30 to 40 percent per decade. The risk of death is 1 percent per year and of serious morbidity, 2 percent per year. AVMs of the posterior fossa have a higher morbidity and mortality if untreated compared to those localized in the supratentorial compartment.[71] Small AVMs with a nidus diameter of less than 3 cm carry a higher risk of bleeding than large AVMs.[72] Contrary to previously held opinions, there is no increased risk of SAH from an AVM dur-

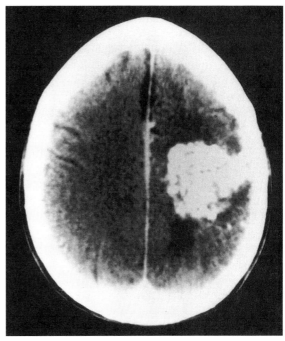

Figure 9-7
Enhanced CT scan showing an area of increased density in the left parietal area. A large arteriovenous malformation causing right-sided partial motor seizures and occasionally generalized seizures.

ing pregnancy. Consequently, surgery for an unruptured AVM should be performed postpartum.

Diagnostic Procedures

As for aneurysm.

Treatment

Seizures should be controlled with adequate anticonvulsant therapy with serial measurements of plasma anticonvulsant levels.

The medical treatment of SAH from rupture of an AVM is the same as the treatment described for aneurysms. Surgical treatment of an unruptured AVM is indicated when the risk of surgical intervention is significantly less than no treatment. The risk can be assessed with a grading system that uses the angiographic characteristics of the malformation to

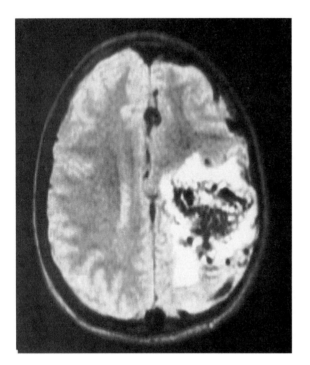
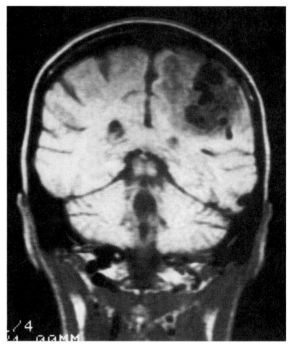
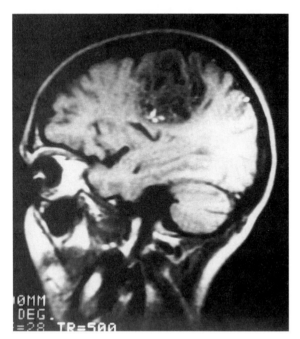

Figure 9-8
MRI scan showing a large arteriovenous malformation in the left parietal area. Dilated vessels can be seen at the periphery and within the substance of the malformation. The same patient is shown in Figure 9-7.

estimate the difficulties of resection. The three criteria are:

1. The size of the nidus in the AVM
   a. Less than 3 cm — 1 point
   b. Between 3 to 6 cm — 2 points
   c. Greater than 6 cm — 3 points
2. Neurological function of the adjacent cortex
   a. Functional — 1 point
   b. Nonfunctional — 0 points
3. Anatomy of venous drainage — drainage into the deep venous system — 1 point

Although some of these points give a grade between 1 and 5, studies have shown that there is no major morbidity associated with resection of grades 1 and 2 AVMs, 4 percent morbidity with a resection of grade 3 lesions, 7 percent morbidity with grade 4 lesions, and 22 percent with grade 5 lesions. The results suggest that resection of all grade 1 to 2 lesions should be recommended unless medically contraindicated, and most grade 4 lesions are resectable.

In some cases, surgical treatment with extubation of an AVM may be preceded by embolization with small plastic beads, injection of a polymerizing glue, or embolization with detractable coils[73] which reduces the size of the malformation and renders the subsequent operation more feasible (see Fig. 9-8).

Venous Angiomas

These malformations consist of anomalous veins providing normal venous drainage from the brain. They are identified frequently by MRI scanning and are benign developmental anomalies that rarely bleed. Consequently, surgical treatment is not indicated.[74]

Cavernous Malformations

Cavernous malformations are circumscribed lesions lying within the brain, composed of multiple thin-walled vessels without smooth muscle, and absence of interposing brain parenchyma. These malformations constitute 10 to 15 percent of vascular malformations in the brain, brainstem, and spinal cord. Some 50 percent of cavernous malformations are familial. Hemorrhage from a cavernous malformation is rare[75] in sporadic cases, and somewhat more common in familial cases. About 50 percent of patients have seizures without evidence of hemorrhage, 45 percent have neurological deficits, and 30 percent have headaches.[76]

Surgical treatment should be considered when seizures are poorly controlled and when there is a progressive neurological deficit.

Dural Arteriovenous Malformations

This subgroup of AVMs with a nidus located within the dura can rupture and cause a devastating SAH. This is more likely to occur when the lesion is located in the anterior cranial fossa or near the incisura of the tentorium cerebelli,[77] or when there is prominent venous drainage with varicocele dilatation or aneurysm formation.[78] Surgical extubation is recommended in such cases, or following SAH, and in patients with unacceptable bruits or intractable headaches.

MYCOTIC ANEURYSMS

Definition

A *mycotic aneurysm* is an aneurysm that results from infection of, and subsequent weakening of, an arterial wall.

Etiology and Pathology

The repeated introduction of bacterial organisms into the bloodstream by drug addicts who use contaminated syringes and needles results in subacute bacterial endocarditis and septic embolism. Septic emboli nearly always lodge in the middle cerebral artery, producing a low-grade infection of the arterial wall with formation of one or more mycotic aneurysms.

Clinical Features

Mycotic aneurysms of the middle cerebral artery were common at the turn of the century, but the incidence decreased with the declining incidence of rheumatic fever and subacute bacterial endocarditis. The condition became rare after the introduction of antibiotics, but identification of mycotic aneurysms in drug addicts has increased in the last 20 years. Most cases of mycotic aneurysm remain undetected until the patient presents with SAH. The symptoms have been described in the discussion of ruptured aneurysms.

Diagnostic Procedures

1. As for ruptured aneurysm
2. The infecting organism may be identified by repeated blood cultures

Treatment

1. As for SAH following rupture of an aneurysm
2. Subacute bacterial endocarditis must be treated with the appropriate antibiotic therapy, and many weeks of antibiotic treatment may be necessary
3. Some aneurysms heal and disappear after antibiotic therapy. If the aneurysm persists, it may be treated surgically. However, in many cases, the surgical approach is difficult and it is preferable to follow the patient with repeated MRI scans[79]

Prognosis

The prognosis of ruptured mycotic aneurysms is poor once SAH has occurred, and most patients die following this complication. Unruptured mycotic aneurysms, however, often respond to antibiotic therapy or can be treated by interval surgery, if they increase in size, with good results.

SUBARACHNOID HEMORRHAGE— CAUSE UNKNOWN

It is not possible to determine the cause of SAH in about 10 percent of cases. The possibility of one of the rarer causes of SAH should be considered[80,81] (see Table 9-1), but investigation will not identify a cause in most cases when arteriography fails to reveal aneurysm or AVM. Because the false-negative rate of four-vessel arteriography is less than 2 percent, repeated studies are usually recommended after re-

bleeding, which occurs in about 10 percent of cases provided that the cerebral arteriogram is technically satisfactory. Subarachnoid hemorrhage of unknown etiology is a relatively benign disease with an early mortality rate of less than 5 percent, and a normal functioning capacity in about 90 percent of cases, after many years of follow-up.[82]

A distinct form of SAH, presenting with headache and a normal neurological examination, in which the bleeding is confined to the perimesencephalic or prepontine cisterns, has been described. The cerebral arteriogram is normal. This perimesencephalic hemorrhage has been regarded as a benign variant of SAH, with an excellent prognosis.[83] Although the bleeding may be venous or capillary in some cases, the hemorrhage can be the result of rupture of a small aneurysm in the vertebrobasilar system, and the perimesencephalic SAH should not be regarded as invariably benign.[84]

ARTERIOSCLEROTIC ANEURYSMS

An arteriosclerotic aneurysm is a dilatation of an arteriosclerotic cerebral vessel. Arteriosclerotic aneurysms usually occur in elderly patients. These aneurysms do not rupture and bleed but may exert pressure on surrounding structures. Arteriosclerotic aneurysms of the basilar artery can compress cranial nerves, particularly the fifth and seventh cranial nerves, producing neurological symptoms. Pressure from an arteriosclerotic aneurysm located on the terminal portion of the internal carotid artery on the optic nerve may cause optic atrophy on one side.

REFERENCES

1. Sahs A, Perret GE, Locksley HB, (eds) et al: *Intracranial aneurysm and subarachnoid hemorrhage:* a cooperative study. Philadelphia, Lippincott, 1969.
2. Locksley HB: Cooperative clinical study of intracranial aneurysms and subarachnoid hemorrhage. Sect 5 P1 natural history of subarachnoid hemorrhage. *Neurology* 2:162, 1961.
3. Sacco RL, Wolf PA, Bharucha NE, et al: Subarachnoid and intracerebral hemorrhage: natural history, progno-

sis, and precursor factors in the Framington study. *Neurology* 34:847, 1984.

4. Bromberg JEC, Rinkel GDE, Algra A, et al: Outcome in familial subarachnoid hemorrhage. *Stroke* 26:961, 1995.

5. Jafar JJ, Weiner HL: Surgery for angiographically occult cerebral aneurysms. *J Neurosurg* 79:674, 1993.

6. Pope FM, Nicholls AC, Narcisi P, et al: Some patients with cerebral aneurysms are deficient in Type III collagen. *Lancet* 1:973, 1981.

7. Adamson J, Humphries SE, Ostergaard MA, et al: Are cerebral aneurysms atherosclerotic? *Stroke* 25:963, 1994.

8. Weir BK, Kongable GL, Kassell NF, et al: Cigarette smoking as a cause of aneurysmal subarachnoid hemorrhage and risk of vasospasm: a report of the Cooperative Aneurysm Study. *J Neurosurg* 89:405, 1998.

9. Asari SS, Ohmoto T: Natural history and risk factors of unruptured serosal aneurysms. *Clin Neurol Neurosurg* 95:205, 1998.

10. Shinton R, Beevers G: Meta analysis of relation between cigarette smoking and stroke. *BMJ* 298:789, 1989.

11. Morris KM, Shaw MD, Foy PM: Smoking and subarachnoid hemorrhage: a case control study. *Br J Neurosurg* 6:429, 1992.

12. Longstreth WT, Nelson LM, Koepsell TD, et al: Cigarette smoking, alcohol use, and subarachnoid hemorrhage. *Stroke* 23:1242, 1992.

13. Juvela S, Hillbom M, Numminen M, et al: Cigarette smoking and alcohol consumption as risk factors for aneurysmal subarachnoid hemorrhage. *Stroke* 24:639, 1993.

14. Linn FH, Wijdicks EF, Vander Graf Y, et al: Prospective study of sentinel headache in aneurysmal subarachnoid hemorrhage. *Lancet* 344:590, 1994.

15. Haykowsky MJ, Findley JM, Ignaszweski AP: Aneurysmal subarachnoid hemorrhage associated with weight training: three case reports. *Clin J Sport Med* 6:52, 1996.

16. Talavera JO, Wacher NH, Laredo F, et al: Predictive value of signs and symptoms in the diagnosis of subarachnoid hemorrhage among stroke patients. *Arch Med Research* 27:353, 1996.

17. Macdonald RL, Wallace MC, Coyne TJ: The effect of surgery on the severity of vasospasm. *J Neurosurg* 80:433, 1994.

18. Kopitnik TA, Samson DS: Management subarachnoid hemorrhage. *J Neurol Neurosurg Psychiatry* 56:947, 1993.

19. Kistler JP, Cromwell RM, Davis KR, et al: The relation of cerebral vasospasm to the extent and location of subarachnoid hemorrhage visualized by CT scan. A prospective study. *Neurology* 33:424, 1983.

20. Macdonald RL, Weir BK: A review of hemoglobin and pathogensis of vasospasm. *Stroke* 22:971, 1991.

21. Suzuki H, Sato S, Suzuki Y, et al: Increased endothelin concentrations in CSF from patients with subarachnoid hemorrhage. *Acta Neurol Scand* 81:553, 1990.

22. Hiroshima Y, Endo S, Olmon T, et al: Platelet activating factor (PAF) concentration and PAF acetylhydroxylase activity in cerebrospinal fluid of patients with subarachnoid hemorrhage. *J Neurosurg* 80:31, 1994.

23. Shen WC, Cho DY, Lee CC: Acute subdural hematoma with subarachnoid hemorrhage caused by an intracranial aneurysm: a case report. *Chung Hua I, Hsueh Tsa Chih* (Taipan) 61:358, 1998.

24. Black P. Hydrocephalus and vasospasm after subarachnoid hemorrhage from rupured intracranial aneurysms, *Neurosurgery* 18:12, 1986.

25. Mayer SA, Fink ME, Homma S: Cardiac injury associated with neurogenic pulmonary edema following subarachnoid hemorrhage. *Neurology* 44:815, 1994.

26. Svigeli V, Grad A, Tekavcic I, et al: Cardiac arrhythmias associated with reversible damage to the insula in a patient with subarachnoid hemorrhage. *Stroke* 23:1053, 1994.

27. Hasan D, Schonck RS, Avezaat CJ, et al: Epileptic seizures after subarachnoid hemorrhage. *Ann Neurol* 33:286, 1993.

28. Adams HP, Kassell NF, Tomer JC: Usefulness of computed tomography in predicting outcome after aneurysmal subarachnoid hemorrhage: a preliminary report of the Cooperative Aneurysm Study. *Neurology* 35:1263, 1985.

29. Hackney DB, Lesnick JE, Zimmerman RA, et al: MR Identification of bleeding site in subarachnoid hemorrhage with multiple intracranial aneurysms. *J Comput Assist Tomogr* 10:878, 1986.

30. Koegh AJ, Vhora S: The usefulness of magnetic resonance angiography in surgery for intracranial aneurysms that have bled. *Surg Neurol* 50:122, 1998.

31. Wasserberg J, Barlow P: Lesson of the week. Lumbar puncture still has an important role in diagnosing subarachnoid hemorrhage. *BMJ* 315:1598, 1997.

32. Komiyama M, Tamura K, Nagata Y, et al: Aneurysmal rupture during angiography. *Neurosurgery* 33:798, 1993.

33. Velthuis BK, Rinkell GJ, Ramos LM, et al: Subarachnoid hemorrhage: aneurysm detection and preoperative

evaluation with CT angiography. *Radiology* 208:423, 1998.

34. Wardlaw JM, Offin R, Teasdale GM, et al: Is routine transcranial Doppler ultrasonography monitoring useful in the management of subarachnoid hemorrhage?. *J Neurosurg* 88:272, 1998.

35. Morgenstern LB, Luna-Gonzales H, Huber JC Jr, et al: Worst headache and subarachnoid hemorrhage: prospective modern computed tomography and spinal fluid analysis. *Ann Emerg Med* 32 (3 Pt 1):297, 1998.

36. Hunt WE, Hess RM: Surgical risk as related to time of intervention in the repair of intracranial aneurysm. *J Neurosurg* 28:14, 1968.

37. Krupp W, Heienbrok W, Muke R: Management results attained by predominantly late surgery for intracranial aneurysms. *Neurosurgery* 34:227, 1994.

38. Bell TE, Kongable GL: Innovations in aneurysmal subarachnoid hemorrhage: intracisternal t-PA for the prevention of vasospasm. *J Neuroscience Nursing* 28:107, 1996.

39. Kassel NF, Torner JC: Aneurysmal rebleeding: a preliminary report from the cooperative aneurysm study. *Neurosurgery* 13:479, 1983.

40. Duke BJ, Kindt GW, Breeze RE: Outcome after urgent surgery for grade IV subarachnoid hemorrhage. *Surg Neurol* 50:169, 1998.

41. Roos YB, Beenen LF, Groen RJ, et al: Timing of surgery in patients with aneurysmal subarachnoid hemorrhage: rebleeding is still the major cause of poor outcome in neurosurgical units that aim at early surgery. *J Neurol Neurosurg Psychiatry* 63:490, 1997.

42. Fogelholm R, Hernesniemi J, Volpalahti M: Impact of early surgery on outcome of aneurysmal subarachnoid hemorrhage: a population based study. *Stroke* 24:1649, 1993.

43. Pichard JD, Murray GD, Illingworth R, et al: Effect of oral nimodipine or cerebral infarction and outcome after subarachnoid hemorrhage: British aneurysm nimodipine trial. *BMJ* 298:636, 1989.

44. van Gijn JV, Hijdra A, Wijdicks EF, et al: Acute hydrocephalus after aneurysmal subarachnoid hemorrhage. *J Neurosurg* 63:335, 1985.

45. Murayama Y, Malisch T, Gugliemi G, et al: Incidence of cerebral vasospasm after endovascular treatment of acutely ruptured aneurysms: report on 69 cases. *J Neurosurg* 87:830, 1997.

46. Darby JM, Yones M, Marks EC, et al: Acute cerebral blood flow response to dopamine-induced hypertension after subarachnoid hemorrhage. *J Neurosurg* 80:857, 1994.

47. Polin RS, Hansen CA, German P, et al: Intra- arterially

adminstered papaverine for the treatment of symptomatic cerebral vasospasm. *Neurosurgery* 42:1256, 1998.

48. Numaguchi Y, Zoarski GH, Clouston JE, et al: Repeat intra-arterial papaverine for recurrent cerebral vasospasm after subarachnoid hemorrhage. *Neuroradiology* 39:751, 1997.

49. Elliott JP, Newell DW, Lam DJ, et al: Comparison of balloon angioplasty and papaverine infusion for the treatment of vasospasm following aneurysmal subarachnoid hemorrhage. *J Neurosurg* 88:277, 1998.

50. Bejjani GK, Bank WO, Olan WJ, et al: The efficacy and safety of angioplasty for cerebral vasospasm after subarachnoid hemorrhage. *Neurosurgery* 42:979, 1998.

51. Gruber A, Ungersbock K, Reinprecht A, et al: Evaluation of cerebral vasospasm after early surgery and endovascular treatment of ruptured intracranial aneurysms. *Neurosurgery* 42:258, 1998.

52. Usui M, Saito N, Hoya K, et al: Vasospasm prevention with postoperative intrathecal thrombolytic therapy: a retrospective comparison of urokinase, tissue plasminogen activator, and cisternal drainage alone. *Neurosurgery* 34:235, 1994.

53. Higashida RT, Smith W, Gress D, et al: Intravascular stent and endovascular coil placement for a ruptured fusiform aneurysm of the basilar artery. Case report and a review of the literature. *J Neurosurg* 87:944, 1997.

54. Casasco AE, Aymard A, Gobin AA, et al: Selective endovascular treatment of 71 intracranial aneurysms with platinum coils. *J Neurosurg* 79:3, 1993.

55. Leber KA, Klein GE, Trummer M, et al: Intracranial aneurysms: a review of endovascular and surgical treatment in 248 patients. *Minim Invasive Neurosurg* 41:81, 1998.

56. McDougall CG, Halback VV, Dowd CF, et al: Causes and management of aneurysmal hemorrhage occurring during embolization with Guglielmi detachable coils. *J Neurosurg* 89:87, 1998.

57. Andreoli A, DePasquale G, Pinelli G, et al: Subarachnoid hemorrhage: frequency and severity of cardiac arrhythmias. *Stroke* 18:558, 1987.

58. Asplin BR, White RD: Subarachnoid hemorrhage: atypical presentation associated with rapidly changing cardiac arrhythmias. *Am J Emerg Med* 12:370, 1994.

59. Wells C, Cujec B, Johnson D, et al: Reversibility of severe left ventricular dysfunction in patients with subarachnoid hemorrhage. *Am Heart J* 129:409. 1995.

60. Allard JC, Hochberg FM, et al: Magnetic resonance imaging in a family with hereditary cerebral arteriovenous malformations. *Arch Neurol* 46:184, 1989.

61. Hop JW, Rinkel GJ, Algra A, et al: Case-fatality rates

and functional outcome after subarachnoid hemorrhage. A systematic review. *Stroke* 28:660, 1997.

62. Schievink WI, Wydicks EFM, Parisi JE, et al: Sudden death after aneurysm subarachnoid hemorrhage. *Neurology* 45:871, 1995.

63. Lanzino G, Kassell NF, Germanson T, et al: Plasma glucose levels and outcome after aneurysmal subarachnoid hemorrhage. *J Neurosurg* 79:885, 1993.

64. Nishioka H, Tomer JC, Graf J, et al: Cooperative study of intracranial aneurysms and subarachnoid hemorrhage. A long-term prognostic study. *Arch Neurol* 41:1142, 1984.

65. Hütter BO, Gilsbach JM: Which neuropsychological deficits are hidden behind a good outcome (Glasgow = 1) after aneurysmal subarachnoid hemorrhage? *Neurosurgery* 33:999, 1993.

66. Ogden J, Mee EW, Henning M: A prospective study of impairment of cognition and memory and recovery after subarachnoid hemorrhage. *Neurosurgery* 33:572, 1993.

67. Stenhouse LM, Knight RG, Longmore BE, et al: Long-term cognitive deficits in patients after surgery on aneurysm of the anterior communicating artery. *J Neurol Neurosurg Psychiatry* 54:909, 1991.

68. Raaymakers T, Rinkel GJ, Limburg M, et al: Mortality and morbidity of surgery for unruptured intracranial aneurysms: a meta analysis. *Stroke* 29:1531, 1998.

69. Allard JC, Hochberg FM, Franklin PD, et al: Magnetic resonance imaging in a family with hereditary cerebral arteriovenous malformation. *Arch Neurol* 46:184, 1989.

70. Sundaram MB, Chow F: Seizures associated with spontaneous subarachnoid hemorrhage. *Canad J Neurol Sci* 13:209, 1986

71. Symon L, Tacconi L, Mendoza N, et al: Arteriovenous malformations of the posterior fossa: a report of 28 cases and review of the literature. *Brit J Neurosurg* 9:721, 1995.

72. Samson DS, Batjer HH: Preoperative evaluation of the risk/benefit ratio for arteriovenous malformations of the brain in Wilkins RH, Rengachary SS (eds): *Neurosurgery 2nd ed Volume II.* New York, McGraw-Hill, 1996, pp 2443–2454.

73. Miller VS, Roach ES: Embolization and radiosurgical treatment of cerebral arteriovenous malformations. *Int Pediatr* 7:173, 1994.

74. Rigamonti D, Spetzler RF, Medina M, et al: Cerebral venous malformations. *J Neurosurg* 73:560, 1990.

75. Del Curling O Jr, Kelly DL Jr, Elster AD, et al: Analysis of the natural history of cavernous angiomas. *J Neurosurg* 75:702, 1991.

76. Robinson JR, Awad IA, Little JR: Natural history of the cavernous angiomas. *J Neurosurg* 75:709, 1991.

77. Awad IA, Little JR, Akrawi WP, et al: Intracranial dural arteriovenous malformation: factors predisposing to an aggressive neurological course. *J Neurosurg* 72:839, 1990.

78. Martin NA, King WA, Wilson CB, et al: Management of dural arteriovenous malformations of the anterior cranial fossa. *J Neurosurg* 72:692, 1990.

79. Ahmadi J, Tung H, Giannotta SL, et al: Monitoring of infectious aneurysms by sequential computed tomographic/magnetic resonance imaging studies. *Neurosurgery* 32:45, 1993.

80. Papa ML, Schisano G, Franco A, et al: Congenital deficiency of Factor VII in subarachnoid hemorrhage. *Stroke* 35:508, 1994.

81. Duke R, Fawcett P, Booth J: Recurrent subarachnoid hemorrhage due to endometriosis. *Neurology* 45:1000, 1995.

82. Endo S, Nishijama M, Nomura H, et al: A pathological study of intracranial posterior circulation dissecting aneurysms with subarachnoid hemorrhage: report of three autopsied cases and review of the literature. *Neurosurgery* 33:732, 1993.

83. Wijdicks EF, Schievink WI, Miller GM: Pretruncal nonaneurysmal subarachnoid hemorrhage. *Mayo Clin Proc* 73:745, 1998.

84. Schievink WI, Parisi JE, Piepgras DG, et al: Intracranial aneurysms in Marfan's syndrome: an autopsy study. *Neurosurgery* 41:866, 1997.

85. Schievink WI, Prendergast V, Zabramski JM: Rupture of previously documented small asymptomatic intracranial aneurysm in a patient with autosomal dominant polycystic kidney disease. *J Neurosurg* 89:479, 1998.

86. Minami H, Hanakita J, Suwa H, et al: Cervical hemangioblastoma with a past history of subarachnoid hemorrhage. *Surg Neurol* 49:278, 1998.

87. Preul MC, Cendes F, Just N, et al: Intracranial aneurysms and sickle cell anemia: multiplicity and propensity for the vertebrobasilar territory. *Neurosurgery* 42:971, 1998.

88. Cruz DN, Segal AS: A patient with Wegener's granulomatosis presenting with a subarachnoid hemorrhage: case report and review of CNS disease associated with Wegener's granulomatosis. *Am J Nephrol* 17:181, 1997.

89. Ozawa T, Sasaki O, Sorimachi T, et al: Primary angiitis of the central nervous system: report of two cases and review of the literature. *Neurosurgery* 36:173, 1995.

Chapter 10

INTRACEREBRAL, PONTINE, AND INTRACEREBELLAR HEMORRHAGE

Although the incidence of primary intracerebral hemorrhage has decreased considerably in the past 20 years, the condition remains a dramatic event, with high mortality, and there has been little improvement in therapy of patients with deeply situated hemorrhage. The decrease in incidence is probably related to improved control of hypertension in the population and is an indication of the success of antihypertensive therapy. This form of preventive medicine can be carried out by every practicing physician and is the keystone to the reduction in nearly all forms of cerebrovascular disease.

PRIMARY INTRACEREBRAL HEMORRHAGE

Definition

Primary intracerebral hemorrhage is a syndrome characterized by spontaneous bleeding into the substance of the brain.

Etiology and Pathology

1. Most cases of primary intracerebral hemorrhage occur in patients with chronic hypertension.[1] This condition results in arteriosclerotic changes of small blood vessels, particularly in those branches of the middle cerebral artery, which penetrate into the substance of the basal ganglia and internal capsule. These vessels become weakened, as reflected in splitting and reduplication of the internal elastic lamina, hyalinization of the media, and the eventual formation of small aneurysms known as Charcot-Bouchard

aneurysms. Similar conditions probably occur in the penetrating vessels of the pons and cerebellum. Rupture of one of the weakened blood vessels results in hemorrhage into the substance of the brain. Patients with other atherosclerotic conditions, for example, chronic lower limb ischemia, hypertension, and insulin-dependent diabetes mellitus receiving oral anticoagulant therapy, are at high risk for intracerebral hemorrhage.[2]

2. In normotensive and elderly patients, nontraumatic primary intracerebral hemorrhage is likely to be the result of cerebral amyloid angiopathy.[3] This condition is the result of a cumulation of amyloid β-protein within the walls of the small and medium-sized leptomeningeal and cortical arteries. The amyloid β-protein deposits displace collagen and contractile elements, producing a brittle and weakened artery, which is subject to increased risk of spontaneous rupture. The lack of contractile elements interferes with vasoconstriction and a massive hemorrhage can occur, with extension into the ventricles or subdural space.[3] Furthermore, lack of contractility predisposes to further bleeding and intermittent enlargement of the hematoma. There is a significant association between the E4 allele of the apolipoprotein gene and cerebral hemorrhage related to amyloid angiopathy.[4]

3. An angiomatous malformation (arteriovenous malformation [AVM] cavernous angioma) located at any site in the brain may rupture and produce an intracerebral hemorrhage of lobular type. Impaired venous drainage owing to stenosis or occlusion of the draining veins increases the risk of bleeding from an AVM.[5]

4. The abnormal vessels within high-grade astrocytomas frequently rupture and may bleed extensively, with the production of an intracerebral hemorrhage. Other tumors, including lymphoma, meningioma, pituitary tumors, and metastatic tumors, can bleed occasionally.[6]

5. Rupture of a congenital or a saccular aneurysm can result in a massive intracerebral hemorrhage if the high-pressure bleed is directed into the brain parenchyma.

6. Recreational amphetamine use can result in a vasculitis followed by arterial rupture and intracerebral hemorrhage.[7]

7. Chronic cocaine use has been associated with intracerebral hemorrhage. The mechanism has not been identified, but could include accelerated atherosclerosis induced by hypertension or the development of cerebral vasculitis.[8,9]

8. Anticoagulant therapy carries a high risk for intracerebral hemorrhage, particularly in patients with the following conditions: venous thrombosis and pulmonary embolism, cerebrovascular disease with transient ischemic attacks or prosthetic heart valves.[10,11] An international normalized ratio (INR) of 2.0 to 3.0 is an adequate level of anticoagulation in all cases except for prevention of embolism from prosthetic heart valves, where the current recommendation is for an INR of 2.5 to 3.5.[12] Other anticoagulants, including heparin, thrombolytic agents, and aspirin, increase the risk of intracerebral bleeding.[13–15] The use of thrombolytic agents after myocardial infarction is followed by intracerebral hemorrhage in several thousand patients each year.[16,17]

9. Moyamoya disease, in which an absent circle of Willis is replaced by a network of collateral vessels running into the brain parenchyma, has a high incidence of intracerebral hemorrhage.[18]

10. The weakened walls of vasculitis-inflamed arteries, such as those found in granulomatous angiitis, systemic lupus erythematosus, and mixed connective tissue disease, may result in an intracerebral hemorrhage.[19] Vasculitis and bleeding can also occur in herpes encephalitis, bacterial cerebritis, and fungal arteritis.

11. Leukemia and leukemic infiltration of the brain parenchyma can be followed by intracerebral hemorrhage.

12. Ingestion of sympathomimetics, including phenylpropanolamine in dietary medication and overdose or abuse of ephedrine or pseudoephedrine, has resulted in intracerebral hemorrhage.[20]

13. Sickle cell disease, which produces a vasculopathy, can be associated with arterial rupture or subarachnoid or intracerebral hemorrhage see page 307).

14. Idiopathic or acquired thrombocytopenia and hypofibrinogenemia are known or putative causes of intracerebral hemorrhage.

15. Disseminated intravascular coagulopathy has been associated with intracerebral hemorrhage.

Risk factors identified in cases of intracerebral hemorrhage include hypertension, recent moderate or heavy alcohol intake, hepatic disease, electrocardio-

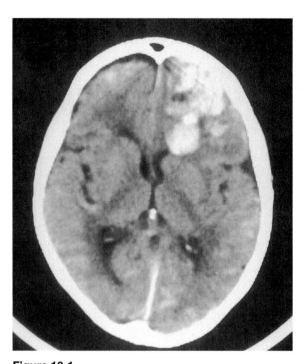

Figure 10-1
CT scan. Intracerebral hemorrhage involving the left frontal lobe.

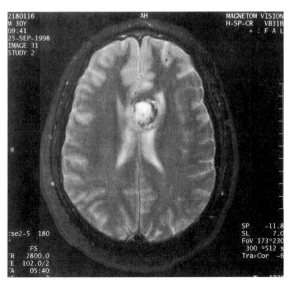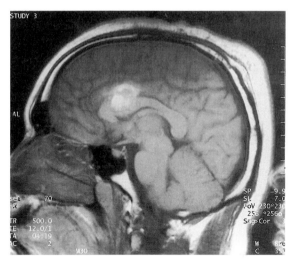

Figure 10-2
MRI scan. Well-circumscribed intracerebral hemorrhage involving the corpus callosum with extension into the left cingulate gyrus.

graphic abnormalities, prior cerebral infarction or hemorrhage, and an abnormally high hematocrit.[21–23]

In the majority of patients, hemorrhage occurs in the area of the thalamus, internal capsule, and basal ganglia (65 percent); brainstem (10 percent); cerebellum (10 percent); and subcortical white matter (15 percent).[24] The advent of computed tomography (CT) scanning has demonstrated that focal hemorrhages situated in the subcortical white matter (Fig. 10-1), deep white matter including the corpus callosum (Fig. 10-2), or restricted to the thalamus are probably more common than has been previously thought (Fig. 10-3).[25,26]

An intracerebral hemorrhage produces direct destruction of tissue and compression of surrounding parenchyma. Deeply situated hemorrhage may rupture into the ventricular system[27] or, rarely, rupture through to the surface of the brain.

Clinical Features

In the majority of patients, there is an acute onset of headache and rapid development of stupor followed by coma. Examination usually reveals systemic evidence of chronic hypertension. The signs and symp-

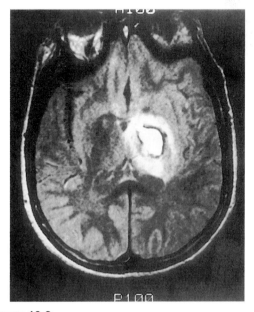

Figure 10-3
MRI scan. Left thalamic hemorrhage in the left thalamus with a surrounding halo of hemosiderin.

toms depend on the location of the hematoma, which acts like a mass lesion. Uncal herniation with rostral-caudal loss of brainstem function may occur. Survivors gradually recover consciousness over a period of several days. Patients with temporal or frontal lobe hematomas may present with sudden onset of seizures followed by some degree of contralateral hemiparesis.[28]

Normotensive elderly individuals with intracerebral or intracerebellar hemorrhage secondary to amyloid angiopathy often suffer from Alzheimer disease or progressive dementia of the Alzheimer type and develop intracerebral hemorrhage with rupture into the subarachnoid space during the night.[29,30]

Diagnostic Procedures

1.   Computed tomography scanning is the most sensitive test for intracerebral hemorrhage during the first few hours after a hemorrhage. The CT scan should be repeated in 24 h to assess stability (Fig. 10-4). Emergency surgery with evacuation of the hematoma is indicated in conscious or obtunded patients who have experienced an increase in the volume of the hematoma.[31]

2.   Magnetic resonance imaging (MRI) will demonstrate an intracerebral hematoma and the age of the hematoma after the first few hours following hemorrhage. Changes in the appearance of the MRI depend on the stages of hemoglobin dissolution—oxyhemoglobin-deoxyhemoglobin-methemoglobin-ferritin and hemosiderin.[32]

Differential Diagnosis

1.   Other causes of acute coma (see Chap. 2) and other cases of mass lesion.

2.   Cerebral infarction caused by thrombus or embolism. The acute onset and the presence of blood in the cerebrospinal fluid (CSF) will establish the diagnosis of intracerebral hemorrhage in the majority of cases. Small hematomas in the frontal or temporal lobes may be difficult to distinguish from cerebral infarction. The diagnosis will be established by MRI or CT scan.

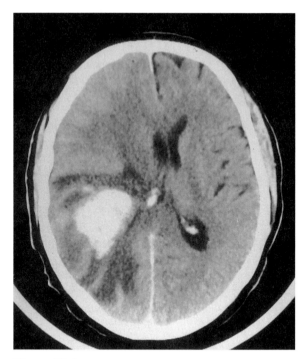

Figure 10-4
CT scan. There is a large right intracerebral hemorrhage. There is marked surrounding edema with obliteration of the right posterior horn of the lateral ventricle and shift of the midline structures to the left side.

3.   Ruptured saccular aneurysm may occasionally present with severe headache, neck stiffness, and bloody CSF without neurological deficits. In contrast, this rarely occurs in intracerebral hemorrhage. The two conditions are difficult to differentiate when bleeding from an aneurysm has caused an intracerebral hematoma. The diagnosis can be established by angiography or MRA scanning.

Treatment

See "Treatment of the Comatose Patient" in Chapter 2. In general, these measures apply to patients with intraparenchymal hemorrhage. Additional measures include:

1.   Assess airway, loss of consciousness, blood pressure, and Glasgow Coma Scale (see page 562).

2. If the Glasgow Coma Scale score is less than 8, intubate the patient using a short-acting barbiturate or lidocaine as anesthesia.[33]

3. As an emergency measure, hyperventilate to reduce $Paco_2$ to levels between 25 and 30 mmHg until mannitol infusion is completed.

4. Administer mannitol 0.5 to 1 g/kg intravenously.

5. Control hypertension with nitroprussides or agents that do not influence intracranial pressure (ICP) such as labetalol intravenously.

6. Check coagulation status:
   a. Patients taking heparin should be treated with protamine 1 mg per 100 units heparin and monitored carefully for hypotension.
   b. Neutralize urokinase or tissue plasminogen activator with 5 g ϵ-aminocaproic acid and 10 to 15 bags of cryoprecipitate.
   c. Warfarin effects can be reversed with 10 mg vitamin K intravenously and treated with frozen plasma. If the prothrombin time remains elevated, repeat in 6 h.

7. Seizures should be controlled with phenytoin 1 g intravenous piggyback or diazepam 10 mg intravenous followed by a diazepam drip at 5 mg/h.

8. If Glasgow Coma Scale score is less than 8, ICP monitoring is desirable.

9. Increased ICP or cerebral edema requires treatment with loop diuretics and replacing urinary and insensible fluid loss with isotonic saline. Mannitol 1 g/kg over 10 to 20 min will reduce ICP and should be repeated in doses of 0.25 g/kg q3–4h. The ICP should be monitored carefully or serum osmolality maintained between 300 and 320 mosmol.

10. Reduction of neural damage in the ischemic area surrounding an intracerebral hematoma using neuroprotective agents such as calcium channel blockers or N-methyl-D-aspartate receptor antagonists may reduce neuronal loss and minimize brain damage.

11. Surgical treatment may be lifesaving in selected patients with signs of rapidly increasing ICP. Frequently, MRI or CT scanning reveals an acute hydrocephalus in these patients, apparently caused by an acute shift of the midline structures, which distorts and blocks the outflow of CSF from the ventricles. There may be dramatic improvement after emergency ventricular drainage, which should be maintained until the patient stabilizes.

Patients with cerebral edema secondary to hematomas in the frontotemporal lobe often improve after surgical evacuation of the hematomas. Intraventricular hematomas are associated with a high mortality rate (Fig. 10-5), which can be reduced by continuous ventricular drainage and intraventricular infusion of urokinase or recombinant tissue plasminogen activator.[34] However, patients who show improvement with hyperbaric oxygen, and those who have improved in serial somatosensory evoked potential recordings or brainstem auditory evoked potential recordings after intravenous mannitol may benefit from surgical evacuation of the hematoma.[35] Recent developments, including stereotactic aspiration and

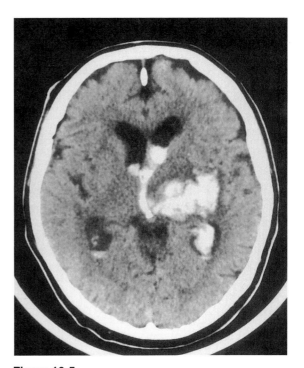

Figure 10-5

CT scan. Intracerebral hemorrhage involving the basal ganglia and the thalamus with extension into the third and lateral ventricles.

installation of fibrinolytic agents have potential for the future.[36]

Cerebral hemorrhage caused by a ruptured AVM in an individual with acute and profound neurological deterioration responds to prompt evacuation of the hematoma and excision of the AVM or later obliteration of the AVM by embolization in a center with excellent postoperative neurosurgical care facilities.[37] Nevertheless, attempts to drain deeply situated hematomas are often unsuccessful.[38]

Prognosis

The advent of MRI and CT scanning has shown that intracerebral hemorrhage is not an inevitably fatal disease (Fig. 10-6). Nevertheless, the mortality rate remains as high as 44 percent,[39] particularly when large hemorrhages involve the basal ganglia, internal

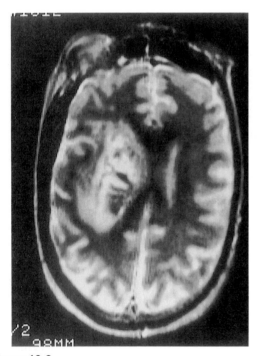

Figure 10-6
MRI scan. Large quadrilateral right intracerebral hemorrhage involving the basal ganglia, internal and external capsule in an individual recovering from the effects of the hemorrhage.

capsule, and thalamus. A Glasgow Coma Scale score of less than 8, a wide pulse pressure, a large hemorrhage, and intraventricular extension indicate poor prognosis.[40,41] Surviving patients usually have persistent neurological deficits, but those who recover from a thalamic or lobar intracerebral hemorrhage often have surprisingly good return of neurological functioning.[26] Every effort should be made to control those factors that lead to arteriosclerosis. In particular, hypertension must always be vigorously controlled.[42]

Thalamic Hemorrhage

Thalamic hemorrhage is a distinct variant of intracerebral hemorrhage and represents about 25 percent of the patients with this condition.

Four clinical types have been described (anterolateral, posterolateral, medial, and dorsal thalamic hemorrhages).[39] When large, all are characterized by a contralateral hemiparesis, hemisensory loss, vomiting, headache, oculomotor disturbances, and dysphasia or aphasia. Posterolateral hemorrhages present with hemiparesis or hemiplegia, hemisensory impairment, and aphasia, with left-sided lesions. Oculomotor disturbances include lack of upward gaze, skew deviation or eye deviation toward the side of the lesion and miotic pupils. Anterolateral thalamic hemorrhage is characterized by severe contralateral motor or sensory deficits. Medial hemorrhage presents with contralateral sensorimotor deficits and dysphasia with left-sided lesions and neglect in patients with right-sided lesions. Dorsal thalamic hemorrhage usually presents with mild contralateral sensorimotor disturbance. When ocular motor signs are present, there may be impaired vertical gaze, miosis, and horizontal gaze palsy. Extension of the hemorrhage into the midbrain results in forced downward convergence of the eyes (tip of the nose syndrome).

Neurobehavioral disturbances are not uncommon in thalamic hemorrhage with disorientation, memory impairment, aphasia, or dysphasia. Right-sided hemorrhage results in anosognosia and visual spatial impairment.

Thalamic pain (central neurogenic pain) may develop, in some cases, a month or more after the hemorrhage.

PONTINE HEMORRHAGE

Definition

A *pontine hemorrhage* is a hemorrhage into the pons. This condition is relatively rare and occurs in about 10 percent of patients with cerebral hemorrhage.

Etiology and Pathology

The most frequent cause of primary pontine hemorrhage is rupture of an arteriosclerotic vessel or rupture of a microaneurysm in a chronically hypertensive patient. Other possible causes include rupture of a small AVM.

The initial hemorrhage usually occurs either at the junction of the tegmentum and basilar portion of the pons or in the tegmentum at the midpontine level. When the hemorrhage involves the junction of the tegmentum and basilar pons, it may extend medially, ventrally, dorsally into the fourth ventricle, or rostrally into the midbrain. When hemorrhage is in the tegmentum at the midpontine level, it tends to have limited extension.

Clinical Features

The onset is sudden with rapid loss of consciousness and coma in the majority of cases; a few patients present with stupor. Comatose patients are usually hypertensive with central neurogenic hyperventilation, and most exhibit decerebrate rigidity. There is extreme miosis in 50 percent of cases, and reflex conjugate eye movements are impaired in horizontal and vertical planes. Anisocoria, conjugate deviation of the eyes, or skewed deviation are occasional occurrences. Most patients are quadriplegic or hemiplegic. Hypothermia is an ominous prognostic sign.[43] Stuporous patients may show similar signs of eye involvement and motor deficits, with additional unilateral or bilateral facial palsy and hemisensory loss. Gastrointestinal hemorrhage can occur in deeply comatose patients with extensive brainstem hemorrhages. Survivors recover to a stage of the locked-in syndrome in some cases. A hemorrhage into the pontine tegmentum can be associated with hearing loss and auditory hallucinations.[44]

Diagnostic Procedures

The MRI or CT scan will demonstrate the hematoma (Fig. 10-7).

Treatment

Treatment is described under intracerebral hemorrhage.

See page 300.

Prognosis

The prognosis is poor. When recovery does occur, severe neurological deficits remain.

CEREBELLAR HEMORRHAGE

Definition

A *cerebellar hemorrhage* originates within the substance of the cerebellum.

Etiology and Pathology

The three major causes of cerebellar hemorrhage include:

1. Rupture of a penetrating artery, usually in the area of the dentate nucleus. In the chronic hypertensive patient, penetrating arteries in the cerebellum undergo the same degenerative changes as the vessels in the cerebral hemispheres.

2. Rupture of an AVM.

3. Bleeding from a cerebellar hemangioblastoma (see page 416)

Hemorrhages followed by hematoma formation are located within the substance of the cerebellum with dissection toward the subarachnoid space or toward the brainstem. An increasing volume of the hematoma distorts the contents of the posterior fossa and produces pressure on the brainstem.

Clinical Features

There are three common clinical presentations of cerebellar hemorrhage. The patient may present with:

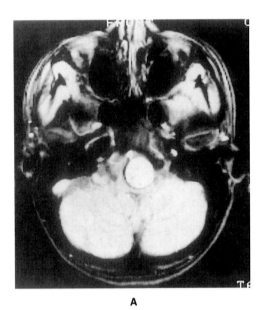

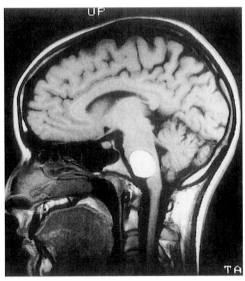

A   B

Figure 10-7
MRI scan. Pontine hemorrhage: axial **(A)** *and lateral* **(B)** *views, showing a well-circumscribed area of increased signal in the pons.*

1. Rapid onset with severe headache followed by clouding of consciousness and rapid progression. Sudden death may occur due to compression of the cardiorespiratory centers in the medulla. Given that there are no localizing neurological findings, these patients are often diagnosed as having an intracerebral hemorrhage or subarachnoid hemorrhage.

2. Abrupt onset of occipital headache, severe vertigo, vomiting, and ataxia. There is progressive diminution of the level of consciousness followed by the appearance of central neurogenic hyperventilation, indicating brainstem compression. These patients die within 2 or 3 days unless the hematoma is evacuated.

3. Approximately 20 percent of patients show slower progression following the development of occipital headache, vomiting, and vertigo. These patients are often conscious or obtunded and dysarthric. There are contralateral deviation of the eyes, ipsilateral cerebellar signs, contralateral hemiparesis and extensor plantar response, and nuchal rigidity. The course is slowly progressive.

Diagnostic Procedures

1. The MRI or CT scan shows the presence of cerebellar hemorrhage with a circumscribed area of increased density lying within the substance of the cerebellum. The MRI scan gives much better detail of the age and extent of the hemorrhage and proximity to or involvement of the brainstem (Fig. 10-8).

2. Arteriography reveals a posterior fossa mass and an AVM in some cases.

Treatment

Criteria for surgical or nonsurgical treatment have been established. Patients with a Glasgow Coma Scale score of 14 or 15 with a hematoma less than 40 mm in diameter are treated conservatively. Those with a score of 13 or less, or with a hematoma of 40 mm or more, require hematoma evacuation and decompressive suboccipital craniotomy. Patients with a low Glasgow Coma Scale score with loss of brainstem reflexes and quadriplegia are not surgical candidates.[45]

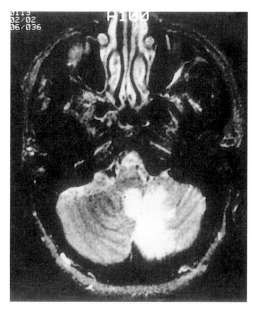

Figure 10-8
MRI scan. Intracerebellar hemorrhage with spread into the fourth ventricle and subarachnoid space.

Prognosis

The prognosis is good if evacuation occurs before signs of severe brainstem compression appear. There may be some residual signs of cerebellar ataxia, but these are often mild.

REFERENCES

1. Brott T, Thalinger K: Hypertension as a risk factor for spontaneous intracerebral hemorrhage. *Stroke* 17:1078, 1986.
2. Dawson I, van Bockel H, Ferrari MD, et al: Ischemic and hemorrhagic stroke in patients on oral anticoagulants after reconstruction for chronic lower limb ischemia. *Stroke* 24:1655, 1993.
3. LeBlanc R, Carpenter S, Stewart J, et al: Subacute enlarging cerebral hematoma from amyloid angiopathy: case report. *Neurosurgery* 36:403, 1995.
4. Greenberg SM, Rebeck GW, VonSattel JPG, et al: Apolipoprotein ε 4 and cerebral hemorrhage associated with amyloid angiopathy. *Ann Neurol* 38:254, 1995.
5. Miyasaka Y, Kurata A, Takiwa K, et al: Draining vein pressure increases and hemorrhage in patients with arteriovenous malformation. *Stroke* 25:504, 1994.
6. Weir B: The clinical problem of intracerebral hematoma. *Stroke* 24(suppl 12):193, 1993.
7. Toffol GJ, Biller J, Adams HP Jr: Nontraumatic intracerebral hemorrhage in young adults. *Arch Neurol* 44:483, 1987.
8. Daras M, Tuchman AJ, Koppel BS, et al: Neurovascular complications of cocaine. *Acta Neurol Scand* 90:124, 1994.
9. Krendel DA, Ditter SM, Frankel MR, et al: Biopsy-proven cerebral vasculitis associated with cocaine abuse. *Neurology* 40:1092, 1990.
10. Hylek EM, Singer DE: Risk factors for intracranial hemorrhage in outpatients taking warfarin. *Ann Intern Med* 120:897, 1994.
11. Mathiesen T, Benediktsdottir K, Johnsson H, et al: Intracranial traumatic and non-traumatic haemorrhagic complications of warfarin treatment. *Acta Neurol Scand* 91:208, 1995.
12. Hirsh J, Dalen JE, Deykin D, et al: Oral anticoagulants. Mechanism of action, clinical effectiveness and optimal therapeutic range. *Chest* 102:(4 suppl):3125, 1992.
13. Levy DE, Brott TG, Haley EC Jr., et al: Factors related to intracranial hematoma formation in patients receiving tissue-type plasminogen activator for acute ischemic stroke. *Stroke* 25:291, 1994.
14. Gore JM, Granger CB, Simoons ML, et al: Stroke after thrombolysis. Mortality and functional outcomes in the GUSTO-1 trial. Global use of strategies to open occluded coronary arteries. *Circulation* 92:2811, 1995.
15. Sloan MA, Price TR, Petito CK, et al: Clinical features and pathogenesis of intracerebral hemorrhage after rt-PA and heparin therapy for acute myocardial infarction: the thrombolysis in myocardial infarction (TIMI) II pilot and randomized clinical trial combined experience. *Neurology* 45:649, 1995.
16. Kaufman HH, McAllister P, Taylor H, et al: Intracerebral hematoma related to thrombolysis for myocardial infarction. *Neurosurgery* 33:898, 1993.
17. Hillegass WB, Jollis JG, Granger CB, et al: Intracranial hemorrhage risk and new thrombolytic therapies in acute myocardial infarction. *Am J Cardiol* 73:444, 1994.
18. Hamada J, Hashimoto N, Tsukahara T: Moyamoya disease with repeated intraventricular hemorrhage due to aneurysm rupture. Report of two cases. *J Neurosurg* 80:328, 1994.
19. Toyoda K, Tsuji H, Sadoshima S, et al: Brain hemorrhage in mixed connective tissue disease. A case report. *Angiology* 45:967, 1994.

20. Kase CS, Foster TE, Reed JE, et al: Intracerebral hemorrhage and phenylpropanolamine use. *Neurology* 37:399, 1987.
21. Calandre L, Arnal C, Fernandez-Ortega JF, et al: Risk factors for spontaneous cerebral hematomas. Case control study. *Stroke* 17:1126, 1986.
22. Bahemuka M: Primary intracerebral hemorrhage and heart weight: a clinicopathological case-control review of 218 patients. *Stroke* 18:531, 1987.
23. Juvela S: Risk factors for impaired outcome after spontaneous intracerebral hemorrhage. *Arch Neurol* 52: 1193, 1995.
24. Jørgensen HS, Nakayama H, Raaschou HO, et al: Intracerebral hemorrhage versus infarction: stroke severity, risk factors, and prognosis. *Ann Neurol* 38:45, 1995.
25. Heiskanen O: Treatment of spontaneous intracerebral and intracerebellar hemorrhage. *Stroke* 24(suppl 12): 194, 1993.
26. Tanaka Y, Furuse M, Iwasa H, et al: Lobar intracerebral hemorrhage: etiology and a long-term follow-up study of 32 patients. *Stroke* 17:51, 1986.
27. Gates PC, Barnett HJ, Vinters HV, et al: Primary intraventricular hemorrhage in adults. *Stroke* 17:872, 1986.
28. Berger AR, Lipton RB, Lesser ML, et al: Early seizures following intracerebral hemorrhage: implications for therapy. *Neurology* 38:1363, 1988.
29. Itoh Y, Yamada M, Hayakawa M, et al: Cerebral amyloid angiopathy: a significant cause of cerebellar as well as lobar cerebral hemorrhage in the elderly. *J Neurol Sci* 116:135, 1993.
30. Silbert PL, Bartleson JD, Miller GM, et al: Cortical petechial hemorrhage, leukoencephalopathy, and subacute dementia associated with seizures due to cerebral amyloid angiopathy. *Mayo Clin Proc* 70:477, 1995.
31. Fujii Y, Tanaka R, Takeuchi S, et al: Hematoma enlargement in spontaneous intracerebral hemorrhage. *J Neurosurg* 80:51, 1994.
32. Bradley WG Jr: MR appearance of hemorrhage in the brain. *Radiology* 189:15, 1993.
33. Diringer MN: Intracerebral hemorrhage: pathophysiology and management. *Crit Care Med* 21:1591, 1993.
34. Kaufman HH: Treatment of deep spontaneous intracerebral hematomas. A review. *Stroke* 24(suppl 12):I107, 1993.
35. Kanno T, Nagata J, Nonomura K, et al: New approaches in the treatment of hypertensive intracerebral hemorrhage. *Stroke* 24(suppl 12):I 96, 1993.
36. Rohde V, Schaller C, Hassler WE: Intraventricular recombinant tissue plasminogen activator for lysis of intraventricular haemorrhage. *J Neurol Neurosurg Psychiatry* 58:447, 1995.
37. Jafar JJ, Rezai AR: Acute surgical management of intracranial arteriovenous malformations. *Neurosurgery* 34:8, 1994.
38. Mendelow AD: Mechanisms of ischemic brain damage with intracerebral hemorrhage. *Stroke* 24(12 suppl): 1–115, 1993.
39. Kumral E, Kocaer T, Ertubey NO, et al: Thalamic hemorrhage. A prospective study of 100 patients. *Stroke* 26:964, 1995.
40. Broderick JP, Brott TG, Duldner JE, et al: Volume of intracerebral hemorrhages. A powerful and easy-to-use predictor of 30-day mortality. *Stroke* 24:987, 1993.
41. Lampl Y, Gilad R, Eshel Y, et al: Neurological and functional outcome in patients with supratentorial hemorrhages. A prospective study. *Stroke* 26:2249, 1995.
42. Chen ST, Chiang CY, Hsu CY, et al: Recurrent hypertensive intracerebral hemorrhage. *Acta Neurol Scand* 91:128, 1995.
43. Kitanaka C, Inoh Y, Toyoda T, et al: Malignant brain stem hyperthermia caused by brain stem hemorrhage. *Stroke* 25:518, 1994.
44. Murata S, Naritomi H, Sawada T: Musical auditory hallucinations caused by a brain stem lesion. *Neurology* 44:156, 1994.
45. Kobayashi S, Sato A, Kageyama Y, et al: Treatment of hypertensive cerebellar hemorrhage—surgical or conservative management? *Neurosurgery* 34:246, 1994.

Chapter 11

STROKES IN CHILDREN AND YOUNG ADULTS

The incidence of cerebrovascular disease in children younger than 15 years of age is 2.5/100,000 per year,[1] rising to 34/100,000 per year in individuals younger than 55 years of age.[2] Although there is a steady rise in the incidence of strokes in children and young adults with increasing age, strokes are encountered less frequently than in the middle-aged and elderly. However, the results of a stroke in a young person can be devastating when permanent deficits affect an individual for life. Although more than 70 percent make a good recovery, cerebral embolism and intracerebral hemorrhage carry a poorer prognosis in younger patients.[3] Therefore, prevention, diagnosis, and treatment are extremely important in susceptible or afflicted individuals. There are many causes of stroke or strokelike symptoms in young persons (Table 11-1), but many of these conditions are treatable and appropriate therapy should reduce the risk of stroke or limit the neurological deficit if a stroke has occurred.

Etiology

The hereditary hemoglobinopathies with a predisposition to stroke include sickle cell disease (hemoglobin S-S), sickle cell trait (hemoglobin S-A), and hemoglobin C and hemoglobin S-C disease. Cerebral infarction occurs in 5 percent of patients with sickle cell disease.[4] This complication is probably the result of a progressive arteriolopathy secondary to intimal abnormalities associated with fibroblastic proliferation in the vessel wall with stasis of lesser importance.[5]

The incidence of cerebral infarction peaks at 10 years of age with older children showing an increased susceptibility to intracerebral hemorrhage,[6] cerebral venous thrombosis, and subarachnoid hemorrhage.[7] However, most children with S-S disease do not develop stroke, but the reason for this outcome is not understood.[8] Cerebral infarction can occur in the territory of the middle cerebral artery distribution, in a more diffuse fashion, with multiple lesions or with "silent strokes" detected by magnetic resonance imaging (MRI) scans[9] or transcranial Doppler ultrasound[10] in children at risk with a normal neurological examination who have never had symptoms. All children with sickle cell disease and stroke have abnormal neuropsychological profiles, with significant impairment of cognitive functioning.[11] Children with anterior lesions show attention deficits, whereas diffuse strokes produce impairment of spatial ability.[12]

Children with S-S disease and stroke are at a higher risk for further events because of progressive arteriolopathy. Treatment should include repeated transfusion therapy to keep the hemoglobin S-S concentration below 50 percent.[13]

Hereditary coagulopathies causing stroke include protein C and protein S deficiency. Protein C is a vitamin K-dependent plasma glucoprotein that functions as an anticoagulant by inactivation of factors V-a and VII-a. Protein S enhances protein C activity by increasing the affinity of activated protein C for cell surfaces. Clinical manifestations of protein C deficiency include phlebothrombosis, pulmonary embolism, and cerebral infarction.[14] All patients under 45 years of age with unexplained stroke should be screened for protein C and protein S deficiency. Treatment consists of infusion of the deficient protein or by prophylaxis with vitamin K antagonists.

Antithrombin III deficiency is also a recognized cause of thrombosis, although of lesser importance than protein C or protein S deficiency. Antithrombin III inactivates thrombin and other coagulation factors on endothelial surfaces and deficiency may lead to thrombosis of the dural venous sinuses or to arterial occlusion and cerebral infarction.[15] It is possible that a number of conditions with a tendency to thrombosis and stroke may have reduced concentrations or func-

Table 11-1

Factors known to contribute to stroke in children and young adults

---

I. **Hereditary**
Sickle cell disease, sickle cell trait, S-C disease, factor V Leiden, factor VII abnormality, factors VIII, IX and X abnormalities, protein C deficiency, protein S deficiency, dysfibrinogenemia, dysplasminogenemia, homocystinuria, ornithine transcarbamylase deficiency, Melas syndrome, isovaleric acidemia, methylmalonic acidemia, propionicacidemia, NADH-CoQ reductase deficiency

II. **Congenital Heart Disease**
Atrial septal defect of paradoxical embolism, ventricular septal defect, atrial myxoma or rhabdomyoma, subaortic stenosis, mitral valve prolapse, mitral stenosis

III. **Other Congenital Abnormalities**
Arteriovenous malformation, cavernous hemangioma, congenital aneurysm, saccular aneurysm, Sturge-Weber syndrome, arterial fibromuscular dysplasia, spontaneous arterial dissection

IV. **Traumatic**
Head trauma, subdural hematoma, subdural hygroma, subarachnoid hemorrhage, traumatic intracerebral hemorrhage, direct trauma to the carotid or vertebral arteries, intraoral trauma, post-traumatic arterial dissection, traumatic carotid-cavernous sinus fistula, fat embolism, air embolism, chiropractic manipulation

V. **Infections in Children**
Pneumonia, cervical adenitis, pharyngitis, retropharyngeal abscess, tonsillitis, sinusitis, cerebral venous thrombosis, infections of face, sinusitis, otitis media, mastoiditis, epidural abscess, cerebral abscess, viral encephalitis, mycoplasma infection, syphilitic arthritis, acute or subacute bacterial endocarditis and mycotic aneurysm, bacterial meningitis, tuberculous meningitis, fungal meningitis, amebic meningitis

VI. **Metabolic**
Hyperlipidemia, hypercholesterolemia, hyperuricemia, hypothyroidism, diabetes mellitus, obesity, smoking, excess alcohol consumption, pregnancy

VII. **Neoplastic**
Primary or metastatic brain tumor, lymphoma in AIDS or other immunosuppressed states

VIII. **Blood dyscrasias**
Antiphospholipid antibodies including anticardiolipin, lupus anticoagulant and antithrombin III, diffuse intravascular coagulation, hemolytic uremic syndrome, liver dysfunction, immune thrombocytopenic purpura, thrombotic thrombocytopenic purpura, polycythemia, pregnancy, postpartum, paroxysmal nocturnal hemoglobinuria, thrombocytosis, vitamin K deficiency, leukemia

IX. **Vascular**
Hypertension, atherosclerosis, lupuserythematosus, vasospasm of subarachnoid hemorrhage

X. **Vasculopathies**
Fabry disease, moyamoya, neurofibromatosis, Ehlers-Danlos syndrome, pseudoxanthoma elasticum, MELAS syndrome, spontaneous dissection of carotid or vertebral arteries

XI. **Acquired Heart Disease**
Atrial fibrillation, atrial fibrillation with valvular heart disease, rheumatic heart disease, bacterial endocarditis, Lippman-Sachs disease, viral myocarditis, idiopathic cardiomyopathy, myocardial infarction, prosthetic heart valves

XIII. **Miscellaneous**
Migraine, unilateral status epilepticus, dehydration, angiography, balloon angioplasty, cardiac surgery, carotid endarterectomy, brain or neck irradiation, chemotherapy inducing thrombocytopenia

---

tion of protein C, protein S, or antithrombin III. This would include the nephrotic syndrome,[16] disseminated intravascular coagulation, liver disease, Crohn's disease, and various cancers.

The antiphospholipid antibody syndrome in which antiphospholipid antibodies bind to phospho-lipids has been recognized as a potent cause of cerebral, venous, and arterial thrombosis in younger patients. Antiphospholipid antibodies, which include anticardiolipin and lupus anticoagulant[17] can occur independently or in association with systemic lupus erythematosus (SLE).[18] It is probable that antiphospholipid antibodies account for thrombotic events in SLE, Sjögren syndrome,[19] rheumatoid arthritis, Sneddon syndrome (lividoreticularis and stroke), and Behçet disease. In addition, it is possible to identify a primary antiphospholipid syndrome in some cases of stroke in young patients, but the antibodies may also be a feature related to stroke in collagen vascular disorders. The abnormal function of the antibodies is unknown, but it is possible that antiphospholipid antibodies alter normal vascular endothelial function mediated by protein C and protein S. Platelet activation and aggregation may be an additional factor and treatment with aspirin or ticlopidine has been suggested for patients with minor symptoms. Long-term anticoagulation with warfarin is indicated in stroke-prone cases.

Lupus Anticoagulant. This serum gamma globulin is associated with an increased risk of both venous and arterial thrombosis. Although the antibody is often associated with SLE and the antiphospholipid syndrome, lupus anticoagulant can occur independently and has been detected in significant numbers of young patients with stroke. Increased risk of stroke with increased levels of lupus anticoagulant is probably the result of an imbalance in the fibrinolytic system, producing hypercoagulability secondary to increased levels of tissue plasminogen activator inhibitor. The role of lupus anticoagulant is not clear.

Factor V Leiden Mutation. The genetic basic for resistance to activated protein C has been defined as a point mutation in the factor V gene at the site where activated protein C cleaves and inactivates factor V procoagulant. Failure to achieve inactivation because of the mutation in the factor V gene—factor V Leiden mutation—results in persistence of the procoagulant properties of factor V. This carries a significant increase in the risk of thrombosis, probably 5 to 10 times the thrombotic risk of the normal population in the heterozygous factor V mutation and an even higher risk for those carrying a homozygous factor V mutation. It is believed that factor V mutation is the most common cause of familial thrombotic disease.

Most patients present with cerebral venous thrombosis,[20] but cerebral arterial thrombosis has been reported.[21]

An increased risk of cerebral thrombosis has

been reported in factor VII gene mutation.[22] This anomaly is rare, in contrast to the factor V Leiden mutation. There is also an increased risk of stroke due to carotid atherosclerosis with high factor VIIIa activity, dyslipidemia, and hypertension.[23]

Elevated levels of lipoprotein A, a low-density lipoprotein related to plasminogen, and which may substitute for plasminogen, have been related to both coronary artery disease and stroke. Lipoprotein A should be regarded as an independent risk factor for stroke in young adults.[24]

Dysfibrinogenemia. Although hyperfibrinogenemia has been recognized as a risk factor for stroke, abnormal fibrinogens, where fibrinogen molecules are resistant to fibrinolysis and bind to platelets with increasing proclivity, can result in thrombosis. Abnormal fibrinogens are genetically determined and result in both cerebral venous thrombosis or cerebral arterial occlusion in children and young adults.[25]

Dysplasminogenemia. There are four possible mechanisms of hypofibrinolysis, where there is a reduction of fibrinolytic activity and increased tendency to thrombosis. The abnormal mechanisms include decreased circulation of plasminogen, abnormal plasminogen with decreased plasminogen activity,[26] increased concentrations of plasminogen activator inhibitor, or decreased levels of plasminogen activator. All of these states appear to be associated with increased risk of venous thrombosis. However, the possibility of a dysplasminogenemia should be considered in young persons with stroke or cerebral venous thrombosis.

The myeloproliferative disorders, which include polycythemia rubra vera with increased blood viscosity, essential thrombothemia with abnormal platelet morphology, and paroxysmal nocturnal hemoglobinuria, in which the erythrocyte membrane proteins are abnormal, are all associated with increased hypercoagulability, venous thrombosis, and cerebral arterial occlusion, often in relatively young adults.

Alterations in Vascular Endothelial Wall Integrity. Homocystinuria, with increased serum concentrations of homocystine, can result in damage to the vascular endothelium, accelerated atherosclerosis, arterial thrombosis, myocardial infarction, and stroke.[27] The risk of venous thrombosis and pulmonary embolism is also increased. These events can occur in individuals with an autosomal recessive deficiency of cystathionine synthetase. About 50 percent of cases present with ocular manifestations and skeletal abnormalities,[28] including dislocation of the lens, cataract, retinal degeneration, corneal opacities, optic atrophy, osteoporosis, arachnodactyly, scoliosis, and pes planus. There is developmental delay, mild-to-moderate mental retardation, proximal muscular weakness, waddling gait, and a high incidence of psychiatric disorders. The remainder are intellectually normal, without stigmata of the disease, and the diagnosis may be delayed in such cases, when elevated homocystine levels are only slightly increased.[29] Nevertheless, young adults who are otherwise asymptomatic but who are heterozygous for homocystinuria have an increased risk of accelerated atherosclerosis and stroke.[30]

Children who are symptomatic for homocystinuria often respond to oral pyridoxine 1000 mg/day, because pyridoxine acts as a coenzyme of cystathionine synthetase. Folate therapy also reduces homocystine levels in some cases and can be added to the treatment regimen with vitamin E, ascorbic acid, vitamin B_6, vitamin B_{12}, and dietary methionine restriction. Young adults with increased homocystine levels and stroke require anticoagulation indefinitely.

Other rare conditions associated with damage to the vascular wall include Fabry disease (page 368), Melas syndrome (page 637), subacute necrotizing encephalopathy of Leigh[31] (page 371), organic acidopathies including methylamine malonic acidemia, propionicacidemia, isovaleric acidemia, glutaric acidemia, and ornithine transcarbamoxylase deficiency.

Migraine. Migraine is a recognized cause of stroke. The complication usually presents with hemiparesis in an individual with an established history of migraine or a family history of migraine.[32] The mechanism is controversial, that is, prolonged vascular spasm versus spreading depression. However, most patients give a history of migraine with aura.[33] The symptoms resolve in most cases, but infarction can occur in migraine with a hemiparesis. Infarction can also occur at other sites, resulting in hemisensory deficits or symptoms of brainstem involvement in rare cases. Complicated migraine-like episodes with severe intermittent unilateral headache associated with hemiparesis, hemisensory loss, and aphasia are reported to follow cranial irradiation and chemotherapy for brain tumor in children.[34]

Miscellaneous. Unilateral generalized status epilepticus is associated with cerebral infarction and hemiparesis if there is a delay in controlling seizure activity (page 113). This process can occur as early as 2 hours after the onset of seizure activity in children or young adults, indicating the urgent need for effective treatment of seizures as soon as possible (page 115).

There is an increased risk of stroke due to cerebral venous thrombosis in the postpartum period in young women. Dehydration, particularly in young children, is sometimes associated with venous sinus thrombosis, cerebral venous thrombosis, and infarction with hemiparesis.

Trauma. Traumas is a potent cause of childhood stroke and hemiparesis and has been reported in closed head injury in children. Damage to the internal carotid artery following trauma to the neck may result in thrombosis and infarction. The internal carotid artery may also be damaged by trauma to the tonsillar fossa by a stick, toothbrush, or pencil held in the mouth.[35] Delayed cerebral infarction has been reported following dog bites in the region of the internal carotid artery.[36]

Injury to the carotid artery in stroke in young adults has been attributed to a sudden blow in the neck by a ski when snow or water skiing. This results in damage to the intima followed by thrombosis and carotid occlusion or occlusion following traumatic dissection of the arterial wall.

Adolescents and young adults can suffer a major stroke following accidental injection of heroin into the carotid artery during the attempt to enter the jugular vein.

Damage to the vertebral arteries in the neck with brainstem infarction has been reported after hyperextension-flexion injuries in high-speed accidents, resulting in fracture, or dislocation of the cervical spine, following chiropractic manipulation, or trauma to the neck.[37] Traumatic vertebral artery lesions at the C1–C2 level are the most common sites of injury in such cases.[38]

Fat embolism is an occasional cause of stroke in children.

Infection.   A number of infectious conditions may be followed by stroke. Infant and childhood hemiparesis has been associated with pneumonia, cervical adenitis, pharyngitis, retropharyngeal abscess, tonsillitis, and sinusitis. The mechanism is presumed to be a local arteritis affecting the carotid artery with thrombosis and cerebral infarction. Cerebral venous thrombosis and cerebral venous sinus thrombosis can occur in the presence of infection of the face, paranasal sinuses, or middle ears.

The development of an epidural abscess or cerebral abscess is occasionally a rapid process producing a progressive hemiparesis and mimicking a stroke.

Viral encephalitis, particularly herpes simplex encephalitis, occasionally presents with hemiparesis when the infection is predominantly in one hemisphere. Infection by the varicella-zoster virus may be followed by an arteritis[39] with vascular occlusion and stroke[40] involving the cerebral hemisphere or brainstem.[41] The onset of infarction may be delayed for several weeks in some cases. A similar condition can occur in syphilitic arteritis in young adults.

Hemiparesis is an occasional feature of an acute bacterial meningitis due to *Haemophilus influenzae*[42] but is more likely to occur in tuberculous meningitis or other chronic forms of chronic meningeal inflammation in syphilis, staphylococcal meningitis, or fungal meningitis. Delayed borrelial encephalomyelitis of Lyme disease is usually seen in Europe and is rare in North America. However, the spirochetal meningovasculitis can result in transient ischemic attacks or stroke.[43] Cysticercosis can cause stroke in persons living in areas where the disease is endemic.[44]

Subacute bacterial endocarditis can cause stroke by embolism and vascular occlusion or rupture of a mycotic aneurysm with subarachnoid hemorrhage. Mycotic aneurysms usually occur in heroin addicts with bacterial endocarditis following numerous intravenous injections of bacteria that have colonized within the lumen of unsterilized needles.

Toxic.   Toxic alcohol abuse increases the risk of stroke in young adults, and heroin, cocaine and "crack" cocaine, a highly potent refined cocaine, can cause a cerebral arteritis or vasospasm resulting in a severe stroke in young adult drug addicts.[45] Intravenous use of sympatheticomimetic drugs has also resulted in stroke.

Metabolic.   A number of metabolic abnormalities, including diabetes mellitus, hyperlipidemia, hypercholesterolemia, hyperuricemia, and hypothyroidism, predispose to cerebral infarction and stroke in young adults.[46] The effect of these conditions may be accentuated by severe hypertension, cardiac disease, obesity, smoking, and frequent alcohol intoxication.[47] Although a milder degree of atherosclerosis is not uncommon in young adults, marked development of atherosclerosis can occur, even in children who are subjected to prolonged action of predisposing factors, mainly hypertension and diabetes. There is an increased incidence of stroke during pregnancy. The causes are probably multiple and include metabolic changes, increased circulating blood volume, increased fibrinogen levels, and increased platelet activation.

Brain Tumors.   Two types of brain tumor, a rapidly growing glioma and primary lymphoma in acquired immunodeficiency syndrome (AIDS), may mimic a stroke with a rapid development of hemiparesis.

Immunodeficiency Virus (HIV) Type 1 Infection.   Children and young adults with acquired human immunodeficiency virus (HIV) type 1 disease (AIDS) are prone to cerebral infarction and cerebral hemorrhage, the latter associated with thrombocytopenia. Infarction can result from aneurysmal dilatation and thrombosis of major cerebral arteries, probably the result of frequent infection.[48] Cerebral embolism secondary to bacterial endocarditis is also a potent factor. The presentation is usually an acute hemiparesis, but silent multiple microinfarction or hemorrhage can occur.[49]

Congenital Abnormalities. Congenital conditions that predispose to stroke in the child or young adult include congenital heart disease with cerebral embolism.[50] Intracerebral arteriovenous malformations are a potent cause of both seizures and strokes in children and young adults. Hemorrhage from a ruptured arteriovenous malformation can cause a large intracerebral hemorrhage and young females are at a higher risk during pregnancy, when there is considerable increase in circulating blood volume.

Fibromuscular dysplasia, in which there is hyperplasia of the arterial intima or median layers, is a disorder of unknown etiology, often affecting the carotid, vertebral, or renal arteries.[50] The development of a stroke in a child or young adult suffering from chronic hypertension suggests the presence of this condition.

Moyamoya, first described in Japanese children, is known to occur worldwide. The cause of moyamoya is not known, but this collateral network of vessels is occasionally seen in association with congenital heart disease and Fanconi anemia, an autosomal recessive disorder characterized by pancytopenia, congenital malformations, and a predisposition to malignancy.[52] Moyamoya has also been described in association with neurofibromatosis, tuberous sclerosis, sickle cell disease, head trauma, bacterial meningitis, including tuberculous meningitis, renal vascular hypertension,[53] atherosclerosis, polyarteritis nodosa, mitochondrial disease and following radiation for optic glioma.[54] There is occlusion of one or both carotid arteries associated with the development of numerous small collateral vessels at the base of the brain and filling of the terminal portions of the internal carotid arteries (Fig. 11-1). Symptoms vary from the asymptomatic to transient ischemic attacks or repeated strokes with hemiplegia and intellectual deficits. The diagnosis is established by magnetic resonance angiography (MRA), which has largely replaced cerebral angiography in the diagnosis of moyamoya disease.[55]

Treatment should be directed to the control of hypertension and the development of cerebral cortical revascularization using split dural grafts applied to the cortical surface[56] to use the middle meningeal circulation as a source of collateral blood supply.[57]

Spontaneous dissection of the internal carotid

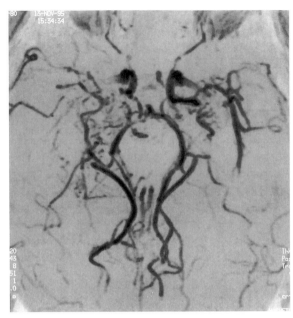

Figure 11-1
Moyamoya. There is occlusion of both internal carotid arteries with the development of numerous collateral channels, leading to restoration of flow in both terminal portions of the internal carotid arteries.

artery has been reported to be a major cause of stroke in persons under age 45 years in some studies. Vertebral artery dissection is also recognized but is a less frequent phenomenon. The cause of nontraumatic dissection is not identified in the majority of cases, but the presence of dissection suggests a congenital defect in the arterial wall. Certainly similar dissections can occur in hereditary conditions such as Marfan's syndrome or Ehlers-Danlos syndrome, which are associated with defects in the structure of the connective tissue.

Other congenital conditions in which there appear to be an increased incidence of stroke, with or without dissection, include neurofibromatosis, tuberous sclerosis, and encephalotrigeminal angiomatosis.

Vasculitis. Inflammation of blood vessels by infection or other vasculopathies is a potent cause of stroke in the younger population. Infectious causes have been discussed. Other vasculopathies, presumably related to an autoimmune process, include polyarteritis nodosa, rheumatoid arthritis, dermatomyositis, Crohn disease, ulcerative colitis,[58] and granulomatous angiitis. SLE, although causing damage to the brain by the laying down of immune complexes, occasionally causes an arteritis. A condition of isolated cranial arteritis has been described, particularly in younger women. All of these conditions are associated with endothelial damage and thrombosis.

Accelerated Atherosclerosis. A mild degree of atherosclerosis is not uncommon in young adults, but marked development of atherosclerosis can occur, even in children who are subjected to prolonged action of predisposing factors such as hypertension and diabetes mellitus. Consequently, strokes in children or young adults may be the result of accelerated atherosclerosis in some cases. This is discussed in detail in Chapter 8.

Heart Disease. Heart disease is a potent cause of stroke in all ages. Congenital heart disease may result in cerebral embolism because of clinically silent atrial septal defects,[59] periodic dysrhythmias, or atrial fibrillation.[60] Another condition associated with congenital heart disease is paradoxical embolism, when there is right-to-left shunt.[61] Subacute bacterial endocarditis is an ever-present risk in congenital heart disease. Rheumatic heart disease has declined in the last several decades but may cause stroke in young adults by embolism, subacute bacterial endocarditis, or paroxysmal fibrillation. Mitral valve prolapse has probably been overestimated as a cause of cerebral embolism, but occasionally this condition can give rise to emboli and it should be borne in mind when embolism is suspected. Ischemic heart disease occasionally occurs in young adults and may be complicated by dysrhythmias, embolism, and stroke.

Cardiac surgery carries a considerable risk of cerebral infarction from embolism due to clots or entrance of particulate matter into the circulation, resulting in air embolism and hypoxia.[62]

Clinical Features

The majority of strokes affecting the cerebral hemispheres are of acute onset and present with hemiparesis in 90 percent of cases. The remainder may show more subtle findings of impaired function of an affected limb or clumsiness of gait. Examination may reveal homonymous hemianopia and hemisensory loss. Dysphasia occurs with involvement of the dominant hemisphere and may be difficult to detect in young children. Seizures are common in young children at the onset of stroke; older children frequently complain of headache. AV malformations may be associated with contralateral involuntary movements.

Children and young adults with subarachnoid hemorrhage complain of headache and frequently have seizures and focal neurological signs, including cranial nerve palsy and hemiparesis. Examination shows the presence of nuchal rigidity and occasionally the presence of subhyaloid hemorrhages.

Differential Diagnosis

1. Trauma. All children who have suffered head trauma with neurological deficits should be closely investigated for the possibility of epidural hematoma, subdural hematoma, cerebral contusion, or intracerebral hemorrhage.

2. Cerebral abscess. In this case, the onset is usually gradual. There are headache, vomiting, and signs of increased intracranial pressure, with the development of focal neurological signs. The temperature is elevated and there may be signs of infection elsewhere, or signs of congenital heart disease.

3. Encephalitis. The onset is usually acute, with fever, headache, neck stiffness and occasionally focal seizures followed by the development of focal neurological signs. In some cases, however, the infection may develop without fever and only minimal headache and rather sudden development of hemiparesis. Such cases present some difficulty in diagnosis. If there is any doubt, a head computed tomography (CT) scan should be obtained, followed by a lumbar puncture. This will reveal an increase in CSF pressure with pleocytosis, elevated protein content, and normal glucose content in viral encephalitis.

4. Bacterial meningitis may present with much the same symptoms of fever, headache, lethargy, seizures, and nuchal rigidity. In this case, however, the lumbar puncture will reveal a polymor-

phonuclear pleocytosis, elevated protein content, and decreased glucose content.

5. Uremia. The presence of hypertension associated with elevated blood urea nitrogen and creatinine and anemia characterizes uremia.

6. Postictal (Todd) paralysis. The acute onset of hemiparesis in a semicomatose child may indicate a postictal state following a seizure. In this case, there will be rapid recovery of consciousness and resolution of the hemiparesis.

7. Migraine. The sudden onset of neurological deficit, usually a hemiparesis associated with a severe headache in a child with a history of previous headaches, suggests hemiplegic migraine. Ophthalmoplegic migraine with third nerve palsy is rare in children but has been reported.

8. Lead encephalopathy. This condition may present acutely. There are signs of increased intracranial pressure with neurological deficits. The diagnosis depends on the demonstration of elevated serum lead levels.

9. Tumors can present with acute neurological deficits, particularly following repeated seizures or status epilepticus. There may be signs of increased intracranial pressure, and the diagnosis can usually be established by MRI or CT scanning.

Diagnostic Procedures

The diagnostic procedures are outlined in Table 11-2.

Treatment

A. In the acute situation:
1. An airway should be established in an obtunded, semicomatose, or comatose patient.
2. Adequate hydration should be maintained. Children become easily dehydrated. The requirement of fluid is 1200 mL/m^2 of body surface per day.
3. Any electrolyte imbalance should be corrected.
4. Any identified medical condition should be treated. For instance, patients with congenital heart disease may have dysrhythmia or heart failure and require appropriate treatment.

5. Seizures should be controlled. If the patient is in status epilepticus, treat as status epilepticus (page 115).
6. In stroke due to cerebral embolism, the patient should be heparinized (page 253).
7. Increased intracranial pressure requires admission to an intensive care unit and intracranial pressure monitoring. Cerebral edema may be reduced by infusion of 20% mannitol in dosage of 1.5 g/kg over a 20-min period. It is then possible to titrate the requirements of mannitol by observing the intracranial pressure monitoring readings. In addition, the serum osmolality should be maintained between 300 and 320 mOsm and periodic mannitol infusion may be given to that end. The use of hyperventilation is controversial. The patient must be intubated and receiving ventilator support, when hyperventilation may be introduced as an emergency measure for a short period of time, and when there is a rapid rise in intracranial pressure. The P_{CO_2} should be reduced to 22 to 24 mmHg during this emergency procedure. The use of dexamethasone is not indicated for reduction of increased intracranial pressure and has little effect in the stroke patient. Dexamethasone is, however, indicated in some cases of bacterial meningitis. Acute surgical procedures are indicated for patients suffering from traumatic events producing epidural hematoma, epidural hemorrhage, or subdural hematoma. Acute hydrocephalus should be treated by ventricular drainage.

B. In the chronic situation:
1. Patients with residual neurological deficits who are suffering from seizures should have adequate seizure control with appropriate anticonvulsants. Frequent determinations of serum levels of anticonvulsants may be necessary to ensure control of seizure activity.
2. Patients with permanent neurological problems require a planned multidisciplinary program to obtain optimum benefit. The emotional impact of the chronic illness on the child and the family should always be considered. A planned program of physical therapy extending over many months is useful. Speech therapy by a

Table 11-2
Strokes in children and young adults: diagnostic procedures

An acute stroke in a child or young adult requires immediate comprehensive investigation to rule out trauma, intracranial infection, intracranial mass lesion, and congenital heart disease. When the patient is a young child, the history obtained from parents must be complete and include details of birth and early development in the child. A family history of stroke, myocardial infarction, lipid disorders, bleeding diathesis, failure to thrive, and early death in siblings or near relatives suggests a hereditary factor. The general physical and neurologic examination must be as complete as possible prior to the use of additional testing.

1. A CT Scan should be obtained in the emergency center to rule out mass lesion, including epidural and subdural hematoma, intracerebral hemorrhage, cerebral edema due to trauma, tumors, and cerebral abscess. A CT scan is superior to MRI scanning in detection of an acute hemorrhage, but the CT scan may have a normal appearance in the presence of an ischemic infarction readily detected by an MRI scan in the early hours following a stroke. Consequently, a CT scan taken without contrast in the emergency center should be followed by an MRI scan if the CT scan is negative and the clinical signs point to an infarction.

2. A CT scan will show involvement of mastoid air cells and paranasal sinuses in mastoiditis or sinusitis.

3. A chest x-ray should be taken to rule out pneumonia or unexpected primary of metastatic tumor.

4. A lumbar puncture should be performed after the CT scan in any case with fever and nuchal rigidity to rule out encephalitis and meningitis. The cerebrospinal fluid should be examined for cells, glucose and protein content. A VDRL and streptococcal antigen should be obtained. A smear should be stained by Gram stain and for tuberculosis and the fluid cultured aerobically and anaerobically for bacteria and appropriately for fungi and viruses.

5. A blood sample should be drawn for a complete blood count and differential, platelet count, sedimentation rate, prothrombin time, partial thromboplastin time, plasma fibrinogen, VDRL, antinuclear antibody, factor V Leiden, and blood culture for bacterial septicemia.

6. It is important to rule out heart disease as the source of embolism. Studies include an electrocardiogram, 24-hour continuous cardiac monitoring, two-dimensional echo, and transesophageal echocardiogram. Additional studies may be suggested by a cardiology consultant, should this be necessary.

7. If all of the above are normal in an unexplained stroke, the following tests should be obtained: anticardiolipin, antithrombin III, lupus anticoagulant, protein C, protein S, plasma homocysteine.

8. When all of the above are negative, additional clotting factors, including factor III, factor VII, factor VIII, factor IX, and factor X should be assayed. In addition, fibrinogen molecular assay, hemoglobin electrophoresis, and erythrocyte osmotic fragility should be determined.

9. Arteriography will be required in all cases of nontraumatic subarachnoid hemorrhages of unknown etiology, to rule out the presence of cerebral aneurysm or a small vascular malformation that has not been detected by MRI or MR angiography. Arteriography is the definitive study for the diagnosis of cerebral arteritis in young adults.

trained speech pathologist is indicated for patients with dysphasia or dysarthria. All children should receive full psychological evaluation and a psychologist should be available for counseling if this is required by the child or family. The psychological evaluation is useful in planning education for the impaired child or adolescent. In addition, the evaluation will detect and measure depression, which is quite common following stroke in the young adult. Treatment with appropriate antidepressants and psychotherapy should be obtained, if indicated. A social worker may also help in counseling and in arranging for available community resources to be used in the rehabilitation process.

Prognosis

Although young children show much better recovery from motor and speech deficits following a stroke than adults, many children are left with obvious neurological deficits. One of the main problems is epilepsy, and almost all children with hemiplegia accompanied by seizures at onset have subsequent epileptic attacks. Many children with motor deficits also have intellectual impairment and hyperkinetic behavior. Language development is often delayed in children, or dysphasia is a problem in the young adult, but recovery is often quite good over a period of 2 years. Permanent aphasia or severe dysphasia is rare if the neurological deficit begins before the age of 4 years.[63]

Some conditions producing stroke have a high risk of recurrence: homocystinuria, sickle cell disease, cerebral embolism from congenital heart disease, and particularly, polyarthritis nodosa. The risk of cerebral embolism can be reduced by the use of long-term anticoagulant therapy. Arteritis often responds to corticosteroids, although immune suppression may be required in some cases.

Intracerebral Hemorrhage in Children and Young Adults

Trauma is the predominant cause of intracerebral hemorrhage in children and young adults. Nontraumatic intracerebral hemorrhage results from platelet disorders such as idiopathic thrombocytopenic purpura[64] or thrombocytopenia secondary to leukemia.

Intracerebral hemorrhage is also related to coagulation defects, particularly hemophilia, where bleeding can occur following trivial head injury. Hemophiliacs should receive prompt replacement of factor VIII [65] or factor IV, according to the defect causing the bleeding.

Subarachnoid Hemorrhage in Children and Young Adults

In the majority of cases, head trauma is the cause of subarachnoid hemorrhage in children and young adults. However, aneurysms of the circle of Willis, pathologically indistinguishable from saccular aneurysms in older adults, can occur at a younger age. Other causes of subarachnoid hemorrhage include bleeding from an arteriovenous malformation or rupture of a mycotic aneurysm, which developed following arterial wall infection by septic emboli in intravenous drug addiction.

Familial occurrence of saccular aneurysm is rare. These aneurysms are usually similar in structure to berry aneurysms occurring in other individuals, but some cases may have an abnormality in type III collagen.[66] Collagen defects also occur in the Ehlers-Danlos syndrome, type I and type IV,[67] pseudoxanthoma elasticum, and fibromuscular dysplasia, predisposing to aneurysm formation. The presumed relationship between symptomatic intracranial aneurysms and Marfan syndrome has not been established.[68]

The prognosis following aneurysmal rupture in children and young adults is similar to that in the older adult population, with a high mortality rate and recurrence in the first several days. It may be possible to reduce mortality by the earliest possible surgical intervention in patients with absence of or mild neurological deficits.[69]

Venous Sinus and Cortical Venous Thrombosis

Cerebral venous thrombosis is a feature of some hemoglobinopathies, coagulation disorders such as factor V Leiden mutation,[70] polycythemia, dehydration, and congestive heart failure. Infections of the paranasal sinuses, chronic otitis media, and facial orbital cellulitis are associated with venous sinus thrombosis.

Occlusion of the anterior superior sagittal sinus results in headache, papilledema, nausea and vomiting, partial or generalized seizures, and focal neurological deficits when there is involvement of cortical veins. Cavernous sinus thrombosis, usually a complication of facial or orbital cellulitis, presents with headache, proptosis, and ipsilateral third, fourth, fifth, and sixth nerve palsies. In contrast, signs of lateral sinus thrombosis are often minimal because of collateral venous drainage but can present the constant headache and hearing loss.[71] Venous sinus thrombosis can be demonstrated by MRA scanning.[72]

Treatment Infection should be treated with intravenous antibiotics and thrombosis by intravenous heparin, then oral warfarin. There is a small risk of hemorrhage when anticoagulant therapy is strictly controlled by International Normalized Ratio.

REFERENCES

1. Powell FC, Hanigan WC, McCluney KW: Subcortical infarction in children. *Stroke* 25:117, 1994.
2. Bogousslavsky J, Pierre P: Ischemic stroke in patients under age 45. *Neurol Clin* 10:113, 1992.
3. Leno C, Berciano J, Combarros O, et al: A prospective study of stroke in young adults in Cantabria, Spain. *Stroke* 24:792, 1993.
4. Balkaran B, Char G, Morris JS, et al: Stroke in a cohort of patients with homozygous sickle cell disease. *J Pediatr* 120:360, 1992.
5. Joist JH: Hypercoagulability: Introduction and perspective. *Semin Throm Hemost* 16:151, 1990.
6. Van Hoff J, Ritchey AK, Shaywitz BA: Intracranial hemorrhage in children with sickle cell disease. *Am J Dis Child* 139:1120, 1985.
7. Coull BM, Clark WM: Abnormalities of hemostasis in ischemic stroke. *Med Clin North Am* 77:77, 1993.
8. Powars D, Chan LS, Schroeder WA: The variable expression of sickle cell disease is genetically determined. *Semin Hematol* 27:360, 1990.
9. Armstrong FD, Thompson RJ Jr, Wang W, et al: Cognitive functioning and brain magnetic imaging in children with sickle cell disease. Neuropsychology Committee of the Cooperative Study of Sickle Cell Disease. *Pediatrics* 97:864, 1996.
10. Siegel MJ, Luker GD, Glauser TA, et al: Cerebral infarction in sickle cell disease: transcranial Doppler U.S. versus neurologic examination. *Radiology* 197:191, 1995.
11. Wasserman AL, Wilimas JA, Fairclough DL, et al: Subtle neuropsychological deficits in children with sickle cell disease. *Am J Pediatr Hematol Oncol* 13:14, 1991.
12. Cohen MJ, Branch WB, McKie VC, et al: Neuropsychological impairment in children with sickle cell anemia and cerebrovascular accidents. *Clin Pediatr* 33:517, 1994.
13. Miller ST, Jensen D, Rao SP: Less intensive long-term transfusion therapy for sickle cell anemia and cerebrovascular accident. *J Pediatr* 120:54, 1992.
14. Brown DC, Livingston JH, Minns RA, et al: Protein C and protein S deficiency causing childhood stroke. *Scot Med J* 38:114, 1993.
15. Graham JA, Daly HM, Carson PJ: Antithrombin III deficiency, and cerebrovascular accidents in young adults. *J Clin Pathol* 45:921, 1992.
16. Fuh JL, Teng MM, Yang WC, et al: Cerebral infarction in young men with nephrotic syndrome. *Stroke* 23:295, 1992.
17. Ferro D, Quintarelli C, Rasura M, et al: Lupus anticoagulant and the fibrinolytic system in young patients with stroke. *Stroke* 24:368, 1993.
18. Dungan DD, Jay MS: Stroke in an early adolescent with systemic lupus erythematosus and coexistent antiphospholipid antibodies. *Pediatrics* 90:96, 1992.
19. Lousa M, Sastre JL, Cancelas JA, et al: Study of antiphospholipid antibodies in a patient with Sneddon's syndrome and her family. *Stroke* 25:1071, 1994.
20. Zuber M, Toulon P, Marnet L, et al: Factor V Leiden mutation in cerebral venous thrombosis. *Stroke* 27:1721, 1996.
21. Ridker PM, Hennekens CH, Lindpaintner K, et al: Mutation in the gene coding for coagulation factor V and the risk of myocardial infarction, stroke, and venous thrombosis in apparently healthy men. *N Engl J Med* 332:912, 1995.
22. Heywood DM, Carter AM, Catto AJ, et al: Polymorphisms of the factor VII gene and circulating FVII: C levels in relation to acute cerebrovascular disease and poststroke mortality. *Stroke* 28:816, 1997.
23. Pan WH, Bai CH, Chen JR, et al: Associations between carotid atherosclerosis and high factor VIII activity, dyslipidemia, and hypertension. *Stroke* 28:88, 1997.
24. Nagayama M, Shinohara Y, Nagayama T: Lipoprotein (a) and ischemic cerebrovascular disease in young adults. *Stroke* 25:74, 1994.
25. Di Minno G, Martinez J, Cirillo A, et al: A role for platelets and thrombin in the juvenile stroke of two siblings with defective thrombin-adsorbing capacity of fibrin. *Arteriosclerosis Thromb* 11:785, 1991.
26. Nagayama T, Tsuda M, Sei Y, et al: DNA analysis of congenital abnormal plasminogen with clinical significance. *Jpn J Stroke* 14:395, 1992.
27. Clarke R, Daly L, Robinson K, et al: Hyperhomocysteinemia: an independent risk factor for vascular disease. *N Engl J Med* 324:1149, 1991.
28. Mereau-Richard C, Muller JP, Faivre E, et al: Total plasma homocysteine determination in subjects with premature cerebral vascular disease. *Clin Chem* 37:126, 1991.
29. Cruysberg JR, Boers GH, Trijbels JM, et al: Delay in diagnosis of homocystinuria: retrospective study of consecutive patients. *BMJ* 313:1037, 1996.
30. Petri M, Roubenoff R, Dallal GE, et al: Plasma homocysteine as a risk factor for atherothrombotic events in systemic lupus erythematosus. *Lancet* 384:1120, 1996.
31. Curless RG: Idiopathic ischemic infarction of the brain stem in children. *Child's Nerv System* 7:305, 1991.

32. Trescher WH: Ischemic stroke syndromes in childhood. *Pediatr Ann* 21:374, 1992.

33. Rothrock J, North J, Madden K, et al: Migraine and migrainous stroke: risk factors and prognosis. *Neurology* 43:2473, 1993.

34. Shuper A, Packer RJ, Vezina LG, et al: Complicated migraine-like episodes in children following cranial irradiation and chemotherapy. *Neurology* 45:1837, 1995.

35. Moriarty KP, Harris BH, Benitez-Marchand K: Carotid artery thrombosis and stroke after blunt pharyngeal injury. *J Trauma* 42:541, 1997.

36. Meuli M, Glarner H: Delayed cerebral infarction after dog bites: case report. *J Trauma* 37:848, 1994.

37. Sheth RD, Jaynes M, Gingold M, et al: Stroke due to a traumatic vertebral artery dissection in a girl. *Clin Pediatr* 33:503, 1994.

38. Garg BP, Ottinger CJ, Smith RR, et al: Strokes in children due to vertebral artery trauma. Neurology 43:2555, 1993.

39. Geny C, Yulis J, Azoulay A, et al: Thalamic infarction following lingual herpes zoster. *Neurology* 41:1846, 1991.

40. Ganesan V, Kirkham FJ: Mechanisms of ischaemic stroke after chickenpox. *Arch Dis Child* 76:522, 1997.

41. Kovacs SO, Kuban K, Strand R: Lateral medullary syndrome following varicella infection. *Am J Dis Child* 147:823, 1993.

42. Taft TA, Chusid MJ, Sty JR: Cerebral infarction in *Hemophilus influenzae* type B meningitis. *Clin Pediatr* 25:177, 1986.

43. Reik L Jr: Stroke due to Lyme disease. *Neurology* 43:2705, 1993.

44. Alarcon F, Hidalgo F, Moncayo J, et al: Cerebral cysticercosis and stroke. *Stroke* 23:224, 1992.

45. Sloan MA, Mattioni TA: Concurrent myocardial and cerebral infarctions after intranasal cocaine use. *Stroke* 23:427, 1992.

46. Barinagarrementeria F, Cantu-Brito C, De La Pena A, et al: Prothrombotic states in young people with idiopathic stroke. A prospective study. *Stroke* 25:287, 1994.

47. Haapaniemi H, Hillbom M, Juvela J: Lifestyle associated risk factors for acute brain infarction among persons of working age. *Stroke* 28:26, 1997.

48. Park YD, Belman AL, Kim TS, et al: Stroke in pediatric acquired immunodeficiency syndrome. *Ann Neurol* 28:303, 1990.

49. Philippet P, Blanche S, Sebag G, et al: Stroke and cerebral infarcts in children infected with human immunodeficiency virus. *Arch Pediatr Adolescent Med* 148:965, 1994.

50. Conti CR: Embolic stroke: are we missing the source in many young patients? *Clin Cardiol* 16:83, 1993.

51. Diez-Tejedor E, Munoz C, Frank A: Cerebellar infarction in children and young adults related to fibromuscular dysplasia and dissection of the vertebral artery. *Stroke* 24:1096, 1993.

52. Pavlakis SG, Verlander PC, Gould RJ, et al: Fanconi anemia and moyamoya: evidence for association. *Neurology* 45:998, 1995.

53. Choi Y, Kang BC, Kim KJ, et al: Renovascular hypertension in children with moyamoya disease. *J Pediatr* 131:258, 1997.

54. Kestle JR, Hoffman HJ, Mock AR: Moyamoya phenomenon after radiation for optic glioma. *J Neurosurg* 79:32, 1993.

55. Hopper KD: Neuroradiology case of the day. Moyamoya disease. *AJR Am J Roentgenol* 162:1479, 1994.

56. Kashiwagi S, Kato S, Yasuhara S, et al: Use of a split dura for revascularization of ischemic hemispheres in moyamoya disease. *J Neurosurg* 85:380, 1996.

57. Dauser RC, Tuite GF, McCluggage CW: Dural inversion procedure for moyamoya disease. Technical note. *J Neurosurg* 86:719, 1997.

58. Calderon A, Wong JW, Becker LE: Multiple cerebral venous thromboses in a child with ulcerative colitis. *Clin Pediatr* 32:169, 193.

59. Harvey JR, Teague SM, Anderson JL, et al: Clinically silent atrial septal defects with evidence for cerebral embolization. *Ann Int Med* 105:695, 1986.

60. Flegel KM, Shipley MS, Rose G: Risk of stroke in non-rheumatic atrial fibrillation. *Lancet* 1:526, 1987.

61. Biller J, Adams HP, Jr, Johnson MR, et al: Paradoxical cerebral embolism: eight cases. *Neurology* 36:1356, 1986.

62. Ferry PC: Neurologic sequelae of cardiac surgery in children. *Am J Dis Child* 141:309, 1987.

63. Bogousslavsky J, Regli F: Ischemic stroke in adults younger than 30 years of age. Cause and prognosis. *Arch Neurol* 44:479, 1987.

64. Lilleyman JS: Intracranial haemorrhage in idiopathic thrombocytopenic purpura. Paediatric Haematology Forum of the British Society for Haematology. *Arch Dis Child* 71:251, 1994.

65. Myers DJ, Moossy JJ, Ragni MV: Fatal clival subdural hematoma in a hemophiliac. *Ann Emerg Med* 25:249, 1995.

66. Pope FM, Limburg M, Schievink WI: Familial cerebral aneurysms and type III collagen deficiency. J Neurosurg 72:156, 1990.

67. North KN, Whiteman DA, Pepin MG, et al: Cere-

brovascular complications in Ehlers-Danlos syndrome type IV. *Ann Neurol* 38:960, 1995.

68. van den Berg JS, Limburg M, Hennekam RC: Is Marfan syndrome associated with symptomatic intracranial aneurysms? *Stroke* 27:10, 1996.

69. Olafsson E, Hauser WA, Gudmundsson G: A population-based study of prognosis of ruptured cerebral aneurysm: mortality and recurrence of subarachnoid hemorrhage. *Neurology* 48:1191, 1997.

70. Martinelli I, Landi G, Merati G, et al: Factor V gene mutation is a risk factor for cerebral venous thrombosis. *Thromb Haemostasis* 75:393, 1996.

71. Crassard I, Biousse V, Bousser M-G, et al: Hearing loss and headache revealing lateral sinus thrombosis in a patient with factor V Leiden mutation. *Stroke* 28:876, 1997.

72. Vogl TJ, Balzer JO, Stemmler J, et al: MR angiography in children with cerebral neurovascular diseases: findings in 31 cases. *AJR Am J Roentgenol* 159:817, 1992.

Chapter 12

VASCULAR DISEASE OF THE SPINAL CORD

When compared to cerebrovascular disease, vascular disease of the spinal cord is uncommon, a fact that does not support the unsubstantiated claim that the spinal cord has a "poor blood supply." The blood supply to the spinal cord is adequate in a healthy individual with ample reserve and the capacity for development of substantial collateral circulation. There are many common factors in vascular disease of the brain and spinal cord (i.e., atherosclerosis). However, because of a unique blood supply, a number of additional factors may produce vascular disease of the cord.

ANATOMY

Arterial Supply of the Spinal Cord

The anterior spinal artery runs the entire length of the spinal cord and is located in the anterior ventral sulcus of the cord. At the cranial end, the anterior spinal artery arises from the fourth portion of the vertebral artery and descends over the ventral surface of the medulla toward the midline to join the anterior spinal artery from the opposite side. The two vessels are usually small but have the capacity for hypertrophy and are a potential source of collateral circulation to the medulla and spinal cord. The anterior spinal artery is reinforced by three anterior, anastomotic (medullary) arteries in the cervical area. These vessels take origin from the vertebral artery, the deep cervical artery, and the costocervical or ascending cervical artery and usually join the anterior spinal artery at the level of C3, C6 and C8, respectively. The thoracic portion receives one or two anastomotic vessels, which arise from intercostal arteries. The most common site is at T4 or T5. The thoracolumbar portion of the anterior spinal artery is joined by the great anterior anastomotic artery of Adamkiewicz, which arises anywhere between the levels of T8 and L4 on the left side in about 80 percent of cases. This vessel receives blood from the aorta via the lower intercostal or lumbar arteries. In its course over the cauda equina the anterior artery is joined by branches from the lumbar, iliolumbar, lateral, and medial sacral arteries.

The anterior spinal artery is not a continuous vessel. Rather, it should be regarded as a series of anastomotic systems fed by anastomotic arteries such as the artery of Adamkiewicz. This physiological concept suggests that the arterial system of the spinal cord is similar to the arterial systems of the brain and brainstem.

The branches of the anterior spinal artery are of two types.

1. Central arteries penetrate the median fissure and branch alternately to the right or to the left with an occasional bifurcating vessel. These branches extend to the anterior horn, where they divide into a rich capillary network and form a plexus involving the anterior horn cells, the gray commissure, the lateral horn, and the base of the posterior horn. The capillaries from this system also penetrate the white matter and anastomose with branches of the centripetal system. There is further anastomosis through intersegmental arterioles, which extend upward and downward in the cord, forming a connection between adjacent segmental arterial systems.

2. The centripetal system arises from the anterior spinal artery and extends around the periphery of the spinal cord as far as the posterior nerve root. These vessels give rise to numerous penetrating radial arteries, which enter the white matter and anastomose with the capillaries of the central system.

The posterior spinal arteries constitute an irregular system that traverses the length of the spinal cord immediately posterior to the entrance of the posterior nerve root. These vessels are reinforced by 12 to 16 small posterior anastomotic arteries. The posterior spinal system anastomoses superiorly with the vertebral arteries and inferiorly with the anterior spinal artery through many fine arterioles surrounding the terminal portion of the spinal cord and cauda equina. The posterior horns of the spinal cord and the posterior columns, which constitute the posterior third of the spinal cord, are supplied by penetrating vessels arising from numerous superficial anastomotic vessels joining the two posterior spinal arteries.

Venous Drainage of the Spinal Cord

The intrinsic drainage of the spinal cord occurs through a central venous system and a radial group of veins.

The central veins of the spinal cord converge toward the anterior median fissure and enter the anterior median spinal vein. The radial veins pass to the surface of the cord, where a plexus is formed. This plexus drains into the anterior median spinal vein.

The posterior one-third of the spinal cord is also drained by a series of radial veins into a posterior plexus. Blood from the anterior medial spinal vein and from the posterior plexus of veins enters a series of anastomotic veins, which penetrate the dura and enter the internal and external vertebral plexi. These systems extend throughout the length of the spinal canal and anastomose with the vena cava, the azygos, and the hemiazygos systems. Such an arrangement allows blood to be channeled into the pelvic plexus of veins and into the dural sinuses and cerebral veins at the level of the foramen magnum.

SPINAL CORD INFARCTION

Definition

Spinal cord infarction results from inadequate blood supply to the spinal cord parenchyma.

Etiology and Pathology

The development of spinal cord infarction is influenced by a number of anatomical, physiological, and pathological factors, including:

1. Site of occlusion. The farther from the cord the occlusion occurs, the better the chance of developing collateral circulation.

2. Anatomical variation. The greater the number of anastomotic vessels to the cord, the better the chance of avoiding infarction should an anastomotic vessel or its parent vessel become occluded.

3. Onset of occlusion. Gradual occlusion of a vessel permits the development of collateral circulation and is less likely to cause infarction than rapid occlusion. A decrease in perfusion pressure in the anastomotic vessels produces spinal cord ischemia and increases the chance of infarction.

4. Systemic blood pressure. Hypotension due to cardiac arrest or acute blood loss decreases perfusion pressure and increases the chance of infarction.

5. Hypoxia. Chronic hypoxia results in lower arterial oxygen tension and increases the chance of infarction. Acute hypoxia caused by cardiac or pulmonary arrest may result in infarction.

6. Atherosclerosis. Progressive atherosclerosis involving the aorta, anastomotic vessels, or the spinal arteries reduces blood flow to the cord and increases the chances of infarction.[1]

7. Inflammation. Arteritis (syphilis, giant cell arteritis, or polyarteritis nodosa) of the anastomotic vessels or the anterior spinal artery and its branches will increase the chance of thrombosis and infarction.

8. Embolism. Emboli can arise from the heart or become detached from atherosclerotic plaques in the aorta, iliac vessels, vertebral, intercostal, or lumbar arteries and enter the circulation of the spinal cord. Cartilaginous embolism from the nucleus pulposus of a herniated intervertebral disc has been reported.[2]

9. Trauma. The spinal arteries and anastomotic vessels are susceptible to trauma. Fracture dislocation, cervical subluxation, spondylosis, and disc protrusion may produce damage to the intercostal, lumbar, or anastomotic vessels.

10. Anastomotic arteries may be occluded by a dissecting aneurysm of the aorta or by surgical procedures for aortoiliac occlusive disease.

11. Sickle cell disease with progressive narrowing and thrombosis of the anastomotic arteries, or anterior spinal arteries, may lead to ischemia and infarction.

The pathology of ischemia shows some variation according to the site of the involved vessel. When the aorta is involved, there may be occlusion at the origin of the intercostal or lumbar arteries due to aortic aneurysm, dissecting aneurysm of the aorta, thrombosis, or surgical procedures of the aorta. The vertebral arteries are susceptible to thrombosis owing to atherosclerosis, after cervical injury or chiropractic manipulation, which can cause occlusion or dissecting aneurysm of the vertebral arteries. Intercostal and lumbar arteries are occasionally injured in thoracoplasty and resection of an aortic aneurysm. An anastomotic artery may be occluded following trauma to the spine or the development of primary or metastatic tumors of the spine. There may be involvement due to osteomyelitis of the spine or tuberculous osteomyelitis (Pott's disease). In addition, the vessel may be involved by an arteritis in syphilis or collagen vascular diseases. Anterior and posterior spinal arteries may be occluded because of trauma with fracture dislocation of the spine or pressure from a herniated lumbar disc. The anterior spinal artery is particularly susceptible to compression in cases of cervical spondylosis.

The pathological changes in infarction of the spinal cord resemble those seen in ischemic infarction of the brain with necrosis of the gray matter followed by astroglial proliferation and formation of a glial scar.

Clinical Features

All of the signs and symptoms of spinal cord infarction can be attributed to a lesion within the distribution of the occluded vessel.

Transient ischemic attacks of the cervical spinal cord may resemble "drop attacks" without loss or impairment of consciousness, and are usually attributed to ischemia of the medullary pyramids. Intermittent attacks can also occur in coarctation of the aorta with an associated "steal" of blood from the spinal cord. Shunting of blood to a low resistance vascular malformation in the spinal cord may produce temporary

ischemia in the surrounding area. Intermittent compression of the spinal cord in patients with spinal stenosis can produce temporary symptoms of cord ischemia.

The onset of transient ischemia may be sudden or gradual, with deficits developing in an hour or less. Motor symptoms can consist of abrupt onset of quadriplegia or paraplegia presenting with sudden loss of tone in all four limbs and a drop attack. The less acute episodes consist of numbness, pain, tingling, aching, and cramping below the level of the cord involvement, with limb weakness and loss of bladder and bowel function followed by recovery over several hours.

When the anterior spinal artery is occluded, infarction may occur some distance from the site of occlusion, in an area of cord that is a boundary zone between two anastomotic arteries. In this case, there is initial flaccid paralysis and loss of reflexes with a sensory level displaying loss of pain and temperature sensation below the area of infarction. Sphincter control is lost, with bladder and bowel paralysis. The initial flaccidity is followed by a gradual development of spasticity, hyperreflexia, and bilateral extensor plantar responses.[3] Occlusion of the cervical anastomotic branch of the anterior spinal artery produces a combination of upper and lower motor neuron abnormalities. There are weakness and wasting of muscles in the upper limb supplied by the appropriate anterior horn cells at the level of the infarct with flaccid quadriparesis progressing gradually to spastic paraparesis and loss of pain and temperature sensation below the level of the lesion.

Infarction in the thoracic cord produces a flaccid paraplegia with gradual progression to spastic paraparesis and impairment or loss of bladder control. This is associated with a dissociated sensory loss and eventually with some return of bladder function.

Lesions of the lumbosacral cord tend to produce flaccid paraparesis because of destruction of the motor neurons of the anterior horn cells at this level. A dissociated sensory loss and incomplete involvement of bowel and bladder function are apparent.

It is not unusual to encounter incomplete infarction of the spinal cord. The effects of infarction depend on the efficiency of the collateral circulation, and only small segments of the anterior two-thirds of the spinal cord may be irreversibly damaged after oc-clusion of the anterior spinal artery or its branches.

Posterior spinal artery occlusion is very rare.[4] Syphilitic arteritis is believed to have been the major cause of this condition in the past. However, trauma, infection, or compression of the posterior spinal ar-teries may compromise the circulation sufficiently to produce infarction of the posterior one-third of the spinal cord. The clinical picture is tabetic-like, with progressive ataxia and loss of vibration and position sense. Tendon reflexes are depressed or absent. There may be retention of urine with painless distention of the bladder. Spinal cord compression should be relieved and infection controlled by appropriate antibiotic therapy. Urinary retention or incomplete emptying can be managed with intermittent self-catheterization. Gait may be improved by physical therapy.

Table 12-1
Differential diagnosis: cord infarction, transverse myelitis, epidural abscess

Infarction	Transverse myelitis	Epidural abscess
Age		
Elderly, unless some unusual easily identifiable condition exists (e.g., syphilis)	Any age	Any age
Pain		
Acute onset, radicular distribution	Yes. Often interscapular with radiation into the abdomen and lower limbs	Yes. At site of abscess
Onset of spasticity		
Acute onset, initially flaccid followed by development of spasticity	May be acute or insidious onset. May be prolonged flaccidity	Insidious onset, spastic lower extremities
Spinal fluid		
Normal	Abnormal. Inflammatory cells and elevated protein content	Abnormal. Xanthochromic if complete block, polymorphonuclear leukocytosis, protein elevated, glucose normal
Peripheral nerve involvement		
None (except diabetic neuropathy)	Yes. Lesion may involve nerve roots	None (except diabetic neuropathy)
Dissociated sensory loss		
Yes	Unusual	No
X-ray spine		
Normal	Normal	Osteomyelitis in some cases
Myelography		
Normal	Normal	Extradural compression, may be a complete block
MRI scan		
Abnormal, round Hypointensity T1 Hyperintensity T2 Areas in acute infarction	Hypointensity T1 Hyperintensity T2 Areas in white matter	Obstructed epidural space by enhancing mass

Diagnostic Procedures

1. Lumbar puncture. The cerebrospinal fluid (CSF) is normal in appearance, and there is little or no cellular response. The protein content may be elevated.
2. Magnetic resonance imaging (MRI) will show a round area of hypointensity of T1-weighted images and hyperintensity on T2-weighted images in an acute ischemic infarction of the spinal cord.[5] This changes to a strand-like abnormality with negative enhancement after infusion of gadolinium several weeks later.

Differential Diagnosis

Table 12-1 differentiates cord infarction, transverse myelitis, and epidural abscess.

Treatment

Treatment is as for cerebral infarction (see page 256).

Prognosis

Many patients with spinal cord infarction show gratifying return of function in the lower limbs and considerable improvement in bowel and bladder function over a period of several months. Prevention of further infarction depends on the control of precipitating factors discussed in Chapter 8. Patients with atherosclerosis run a high risk of coronary artery disease and cerebral thrombosis.

INTERMITTENT CLAUDICATION OF THE SPINAL CORD

Intermittent ischemia of the spinal cord or cauda equina may result in transient pain, weakness, and numbness in one or both lower limbs during exercise. The disorder is believed to result from narrowing of the spinal canal, herniation of a lumbar disc, or lumbar spondylosis, leading to spinal stenosis that results in pressure on the spinal cord or cauda equina. A similar ischemic effect can occur in aortoiliac occlusive disease.[6] Patients with this condition develop aching in one or both calves followed by paresthesias of one or both feet while walking. Continued walking may result in foot drop. Examination reveals that the circulation of both lower limbs is adequate. There is exaggeration of tendon reflexes if the spinal cord is involved. Radiography, MRI, or computed tomography (CT) scanning of the lumbosacral spine will show the presence of osteoarthritis and narrowing of intervertebral disc spaces. Surgical removal or herniated discs and decompression of the spinal stenosis will result in improvement.

CHRONIC ISCHEMIA OF THE SPINAL CORD

It is likely that change in the cervical cord in some individuals with cervical spondylosis are due to a combination of compression of the cord and ischemia of the cord due to compression of the vasculature. This would account for the development of symptoms indicating damage to the cord above and below the site of the lesion.

ARTERIOVENOUS MALFORMATION OF THE SPINAL CORD

Definition

Most arteriovenous malformations (AVMs) involving the spinal cord are low-flow conditions. Symptoms are probably the result of increased venous pressure and cord ischemia.

Pathology

Spinal AVMs are categorized into four types.[7] Type 1 (dural arteriovenous fistula) is divided into types 1a and 1b.

Type 1a, the most common type of spinal AVM, is usually found on the dorsal aspect of the thoracic spinal cord or the conus medullaris. There is a single arterial feeder entering the dura at the dural root sleeve. The arteriovenous fistula lies within the dura and the venous outflow drains intradurally into an arterialized vein extending several segments above and below, draining into the venous plexus on the dorsal surface of the spinal cord. Type 1b AVMs are similar to 1a AVMs but have multiple additional feeders at one or two adjacent levels that communicate with the dural nidus. Type 2 (glomus) AVMs have a nidus lying within the spinal cord and are fed by multiple feeders from the anterior spinal and posterior spinal arteries. Type 3 (juvenile) AVMs are rare. They are intermedullary but have extramedullary and occasional extraspinal extensions. Type 4 AVMs (intra- or perimedullary fistulae) are intradural extramedullary fistulas fed by the anterior and posterior spinal arteries and are found outside the spinal cord. There are three subdivisions: type 4a, simple extramedullary fistulae; type 4b, intermediate in size extramedullary and supplied by one or more feeders; and type 4c, giant AVMs fed by the anterior spinal artery and draining into a greatly dilated and tortuous plexus of veins. The high-flow shunting may lead to a form of vascular steal from the intrinsic spinal cord arterial supply and cause ischemia of the spinal cord.

Clinical Features

Most patients with an AVM of the spinal cord experience pain at the level of the lesion or in the lower limbs. The pain may be constant or episodic and is often of an unpleasant burning quality. Some patients show progressive spastic paraparesis with or without evidence of a lower motor neuron lesion. This is typical of the type 1a dural arteriovenous fistula, which produces a chronic myelopathy secondary to increased venous pressure and impaired venous drainage from the spinal cord.[8] Urgency, frequency, and incontinence are present in about two-thirds of patients. Sensory deficits occur below the level of the lesion and affect all sensory modalities. The neurological deficits tend to progress in a stepwise fashion over a period of months or years. Sudden paraplegia from hemorrhage or infarction may occur at any time. Rupture of an AVM with spinal subarachnoid hemorrhage is unusual but has been reported.[9]

Diagnostic Procedures

1. The MRI will demonstrate the site of the malformation and the presence of any hemorrhage.
2. Superselective arteriography is needed to demonstrate the extent of the AVM, its feeding vessels, and its type.

Treatment

Direct removal of the AVM is the treatment of choice in type 1 malformations. The best results with type 2 AVMs are probably obtained with preoperative embolization and subsequent surgical resection. Because type 3 AVMs are intermedullary and extramedullary, they require feeder ligation embolization and partial resection.[10]

A small type 4 AVM can be removed surgically; those of medium size require embolization and surgical excision, whereas large type 4 AVMs are treated by embolization alone. Embolization is, however, followed by a recanalization in some cases.[11]

VENOUS SPINAL CORD INFARCTION

Three types of venous infarction of the spinal cord have been recognized: embolic, hemorrhagic, and nonhemorrhagic. *Embolic infarctions* are associated with venous embolism elsewhere, such as pulmonary embolism, and produce sudden back pain with symmetrical dysfunction and dissociate sensory loss. *Hemorrhagic infarctions* have equally sudden onset with back pain or radicular pain, progressive neurological dysfunction, and a high mortality rate. *Nonhemorrhagic infarction* is more gradual and painless, with neurological signs evolving over several weeks.

Venous spinal cord infarction is often diagnosed as a transverse myelitis. Angiography may be helpful and MRI scanning will help to rule out hemorrhage. Nonhemorrhagic cases should be treated with anticoagulation.

TRANSVERSE MYELITIS (MYELOPATHY)

Definition

Transverse myelitis is a syndrome characterized by acute spinal cord dysfunction involving both halves of the cord in transverse section.

Etiology and Pathology

The various etiologies of transverse myelitis are outlined in Table 12-2. The condition may be a peri-infectious or postinfectious process and has been associated with many viral infections, including poliovirus, echovirus, and Coxsackieviruses.[12] In some patients, there is direct viral involvement of the spinal cord, whereas others present with a postinfectious process, probably the result of inflammation, edema, or an autoimmune response to viral infection. Transverse myelitis has been associated with measles, varicella, mumps, rabies, typhoid, systemic lupus erythematosus, and a reaction to sulfonamides. Transverse myelitis has also followed vaccination and immunization against rubella, diphtheria, and poliomyelitis. Vascular occlusion with softening of the cord may occur in syphilitic arteritis and in the arteritis associated with collagen vascular diseases. Arterial occlusion due to a dissecting aneurysm of the aorta or after surgical resection of an aortic aneurysm are other possible causes. Acute transverse myelitis in

Table 12-2
Etiologies of transverse myelitis

1. Congenital—vascular malformation
2. Infectious—viral infection
3. Autoimmune—peri-infectious, postinfectious, or vaccinial myelitis
4. Multiple sclerosis
5. Neoplastic—paraneoplastic necrosis
6. Toxic—secondary to heroin injections
7. Vascular—vascular insufficiency—arteritis, dissecting aneurysm, aorta resection, aortic aneurysm
8. Degenerative—irradiation
9. Idiopathic

heroin addicts is probably due to focal arteritis. Transverse myelitis may occur as an acute demyelinating process in multiple sclerosis and a severe acute myelitis as a remote effect of carcinoma. The increasing survival of patients with treated neoplasms has led to the recognition of increasing numbers of cases of acute transverse myelitis secondary to radiation therapy.

Sudden bleeding from vascular malformations or capillary telangiectasia may produce a similar picture.

The pathological changes vary. In most cases, there is necrosis of the cord, often involving several segments. The necrosis is maximal in the center of the cord and even in severe cases, there is always a thin rim of surviving tissue at the periphery. The posterior nerve roots and posterior root ganglia are occasionally involved in the process. In cases of vascular etiology, there is infarction of the spinal cord.

Clinical Features

A history of recent acute illness suggesting a viral or bacterial infection may be obtained in about one-third of the patients. The most common complaint is a history of upper respiratory tract infection or a flu-like illness. Transverse myelitis is occasionally preceded by a gastrointestinal illness. Patients with transverse myelitis occurring as a paraneoplastic condition have a history of pre-existing neoplasia that is frequently metastatic. Radiation transverse myelitis occurs several months to a year after radiation therapy.

Transverse myelitis presents with symptoms and signs indicating involvement of gray matter and the corticospinal and spinothalamic tracts.

1. Paresthesias, which are often described as numbness, tingling, or pins and needles, usually begin in the toes or the feet and extend up the lower limbs into the trunk, with eventual involvement of the upper limbs in cervical transverse myelitis.

2. Pain is of sudden onset, usually severe and corresponding to the level of the cord involvement. Consequently, the pain is often in the intrascapular region.

3. Progressive lower limb weakness is noted, often presenting with "stumbling or weakness of one leg."

4. Urinary retention occasionally occurs as the initial complaint and is usually followed by lower limb weakness in a short period of time.

The course of transverse myelitis may vary:

1. A smooth progressive course often begins with involvement of the lower limbs followed by ascending paresthesias and weakness over a period of 2 weeks, at which time the condition stabilizes with paraplegia or quadriplegia and a well-defined sensory level.

2. In subacute progression the symptoms appear intermittently over a 10-day to 4-week period. During this time, the illness may appear to stabilize, only to be followed by the appearance of new symptoms after several days of apparent stabilization.

3. Progressive limb weakness often presents with stumbling or asymmetrical weakness of a lower limb[13] or with upper limb paresthesias when there is cervical cord involvement.

4. An acute catastrophic illness with all symptoms develops within 12 h and sometimes in less than an hour after onset. This type of presentation is usually preceded by marked back pain. Recovery is slow and incomplete.

Examination of the patient reveals a flaccid paresis or paralysis with depressed or absent tendon reflexes suggesting involvement of anterior horn cells. There is bilateral symmetrical sensory loss extending to the upper level of cord involvement. This site commonly lies between T6 and T12, but there may be extension of the cervical cord in some cases. The sensory loss is usually total, involving touch, pinprick, vibration, and proprioception, or the loss may be dissociated, with loss of pinprick and preservation of posterior column functions. Bladder distention occurs early in the illness in the majority of patients and is followed by overflow incontinence. Fecal incontinence is less frequently encountered.

Diagnostic Procedures

1. The T2-weighted MRI scan shows areas of increased signal intensity involving gray matter and surrounding white matter.
2. Electromyography performed after 2 weeks will demonstrate motor axonopathy in keeping with anterior horn cell involvement.
3. Lumbar puncture. The CSF is abnormal with a pleocytosis in about 50 percent of cases, which varies from a mild increase in leukocytes to a white count as high as 300 cells per cubic millimeter. The cells are predominantly monocytic. Protein content is elevated in about 40 percent of cases.

Differential Diagnosis

See Table 12-1.

Treatment

The patient should be placed on bed rest and turned every 2 h to prevent the development of decubiti and also to promote drainage of the dependent portions of the lungs. The bladder should be catheterized and the urine cultured periodically to detect any infection. Appropriate antibiotics are inducted if infection occurs. The bowels should be moved once every 2 days and a diet with adequate bulk content given as soon as possible to prevent fecal impaction. Physical therapy with passive movements of all joints should be performed twice a day. Application of foam rubber splints to the lower limbs helps to prevent contraction deformities. Patients with involvement of the upper limbs require adequate splinting of the forearms, wrists, and hands.

As recovery occurs, efforts should be made to remove the bladder catheter as soon as possible and urological evaluation should be obtained to determine bladder function. Stimulants such as bethanechol chloride, a parasympathetic stimulant, 10 to 50 mg three or four times a day may help to initiate micturition and empty the bladder in patients with persistent bladder paralysis.

Spasticity involving the lower limbs can be relieved by baclofen (Lioresal) 10 mg q6h, increasing slowly to as high as 100 to 120 mg/day. Severe spasticity will require the use of a baclofen pump with intrathecal injection of baclofen.[14]

Physical therapy, beginning with passive therapy in the acute phase, should be changed gradually to a more active program as the patient recovers.

Prognosis

The majority of patients with transverse myelitis show some degree of recovery, which varies from complete to minimal. More than 50 percent of patients with the idiopathic form of the disease regain the ability to walk within a year, although a number will be dependent on orthopedic appliances. Twenty-five percent of patients show poor recovery and the majority of these give a history of severe back pain preceding a rapid catastrophic onset of transverse myelitis.

NONTRAUMATIC SUBDURAL HEMATOMA OF THE SPINAL CORD

Definition

Nontraumatic subdural hematoma of the spinal cord is a rare condition in which blood accumulates in the spinal subdural space.

Etiology and Pathology

The majority of cases of nontraumatic spinal subdural hematoma occur in patients with an underlying hematological disorder such as hemophilia, leukemia, or thrombocytopenic purpura. Many cases have been reported following lumbar puncture and anticoagulant therapy. Blood accumulates in the spinal subdural space with compression of the underlying spinal cord.

Clinical Features

The patient typically presents with a gradual onset of low back pain, followed by the development of progressive paraparesis over a period of several days.

Diagnostic Procedures

An MRI scan will show the presence of an extradural lesion with compression of the spinal cord.

Treatment

1. Dexamethasone (Decadron) should be administered immediately, 12 mg intravenously and then 4 mg q6h.
2. The subdural hematoma should be surgically evacuated as soon as possible.

Prognosis

Patients who have surgical relief of a cord compression before the development of complete paraplegia may show considerable improvement in weakness of the lower limbs.

REFERENCES

1. Gloviczki P, Cross SA, Stanson AW, et al: Ischemic injury to the spinal cord or lumbosacral plexus after aorto-iliac reconstruction. *Am J Surg* 162:131, 1991.
2. Moorhouse DF, Burke M, Keohane C, et al: Spinal cord infarction caused by cartilage embolus to the anterior spinal artery. *Surg Neurol* 37:448, 1992.
3. Satran R: Spinal cord infarction. *Stroke* 19:529, 1988.
4. Kaneki M, Inoue K, Shimizu T, et al: Infarction of the unilateral posterior horn and lateral column of the spinal cord with sparing of posterior columns: demonstration by MRI. *J Neurol Neurosurg Psychiatry* 57:629, 1994.
5. Nagashima C, Nagashima R, Morota N, et al: Magnetic resonance imaging of human spinal cord infarction. *Surg Neurol* 35:368, 1991.
6. Newcombe DS: Intermittent spinal ischemia. A reversible cause of neurologic dysfunction and back pain. *Arthritis Rheum* 37:142, 1994.
7. Anson JA, Spetzler RF: Classification of spinal arteriovenous malformations and implications for treatment. *BNI Q* 8:2, 1992.
8. Hurst RW, Kenyon LC, Lavi E, et al: Spinal dural arteriovenous fistula: the pathology of venous hypertensive myelopathy. *Neurology* 45:1309, 1995.
9. Gueguen B, Merland JJ, Riche MC, et al: Vascular

malformations of the spinal cord: intrathecal peri-medullary arteriovenous fistulas fed by medullary arteries. *Neurology* 37:969, 1987.

10. Touho H, Karasawa J, Shishido H, et al: Successful excision of a juvenile-type spinal arteriovenous malformation following intraoperative embolization. Case report. *J Neurosurg* 75:647, 1991.

11. Hall WA, Oldfield EH, Doppman JL: Recanalization of spinal arteriovenous malformations following embolization. *J Neurosurg* 70:714, 1989.

12. Jadoul C, Van Goethem J, Martin JJ: Myelitis due to coxsackievirus B infection. *Neurology* 45:1626, 1995.

13. Yui LA, Gledhill RF: Limb paralysis as a manifestation of coxsackie B virus infection. *Dev Med Child Neurol* 33:427, 1991.

14. Loubser PG, Narayan RK, Sandin KJ, et al: Continuous infusion of intrathecal baclofen: long-term effects on spasticity in spinal cord injury. *Paraplegia* 29:48, 1991.

Chapter 13

SYNCOPE AND SLEEP DISORDERS

There are relatively few causes of sudden loss of consciousness. These are outlined in Table 13-1. There is a common misconception that conditions such as myocardial infarction and intracerebral hemorrhage can produce a sudden loss of consciousness. This is incorrect and emphasizes the importance of obtaining an accurate history when faced with the problems of loss of consciousness.

SYNCOPE

Syncope is a loss of consciousness associated with a loss of postural tone and spontaneous recovery. The event is a result of transient cortical reduction of blood flow to the brain or brainstem (Table 13-2). There are three basic causes for syncope[1]:

1. Vasomotor instability with a decrease in systemic vascular resistance resulting in an increase in peripheral vascular volume and decreased venous return to the heart

2. Decrease in cardiac output owing to arrhythmias or obstruction of blood flow within the heart or pulmonary circulation

3. Sudden focal or generalized decrease in cerebral blood flow in individuals with loss of or impaired cerebral autoregulation owing to cerebrovascular disease

The importance of the history in the diagnosis of syncope cannot be overemphasized. In the majority of cases, the diagnosis will be apparent following a detailed description of events accompanying a typical syncopal episode obtained from the patient and from an observer. The approach is the same as that recommended in patients with suspected epilepsy and has been outlined in Chapter 1. A drug history should be taken at the end of the interview and may uncover a drug-induced syncope.

The physical examination is particularly important in revealing cardiac abnormalities that might contribute to syncope or in detecting orthostatic hypotension. All patients should have a blood pressure measurement performed in the supine position, then repeated with the patient standing after a period of 5 minutes, supine.

If ancillary tests are required, they are a logical extension of the history and examination and should be confirmatory rather than diagnostic in most cases.

Cardiac Syncope

Cardiac syncope is the result of an abrupt decrease in cardiac output. The episodes are charateristically sudden in onset and brief in duration. Loss of consciousness occurs without warning and the patient falls to the ground. On examination, the patient is pale and feels weak; the respirations are shallow and the pulse

Table 13-1
Causes of sudden loss of consciousness

I. Cardiac causes
  a. Cardiac asystole
  b. Cardiac arrhythmias
  c. Obstruction of left ventricular blood flow
    1. Aortic stenosis
    2. Idiopathic subaortic stenosis
    3. Atrial myxoma

II. Reflex cardiac causes
  a. Carotid sinus sensitivity
  b. Deglutition syncope
  c. Micturition syncope

III. Cerebral causes
  a. Epilepsy
  b. Transient ischemic attacks
  c. Trauma—concussion

Table 13-2
Causes of syncope

I . Cardiovascular syncope
  a. Impaired cardiac output
    1. Arrhythmias
    2. Extensive myocardial infarction
    3. Obstruction to left ventricular output
      a. Aortic stenosis
      b. Atrial myxoma — left atrium
      c. Idiopathic hypertrophic subaortic stenosis
    4. Obstruction to right ventricular output
      a. Pulmonary embolism
      b. Pulmonary stenosis
      c. Pulmonary hypertension
    5. Impaired venous return to the heart
      a. Atrial myxoma, right atrium
      b. Orthostatic hypotension

II. Reflex cardiac syncope
  a. Carotid sinus sensitivity
  b. Cough syncope
  c. Deglutition syncope
  d. Vasovagal syncope
  e. Micturition syncope
  f. Defecation syncope

III. Decreased oxygen supply in blood
  a. Hypoxia/anoxia
  b. Anemia

IV. Cerebral causes
  a. Transient ischemic attacks
  b. Subclavian steal syndrome

V. Drug-induced syncope

may be irregular. Recovery is rapid without confusion or fatigue.[2]

Diagnostic Procedures The electrocardiogram may be abnormal, or a cardiac monitor may reveal an abnormality as the patient is observed in the hospital. Further testing, such as an exercise treadmill test in case of exertional syncope, may be ordered at the discretion of the cardiologist.

Cardiac syncope is occasionally encountered in glossopharyngeal neuralgia, probably due to impulses arising from the irritated glossopharyngeal nerve reaching the dorsal nucleus of the vagus with a resulting bradycardia or asystole.[3]

Carotid Sinus Sensitivity

Stimulation of the carotid sinus results in a cardioinhibitory response or an abnormal vasodepressor response, resulting in bradycardia, a decrease in systolic blood pressure, and syncope.[6] The diagnosis is established by carotid sinus massage and concurrent electrocardiographic (ECG) and blood pressure monitoring. A cardiac asystole of greater than 3 s indicates a cardioinhibitory response. A decline in systolic pressure of 50 mm Hg or more is compatible with a vasodepressor response. The disorder can be controlled by the use of anticholinergic drugs in most cases. Those who experience a vasodepressor response may respond to ergotamine tartrate 2 mg q12h orally.[7] Refractory carotid sinus sensitivity may require a permanent pacemaker.[8]

Cough Syncope

The condition is probably caused by a transient elevation of intracranial pressure during coughing and cortical impairment of cerebral blood flow.[9]

Deglutition Syncope

Deglutition sycope is characterized by the occurrence of a syncopal episode after swallowing. The mechanisms are probably much the same as those of carotid sinus sensitivity. The diagnosis can be established as outlined under carotid sinus sensitivity. The treatment is the same.

Vasovagal Syncope

The vasovagal syncopal episode is usually, but not invariably, preceded by various precipitating factors such as apprehension, pain, or instrumentation. However, attacks may occur in the absence of identifiable precipitants and can occur with little or no warning. Light-headedness is the most common prodromal symptom, while nausea, warmth, diaphoresis, and palpitations occur in 25 to 50 percent of cases. Fatigue is a prominent symptom on recovery.

The attack is triggered by a sudden hypotension. This leads to a decrease in the volume of blood returning to the heart, causing stimulation of mechanoreceptors in the wall of the left ventricle. In response to increased impulses to the brainstem via vagal afferents, there is a sudden rise in parasympathetic activity and bradycardia. At the same time, there is peripheral sympathetic inhibition with arterial dilatation, hypotension, and a further fall in blood pressure and in blood flow to the heart. Cardiac output decreases precipitously, cerebral perfusion is suddenly impaired, and there is transient loss of consciousness.[10] There is immediate improvement in venous return to the heart as soon as the patient assumes a horizontal position, and recovery occurs.

Diagnostic Procedures   Diagnosis is established by history in most cases. The patient with syncope of unknown origin who has no heart disease should receive upright tilt testing, which is positive in approximately 90 percent of cases of individuals who have vasovagal syncope.[11]

Treatment   Recurrent vasovagal syncope often responds to treatment with beta blockers. Propranolol 30 mg to 120 mg per day is effective in most cases.[12] A permanent pacemaker may be required in recurrent refractory cases with a predominantly cardioinhibitory vasovagal response.

Micturition Syncope

Micturition syncope is a sudden loss of consciousness that occurs immediately after completion of micturition in men.

Micturition syncope is believed to result from a combination of the following factors:

1.   Rapid emptying of a distended bladder excites mechanoreceptors in the bladder wall. Afferent impulses travel through the vagus nerve to the brainstem and trigger excess parasympathetic activity and bradycardia with inhibition of sympathetic activity producing arterial dilatation and hypotension.

2.   Straining with the glottis closed resulting in a Valsalva maneuver will reduce venous return to the heart.

3.   The emptying of the distended bladder results in pooling of venous blood in the abdominal and pelvic organs.

The condition occurs in middle-aged or elderly men who usually admit to heavy alcohol intake before the syncopal episode. The patient arises to empty the bladder in the middle of the night and suddenly loses consciousness without warning immediately after emptying the bladder. There may be a precipitous fall and injuries to the head. Recovery occurs in a few seconds.

The diagnosis can be established by the characteristic history.

Treatment   The patient should avoid the precipitating factors of heavy alcohol intake, excessive straining, and standing while urinating.

Orthostatic Hypotension

Definition   Orthostatic hypotension is a condition characterized by increasing light-headedness, blurring of vision, tinnitus, weakness, and ataxia, which is occasionally followed by syncope.

Etiology   There are many causes of orthostatic hypotension. The common causes are listed in Tables 13-3 and 13-4.

In neurogenic orthostatic hypotension, the major abnormality is the lack of neurally mediated vasoconstriction in large vascular beds, particularly those supplying skeletal muscle and the viscera. This is compromised by a gravitational effect increasing pooling in the periphery. There is a failure of venous return to the heart, hypotension, decreased cerebral perfusion, which can no longer be compensated by autoregulation, and syncope.[13]

Clinical Features   The patient with orthostatic hypotension experiences symptoms on arising from a lying or sitting position. Progressive light-headedness, blurring of vision, tinnitus, weakness, and ataxia occur and may culminate in syncope if the patient does not sit or assume a supine position. Examination reveals cold, clammy skin and a weak, shallow pulse. Orthostatic hypotension may result in the typical symptoms of a transient ischemic attack in patients with a hemodynamically significant stenosis of an internal carotid artery or vertebral arteries.

Table 13-3
Neurogenic orthostatic hypotension

Primary autonomic failure

1. Pure autonomic failure
   (Idiopathic orthostatic hypotension)

2. Multisystem atrophy
   (Shy-Drager)
   (Olivopontocerebellar atrophy)

3. Hereditary

Secondary autonomic failure

1. Hereditary
   Hereditary sensorimotor neuropathy, Type V (Reilly-Day syndrome)
   Dopamine B hydroxylase deficiency
   Familial amyloidosis

2. Congenital
   Syringomyelia
   Syringobulbia
   Holmes-Adie syndrome

3. Infectious
   Guillain-Barré syndrome
   Chronic inflammatory demyelinating polyneuropathy
   Tabes dorsalis

4. Metabolic diabetes mellitus, amyloidosis

5. Neoplastic brainstem glioma

6. Vascular vertebral basilar insufficiency, collagen vascular diseases

7. Renal failure

8. Reflex disorders
   Vasovagal syncope
   Carotid sinus sensitivity
   Micturition syncope
   Deglutition syncope
   Glossopharyngeal neuralgia and syncope

Table 13-4
Non-neurogenic orthostatic hypotension

1. Cardiac causes
   a. Contractility
      Myocardial infarction
      Myocarditis
   b. Impaired ventricular filling
      Constrictive pericarditis
      Atrial myxoma
   c. Impaired cardiac output
      Aortic stenosis
      Subaortic stenosis
      Hypertrophic obstructive cardiomyopathy

2. Hereditary
   Cardiomyopathy of the muscular dystrophies
   Amyloidosis

3. Infection
   Myocarditis

4. Metabolic
   Hypothyroidism
   Diabetes insipidus
   Adrenal insufficiency

5. Toxic with vasodilatation
   Nitrites
   Alcohol

6. Impaired venous return
   Varicose veins
   Vena caval compression
   Valsalva maneuver
   Micturition syncope

7. Reduced circulating volume
   Dehydration
   Vomiting
   Diarrhea
   Inadequate intake of water

8. Renal salt-losing nephropathy
   Diuretics

9. Blood and plasma loss
   Hemorrhage
   Burns
   Hemodialysis

10. Shock
    Sepsis
    Endotoxic shock

Diagnostic Procedures The diagnosis is established by demonstrating a drop in blood pressure when the patient stands after lying or sitting for a few minutes. Patients with idiopathic orthostatic hypotension fail to show the expected rise in pulse rate on standing.

Treatment Prevention: blood pressure is higher later in the day, indicating that activities should be scheduled in the afternoon rather than the morning. Food and exercise lower blood pressure; consequently, activities should be preprandial. Swimming is the ideal exercise because the hydrostatic pressure of water inhibitis hypotension. Hot weather, hot showers, or hot baths lower blood pressure. Lifting, coughing, or straining at stool should be avoided. A liberal water and salt intake may improve blood volume.[14]

Drug Therapy

1. Fludrocortisone therapy results in sodium retention, which develops over time and maximum benefits are delayed for about 2 weeks. Potassium and magnesium depletion occur and should be treated with appropriate supplements. Fludrocortisone therapy begins with 0.1 mg q.d., increasing by 0.1-mg increments at 2-week intervals. The effective dose usually lies between 0.1 to 0.4 mg per day.

2. Milodione, an alpha-adrenoreceptor agonist, produces arterial and venous constriction, thus raising blood pressure. Therapy begins with 2.5 mg q. a.m., increasing by 2.5-mg increments to as high as 30 mg given in divided doses in the morning and at lunch. Adverse effects include piloerection, paresthesias, and pruritus.

3. Erythropoietin is available in recombinant form and can be administered intravenously or subcutaneously 25 to 75 Ukg three times a week. The drug corrects anemia and also raises blood pressure by unknown mechanisms. Supplemental iron therapy may be required.

Treatment of autonomic failure in Parkinson disease and multiple system atrophy is discussed elsewhere.

SLEEP DISORDERS

Narcolepsy

Definition Narcolepsy is a disorder of unknown etiology characterized by excessive sleepiness that typically is associated with cataplexy and other rapid eye movement (REM) sleep phenomena such as sleep paralysis and hypnagogic hallucinations.[15]

Etiology and Pathology The etiology is unknown. Human leukocyte antigen testing shows (HLA-DR2) positivity for DQW6 or DRW15 (HLADR2) in 98 percent of patients.[16] Narcolepsy is believed to result from the intrusion of REM sleep into the waking state.

The reported pontine lesions in magnetic resonance images in patients with narcolepsy[17] have not been confirmed.[18] However, narcolepsy is believed to be associated with dysfunction of neural structures in the brainstem and thalamus.[19]

Clinical Features Narcolepsy is not uncommon and may affect as many as 200,000 people in the United States. Unfortunately, many cases are misdiagnosed as inattention in class, since most individuals experience their first symptoms in their teens or twenties, although narcolepsy has been described infrequently in prepubertal children.[15,20] Cataplexy usually develops later than the sleep attacks and may occasionally precede them.

The first symptom is usually excessive daytime sleeping, which develops over a period of years. The patient begins to fall asleep in situations of monotony such as a monotonous lecture, working alone at a repetitive task, or sitting in a warm room after a meal. The attacks gradually become more frequent and less appropriate, until the individual falls asleep in an obviously inappropriate or hazardous situation such as driving a car[21] or working with machinery. In most cases, the episodes are preceded by an intense feeling of fatigue and an irresistible urge to sleep. However, some patients fall asleep without any warning and at times do not realize that a short period of sleep has occurred. In most cases, attacks last for a few seconds to about 30 minutes. The patient often awakens refreshed and alert, but some individuals complain of constant fatigue and the distress of attempting to suppress the urge to sleep.

Cataplexy may be defined as laughter-induced loss of facial and jaw control, spreading to involve the trunk and other body areas, accompanied by muscle jerking around the mouth. The presence of cataplexy is considered essential to the diagnosis of narcolepsy by many but not all authorities, and the interval between the onset of excessive daytime sleepiness and cataplexy is usually no more than 2 years.[22]

Cataplexy is usually mild at the onset with no more than a sudden brief feeling of weakness. However, attacks often increase in frequency and severity until the patient falls to the ground. At that stage, the mere thought of an amusing or stressful situation may provoke a cataplectic attack.

Sleep paralysis and hypnagogic hallucinations, although frequent in narcolepsy, are not essential to the diagnosis of narcolepsy, since they are frequently experienced independently and recognized as REM sleep parasomnias (see page 338).

Some patients with narcolepsy experience disruptive sleep and report they usually awaken several times during the night. About 20 percent of men with narcolepsy have an associated sleep apnea. It is not unusual for a patient with narcolepsy to automatically perform repetitive tasks and have no recollection of the passage of time. Automatic behavior is occasionally inappropriate and the patient may interject comments that are completely out of context with the conversation.

Diagnostic Procedures Polysomnographic findings show sleep latency less than 7 min and REM sleep latency less than 20 min. Multiple sleep latency test findings show a mean sleep latency of less than 5 min and two or more sleep onset REM periods.

Differential Diagnosis

1. Idiopathic hypersomnia. The essential feature is the absence of cataplexy. Multiple sleep latency test findings show a mean sleep latency less than 7 min and the occurrence of two or more sleep-onset REM periods in a two nap protocol. However, there is an overlap in polysomnographic findings in narcolepsy and idiopathic hypersomnia. The essential feature is the lack of cataplexy in the latter condition.

2. Partial complex seizures. The description of automatic behavior or frightening hallucinations may suggest the possibility of partial complex seizure activity. However, the history of excessive daytime sleeping and cataplexy helps to differentiate the narcoleptic patient.

3. Transient global amnesia. Episodes of automatic behavior are a feature of transient global amnesia, but this disorder is not associated with other symptoms of narcolepsy.

4. Sleep apnea. This condition may lead to excessive daytime sleepiness suggesting narcolepsy.

Treatment

1. Modafinil 200 to 400 mg once daily is a well tolerated and effective wake-promoting agent in the treatment af excessive daytime sleepiness associated with narcolepsy.[23] Adverse effects are few particularly with doses of 200 mg per day.[24]

2. Methylphenidate (Ritalin) remains the drug of choice in most cases of narcolepsy.[25] The initial dose of 10 mg in the morning and at noon may be increased to 80 to 100 mg per day. Methylphenidate can be used in combination with other drugs used in the treatment of cataplexy.

3. Amphetamines are also useful and often very effective in treatment of excessive daytime sleeping but can have a number of unpleasant adverse effects. These include progressive hypertension or personality changes ranging from emotional lability and mild depression to frank psychosis.

4. Selegiline 20 to 40 mg in divided doses daily, in combination with a low-tyramine diet, is an effective treatment for narcolepsy with few side effects.[26]

5. Pemoline and yohimbine are also reported to significantly increase sleep latency in narcolepsy.[27]

Cataplexy

Imipramine (Tofranil) is widely used in the control of cataplexy. Imipramine is well-tolerated in the majority of cases but may become less effective with the passage of time. This requires a gradual increase in dosage. An initial effective dose of 25 mg three times a day may rise to 50 mg three times a day over a 2-year period. Imipramine may also produce somnolence in some cases and has caused impotence and urine retention. It is recommended that one begin imipramine with a 10-mg dose at night and gradually increase by 10-mg increments to the initial dose of 25 mg three times a day.

Prognosis Narcolepsy is a lifelong affliction that tends to increase slowly in severity until about the age of 50. Symptoms may become less disabling in older patients.

Sleep Apnea

Definition There are two types of sleep apnea: (1) obstructive sleep apnea characterized by intermittent obstruction of the airway with cessation of breathing and interruption of sleep, and (2) central sleep apnea due to a loss of sensitivity of central respiratory control mechanisms.

Obstructive Sleep Apnea

Etiology and Pathology Obstructive sleep apnea is a common sleep disorder second only to insomnia in frequency. Approximately 20 million people in the United States have obstructive sleep apnea with a male-to-female ratio of 2:1. The condition has a strong family component[28] and has been underdiagnosed in women in the past.[29] It is associated with arterial hypertension,[30] coronary artery disease, myocardial infarction, pulmonary hypertension, congestive heart failure, transient ischemic attacks, and stroke.[31] Excessive daytime sleepiness results in professional, social, and emotional problems as well as a threat to life because of a significantly higher incidence of motor vehicle accidents owing to the increased risk of falling asleep when driving.[32]

The cause of obstructive sleep apnea is recurrent occlusion of the airway during sleep, at the level of the soft palate. The upper airway muscles contract during inspiration, pulling the airway open when the patient is awake. However, this mechanism fails during sleep in the sleep apnea sufferer, and airway patency is lost.[33] This results in snoring as the airway is compromised, and occlusion with apnea in some cases.[34]

Clinical Features The sufferers are known to snore loudly during sleep. This is interrupted by sudden cessation of breathing followed by restlessness, gasping respiratory sounds, and brief awakening. However, the patient has no recollection of the episodes. The condition occurs many times during the night, resulting in daytime sleepiness, suddenly falling asleep if alone or lacking stimulation, and impaired performance when awake. Intermittent airway obstruction produces intermittent hypoxia and hypercapnia, which increases the risk of systemic hypertension, cardiac arrhythmias, and epilepsy.[35] There is a significant association with narcolepsy.

Predisposing factors to obstructive sleep apnea include obesity, a positive family history, acromegaly or hypothyroidism, and the use of alcohol or sedatives.

Diagnostic Procedures The diagnosis is established by polysomnography.

Treatment

1. When obesity is a contributing factor, weight reduction reduces upper respiratory obstruction and daytime hypersomnolence. Nocturnal oxygenation is improved.

2. Surgical procedures to promote weight reduction, such as gastroplasty and gastric bypass, can be used to treat morbidly obese patients who fail to respond to weight reduction programs.

3. Orthodontic appliances designed to prevent upper respiratory collapse by altering the position of the jaws and soft tissue components of the pharynx may be of help during weight reduction.

4. Nasal continuous positive airway pressure (CPAP) increases pharyngeal airway pressure and prevents pharyngeal collapse. This is a successful procedure, but patient compliance is a major problem.

5. Surgical procedures such as uvulopalatopharyngoplasty have had limited success.[36]

6. Other surgical procedures that attempt to modify each site of potential pharyngeal occlusion, using modern maxillofacial techniques, may be more successful.

Central Sleep Apnea This condition is not as common as obstructive sleep apnea and is believed to be due to a decreased sensitivity of central respiratory control and change in sensitivity of CO_2 chemoreceptors during sleep.

Central sleep apnea occurs in some cases at high altitudes. Others suffer from obesity-hyperventilation-hypersomnia (pickwickian) syndrome in which patients often have a combination of obstructive and central sleep apnea. Multisystem atrophy may be associated with central sleep apnea.[37]

Diagnostic Procedures

1. Pickwickian patients have a waking hypercapnia.
2. Hypothyroidism must be excluded.
3. Diagnosis is established by polysomnography.

Treatment

1. Acetazolamide 250 mg four times a day is effective in some patients with central sleep apnea.

2. Medroxyprogesterone acetate is effective in patients with pickwickian syndrome.

3. Trazodone 50 mg q.h.s. is also effective in central sleep apnea.

PARASOMNIAS

Parasomnias are undesirable phenomena that occur predominantly during sleep. Some, such as sleep paralysis and REM sleep behavior disorder, are seen during REM sleep. Others, which include confusional arousals, sleepwalking, and sleep terrors, are associated with impairment of arousal from slow wave sleep. A third group of sleep/wake transition disorder includes rhythmic movement disorder, sleep starts, sleep talking, and nocturnal leg cramps. A final group of parasomnias can occur at any stage of sleep and include nocturnal paroxysmal dystonia, bruxism, enuresis, panic disorder, and nocturnal dissociative disorder.

REM Sleep Parasomnias

Sleep Paralysis Sleep paralysis consists of episodes of limb paralysis occurring at the onset of sleep or on awakening, lasting from a few seconds to several minutes, occasionally as long as 20 minutes. Some 50 percent of adults have at least one attack of sleep paralysis.[38] The condition is much more com-

mon in narcolepsy. Respiratory and eye muscles are spared. Patients may experience a sensation of struggling to move, accompanied by fear and occasional vivid hallucinations at first. Subsequent episodes are more benign and are regarded as an annoyance. The patient usually responds to a mild stimulus. The cause is probably REM sleep intrusion into arousal. Sleep paralysis is associated with muscle atonia, H-reflex suppression, and an EEG pattern of alpha activity or drowsiness.

REM Sleep Behavior Disorder (RBD) This condition consists of sudden episodes of violent behavior occurring several times a night or once every few weeks and consisting of punching, kicking, and jumping out of bed. The patient or bed partner may be injured.[28] The muscle atonia of REM sleep is incomplete and patients have brief violent motor automatisms during vivid dreams. RBD occurs in middle-aged and elderly persons, and about one-third have Parkinson disease, multi-infarct dementia, or multiple system disease. Medications with anticholinergic properties exacerbate RBD. Clonazepam 0.5 to 2 mg q.h.s. is effective in the great majority of cases,[40] the remainder responding to levodopa, other benzodiazepines, or carbamazepine.

Confusional Arousal

Affected individuals with this problem show incomplete alertness on sudden arousal from sleep. There is disorientation, confusion with slowed speech and response. Arousal is usually from stage III or IV sleep and the EEG shows synchronous or asynchronous delta activity. Episodes last for a short period, ranging from a few seconds to no more than 10 minutes.

Sleepwalking

This disorder may be regarded as one of the complex automatisms associated with getting out of bed and walking. This occurs in stage III or IV of sleep, during the first third of the night. Injury can occur from tripping over objects or falling; violent behavior may be directed at those trying to help the sleepwalker. Children and adolescents are more commonly affected. The EEG shows hypersynchronous delta activity of stage III or IV sleep.[41] Symptoms consist of screaming, agitation, tachycardia, sweating, mydriasis, inconsolabilty, amnesia, and attempts to leave the bed or the room. In most cases, morning recall is absent, but some recall vivid dreams of threatening situations. There is an increased association of psychopathology in adults[42] and Tourette syndrome in children. Treatment with imipramine 0.5 to 1 mg/kg q.h.s., diazepam 5 mg q.h.s., or clonazepam 0.5 to 1 mg q.h.s. is usually successful.

Rhythmic Movement Disorder

This condition usually occurs in children and consists of stereotyped, repetitive movements such as head banging, head rolling, body rocking, or body rolling. Some children hum or chant during the episode. Episodes last up to 20 minutes and are associated with stage I sleep. The majority of children cease rhythmic movements after the age of 4 years.

Sleep Onset Myoclonus

This is a sudden violent myoclonic jerk affecting arms or legs, or both upper and lower limbs. The episode can occur as the individual is in the transitional stage from wakefulness to sleep.

Sleep Talking

Brief episodes of speaking can occur during arousal from non-REM sleep or occasionally from REM sleep. Sleep talking is often associated with sleep deprivation, stress or febrile illness, sleep apnea, or sleep walking.

Nocturnal Leg Cramps

Painful muscle spasms affecting the calf or foot can occur during sleep or, more frequently, during arousal from sleep. They tend to be precipitated by unaccustomed exercise, pregnancy, metabolic disorders, particularly diabetes mellitus, and fluid or electrolyte disturbances. Affected muscles have palpable cramping. Treatment with quinine, verapamil, or vitamin E is usually effective.

Nocturnal Paroxysmal Dystonia

Dystonic posturing with ballistic choreoathetoid movements can occur during stage II of sleep and last from 15 to 60 s, often recurring repetitively during the night. The patient is usually awake. The disorder is believed to be a partial seizure originating in the supplementary motor area of the frontal lobe and responds to carbamazepine therapy.[32]

Bruxism

Grinding of the teeth can occur in any stage of sleep and may be loud enough to awaken a bed partner. The condition is often precipitated by stress. Tooth damage can be prevented by use of a mouth guard.

Enuresis

Most children achieve total bladder control by the age of 3 years, but 10 percent have episodes of enuresis up to the age of 6 years, and 3 percent have episodes at age 12 years. There may be a genetic predisposition in some cases with a family history of enuresis. Urologic evaluation is negative. Treatment with bladder training exercises and conditioning devices may be beneficial. Desmopressin or imipramine is usually effective in most refractory cases.

Panic Disorder

Nocturnal episodes of panic can occur during stage II of sleep. Attacks are associated with fear or terror, palpitations, and sweating. There is absence of dreaming. Daytime panic episodes are usually present.

Nocturnal Dissociative Disorder

Complex behavior and violent activity suggesting REM sleep behavior occasionally occur as a nocturnal fugue state. There is usually a history of physical or sexual abuse and the condition may be an acting out of a previous assault. The EEG shows patterns of wakefulness before and during the episode.

Sudden Unexpected Nocturnal Death (SUND)

This condition affects men, primarily who have emigrated to the United States from certain Far Eastern countries where it is not an unusual phenomenon. Gasping, groaning, choking, or difficulty breathing may occur just prior to death, which is believed to be the result of ventricular fibrillation. SUNDs may be an excessive sympathetic discharge during REM sleep.[44] Treatment for those successfully resuscitated includes antiarrhythmics and implanted defibrillators.

Epilepsy

Many parasomnias resemble—and therefore, have to be distinguished from—nocturnal epilepsy. This group includes primary generalized epilepsy with tonic-clonic seizures, absence seizures, benign rolandic epilepsy, primary generalized epilepsy with myoclonus, and partial complex seizures of temporal lobe and frontal lobe origin.

Diagnosis depends on a good history from an observer, polysomnography, and positron emission tomography scanning, if available.

REFERENCES

1. Kapoor WN: Workup and management of patients with syncope. *Med Clin North Am* 79:1153, 1995.
2. Calkins H, Shyr Y, Frumin H, et al: The value of the clinical history in the differentiation of syncope due to ventricular tachycardia, atrioventricular block, and neurocardiogenic syncope. *Am J Med* 98:365, 1995.
3. Ferrante L, Artico M, Nardacci B, et al: Glossopharyngeal neuralgia with cardiac syncope. *Neurosurgery* 36:58, 1995.
4. Devinsky O, Pacia S, Tatambhotla G: Bradycardia and asystole induced by partial seizures: a case report and literature review. *Neurology* 48:1712, 1997.
5. Iani C, Colicchio G, Attanasio A, et al: Cardiogenic syncope in temporal lobe epileptic seizures. *J Neurol Neurosurg Psychiatry* 63:259, 1997.
6. Gaggioli G, Brignole M, Menozzi C, et al: Reappraisal of the vasodepressor reflex in carotid sinus syndrome. *Am J Cardiol* 75:518, 1995.
7. Costa F, Biaggioni I: Microneurographic evidence of sudden sympathetic withdrawal in carotid sinus syncope: treatment with ergotamine. *Chest* 106:617, 1994.
8. Benditt DG, Petersen M, Lurie KG, et al: Cardiac pacing for prevention of recurrent vasovagal syncope. *Ann Intern Med* 122:204, 1995.
9. Mattle HP, Nirkko AC, Baumgartner RW, et al: Transient cerebral circulatory arrest coincides with fainting in cough syncope. *Neurology* 45:498, 1995.
10. Kaufmann H: Neurally mediated syncope: pathogenesis, diagnosis, and treatment. *Neurology* 45 (Suppl 5):S12, 1995.
11. Hargreaves AD, el Hag O, Boon NA: Head up tilt testing. The balance of evidence. *Br Heart J* 72:216, 1994.
12. Abe H, Kobayashi H, Nakashima Y, et al: Effect of beta adrenergic blockage on vasodepressor reaction in patients with vasodepressor syncope. *Am Heart J* 128:911, 1994.
13. Mathias CJ: Orthostatic hypotension: causes, mechanisms, and influencing factors. *Neurology* 45 (Suppl 5):S6, 1995.
14. Robertson D, Davis TL: Recent advances in the treatment of orthostatic hypotension. *Neurology* 45 (Suppl 5):S26, 1995.
15. *International classification of sleep disorders. Diagnostic and coding manual.* Diagnostic Steering Committee. Thorpe MJ, Chairman. Rochester, Minnesota: American Sleep Disorders Association p 38, 1990.
16. Rogers AE, Meehan J, Guilleminault C, et al: HLA DR15 (DR2) and DQB1*0602 typing studies in 188 narcoleptic patients with cataplexy. *Neurology* 48:1550, 1997.
17. Plazzi G, Montagna P, Provini F, et al: Pontine lesions in idiopathic narcolepsy. *Neurology* 46:1250, 1996.
18. Frey JL, Heiserman JE: Absence of pontine lesions in narcolepsy. *Neurology* 48:1097, 1997.
19. Aldrich MS: The clinical spectrum of narcolepsy and idiopathic hypersomnia. *Neurology* 46:393, 1996.
20. Guilleminault C, Pelayo R: Narcolepsy in prepubertal children. *Ann Neurol* 43:135, 1998.
21. Findley L, Unverzagt M, Guchu R, et al: Vigilance and automobile accidents in patients with sleep apnea or narcolepsy. *Chest* 108:619, 1995.
22. Parkes JD, Crift SJ, Dahlitz MJ, et al: The narcoleptic syndrome—editorial. *J. Neurol Neurosurg Psychiatry* 59:221, 1995.
23. U.S. Modafinil in Narcolepsy Multicenter Study Group. Randomized trial of modafinil for the treatment of pathological somnolence in narcolepsy. *Ann Neurol* 43:88, 1998.
24. Broughton RJ, Fleming JA, George CF, et al: Random-

ized, double-blind, placebo-controlled crossover trial of modafinil in the treatment of excessive daytime sleepiness in narcolepsy. *Neurology* 49:444, 1997.

25. Mitler MM, Hajdukovic R: Relative efficacy of drugs for the treatment of sleepiness in narcolepsy. *Sleep* 14:218, 1991.

26. Hublin C, Partinen M, Heinonen EH, et al: Selegiline in the treatment of narcolepsy. *Neurology* 44:2095, 1994.

27. Wooten V: Effectiveness of yohimbine in treating narcolepsy. *South M J* 87:1065, 1994.

28. Mathur R, Douglas NJ: Family studies in patients with the sleep apnea-hypopnea syndrome. *Ann Intern Med* 122:174, 1995.

29. Guilleminault C, Stoohs R, Kim YD, et al: Upper airway sleep-disordered breathing in women. *Ann Intern Med* 122:493, 1995.

30. Fletcher EC: The relationship between systemic hypertension and obstructive sleep apnea: facts and theory. *Am J Med* 98:118, 1995.

31. Bassetti C, Aldrich MS, Chervin RD, et al: Sleep apnea in patients with transient ischemic attack and stroke: a prospective study of 59 patients. *Neurology* 47:1167, 1996.

32. Wu H, Yan-Go F: Self-reported automobile accidents involving patients with obstructive sleep apnea. *Neurology* 46:1254, 1996.

33. Sher AE: Treating obstructive sleep apnea syndrome—a complex task. *West J Med* 162:170, 1995.

34. Riley RW, Powell NB, Guilleminault C, et al: Obstructive sleep apnea. Trends in therapy. *West J Med* 165:143, 1995.

35. Britton TC, O'Donoghue M, Duncan JS, et al: Exacerbation of epilepsy by obstructive sleep apnoea. *J Neurol Neurosurg Psychiatry* 63:808, 1997.

36. Doghramji K, Jabourian ZH, Pilla M, et al: Predictors of outcome for uvulopalatopharyngoplasty. *Laryngoscope* 105:311, 1995.

37. Tachibana N, Kimura K, Kitajima K, et al: REM sleep motor dysfunction in multiple system atrophy: with special emphasis on sleep talk as its early clinical manifestation. *J Neurol Neurosurg Psychiatry* 63:678, 1997.

38. Fukuda K, Miyasita A, Inugami M, et al: High prevalence of isolated sleep paralysis: kanashibari phenomenon in Japan. *Sleep* 10:279, 1987.

39. Schenck CH, Milner DM, Hurwitz TD, et al: A polysomnographic and clinical report on sleep-related injury in 100 adult patients. *Am J Psychiatry* 146:1166, 1989.

40. Schneck CM, Manowald MW: A polysomnographic neurologic, psychiatric and clinical outcome report on 70 consecutive cases with REM sleep behavior disorder (RBD): sustained clonazepam efficacy in 89.5% of 57 treated patients. *Clev Clin J Med* 57 (Suppl):9, 1990.

41. Blatt I, Peled R, Gadoth N, et al: The value of sleep recording in evaluating somnambulism in young adults. *Electroencephalogr Clin Neurophysiol* 78:407, 1991.

42. Llorente MD, Currier MB, Norman SE, et al: Night terrors in adults: phenomenology and relationship to psychopathology. *J Clin Psychiatry* 53:392, 1992.

43. Meierkord H, Fish DR, Smith SJ, et al: Is nocturnal paroxysmal dystonia a form of frontal lobe epilepsy? *Mov Disord* 7:38, 1992.

44. Pressman MR, Marinchak RA, Kowey PR, et al: Polysomnographic and electrocardiographic findings in a sudden unexplained nocturnal death syndrome (SUNDS) survivor. *Sleep Res* 22:213, 1993.

Chapter 14

DEGENERATIVE DISEASES

Degenerative diseases of the central nervous system (CNS) can affect gray matter, white matter, or both. Involvement is often diffuse but usually affects one area or system more than another, which permits an anatomical classification of these conditions.

DISEASES OF THE GRAY MATTER

Diseases of the Cerebral Cortex: The Dementias

Dementia may be defined as a progressive deterioration of intellectual capacity resulting from diseases of the brain. Although Alzheimer disease and multi-infarct dementia account for 80 percent of the dementias of old age, many neurological diseases are associated with dementia. The dementias as a group constitute one of the most common problems presented to neurologists and psychiatrists and comprise the third leading cause of death.[1] At least two domains of function, one of which is memory, are affected; language, perception, visual-spatial function, calculation, judgment, abstraction, and problem-solving skills may also be impaired.[2] Consequently, any condition that damages the brain, including trauma, CNS infections, toxins, metabolic abnormalities, tumors, infarctions, or hemorrhages may result in dementia. These conditions all have an identifiable and often treatable cause of dementia, in contrast to a group of degenerative diseases of unknown etiology, in which dementia is a predominant sign. This latter group of diseases includes Alzheimer disease, Pick disease, multisystem disease, progressive supranuclear palsy, Huntington disease, Lewy body disease, cortical basal degeneration, Creutzfeldt-Jakob disease, frontotemporal dementia, normal pressure hydrocephalus, and the vascular dementias, including multi-infarct dementia and cerebral arteritis. Such conditions constitute the majority of cases of progressive dementia encountered in clinical practice.

Dementia occurs predominantly in older people and it is estimated that less than 1 percent of individuals under the age of 65 have dementia. Nevertheless, while dementia is an increasing problem in our aging population, it should never be accepted as an inevitable concomitant of aging. There is increasing recognition of the treatable causes of dementia, and each patient deserves full evaluation and correct diagnosis. This approach will obviate the use of such terms as "presenile dementia," "senile dementia," "senility," "organic brain syndrome," and "hardening of the arteries," which imply failure to establish a diagnosis and consequently, lead to delay in—or lack of—treatment. It is possible that some of the dementias are due to chronic (slow) virus infection. The evidence for this has evolved from studies of such neuronal diseases as kuru and Creutzfeldt-Jakob disease.

At present, about 20 percent of patients with dementia have a treatable condition. Consequently, it is incorrect to assume that a patient suffering from dementia is destined to a course of progressive intellectual deterioration. Table 14-1 lists the more common causes of reversible or treatable dementia.

Evaluation of Patients with Dementia

1. *The history obtained from the patient*

In early cases of dementia, the history is likely to be punctuated by denial, including the statement that the patient has no desire to be seen by the physician and is only keeping the appointment to please the family. In more advanced cases, answers to questions are often sparse, fragmented, hesitant, or posed in the series of questions directed by the patient to the spouse, relative, or those in attendance. This, in itself, is important in that it permits an assessment of the patient's memory, rationalization, denial, delusions, and emotional state and the family's reaction to the illness. An individual who volunteers the information that the memory is failing is unlikely to have

Table 14-1
Causes of treatable dementia

Therapeutic drug use: anticholinergics—atropine and related compounds; anticonvulsants—phenytoin, mephenytoin, barbiturates; antihypertensives—clonidine, methyldopa, propranolol; psychotropics—haloperidol, lithium carbonate, phenothiazines; miscellaneous—disulfiram, bromides, paraldehyde, quinidine

Metabolic–systemic disorders: electrolyte or acid-base disorders; hypo-, hyperglycemia; severe anemia; polycythemia vera; hyperlipidemia; hepatic failure; uremia; pulmonary insufficiency; hypopituitarism; thyroid, adrenal, or parathyroid dysfunction; cardiac dysfunction; hepatolenticular degeneration

Intracranial disorders: cerebrovascular insufficiency, chronic meningitis or encephalitis, neurosyphilis, HIV, epilepsy, tumor, abscess, subdural hematomas, multiple sclerosis, normal pressure hydrocephalus

Deficiency states: vitamin B_{12} deficiency, folate deficiency, pellagra (niacin)

Collagen-vascular disorders: systemic lupus erythematosus, temporal arteritis, sarcoidosis, Behçet's syndrome

Exogenous intoxication: alcohol, carbon monoxide, organophosphates, toluene, trichloroethylene, carbon disulfide, lead, mercury, arsenic, thallium, manganese, nitrobenzene, anilines, bromine hydrocarbons

Alzheimer disease, where insight into memory failure is lacking.

2. *The history obtained from the spouse, relative, or attendant*

The examiner should attempt to obtain a history from one individual, preferably the spouse, in the absence of the patient. This avoids embarrassment and encourages frankness. Under these circumstances, the surrogate should be approached as though he or she was the patient and a full history obtained, followed by a neurological review (see Chapter 1). The past history and family history are then recorded, followed by an expanded social history, to include the usual questions about employment, habits, and marital status and an expanded section to cover activities of daily living, including sleeping habits, awakening at night, wandering in the home, toileting, dressing, eating, hygiene, driving, shopping, working, and changes in attitude toward family members and friends. Symptoms suggesting depression are important, in that memory failure may be the result of a pseudodementia in a depressed individual who has withdrawn from contact with friends and no longer indulges in previously enjoyable activities.

3. *The neurological examination*

The neurological examination should be performed as described in Chapter 1, using the Mini-Mental Status Examination as a test of cognitive function (mentation). The same test can be given at 6-month intervals to assess deterioration in affected individuals.

The cranial nerve examination may reveal subtle changes such as saccadic eye movements, impersistence, or a positive glabellar sign, even in the early stages of dementia. There may be slight differences of tone on the two sides or early paratonia on passive movements of the limbs. Rapid alternating movements are often slowed early in dementia, and dyspraxia of the nondominant hand is not unusual. The tendon reflexes are often exaggerated and slightly asymmetrical, even though there are normal plantar responses in the early stages of dementia.

4. *The general physical examination*

The general physical examination is equally important to exclude signs of hypothyroidism or hyperthyroidism, vascular disease with hypertension, cardiac murmurs, and carotid bruits. Peripheral neuropathy may be present in B_{12} deficiency, which is a potent cause of dementia.

5. *Diagnostic procedures*[3,4] (Fig. 14-1 and Table 14-2).

Alzheimer Disease

Definition Alzheimer disease is the most common form of dementia. The disease, caused by progressive neuronal degeneration, primarily affects middle-aged and elderly individuals in whom it is the cause of 70 percent of cases of dementia. However, the incidence is about 1 percent in people aged 50 to 70 years, with a dramatic rise to 50 percent in very elderly people.[5]

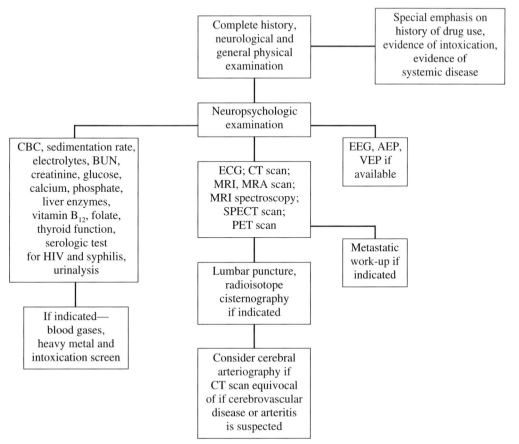

Figure 14-1
Evaluation of the patient with dementia.

Etiology and Pathology The etiology of Alzheimer disease is unknown. The salient pathological features are the presence of amyloid plaques and neurofibrillary tangles. Plaques consist of β-amyloid peptide, a fragment of amyloid precursor protein. Neurofibrillary tangles contain a core of an abnormally phosphorylated form of the microtubule binding protein tau.

The relationship of apolipoprotein E (apo E) to Alzheimer disease is the subject of intense research and speculation. Apo E plasma lipoprotein is synthesized primarily in the liver and brain. The role of apo E is diverse. It regulates lipid metabolism in the transfer of cholesterol from cells carrying high levels of cholesterol to cells with inadequate levels of cholesterol. Consequently, apo E plays a part in the ath-

erosclerotic process. However, the function of apo E in the brain is unique, in that apo E is synthesized in astrocytes and has a role in dendritic remodeling and synaptogenesis after brain tissue injury. There are three isoforms of apo E—apo E2, apo E3, apo E4—encoded by a gene located on chromosome 19. The apo E gene has three alleles—apo Ee2, apo Ee3, and apo Ee4—and about 77 percent of all apo E variants are E3, 15 percent are E4, and 8 percent are E2. All isoforms encoded by the varying alleles differ by only one or two amino acids.[6] The apo Ee4 allele has been associated with high- or low-density lipoprotein cholesterol and an increased risk of cardiovascular disease,[7] cerebrovascular disease,[8] Alzheimer disease,[9] and cognitive decline.[10,11] The apo Ee4 allele is considered a major inherited risk factor for

Table 14-2
Diagnostic procedures in the evaluation of dementia

A. Basic evaluation
1. Complete blood count to detect anemia or polycythemia; sedimentation rate—infection or vasculitis
2. Biochemical studies for impaired liver function or renal function, electrolyte imbalance, hypercalcemia, glucose level
3. Thyroid function tests to exclude hyperthyroidism or hypothyroidism
4. Vitamin B_{12} determination; folate determination if patient anemic
5. Testing for human immunodeficiency virus (HIV)
6. Serologic tests for syphilis
7. Chest x-ray for infection or primary or metastatic tumors
8. Magnetic resonance imaging (MRI) or computed tomography (CT) scanning of head to exclude tumors, subdural hematoma, multiple infarcts, or normal pressure hydrocephalus

B. Additional tests if indicated
9. Lumbar puncture in suspected cases of meningoencephalitis, chronic meningitis, or cerebral vasculitis. Cerebrospinal fluid (CSF) examination should be performed in a dementing illness of acute or subacute onset, atypical or rapidly progressive initial symptoms, dementia in patients younger than 55 years of age, or suspected syphilis or HIV infection.
10. Drug screen for heavy metals, illicit drug levels, benzodiazepines, barbiturates, alcohol
11. An electroencephalogram (EEG) is often normal in the early stages of dementia. Occasionally the record shows bursts of seizure activity indicating subclinical seizures in an elderly patient with recent onset of dementia.
12. The single photon emission computed tomography (SPECT) scan often shows a decrease in tissue blood flow in the temporal and parietal regions bilaterally in Alzheimer disease. The pattern in multi-infarct dementia is one of a patchy decrease of cerebral blood flow in an asymmetrical fashion.
13. Screening for collagen vascular disease is indicated in suspected cases of cerebral lupus or cerebral arteritis.
14. Neuropsychological evaluation is appropriate when there is a question of competence particularly in managing financial affairs, or in assessing ability to continue to drive or to remain in an occupation. Neuropsychological evaluation is useful in differentiating between depression and dementia.
15. Psychiatric evaluation—depression versus dementia, paranoia, delusions, hallucinations, or combativeness

---

Alzheimer disease, with a moderate risk of developing the disease with one apo Ee4 allele and a higher risk with two apo Ee4 alleles. This translates into individuals with two copies of the apo Ee4 allele having a risk of an average age of onset before age 70 years, whereas individuals with no copies of the Ee4 allele carry an average age of onset later than 85 years.[12] The apo Ee2 gene appears to have a protective effect against sporadic Alzheimer disease, and the apo Ee3 gene does not influence the age of onset of the disease.

The current hypothesis proposes that apo Ee4 may have a role in Alzheimer disease by acting as a carrier for β-amyloid in the formation of amyloid plaques.[13] Another role may be the failure of apo Ee4 to bind to tau, the protein located within the neurofibrillary tangles in the brains of patients with Alzheimer disease, leading to a failure of phosphorylation of tau, a prerequisite step in the formation of neurofibrillary tangles.[14] The number of neurofibrillary tangles correlates with the severity of the disease,[15] but neuronal loss in the cortex is far greater than the number of neurofibrillary tangles.[8] This suggests that other factors are promoting neuronal loss in Alzheimer disease, particularly amyloid deposition, neuronal death, and plaque formation, which correlates with apo Ee4 dose, the highest numbers in plaque densities occurring in apo Ee4 homozygotes.[16]

The apo E gene is located on chromosome 19 and is associated with risk and age of onset of Alzheimer disease. Each Ee4 allele lowers the age of onset by 3 to 7 years in sporadic Alzheimer disease.[17] However, the lifetime risk of developing Alzheimer disease in those with one Ee4 allele remains below 30 percent,[18] but patients with no Ee4 alleles are still at risk for the disease.[19] About 2 percent of the population are Ee4/Ee4 homozygotes and have approximately a 30 percent lifetime risk of developing Alzheimer disease.[20] Other forms of dementia, such as Lewy body disease, multi-infarct dementia, and Pick disease, may be associated with Ee4, whereas 30 to 50 percent of patients with Alzheimer disease have no apo Ee4 allele.[21]

Individuals who are Ee4 homozygotes, in whom dementia is most likely a result of Alzheimer disease, can develop other forms of dementia and should be investigated for treatable causes of dementia.[22] Apo E testing however may be valuable as an adjuvant to other forms of testing in persons with dementia,[23] because clinically typical patients with Alzheimer disease who are Ee4/Ee4 homozygotes have a 90 to 100 percent chance of having Alzheimer disease at autopsy.[24] However, knowledge of apo E genotype alone in elderly individuals with memory impairment is not sufficient to predict the development of Alzheimer disease.[25]

Although nonfamilial Alzheimer disease is the most common form of dementia, familial forms of the disease, which are clinically and pathologically indistinguishable from the sporadic nonfamilial disease, have been recognized.[26] Familial Alzheimer disease is being classified into early onset—mean onset at age less than 60 years—and late onset, which has a significantly increased risk in women.[27] Three causative genes have been identified in familial Alzheimer disease and are quite distinct from the apo E susceptibility gene on chromosome 19. The causative genes in familial Alzheimer disease are the amyloid precursor protein gene (APP gene) on chromosome 21[28] and genes on chromosome 14[29] and on chromosome 1.[30]

Clinical Features   There are probably 4 million people over age 65 years with Alzheimer disease in the United States, the majority of cases occurring in the over 85 age group. The disease can occur in both sexes and can begin at any age after the early thirties, although less than 1 percent of cases occur in the group under age 70, with a dramatic rise to over 50 percent in very elderly people.[5]

Clinically, loss of operational judgment and subjective complaints of failure of recent memory may antedate the development of dementia by as much as 3 years.[31] The patient resorts to keeping written notes to circumvent the failure of recent memory. Apathy is the most common change in behavior, followed by agitation and physical aggression.[32] In order of decreasing frequency, anxiety, irritability, dysphoria, aberrant motor behavior, disinhibition, delusions, and hallucinations occur.[33] Agitation, dysphoria, apathy, and aberrant motor behavior are significantly correlated with cognitive impairment. The dominant symptom often reflects the premorbid personality of the patient. Focal signs, including dysphasia, dyscalculia, dyslexia, dysgraphia, dyspraxia, and oral-facial dyskinesia, can develop at any time.[34]

Parkinsonian features, with rigidity and bradykinesis, are not uncommon. The early appearance of bradykinesis and rigidity seems to be associated with a faster progression of cognitive decline and disability. Similarly, more rapid cognitive decline occurs in early onset Alzheimer disease, and a disproportionate language and concentration impairment appears in younger patients.[35]

Muscle tone is often increased, with rigidity, paratonia, or spasticity. Resting and intention tremor is not uncommon. Patients may exhibit normal gait, short-stepped bradykinetic gait, or apraxia of gait—an inability to initiate gait, with the patient apparently "glued to the floor." The presence of apraxia of gait also creates a spurious impression of parkinsonism; however, once the patient with Alzheimer disease is able to initiate gait, it does not have the hesitant quality of parkinsonism. Myoclonus and seizures occur in about 10 percent of patients with Alzheimer disease. Sensory testing often reveals astereognosis or graphesthesia. More than 50 percent of patients have increased tendon reflex or exhibit release signs such as glabellar sign and snout, palmomental, and grasp reflexes.

Diagnostic Procedures

1. A detailed history should be obtained from the patient and an informant. The latter is essential to document the patient's deficits, which are unrecognized, denied, or forgotten by the patient.[36]
2. A general physical examination and evaluation for treatable causes of dementia are all negative (see Table 14-1).
3. The presence of criteria outlined in Table 14-3 suggests the diagnosis of Alzheimer disease.
4. An MRI, which is preferable to CT scanning of the brain, shows the presence of diffuse atrophy, with ventricular enlargement and enlarged cortical sulci. In the early stages, there may be little evidence of cortical atrophy.
5. The SPECT scans may show the typical appearance of reduced tissue perfusion in the temporoparietal regions bilaterally, which is the usual finding in Alzheimer disease.
6. A positron emission tomography (PET) scan may show reduced metabolic activity in the temporoparietal regions bilaterally.
7. The EEG shows progressive deterioration with loss of alpha activity and gradual development of generalized theta activity. The slowing may not be entirely symmetrical and focal slowing or focal seizure activity may be recorded.
8. Neuropsychological evaluation, which includes two tests, the Rey Auditory Verbal Learning Test and the Mental Control Subtest of the Weschler Memory Scale, can predict a probable diagnosis of Alzheimer disease with a high degree of accuracy.[37]

Treatment

1. Diet. Many patients with Alzheimer disease develop the habit of taking a very restricted diet and may have an associated vitamin deficiency. It is important to ensure that the patient has an adequate diet with vitamin supplementation.
2. Adequate care. When the spouse of an elderly patient is infirm or incapable of providing care for the patient, a search should be made for an aide through community resources. Many communities will provide services to patients with chronic ill-

Table 14-3
DSM-IV diagnostic criteria for Alzheimer dementia

A. The development of multiple cognitive deficits manifested by both 1) memory impairment (impaired ability to learn new information or to recall previously learned information); 2) one (or more) of the following cognitive disturbances: a) aphasia (language disturbance), b) apraxia (impaired ability to perform motor activities, despite intact motor function, c) agnosia (failure to recognize or identify objects, despite intact sensory function), d) disturbance in executive functioning (that is, planning, organization, sequencing, abstracting).

B. The cognitive deficits in criteria A1 and A2 each cause severe impairment in social or occupational functioning and represent a major decline from a previous level of functioning.

C. The course is characterized by gradual onset and continuing cognitive decline.

D. The cognitive deficits in criteria A1 and A2 are not due to any of the following: 1) other central nervous system conditions that cause progressive deficits in memory and cognition (for example, cerebrovascular disease, Parkinson's disease, Huntington's disease, subdural hematoma, normal-pressure hydrocephalus, brain tumor); 2) systemic conditions known to cause dementia (for example, hypothyroidism, vitamin B_{12} and folic acid deficiency, niacin deficiency, hypercalcemia, neurosyphilis, HIV infection).

E. The deficits do not occur exclusively during the course of a delirium.

F. The disturbance is not better accounted for by any other Axis I disorder (for example, major depressive disorder, schizophrenia).

Source: American Psychiatric Association (APA): *Diagnostic and Statistical Manual of Mental Disorders,* 4th ed. Washington, DC, APA, 1994.

nesses of all types. These resources should always be identified and the family made fully aware of their existence.
3. Planning with the family. It is important to discuss all aspects of the disease with the family and to indicate that symptoms progress. The physician

should be available to discuss the many problems of management with the family and refer them to the appropriate agency when they decide to transfer the patient to a chronic care institution. The services of a social worker are invaluable at that time. When it is apparent that the patient is no longer competent to take care of his or her affairs, the family should be informed and advised that the patient should be declared mentally incompetent according to the laws of the state.

4. Sedation. Many patients with Alzheimer disease require some form of sedation because of impulsive or combative behavior. Daytime sedation can be managed with a phenothiazine such as thioridazine (Mellaril). This should be given in small doses beginning with 25 mg 12h followed by the addition of 25 to 50 mg q3d until there is a satisfactory change in the patient's behavior. This usually requires between 100 and 450 mg daily. When a family complains that the patient is unable to sleep at night, the physician should determine whether the patient is sleeping during the day. The correction of this practice is often difficult but usually leads to restoration of a normal sleep pattern. However, if the patient remains restless at night, a simple sedative such as temazepam 15 mg at bedtime, which may be repeated an hour or so later, if the patient is still awake, is usually effective.

5. Signs and symptoms of depression may be treated with either fluoxetine hydrochloride (Prozac) 20 mg q.d., or sertraline hydrochloride (Zoloft) 50 mg q.d., or paroxetine hydrochloride (Paxil) 20 mg q.d.

6. Drug therapy
   i. Tacrine (Cognex), an acetylcholine esterase inhibitor, is moderately effective in improving cognitive performance in mild-to-moderate Alzheimer disease.
   ii. Donepezil hydrochloride (Aricept), a reversible inhibitor of the enzyme acetylcholine esterase, is also effective in improving cognition and memory in some patients over a 30-week period. The usual dose is 5 mg daily. Additional benefit may accrue following an increase to 10 mg daily after 6 weeks of therapy. Adverse reactions to this drug are unusual. The effectiveness of the medication for a longer

period than 30 weeks has not yet been established.

Apo E Genotype Testing The determination of apo E genotype is available, and the indication for testing has been subject to some controversy. Testing seems to be justified in the context of diagnosis, when it can be used as an adjuvant to the evaluation of a patient with progressive dementia who exhibits clinical features compatible with Alzheimer disease. Under these circumstances, the detection of one or two apo Ee4 alleles adds to the probability that the condition is Alzheimer disease. The test does not confirm Alzheimer disease. Confirmation depends on a positive result at autopsy.

The use of the apolipoprotein genotype for prediction of Alzheimer's disease in an asymptomatic individual is not supported because of the low positive predictive value of this marker.[38] Many asymptomatic individuals with an E4/E4 genotype never develop the disease; they are more likely to get the disease, but when—if at all—is unpredictable. When an asymptomatic individual obtains genotyping indicating the presence of an A4 allele, the testing must be followed by careful counseling to place the results in perspective.

Prognosis Patients with Alzheimer disease have a mean survival of 5 to 10 years after diagnosis and usually die secondary to intercurrent infection.

Pick Disease

Definition Pick disease is a rare type of dementia characterized by selective atrophy of the frontal and temporal lobes of the brain.

Etiology and Pathology The cause of the neuronal degeneration is unknown. The brain shows a marked atrophy of the frontal and temporal lobes, with sparing of the superior temporal gyrus. The atrophy is usually symmetrical but asymmetrical atrophy or unilateral atrophy has been described.[39] There is compensatory dilatation of the frontal and temporal horns of the lateral ventricles. The affected areas show loss of neurons maximal in the outer three layers of the cortex. Surviving neurons are small with argentophilic inclusions; because of their characteristic appearance, these cells have been called Pick cells. Senile plaques and neurofibrillary tangles are not a characteristic feature of Pick disease.

Clinical Features   The clinical features are those of a progressive dementia (see Alzheimer disease). The progressive decline in cognitive performance is associated with a steadily increasing antegrade amnesia for verbal and nonverbal material.[40] Some patients show a progressive dysphasia and Pick disease may be one of the causes of primary progressive aphasia or primary progressive apraxia.[41] Other cases can mimic corticobasal degeneration.[42]

Diagnostic Procedures

1. MRI or CT scanning shows dilation of the frontal and temporal horns of the lateral ventricles. There is marked widening of the cortical sulci in the same areas, indicating maximal atrophic changes in the frontal and temporal lobes, with sparing of the superior temporal gyrus readily identified by MRI scanning.
2. The SPECT scan is abnormal, with decreased tracer uptake in the frontal and anterior temporal areas.[43]
3. The PET scan shows a marked decrease in metabolic rate for glucose in the frontal lobes, sufficiently distinctive to distinguish Pick disease from Alzheimer disease.[44]

Treatment   There is no specific treatment for Pick disease. The patient should be treated with the general measures, as outlined for Alzheimer disease.

Dementia with Lewy Bodies

Definition   Dementia with Lewy bodies (DLB) is a progressive dementia occurring in the elderly characterized by the presence of Lewy bodies in the neurons of the brainstem and cerebral cortex.

Etiology and Pathology   The etiology is unknown. The salient feature is the presence of Lewy bodies—intracytoplasmic spherical eosinophilic neuronal inclusion bodies in the brainstem, subcortical nuclei, and limbic cortex and in the neocortex of the temporal, frontal, and parietal lobes. Some changes are similar to the pathology of Alzheimer disease, including β-amyloid deposition and diffuse plaque formation in most—but not all—cases of DLB. Neurofibrillary tangles occur in a minority.[45]

Clinical Features   This type of dementia occurs in 15 to 20 percent of elderly demented patients and is probably second in frequency as a cause of dementia, after Alzheimer disease.

The central feature of DLB is progressive cognitive decline and prominent deficits in tests of executive function and problem solving, and visual-spatial performance.[46] There may be marked fluctuation in cognitive functioning in the early stages and obvious deficits, alternating with normal or near-normal performance.[47] Episodic somnolence, with reduced awareness of surroundings and confusion, is prominent in some cases. Recurrent visual hallucinations, often complex in nature, associated with fear, amusement, or indifference, are a common feature. Auditory hallucinations are a less likely occurrence. Delusions based on recollection of hallucinations often have a fixed, complex, and bizarre context, in contrast to the poorly formed persecutory ideas seen in Alzheimer disease. Depression is a significant factor in 50 percent of individuals with DLB.[48]

A mild parkinsonism with rigidity and bradykinesis,[49] hypophonic speech, masked facies, stooped posture and a slow, shuffling gait, and a mild or absent resting tremor is characteristic of DLB but may be delayed in appearance in some cases.

Other factors include repeated falls, syncopal episodes with transient loss of consciousness and increased muscle tone.[50] Neuroleptic sensitivity or an adverse reaction to standard neuroleptic medications is a prominent feature.[51]

Diagnostic Procedures

1. The MRI or CT scans may show generalized cortical atrophy.
2. The SPECT scan shows reduced cerebral blood

flow in a similar pattern to that seen in Alzheimer disease.

3. The EEG is abnormal, with background slowing, paroxysmal activity in the temporal leads, and a frontal dominant burst pattern.[52]

Treatment   Essentially supportive. The response to levodopa is unpredictable, unlike Parkinson disease.

Prognosis   There is a steady decline to death from intercurrent infection. Men are more susceptible and carry a worse prognosis than women.

Corticobasal Degeneration

Definition   This is a slowly progressive condition with a unilateral, tremulous, akinetic rigid apraxic upper limb held in a fixed dystonic posture and displaying the alien limb syndrome.[53]

Etiology and Pathology   The etiology is unknown. The brain shows mild atrophy of the gyri. Microscopic examination reveals pale, swollen neurons with eccentric nuclei scattered throughout the cerebrum, most numerous in the medial frontal area. The substantia nigra shows severe neuronal loss and there is achromasia of surviving neurons in the substantia nigra and caudate nucleus.[54]

Clinical Features   The disease presents in the sixth or seventh decade with unilateral rigidity and dyspraxic clumsiness gradually involving an upper limb or occasionally a lower limb, or both. The condition remains unilateral for many years. Additional symptoms include a tonic, predominantly flexor dystonia, stimulus-sensitive myoclonus, abnormal saccadic eye movements, and the development of an alien hand.[55] This is a hand that assumes a posture or grasps an object unperceived by the patient. Dementia, dysarthria, dysphasia, and corticospinal tract signs are late features.[56]

Treatment   There is no effective treatment for this condition, which is slowly progressive, with late appearance of impairment of function on the initially unaffected side.

Progressive Aphasia Without Dementia

Definition   This is a rare condition often mistaken for Alzheimer disease, in which there is progressive failure of language without dementia.

Etiology and Pathology   The etiology is unknown. Autopsy studies have shown atrophy of the temporal poles with dilatation of the temporal horns, associated with mild frontal lobe atrophy.[57] Microscopic examination reveals severe neuronal loss and intense gliosis throughout the cortex of the temporal poles. There is mild neuronal loss in the frontal and parietal cortex. In other cases, the brain shows generalized atrophy accentuated over the inferior left frontal lobe and superior left parietal areas[58] with microscopic changes of ballooned neurons or Pick cells. There is persuasive evidence that primary progressive aphasia without dementia may be a variant of Pick disease in some cases.

Clinical Features   The disease presents with an insidious onset and gradual deterioration of selective language skills.[59] There is a progressive language disturbance with reduced verbal output, agrammatism and phenomic paraphasic errors but preserved language comprehension and nonverbal cognition.[60] Writing is slowed and shows mild spelling dysgraphias. Anomic dysphasia may be a prominent and early sign, and the overall impression is that of a nonfluent dysphasia. Despite the profound involvement of language function, other cognitive and behavioral functions are relatively spared. This contrasts with cases of Alzheimer disease, which can likewise present with dysphasia, in that other signs of deterioration in judgment, insight, memory, cognition and perception appear at an early stage in Alzheimer disease.

Treatment   There is no treatment for progressive aphasia without dementia, but recognition of the condition is important, because the patient can maintain independent living but may require help in developing alternative methods of communication.

Frontotemporal Dementia

Definition   This insidious and slowly progressive dementia is associated with cerebral atrophy, involving the frontal and temporal lobes, and occasionally accompanied by clinical signs of amyotrophic lateral sclerosis (ALS).

Etiology and Pathology   The brain shows atrophy of the frontal and temporal lobes with dilatation of the frontal horns of the ventricles. Pathological changes consist of neuronal loss and spongiform changes in the affected areas, with moderate to severe astrocytic gliosis, without evidence of the intranuclear inclusions characteristic of Pick disease.

Clinical Features   The onset is insidious and the progression slow.[61] The individual becomes careless in dress, hygiene, and grooming, lacks social tact, and may be involved in misdemeanors such as shoplifting. There are early signs of disinhibition, such as restlessness, violent behavior, inappropriate jocularity, and unrestrained sexuality, and at the same time, there is mental rigidity and inflexibility. The diet may change because of food fads and there may be overeating and excessive smoking and alcohol consumption. Behavior may be stereotyped, manifested by wandering, repetitive mannerisms, and a preoccupation with hoarding objects, toileting, or dressing. There is a tendency to unrestrained exploration of objects in the environment, distractibility, and impulsivity, with loss of insight.

Depression, anxiety, excessive sentimentality, delusions, and suicidal thoughts may be noted by observers, and the patient may be hypochondrial or express bizarre somatic complaints. At the same time, there is lack of empathy, emotional unconcern, or apathy. Language content may be reduced and stereotyped, until there is a limited repertoire of words. Asymmetrical involvement of the left dominant frontotemporal lobe is associated with progressive nonfluent dysphasia.[62] Echolalia is a late phenomenon leading to mutism. Incontinence is often an early symptom.

Examination shows rigidity, paratonia, and early appearance of primitive reflexes, including glabellar, snout, and grasp reflexes. Signs of bulbar

palsy, muscle wasting and weakness and fasciculations (ALS) are present in some cases.[63]

Diagnostic Procedures

1. The EEG shows progressive symmetrical slowing in the later stages of the disease.
2. The CT and MRI scans are abnormal, with frontotemporal atrophy and dilatation of the frontal horns of the lateral ventricles.

Treatment   General measures, as for other dementias.

Diseases of the Basal Ganglia

The majority of degenerative diseases that affect the basal ganglia are associated with involuntary movements and are discussed in Chapter 6.

Progressive Supranuclear Palsy

Definition   Progressive supranuclear palsy (PSP) is a chronic progressive brain disease characterized by supranuclear ophthalmoplegia affecting chiefly vertical gaze, pseudobulbar palsy, prominent neck dystonia, behavioral and cognitive disturbances, parkinsonism, axial dystonia, gait disturbances, impaired equilibrium and falls.[64]

Etiology and Pathology   The etiology is unknown, but the condition may be related to exposure to an exogenous toxin.[65]

The brain shows evidence of atrophy. There is decreased pigment in the substantia nigra and locus ceruleus and loss of neurons in the basal ganglia, brainstem and cerebellum. Neurofibrillary tangles are present in the cerebral cortex, caudate nucleus, putamen, globus pallidus, subthalamic nucleus, brainstem, and cerebellum.[66]

Clinical Features   The prevalence of PSP is 1.4 cases per 100,000, with an annual incidence of 3 to 4 per million. The disease is usually sporadic, but familial cases have been described, suggesting an autosomal dominant trait.[67] The symptoms begin in the early sixties and are seen in all ethnic groups. Survival following the onset of overt symptoms is from 6 to 9 years. Early symptoms consist of bradykinesia and supranuclear gaze palsy, with voluntary down gaze less than 15°, impaired optokinetic nystagmus, stimulus downward, and horizontal square wave jerks. This is followed by the development of rigidity affecting the axilla muscles more than the limb muscles, in the lower limbs more than the upper limbs. Parkinsonian features, including paucity of blinking and a fixed facial expression, occur early in the course of the disease. Progressive dysarthria, increased reflexes, and extensor plantar responses are constant features. The head and neck are held in extension, and there are frequent falls in a patient with a relatively well-preserved gait. Torticollis, blepharospasm, and stuttering speech have been described. The dementia associated with PSP is often mild, with cognitive slowing,[68] but almost all patients suffer from apathy and disinhibition occurs in about one-third of cases.[69] Eventually the patient becomes bedridden and dies from intercurrent infection.

Diagnostic Procedures The diagnosis depends largely on clinical presentation and the characteristic progression of the disease.

The MRI scan shows diffuse brain atrophy, including cerebellar atrophy, atrophy of the midbrain, a widening of the posterior third ventricle, and increased signal intensity in the periaqueductal region in the T2-weighted images.

Differential Diagnosis In the early stages of PSP, the condition is frequently misdiagnosed as Parkinson disease. Other conditions that might be considered include multisystem atrophy, including striatonigral degeneration, Shy-Drager syndrome, and olivopontocerebellar atrophy.

Treatment Carbidopa-levodopa therapy may produce some improvement in the early stages of the disease and at relatively high doses. Levodopa content up to 1500 mg 24 h can be used without producing adverse effects. Amitriptyline beginning at 10 mg q.h.s. and increased by 10 mg q5d, up to 100 mg q.h.s., is of established benefit. Amantadine and selegiline may produce temporary improvement.

Multiple System Atrophy   Multiple system atrophy (MSA) is a sporadic, progressive adult-onset disorder characterized by autonomic dysfunction, parkinsonism, and ataxia in any combination.[70] MSA encompasses conditions described previously under the heading of striatonigral degeneration (SND), sporadic olivopontocerebellar atrophy (OPCA), and Shy-Drager syndrome (SDS),[71] presenting with any combination of extrapyramidal corticospinal cerebellar and autonomic signs and symptoms.[72]

Etiology and Pathology The etiology is unknown. Pathological changes consist of neuronal loss and gliosis in the striatal, nigral, and olivopontocerebellar systems, with the presence of oligodendroglial and neuronal intracytoplasmic and intranuclear argyrophilic inclusions[73] containing accumulations of tubular structures.[74]

Clinical Features Initial symptoms consist of parkinsonism (SND type), or cerebellar ataxia (OPCA type), or autonomic dysfunction (SDS).

Parkinsonism consisting of akinesia and rigidity is an early feature of SND, accompanied by a jerky irregular tremor in some cases. Cerebellar signs with intention tremor or heal-to-shin ataxia occur in the early stages of OPCA, with later development of postural instability and gait ataxia.

Autonomic failure is a feature of SND and OPCA or SDS and may be the presenting symptom or develop later in the course of the disease. Symptoms consist of impotence, mild-to-moderate postural hypotension, urinary incontinence or retention, and syncopal episodes. Corticospinal tract involvement, with increased tendon reflexes and extensor plantar responses, are usual, but spasticity and lower limb weakness are uncommon.

Many patients develop nystagmus, saccadic eye movements, and dysarthria, which can be severe in some cases. Upward, downward, or horizontal gaze may be limited. Respiratory stridor is a later feature, and stimulus-sensitive myoclonus occurs in about one-third of cases. Sensory changes are minor, with some impairment of vibration and position sense in the toes.

Patients presenting with prominent autonomic dysfunction and labeled SDS ultimately develop parkinsonism or cerebellar dysfunction, or both. Consequently, SDS is probably a variant of MSA, with later development of the features of SND or OPCA.

Diagnostic Procedures An MRI scan may show brainstem and cerebellar atrophy in the later stages of OPCA.

Treatment Parkinsonism responds to levodopa preparations in about one-third of cases. Response to dopamine agonists is poor.

Orthostatic hypotension often responds to head uptilt at night, elastic support stockings, or an elastic leotard and an increased salt intake. When syncope is a feature, additional treatment is indicated (see Chap. 13).

Prognosis Life expectancy is reduced to a considerable degree. The mean survival time is approximately 10 years.

Olivopontocerebellar Atrophy

Definition The OPCAs are a group of inherited degenerative disorders characterized by a predominant involvement of the brainstem and cerebellum.

Etiology and Pathology The disorders may be inherited as an autosomal dominant[75] or autosomal recessive trait and have in common neuronal degeneration and gliosis in the cerebellum, brainstem, spinal cerebellar tract, and dorsal columns.[76] Histopathological changes typical of MSA have been described in some cases, indicating a close relationship between inherited OPCA and MSA. However, the inclusion bodies of MSA are usually absent in inherited OPCA.

Clinical Features One of the characteristics of olivopontocerebellar degeneration is the wide variety of presenting symptoms. Affected members of the same family may present with a totally different clinical picture. Eventually, however, the affected members of the family will develop ataxia, nystagmus, intention tremor, and titubation of the head. There may

be generalized rigidity and parkinsonian features in some cases. The speech becomes severely dysarthric. The tendon reflexes may be hyperactive or hypoactive, and there is a bilateral extensor plantar response. Some patients develop signs of dementia as a late feature of the disease. Others have prominent autonomic symptoms, with incontinence and orthostatic hypotension and can be regarded as a form of multiple system disease. Sleep disorders, including hyposomnia, rapid eye movement sleep without atonia, and sleep apnea are present in some cases.[77]

Diagnostic Procedures Magnetic resonance imaging and CT scanning may show atrophy of the brainstem and atrophy of the cerebellum with enlargement of the fourth ventricle, ambiens, and prepontine cisterns.

Treatment Treatment is symptomatic. Sleep apnea may respond to trazodone 50 mg q.h.s.

Prognosis There is typically a relentless progression of the disease with death occurring from intercurrent infection approximately 20 years after the development of initial symptoms.

Familial Spinocerebellar Ataxias The autosomal dominant spinal cerebellar ataxias (SCAs) are a heterogeneous group of multisystem neurodegenerative diseases that have been mapped to five chromosomes.[78]

The clinical features, pathological changes, and gene location are listed in Table 14-4.

Families diagnosed with SCA-3 may be examples of Machado-Joseph disease, exhibiting the type 2 phenotype.[79]

Treatment No therapeutic measures are available to treat these diseases. Patients require aids to maintain ambulation and prevent falling.

Friedreich's Ataxia

Definition Friedreich's ataxia is a degenerative disease of childhood and early adult life that primarily involves the long tracts of the spinal cord. The disease is inherited as an autosomal recessive trait in

Table 14-4

Familial spinocerebellar ataxias

Type	Clinical features	Pathology	Gene location
SCA-I	Ataxia, optic atrophy, ophthalmoplegia, corticospinal tract involvement, extrapyramidal features	Neuronal loss, Purkinje cells, pontine nuclei, inferior olivary nuclei	6p23-24
SCA-2	Ataxia, slow saccades, ophthalmoplegia, peripheral neuropathy	Neuronal loss, Purkinje cells, inferior olivary nuclei, substantia nigra, degeneration of posterior columns of spinocerebellar tracts	12q23-24
SCA-3	Ataxia, nystagmus, corticospinal tract involvement, dystonia, hyporeflexic tendon reflexes ankles	Neuronal loss, molecular layer cerebellum, pontine nuclei	14q24-q32
SCA-4	Ataxia, sensory axonal neuropathy, corticospinal tract involvement	Unknown	16q24ter
SCA-5	Benign ataxic course, later appearance of corticospinal tract involvement	Unknown	11
SCA-7	Ataxia, macular dystrophy, retinal degeneration	Unknown	3p14-21.1
Machado-Joseph disease Type 1, early onset	Ataxia, ophthalmoplegia Plus dystonia corticospinal tract involvement	Lost neurons, substantia nigra, subthalamic nuclei, pontine nuclei, dentate nuclei, anterior horn cells, posterior root ganglia, degeneration, Clarke's column, spinocerebellar tract	14q32.1
Type 2, onset middle age Type 3, onset fifth decade	Corticospinal tract involvement Amotrophy		
Dentatorubropallidoluysian atrophy	Ataxia, choreoathetosis, myoclonus, epilepsy, dementia	Lost neurons, dentate nucleus, red nucleus, globus pallidus, subthalamic nucleus, Purkinje cells, brainstem tegmentum, corticospinal tracts	12p12ter

which the Friedreich's ataxia gene has been mapped to the proximal long arm of chromosome 9 (9q13-q21).[80a] This mutation consists of an unstable expression of GAA repeats in the first intron of the frataxin gene on chromosome 9, which encodes a protein of unknown function.[81a] Larger GAA expansions corre-late with earlier age of onset and shorter time to loss of ambulation.[82a]

Pathological changes consist of atrophy with demyelination involving the posterior columns and the spinocerebellar, and corticospinal tracts of the spinal cord. The areas of degeneration show a loss of axons and myelin with secondary gliosis. The degenerative changes begin in the neurons of the dorsal root ganglia and are followed by a dying back of axons of large myelinated fibers in the peripheral nerve and in the posterior columns of the spinal cord. Similar neuronal changes eventually involve the nucleus gracilis and cuneatus, with degenerative changes in the medial lemniscus. The dorsal and ventral spinocerebellar tracts are similarly involved. The corticospinal tract shows demyelination with increased involvement in a caudal direction. Loss of Purkinje cells in the cerebellum and degeneration of the dentate nucleus with axonal loss and demyelination of the superior cerebellar peduncle also occur.

Cardiac hypertrophy and diffuse myocardial fibrosis with degeneration of cardiac muscle cells are an invariable finding.

Clinical Features The first symptoms of ataxia and easy fatigability develop before 10 years of age in about half the cases, and the majority have well-established signs before the age of 20. The ataxia is progressive, beginning in the lower limbs and gradually involving the trunk and upper limbs. Cranial nerve examination reveals reduced visual acuity in some cases, horizontal nystagmus, saccadic pursuit eye movements, hearing loss, dysarthria, and dysphagia. The motor system shows wasting of muscles and weakness of all four limbs. Rapid alternating movements are slowed, with overflinging and past pointing on finger-to-nose testing and bilateral intention tremor. The gait is wide based due to a combination of posterior column dysfunction, spasticity, and cerebellar ataxia. Involvement is symmetrical in most cases, but some asymmetry is not unusual. Sensation is abnormal, with preservation of touch but impairment of temperature, vibration, and position sense in hands and feet. Tendon reflexes are depressed or absent, but there is a bilateral extensor plantar response. Early onset ataxia with cardiomyopathy and retained reflexes has been described.[83a] The fully developed syndrome is characterized by a mild degree of dementia. Optic atrophy with visual failure is not unusual and many patients have a progressive hearing loss. Speech is slow, staccato, and explosive in more developed cases but may eventually become unintelligible in the later stages of the disease.

Examination of the spine shows scoliosis in the majority but not all cases and there is deformity of the feet with pes cavus and extension of the metacarpophalangeal joints and flexion of the interphalangeal joints in about 90 percent of patients.

Cardiomyopathy occurs in about two-thirds of the cases and electrocardiographic (ECG) abnormalities can occur early in the disease and are present in most cases.[84a] Death from congestive heart failure or cardiac arrhythmia is common.

Diagnostic Procedures

1. Clinical diabetes mellitus due to insulin-resistant B cell deficiency and type 1 diabetes are present in about 20 percent of cases.
2. Serum bilirubin levels are frequently elevated.
3. Pulmonary function tests show progressive impairment due to progressive kyphoscoliosis.
4. The ECG is abnormal and many patients have obstructive hypertrophic cardiomyopathy.
5. The EEG shows mild nonspecific abnormalities in most cases.
6. Motor nerve conduction velocities are normal, but sensory conduction velocities are prolonged or absent in the lower limbs.
7. Somatosensory evoked potentials recorded after peroneal nerve stimulation are abnormal, indicating spinal cord involvement.

Differential Diagnosis

1. Other forms of spinal cerebellar degeneration. The characteristic finding of moderately rapid progression and cardiac involvement differentiate Friedreich's ataxia from other spinocerebellar degenerations.
2. Congenital abnormalities. The Arnold-Chiari malformation, platybasia, and odontoid compression can be excluded by MRI studies.
3. Arteriovenous (AV) malformation of the spinal cord. Increased tone and hyperreflexia occur only below the level of the malformation. There are progressive urgency of micturition and a sensory level. The AV malformation can be demonstrated by MRI scanning.
4. Syphilis. Syphilitic pachymeningitis is rare. The

condition is associated with a CSF pleocytosis and increased protein content. The serological test for syphilis is positive.

5. Subacute combined degeneration can cause confusion if it occurs before overt signs of pernicious anemia. Serum vitamin B_{12} levels are depressed.
6. Spinal cord tumors tend to cause pain, particularly nerve root pain. There is progressive spasticity below the level of the lesion and progressive urgency of micturition. Examination shows a sensory level. The diagnosis can be established by MRI scanning.
7. Multiple sclerosis. The spinal cord form of multiple sclerosis can cause some confusion with Friedreich's ataxia. There tends to be a relapsing and remitting course in multiple sclerosis, with bladder involvement and patchy sensory loss. Visual evoked potentials and auditory evoked potentials may be abnormal in multiple sclerosis. The CSF may show an elevated protein, increased gamma globulin content, and the presence of oligoclonal bands in the CSF, which are not present in the serum. An MRI scan of the brain is usually abnormal.
8. Vitamin E deficiency is a condition closely resembling Friedreich's ataxia. Serum vitamin E levels are normal in Friedreich's ataxia.

Treatment   The treatment is symptomatic. Cardiac and pulmonary complications should receive prompt attention in advanced cases because they are frequently fatal.

Prognosis   The disease runs a progressive course and most patients are unable to walk 5 years after the appearance of symptoms. Death occurs 10 to 20 years after onset from pulmonary or cardiac complications.

Familial Spastic Paraplegia

Definition   This is a slowly progressive spastic paraparesis, without involvement of other cerebrospinal or cerebellar systems.

Etiology and Pathology   The condition is inherited as an autosomal dominant or autosomal recessive trait but occasionally appears to be a sex-linked recessive trait and occurs more frequently in males.

In some cases, the disease may represent a forme fruste of an inherited spinocerebellar degeneration.

Clinical Features   The first symptoms begin in the first two decades of life, although a rare form with later onset has been described. There is a slowly progressive spastic paraparesis evolving to spastic paraplegia, with increasing weakness and spasticity of the lower limbs, increasing tendon reflexes and extensor plantar responses.

Treatment   It is important to rule out compressive conditions of the spinal cord, particularly cervical spondylosis in all cases. Because the condition is slowly progressive, most cases are not associated with the reduction of a normal life span.

There is no definitive treatment for this condition. The use of a baclofen pump should be considered in those with advanced disease and severe spasticity.

Familial Episodic Ataxia   This uncommon condition is characterized by episodic ataxia, which occurs in two distinct forms, familial episodic ataxia with interictal myokymia (EA1) and familial episodic ataxia with interictal nystagmus (EA2). In EA1, the result of a genetic defect located on chromosome 12p13,[80] the attacks are brief, lasting no more than several minutes. EA2, the result of a genetic defect on chromosome 19p,[81] is characterized by longer episodes of ataxia of several hours' duration. In EA2, symptoms vary from pure ataxia to signs suggesting involvement of the cerebellum, brainstem, and cerebral cortex, and some individuals exhibit a progressive ataxia indistinguishable from dominantly inherited spinal cerebellar ataxia. About 50 percent of patients with EA2 experience basilar migraine or hemiplegic migraine, the latter linked to a genetic defect on chromosome 19[82] in the same region as EA2.

Both EA1 and EA2 respond to acetazolamide therapy.[83]

Motor Neuron Disease (Amyotrophic Lateral Sclerosis)

Definition   Motor neuron disease (amyotrophic lateral sclerosis—ALS) is a chronic disease characterized by progressive degeneration of motor neurons of the anterior horn of the spinal cord, motor nuclei in the brainstem, and neurons in the motor area of the posterior aspect of the frontal lobe.

Etiology and Pathology The etiology is unknown. The disease is familial in 10 percent of cases, when it is inherited as an autosomal dominant or autosomal recessive trait. Dominant familial ALS has a penetrance of less than 100 percent by age 70 years[84] and may be lower than 50 percent by age 63.[85] This is the most common form of familial ALS, with the responsible gene located on chromosome 21,[86] whereas some families with recessive ALS show linkage to markers on chromosome 2 or 21. The mutations are associated with an abnormality in the superoxide dismutases, which are a group of isoenzymes that catalyze the conversion of superoxide free radical ions to hydrogen peroxide and oxygen. Failure of this reaction permits free radicals, which are highly toxic, to accumulate in motor neurons, producing free radical toxicity and accelerated cell death.

Some 90 percent of patients with ALS are without evidence of chromosomal abnormality[87] with superoxide dismutases mutations present in a small percentage.[88] In the majority, however, the disease may be the result of exotoxicity. This process postulates overactivity of the glutamate system, in which the normal amino acid is converted into an exotoxin which produces glutamate overstimulation of the five subtypes of the glutamate receptors on the neuronal membrane,[89] resulting in increased calcium entry into neurons, overproduction of free radicals, and premature cell death.

Evidence for an autoimmune mechanism producing neuronal loss[90] or the role of positive viral agents such as the poliovirus[91] are unproven. Failure of axonal transport with accumulation of neurofilaments, which are known to be increased in ALS, could indicate a failure of axonal transport, leading to dendritic atrophy and death of the perikaryon.[92]

Pathological changes consist of loss of motor neurons in the spinal cord, brainstem, and cerebral cortex. Surviving neurons are atrophic with abnormalities of dendritic pattern on Golgi staining and show reduced levels of RNA. Inclusion bodies, identified as hyalin inclusions, Lewy bodies, basophilic inclusions, and Bunani bodies, occur in motor neurons in familial and nonfamilial ALS. A filamentous neuronal inclusion body has been identified in nonfamilial ALS in both motor and nonmotor neurons in the brain, suggesting that ALS should be considered a multisystem disease.[93]

Clinical Features Amyotrophic lateral sclerosis is a rare disease with a prevalence of approximately 2 per 100,000 and a male-to-female ratio of 1.1:1. The median age of onset is 66 years.

The fundamental disease process in ALS involves loss of motor neurons in the cerebral cortex, the motor nuclei of the cranial nerves, and the anterior horn cells of the spinal cord.[94] Consequently, the classical division of ALS into those with bulbar onset (progressive bulbar palsy) and those with involvement of the spinal cord motor neurons (progressive muscular atrophy) may well be artificial because careful neurological examination will reveal evidence of lower motor neuron involvement in patients with predominantly bulbar symptoms, whereas those with spinal motor neuron signs of wasting and fasciculations usually present with increased tendon reflexes and extensor plantar responses, indicating that the pathological process includes the corticospinal tracts. It is probable that ALS consists of a spectrum of disease extending from primary lateral sclerosis to spinal muscular atrophy and that ultimately, if the patient survives, signs of both upper and lower motor neuron disease will be apparent.

The disease often begins with progressive loss of motor neurons in the anterior horns of the spinal cord. When the neurons of the cervical cord are involved, there will be progressive weakness, wasting, and fasciculations involving the small muscles of the hands. However, the loss may occur at any site in the spinal cord. The sensory examination is normal. Initially, there may be no clinical evidence of corticospinal tract or bulbar involvement, which will inevitably develop later as the disease progresses.

Alternatively, the disease may begin with involvement of the motor neurons of the cranial nerve nuclei. Under these circumstances, there is progressive weakness and wasting involving the pharyngeal musculature, the tongue, and the facial muscles. The patient develops progressive dysarthria and dysphagia. Fasciculations of the tongue are usually prominent and can be seen when the tongue is examined, lying quietly on the floor of the mouth. The oculomotor nuclei are usually not involved.

Signs indicating spinal motor neuron disease with wasting, fasciculations, the development of corticospinal tract dysfunction, increased tendon reflexes and extensor plantar responses, ultimately occur in patients who survive for more than a few months.

A combined form of upper motor neuron disease and anterior horn cell involvement, plus corticospinal tract dysfunction, is the most common form of ALS. The patient complains of increasing weakness and examination reveals atrophy, fasciculations, and wasting of the muscles in both upper and lower limbs, associated with increased reflexes and extensor plantar responses. Eventually the brainstem nuclei are involved, resulting in dysphagia, dysarthria, and facial weakness. There are no sensory changes.

Diagnostic Procedures

1. Electromyography (EMG) as an extension of the clinical examination, is the single most useful test in evaluating disease of the lower motor neurons.[94] The EMG will demonstrate abnormalities in upper and lower extremities and thoracic paraspinal muscles and the presence of normal nerve conduction velocities.
2. Muscle biopsy shows the typical appearance of denervation atrophy with atrophic fascicles coexisting with normal fascicles.
3. Muscle enzymes such as creatinine phosphokinase (CK) may be elevated in rapidly progressive cases.
4. The CSF is normal.
5. There are no MRI, CT, or myelographic abnormalities.

Differential Diagnosis

1. With mass lesions impinging on the spinal cord (e.g., tumors, spondylosis, abscess), the weakness, wasting, and fasciculations are confined to one or more myotomes, and there is appropriate sensory loss in the affected dermatomes.
2. Multifocal motor neuropathy with conduction block can be differentiated by EMG and the presence of GM_1 antibodies in this disease.[95]
3. Combined cervical myeloradiculopathy and lumbosacral radiculopathy with both upper and lower motor neuron signs can be excluded if brainstem cervical, thoracic, and lumbosacral areas are included in the EMG evaluation.
4. Benign fasciculations, myokymia. Benign fasciculations are not at all uncommon and are often diffuse. There are no other signs of neurological involvement, and the general physical examination and neurological examination are perfectly normal. Follow-up examinations remain normal.
5. Chronic inflammation of the meninges or spinal cord (e.g. adhesive arachnoiditis). In this condition, the CSF is abnormal. The MRI and CT scans with myelography may be abnormal.

Treatment   There is no effective treatment for this disease and the course is one of progressive deterioration, with a mean survival of 3 years. Immunosuppressant[96] and intravenous immunoglobulin[97] therapies are not effective. Selegiline does not modify the progression of ALS.[98] Ceftriaxone is without benefit.[99] Lamotrigine[100] and gabapentin,[101] which inhibit glutamate release, do not alter the course of this disease. Neither dextromethorphan,[102] physostigmine,[103] branch-chain amino acids,[104] 3,4-aminopyridine,[105] nor acetylcysteine[106] has had a significant effect on ALS. Recombinant human insulin-like growth factor-1 is reported to slow the progression of ALS and deterioration in the quality of life.[107]

Riluzole, a glutamate antagonist, is reported to increase survival in ALS[108] and appears to be most effective in patients with disease of bulbar onset.[109] The drug is taken by mouth, 50 mg q12h, 1 h before or 2 h after a meal. Adverse effects include nausea, weight loss, and headache.

There should be close support by physicians, nurses, social workers, and psychologists to help the patient face the ravages of this disease. The family should be informed of the course complications and prognosis of the disease. Community resources should be obtained through the help of a social worker because the family will require increasing support as the patient becomes increasingly dependent. When dysphagia prevents normal feeding, feedings should be continued through a plastic naso-gastrostomy or jejunostomy tube, using a pureed diet and ultimately the use of a percutaneous gastronomy (PEG) tube. The weakness and wasting often produce painful subluxation of the scapulohumeral joints, and the arms should be supported by hemiplegic slings. Adequate analgesia for pain control is essential. Aggressive symptomatic treatment should focus on the goal of maintaining the patient's functional independence as long as possible.[110] This requires an ongoing program of physical rehabilitation, including physical and occupational therapies, the use of assistive devices, the provision of home equipment, and nutritional, communication, respiratory, and psychological support.

When respiratory failure occurs, the family should be assured that the patient will pass quietly into a carbon dioxide narcosis, followed by coma and death, and should be urged to avoid the use of a mechanical respirator in most cases. However, a number of patients develop respiratory failure at an early stage, when there is still adequate function in the upper limbs. These individuals may lead a useful life of 2 or more years, in some cases, with portable mechanical ventilator support. Death occurs from pulmonary infection as the patient becomes immobilized by muscle weakness.

The bulbar musculature tends to lose function at a slower rate than the muscles of the upper limbs, but bulbar involvement is more critical because of the dangers of aspiration pneumonia.

Prognosis   The course is one of steady progression until death. Life expectancy of patients with dysphagia is less than that of patients with limb weakness, presumably because of the higher risk of aspiration pneumonia in the dysphagia group.[111] Occasionally, the process seems to be arrested for a period of several months before continuing a downhill course. Mean survival in the familial form of ALS is 3 years, with mean survival of 4 years in sporadic cases of ALS.

Primary Lateral Sclerosis

Definition   This is a slowly progressive disorder of nonfamilial form, in which there is a gradual development of spastic paraparesis over a period of many years.

Etiology and Pathology   The etiology is unknown. Pathological changes consist of frontal lobe atrophy with neuronal loss and corresponding reduction in subcortical white matter, involving the precentral gyrus, the premotor areas, and the supplementary motor areas, with degeneration of the corticospinal and corticobulbar axons.[112] The pathological changes suggest that there may be an overlap with ALS and frontotemporal dementia.

Clinical Features   The condition presents in adults with a gradual development of spasticity in the lower limbs, producing progressive impairment of gait and eventual requirement of a cane or walker. The upper limbs are spared but show hyperreflexia. The tendon reflexes are increased in the lower limbs, and bilateral extensor plantar responses are present. Spastic dysarthria and mild dysphagia are late developments. There is no evidence of amyotrophy, fasciculations, optic atrophy, hearing loss, sensory change, or pes cavus. There are no sphincter problems, no urgency of micturition, and absence of any evidence of a segmental lesion.

The clinical course is slow, with a median survival of several years. Some patients show evidence of muscle wasting late in the course of the disease, suggesting that primary lateral sclerosis is a forme fruste of ALS[113] or frontotemporal dementia.

Diagnostic Procedures

1. An MRI or CT scan should be obtained to exclude malformations at the craniocervical junction, cervical spondylosis, spinal canal or canal tumors, and multiple sclerosis.
2. The CSF is normal.
3. A SPECT or PET scan shows bilateral posterior frontal lobe hypoperfusion/hypometabolism.
4. Neuropsychological testing may reveal minor cognitive deficits that escape detection in a brief mental status evaluation.

Treatment   Oral baclofen or a baclofen pump may be useful in reducing spasticity. Adequate evaluation will avoid unnecessary surgery for higher cervical cord compression.

Spinomuscular Atrophies

Definition The spinomuscular atrophies are a group of diseases of unknown etiology that result from degeneration of motor neurons in the spinal cord and occasionally in the brainstem.

Etiology and Pathology The etiology is unknown. In most cases, the condition is inherited as an autosomal recessive trait, and rarely as an autosomal dominant condition, with linkage to chromosome 5.[114] Major deletions of 5q11.2-13.3 have been described in severe infantile spinal muscular atrophy, unlike patients with mild disease who have smaller deletions.[115] Genes for neuronal apoptosis inhibitory protein and the spinal muscular atrophy motor determining gene also map to 5q13 and one or both of these genes may be implicated in spinomuscular atrophy.[116,117]

The primary pathological process appears to be degeneration and atrophy of the anterior horn cells. However, chromatolytic changes with enhanced mitochondrial and oxidative activity in surviving neurons suggest that the primary change may be distal in the axons.

The muscle shows evidence of denervation atrophy with atrophic motor units surrounded by normal-appearing muscle fibers. However, histochemical studies show that the surrounding fibers are all of one histochemical fiber type, because of reinnervation of denervated fibers by sprouting collaterals from axons of surviving anterior horn cells. Other helpful findings include the presence of angular fibers and target or targetoid fibers.

Clinical Features There are four clinical forms based on age and onset of signs and symptoms.

INFANTILE FORM (WERDNIG-HOFFMAN) The

condition is present at birth and the mother frequently reports diminution of the child's movements *in utero* in the later weeks of pregnancy. The infant is weak at birth and shows progressive muscular weakness and hypotonia (floppy infant). This produces a characteristic "frog" position when the baby is prone. The arm is abducted at the shoulder and flexed at the elbow, and the lower limbs are abducted and externally rotated at the hips and flexed at the knees. There is progressive weakness of respiratory muscles, paradoxical respirations leading to respiratory insufficiency, pneumonia, and death within 12 to 18 months.

LATE INFANTILE FORMS These children have

normal movements at birth but develop progressive muscle weakness and hypotonia within 2 months. The lower limbs are weaker than the upper limbs and the child is never able to stand or crawl. Fasciculations of the tongue occur in about 50 percent of cases. Death usually occurs within 2 years, but some children survive for several years.

CHILDHOOD FORM Children with this form of

spinomuscular atrophy develop normally up to or beyond the first birthday and are able to stand and crawl. Many are able to walk for a short period of time, but progressive weakness, wasting, hypotonia, and hyporeflexia, with proximal or distal preponderance, impose increasing restriction of activities. Fasciculations are unusual in limb muscles but may be present in the tongue. Focal or even diffuse muscle hypertrophy can occur due to hypertrophy of surviving motor units. There may be a fine asynchronous tremor of the outstretched hands due to the firing of large motor units; this results from reinnervation of denervated muscles by surviving nerve fibers. Voluntary contraction fasciculation, which disappear on relaxation, may be present. Palpation of the contracting muscle may yield a vibration-like sensation. Auscultation may reveal a low-pitched rumbling. Late changes include joint contractures and scoliosis. Severe scoliosis may lead to spinal cord compression and result in hyperreflexia and extensor plantar responses. The combination of scoliosis and respiratory muscle involvement can produce severe respiratory insufficiency.

ADOLESCENT FORM (FAMILIAL SPINAL MUSCULAR ATROPHY—KUGELBERG-WELANDER SYNDROME)

This is a more benign form of spinomuscular atrophy that is inherited as an autosomal dominant or autosomal recessive trait and begins at about 2 years of age. Wasting and weakness may be confined to the proximal limb-girdle musculature. There may be fasciculations in the limb-girdle muscles and the tongue, and some hypertrophy of muscles can occur. Both hyporeflexia and hyperreflexia are reported. The disease is often confused with the limb-girdle type of muscular dystrophy but can be distinguished by muscle biopsy. This is the most benign form of generalized spinomuscular atrophy. The patient survives into adult life, at which time there is slowing or apparent arrest of the muscle weakness.

Focal forms of the disease present with:

1. Scapulohumeral distribution. This form is usually benign but may present as a rapidly progressive disease in adults, with death from respiratory failure within 3 years.
2. Scapuloperoneal distribution. This form also occurs in adolescents and adults. The atrophy involves muscles of the scapular and periscapular region and the anterior compartment of the leg.
3. Ocular and facial muscle involvement. This form occurs in children and adults and constitutes one of the conditions in the syndrome of "oculomyopathy."
4. Bulbar involvement (Fazio-Londe disease). This rapidly progressive form of muscular atrophy involves bulbomotor neurons and begins in early childhood. The atrophy is most marked in the bulbar musculature with weakness and wasting of the extraocular facial and pharyngeal muscles. Death occurs from respiratory insufficiency and pneumonia.

Diagnostic Procedures

1. It is possible to produce fasciculations in suspected cases by intramuscular injection of 1 mg Prostigmin.
2. The EMG may show the presence of fasciculations and fibrillations.
3. Muscle biopsy with histochemistry is abnormal. The findings are outlined under etiology and pathology.

Treatment The infantile form of spinomuscular atrophy runs a rapid course, with death from respi-

ratory failure 12 to 18 months after birth. Patients with the more chronic forms of the disease should receive:

1. Treatment directed toward maintaining ambulation as long as possible. This includes physical therapy, orthopedic consultation, bracing, and surgical procedures.
2. Prompt treatment of all respiratory tract infections that may lead to pneumonia, pulmonary insufficiency, and death.
3. The intelligence is not affected and patients benefit from an appropriate education.

Prognosis The life span is reduced in all forms of generalized spinomuscular atrophy, but a normal life span is possible in some patients, with focal forms of the disease.

HEREDITARY DISEASES OF WHITE MATTER

The Leukodystrophies

The leukodystrophies are a rare group of genetically determined conditions characterized by metabolic defects in the formation or breakdown of myelin (Table 14-5). Metachromatic leukodystrophies are the most frequently encountered in this group of rare metabolic disorders.

Metachromatic Leukodystrophy

Definition Metachromatic leukodystrophy is characterized by a degeneration of myelin in the central and peripheral nervous systems due to lack of the enzyme arylsulfatase A. The condition is transmitted as an autosomal recessive trait and the mutated gene is located on chromosome 22.

Etiology and Pathology There is a disturbance of the sphingolipid metabolism in which galactosyl-3-sulfate ceramide (sulfatide) is metabolized. The decreased activity of arylsulfatase A in metachromatic leukodystrophy leads to accumulation of sulfatide in the central and peripheral nervous systems.

Table 14-5
Disorders of sphingomyelin metabolism

Disease	Inheritance	Enzyme deficiency	Metabolite that accumulates
Metachromatic leukodystrophy	Autosomal recessive	Sulfatidase	Sulfatide
Globoid cell leukodystrophy (Krabbe)	Autosomal recessive	Galactocerebroside-β-galactosidase	Galactocerebroside
GM$_1$ gangliosidoses (generalized)	Autosomal recessive	Ganglioside GM$_1$-β-galactosidase	Ganglioside GM$_1$
Tay-Sachs disease (infantile)	Autosomal recessive	Hexosaminidase A	Ganglioside GM$_2$
Tay-Sachs disease (juvenile)	Autosomal recessive	Hexosaminidase B	Ganglioside GM$_2$
Tay-Sachs disease (Sandhoff-Jatzkewitz)	Autosomal recessive	Hexosaminidase A, B	Ganglioside GM$_2$
Fabry disease	X-linked recessive	Ceramidetrihexoside-α-galactosidase	Ceramidetrihexoside
Gaucher disease	Autosomal recessive	Glycocerebroside β-galactosidase	Glucocerebroside
Niemann-Pick disease	Autosomal recessive	Sphingomyelinase	Sphingomyelin

The brain is normal in size and weight. The white matter is firm and brownish in appearance, with occasional cavitation. Microscopic abnormalities include loss of myelin sheaths, axonal degeneration, loss of oligodendrocytes, and accumulation of lipid lying free within macrophages and neurons. The peripheral nerves show myelin degeneration and axonal loss, with accumulation of lipid. Lipid deposits are also present in the Kupffer cells of the liver and the renal tubules. The ganglion cells of the retina are heavily involved.

Clinical Features There are three clinical forms of metachromatic leukodystrophy:

LATE INFANTILE FORM This form has its onset at 12 to 18 months of age, with progressive weakness of the lower limbs. The gait is abnormal because of spasticity and ataxia or hypotonia due to peripheral neuropathy. There is progressive visual loss and optic atrophy. Occasionally, macular degeneration and a "cherry-red spot" appearance occur. Progressive dementia, loss of speech, ataxia, spasticity and tremors are seen. Seizures occur in about 50 percent of cases. The condition progresses to severe dementia, blind-

ness, and spastic tetraplegia, with decerebration in the terminal stages. Death occurs 2 to 10 years after onset.

JUVENILE FORM In this form, symptoms do not appear until 5 to 10 years of age. The initial symptoms consist of a declining performance in school, behavioral changes, and gait disturbance. Older children show cognitive decline and abnormal behavior before the gait is affected. The early symptoms are followed by progressive spasticity, rigidity, and ataxia with a somewhat slower progression than the late infantile form of the disease. Peripheral neuropathy may develop but is usually mild. Seizures occur in 80 percent of patients. Life expectancy is 3 to 15 years from time of onset.

ADULT FORM Symptoms begin in the early twenties with mental deterioration and behavior abnormalities, followed by ataxia. The disease is slowly progressive, with the development of dementia and polyneuropathy progressing to death after several years. Psychiatric illness with psychosis, personality change, emotional lability, abnormal behavior, and dementia occur in the late teens. Neurological findings are similar to the younger onset types but evolve slowly. The course is prolonged, with eventually profound dementia, but survival into the fifth or sixth decades is possible. An adult pseudodeficiency of arylsulfatase A, with progressive neurological and psychiatric symptoms, has been described, in which arylsulfatase A levels are low, but there is no accumulation of sulfatides in the nervous system or in other organs.[118]

Diagnostic Procedures

1. Metachromatic bodies can be seen in frozen sections of the sural nerve after biopsy.
2. Metachromatic bodies or abnormal urinary lipids can be demonstrated in the urine.
3. A deficiency of arylsulfatase A can be demonstrated in the urine and leukocytes and in cultured skin fibroblasts.
4. Visual, brainstem, auditory, and somatosensory evoked responses are abnormally prolonged or absent.
5. Peripheral nerve conduction velocities are slowed to less than 30 m/s.
6. The MRI scan shows cortical atrophy, ventricular enlargement, and abnormal signal intensity in the periventricular white matter on T2-weighted images. CT scanning shows scattered areas of decreased attenuation in the central white matter or decreased white matter attenuation near the frontal and occipital horns.
7. The CSF protein is elevated in 90 percent of patients, sometimes greater than 2000 mg/dL.
8. The diagnosis should be confirmed by leukocytic genomic DNA analysis.
9. Prenatal diagnosis is possible by demonstrating lack of arylsulfatase A in the amniotic fluid.

Treatment   A bone marrow transplant may slow the progression of the disease in some patients with the infantile form of the disease, but treatment is usually symptomatic.

Globoid Cell Leukodystrophy

Definition   Globoid cell leukodystrophy is a rare demyelinating disorder of the central and peripheral nervous systems in which there is a deficiency of the lysosomal enzyme galactosylceramide-β-galactoside. The disorder is inherited as an autosomal recessive trait that maps to chromosome 14q31.[120]

Etiology and Pathology   The deficiency of the enzyme leads to an abnormal accumulation of galactosyl sphingosine, which is cytotoxic to oligodendrocytes resulting in impaired myelin formation in the brain (see Table 14-5). The brain is small and there is a diffuse loss of myelin. Microscopic examination shows the presence of multinucleated histiocyte (globoid) cells in the white matter. The globoid cells contain galactosyl sphingosine. The cortex remains remarkably normal in appearance, despite isolation from subcortical centers and loss of interhemispheric connections.

Clinical Features   Globoid cell leukodystrophy usually occurs in the infantile form. Rare juvenile and adult variants have been described.[121] In the infantile form, there is loss of ability to sit, hold up the head, and reach other developmental milestones. Hyperirritability, hyperesthesia, and episodic fever occur. There are gradual development of optic atrophy, deafness, and progression to hypotonic or spastic quadriparesis. Seizures may occur. Terminal decerebration and death occur within a year of onset.

Diagnostic Procedures

1. There is diminished activity of the enzyme galactosylceramide-β-galactosides in leukocytes or cultured fibroblasts.
2. The MRI scan shows areas of increased signal intensity in T2-weighted images in the white matter of the cerebral hemispheres and cerebellum and occasionally in the thalamus and posterior limb of the internal capsule and corona radiata.
3. The CT scan will show areas of low attenuation in the white matter in similar areas.
4. Nerve conduction velocities are slowed.
5. The CSF protein may be elevated.
6. Antenatal diagnosis can be made by amniocentesis and demonstration of deficient galactosylceramide-β-galactoside in cultured amniotic fluid cells.

Treatment   Treatment is symptomatic.

Adrenoleukodystrophy

Definition   Adrenoleukodystrophy is a sex-linked recessive disorder owing to a mutation of a gene located in Xq28 that encodes a peroxisomal transporter protein of unknown function.[122] The disorder is characterized by degeneration of myelin and adrenal insufficiency.

Etiology and Pathology   The etiology is unknown. There is accumulation of very long chain fatty acids, particularly hexacosanoate in the tissues. There is symmetrical demyelination of the cerebrum, brainstem, cerebellum and spinal cord. Microscopic examination shows sudanophilic lipids within macrophages lying in the perivascular spaces of the white matter. The adrenal glands are atrophic and contain balloon cells with eccentric nuclei.

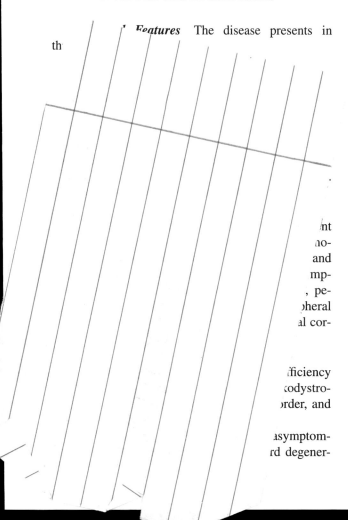

Features   The disease presents in
th

nt
no-
and
mp-
, pe-
pheral
al cor-

ficiency
codystro-
order, and

asymptom-
rd degener-

Diagnostic Procedures

1. Elevated plasma concentrations of long chain fatty acids can be demonstrated in some, but not all, cases of adrenoleukodystrophy.
2. An MRI scan shows diffuse areas of increased signal intensity in the white matter cerebrum and spinal cord. They appear as areas of decreased attenuation in the CT scan.
3. An EMG and nerve conduction studies are compatible with a primary axonal degeneration in peripheral nerves.[124]
4. The EEG shows symmetrical slowing that increases as the disease progresses.
5. The corticotropin infusion test is abnormal, indicating primary adrenal insufficiency.
6. The CSF protein content may be elevated.
7. Adrenocortical biopsy will reveal the characteristic balloon cells and establish the diagnosis.

Treatment

1. Dietary therapy with a mixture of glyceryl trioleate and glyceryl trierucate oil (Lorenzo's oil) is controversial but has been reported to show a slight slowing in clinical progression and delay of death.[125]
2. Bone marrow transplantation offers significant improvement in the clinical course of the disease and a better quality of life.[126]

Pelizaeus-Merzbacher Disease

Definition   Pelizaeus-Merzbacher disease is a rare, sex-linked disorder characterized by degeneration of myelin in the CNS.

Etiology and Pathology   The disorder is associated with mutations in the proteolipid protein (PLP) gene. There is no reproduction or expression of a truncated form of PLP resulting in death of oligodendrocytes, because of accumulation of PLP in the endoplasmic reticulum and progressive demyelination.[127]

A severe degree of atrophy of the brain, which shows irregular areas of demyelination in the cerebral hemispheres, cerebellum, and brainstem, gives it a so-called tigroid appearance. The cerebellum shows loss of Purkinje cells and granular cells in addition to demyelination. Subcortical U fibers are frequently spared.

Clinical Features   The condition is apparent shortly after birth, with failure to attain expected developmental milestones. Progressive spasticity, cerebellar ataxia, coarse nystagmus, choreoathetosis, optic atrophy, and mental retardation occur. Death occurs from intercurrent infection after several years. A few cases show slow progression and survive to adolescence. A rare adult form of the disease has been described.

Diagnostic Procedures

1. The MRI scan shows irregular areas of increased signal intensity in T2-weighted images, compatible with demyelination in the white matter of the cerebrum and cerebellum. The CT scan has similar irregular areas of decreased attenuation in the white matter.
2. Serial EEGs show progressive slowing as the disease progresses.
3. Auditory, visual, and somatosensory evoked potentials are all prolonged.

Treatment   There is no treatment for this condition.

Leukodystrophy with Diffuse Rosenthal Fiber Formation (Alexander Disease)

Definition   Leukodystrophy with diffuse Rosenthal fiber formation is a sex-linked recessive disorder characterized by demyelination and progressive deterioration.

Etiology and Pathology   The etiology is unknown. Rosenthal fibers are inclusion bodies within the astrocytes in which stress protein inclusions consisting of α-B-crystallin and small heat shock protein, HSP-27, are formed as part of a chronic stress response to an unknown stimulus.[128] The brain is normal in size or enlarged. There is diffuse demyelination, occasionally accompanied by cavitation, with proliferation of astrocytes containing granular eosinophilic deposits within astrocytic processes and cell bodies.[129]

Clinical Features   There are three clinical forms of presentation of this disorder.

INFANTILE ONSET   This form occurs in boys and is characterized by progressive psychomotor retardation, spasticity, megalocephaly, and seizures at approximately 6 months of age. Death occurs by age 3.

JUVENILE ONSET   This form of the disorder occurs equally in boys and girls; it begins in late childhood and is characterized by progressive paresis, bulbar signs, and hyperreflexia. The patient dies in the late teens.

ADULT ONSET   The adult-onset form may resemble multiple sclerosis[130] presenting with a remittent course with ataxia, nystagmus, and spastic paraparesis or quadriparesis.

Sensory symptoms are not significant in any of the clinical presentations.

Diagnostic Procedures   The diagnosis is established by brain biopsy or autopsy, with demonstration of a profusion of refractile Rosenthal fibers within astrocytes.

Treatment   Treatment is symptomatic.

Spongy Degeneration (Canavan)   Spongy degeneration is an autosomal recessive disorder that occurs predominantly in Ashkenazi Jewish families and is characterized by demyelination and progressive deterioration, caused by the deficiency of aspartoacyclase (ASPA). The human ASPA gene has been localized to chromosome 17.[131]

Clinical Features   The etiology is unknown. There is progressive megalencephaly spasticity and developmental delay. The disease runs a progressively deteriorating course with death in childhood.

Diagnostic Procedures

1. There are high levels of *N*-acetylaspartic acid in the urine, serum, and CSF and absence of ASPA activity in fibroblasts.

2. The MRI and CT scans show findings compatible with leukodystrophy.
3. DNA analysis of amniotic cells is probably a reliable method for prenatal diagnosis.[132]
4. Screening for the mutation is warranted among Ashkenazi Jewish couples.[133]

GM₁ Gangliosidosis (Generalized) The GM$_1$ gangliosidoses are autosomal recessive degenerative disorders characterized by a deficiency of the enzyme ganglioside GM$_1$-β-galactoside (see Table 14-5). GM$_1$ gangliosides accumulate in the nervous system, liver, spleen, and bone marrow. There are three clinical variants of GM$_1$ gangliosidoses. In the infantile form, the patient presents with coarse facial features, bony abnormalities, hepatosplenomegaly, seizures, an exaggerated startle reflex, and progressive visual, motor, and intellectual deterioration. The patient usually dies by the age of 3 years. A cherry-red spot is seen in the area of the fovea, owing to retinal degeneration. This is caused by accumulation of GM$_1$ ganglioside in the ganglion cells of the retina, producing a grayish appearance. Because the fovea is devoid of ganglion cells, it appears as a dark red area. Patients with juvenile-onset GM$_1$ gangliosidosis are normal at birth and develop ataxia, progressive motor and intellectual deterioration, and seizures late in childhood. Cherry-red spots, visual disturbances, hepatosplenomegaly, and bony abnormalities are not seen in the juvenile form of the disease.

An adult form of the disease, presenting with progressive dementia, dysarthria, rigidity, myoclonus, and choreoathetosis has been described. This appears to be the result of a combined deficiency of β-*D*-galactosidase deficiency and β-*D*-fucosidase deficiency.[134]

The diagnosis in the gangliosidoses is established by demonstration of a deficiency of ganglioside GM$_1$-β-galactosidase in cultured white blood cells or skin fibroblasts. Prenatal diagnosis is possible, and treatment is symptomatic.

Tay-Sachs Disease — GM₂ Gangliosidosis

Definition Tay-Sachs disease is an autosomal recessive disturbance of sphingomyelin metabolism in which the enzyme *N*-acetyl-hexosaminidase-A is deficient (see Table 14-5).

Etiology and Pathology There are two forms of the enzyme. Hexosaminidase A is lacking in Tay-Sachs disease, but hexosaminidase B is increased. GM$_2$ ganglioside is cleaved only by hexosaminidase A in the presence of an activator protein that binds to GM$_2$ ganglioside. Hexosaminidase A is also absent in the juvenile variant of GM$_2$ gangliosidosis. Both A and B hexosaminidase are decreased in the Sandhoff form of Tay-Sachs disease. Deficiency has also been identified in infants, children, and adults with cerebellar ataxia, spinomuscular atrophy, dementia, and basal ganglia deficits.[135]

Pathological changes in the CNS consist of diffuse demyelination, astrocytosis, and accumulation of GM$_2$ ganglioside within the neurons of the brain and spinal cord. The optic nerves show marked demyelination.

Clinical Features The disorder occurs predominantly in patients of Ashkenazi Jewish descent. There are two clinical forms of the disease based on age of onset. In the infantile form, the patient develops loss of interest in surroundings and progressive visual impairment, beginning at approximately 6 months of age. Progressive weakness, spasticity, intellectual impairment, and seizures are apparent; death occurs in early childhood. Examination of the fundus reveals the presence of a cherry-red spot. The juvenile form of the disease (Sandhoff variant — gangliosidosis type 2) is rather rare and begins at 2 to 4 years of age. It is also characterized by progressive deterioration, but the cherry-red spot is absent.

Diagnostic Procedures

1. The diagnosis depends on demonstration of decreased hexosaminidase activity in serum or cultured fibroblasts. Amniocentesis allows identification of an affected fetus when therapeutic abortion is still possible.
2. The MRI or CT scans reveal cortical atrophy and ventricular dilatation.
3. Brain biopsy or retinal biopsy reveals neurons distended with lipid.

Treatment Intrathecal injections of hexosaminidase A have been attempted but have not proved beneficial at this time.

Fabry Disease

Definition   Fabry disease is an X-linked recessive disorder of glycosphingolipid metabolism, caused by a deficiency of a lysosomal hydrolase, α-galactosidase A, with accumulation of ceramide trihexoside in the tissues, primarily in the lysosomes of vascular endothelium.[136]

Clinical Features   The majority of the neurological manifestations are caused by cerebral ischemia and infarction, the result of progressive accumulation of glycophospholipids in the vascular endothelium. The vertebrobasilar system is involved more than the carotid middle cerebral system and symptoms and signs indicate brainstem infarction in most cases. Intracerebral hemorrhage is an occasional occurrence. Recurrence of infarction in a young patient without risk factors for atherosclerosis should indicate the possibility of Fabry disease.[137]

The diagnosis should be considered when dermatologic abnormalities consisting of elevated brownish red zones are associated with excruciating burning pains in the extremities, inability to sweat, and disturbance of renal and cardiac function.[138] Other signs that may be present include corneal and lens opacities, vascular lesions of the retina, and ischemic CNS signs and symptoms of spasticity and hemiplegia.

Diagnostic Features   The diagnosis is established by demonstration of deficient α-galactosidase. Prenatal diagnosis has been made by demonstration of α-galactosidase deficiency in the chorionic villi or in amniotic fluid cells.

Treatment   Treatment is symptomatic. The patient usually dies of renal disease. Heterozygous females may show corneal opacities and ECG abnormalities.

Gaucher Disease

Definition   Gaucher disease is an autosomal recessive disorder of glycosphingolipid metabolism, owing to a mutation in the gene encoding glucocerebroside.[139] This results in the accumulation of gluco-cerebroside in various tissues, including cells of the reticular endothelial system and neurons.[140]

Etiology and Pathology   There are three types of Gaucher disease. In type 1 (the adult form), the liver, spleen, lungs, and bones are affected and the CNS is spared. However, in the type 2 and type 3 forms of the disease, neurons are affected, with involvement of both the CNS and peripheral nervous system.[141]

Clinical Features   In type 1 Gaucher disease, the patient presents with episodic pain in the limbs or spine in the first or second decade of life, followed by the development of aseptic necrosis of bone, hepatosplenomegaly, pancytopenia, and a hemorrhagic diathesis. Abdominal distention due to a hypotonic colon, respiratory difficulties, and a dark yellow discoloration of the skin over the face and lower limbs are noted.

In addition to systemic features, the CNS is affected in the type 2 and 3 forms of the disease, with seizures, myoclonus, ataxia, and intellectual and motor function deterioration. Type 2 patients (infantile form) develop symptoms by age 3 months and typically die in 2 years. Type 3 patients (the juvenile form) have a course similar to type 1 patients but later develop neurological abnormalities. Patients who appear to have a type 1 form of the disease, but actually have type 3, may be distinguished by an EEG. These patients are more likely to have EEG abnormalities and eventually may develop characteristic 6 to 10 per second multiple rhythmic spike and wave discharges that are more prominent over the posterior head region.

Diagnostic Procedures

1. Glucocerebrosidase is decreased in leukocytes, skin fibroblasts, and amniotic fluid; thus, prenatal diagnosis may be established.
2. There may be diffuse increase in immunoglobulins without a monochromal gammopathy, indicating a B-lymphocyte disorder in this disease.
3. The EMG and nerve conduction studies indicate a sensory neuropathy with axonal loss.

4. Sural nerve biopsy indicates the presence of an axonopathy.

Treatment

1. Splenectomy may be necessary for hypersplenism.
2. Enzyme replacement has not produced a sustained benefit in type 1 disease, and intravenous, intrathecal, or intrasternal therapy has not been effective in neuronal involvement in type 2 or type 3 disease.

Niemann-Pick Disease

Definition Niemann-Pick disease is an autosomal recessive disorder of sphingomyelin metabolism, with accumulation of sphingomyelin and other lipids, mainly in the reticuloendothelial system.

Etiology and Pathology Type 1 disease is a result of lysosomal sphingomyelinase deficiency in which there is a massive accumulation of sphingomyelin and other lipids, including bis(AAG)P glycolipids and cholesterol, in the liver and spleen, and smaller amounts in the brain.[142] In type 1a disease, the lipids accumulate in cells of the reticuloendothelial system and have a foamy appearance. Cells stained with Wright or Giemsa stain exhibit blue-green homogeneous granules in the cytoplasm and have been termed "sea-blue histiocytes." There is prominent involvement of the CNS in type 1a disease with widespread accumulation of lipid in neurons in the cerebral and cerebellar cortex. Type 1b (type b variant) presents with marked visceral involvement but mild or absent involvement of the CNS. Type 2 Niemann-Pick disease (type c variant) is a milder form of the disease and presents with marked heterogeneity in the pattern of organ system involvement.[142a]

Clinical Features Type 1a, the severe infantile form of the disease, is a severe neurological disorder presenting in infancy with hepatosplenomegaly and a severe neurodegenerative course. Symptoms consist of feeding problems, vomiting, diarrhea, pyrexia, failure to thrive, and progressive loss of motor and intellectual skills developing during the first

year of life. As the disease progresses, the child shows hypotonia, psychomotor retardation, and progressive failure of vision and hearing. Cherry-red spots are present in 50 percent of cases. Death occurs before the age of 5 years. Type 1b (type b variant) presents with marked hepatosplenomegaly in infancy, recurrent respiratory infection, osteoporosis, failure to grow, and delayed puberty.

Type 2 (type C variant) Niemann-Pick disease is a milder form of the disease occurring in children, adolescence, and adults. This type has been linked to chromosome 18[143] and accounts for 50 percent of cases of Niemann-Pick disease.[144] Three phenotypes are described: a rapidly progressive form appearing in infancy; a delayed-onset, slowly progressive form appearing in childhood; and a late-onset, slowly progressive form appearing in adolescence or in adulthood. The major clinical features are dementia, dysarthria, ataxia, vertical supranuclear ophthalmoplegia, dystonia and choreoathetosis, followed by seizures, spasticity, and dysphagia. Adult presentation with chronic psychosis can occur.[145]

Diagnostic Procedures The diagnosis is based on the characteristic clinical findings and reduced fibroblast esterification of low-density lipoprotein-derived cholesterol. Prenatal diagnosis is possible.

Treatment

1. Cholesterol lowering agents—a combination of cholestyramine, lovastatin, and nicotinic acid—will lower cholesterol levels in the liver and blood and may be of benefit.[146]
2. Orthotopic liver transplantation has produced improvement in adult forms of the disease.[147]

Neuronal Ceroid Lipofuscinoses
The neuronal ceroid lipofuscinoses are rare, genetically determined disorders of metabolism characterized by accumulation of autofluorescent lipopigments.

Etiology and Pathology The disorder is inherited as an autosomal recessive trait with molecular heterogeneity. The gene for the infantile form of the disease (CLN1) is assigned to 1p32; the gene for the juvenile form (Batten) (CLN3) has been localized to 16p12.[148] The genetic defect in the late infantile variety (CLN2) is unknown.

Evidence suggests that the disease process may involve failure in the degradation of subunit C after its accumulation in mitochondria and lysozymes. This defect could result in suboptimal mitochondrial function, γ-aminobutyric acid, (GABA)-ergic (inhibitory) cell loss, and neuron death caused by exotoxicity,[149] the result of excessive peroxidation and accumulation of insoluble lipopigments in the central and peripheral nervous system skeletal muscle, visceral organs, and circulating lymphocytes.

Clinical Features   The infantile onset form (Bielschowsky-Jansky) is characterized by onset at 2 to 4 years of age of progressive visual loss, seizures, and intellectual and motor function deterioration. In the juvenile onset form (Batten, Vogt-Spielmeyer, or Spielmeyer-Sjögren), the patient develops visual loss at 4 to 8 years of age, followed by more gradual development of intellectual and motor function deterioration. Macular degeneration, retinitis pigmentosa, and seizures may be present. An adult form of the disease (Kufs) has been described,[150] beginning after age 20 and characterized by intellectual deterioration, ataxia, involuntary movements, spasticity, and seizures. Visual loss is unusual in this form of the disease.

Serious, often fatal, infections may occur during the course of all three forms. The diagnosis is established by detection of cytoplasmic lipopigment inclusions in lymphocytes or epithelial cells in the sediment. Skin, muscle, or nerve biopsy can also contain cells with characteristic inclusion bodies in the neuronal-lysosomal storage compartment.

Treatment   There is no effective treatment for this disease.

Cerebrotendinous Xanthomatosis   Cerebrotendinous xanthomatosis is a rare degenerative disorder of deranged cholestanol metabolism that is inherited as an autosomal dominant trait. The disease is characterized by a defect of sterol-27 hydroxylase resulting in high cholestanol concentrations in xan-

thomas involving multiple tissues, including the CNS, particularly the brainstem and cerebellum. The cornea, lungs, tendons, and peripheral nerves are involved. The disorder presents with progressive visual loss in the second to third decade, large Achilles tendons, and progressive cerebellar ataxia and dementia beginning in the sixth decade. The diagnosis is established by demonstration of increased excretion of bile alcohols in the urine[151] and high cholestanol concentration in biopsied material. Treatment with chenodeoxycholic acid 750 mg q.d. and simvastatin 40 mg q.d. will significantly lower plasma cholestanol levels.[152]

AMINOACIDURIAS

Phenylketonuria

Definition   The phenylketonurias are a heterogeneous group of conditions characterized by the development of hyperphenylalaninemia in response to a normal diet.

Etiology and Pathology   Phenylketonuria (PKU) is inherited as an autosomal recessive trait and is an inborn error of metabolism in which there are large numbers of mutations at the phenylalanine hydroxylase locus, which maps to chromosome 12. The mutant allele is expressed in an environment containing an abundance of the amino acid L-phenylalanine. There are three biochemical phenotypes, including absent or reduced phenylalanine hydroxylase, absent or reduced dihydropteridine reductase, and deficient biopterin synthetase. The latter phenotype has additional involvement in the hydroxylation of tyrosine. The exact metabolic abnormalities leading to brain damage are not clearly understood at this time.

Clinical Features   Phenylketonuria has a prevalence of 1 per 10,000 births. There is progressive delay in development, beginning shortly after birth, with failure to achieve expected normal developmental milestones, and IQ levels generally below 60. Seizures occur in about one-third of the cases, and two-thirds become severely retarded, with microcephaly, spasticity, hyperreflexia, and gait disturbances. Parkinsonian features may develop in the teens. Examination shows an irritable, hyperactive, retarded child. Eczema occurs in 30 percent of cases.

Diagnostic Procedures

1. A filter paper sample of capillary blood should be analyzed for phenylalanine content by fluorometric or microbiologic techniques. The sample should be obtained in full-term infants at least 24 hours after milk feeding has begun or from the premature infant between the fifth and seventh day of life.
2. Infants with elevated phenylalanine levels should be tested to determine the biochemical phenotype of PKU.
3. The MRI scan shows areas of demyelination in the white matter of the brain in individuals who are not taking a strict low-phenylalanine diet. These changes are often reversible and are closely related to the phenylalanine status at the time of examination.[153]
4. The EEG shows generalized slowing in untreated patients with spike wave or epileptic discharges in many cases. Seizure activity correlates with high blood phenylalanine levels. Dietary restriction of phenylalanine results in EEG improvement.
5. Visual evoked responses are sensitive to phenylalanine levels with delay in the P100 waves when there is hyperphenylalaninemia, reverting to normal latency of the P100 when phenylalanine levels are reduced.

Treatment The classical form of PKU should be treated with a low-phenylalanine diet. The diet should be adjusted to maintain blood phenylalanine levels within the normal range. Dietary treatment should be maintained as long as possible but may be relaxed although still restricted in older children and adults. The deficient biopterin synthetase phenotype requires a low-phenylalanine diet and additional treatment with L-dopa, 5-hydroxytryptophan, and dopadecarboxylase.

Pregnant women with PKU should be treated with a phenylalanine-restricted diet to achieve biochemical control and prevent the teratogenic effects of PKU on the fetus. The maternal phenylalanine syndrome consists of mental retardation, microcephaly, congenital heart disease, and intrauterine growth retardation. Bearing a normal or near-normal offspring is possible if the woman complies with a difficult diet.[154]

Prognosis The dietary treatment of PKU has produced a remarkable change in the prognosis of this disease. Early treatment prevents mental retardation and allows normal or near-normal development. Nevertheless, learning disabilities and a decline in IQ are common, even in individuals treated early, who show impairment in problem-solving, abstract reasoning, and executive functions.[155]

Diseases Involving the Tricarboxylic Acid Cycle

Leigh Disease—Subacute Necrotizing Encephalopathy

Definition Subacute necrotizing encephalopathy is a rare disease characterized by symmetrical areas of necrosis in the neuropil of the brainstem, with lesser involvement of the cerebral hemispheres and cerebellum.

Etiology and Pathology Subacute necrotizing encephalopathy is believed to be caused by more than one biochemical defect, the most common being cytochrome c oxidase deficiency[156] inherited as an autosomal recessive trait. Pyruvate dehydrogenous deficiency has been established in some cases. Others are the result of a mutation in the adenosine triphosphatase sloth gene,[157] a mitochondrial DNA mutation,[158] or a deficiency of complex 1 of the respiratory chain.[159]

The pathological changes are similar in all types of Leigh disease and resemble those seen in Wernicke encephalopathy. However, the pattern of distribution is different, and the mammillary bodies are usually spared. The brain is normal in appearance, but the brainstem shows the presence of widespread symmetrical necrosis involving the periaqueductal gray, inferior colliculi, cranial nerve nuclei, inferior olives, superior olives, and nuclei gracilis and cuneatus. Microscopic examination shows vacuolization of the white matter with loss of myelin and preservation of neuronal cell bodies. There are capillary proliferation and reactive gliosis.

Clinical Features The disease may run a rapidly fatal course in children under 5 years of age but has a more chronic course extending over a period of many years in older children and adults. The acute onset in infants and children is characterized by progressive cerebellar ataxia, cranial nerve palsies, hemiparesis, pseudobulbar palsy, quadriplegia, and death from respiratory failure within a few weeks. The more chronic form presents with mental deterioration, involuntary movements, ataxia, seizures, and a slow progression to quadriparesis and death from intercurrent infection.

Diagnostic Procedures Lactic acidosis is present in more than 90 percent of cases, and there is increased lactate in the CSF. The diagnosis should be confirmed by the demonstration of a decrease in adenosine triphosphate (ATP) synthesis in cultured fibroblast mitochondria in all types of Leigh disease.[160]

In the early stages of the illness, the MRI scan shows increased signal intensity surrounding the aqueduct and involving the tectum of the midbrain. Serial MRI scans show the lesions extending symmetrically into the substantia nigra, globus pallidus, putamen, and caudate nucleus.

Diseases of Purine Metabolism

Lesch-Nyhan Syndrome The Lesch-Nyhan syndrome is a sex-linked recessive disorder of purine metabolism. The enzyme hypoxanthine guanine phosphoribosyltransferase (HPRT) is deficient, resulting in a buildup of the purine-based hypoxanthine. In addition, there is a deficiency of dopaminergic nerve terminals and cell bodies throughout the brain, which may account for the neuropsychiatric manifestations of the disease.[161]

The pathological changes consist of thickening of blood vessel walls, perivascular demyelination, and marked degeneration of cerebellar granular cells.

Clinical Features The progressive intellectual deterioration results in moderate-to-low average re-

tardation.[162] Areas of weakness include attention deficit, manipulation of complex visual images, comprehension of complex speech, mathematical ability, and multistep reasoning. The affected individual shows progressive spasticity associated with choreoathetosis, dystonia, aggressive behavior with biting and scratching, and in some cases, self-mutilation and macrocytic anemia.[163]

Diagnostic Procedures

1. Serum uric acid levels are elevated.
2. There is marked deficiency of the enzyme HPRT, which can be demonstrated in red blood cells and T lymphocytes.

Treatment Increasing serum uric acid levels can be reduced with allopurinol 10 mg/kg per day. Methods should be devised to prevent self-mutilation through biting and scratching. Dental intervention may be necessary in many cases.

Prognosis Most patients die from respiratory infection between 15 and 20 years of age.

NEUROECTODERMAL DEGENERATIONS—PHAKOMATOSES

The neuroectodermal degenerations are hereditary diseases characterized by lesions involving the skin and nervous system. They include:

1. Neurofibromatosis (von Recklinghausen disease)
2. Tuberous sclerosis (Bourneville disease)
3. Sturge-Weber disease (encephalotrigeminal vascular syndrome)
4. von Hippel-Lindau syndrome (retinocerebellar angiomatosis)
5. Ataxia telangiectasia (Louis-Barr syndrome)

Neurofibromatosis (von Recklinghausen Disease) Neurofibromatosis is a neuroectodermal degeneration characterized by localized overgrowth of both mesodermal and ectodermal elements in the skin and nervous system.

Etiology and Pathology Neurofibromatosis is inherited as an autosomal dominant trait, the gene responsible located on chromosome 17 in the common NF-1 type of the disease. The gene responsible for the rarer central NF-2 type of the disease is located on chromosome 22.

The condition consists of hyperpigmented lesions (café au lait patches) and multiple neurofibromas involving the skin and deeper structures. The tumors are usually multiple. There is an increased incidence of CNS tumors, including astrocytomas of the optic nerve and chiasm, ependymomas, meningiomas, primitive neuroectodermal tumors, and astrocytomas in the brainstem, predominantly located in the medulla.[161]

Clinical Features The NF-1 type is characterized by multiple café au lait spots and subcutaneous neurofibromatosis and can be associated with the development of more deeply located neurofibromata. In the NF-1 type of the disease, the cutaneous lesions include pigmentary nevi, café au lait spots, and sessile or pedunculated neurofibromas. The café au lait spots are brown in color, greater than five in number, and are usually located on the trunk. Neurofibromas are of two types: smooth tumors that can be palpated along the course of peripheral nerves and pedunculated neurofibromas scattered over the trunk, head, and extremities. These tumors may produce pain and muscle weakness by compression of the brachial plexus or lumbosacral plexus and by pressure on individual nerves or nerve roots. A neurofibroma developing on a spinal nerve root may extend through the intravertebral foramen in dumbbell fashion to compress the spinal cord. These tumors may attain considerable size in the posterior mediastinum or retroperitoneal space.

The majority of patients with neurofibromatosis type 1 show the presence of Lisch nodules (pigmented iris hematomas). Other occasional features include macrocephaly, short stature, pseudoarthrosis, kyphoscoliosis, intellectual decline, speech impediments, headache, seizures, syringomyelia, learning disorders, attention deficit disorder, intracranial tumors, spinal cord tumors, ganglioneuromas, and pheochromocytomas. Brainstem tumors located in the medulla usually produce headache and examination shows, in order of frequency, poor coordination, cranial neuropathies, dysarthria, hemiparesis, papilledema, ataxia, head tilt, and seizures. An increased incidence of stroke, often the result of internal carotid artery occlusion, has been reported. A number of congenital abnormalities may be associated with NF-1, including bony malformations of the spine, syringomyelia, aqueductal stenosis, cortical dysplasia, and heterotopias.

The NF-2 type of neurofibromatosis consists of bilateral acoustic neurinomas and the presence of one or more café au lait spots and subcutaneous neurofibromas. The neurinomas develop on the eighth cranial nerve in most cases, although other cranial nerves are occasionally involved. The tumors may be bilateral or multiple and are associated with signs of cutaneous neurofibromatosis.

Diagnostic Procedures The diagnostic criteria for NF-1 type of neurofibromatosis are met when an individual shows two or more of the following conditions[162]:

1. Six more café au lait macules more than 5 mm in greatest diameter in prepubertal individuals and over 15 mm in diameter in postpubertal individuals
2. Two or more neurofibromas of any type or one plexiform neurofibroma
3. Freckling in the axillary or inguinal regions
4. Optic glioma
5. Two or more Lisch nodules (iris hematomas)
6. Distinctive osseous lesions such as sphenoid dysplasia or thinning of long bone cortex with or without pseudoarthrosis
7. A first-degree relative (parents, sibling, or offspring) with NF-1 by the above criteria.

The MRI scan shows the presence of scattered lesions of increased signal intensity on T2-weighted images, usually located in the basal ganglia, thalamus, brainstem, cerebellum, and subcortical white matter, which represent vacuolar or spongiform change.[163] These lesions may be distinguished from tumors in that the lesions do not enhance after gadolinium infusion and do not exhibit mass effect.[164] Brainstem tumors are usually located in the medulla with contiguous involvement of the pons or upper cervical spinal cord in some cases. The majority are associated with hydrocephalus and show contrast enhancement.

The criteria for NF-2 neurofibromatosis are met by an individual who has:

1. Bilateral eighth nerve masses seen by appropriate imaging techniques (CT or MRI scanning)
2. A first-degree relative with NF-2 and either unilateral eighth nerve mass or two of the following: neurofibromata, meningioma, glioma, schwannoma, or juvenile posterior subcapsular lenticular opacity

Treatment   Neurofibromas producing peripheral nerve or spinal cord compression require surgical removal. This is often incomplete and symptoms may recur years later. The treatment of acoustic neuroma is discussed in Chapter 15 page 413. Brainstem tumors with hydrocephalus should be treated by ventricular peritoneal shunting. Intervention by radiation therapy or chemotherapy should be avoided unless there is evidence of tumor progression.

Prognosis   The majority of patients with neurofibromatosis do not suffer any serious complications. Treatment of brain tumors is discussed elsewhere. Brainstem gliomas are usually more benign than non-NF-1 pontine gliomas.[165]

Tuberous Sclerosis (Epiloia Bourneville Disease)

Definition   Tuberous sclerosis is a neuroectodermal degeneration characterized by epileptic seizures, mental retardation, and adenoma sebaceum. Genetic linkage analysis indicates that about half of all patients with tuberous sclerosis show linkage to chromosome 9q34 and about half to chromosome 16p13.[166]

Pathology   The brain is normal in size and may show the presence of tubers on the cortical and ventricular surfaces. Microscopically, the cortex shows a diffuse disturbance of structure, with gliosis and atypical monster, or giant cell, forms of glial cells. Nodules composed of masses of subependymal glial cells, with incorporation of distorted neurons, or giant glial cells, protrude into the ventricles. Calcification may occur.

Adenoma sebaceum is a cutaneous disorder in which hyperplasia of connective and vascular tissue results in small, approximately 2 mm, pinkish yellow wartlike lesions. Other skin changes include café au lait spots and shagreen patches of thick yellowish skin over the lower trunk.

There are increased incidents of glial tumors; rhabdomyomas of the skeletal muscle and heart; endocrine tumors; cyst formation in the kidneys, pancreas, and liver; and honeycomb appearance of the lungs in tuberous sclerosis.

Clinical Features   Patients with tuberous sclerosis present with a progressive mental deterioration and seizures usually beginning in childhood. The seizures may be partial or generalized and are often difficult to control. Focal neurological deficits may occur, resulting from the local growth of tubers in the brain. Dystonia and athetosis may develop in some cases.

Adenoma sebaceum typically occurs in a butterfly distribution over the bridge of the nose and cheeks. Some patients may present with only a few lesions in the nasolabial folds. These patients often have subungual fibromas beneath the fingernails. Ophthalmoscopic examination may reveal the presence of white nodules (phakomata) in the retina. There is an increased incidence of cerebral cortical dysgenesis[167] and glial tumors, particularly subependymal astrocytomas, in tuberous sclerosis. Rhabdomyomas can occur in skeletal muscle in the heart, and may be associated with ventricular preexcitation syndrome and supraventricular tachycardia in infants.[168]

Endocrine tumors, renal or uterine angiomyolipomas, cysts of the kidney, hemartomas, or cysts of the liver, pancreatic cysts, thyroid hemartomas or cysts, pulmonary lymphangioleiomyomatosis, honeycomb appearance of the lungs, and retroperitoneal lymphangiomatous cysts have been described.

Diagnostic Procedures   The diagnosis may be established by the typical clinical appearance and the

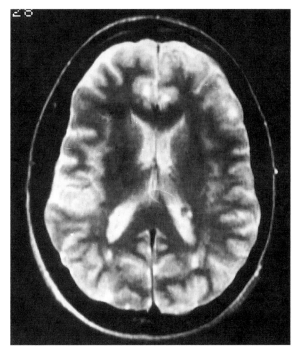

Figure 14-2
An MRI scan showing multiple areas of increased signal intensity in both gray and white matter in tuberous sclerosis.

occurrence of periventricular calcifications on skull x-ray or by MRI or CT scanning (Fig. 14-2). The MRI with gadolinium enhancement is the method of choice for diagnosing tuberous sclerosis and for following patients or screening family members.[169]

Treatment   Treatment is symptomatic.

Prognosis   Some patients show a slow progression and death occurs in adolescence or early adult life. Incomplete or abortive forms of tuberous sclerosis have a better prognosis, and there is a tendency for seizures to decrease with age.

von Hippel-Lindau Syndrome (Retinocerebellar Angiomatosis)

Definition   von Hippel-Lindau syndrome is a rare neuroectodermal degeneration characterized by the presence of a hemangiomatous malformation of the retina, associated with retinal hemangioblastomas, hemangioblastomas of the CNS, particularly the cerebellum, endolymphatic sac tumors, renal cell carcinomas, cysts of the liver, kidney and adrenals, pancreatic cysts and tumors, pheochromocytomas, and epididymal cyst adenomas.[170] The condition is inherited as an autosomal dominant trait and the von Hippel-Lindau gene has been identified at the chromosome 3p25.5.[171] The gene appears to be a tumor suppressor gene and its absence or a defect in its structure is responsible for the predisposition to the disease.[172]

Treatment

1. The hemangioblastoma of the cerebellum should be removed surgically if possible.
2. The retinal lesion may be treated by photocoagulation, using a laser technique.
3. Patients with von Hippel-Lindau disease and their at-risk relatives should be screened with annual indirect ophthalmoscopy from age 5 years. Urine VA and metadrenaline estimation should be introduced at 10 years of age. Biannual MRI or CT scans of the abdomen to visualize kidneys, adrenals, and the pancreas are recommended from the age of 20 years.
4. All renal lesions, whether solid or cystic, should be excised when detected utilizing nephron-sparing surgery for cystic and small solid lesions and radical nephrectomy for patients with diffuse disease.[173]

Ataxia Telangiectasia (Louis-Barr Syndrome)

Definition   Ataxia telangiectasia is a neuroectodermal degeneration characterized by progressive cerebellar ataxia, oculocutaneous telangiectasias, mental retardation, a defective cell-mediated and humoral immunity, and recurrent infections due to IgA and IgE deficiency. There is an increased incidence of malignancies and an unusual sensitivity to the effects of ionizing radiation.[174]

Etiology and Pathology   The etiology is unknown. The disease is inherited as an autosomal recessive trait with chromosomal instability resulting in the frequent occurrence of cells with translocations involving chromosomes 7 and 14.

There are extensive loss of Purkinje cells in the cerebellar cortex and degeneration of neurons in the cerebral cortex, basal ganglia, brainstem, and anterior horns of the spinal cord.

Clinical Features   The condition presents in childhood with progressive cerebellar ataxia, often labelled "clumsiness" by the parents. Other stigmata of the disease may be absent at that time but gradually develop as the neurological condition deteriorates. The child has a characteristic facial appearance, which has been described as "sad." Many affected children have strabismus. Telangiectasias first appear in the conjunctivae with later development on the cheeks and across the bridge of the nose in a butterfly distribution. The eyelids and pinnae may also be involved. Oropharyngeal telangiectasias of the hard and soft palate and nasal mucosa and infraoral hemangiomas of the tongue and buccal mucosae have been described.[175] There is an increased incidence of cancer, approximately 1000 times higher than in an age-matched control population.[176] The most frequent malignancies are Hodgkin and non-Hodgkin lymphoma, and acute lymphoblastic leukemia, and to a lesser degree, carcinomas of the stomach, liver, ovary, salivary glands, mouth, and breast in patients with ataxia telangiectasia and heterogeneous carriers. About 10 percent of all ataxia telangiectasia homozygotes develop a malignancy in childhood or early adolescence.[177]

Many children have repeated attacks of sinusitis and pneumonia because of altered resistance to infection leading to chronic bronchitis and bronchiectasis. Endocrine disturbances, including insulin-resistant diabetes, hypogonadism, and delayed development of secondary sex characteristics have been described. Most children show some degree of mental retardation, usually mild, and progressive cerebellar ataxia, with impaired coordination, dysmetria, intention tremor, truncal ataxia, and ataxia of gait. Speech becomes progressively dysarthric and there may be excessive drooling. Choreoathetosis appears in adolescence. There is generalized hypotonia with depression of tendon reflexes.

Diagnostic Procedures

1. Depression of IgA and IgE indicate an alteration in the normal immune system, with increased susceptibility to infection.
2. Serum α-fetoprotein levels are elevated for unknown reasons.[178]
3. The CT scans show the presence of chronic sinusitis.
4. Chest radiographs may show the presence of pneumonia or increased markings associated with chronic bronchitis and bronchiectasis.
5. Cytogenic abnormalities can be demonstrated in cultured cells such as lymphocytes with excessive chromosomal breaks and rearrangement and clonal abnormalities in freshly isolated lymphocytes.[179]
6. The MRI or CT scan shows the presence of cerebellar atrophy in older children and adolescents.

Treatment

1. Infection should be controlled with appropriate antibiotic therapy.
2. Most children require special schooling because of mental retardation and the associated ataxia.
3. Ongoing physical therapy will help to keep children ambulatory although the majority will be confined to a wheelchair by the time they reach adolescence.

Prognosis   The majority of children with ataxia telangiectasia die from intercurrent infection in late childhood or early adolescence.

Sturge-Weber Disease (Encephalotrigeminal Vascular Syndrome)

Definition   Sturge-Weber disease is a neuroectodermal degeneration characterized by a unilateral cavernous or capillary cutaneous hemangioma in the distribution of the ophthalmic division of the trigeminal nerve, a venous hemangioma of the meninges, and gliosis and calcification of the underlying cortex.

Pathology   The changes consist of a hemangiomatous malformation involving the ophthalmic division of the trigeminal nerve. The hemangioma may spread to involve other divisions of the trigeminal nerve in some cases. When the ophthalmic division is involved, the occipital lobes are usually the site of the venous hemangioma and cortical degeneration. The brain on the side of the lesion is atrophied, with a venous hemangioma in the parietal-occipital region and calcification of the second and third layers of the cortex.

Clinical Features The condition is associated with seizures that usually begin in infancy or early childhood. There is some degree of mental retardation and a contralateral hemiparesis in severe cases. The eye on the side of the lesion is often involved, with diffuse choroidal hemangioma,[180] protrusion (buphthalmos), and later development of glaucoma and blindness. Megencephaly has been reported. Migraine headaches occur in 28 percent of patients with Sturge-Weber disease, often associated with transient neurological deficits.[181]

Diagnostic Procedures The diagnosis is established by the typical appearance of the port-wine stain in the ophthalmic division of the trigeminal nerve, leptomeningeaal vascular anomalies demonstrated by CT or MRI scanning, and the presence of choroidal vascular lesions. The MRI is the imaging modality of choice,[182] with better definition of leptomeningeal angiomatosis, hemiatrophy, cortical calcifications, patchy gliosis, demyelination, and enlarged choroid plexus.

Treatment Seizures are usually controlled by administration of adequate doses of anticonvulsant drugs and monitoring plasma anticonvulsant levels. Hemispherectomy should be considered in infants with intractable seizures who do not respond to anticonvulsants.

DISEASES OF MITOCHONDRIA

Leber's Optic Atrophy

Definition Leber's optic atrophy is a hereditary condition associated with pathological mutation of mitochondrial DNA at base pair 11778; 14484; or 3460.[183]

Pathological changes consist of loss of ganglion cells in the retina with secondary demyelination of the optic nerve. After an interval, patients develop neuronal loss and demyelination in the CNS.

Clinical Features This disease is a maternally transmitted condition of mitochondrial DNA mutation. The onset of visual failure usually occurs between ages of 11 and 30 years with a range of 6 to 62 years.[184] Visual loss may be unilateral or bilateral and is particularly severe in women but tends to stabilize in the majority.[185] Improvement can occur in younger patients below age 20 years with return of adequate vision as long as four years after onset of visual failure.

Symptoms suggesting multiple sclerosis develop following visual loss in about half the patients. The Wolff-Parkinson-White pre-excitation syndrome occurs in about 10 percent of patients with Leber's optic atrophy and in their symptom-free maternal relatives.[186]

Diagnostic Procedures

1. The diagnosis is established by mitochondrial DNA analysis.
2. Serial visual evoked potential determination is useful in assessing the progression of optic atrophy.
3. All patients should be thoroughly investigated to exclude the possibility of pituitary or parapituitary tumors producing pressure on the optic chiasm.

Differential Diagnosis

1. Mass lesions with pressure on the optic chiasm. Compressive lesions of the optic chiasm typically produce bitemporal hemianopia, whereas Leber's optic atrophy presents with large bilateral central scotomata in the early stages.
2. Multiple sclerosis. The onset with rapidly progressive optic atrophy followed by signs and symptoms of patchy involvement of the CNS in later life may mimic multiple sclerosis.

Treatment

1. Because increased serum cyanide levels are believed to enhance optic atrophy, conditions associated with raised serum cyanide should be avoided. These include tobacco smoking and certain bacterial infections, particularly urinary tract infections caused by *Escherichia coli* and *Pseudomonas aeruginosa,* which increase serum cyanide levels. Consequently, infections by these organisms should be treated promptly with appropriate antibiotics.
2. Large doses of vitamin B_{12} (hydroxocobalamin) are said to be helpful because this vitamin has cyanide-binding properties.

MELAS Syndrome

Definition   This is a familial disease characterized by mitochondrial encephalomyelopathy, lactic acidosis, and stroke (MELAS).

Etiology and Pathology   The condition is a result of a defect in one or more enzymes in the mitochondrial respiratory chain[187] and is maternally transmitted in a nonmendelian fashion.

Clinical Features   Both childhood and adult forms of the disease are recognized. The patient often exhibits short stature and sensorineural hearing loss. There is a gradual decline in intellectual functioning and memory, associated with seizures, interictal myoclonus, episodic confusion, severe migraine attacks, nausea, vomiting, heart block, and cerebellar ataxia. Recurrent cerebral infarction with hemianopia or cortical blindness, ophthalmoplegia, retinitis pigmentosa, and hemiplegia occurs in some cases.

Diagnostic Procedures

1. The serum and CSF lactate values are persistently elevated.
2. The MRI or CT scan shows bilateral basal ganglia calcifications.
3. Muscle biopsy is positive for mitochondrial myopathy with ragged red fibers on trichrome acid or red-O staining.

Treatment   Combination of methylprednisolone and chlorpromazine may produce clinical improvement. Seizures respond to anticonvulsant medication.

MERRF Syndrome

Definition   This syndrome is maternally transmitted because all mitochondrial DNA is inherited in this fashion and is the result of a defect in respiratory enzyme complexes within mitochondria. This can lead to accumulation of metabolic intermediates and inadequate or inefficient ATP generation.[188] This results in the generation of oxidants, which can cause cellular damage and premature cell death.

Clinical Features   Development is normal in early childhood, with the gradual appearance of myoclonus and cerebellar ataxia in late childhood or adolescence. This state is followed by seizures, intellectual deterioration, optic atrophy, and hearing loss. There may be evidence of myopathy with proximal weakness, but there are no episodes of hemiparesis, indicating an absence of infarction, ophthalmoplegia, retinitis pigmentosa, or heart block, unlike patients with the MELAS syndrome.

Diagnostic Procedures

1. There are abnormalities in respiratory chain metabolism with deficiency of enzyme complexes in mitochondria, including deficiency of cytochrome oxidase complex A.[189]
2. The muscle biopsy is abnormal, with ragged red fibers by light microscopy.

Treatment   A temporary improvement has been reported following administration of L-5-hydroxytryptophan.

DISORDERS OF CEREBROSPINAL FLUID AND CIRCULATION

Hydrocephalus

Definition   Hydrocephalus is an excessive accumulation of CSF within the cranial cavity.

Etiology and Pathology The classical concept of CSF circulation is based on the belief that CSF is secreted by the cells of the choroid plexus of the lateral, third and fourth ventricles and flows through the ventricular system and the foramina Luschka and Magendie into the subarachnoid space. The fluid then flows up and over the cerebral convexities and is absorbed, principally through the arachnoid granulations along the superior sagittal sinus. Part of the fluid passes into the central canal of the spinal cord and is absorbed into the general circulation. In addition, the CSF must also communicate with the interstitial fluid in the brain, across the ependymal layer and pial surface of the brain.[190] Thus, water and small molecules may be exchanged in a bidirectional fashion through the intracellular spaces in the CNS and this communication may play an important role in brain volume control. However, because the brain does not have a lymphatic system, the passage of interstitial fluid from the CNS will depend on absorption at the capillary level and drainage through the venous system. Consequently, volume control is a complex matter involving not only the classical concept of CSF production by the choroid plexus and absorption through the arachnoid villi, but also bidirectional flow through the intracellular spaces and absorption into the venous system. The several channels of cerebrospinal flow are usually in a state of dynamic equilibrium, which can be disturbed by a variety of factors leading to hydrocephalus, which should be regarded as a multifactorial disease with diverse pathogenesis.[191]

Hydrocephalus may occur under the following conditions:

1. Cerebral malformation. A failure or arrest in development of a part of the brain is associated with accumulation of CSF in the area of the abnormality. These defects vary from failure of development of the cerebral hemispheres (anencephaly) to minor developmental abnormalities.
2. Increased production of CSF. This rare condition occurs with papilloma of the choroid plexus and resolves following excision of the tumor.
3. Obstruction of CSF circulation
   a. Tumors of the lateral ventricles
   b. Obstruction of the third ventricle by tumors, colloid cysts, or parasitic cysts
   c. Pressure on the third ventricle by pineal tumors posteriorly or pituitary tumors, cranial pharyngiomas, hypothalamic tumors, optic nerve gliomas or metastatic tumors from below
   d. Aqueductal narrowing by congenital stenosis, forking or septum formation, or by pressure from a pontine glioma
   e. Obstruction in the fourth ventricle by tumors or parasitic cysts
   f. Occlusion of the foramina of Luschka and Magendie by cerebellopontine angle tumors or by fibrosis following meningitis or subarachnoid hemorrhage
   g. Impaired circulation of CSF in the subarachnoid space at the base of the brain or over the convexities, following subarachnoid hemorrhage with fibrosis, chronic meningitis, other granulomatous diseases, following trauma with brain injury, or by the presence of fibrinogen in the CSF and its transformation into fibrin, and the presence of intramedullary spinal cord tumors[192]
4. Reduced absorption of CSF. The absorptive capacity of the arachnoid granulations may be damaged following meningitis or subarachnoid hemorrhage. A thrombosis of the major venous sinuses may also decrease CSF absorption.
5. Compensation for cerebral atrophy. Loss of brain substance leads to accumulation of increased amounts of CSF in the ventricular system and over the surface of the brain. This is termed hydrocephalus *ex vacuo.*

Clinical Features Hydrocephalus is a frequent accompaniment of meningitis, encephalitis, or subarachnoid hemorrhage when the signs of increased intracranial pressure (ICP) are masked by the acute disease progress. In some cases, however, symptoms of hydrocephalus are delayed for weeks or months after the acute event and present as classical features of increasing ICP. Similarly, hydrocephalus may be the sole manifestation of a brain tumor or parasitic cyst. More chronic presentation of hydrocephalus consists of headache, nausea, vomiting, visual impairment, and ataxia. Headache is intermittent at first, often awakening the patient in the early hours of the morning and persisting in the morning, and then gradually resolving. This may be the result of higher P_{CO_2} during sleep, which increases cerebral blood volume and ICP. Eventually the headache becomes constant. Vomiting is usually a later feature of hydrocephalus when headache is severe. Seizures may occur at any time. Progressive ataxia involving trunk and limbs produces a broad-based gait. Visual disturbances consist of intermittent blurring of vision progressing to visual failure as hydrocephalus and ICP increase. There is usually papilledema bilaterally at this stage and diplopia due to stretching of the sixth nerve, owing to downward pressure on the brainstem.

Diagnostic Procedures

1. The MRI and CT scans will demonstrate hydrocephalus and frequently identify the cause.
2. Lumbar puncture should be delayed or avoided, if possible, in the presence of hydrocephalus and symptoms of increased ICP because of the risk of cerebellar tonsillar herniation or increased downward pressure on the brainstem.

Treatment

1. Tumors or cysts causing hydrocephalus should be removed surgically if possible.
2. Ventriculostomy and ventricular drainage may be required in emergency situations.
3. In less emergent situations, a ventricular peritoneal shunt can be used initially to reduce increased ICP before attempting more definitive procedures to remove a tumor or cyst.

Infantile Hydrocephalus

Definition Infantile hydrocephalus is a progressive hydrocephalus that develops in infants and children.

Etiology and Pathology One of the more common causes of infantile hydrocephalus is obstruction of the sylvian aqueduct at the level of the midbrain. The aqueduct may show the presence of stenosis with or without gliosis; "forking" in which the aqueduct is replaced by a number of small, inefficient channels; or septum formation. Certain inherited or dysgraphic malformations are associated with hydrocephalus, including Arnold-Chiari malformation, the Dandy-Walker syndrome in which atresia of the foramen of Magendie is associated with failure of development of the vermis of the cerebellum, and the presence of a cranial or spinal encephalocele. Other conditions producing infantile hydrocephalus include prenatal intraventricular hemorrhage, prenatal viral infections, and possible exposure to toxins or drugs during pregnancy.[193] Meningitis with an inflammatory exudate and subsequent fibrosis can block the sylvian aqueduct, the foramina of Luschka and Magendie, or the subarachnoid space at the base of the brain. Subarachnoid hemorrhage, which usually results from trauma in children, produces the same effect. Posterior fossa tumors are a rare but potent cause of hydrocephalus in children.

Infantile hydrocephalus is characterized by dilatation of the ventricular system and compression of the brain. The width of tissue between the dilated ventricles and the surface of the brain may be less than 2 cm in some cases. Increased ICP results in enlargement of the skull and separation of the cranial sutures.

Clinical Features Hydrocephalus is unusual at birth but can cause difficult labor, which may require cesarean section. The great majority of hydrocephalic children appear normal at birth and signs and symptoms do not appear until later in infancy or early childhood. The head gradually enlarges and the normal proportions of the cranial cavity are distorted. The face has an abnormal appearance, but there may be some degree of exophthalmus and prominence of the sclerae, due to anterior displacement of orbital contents. The children are often surprisingly alert but eventually fall behind in developmental milestones. Examination reveals an enlarged head, prominent scalp veins, and enlarged fontanelles. There may be progressive visual loss and optic atrophy, with a poor pupillary reaction to light, failure of upward gaze, impairment of lateral gaze, strabismus, nystagmus, paralysis or spasm of convergence and absence of visual fixation. Percussion of the skull produces a typical "cracked pot" sound. In advanced cases, the head may be so enlarged that the child is unable to lift the head from the pillow. Increased intraventricular pressure results in damage to the corticospinal tracts, with increased tendon reflexes and a bilateral extensor plantar response.

Untreated children eventually develop necrosis of the scalp with leakage of CSF, followed by infection, and death. A minority of patients used to survive before shunting procedures were available, and the child with arrested hydrocephalus would show enlargement of the head, some degree of mental retardation, spasticity of the limbs, and impairment of bladder function.

Diagnostic Procedures

1. The MRI or CT scan will clearly define the extent of the hydrocephalus and the presence or absence of any cerebral malformations.
2. Transcranial Doppler ultrasound will demonstrate hemodynamic changes in infants with progressive hydrocephalus. The value of this technique has been questioned[194] but endorsed by others.[195]
3. The skull should be measured at each visit to record the progression of the hydrocephalus.
4. The fundi should be examined for the development of optic atrophy. The presence of papilledema is unusual. All infants should receive transillumination to exclude hydroencephaly and subdural hygroma.

Treatment All cases of infantile hydrocephalus should have a ventriculoperitoneal or lumboperitoneal shunting procedure. The procedure is not without complications, which include shunt occlusion, infection of the shunt or valves, subdural hematoma, low pressure headaches, and thromboembolism.

Prognosis More than 80 percent of children with infantile hydrocephalus will benefit from a shunting procedure. Irreversible damage from previous meningitis, subarachnoid hemorrhage, or cerebral trauma may produce permanent neurological deficits. Shunting should be performed as soon as possible to avoid the development of permanent neu-

rological deficits, such as visual impairment and mental retardation.

Normal Pressure Hydrocephalus

Definition Normal pressure hydrocephalus is a chronic hydrocephalus that occurs in children and adults and is associated with a delay in circulation or absorption of CSF and progressive neurological deficits.

Etiology and Pathology In the majority of cases, the etiology cannot be determined, but when cause can be established, it is apparent that normal pressure hydrocephalus is a syndrome. Obstruction of the subarachnoid space may occur months or years after subarachnoid hemorrhage, chronic meningoencephalitis, or trauma. It is possible that some cases are due to aqueductal stenosis, which slowly decompensates as the patient ages. Other causes include obstruction of the third ventricle by slowly growing tumors or cysts, or by enlargement of the basilar artery. Dural sinus thrombosis is another factor in this syndrome.[196] It has been postulated that the condition is the result of altered CSF dynamics in the subcortical and periventricular white matter, possibly the result of subcortical arteriosclerotic encephalopathy,[197] because there is a significant association with hypertension, diabetes mellitus, and normal pressure hydrocephalus.[198] Other white matter diseases, such as Lyme disease, might produce the same effect.[199]

Pathological changes consist of dilatation of all of the ventricles, without cortical atrophy.

Clinical Features This syndrome presents with increasing clumsiness of gait. The gait disturbance is followed by urgency of micturition and eventually by incontinence. After a period of several months or a year or two, definite evidence of dementia appears. The patient shows progressive unsteadiness and frequent falls due to a mixture of ataxia, spasticity, and dyspraxia of gait. There is a general slowing of function, with complaints of weakness and fatigue. The patient may develop dysesthesias of the feet and lower legs. There may be psychotic-like symptoms or obsessive-compulsive disorder in a minority of cases.[200,201]

Diagnostic Procedures

1. The MRI or CT scan shows the presence of ventricular dilatation, with enlargement of the third, fourth, and lateral ventricles. Cortical atrophy is often absent, but the presence of cortical atrophy does not rule out the diagnosis of normal pressure hydrocephalus.
2. The CSF is under normal pressure. The appearance, cell count, and chemical composition are normal. Improvement in gait after removal of 50 mL CSF correlates with a good outcome following a shunting procedure.[202]
3. Radioactive cisternography, which is performed by injecting a radiopharmaceutical into the lumbar subarachnoid space, shows prolonged retention of the radioactive material within the ventricular system and impaired diffusion of radioactive material over the cerebral convexities.
4. A demonstrable increase in regional cerebral blood flow, following the administration of glycerol, predicts a successful response to a shunting procedure.[203]

Differential Diagnosis

The main problem in an elderly patient is the separation of Alzheimer disease from normal pressure hydrocephalus. Patients with Alzheimer disease present with progressive cognitive decline, with a characteristic pattern of cerebral atrophy by MRI, and a distinctive pattern on the SPECT scan. This contrasts with normal pressure hydrocephalus, where there is progressive impairment of gait associated with ataxia and incontinence, with initial mild cognitive impairment.[204]

Treatment

1. There may be transient improvement in the early stages of normal pressure hydrocephalus by repeated lumbar puncture, with removal of 15 to 20 mL CSF.
2. A ventriculoperitoneal shunt procedure can produce dramatic improvement in some cases. Improvement in postoperative cognitive function is more likely if there is a known cause for the condition. However, most patients with normal pressure hydrocephalus of unknown etiology, who present primarily with gait disorder, experience significant improvement in gait.[205] Complications of the shunting procedure consist of infection of the catheter or valve and an occasional occurrence of subdural hematomas. These complications have decreased over the years as technique has improved.
3. A lumboperitoneal shunt is an alternative method of treatment with similar results and complications.

Syringomyelia, Syringobulbia

Definition Syringomyelia is a cavitation of the spinal cord. It is a rare and destructive condition involving the cord and occasionally the brainstem (syringobulbia).

Etiology and Pathology Syringomyelia is a syndrome. The common factor is cavitation within the substance of the spinal cord. Three types of cavity can be identified.[206]

1. A tubular dilatation of the central canal of the spinal cord communicates with the fourth ventricle. This abnormality has been termed hydromyelia or communicating syringomyelia and is associated with hydrocephalus and may follow meningitis or subarachnoid hemorrhage, where the aqueduct of Sylvius is obstructed and the outlets from the fourth ventricle occluded by arachnoid adhesions. Other conditions associated with communicating syringomyelia include Chiari type 2 malformation.

The syrinx consists of a dilatation of the central canal lined by ependyma, surrounded by glial tissue. There is no communication with the subarachnoid space, but communicating syringomyelia with Chiari type 2 malformation may be associated with myelomeningocele.

2. The second type of syringomyelia consists of a focal dilatation of the central canal separated from the fourth ventricle by syrinx-free spinal cord. There are Chiari type 1 malformations in about 50 percent of cases, cervical canal stenosis, arachnoiditis, basilar impression, and occipital encephalocele; congenital cysts of the fourth ventricle occur in some cases. This type of syrinx is closed at the upper end by a canal stenosis; the rostral proportion communi-

cations with a normal or occasionally stenosed central canal. This type of syrinx frequently dissects into the parenchyma of the spinal cord and occasionally communicates with the subarachnoid space. Dissection into the parenchyma of the lower brainstem causing syringobulbia has been described.

3. A third type of syringomyelia consists of a cavity within the parenchyma of the spinal cord, which does not communicate with a central canal. This condition, which is an extracanalicular syrinx, is usually found in central gray matter, dorsal and lateral to the central canal. Etiologic factors include trauma,[207] ischemic infarction, postmeningitic infarction, intramedullary hemorrhage, transverse myelitis, and radiation necrosis. Extracanalicular syringomyelia is associated with as many as 45 percent of intramedullary tumors, with 49 percent presenting above the tumor, 11 percent below the tumor, and 40 percent above and below the tumor. Ependymomas, hemangioblastomas, and astrocytomas, in that order, have the highest association with syringomyelia.[208] Syrinx formation probably results from partial obstruction of the subarachnoid space by arachnoiditis, with passage of pressure waves of CSF through extracellular spaces in the spinal cord, into the parenchyma of the cord, with subsequent cavity formation.[209]

Clinical Features   Syringomyelia occurs most commonly in the cervical area of the cord, and the clinical features can be explained by the anatomic location of the tract of the spinal cord (Fig. 14-3).

Extension of the cavity in an anterolateral direction produces pressure on and destruction of the anterior horn cells, resulting in weakness and wasting of the small muscles of the hand. Fasciculations may be seen. Expansion laterally exerts pressure on the corticospinal tracts, producing spasticity, increased tendon reflexes below the level of the lesion, and extensor plantar responses. Lateral extension involves the lateral spinothalamic tract, with subsequent loss of pain and temperature sensation on the opposite side of the body. When the cavity expands anteriorly, it interrupts the decussating fibers of the lateral spinothalamic tracts and results in bilateral loss of pain and temperature sensation. Loss of pain sensa-

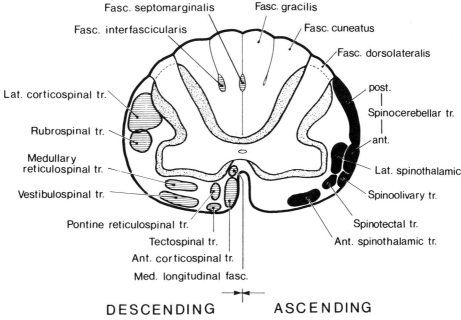

Figure 14-3
Ascending and descending tracts of the spinal cord.

tion results in undetected injury of the affected areas of the hands and fingers. Infection and joint deformities may result. The presence of Charcot joints in the shoulders is nearly always due to syringomyelia and only occasionally occurs in other conditions such as chronic diabetic peripheral neuropathy. Involvement of the descending sympathetic fibers may result in an ipsilateral Horner syndrome.

In syringobulbia the patient usually presents with weakness and wasting of the tongue or dysphagia and dysarthria due to involvement of the vagal complex. Lateral extension may involve the spinal tract of the trigeminal nerve, producing loss of pain and temperature sensation of the ipsilateral face. If the decussating fibers of the medial lemniscus are involved, ipsilateral loss of touch, vibration, and proprioception may result. Involvement of the medial longitudinal fasciculus may result in nystagmus or in-

ternuclear ophthalmoplegia. With more rostral extension, diplopia and ptosis may occur.

Diagnostic Procedures

1. An MRI scan will usually demonstrate the presence of the syrinx within the spinal cord and the extent of the abnormality on sagittal sections (Fig. 14-4). Extracanalicular syringomyelia, including post-traumatic syringomyelia, presents with a centrally located cavity caudally, extending to a rostral cavity, markedly off-center.[207] Extension into the brainstem can be demonstrated in most cases of syringobulbia by MRI scans.

2. Electrophysiologic studies show reduction in hypothenar compound muscle action potentials in the presence of a cervical syrinx, with fibrillations and reduced motor potentials in the small muscles

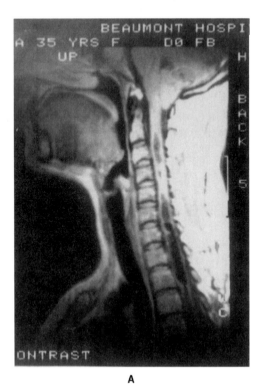
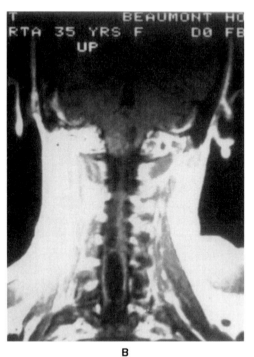

A   B

Figure 14-4
Syringomyelia. MRI scan. Anteroposterior and lateral views. There is widening of the cervical portion of the spinal cord which contains an irregular cavity or syrinx, which extends into the thoracic spinal cord.

of the hand. Ulnar and median somatosensory evoked potentials are normal in the presence of dissociated sensory loss but abnormal when all sensory modalities are impaired. The tibial nerve somatosensory evoked potentials are usually abnormal.[210]

Differential Diagnosis

1. In hematomyelia, there is a sudden onset of pain in the involved area and a history of trauma. The MRI scan reveals the presence of blood within the substance of the spinal cord.
2. An intermedullary tumor tends to have a more rapid course, and the CSF protein is elevated. However, intermedullary tumors can present as a syrinx or in association with syringomyelia.
3. An extramedullary tumor is more likely to present with root pain and obstruction or block of the subarachnoid space. CSF protein is elevated.
4. Amyotrophic lateral sclerosis. There is no sensory abnormality, and there are generalized increased tendon reflexes in ALS.
5. Cervical spondylosis. The sensory loss is confined to involved nerve roots and cervical spondylosis.

Treatment   A small syrinx with very slow deterioration does not require treatment. However, when there are increasing neurological deficits, a communicating syringomyelia associated with hydrocephalus might benefit from a ventricular drainage procedure, whereas a noncommunicating syrinx or extracanalicular syrinx would require a direct shunting procedure or reconstruction of the subarachnoid space to remove obstruction of the CSF flow and relieve pressure waves passing through the cord parenchyma into the syrinx cavity.[211]

Pain associated with syringomyelia may fail to respond to simple analgesics but may respond to carbamazepine, amitripityline, gabapentin, or transcutaneous nerve stimulation.

Prognosis   Syringomyelia and syringobulbia are usually slowly progressive diseases but can eventually prove to be severely disabling. Some patients show remission with no further deterioration for many years.

REFERENCES

1. Rossor MN: Management of neurological disorders: dementia. *J Neurol Neurosurg Psychiatry* 57:1451, 1994.
2. Fleming KC, Adams AC, Petersen RC: Dementia: diagnosis and evaluation. *Mayo Clin Proc* 70:1093, 1995.
3. Corey-Bloom J, Thal LJ, Galasko D, et al: Diagnosis and evaluation of dementia. *Neurology* 45:211, 1995.
4. Sui AZ: Screening for dementia and investigating its causes. *Ann Intern Med* 115:122, 1991.
5. Skoog I, Nilsson L, Palmertz BB, et al: A population-based study of dementia in 85-year-olds. *N Engl J Med* 328:153, 1993.
6. Strittmatter WJ, Saunders AM, Schmechel DE, et al: Apolipoprotein E. high avidity binding to β-amyloid and increased frequency of type 4 allele in late onset familial Alzheimer's disease. *Proc Natl Acad Sci USA* 90:1977, 1993.
7. Jarvik GP, Wijsman EM, Kukull WA, et al: Interactions of apolipoprotein E genotype, total cholesterol level, age and sex in prediction of Alzheimers: disease: a case-control study. *Neurology* 45:1092, 1995.
8. Terry RD: The pathogenesis of Alzheimer disease: an alternative to the amyloid hypothesis. *J Neuropathol Exp Neurol* 55:1023, 1996.
9. Liddell M, Williams J, Bayer A, et al: Confirmation of association between the e4 allele of apolipoprotein E and Alzheimer's disease. *J Med Genet* 31:197, 1994.
10. Reed T, Carmelli D, Swan GE, et al: Lower cognitive performance in normal older adult male twins carrying the apolipoprotein E epsilon 4 allele. *Arch Neurol* 51:1189, 1994.
11. Feskens EJ, Havekes LM, Kalmijn S, et al: Apolipoprotein e4 allele and cognitive decline in elderly men. *BMJ* 309:1202, 1994.
12. Cotton P: Alzheimer's/apo E link grows stronger. *JAMA* 272:1483, 1994.
13. Schmechel DE, Saunders AM, Strittmatter WJ, et al: Increased amyloid beta-peptide deposition in cerebral cortex as a consequence of apolipoprotein E genotype in late-onset Alzheimer disease. *Proc Natl Acad Sci USA* 91:9649, 1993.
14. Strittmatter WJ, Saunders AM, Goedert M, et al: Isoform specific interactions of apolipoprotein E with microtubule-associated protein tau: implications for Alzheimer disease. *Proc Natl Acad Sci USA* 91:11183, 1994.

15. Terry RD: The pathology of Alzheimer's disease: numbers count. *Ann Neurol* 41:7, 1997.

16. Rebeck GW, Reiter JS, Strickland DK, et al: Apolipoprotein in sporadic Alzheimer's disease: allelic variations and receptor interactions. *Neuron* 11:575, 1993.

17. Poirier J, Davignon J, Bouthillier D, et al: Apolipoprotein E polymorphism and Alzheimer's disease. *Lancet* 342:697, 1993.

18. Seshadri S, Drachman DA, Lippa CF: Apolipoprotein E epsilon 4 allele and the lifetime risk of Alzheimer's disease. What physicians know and what they should know. *Arch Neurol* 52:1074, 1995.

19. American College of Medical Genetics/American Society of Human Genetics Working Group on ApoE and Alzheimer Disease. Statement on use of apolipoprotein E testing for Alzheimer disease. *JAMA* 274:1627, 1995.

20. Breitner JCS: ApoE genotyping and Alzheimer's disease. *Lancet* 347:1184, 1996.

21. Levy-Lahad E, Bird TD: Genetic factors in Alzheimers disease: a review of recent advances. *Ann Neurol* 40:829, 1996.

22. Bird TD: Apolipoprotein E genotyping in the diagnosis of Alzheimers disease: a cautionary view. *Ann Neurol* 38:2, 1995.

23. Roses AD: Apolipoprotein E genotyping in the differential diagnosis, not prediction, of Alzheimer's disease. *Ann Neurol* 38:6, 1995.

24. Saunders AM, Hulette O, Welsh-Bohmer KA, et al: Specificity, sensitivity and predictive value of apolipoprotein-E genotyping for sporadic Alzheimer's disease. *Lancet* 348:90, 1996.

25. Tierney MC, Szalai JP, Snow WG, et al: A prospective study of the clinical utility of ApoE genotype in the prediction of outcome in patients with memory impairment. *Neurology* 46:149, 1996.

26. Lippa CF, Saunders AM, Smith TW, et al: Familial and sporadic Alzheimer's disease: neuropathology cannot exclude a final common pathway. *Neurology* 46:406, 1996.

27. Payami H, Montee K, Grimslid H, et al: Increased risk of familial late-onset Alzheimer's disease in women. *Neurology* 46:126, 1996.

28. Goate A, Chartier-Harlin ML, Mullan M, et al: Segregation of a missense mutation in the amyloid precursor protein gene with familial Alzheimer's disease. *Nature* 349:704, 1991.

29. Sherrington R, Rogaev EI, Liang Y, et al: Cloning of a gene bearing missense mutations in early-onset familial Alzheimer's disease. *Nature* 375:754, 1995.

30. Levy-Lahad E, Wasco W, Poorkaj P, et al: Candidate gene for the chromosome 1 familial Alzheimer's disease locus. *Science* 269:973, 1995.

31. Schmand B, Jonker C, Hooijer C, et al: Subjective memory complaints may announce dementia. *Neurology* 46:121, 1996.

32. Victoroff J, Zarow C, Mack WJ, et al: Physical aggression is associated with preservation of substantia nigra pars compacta in Alzheimer disease. *Arch Neurol* 53:428, 1996.

33. Mega MS, Cummings JL, Fiorello T, et al: The spectrum of behavioral changes in Alzheimer's disease. *Neurology* 46:130, 1996.

34. Lehtovirta M, Soininen H, Helisalmi MA, et al: Clinical and neuropsychological characteristics in familial and sporadic Alzheimer's disease: relation to apolipoprotein E polymorphism. *Neurology* 46:413, 1996.

35. Koss E, Edland S, Fillenbaum G, et al: Clinical and neuropsychological differences between patients with earlier and later onset of Alzheimer's disease: A CERAD Analysis part XII. *Neurology* 46:136, 1996.

36. Tierney MC, Szalai JP, Snow WG, et al: The prediction of Alzheimer disease. The role of patient and informant perceptions of cognitive deficits. *Arch Neurol* 53:423, 1996.

37. Tierney MC, Szalai JP, Snow WG, et al: Prediction of probable Alzheimer disease in memory-impaired patients. A prospective longitudinal study. *Neurology* 46:661, 1996.

38. Myers RH, Schaefer EJ, Wilson PW, et al: Apolipoprotein E epsilon 4 association with dementia in a population-based study. The Framingham study. *Neurology* 46:673, 1996.

39. Fukui T, Sugita K, Kawamara M, et al: Primary progressive apraxia in Pick's disease: a clinicopathologic study. *Neurology* 47:467, 1996.

40. Beeson PM, Rubens AB, Kaszniak AW: Anterograde memory impairment in Pick's disease. *Arch Neurol* 52:742, 1995.

41. Caselli RJ, Jack CR Jr, Petersen RC, et al: Asymmetric cortical degenerative syndromes: clinical and radiologic correlations. *Neurology* 42:1462, 1992.

42. Lang AE, Bergeron C, Pollanen MS, et al: Parietal Pick's disease mimicking cortical-basal ganglionic degeneration. *Neurology* 44:1436, 1994.

43. Neary D, Snowden JS, Shields RA, et al: Single photon emission tomography using 99m Tc-HM-PAO in the investigation of dementia. *J Neurol Neurosurg Psychiatry* 50:1101, 1987.

44. Talbot PR, Testa HJ: The value of SPET imaging in dementia. *Nuclear Med Commun* 16:425, 1995.

45. McKeith IG, Galasko D, Kosaka K, et al: Consensus guidelines for the clinical and pathologic diagnosis of dementia with Lewy bodies (DLB): report of the consortium on DLB international workshop. *Neurology* 47:1113, 1996.

46. Salmon DP, Galasko D: Neuropsychological aspects of Lewy body dementia, in Perry RH, McKeith IG, Perry EK (eds): *Dementia with Lewy bodies.* New York, Cambridge University Press, 1996, pp 99-113.

47. Byrne EJ, Lennox G, Lowe J, et al: Diffuse Lewy body disease: clinical features in 15 cases. *J Neurol Neurosurg Psychiatry* 52:709, 1989.

48. Klatka LA, Louis ED, Schiffer RB: Psychiatric features in diffuse Lewy body disease: a clinicopathologic study using Alzheimer's disease and Parkinson's disease comparison groups. *Neurology* 47:1148, 1996.

49. Hansen LA, Galasko D: Lewy body disease. *Curr Opin Neurol Neurosurg* 5:889, 1992.

50. McKeith IG, Perry RH, Fairbairn AF, et al: Operational criteria for senile dementia of Lewy body type (SDLT). *Psychol Med* 22:911, 1992.

51. McKeith I, Fairbairn A, Perry R, et al: Neuroleptic sensitivity in patients with senile dementia of Lewy body type. *BMJ* 305:673, 1992.

52. Kosaka K: Diffuse Lewy body disease in Japan. *J Neurol* 237:197, 1990.

53. Litvan I, Agid Y, Goetz C, et al: Accuracy of the clinical diagnosis of corticobasal degeneration: a clinicopathologic study. *Neurology* 48:119, 1997.

54. Riley DE, Lang AE, Lewis A, et al: Cortical-basal ganglionic degeneration. *Neurology* 40:1203, 1990.

55. Massman PJ, Kreiter KT, Jankovic J, et al: Neuropsychological functioning in cortical-basal ganglionic degeneration: differentiation from Alzheimer's disease. *Neurology* 46:720, 1996.

56. Rinne JO, Lee MS, Thompson PD: Corticobasal degeneration. A clinical study of 36 cases. *Brain* 117:1183, 1994.

57. Scheltens P, Ravid R, Kamphorst W: Pathologic findings in a case of primary progressive aphasia. *Neurology* 44:279, 1994.

58. Kertesz A, Hudson L, Mackenzie IR, et al: The pathology and nosology of primary progressive aphasia. *Neurology* 44:2065, 1994.

59. Kartsounis LD, Crellin RF, Crewes H, et al: Primary progressive non-fluent aphasia: a case study. *Cortex* 27:121, 1991.

60. Karbe H, Kertesz A, Polk M: Profiles of language impairment in primary progressive aphasia. *Arch Neurol* 50:193, 1993.

61. Clinical and neuropathological criteria for frontotemporal dementia. The Lund and Manchester Groups [Review]: *J Neurol Neurosurg Psychiatry* 57:416, 1994.

62. Neary D: Neuropsychological aspects of frontotemporal degeneration. *Ann N Y Acad Sci* 769:15, 1995.

63. Muller M, Vieregge P, Reusche E, et al: Amyotrophic lateral sclerosis and frontal lobe dementia in Alzheimer's disease. Case report and review of the literature. *Eur Neurol* 33:320, 1993.

64. Valldeotiola F, Tolosa E, Valls-Sole J: Differential diagnosis and clinical diagnostic criteria of progressive supranuclear palsy. *Adv Neurol* 69:405, 1996.

65. Golbe LI: The epidemiology of progressive supranuclear palsy. *Adv Neurol* 69:25, 1996.

66. Daniel SE, de Bruin VM, Lees AJ: The clinical and pathological spectrum of Steele-Richardson-Olszewski syndrome (progressive supranuclear palsy): a reappraisal. *Brain* 118 (Pt 3):759, 1995.

67. de Yebenes JG, Sarasa JL, Daniel SE, et al: Familial progressive supranuclear palsy. Description of a pedigree and review of the literature. *Brain* 118 (Pt 5):1095, 1995.

68. Dubois B, Deweer B, Pillon B: The cognitive syndrome of progressive supranuclear palsy. *Adv Neurol* 69:399, 1996.

69. Litvan I, Mega MS, Cummings JL, et al: Neuropsychiatric aspects of progressive supranuclear palsy. *Neurology* 47:1184, 1996.

70. Committee of the American Autonomic Society and the American Academy of Neurology. Consensus statement on the definition of orthostatic hypotension, pure autonomic failure and multiple system atrophy. *Neurology* 46:1470, 1996.

71. Quinn NP, Wenning G, Marsden CD: The Shy-Drager syndrome. What did Shy and Drager really describe? *Arch Neurol* 52:656, 1995.

72. Quinn N: Multiple system atrophy—the nature of the beast. *J Neurol Neurosurg Psychiatry Special Suppl* 78, 1989.

73. Papp MI, Lantos PL: Accumulation of tubular structures in oligodendroglial and neuronal cells as the basic alteration in multiple system atrophy. *J Neurol Sci* 107:172, 1992.

74. Lantos PL, Papp MI: Cellular pathology of multiple system atrophy: a review. *J Neurol Neurosurg Psychiatry* 57:129, 1994.

75. Gilman S, Sima AA, Junck L, et al: Spinocerebellar

ataxia type I with multiple system degeneration and glial cytoplasmic inclusions. *Ann Neurol* 39:241, 1996.

76. Gilman S, Quinn NP: The relationship of multiple system atrophy to sporadic olivopontocerebellar atrophy and other forms of idiopathic late-onset cerebellar atrophy. *Neurology* 46:1197, 1996.

77. Salazar-Greuso EF, Rosenberg RS, Roos RP: Sleep apnea in olivopontocerebellar degeneration: treatment with trazodone. *Ann Neurol* 23:399, 1988.

78. Higgins JJ, Nee LE, Vasconcelos O, et al: Mutations in American families with spinocerebellar ataxia (SCA) type 3: SCA 3 is allelic to Machado-Joseph disease. *Neurology* 46:208, 1996.

79. Junck L, Fink JF: Machado-Joseph disease and SCA- 3. The genotype meets the phenotypes. *Neurology* 46:4, 1996.

80a. Hanauer A, Chery M, Fujita R, et al: The Friedreich ataxia gene is assigned to chromosome 9q13-q21 by mapping of tightly linked markers and shows linkage disequilibrium with D9S15. *Am J Hum Genet* 46:133, 1990.

81a. Campuzano V, Montermini L, Molto MD, et al: Friedreich's ataxia: autosomal recessive disease caused by an intronic GAA triplet repeat expansion. *Science* 271:1423, 1996.

82a. Durr A, Cossee M, Agid Y, et al: Clinical and genetic abnormalities in patients with Friedreich's ataxia. *N Engl J Med* 335:1169, 1996.

83a. Palau F, De Michele G, Vilchez JJ, et al: Early onset ataxia with cardiomyopathy and retained tendon reflexes maps to the Friedreich's ataxia locus on chromosome 9q. *Ann Neurol* 37:359, 1995.

84a. Klockgether T, Zuhlke C, Schulz JB, et al: Friedreich's ataxia with retained tendon reflexes: molecular genetics, clinical neurophysiology and magnetic resonance imaging. *Neurology* 46:118, 1996.

80. Litt M, Kramer P, Browne D, et al: A gene for episodic ataxia/myokymia maps to chromosome 12p13. *Am J Hum Genet* 55:702, 1994.

81. Baloh RW, Yue Q, Furman JM, et al: Familial episodic ataxia: clinical heterogeneity in four families linked to chromosome 19p. *Ann Neurol* 41:8, 1977.

82. Joutel A, Bousser MG, Biousse V, et al: A gene for familial hemiplegic migraine maps to chromosome 19. *Nature Genet* 5:40, 1993.

83. Lubbers WJ, Brunt ER, Scheffer H, et al: Hereditary myokymia and paroxysmal ataxia linked to chromosome 12 is responsive to acetazolamide. *J Neurol Neurosurg Psychiatry* 59:400, 1995.

84. Siddique T, Figlewicz DA, Pericak-Vance MA, et al: Linkage of a gene causing familial amyotrophic lateral sclerosis to chromosome 21 and evidence of genetic-locus heterogeneity. *N Engl J Med* 324:1381, 1991.

85. Suthers G, Laing N, Wilton S, et al: "Sporadic" motoneuron disease due to familial SOD1: mutation with low penetrance. *Lancet* 344:1773, 1994.

86. Figlewicz DA, McInnis MG, Goto J, et al: Identification of flanking markers for the familial amyotrophic lateral sclerosis gene ALS1 on chromosome 21. *J Neurol Sci* 124 (Suppl):90, 1994.

87. Kaneko K, Saito F, Sunohara N, et al: Cytogenetic analysis of 23 Japanese patients with amyotrophic lateral sclerosis. *Clin Genet* 47:158, 1995.

88. Jones CT, Swingler RJ, Simpson SA, et al: Superoxide dismutase mutations in an unselected cohort of Scottish amyotrophic lateral sclerosis patients. *J Med Genet* 32:290, 1995.

89. Hollander D, Pradas J, Kaplan R, et al: High dose dextromethorphan in amyotrophic lateral sclerosis: phase 1 safety and pharmacokinetic studies. *Ann Neurol* 36:920, 1994.

90. Fishman PS, Drachman DB: Internalization of IgG in motoneurons of patients with ALS: selective or nonselective? *Neurology* 45:1551, 1995.

91. Okumura H, Kurland LT, Waring SC: Amyotrophic lateral sclerosis and polio: is there an association? *Ann N Y Acad Sci* 753:245, 1995.

92. Eisen A, Krieger C: Pathogenic mechanisms in sporadic amyotrophic lateral sclerosis. *Can J Neurol Sci* 20:286, 1993.

93. Rowland LP: Riluzole for the treatment of amyotrophic lateral sclerosis—too soon to tell? (Editorial): *N Engl J Med* 330:636, 1994.

94. Denys EH: AAEM case report 5: amyotrophic lateral sclerosis. *Muscle Nerve* 17:263, 1994.

95. Sanders KA, Rowland LP, Murphy P, et al: Motor neuron diseases and amyotrophic lateral sclerosis: GM1 antibodies and paraproteinemia. *Neurology* 43:418, 1993.

96. Smith SA, Miller RG, Murphy JR, et al: Treatment of ALS with high dose pulsed cyclophosphamide. *J Neurol Sci* 124 (Suppl):84, 1994.

97. Dalakas MC, Stein DP, Otero C, et al: Effect of high dose intravenous immunoglobulin on amyotrophic lateral sclerosis and multifocal motor neuropathy. *Arch Neurol* 51:861, 1994.

98. Mazzini L, Testa D, Balzarini C, et al: An open-randomized clinical trial of selegiline in amyotrophic lateral sclerosis. *J Neurol* 241:223, 1994.

99. Norris FH: Ceftriaxone in amyotrophic lateral sclerosis. *Arch Neurol* 51:447, 1994.

100. Eisen A, Stewart H, Schulzer M, et al: Anti-glutamate therapy in amyotrophic lateral sclerosis: a trial using lamotrigine. *Can J Neurol Sci* 20:297, 1993.

101. Taylor CP: Emerging perspectives on the mechanism of action of gabapentin. *Neurology* 44 (Suppl 5):S10, 1994.

102. Askmark H, Aquilonius SM, Gillberg PG, et al: A pilot trial of dextromethorphan in amyotrophic lateral sclerosis. *J Neurol Neurosurg Psychiatry* 56:197, 1993.

103. Norris FH, Tan Y, Fallat RJ, et al: Trial of oral physostigmine in amyotrophic lateral sclerosis. *Clin Pharmacol Ther* 54:680, 1993.

104. Tandan R, Bromberg MB, Forshew D, et al: A controlled trial of amino acid therapy in amyotrophic lateral sclerosis: I clinical, functional, and maximum isometric torque data. *Neurology* 47:1220, 1996.

105. Aisen ML, Sevilla D, Gibson G, et al: 3,4-diaminopyridine as a treatment for amyotrophic lateral sclerosis. *J Neurol Sci* 129:21, 1995.

106. Louwerse ES, Weverling GJ, Bossuyt PM, et al: Randomized double-blind, controlled trial of acetylcysteine in amyotrophic lateral sclerosis. *Arch Neurol* 52:559, 1995.

107. Lange DJ, Felice KJ, Festoff BW, et al: Recombinant human insulin-like growth factor-I in ALS: description of a double-blind placebo-controlled study. North American ALS/IGF-I study group. *Neurology* 47 (Suppl 2):S93, 1996.

108. Bensimon G, Lacomblez L, Meininger V, et al: A controlled trial of riluzole in amyotrophic lateral sclerosis.ALS/Riluzole Study Group. *N Engl J Med* 330:585, 1994.

109. Miller RG, Bouchard JP, Duquette P, et al: Clinical trials of riluzole in patients with ALS. ALS/Riluzole Study Group-II. *Neurology* 47 (Suppl 2):S86, 1996.

110. Gutmann L, Mitsumoto H: Advances in ALS. *Neurology* 47 (Suppl 2):S17, 1996.

111. Wiles CM: Neurogenic dysphagia. *J Neurol Neurosurg Psychiatry* 54:1037, 1991.

112. Kiernan JA, Hudson AJ: Frontal lobe atrophy in motor neuron diseases. *Brain* 117 (Pt 4):747, 1994.

113. Bruyn RP, Koelman JH, Troost D, et al: Motor neuron disease (amyotrophic lateral sclerosis) arising from longstanding primary lateral sclerosis. *J Neurol Neurosurg Psychiatry* 58:742, 1995.

114. Gilliam TC, Brzustowicz LM, Castilla LH, et al: Genetic homogeneity between acute and chronic forms of spinal muscular atrophy. *Nature* 345:823, 1990.

115. Melki J, Lefebvre S, Burglen L, et al: De novo and inherited deletions of the 5q13 region in spinal muscular atrophies. *Science* 264:1474, 1994.

116. Lefebvre S, Burglen L, Reboullet S, et al: Identification and characterization of a spinal muscular atrophy-determining gene. *Cell* 80:155, 1995.

117. Roy N, Mahadevan MS, McLean M, et al: The gene for neuronal apoptosis inhibitory protein is partially deleted in individuals with spinal muscular atrophy. *Cell* 80:167, 1995.

118. Hageman AT, Gabreels FJ, de Jong JG, et al: Clinical symptoms of adult metachromatic leukodystrophy and arylsulfatase A pseudodeficiency. *Arch Neurol* 52:408, 1995.

119. Krivit W, Shapiro E, Kennedy W, et al: Treatment of late infantile metachromatic leukodystrophy by bone marrow transplantation. *N Engl J Med* 322:28, 1990.

120. Cannizzaro LA, Chen YQ, Rafi MA, et al: Regional mapping of the human galactocerebrosidase gene (GALC) to 14q31 by in situ hybridization. *Cytogenet Cell Genet* 66:244, 1994.

121. Bernardini GI, Herrera DG, Carson D, et al: Adult onset Krabbe's disease in siblings with novel mutations in the galactocerebrosidase gene. *Ann Neurol* 41:111, 1997.

122. Laureti S, Casucci G, Santeusanio F, et al: X-linked adrenoleukodystrophy is a frequent cause of idiopathic Addison's disease in young adult male patients. *J Clin Endocrinol Metab* 81:470, 1996.

123. van Geel BM, Assies J, Weverling GJ, et al: Predominance of the adrenomyeloneuropathy phenotype of X-linked adrenoleukodystrophy in The Netherlands: a survey of 30 kindreds. *Neurology* 44:2343, 1994.

124. van Geel BM, Koelman JH, Barth PG, et al: Peripheral nerve abnormalities in adrenomyeloneuropathy: a clinical and electrodiagnostic study. *Neurology* 46:112, 1996.

125. Moser HW: Komrower Lecture. Adrenoleukodystrophy: natural history, treatment, and outcome. *J Inherit Metabol Dis* 18:435, 1995.

126. Krivit W, Lockman LA, Watkins PA, et al: The future for treatment by bone marrow transplantation for adrenoleukodystrophy, metachromatic leukodystrophy, globoid cell leukodystrophy and Hurler syndrome. *J Inherit Metabol Dis* 18:398, 1995.

127. Sistermans EA, de Wijs IJ, de Coo RF, et al: A (G-to-A) mutation in the initiation codon of the proteolipid protein gene causing a relatively mild form of Pelizaeus-Merzbacher disease in a Dutch family. *Hum Genet* 97:337, 1996.

128. Head MW, Corbin E, Goldman JE: Overexpression and abnormal modification of the stress proteins al-

pha B-crystallin and HSP27 in Alexander disease. *Am J Pathol* 143:1743, 1993.

129. Klein EA, Anzil AP: Prominent white matter cavitation in an infant with Alexander's disease. *Clin Neuropathol* 13:31, 1994.

130. Schwankhaus JD, Parisi JE, Gulledge WR, et al: Hereditary adult-onset Alexander's disease with palatal myoclonus, spastic paraparesis, and cerebellar ataxia. *Neurology* 45:2266, 1995.

131. Kaul R, Balamurugan K, Gao GP, et al: Canavan's disease: genomic organization and localization of human ASPA to 17p13-ter and conservation of the ASPA gene during evolution. *Genomics* 21:364, 1994.

132. Matalon R, Kaul R, Gao GP, et al: Prenatal diagnosis of Canavan disease: the use of DNA markers. *J Inherit Metabol Dis* 18:215, 1995.

133. Elpeleg ON, Anikster Y, Barash V, et al: The frequency of the C854 mutation in the aspartoacyclase gene in Ashkenazi Jews in Israel. *Am J Hum Genet* 55:287, 1994.

134. Chakraborty S, Rafi MA, Wenger DA: Mutations in the lysosomal beta-galactosidase gene that cause the adult form of GM1 gangliosidosis. *Am J Hum Genet* 54:1004, 1994.

135. Adams C, Green S: Late-onset hexosaminidase A and B deficiency—family study and review. *Dev Med Child Neurol* 28:236, 1986.

136. Mitsias P, Levine SR: Cerebrovascular complications of Fabry's disease. *Ann Neurol* 40:8, 1996.

137. Grewal RP, Barton NW: Fabry's disease presenting with stroke. *Clin Neurol Neurosurg* 94:177, 1992.

138. Fisher EA, Desnick RJ, Gordon RE, et al: Fabry disease: an unusual cause of severe coronary artery disease in a young man. *Ann Intern Med* 117:221, 1992.

139. Grabowski GA: Gaucher disease. Enzymology genetics and treatment. *Adv Human Genet* 21:377, 1993.

140. Grafe M, Thomas C, Schneider J, et al: Infantile Gaucher's disease: a case with neuronal storage. *Ann Neurol* 23:300, 1988.

141. McAlarney T, Pastores GM, Hays AP, et al: Antisulfatide antibody and neuropathy in a patient with Gaucher's disease. *Neurology* 45:1622, 1995.

142. Weisz B, Spirer Z, Reif S: Niemann-Pick disease: newer classification based on genetic mutations of the disease. *Adv Pediatr* 41:415, 1994.

142a. Natowicz MR, Stoler JM, Prence EM, et al: Marked heterogeneity in Niemann-Pick disease type C Clinical and ultrastructural findings. *Clin Pediatr* 34:190, 1995.

143. Carstea ED, Polymeropoulos MH, Parker CC, et al: Linkage of Niemann-Pick disease type C to human chromosome 18. *Proc Natl Acad Sci U S A* 90:2002, 1993.

144. Vanier MT, Rodriguez-Lafrasse C, Rousson R, et al: Type C Niemann-Pick disease: spectrum of phenotypic variation in disruption of intracellular LDL-derived cholesterol processing. *Biochim Biophys Acta* 1096:328, 1991.

145. Shulman LM, David NJ, Weiner WJ: Psychosis as the initial manifestation of adult-onset Niemann-Pick disease type C. *Neurology* 45:1739, 1995.

146. Patterson MC, Di Bisceglie AM, Higgins JJ, et al: The effect of cholesterol-lowering agents on hepatic and plasma cholesterol in Niemann-Pick disease type C. *Neurology* 43:61, 1993.

147. Smanik EJ, Tavill AS, Jacobs GH, et al: Orthotopic liver transplantation in two adults with Niemann-Pick and Gaucher's diseases: implications for the treatment of inherited metabolic disease. *Hepatology* 17:42, 1993.

148. Dooley TP, Probst P, Obermoeller RD, et al: Phenol sulfotransferases: candidate genes for Batten disease. *Am J Med Genet* 57:327, 1995.

149. Walkley SU, March PA, Schroeder CE, et al: Pathogenesis of brain dysfunction in Batten disease. *Am J Med Genet* 57:196, 1995.

150. Wisneiwski KE, Kida E, Patxot OF, et al: Variability in the clinical and pathological findings in the neuronal ceroid lipofuscinoses: review of data and observations. *Am J Med Genet* 42:525, 1992.

151. Siebner HR, Berndt S, Conrad B: Cerebrotendinous xanthomatosis without tendon xanthomas mimicking Marinesco-Sjöegren syndrome: a case report. *J Neurol Neurosurg Psychiatry* 60:582, 1996.

152. Watts GF, Mitchell WD, Bending JJ, et al: Cerebrotendinous xanthomatosis: a family study of sterol 27-hydroxylase mutations and pharmacotherapy. *Q J Med* 89:55, 1996.

153. Smith I: Treatment of phenylalanine hydroxylase deficiency. *Acta Paediatr Suppl* 407:60, 1994.

154. Levy HL, Ghavami M: Maternal phenylketonuria: a metabolic teratogen. *Teratology* 53:176, 1996.

155. Waisbren SE, Brown MJ, de Sonneville LM, et al: Review of neuropsychological functioning in treated phenylketonuria: an information processing approach. *Acta Paediatr Suppl* 407:98, 1994.

156. Adams PL, Lightowlers RN, Turnbull DM: Molecular analysis of cytochrome c oxidase deficiency in Leigh's syndrome. *Ann Neurol* 41:268, 1997.

157. Matthews PM, Marchington DR, Squier M, et al:

Molecular genetic characterization of an X-linked form of Leigh's syndrome. *Ann Neurol* 33:652, 1993.

158. Santorelli FM, Shanske S, Jain KD, et al: A T→C mutation at nt 8993 of mitochondrial DNA in a child with Leigh syndrome. *Neurology* 44:972, 1994.

159. Morris AA, Leonard JV, Brown GK, et al: Deficiency of respiratory chain complex I is a common cause of Leigh disease. *Ann Neurol* 40:25, 1996.

160. Vazquez-Memije ME, Shanske S, Santorelli FM, et al: Comparative biochemical studies in fibroblasts from patients with different forms of Leigh syndrome. *J Inherit Metabol Dis* 19:43, 1996.

161. Molloy PT, Bilaniuk LT, Vaughan SN, et al: Brainstem tumors in patients with neurofibromatosis type 1: a distinct clinical entity. *Neurology* 45:1897, 1995.

162. Neurofibromatosis Conference statement. National Institutes of Health Consensus Development Conference. *Arch Neurol* 45:575, 1988.

163. Di Paulo DP, Zimmerman RA, Rorke LB, et al: Neurofibromatosis type 1: pathologic substrate of high-signal-intensity foci in the brain. *Radiology* 195:721, 1995.

164. DiMarco FJ Jr, Ramsby G, Greenstein R, et al: Neurofibromatosis type 1: magnetic resonance imaging findings. *J Child Neurol* 8:32, 1993.

165. Packer RJ, Nicholson HS, Vezina LG, et al: Brainstem gliomas. *Neurosurg Clin North Am* 3:863, 1992.

166. Kwiatkowski DJ, Short MP: Tuberous sclerosis. *Arch Dermatol* 130:348, 1994.

167. Raymond AA, Fish DR, Sisodiya SM, et al: Abnormalities of gyration, heterotopias, tuberous sclerosis, focal cortical dysplasia, microdysgenesis, dysembryoplastic neuroepithelial tumour and dysgenesis of the archicortex in epilepsy. Clinical, EEG, and neuroimaging features in 100 adult patients. *Brain* 118 (Pt 3):629, 1995.

168. Mehta AV: Rhabdomyoma and ventricular preexcitation syndrome. A report of two cases and review of literature. *Am J Dis Child* 147:669, 1993.

169. Braffman BH, Bilaniuk LT, Naidich TP, et al: MR imaging of tuberous sclerosis: pathogenesis of this phakomatosis, use of gadopentetate dimeglumine and literature review. *Radiology* 183:227, 1992.

170. Choyke PL, Glenn GM, Walther MM, et al: von Hippel-Lindau disease: genetic, clinical, and imaging features. *Radiology* 194:629, 1995.

171. Gnarra JR, Lerman MI, Zbar B, et al: Genetics of renal cell carcinoma and evidence for a critical role for

von Hippel-Lindau in renal tumorigenesis. *Semin Oncol* 22:3, 1995.

172. Karsdorp N, Elderson A, Wittebol-Post D, et al: Von Hippel-Lindau disease: new strategies in early detection and treatment. *Am J Med* 97:158, 1994.

173. Nelson JB, Oyasu R, Dalton DP: The clinical and pathological manifestations of renal tumors in von Hippel-Lindau disease. *J Urol* 152 (6P+2):2221, 1994.

174. Taylor AM, Jaspers NG, Gatti RA: Fifth International Workshop on Ataxia-Telangiectasia. *Cancer Res* 53:438, 1993.

175. Moghadam BK, Zadeh JY, Gier RE: Ataxia-telangiectasia. Review of the literature and a case report. *Oral Surg Oral Med Oral Pathol* 75:791, 1993.

176. Willems PJ, Van Roy BC, Kleiger WJ, et al: Atypical clinical presentation of ataxia telangiectasia. *Am J Med Genet* 45:777, 1993.

177. Taylor AM: Ataxic telangiectasia genes and predisposition to leukaemia, lymphoma and breast cancer. *Br J Cancer* 66:5, 1992.

178. Gatti RA: Candidates for the molecular defect in ataxia telangiectasia. *Adv Neurol* 61:127, 1993.

179. Swift M, Heim RA, Lench NJ: Genetic aspects of ataxia telangiectasia. *Adv Neurol* 61:115, 1993.

180. Griffiths PD, Boodram MB, Blaser S, et al: Abnormal ocular enhancement in Sturge-Weber syndrome: correlation of ocular MR and CT findings with clinical and intracranial imaging findings. *Am J Neuroradiol* 17:749, 1996.

181. Klapper J: Headache in Sturge-Weber syndrome. *Headache* 34:521, 1994.

182. Marti-Bonmati L, Menor F, Mulas F: The Sturge-Weber syndrome: correlation between the clinical status and radiological CT and MRI findings. *Childs Nerv Syst* 9:107, 1993.

183. Charlmers RM, Harding AE: A case-control study of Leber's hereditary optic neuropathy. *Brain* 119 (Pt 5):1481, 1996.

184. Riordan-Eva P, Sanders MD, Govan GG, et al: The clinical features of Leber's hereditary optic neuropathy defined by the presence of a pathogenic mitochondrial DNA mutation. *Brain* 118 (Pt 2):319, 1995.

185. Fulton AB, Hansen RM, Mayer DL: Vision in Leber congenital amaurosis. *Arch Ophthalmol* 114:698, 1996.

186. Nikoskelainen EK, Savontaus ML, Huoponen K, et al: Pre-excitation syndrome in Leber's hereditary optic neuropathy. *Lancet* 344:857, 1994.

187. Hirano M, Pavlakis SG: Mitochondrial myopathy,

encephalopathy, lactic acidosis and strokelike episodes (MELAS): current concepts. *J Child Neurol* 9:4, 1994.

188. Luft R, Landau BR: Mitochondrial medicine. *J Intern Med* 238:405, 1995.

189. Shoffner JM, Lott MT, Lezza AM, et al: Myoclonic epilepsy and ragged red fiber disease (MERRF) is associated with a mitochondrial DNA tRNA mutation. *Cell* 61:931, 1990.

190. Sato O, Takei F, Yamada S: Hydrocephalus: is impaired cerebrospinal fluid circulation only one problem involved? *Childs Nerv Syst* 10:151, 1994.

191. Mori K: Current concept of hydrocephalus: evolution of new classifications. *Childs Nerv Syst* 11:523, 1995.

192. Cinalli G, Sainte-Rose C, Lellouch-Tubiana A, et al: Hydrocephalus associated with intramedullary low grade-glioma. Illustrative cases and review of the literature. *J Neurosurg* 83:480, 1995.

193. Guiffre R, Pastore FS, De Santis S: Connatal (fetal) hydrocephalus: an acquired pathology? *Childs Nerv Syst* 11:97, 1995.

194. Hanlo PW, Gooskens RH, Nijhuis IJ, et al: Value of transcranial Doppler indices in predicting raised ICP in infantile hydrocephalus. A study with review of the literature. *Childs Nerv Syst* 11:595, 1995.

195. Goh D, Minns RA: Intracranial pressure and cerebral arterial flow velocity indices in childhood hydrocephalus: current review. *Childs Nerv Syst* 11:392, 1995.

196. Gideon P, Thomsen C, Gjerris F, et al: Measurement of blood flow in the superior sagittal sinus in healthy volunteers, and in patients with normal pressure hydrocephalus and idiopathic intracranial hypertension with phase-contrast cine MR imaging. *Acta Radiol* 37:171, 1996.

197. Kristensen B, Malm J, Fagerland M, et al: Regional cerebral blood flow, white matter abnormalities, and cerebrospinal fluid hydrodynamics in patients with idiopathic hydrocephalus syndrome. *J Neurol Neurosurg Psychiatry* 60:282, 1996.

198. Krauss JK, Regel JP, Vach W, et al: Vascular risk factors and arteriosclerotic disease in idiopathic normal-pressure hydrocephalus of the elderly. *Stroke* 27:24, 1996.

199. Danek A, Uttner I, Yoursry T, et al: Lyme neuroborreliosis disguised as normal pressure hydrocephalus. *Neurology* 46:1743, 1996.

200. Bret P, Chazal J: Chronic ("normal pressure") hydrocephalus in childhood and adolescence. A review of 16 cases and reappraisal of the syndrome. *Childs Nerv Syst* 11:687, 1995.

201. Abbruzzese M, Scarone S, Colombo C: Obsessive-compulsive symptomatology in normal pressure hydrocephalus: a case report. *J Psychiatry Neurosci* 19:378, 1994.

202. Sand T, Bovim G, Grimse R, et al: Idiopathic normal pressure hydrocephalus: the CSF tap-test may predict the clinical response to shunting. *Acta Neurol Scand* 89:311, 1994.

203. Shimoda M, Oda S, Shibata M, et al: Change in regional cerebral blood flow following glycerol administration predict clinical results from shunting in normal pressure hydrocephalus. *Acta Neurochir* 129:171, 1994.

204. George AE, Holodny A, Golomb J, et al: The differential diagnosis of Alzheimer's disease. Cerebral atrophy versus normal pressure hydrocephalus. *Neuroimaging Clin N Am* 5:19, 1995.

205. Weiner HL, Constantini S, Cohen H, et al: Current treatment of normal-pressure hydrocephalus: comparison of flow-regulated and differential-pressure shunt valves. *Neurosurgery* 37:877, 1995.

206. Milhorat TH, Capocelli AL Jr, Anzil AP, et al: Pathological basis of spinal cord cavitation in syringomyelia: analysis of 105 autopsy cases. *J Neurosurg* 82:802, 1995.

207. Hida K, Iwasaki Y, Imamura H, et al: Posttraumatic syringomyelia: its characteristic magnetic resonance imaging findings and surgical management. *Neurosurgery* 35:886, 1994.

208. Samii M, Klekamp J: Surgical results of 100 intramedullary tumors in relation to accompanying syringomyelia. *Neurosurgery* 35:865, 1994.

209. Di Lorenzo N, Maleci A, Williams BM: Severe exacerbation of post traumatic syringomyelia after lithotripsy. Case report. *Paraplegia* 32:694, 1994.

210. Veilleux M, Stevens JC: Syringomyelia: electrophysiologic aspects. *Muscle Nerve* 10:449, 1987.

211. Sgouros S, Williams B: A critical appraisal of drainage in syringomyelia. *J Neurosurg* 82:1, 1995.

Chapter 15

TUMORS

Neoplasia can affect the central nervous system (CNS) in three ways. Primary tumors may develop in the brain, spinal cord, or surrounding structures; metastatic tumors may spread to the CNS from primary cancer elsewhere; or the brain and spinal cord may be damaged indirectly by the presence of a tumor elsewhere in the body. This latter condition is discussed under the remote effects of cancer (see Chap. 17).

Tumors arising within the CNS or from surrounding structures, including the meninges, blood vessels, embryonic cell rests, and bone, constitute approximately 10 percent of all tumors and account for 1.7 percent of deaths from cancerous tumors.

Approximately 80 percent of all tumors are primary tumors; 20 percent are metastatic. The gliomas are the most common tumor type with astrocytomas and glioblastoma multiforme exceeding the oligodendrogliomas and ependymomas in frequency. Nongliomatous tumors consist of meningiomas (10 percent), pituitary adenomas (10 percent), and acoustic neuromas (5 percent), with a large group of miscellaneous tumors making up another 5 percent. There is some difference in the frequency and distribution of tumors affecting the brain and spinal cord. The gliomas are the most common brain tumors, followed by meningiomas and pituitary adenomas. In contrast, neuromas are the most common tumors affecting the spinal cord, followed by meningiomas and gliomas.

In general, tumors that arise from embryonic tissue such as the primitive neuroectodermal tumors tend to occur early in life, but identification may be delayed until adolescence or adult life in some cases. Gliomas occur at all ages with increasing frequency up to 65 years of age. Metastatic tumors are usually seen among older patients with a steady increase in incidence after the age of 50.

ETIOLOGY

It is not possible to identify etiological factors in the great majority of brain tumors. Heredity plays a relatively minor role, although there are occasional reports of gliomas, meningiomas, and medulloblastomas in siblings. There is an increased incidence of brain tumors in neurofibromatosis and tuberous sclerosis, but these conditions are relatively uncommon. Congenital abnormalities, particularly incorporation of embryonic tissue in the developing brain or cranial cavity, are believed to be responsible for craniopharyngiomas, chordomas, colloid cysts of the third ventricle, and some pineal tumors. Inclusion of dermal elements may be followed by the development of dermoid and epidermoid tumors. The effects of trauma, infection, and carcinogenic viruses or agents are unclear, and there is little evidence that they play a major role in the development of brain tumors. Radiation treatment for scalp ringworm or malignant brain tumors in children is, however, associated with an increased rate of developing brain or spinal cord[1] tumors including meningiomas[2] later in life.[3]

Genetic factors appear to play a key role in the development of primary brain tumors.[4] At the present time, it is believed that cell nuclei contain genes that regulate cell proliferation. Amplification of these genes can lead to excessive production of positive regulators or proto-oncogenes with conversion into oncogenes. The presence of oncogenes within a cell leads to nuclear proliferation, which, if unchecked, becomes a neoplastic process. There are, however, tumor suppressor genes that inhibit cellular division. The loss of tumor suppressor gene activity by mutation, deletion, or reduced expression is associated with an imbalance of the normal equilibrium that exists between proto-oncogenes and tumor suppressor genes, thus disturbing the balance of cell integrity in favor of uninhibited growth and neoplastic proliferation.[5] Primary glioblastomas occurring in older patients exhibit epidermal growth factor complication. Secondary glioblastomas developing from astrocytomas contain p53 mutations and both types show deletions of chromosome 10. Oligodendrogliomas have genetic abnormalities involving chromosomes 1p and 19q. Meningiomas exhibit loss of chromosome 22q and mutations of the neurofibromatosis type 2 gene with loss of chromosome 14q and 10q in malignant transformation.[6] Primitive neuroectodermal tumors are associated with an abnormality i (17q).[7] Oncogenesis can then be regarded as a blocking or short-circuiting of the differentiation process in adult glial progenitor cells or a dedifferentiation of previously mature cells.[8]

ASTROCYTOMAS

Definition   *Astrocytomas* are neoplasms of astrocytic origin and are the most common type of intracranial tumor in children and in patients who are between 20 and 40 years of age. Although slow growing, they are not benign, because of their invasive quality and location within the confines of the bony calvarium.[9] Anaplastic astrocytomas are found in increasing numbers in patients between 30 and 50 years of age and glioblastoma multiforme, the most malignant astrocytoma, predominates in patients 50 years and older but can be encountered at any age.

There have been several attempts to classify astrocytomas based on the histological subtypes of the astrocyte that normally exists. However, some astrocytomas cannot be categorized in this fashion because they contain not only several histological subtypes of astrocytes but also other glial cells, particularly oligodendrocytes. It is probably better, therefore, to base a description of astrocytomas on their location within the CNS.

Pilocytic Astrocytoma

This tumor is the most benign form of astrocytoma. It occurs predominantly in children and young adults involving the cerebellar hemisphere, third ventricle, hypothalamic region, or optic pathway. Pilocytic astrocytomas may be solid or cystic structures with a mural nodule. The tumor is composed of loosely interwoven astrocytes with a fine fibrillary background and very few mitoses. There may be microcysts and Rosenthal fibers.[10] This tumor is well circumscribed and should be treated by total resection whenever possible. This procedure is usually curative with a survival rate approximating 100 percent. When it is only possible to perform a partial or incomplete resection, patients can be followed with regular magnetic resonance imaging (MRI) scans to detect any further growth. If this occurs, a second partial resection should be followed by radiation therapy. Tumors of the optic nerve, optic chiasm, and hypothalamus should be treated with systemic chemotherapy.

Cerebral Astrocytoma

Pathology   The tumor presents as a solid, slightly discolored yellow or gray mass with indistinct boundaries, often blurring the discrete junction between cerebral white matter and gray matter. Microscopic examination shows the presence of fibrillary astrocytes with a glassy eosinophilic cytoplasm and cell processes. Cells with unusually plump cytoplasm are occasionally encountered and are termed gemistocytes. Mitotic figures, vascular endothelial proliferation, and necrosis are absent, but microcalcification occurs in 15 percent of cases. The spectrum of differentiation runs from well-differentiated tumors to more anaplastic tumors. Astrocytomas may undergo a malignant transformation to glioblastoma multiforme at any time.

Clinical Features   The peak incidence of cerebral astrocytomas occurs during the third and fourth decades of life, but astrocytomas can also develop in childhood. The frontal lobes are the most common site for astrocytomas, followed by the temporal lobes (Fig. 15-1), parietal lobes, basal ganglia, and occipital lobes, in decreasing order of frequency. Thalamic astrocytomas are occasionally seen in children.

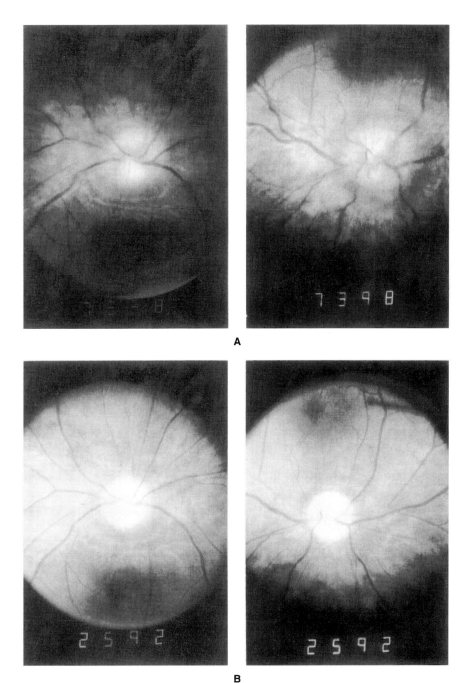

Figure 15–1
A. *Bilateral papilledema in a 17-year-old man with an astrocytoma in the posterior third ventricle obstructing the outflow of cerebral spinal fluid.* **B.** *Postpapilledema optic atrophy 3 months later after radiation therapy relief of hydrocephalus.*

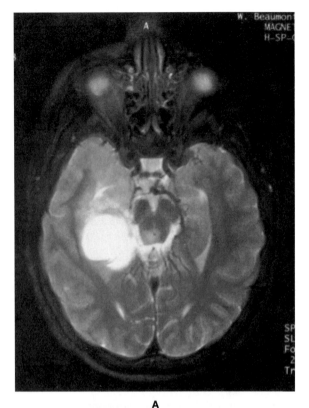

A

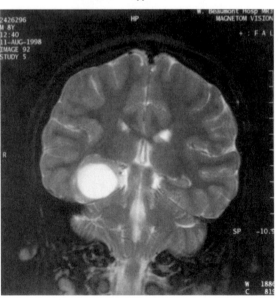

B

The patient often complains of unilateral or focal headache that becomes generalized with the development of papilledema indicating increased intracranial pressure (ICP) (Fig. 15-1). Some cases present with focal or generalized seizures. Other signs depend on the location of the tumor (Fig. 15-2 and Table 15-1).

Diagnostic Procedures   An MRI scan with demonstration of the tumor in axial coronal and sagittal planes is the method of choice in cases of suspected astrocytoma. An MRI gives a more accurate delineation of tumor boundaries than CT, and regular MRI scans can be obtained in follow-up, without risk to the patient (Fig. 15-3). With CT scanning, astrocytomas usually present as areas of increased density and show enhancement after infusion of contrast material. Displacement of midline structures and effacement of the wall of the lateral ventricle on the side of the tumor are seen.

Treatment   Astrocytoma should be surgically excised whenever possible. Radiation therapy is advised when total excision cannot be accomplished, or when the tumor recurs.

The pathology of deep nonresectible tumors can be established using an MRI or CT-guided stereotactic biopsy. A low-grade astrocytoma can then be treated by partial resection, removing as much tumor as possible and any epileptogenic foci without causing neurological deficits. However, patients who are neurologically intact, with well-controlled seizures, can be monitored without surgery, with the intention to intervene surgically if the tumor shows progression symptomatically or by serial imaging.

Prognosis   Approximately 40 percent of adults with cerebral astrocytoma are alive 10 years after total excision of the tumor. Children have a survival rate of 85 percent 10 years after surgery.

Figure 15–2
A. *Axial and* **B.** *Coronal views. MRI scan showing an astrocytoma mesial mid-temporal region right temporal lobe.*

Table 15-1

Signs associated with localized lesions

Location of lesion	Associated signs
Prefrontal area	Loss of judgment, failure of memory, inappropriate behavior, apathy, poor attention span, easily distractible, release phenomena
Frontal eye fields	Failure to sustain gaze to opposite side, saccadic eye movements, impersistence, seizures with forced deviation of the eyes to the opposite side
Precentral gyrus	Partial motor seizures, jacksonian seizures, generalized seizures, hemiparesis
Superficial parietal lobe	Partial sensory seizures, loss of cortical sensation including two-point discrimination, tactile localization, stereognosis and graphism
Angular gyrus	Agraphia, acalculia, finger agnosia, allochiria (right-left confusion) (Gerstmann syndrome)
Broca's area	Motor dysphasia
Superior temporal gyrus	Receptive dysphasia
Midbrain	Early hydrocephalus; loss of upward gaze; pupillary abnormalities; third nerve involvement—ptosis, external strabismus, diplopia; ipsilateral cerebellar signs; contralateral hemiparesis; parkinsonism; akinetic mutism
Cerebellar hemisphere	Ipsilateral cerebellar ataxia with hypotonia, dysmetria, intention tremor, nystagmus to side of lesion
Pons	Sixth nerve involvement—diplopia, internal strabismus; seventh nerve involvement—ipsilateral facial paralysis; contralateral hemiparesis; contralateral hemisensory loss; ipsilateral cerebellar ataxia; locked-in syndrome
Medial surface of frontal lobe	Apraxia of gait, urinary incontinence
Corpus callosum	Left-hand apraxia and agraphia, generalized tonic-clonic seizures
Thalamus	Contralateral "thalamic pain," contralateral hemisensory loss
Temporal lobe	Complex partial seizures, contralateral homonymous upper quadrantanopsia
Paracentral lobule	Progressive spastic paraparesis, urgency of micturition, incontinence
Deep parietal lobe	Autotopagnosia, anosognosia, contralateral homonymous lower quadrantanopsia
Third ventricle	Paroxysmal headache, hydrocephalus
Fourth ventricle	Hydrocephalus, progressive cerebellar ataxia, progressive spastic hemiparesis or quadriparesis
Cerebellopontine angle	Hearing loss, tinnitus, cerebellar ataxis, facial pain, facial weakness, dysphagia, dysarthria
Olfactory groove	Ipsilateral anosmia, ipsilateral optic atrophy, contralateral papilledema (Foster-Kennedy syndrome)
Optic chiasm	Incongruous bitemporal field defects, bitemporal hemianopsia, optic atrophy
Orbital surface frontal lobe	Complex partial seizures, Paroxysmal atrial tachycardia
Optic nerve	Visual failure of one eye, optic atrophy
Uncus	Partial complex seizures with olfactory hallucinations (uncinate fits)
Basal ganglia	Contralateral choreoathetosis, contralateral dystonia
Internal capsule	Contralateral hemiplegia, hemisensory loss, and homonymous hemianopsia
Pineal gland	Loss of upward gaze (Parinaud syndrome), early hydrocephalus, lid retraction, pupillary abnormalities
Occipital lobe	Partial seizures with elementary visual phenomena, homonymous hemianopsia with macular sparing
Hypothalamus/pituitary	Precocious puberty (children), impotence, amenorrhea, galactorrhea, hypothyroidism, hypopituitarism, diabetes insipidus, cachexia, diencephalic autonomic seizures

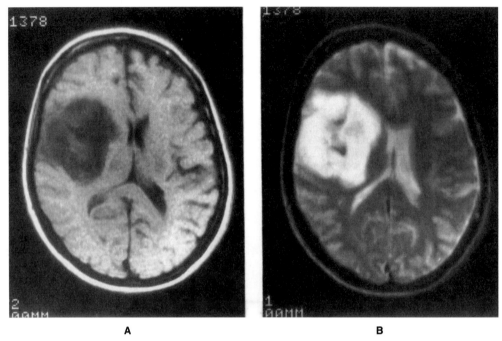

Figure 15–3
An MRI T1-weighted (A) and T2-weighted image (B). There is an abnormality in the right cerebral hemisphere, compatible with a low-grade astrocytoma or an oligodendroglioma. The patient has been asymptomatic for many years apart from occasional left-side simple partial seizure activity.

Anaplastic Astrocytoma

The growth and histologic appearance of the anaplastic astrocytoma is similar to that of a low-grade astrocytoma. However, there is increased cellularity with pleomorphism, hyperchromatic nuclei, and occasional mitoses, but no evidence of necrosis in the tumor. In some cases, astrocytes present with abundant eosinophilic cytoplasm and small nuclei. The presence of more than 20 percent of these cells, termed gemistocytes, is indicative of a poorer prognosis.[11] Another feature of the anaplastic astrocytoma is microvascular proliferation of vascular endothelium in blood vessel walls, often obliterating the lumen.

Cerebellar Astrocytoma

Cerebellar astrocytomas are the most common infratentorial tumors in childhood and carry a more favorable prognosis than most brain tumors because

these neoplasms are usually histologically benign and amenable to extensive resection.[12] The classical juvenile pilocytic astrocytoma tends to arise within the cerebellar hemisphere, presenting as a cyst with a mural nodule or as a solid tumor. The diffuse fibrillary astrocytoma usually occurs in the vermis.

Pathology The pilocytic astrocytoma is composed of loosely interwoven astrocytes with a fine fibrillary background and has few mitoses. There may be microcytes and Rosenthal fibers. The diffuse fibrillary astrocytoma resembles the low-grade astrocytoma of the cerebral hemisphere.

Clinical Features The hemispheric pilocytic astrocytoma presents with a slowly progressive unilateral cerebellar ataxia involving limbs and trunk, followed by increased ICP caused by displacement and obstruction of the fourth ventricle. The diffuse fibrillary astrocytoma situated in the midline results in a truncal ataxia followed by increased ICP.

Diagnostic Procedures The MRI and CT scans will reveal a cystic cerebellar mass (Fig. 15-4) in one cerebellar hemisphere or a solid midline tumor. The much greater detail of the MRI scan is an advantage in delineating the boundaries of the cystic mass and the mural nodule, which may appear in the CT scan only after contrast enhancement. The use of gadolinium enhancement with the MRI scan provides even better definition of tumors and their anatomic relationship. The hemispheric pilocytic tumor should be excised whenever possible, because virtually 100 percent of patients are alive 10 years after total removal.[13] The midline astrocytoma should also be excised whenever possible, but tumors showing anaplasia tend to disseminate in the neuraxis, and further treatment ranging from local radiation therapy to craniospinal radiation therapy plus chemotherapy has been recommended.

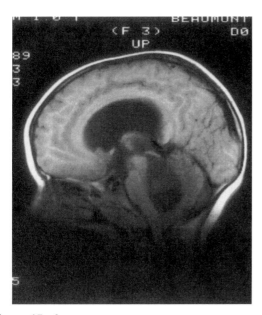

Figure 15—4
MRI scan. There is compression of the fourth ventricle by a cystic astrocytoma with distortion of the brainstem, compression of the cerebral aqueduct, and obstruction of the foramina of Luschka and Magendie producing a marked hydrocephalus.

Glioblastoma Multiforme

This tumor is the highest grade malignant tumor of the astrocytic line, accounting for 20 percent of intracranial tumors and 50 percent of those of astrocytic origin. Although it is possible that some glioblastomas arise from oligodendrogliomas, the majority develop by transformation of astrocytes through progressively higher grades of malignancy from low-grade astrocytoma to glioblastoma multiforme. However, direct malignant transformation from astrocytes is possible.

Pathology The brain is swollen and the neoplasm appears as a pinkish gray, well-demarcated mass with scattered areas of hemorrhage within its substance. Areas of cystic degeneration and a central area of creamy necrosis may be present. Microscopically, the tumor is characterized by hypercellularity and pleomorphism, and the cells show hyperchromatic nuclei and occasional mitoses. Multinucleated giant cells are a feature of the more anaplastic tumors. There are few normal astrocytes. The numerous blood vessels show endothelial proliferation. Despite the presence of a well-demarcated border, the tumor infiltrates the surrounding brain and is associated with considerable edema.

Clinical Features Glioblastoma multiforme occurs most commonly in the fifth and sixth decades and is somewhat more common in men. The incidence is increasing in the elderly.[14] The tumor is found most frequently in one frontal lobe and may spread through the corpus callosum to the opposite side. Glioblastomas also occur in the temporal, parietal, and occipital lobes and in the basal ganglion and thalamus. The tumor is the most common glioma of the pons.

Signs and symptoms usually progress rapidly. The patient may present with unilateral headache over the site of the tumor, but this is rapidly followed by generalized headache, indicating an increase in ICP due to tumor mass, edema, or hydrocephalus (Fig. 15-5). Onset with focal or generalized seizures or the development of seizures early in the course of the illness is not unusual. Additional signs and symptoms depend on the location of the neoplasm (see Table 15-1).

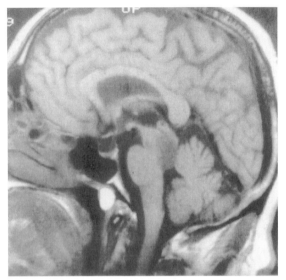

Figure 15–5
Sagittal MRI scan showing a glioma of the midbrain compressing the cerebral aqueduct and extending into the upper fourth ventricle.

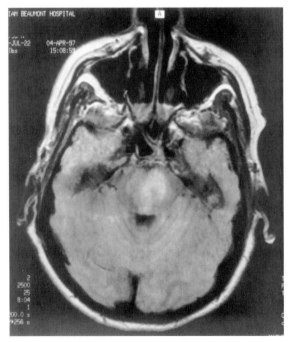

Figure 15–6
Pontine glioma. MRI scan. The pons is enlarged significantly by an astrocytoma.

Diagnostic Procedures

1. The MRI scan is the most sensitive imaging technique in the detection of glioblastoma multiforme and the delineation of the boundaries of the tumor (Fig. 15-6). The volume of the tumor is usually greater than that identified by the MRI scan.[15]

2. The CT scan shows a mass with irregular margins containing areas of high and low density. There are usually significant mass effects and marked surrounding edema. There is usually a homogeneous irregular or ring pattern of enhancement following infusion of contrast material. Calcification occurs in about 15 percent of cases, and there may be areas of cystic, necrotic, or hemorrhagic change within the tumor substance.

3. MR spectroscopy produces a distinctive pattern differentiating tumor from infarction, demyelination, or radiation necrosis.[16]

Treatment

Preoperative Treatment

1. Dexamethasone 4 mg q6h to reduce cerebral edema.[7]

2. Hyperosmolar agents such as mannitol may be required to reduce ICP if the patient is showing signs of rapid progression.

3. Seizures should be controlled with a loading dose of 1 g phenytoin by intravenous piggyback (IVPB) at 50 mg/min followed by 500 mg q12h IVPB until free Dilantin level is 2 µg/mL. At that juncture, the dose can be adjusted to maintain a therapeutic level at 2 µg/mL.

Biopsy Indications for biopsy of a suspected malignant glioma include:

1. Diagnosis in doubt despite adequate MRI studies.

2. Medical and anesthetic risks too great to permit craniotomy.

3. Lesion located in the corpus callosum, thalamus, hypothalamus, brainstem, or cerebellar peduncles.

4. To distinguish between radiation necrosis and tumor recurrence.

5. To verify tumor progression in a known low-grade glioma when there are signs of change in serial imaging studies.

Closed biopsy is intended to obtain a small sample with minimal risk to the patient, the greatest risk being hemorrhage.

Techniques for closed biopsy include CT guidance, ultrasound localization, and the use of CT- or MR-coupled stereotactic frames.

Angiosarcoma

Primary or metastatic angiosarcoma is a rare malignant tumor that usually arises from endothelial cells of arteries or lymphatics in the skin or superficial tissues. There are few reports of primary or metastatic brain involvement. The tumor presents as a unilateral mass, producing a contralateral hemiparesis with hyperreflexia and an extensor plantar response. Clinically, the tumor resembles a glioblastoma.

The CT scan demonstrates an enhancing mass resembling meningioma; MRI scanning will show low-intensity extra-axial tumor on T2-weighted imaging, with marked surrounding edema.[17]

Treatment consists of excision followed by radiotherapy. Prognosis is poor.

Radical Tumor Resection

The role of surgery in the treatment of glioblastoma multiforme is controversial, particularly in the extent of tumor removal. It is clear that cytoreductive procedures are indicated to alleviate increased ICP or to reduce mass effect, producing focal neurological deficits. However, attempts at total tumor removal are hampered by the definition of boundaries, despite advances in imaging techniques. Nevertheless refinement in surgical technique suggests that gross total resection can be performed in many cases one considered inoperable with acceptable neurological deficits.[18] Refinement in procedures such as neurophysiological mapping of the adjacent brain reduces postoperative deficits while electrocorticography will define seizure foci that should be resected. Enhanced optic imaging using a contrast enhancing dye provides a means of differentiating between normal brain and tumor tissue at the resection margins.[19] A gadolinium-enhanced MRI scan should be obtained within 3 days postoperatively after attempting complete extirpation of a glioblastoma multiforme or anaplastic astrocytoma. This study permits the detection of any residual tumor and is valuable in planning additional therapy.[20] All patients will require postoperative radiation therapy and chemotherapy after tumor resection.

Postoperative Management

Following surgery, all patients with an uncomplicated course should be transferred from the postoperative recovery area to an intensive care unit for 48 h. Dexamethasone should be maintained at 4 mg q4h then tapered slowly, depending on the clinical findings and residual mass effect on the postoperative scan. Antiepileptic drugs should be maintained at a high normal therapeutic level. Antibiotics should be given for a 48-h period to minimize infection. Although craniotomy is not usually a painful procedure, patients may have pain for other reasons and may require treatment with intramuscular codeine 60 mg q4h p.r.n. or morphine sulphate 10 mg q4–q6h p.r.n. Insomnia can be a problem and will respond to a short-acting benzodiazepine preparation.

Reoperative Procedures

Although most patients with cerebral gliomas have a poor prognosis following all modalities of treatment, including surgical excision, radiation therapy, and chemotherapy, there does appear to be a limited place for further surgical treatment in some cases (Fig. 15-7). The single factor when considering retreatment is improvement of quality of life, and careful selection of cases may attain this goal. Currently, retreatment may be of benefit when neurological deterioration is related to pressure effects. This situation may be improved by debulking of recurrent tumor, cyst evacuation, or ventricular atrial shunting.[21] Chemotherapy is of questionable value, but brachytherapy may extend survival.[22]

Chemotherapy

Chemotherapy provides limited improvement in survival following surgical excision of a glioblastoma multiforme and radiation therapy.[23] The addition of chemotherapy to surgical excision and radiation improves the median survival from 9.4 to 12 months.[24] This is, in part, due to the integrity of the blood-brain barrier, which limits passage of water-soluble compounds or compounds bound to plasma proteins into the brain.

The limited effect of intermittent systemic chemotherapy has led to the development of a number of techniques to increase drug concentration within the brain. These techniques include continuous infusion chemotherapy, high-dose chemotherapy with stem cell rescue,[25] autogenous marrow transplantation, intraventricular or intrathecal therapy[26] intra-arterial chemotherapy, intra-arterial chemotherapy with blood-brain barrier disruption, interstitial chemotherapy and techniques to modify the blood-brain barrier or blood tumor barrier to improve delivery of agents to the brain.[27] Despite these advances, improvement in chemotherapy is likely to be limited by the fact that malignant cells are dispersed far beyond the boundaries of a glioblastoma multiforme, having tracked along white matter tracts to other areas of the brain, including the noninvolved hemisphere. The challenge would appear to be the development of chemotherapeutic methods to treat the entire brain and meninges without diffuse neurotoxicity.

Radiotherapy

Treatment of glioblastoma multiforme and anaplastic astrocytoma with postoperative radiation therapy produces a modest improvement in survival, compared to surgery alone. Median survival is 14 to 22 weeks postoperatively for those treated with excision of the tumor and 36 to 47 weeks for patients receiving surgery followed by external beam conventional irradiation.[28] However, the median survival time for patients with glioblastoma multiforme is only 10 months, whereas the median survival time for those with anaplastic astrocytoma is 36 months. Although studies have clearly demonstrated the benefit of radiation therapy,[29] the results are far from satisfactory. Research into several innovative techniques indicates that the prognosis can be expected to improve.[30] Proposed therapeutic approaches include combining ra-

diation therapy and chemotherapy, which may increase survival by 10 percent at 1 year.[31] However, this is only a modest improvement. Consequently, several other strategies are under investigation, including hyperfractionation, brachytherapy, stereotactic radiosurgery using gamma knife units of multiple cobalt beams,[32] and three-dimensional conformational photon radiation therapy. Additional techniques, based on the assumption that tumor cells in glioblastoma multiforme are hypoxic include the use of hypoxic cell sensitizers such as nitroimidazole compounds. However, evidence suggests that whole brain irradiation can produce diffuse neuronal damage with impairment of cognitive functioning, including memory.[33] This crucial adverse effect imposes unquestionable caution in the development of newer techniques.

Oligodendrogliomas

Definition   Oligodendrogliomas constitute approximately 5 percent of all gliomas. These tumors usually occur in adults and are located predominantly in the cerebral hemispheres. More than half the patients with oligodendroglioma fail to live for more than 5 years after surgery.[34]

Pathology   The neoplasm presents as a gray-pink to red cystic area in the brain. Microscopic examination reveals a honeycomb appearance at low power caused by the presence of fibrovascular stroma. At higher power, the cells have a uniform appearance with a central nucleus surrounded by clear cytoplasm. The presence of some mitoses is not unusual. Approximately 70 percent of these tumors show some evidence of calcification. The neoplasm expands toward the cortex and may spread through it to eventually attach to the dura.

Clinical Features   Oligodendrogliomas are more common during the third and fourth decades and usually occur in the frontal lobes. Chronic headaches and partial or generalized seizures often constitute the only complaints for several years. Additional signs and symptoms depend on the location of the tumor (Table 15-1).

Diagnostic Procedures

1. The MRI scan will clearly define the oligodendroglioma and its boundaries. The nonenhanced CT scan shows clusters of dense calcification lying within an area of decreased density. There are some surrounding edema and ventricular displacement. There may be little change on contrast enhancement or slight enhancement of the surrounding area.

2. Tissue diagnosis can be established by stereotactic tumor biopsy.

Treatment Because the boundaries of the tumor can often be defined by MRI scanning in three planes, resection may be possible by stereotactic radiosurgery.

Prognosis With the standard procedure, a partial resection followed by irradiation therapy, the mean postoperative survival is between 5 and 7 years. Patients undergoing complete resection have survived beyond 10 years.

Ependymoma

Definition *Ependymomas* are neoplasms derived from the ependymal cell lining of the ventricular system and the central canal of the spinal cord. These tumors are common in childhood and have a 50 percent, 5-year survival rate.

Pathology Ependymomas are usually reddish, lobulated, and well-circumscribed tumors said to resemble a cauliflower in shape. There are two histological types. Epithelial ependymomas contain ependymal cells that form true rosettes. This histological type is most common in tumors involving the cerebral hemispheres and posterior fossa. Papillary ependymomas consist of ependymal cells that resemble simple epithelium or glial fibrillary stroma arranged in papillary configuration. This type is most common in the spinal cord and filum terminale. There may be cystic areas and calcification within the tumor. The tumor is usually benign, but 10 to 20 percent are malignant, with a tendency

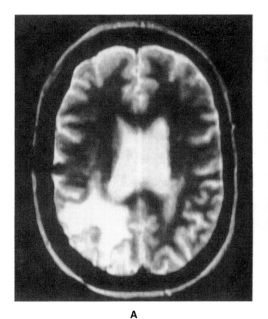
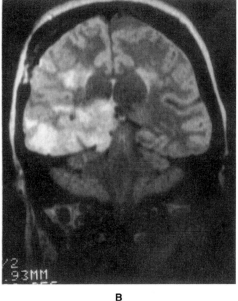

A   B

Figure 15–7
Axial (A) and sagittal (B) scans of a recurrent glioblastoma multiforme in the right posterior temporal, parietal, and occipital areas. The abnormal signal in the central white matter may represent radiation changes.

toward extension and spread through the subarachnoid space.

Clinical Features Ependymomas are the third most frequent posterior fossa neoplasm in childhood. Supratentorial ependymomas are usually found in the parietal occipital area and are more aggressive tumors often growing to a considerable size before detection. Ependymomas of the third ventricle are rare tumors with presenting symptoms of headache, ataxia, vertigo, hydrocephalus, and Parinaud syndrome.[35]

Posterior fossa ependymomas arise in three locations: midline tumors arising from the caudal half of the fourth ventricle and extending through the foramen of Magendie to the upper cervical region; laterally located tumors arising in the lateral recess and extending inferiorly and laterally; and roof tumors arising from the inferior medullary velum. Spinal cord ependymomas commonly involve the lumbosacral area and filum terminale and are often relatively benign.

The signs and symptoms of this neoplasm depend on the location. Ependymomas involving the fourth ventricle are likely to be detected in an early stage because of the signs and symptoms of increased ICP, including headache, nausea, vomiting, and papilledema, followed by lower cranial nerve involvement and cerebellar ataxia.

Diagnostic Procedures The MRI and CT scans show displacement, distortion, or obliteration of the fourth ventricle by a mass that may show cystic areas and foci of calcification (Fig. 15-8). However, the boundaries of the mass are shown in much greater detail by the MRI scan. Supratentorial ependymomas have features similar to those of the glioblastoma multiforme.

Treatment The treatment of choice is resection with removal of as much of the tumor as possible, followed by radiation therapy.[36] Third ventricular tumors are treated by microsurgical resection followed by radiation therapy. Hydrocephalus should be treated by a ventricular shunting procedure.

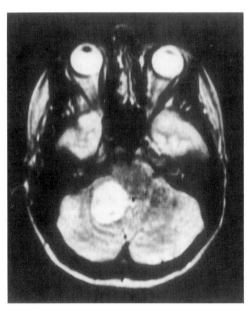

Figure 15–8
MRI scan. Tumor mass within the right cerebellar hemisphere exerting pressure on and displacing the brainstem to the left.

Prognosis The mean survival rate is 62 percent at 5 years postoperatively for ependymomas of the fourth ventricle. Patients with tumors arising in the lateral recess have a poorer survival rate at 5 years than those with midline tumors. Supratentorial ependymomas carry a poor prognosis.

CHOROID PLEXUS PAPILLOMA

The choroid plexus papilloma is a low-grade neoplasm of the choroid plexus that bears a close structural resemblance to normal choroid plexus. This is a rare neoplasm and is usually found in children, where it is often associated with overproduction of cerebrospinal fluid (CSF) and hydrocephalus. The hydrocephalus and the tumor can be demonstrated by MRI or CT scan (Fig. 15-9).

The papilloma can usually be completely removed with subsequent resolution of the hydrocephalus.

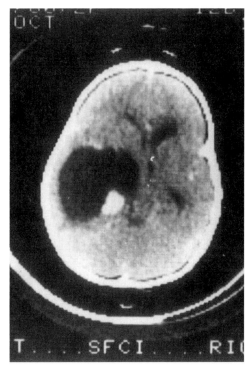

Figure 15–9
CT scan of a choroid plexus papilloma associated with a large cyst containing CSF. There is presssure on the ventricles and displacement to the left.

CHOROID PLEXUS CARCINOMA

Choroid plexus carcinoma is the malignant counterpart of the choroid plexus papilloma. This tumor, which is usually found in children, grows rapidly, producing macrocrania, a bulging fontanelle, and hydrocephalus. Treatment consists of partial tumor resection and placement of a ventricular peritoneal shunt. This should be followed by chemotherapy and delayed radiation therapy.[37]

INTRAVENTRICULAR MASS LESIONS

Many masses impinge on or appear to arise within the ventricular system. When extraventricular, intraventricular masses are excluded, those arising entirely within the ventricular system constitute a variety of conditions, of which the colloid cyst of the third ventricle is the most common often presenting with episodic headache and subtle signs of increased intracranial pressure[38] (Table 15-2). Correlation of patient age and classical features with a CT scan and MRI appearance will frequently narrow the differential diagnosis.[39] Meningioma is the most common cause of a mass in the area of the trigone after the first decade of life, with the highest incidence in the

Table 15-2
Intraventricular mass lesions

1. Cysts
   a. Colloid cyst
   b. Intraventricular CSF cyst
   c. Epidermoid cyst
   d. Dermoid cyst

2. Tumors of the choroid plexus
   a. Choroid plexus papilloma
   b. Choroid plexus carcinoma

3. Meningioma

4. Lipoma choroid plexus

5. Glial tumors
   a. Ependymoma
   b. Astrocytoma

6. Other tumors
   a. Neurocytoma
   b. Neuroblastoma
   c. Primitive neuroectodermal tumor
   d. Lymphoma
   e. Hemangioblastoma
   f. Intraventricular craniopharyngioma

7. Metastatic tumor
   a. Lung
   b. Breast
   c. Melanoma
   d. Gastrointestinal
   e. Genitourinary

8. Malformations
   a. Arteriovenous malformations
   b. Cavernous malformation
   c. Tuberous sclerosis

9. Nonneoplastic cysticercosis

fifth decade. However, many tumors can present as intraventricular mass lesions.

PRIMITIVE NEUROECTODERMAL TUMORS

Medulloblastoma

Definition Primitive neuroectodermal tumors (PNETs) include the medulloblastoma, retinoblastoma, pinealoblastoma, and cerebral neuroblastoma,[40] all of which have common microscopic features and are probably derived from neoplastic transformation occurring within a primitive undifferentiated neuroectodermal cell.[41] The PNETs are the most common malignant primary posterior fossa tumor of childhood, constituting 13 to 20 percent of pediatric brain tumors and 33 percent of posterior fossa tumors in childhood.[42] About 50 percent of PNETs occur in the first decade of life. These tumors are highly malignant, usually develop in the vermis of the cerebellum, and exert pressure on or occlude the fourth ventricle.

Pathology The PNETs present as well-circumscribed soft reddish-gray tumors. Microscopic examination reveals closely packed cells with deeply stained nuclei and scant cytoplasm. The cells occur in random formation but occasionally form pseudorosettes or appear in rows. The tumor is highly vascular and there is a higher incidence of systemic metastasis with PNETs than other gliomas. Seeding into the subarachnoid space is a frequent complication.

Clinical Features The PNETs are more common in males with a male:female ratio of 2:1 to 3:1. The tumors usually develop in the cerebellar vermis but have been described in other sites, including the retina, pineal gland, cerebral hemispheres, brainstem, and cerebellar hemispheres. The younger the patient, the more aggressive the tumor and the higher the incidence of metastasis at presentation.[43] The presence of a PNET close to the fourth ventricle results in the early development of hydrocephalus with signs of increased ICP (headache, vomiting, ataxia), accompanied by cerebellar dysfunction, usually presenting as truncal ataxia (Fig. 15-10).

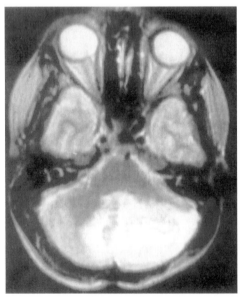 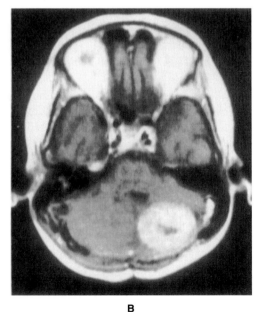

Figure 15-10   **A**   **B**
Primitive neuroectodermal tumor (Medulloblastoma). MRI scan of a medulloblastoma in the left cerebellar hemisphere before (A) and after (B) gadolinium enhancement.

Diagnostic Procedures

1. The CT scan shows a well-defined homogeneous mass with moderate uniform contrast enhancement. Ten percent show cystic change or calcification.

2. The MRI scan is clearly superior to CT scanning in demonstrating the posterior fossa mass with distortion and compression of the fourth ventricle (Fig. 15-11). The tumor is usually hypointense on T1-weighted images and hyperintense on T2-weighted images, with uniform enhancement with gadolinium.

3. A lumbar puncture should be performed with examination of the CSF for cells indicating dissemination of the PNET throughout the subarachnoid space.

4. A contrast-enhanced craniospinal MRI scan, which includes the whole of the neuraxis, is necessary to detect metastatic spread through the subarachnoid space.[44]

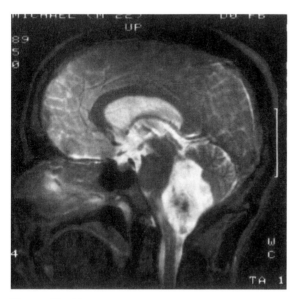

Figure 15–11
Medulloblastoma MRI scan demonstrating involvement of the anterior cerebellum and brainstem with compression of the fourth ventricle and hydrocephalus.

Treatment The tumor should be resected completely if possible. This should be followed by craniospinal radiotherapy and chemotherapy.[45]

Prognosis The postoperative survival is 6 to 12 months for patients treated by surgery alone. Combined surgery and radiation therapy has a 10-year survival rate of 40 to 50 percent. The addition of chemotherapy increases the 5-year rate of survival. Reoperation of recurrent tumors is a useful procedure.[46] Deficiencies of growth hormone and thyrotropin induced by chemotherapy should be corrected by replacement therapy.

Pinealoma

Definition Pinealomas are a heterogeneous group of tumors found in the area of the pineal gland. True neoplasms of the pineal gland constitute less than 1 percent of all intracranial tumors.

Pathology A large number of tumors arise in the pineal area, including benign cysts (dermoid, glial, epidermoid, arachnoid, colloid), hamartomas (lipoma, arteriovenous malformation, cavernous angioma), teratomas, pinealocytoma, astrocytoma, meningioma, oligodendroglioma, granuloma, germinoma, embryonic carcinoma, yolk sac tumor, and pinealoblastoma.

Pinealocytomas are soft masses that replace the pineal gland and are often the site of necrosis, hemorrhage, or cyst formation. Pinealocytomas consist of cells resembling normal pineal tissue. Pinealoblastomas have an appearance similar to primitive neuroectodermal tumors (medulloblastomas). Teratomas contain mixtures of hair, bone, cartilage, and muscle and are the most common brain tumor presenting or producing symptoms at birth occurring in supratentorial locations frequently, but not exclusively, in the pineal region.[47] Germinomas have the microscopic appearance of germinomas of the testes.

Clinical Features Pineal tumors produce symptoms due to pressure on the midbrain at the level of the quadrigeminal plate. Symptoms of increased ICP, including occipital headache, nausea and vomiting, appear at an early stage, because of distortion of the cerebral aqueduct and resultant hydrocephalus. Examination frequently shows the loss of vertical upward gaze (Parinaud syndrome) due to pressure on the superior colliculi. Other signs include lid retraction and pupillary abnormalities such as poor reaction to light or Argyll Robertson pupils when there is pretectal involvement. More severe compression of the midbrain causes ataxia and nystagmus. There may be bilateral signs of corticospinal tract involvement caused by forward displacement of the midbrain with compression of the cerebral peduncles.

Diagnostic Procedures

1. A chest film should be obtained to exclude metastasis from germinoma, pinealoblastoma, choriocarcinoma, or malignant teratoma.

2. Lumbar puncture with examination of the CSF for cytology, chemistry, and tumor markers is indicated in all malignant tumors of the pineal region.

3. Some tumor markers (human chorionic gonadotropin, α-fetoprotein) may be present.

4. Yolk sac tumors are associated with elevated levels of α-fetoprotein in serum and CSF.

5. The MRI scan shows the presence of a pineal tumor in multiple planes and demonstrates the precise anatomical relationships of the tumor, including vascular structures such as the internal cerebral veins, vein of Galen, and straight sinus. The presence of fat within the tumor, shown by MRI or CT scan, suggests the presence of a teratoma or epidermoid or dermoid tumor and excludes germinoma.

6. Arteriography. With the demonstration of vascular structures by MRI scanning, arteriography is necessary only if it is believed that the mass is a vascular tumor.

Treatment   Mature teratomas, pinealocytomas, dermoid or epidermoid cysts, low-grade astrocytomas, oligodendrogliomas, meningiomas, and well-differentiated ependymomas should be resected. Partially resected benign tumors require long-term observation without further treatment, unless recurrence develops.[48]

Isolated pineal germinoma with suprasellar involvement requires excision followed by local radiation therapy. More extensive germinomas and pinealblastomas will require excision followed by whole brain radiation and craniospinal radiation therapy in cases with dissemination in the spinal fluid. Teratomas, embryonic carcinoma, yoke sac tumors, and choriocarcinomas are more malignant and should be treated with subtotal resection, radiation therapy, and chemotherapy.

Prognosis   Shunting and radiation therapy are associated with 60 to 70 percent 5-year survival for germinomas. The more malignant tumors, such as yolk sac tumor, have a very poor prognosis.[49]

Brainstem Glioma

Brainstem gliomas constitute approximately 20 percent of all posterior fossa tumors in children.

Pathology   The majority of brainstem gliomas are diffuse infiltrative lesions arising in the pons. These tumors are low-grade gliomas containing foci of more anaplastic gliomas.

A second type of low-grade, often indolent, glioma occurs in the upper midbrain and grows very slowly.

About 10 percent of brainstem gliomas arise in the cervical medullary region and extend dorsally into the cerebellum.

Clinical Features   The pontine gliomas present with sixth and seventh cranial nerve palsies followed by involvement of lower cranial nerves. Hydrocephalus is a later development. Midbrain gliomas involve the tectum, producing hydrocephalus as the first symptom. Cervical medullary tumors are associated with ataxia and later development of lower cranial nerve symptoms.

Diagnosis is established by MRI.

Treatment   Cervical medullary tumors can be excised in some cases. Midbrain gliomas require ventricular peritoneal shunting procedures. Diffuse pontine gliomas should be treated by hyperfractionated radiotherapy, but the overall survival rate is less than 10 percent in pediatric patients with infiltrating brainstem gliomas at 3 years posttreatment.[50]

Diencephalic Gliomas

Gliomas affecting the optic nerve, optic chiasm, hypothalamus, or thalamus constitute 20 percent of pediatric low-grade gliomas. A large number of children with neurofibromatosis have visual pathway gliomas demonstrated by MRI. These tumors are asymptomatic or have apparently static visual impairment. Low- or high-grade diencephalic gliomas occurring in adults are rare.

Pathology Most diencephalic gliomas in children consist of fibrillary or pilocytic astrocytomas. Despite their low-grade state, the proximity of the ventricular system permits dissemination throughout the subarachnoid space in some cases.[51] Adult tumors, which include anaplastic astrocytoma and glioblastoma multiforme, can develop in the optic pathways and infiltrate the hypothalamus or adjacent structures.

Diagnostic Procedures

1. The MRI scan readily demonstrates diencephalic tumors. Pilocytic astrocytomas may be quite large and show marked enhancement with gadolinium. Cystic components and calcification may be present in the tumor. Thalamic tumors show clear separation from the optic chiasm. Bilateral optic nerve involvement usually indicates a chiasmatic tumor.

2. Hypothalamic tumors are associated with hypertension, euphoria, hyperkinesis, hypoglycemia, hyperhidrosis, and failure to thrive, with elevation of growth hormone levels and corticotropin.

3. Optic chiasmatic involvement produces incongruous field defects. The classical bitemporal hemianopia is a late phenomenon.

Treatment Children with low-grade gliomas with bulky necrotic or cystic components can be managed with partial resection and observation.[52] Patients with rapidly progressive disease should be treated with radiation therapy. However, the effect of radiation on the surrounding brain limits radiation therapy in young children, who may have better results with chemotherapy.[53]

PITUITARY ADENOMA

Definition Pituitary adenomas are tumors derived from cells of the anterior portion of the pituitary gland and represent approximately 10 to 15 percent of all intracranial tumors.

Pathology Pituitary tumors can be classified as follows:

Stage 1: Microadenoma—a tumor less than 10 mm in diameter confined to the pituitary fossa

Stage 2: Macroadenoma—a tumor greater than 10 mm in diameter confined to the pituitary fossa

Stage 3: Macroadenoma with extracellular extension outside the pituitary fossa by invasion of the floor of the sella or by suprasellar extension.

Clinical Features Symptoms may be produced by:

1. The mass of the tumor.
   a. Suprasellar extension often causes compression of the optic chiasm and visual field defects.
   b. Midline extension may produce hypothalamic dysfunction with hyperphagia, weight gain, abnormal temperature regulation, and somnolence. There may be damage to gonadotrophin-releasing cells in the hypothalamus or interference with the delivery of gonadotrophic releasing hormones through the hypophyseal portal system.[54]
   c. Tumor growth into the third ventricle results in hydrocephalus.
   d. Caudal extension can produce pressure on the brainstem.
   e. Lateral extension can involve the cavernous sinus and the third, fourth, fifth, and sixth cranial nerves.
   f. Temporal lobe involvement produces complex-partial seizures.
   g. Acute hemorrhage into a pituitary adenoma causes pituitary apoplexy with acute swelling of the tumor, producing severe headache, vomiting, impaired consciousness, ophthalmoplegia, pupillary abnormalities, visual disturbance, meningismus, and occasionally, subarachnoid

hemorrhage. Symptoms vary. Transient hypopituitarism is common and pituitary function may improve.[55]

   h. Intracranial and spinal dissemination is a rare complication of a pituitary tumor.[56]

2. Oversecretion of pituitary hormones. Excess hormone production occurs in 75 percent of pituitary adenomas.

   a. Prolactin-secreting tumors are the most common hormone-producing adenomas.[57] Symptoms consist of galactorrhea, amenorrhea, anovulation, and infertility in women, and hypogonadism, depressed libido, impotence or infertility in men.

   b. Growth hormone-secreting tumors produce gigantism in the adolescent and acromegaly in the adult. Acromegaly is characterized by hypertrophy of bone and connective tissue, producing progressive enlargement of the hands, feet, thorax, skull, and jaw, leading to "coarsening" of the features.

   c. Corticotrophin overproduction results in Cushing syndrome. This condition is characterized by hypertension, facial and truncal obesity, osteoporosis, abnormal carbohydrate metabolism, muscle weakness, menstrual abnormalities, and hirsutism.

   d. Thyrotropin-secreting hormones present with hyperthyroidism.

   e. Leutinizing hormone and follicle-stimulating hormone adenomas do not produce symptoms, but many of the clinically nonfunctioning tumors are gonadotrophin producing.

   Patients who are found to have a pituitary adenoma should be investigated for the multiendocrine adenoma (MEA1) syndrome, a genetically determined syndrome of pituitary adenoma, pancreatic tumor, and hyperparathyroidism.

Diagnostic Procedures

   1. The MRI or CT scan in the axial, coronal, and sagittal planes will display pituitary adenomas and the relationship of the tumor to the surrounding structures—cavernous sinus, optic chiasm, ca-

rotid arteries, hypothalamus, and third ventricle (Fig. 15-12). The majority of microadenomas are revealed by MRI with contrast enhancement, which shows a focal signal abnormality in the pituitary. Detection may be increased using three-dimensional gradient echo acquisition sequences.[59] Asymptomatic nonsecreting tumors should have repeated MRI studies at 6 months, and 1, 3, and 5 years.

   2. Because pituitary adenoma is the most common tumor in the sella, all patients should be evaluated endocrinologically for hypersecretion or hyperfunction.[60] This will entail determination of prolactin, growth hormone, corticotropin, thyrotropin, luteinizing hormone, and follicle-stimulating hormone.

   3. Patients with tumors greater than 1 cm in diameter require visual field determination.

Treatment   Prolactin-secreting tumors of all sizes can be treated with bromocriptine, the dopamine agonist, 1.25 mg q.h.s., increasing to 2.5 mg q8h. Macroadenomas with visual field defects often shrink with improvement in visual field abnormalities.

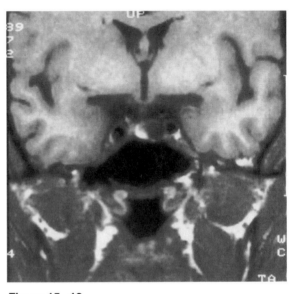

Figure 15–12
MRI scan. Pituitary tumor with suprasellar extension. The upward displacement of the internal carotid arteries is clearly demonstrated.

Bromocriptine therapy may be continued indefinitely. Dopamine receptor agonist-resistant tumors are occasionally encountered.[61]

Other hyperfunctioning adenomas should be treated surgically. Small and medium-sized tumors can be removed by the transphenoidal route.[62] Larger tumors may require a transfrontal approach.

Some clinically nonfunctioning tumors respond to bromocriptine with shrinkage of the mass. If visual field defects persist, the tumor should be removed surgically. Those without visual field defects usually follow a benign course[63] and can be followed with repeated MRI studies at 1, 2, and 5 years.

Postoperative complications include CSF rhinorrhea, hypopituitarism, diabetes insipidus, permanent visual field defects, and cranial nerve palsies.

Hypopituitarism can be treated with appropriate replacement therapy.

MENINGIOMA

Definition *Meningiomas* are benign, slow-growing tumors that are believed to be derived from the cells and vascular elements of the meninges. Evidence indicates that development of a meningioma is related to loss of function of a tumor suppressor gene located on chromosome 22.[64]

Pathology The majority of meningiomas are of four basic types. *Meningothelial meningiomas* are derived from arachnoid cap cells and are composed of sheets of cells with large vesicular nuclei. *Fibrous meningiomas* are derived from connective tissue elements of the arachnoid and consist of strands of interlacing spindle cells with long fibrils. *Psammomatous meningiomas* consist of whorls of spindle cells with a central area that degenerates, calcifies, and forms a concretion or psammoma body. *Angiomatous meningiomas* contain numerous vascular spaces lined by endothelial cells. Many meningiomas undergo secondary xanthomatous or myxomatous change, whereas others calcify or contain melanin, bone, or cartilage. Most meningiomas grow as well-capsulated tumors, but others develop in relatively thin sheets along the dura. The latter type of tumor has been termed "meningioma en plaque."

Clinical Features Meningiomas constitute 10 percent of intracranial tumors. They are most common in the latter years of life and are more frequent in women, particularly in those who have breast cancer.[65] Sex hormones stimulate the growth of meningiomas, which may progress more rapidly in the second half of pregnancy. Meningiomas can be found wherever arachnoid cap cells or connective tissue portions of arachnoid are located. These areas include the convexity of the cerebral hemispheres, the basal skull areas, sphenoid ridge, olfactory groove, sella and parasellar areas, tentorium cerebelli, posterior fossa, choroid plexus, and, rarely, the spinal canal. Because meningiomas are slow-growing tumors producing compression of the brain, abnormal signs and symptoms may evolve over a period of many years. Neurological abnormalities depend on the location of the tumor (see Table 15-1).

Diagnostic Procedures

1. Skull films. Changes in the skull are not infrequent, due to the proximity of the tumor to the inner table of the skull. Radiographic abnormalities consist of thinning or thickening of bone and widening of vascular bone shadows. The tumor may contain calcification in 30 to 60 percent of cases.

2. On MRI scanning, the tumor usually appears as a dense, sharply demarcated mass located near the bone or in close relationship to the falx or tentorium cerebelli. The majority exhibit a heterogeneous intensity pattern that may be related to the presence of calcification, areas of necrosis or hemorrhage, cyst, or tumor vascularity[66] (Fig. 15-13). There is dense enhancement following infusion of contrast material (Fig. 15-14).

Treatment Meningiomas should be excised. Complete removal offers the greatest likelihood of cure.

Prognosis Complete removal is usually followed by resolution of neurological deficits and permanent recovery. Tumor recurrence is not unusual following incomplete excision, and a second operation may be necessary several years later. Radiation therapy prevents or delays recurrence of tumor in most cases.[67]

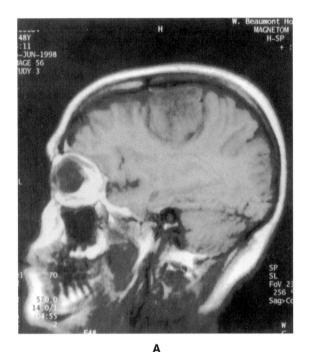

A

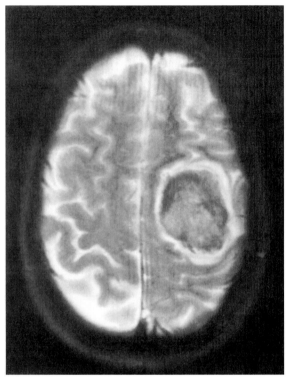

B

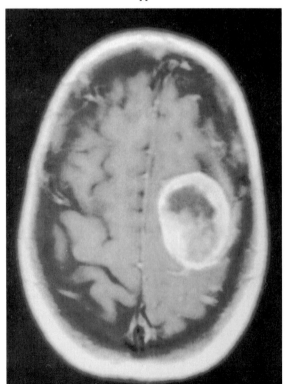

C

Figure 15–13
MRI scan. Meningioma. The tumor is associated with very little edema and the slow growth displaces the cortex and subcortical tissues (A). There is minimal displacement of the midline structures (B) and enhancement of the periphery following the IV injection of contrast material (C).

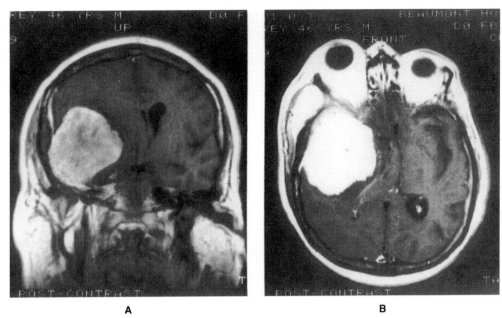

Figure 15-14
MRI scan. Meningioma. A) Precontrast B) Postcontrast studies.

NEUROMA
(NEURINOMA; SCHWANNOMA)

Definition *Neuromas* are slow-growing benign tumors that originate from Schwann cells and most commonly develop on the vestibular portion of the eighth cranial nerve (acoustic neuroma). There are between 2000 and 3000 new cases of acoustic neuromas in the United States each year. Acoustic neuromas also account for 90 to 95 percent of neoplasms in the cerebellopontine angle.

Pathology Grossly, the tumor is thickly encapsulated and lobulated. Microscopic examination shows that it consists of spindle-shaped cells with rod-shaped nuclei that often lie in parallel rows. The tumor is often highly vascular and may contain areas of cystic granulation or loose reticular tissue. Axons are found only in the capsule of this tumor, in contrast to the neurofibroma, where axons are often contained in the substance of the tumor.

Clinical Features The acoustic neuroma is the most common cerebellopontine angle tumor. It presents with the following symptoms, in order of decreasing frequency: progressive hearing loss, tinnitus, ataxia, vertigo, headache, trigeminal nerve dysfunction including hyperesthesia, paresthesias or facial pain, and progressive facial weakness.[68]

Neuromas are often found attached to other cranial nerves and to nerve roots of the spinal nerves, usually in the thoracic area, where they are subdural in location and involve the dorsal sensory nerve root. These tumors may grow out of the intervertebral foramen into the mediastinum in so-called dumbbell fashion.

Bilateral acoustic neuromas are occasionally encountered in patients with the subcutaneous nodules and café au lait lesions of neurofibromatosis.

Diagnostic Procedures

1. Audiologic tests show a high-tone hearing loss and impaired speech discrimination.

2. Impedance audiometry is abnormal, with absence of the acoustic reflex on the affected side.

3. Brainstem auditory evoked potentials are abnormal, with absence of wave 1 or prolongation of all absolute latencies.

4. Caloric tests show diminished or absent response on the affected side.

5. The MRI scan clearly outlines even the smallest tumor in axial, coronal, and sagittal planes. The MRI scan is particularly useful for the diagnosis of intracanalicular tumors (Fig. 15-15).

6. Polytomes of the skull may reveal enlargement of the internal auditory meatus. Polytomes of the thoracic vertebrae may reveal enlargement of the intervertebral foramina in the case of a neuroma developing on a spinal nerve root.

7. A CT scan with enhancement reveals a sharply marginated homogeneous, dense mass in the cerebellopontine angle. Hydrocephalus is often present in long-standing tumors.

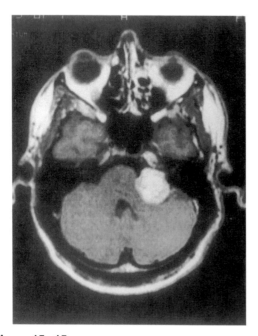

Figure 15-15
MRI scan with gadolinium enhancement. There is a large left cerebellopontine angle mass extending into the internal auditory canal.

Treatment   Surgical removal using a suboccipital transmeatal approach is the treatment of choice in most cases.[69] The tumor has a tendency to recur unless there has been complete removal. Stereotactic radiosurgery is an effective alternative, which has less morbidity with better preservation of hearing and facial nerve function.[70] Transtemporal access is another technique favored by some surgeons.[71]

Elderly patients with minimal symptoms and small tumors can be followed annually with MRI studies. The minority, who develop symptoms of brainstem or cerebellar involvement, can be treated by subtotal resection or cyst drainage.[72]

CRANIOPHARYNGIOMA

Definition   The *craniopharyngioma* is a tumor of congenital origin that develops from remnants of Rathke's pouch. It is histologically benign and occurs most commonly in the suprasellar region in children and adults.

Etiology and Pathology   The neoplasm is believed to develop from squamous cell remnants of Rathke's pouch. The tumor is yellow-brown in color, encapsulated, nodular in appearance, and frequently cystic. Microscopically, it is characterized by interlacing trabeculae of squamous epithelial cells with a peripheral layer of palisading columnar epithelial cells. Keratinization results in formation of squamous "horny pearls" that frequently calcify. Cystic components are lined by stratified squamous epithelium and the contents are oily brown in consistency and contain cholesterol crystals. There is intense gliosis in the surrounding brain.

Clinical Features   The craniopharyngioma is the most common supratentorial tumor of childhood, some 55 percent occurring in children, 45 percent after the age of 20 years. The tumor accounts for 2 to 3 percent of all intracranial tumors. It occurs in a $3:2$ male:female ratio. Clinically, the tumor can present with a variety of signs and symptoms. These include increased ICP, visual field defects, headache, and neuroendocrine disorders resulting in diabetes insipidus, short stature, delayed sexual development, and hypogonadism. Larger tumors may produce hypothalamic involvement, cranial nerve palsies, hydrocephalus because of pressure on the third ventricle, and progressive dementia. There may be evidence of recurrent aseptic chemical meningitis, where the cystic contents are discharged into the subarachnoid space. Diabetes insipidus may precede the appearance of other symptoms for some years in children with occult craniopharyngiomas, pituitary tumors, or hypothalamic tumors.

Diagnostic Procedures

1.   Skull films may reveal thickening, erosion, or enlargement of the sella. There may be evidence of bony invasion. Suprasellar calcifications are present in 80 percent of children with craniopharyngiomas but only in 40 to 50 percent of adult patients with this tumor.

2.   The MRI scan with contrast medium enhancement[73] will clearly delineate the tumor in axial, coronal, and sagittal planes (Fig. 15–16).

3.   The CT scan is characterized by the presence of a calcified high-density mass or an isodense lesion in the case of intrasellar craniopharyngiomas.

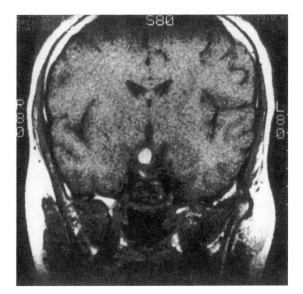

Figure 15–16
MRI scan. Craniopharyngioma with upward extension into the hypothalamus and third ventricle.

Cystic tumors show a well-defined capsule containing high-density areas of calcification surrounding a low-density core. The capsule often shows dense contrast enhancement. Hydrocephalus may be present if the tumor extends into the area of the third ventricle.

4.   Endocrine studies should be obtained to establish the function of the pituitary and hypothalamus. A moderate hyperprolactinemia is not uncommon. Levels greater than 150 ng/mL (normal 1 to 25 ng/mL) suggest the presence of associated pituitary microadenoma.

5.   Arteriography is useful in the preoperative period to delineate the blood supply to the tumor.

6.   Lumbar puncture is indicated in patients with clinical evidence of meningeal involvement. The CSF shows a polymorphonuclear leukocytosis. Glucose content is normal or slightly decreased and protein content is elevated.

Treatment   The treatment of choice is surgical removal of all neoplastic tissue. However, total removal is not always feasible because of adherence to vital structures such as the optic chiasm, hypothalamus, and circle of Willis. In these cases, as much tumor as possible is removed, the cystic contents are aspirated, and the patient is treated with postoperative radiotherapy. Some patients may require repeated stereotactic percutaneous drainage of cysts. Others may be treated by insertion of an Ommaya reservoir for intermittent aspiration of cysts. Gross total resection is associated with a less than 20 percent recurrence, whereas more than 50 percent recur after subtotal resection.[74]

Prognosis   The overall 10-year survival rate is approximately 60 percent. The rate is higher in the pediatric population than in adults. Death is the result of tumor recurrence, which seems to be low in those who survive more than 10 years.[75] Hormone deficiencies may be permanent and should be corrected by appropriate substitution therapy.

RATHKE'S CLEFT CYSTS

Rathke's cleft cysts arise from a remnant of the stomodeum and are enlarged by an accumulation of mucus secreted by cyst wall cells. Small, asymptomatic Rathke's cleft cysts are occasionally found by CT or MRI scanning. Symptomatic Rathke's cleft cysts are rare and can compress the pituitary gland, optic chiasm, and hypothalamus and must be distinguished from cystic pituitary adenomas or craniopharyngiomas. One fact that helps differentiate Rathke's cleft cysts is that the pituitary fossa is not enlarged on plain radiographs. The MRI scans usually show high-intensity T1- and T2-weighted images.[76]

Treatment is by resection of symptomatic cleft cysts.

HEMANGIOBLASTOMA

Definition   The *hemangioblastoma* is believed to be a tumor of capillary endothelial origin and is commonly located in the cerebellum.

Etiology and Pathology   The tumor is most frequently located in the cerebellar hemisphere or vermis. It may also develop in the brainstem or in the spinal cord,[77] where it may be associated with a syrinx formation or supratentorially, where it is frequently attached to the dura. The association of a cerebellar hemangioma with angiomas and cysts of the liver, pancreas, and kidney, and occasionally with tumors of the kidney, epididymis, or adrenals, has been termed Lindau syndrome. The association of a retinal angioma and Lindau syndrome is often referred to as the von Hippel-Lindau syndrome. Hemangioblastomas are yellowish red in color, well circumscribed, lobulated, and cystic in appearance. Small mural nodules of tumor may be located in the cyst walls. Microscopically, the tumor is composed of an endothelial portion and a stromal portion, which is frequently distended with lipid. Reticular fibers separate the two portions. Polycythemia secondary to tumor production of erythropoietin can occur.

Clinical Features   Hemangioblastomas usually develop during the third or fourth decade in men and frequently present as a posterior fossa mass with evidence of increased ICP and signs of cerebellar dysfunction. Brainstem involvement produces cranial

nerve palsies and long tract signs. Polycythemia or evidence of von Hippel-Lindau syndrome may be present. Cerebellar tonsillar herniation can cause sudden death. Subarachnoid hemorrhage is a rare complication of hemangioblastoma.[78]

Diagnostic Procedures

1. The MRI or CT scan reveals a well-circumscribed, solid or cystic mass in the posterior fossa, which may contain calcifications (Fig. 15–17). Solid tumors show enhancement after injection of contrast material.

2. Arteriography usually shows the presence of abnormal blood supply to the vascular nodule in cystic tumors.

Treatment   In the case of cystic hemangioblastomas, the cyst and mural nodule should be removed because this is usually curative. Solid tumors can

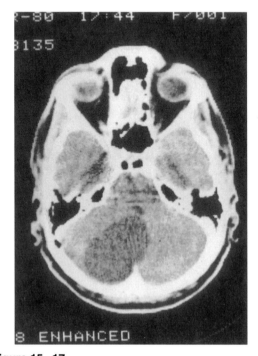

Figure 15–17
CT scan with enhancement showing a cystic cerebellar hemangioblastoma.

only be partially resected. Multiple tumors or inaccessible tumors may benefit from radiotherapy or radiosurgery.[79]

COLLOID CYSTS OF THE THIRD VENTRICLE

A colloid cyst is a rare congenital lesion derived from an outpouching of the ependyma at the site of the paraphysis. The cyst enlarges and contains a clear gelatinous substance. Symptoms occur when the cyst causes intermittent obstruction of the flow of CSF through the third ventricle. The patient experiences intermittent headache that is relieved by change in posture. Sudden death may occur.

An MRI or CT scan will show the presence of a midline cystic lesion in the third ventricle with associated hydrocephalus (Fig. 15–18). The treatment of

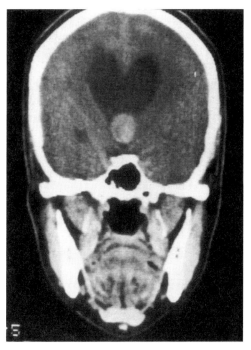

Figure 15–18
CT scan with enhancement. There is a midline colloid cyst in the third ventricle blocking the outflow from the lateral ventricles causing hydrocephalus.

choice is total surgical removal. If this is not possible, the cyst may be drained stereotactically or a bilateral ventricular shunting procedure may be necessary.

DERMOIDS AND EPIDERMOID CYSTS (PEARLY TUMORS)

Dermoids and epidermoid cysts are believed to result from incorporation of a portion of the ectoderm in the developing neural tube. The cysts have a thin capsule of epidermis or dermis and enlarge when desquamation occurs. Dermoid cysts may contain hair or sebaceous glands and are often calcified. They are usually associated with a dermal sinus or an occipital bone defect. The cysts are located in the midline in the posterior fossa, or in the cerebellar pontine angle, intra- and suprasellar region, or the lumbosacral region. Dermoid cysts occasionally develop in the temporal lobe of the brain. These tumors present as a slowly growing intracranial mass, producing partial or generalized seizures, and increased ICP. Cerebellopontine angle cysts present with symptoms suggesting an acoustic neuroma. Intra- and suprasellar dermoid cysts may compress the pituitary gland and cause hypopituitarism. An MRI scan is the procedure of choice. The CT scan shows a cystic lesion, often with negative density values. Peripheral calcification may be present. Total excision should be attempted whenever possible,[80] but dermoid and epidermoid cysts should be excised with care because contamination of the subarachnoid space can result in a severe chemical meningitis, which may be fatal.

CHORDOMA

Definition A *chordoma* is a congenital neoplasm that may arise wherever notochordal tissue is present during embryonic development.

Etiology and Pathology The chordoma is believed to arise from remnants of notochordal tissue and is most commonly located in the sacrococcygeal area or in the vicinity of the clivus. A rare variant of an intradural chordoma, arising from ectopic notochordal tissue, can occur in the prepontine region.[81]

The tumor appears as a whitish or reddish brown lobulated structure containing gelatinous material. In some areas, the cells are grossly distorted by vacuolation and have indistinct boundaries. These have been termed physaliphorous cells. This tumor has local invasive tendencies, and rarely metastasizes to the lung.

Clinical Features   The chordoma is most frequently encountered in the third to seventh decades and is twice as common in men. Signs and symptoms depend on the site of the tumor. When the tumor is in the area of the clivus, it may extend forward to the suprasellar region to involve the optic chiasm or laterally into the middle cranial fossa. There may be progressive cranial nerve involvement, usually beginning with the sixth cranial nerve and followed by hemiparesis or quadriparesis.

Diagnostic Procedures

1. Skull films may reveal sella enlargement, bony erosion, or calcification in the area of the tumor. Separation of the cranial sutures and enlargement of the skull can occur in children.
2. MRI and CT scans are required to clearly delineate the boundaries of the chordoma and to assist in the planning of radiation therapy.[82]

Treatment   Most tumors cannot be resected and should be treated by radiation therapy in an attempt to slow tumor growth. Partial resection by the transpharyngeal route, combined with retromastoid craniotomy, may be possible in selected cases. This should be followed by charged particle radiation therapy, which is only available in major centers. Combined treatment produces a local control rate of 63 percent at 5 years.[83]

ARACHNOID CYSTS

Definition   Arachnoid cysts are encapsulated cysts containing CSF lying within the arachnoid space. The cysts may cause compression of the brain or spinal cord.

Etiology and Pathology   The majority of arachnoid cysts are of developmental origin and result from failure of fusion of the two layers of the arachnoid in early fetal life, followed by accumulation of CSF and cyst formation. Between 20 and 30 percent of arachnoid cysts are associated with other congenital abnormalities, including aqueductal stenosis, agenesis of the corpus callosum, and hamartomas. A number of cases follow head trauma with herniation of the arachnoid between the two layers of the dura, resulting in cyst formation. It is also possible that arachnoid cysts develop after subarachnoid inflammation and the formation of arachnoid adhesions.

Arachnoid cysts are thin-walled structures bounded by arachnoid. The cyst compresses the brain or spinal cord, producing deformity and atrophy.

Clinical Features   Arachnoid cysts are more common in infants and young children and may present with a local bulging of the skull. The cysts may occur in any part of the cranial cavity but are somewhat more common in the posterior fossa. Older children and adults usually complain of increasing headache and other symptoms suggesting an expanding intracranial mass lesion.

Arachnoid cysts of the spinal canal are usually located posteriorly and produce progressive paraparesis without pain. Examination shows a well-demarcated sensory level at the site of compression.

Diagnostic Procedures

1. Radiography of the skull may reveal asymmetry and local bulging and thinning of the bone.
2. The MRI and CT scans reveal a lucent area with the density of CSF and a clearly defined border (Fig. 15–19).
3. Arachnoid cysts in infants may be demonstrated by ultrasound.

Treatment   Treatment consists of cyst peritoneal shunting when cyst compression is present. Many cases require a ventricular peritoneal shunting procedure because of associated hydrocephalus.

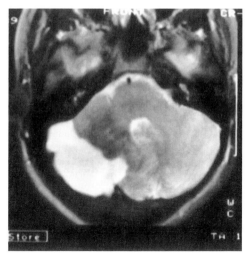

Figure 15–19
MRI scan. There is a large arachnoid cyst compressing the right cerebellar hemisphere.

LYMPHOMA

Primary lymphoma of the CNS has increased in incidence in the last decade. This increase can be explained in part by the rising number of immunosuppressed individuals who are receiving immunosuppressant drugs after organ transplantation or from infection by the human immunodeficiency virus.

Pathology   Most primary CNS lymphomas are almost exclusively large B-cell lymphomas.[84]

Clinical Features   Most primary lymphomas of the CNS are parenchymal lesions that involve the deep white matter and basal ganglia and are a frequent complication of HIV-1 infection in children and adults with AIDS.[85] These lesions are often periventricular and may be multifocal. Posterior fossa involvement occurs in approximately 15 percent of patients and isolated spinal cord lymphoma is rare.[86] Leptomeningeal involvement occurs in 42 percent of cases.[87]

Diagnostic Procedures

1. The MRI scan shows isointensity on T1- and T2-weighted images with intense enhancement after intravenous administration of gadolinium.

2. The CT scan shows an intensely enhancing parenchymal mass.

3. The CSF contains a mononuclear pleocytosis and increased protein content. The fluid should be examined by flow cytometry for the presence of abnormal lymphocytes. The fluid should also be examined for tumor markers, including β_2- microglobulin.

Treatment   Short intensive primary chemotherapy, followed by whole brain radiation therapy, is recommended.[88]

METASTATIC BRAIN TUMOR

Definition   More than 100,000 cancer patients develop brain metastases each year in the United States. The most common primary site is the lung and 10 percent of bronchial carcinomas present with neurological symptoms before evidence of lung involvement appears. Other common primary sites for brain metastasis are cancer of the breast and malignant melanoma. Metastatic brain tumors are most frequent in the sixth and seventh decades.[89]

Etiology and Pathology   The great majority of metastases reach the CNS through the arterial system. A smaller number arise by direct extension from extracranial sites such as the pharynx, neck, or paranasal sinuses. There is a theoretical pathway from the pelvis through the vertebral venous plexus, but it is doubtful that metastases in the brain originate in this manner. Most metastatic tumors develop in the cerebral hemispheres in the distribution of the middle cerebral artery at the junction of the gray and white matter. Approximately 35 percent of metastatic brain tumors arise from a primary lung tumor, 20 percent are associated with carcinoma of the breast, and 10 percent from melanomatous tumors of the skin, with a further 10 percent from gastrointestinal carcinoma,

5 percent from carcinoma of the kidney, and the remainder from the genitourinary system and the endocrine glands. Most metastases present as multiple spherical gray-pink tumors with sharply defined margins but without encapsulation, and are typically associated with large areas of edema in the surrounding brain (Fig. 15-20). It is not unusual to see a small tumor measuring 1 cm in diameter associated with massive cerebral edema. This edema is believed to arise as a transudate from abnormal capillaries within the tumor. Massive hemorrhage into tumors is rare and usually occurs with melanoma.

It is not always possible to determine the location of the primary lesion from the study of histological characteristics of a metastatic tumor.

Clinical Features   Most metastatic tumors present with headache and partial or generalized seizures. Other signs and symptoms depend on the location of

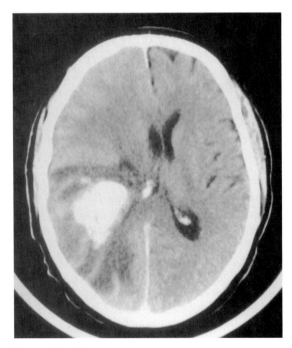

Figure 15-20
CT scan with contrast enhancement showing a metastatic tumor with prominent edema, an area of hemorrhage, marked displacement of the middle structures, and obliteration of the posterior horn of the right lateral ventricle.

the tumor and the rapidity of development of the tumor (Table 15-1).

Diagnostic Procedures

1.   An MRI scan is the procedure of choice in metastatic disease (Fig. 15-21). The MRI scan is more sensitive than the CT scan and will often reveal multiple metastases that have escaped detection by CT scanning (Fig. 15-22).

2.   A CT scan should be performed with both nonenhancing and contrast-enhanced studies. If only one scan can be performed, a contrast-enhanced scan is recommended, although it is not possible to differentiate between hemorrhage or tumor enhancement in contrast-enhanced scans. Metastatic tumors most often appear as high-density nodular or spherical masses, often surrounded by frond-like areas of lucency representing edema. There is increased density on contrast enhancement, often appearing as a ring-shaped area.

3.   Radiographs of the chest will reveal one or more lesions indicating the presence of primary or metastatic tumors in the lung, in most cases.

4.   The presence of carcinoembryonic antigen (CEA) in the CSF in a patient with a solitary mass le-

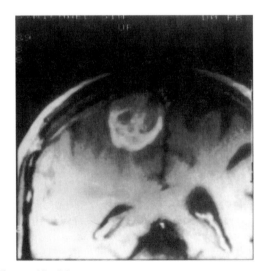

Figure 15-21
MRI scan. There is a well-defined metastatic tumor in the right parietal area.

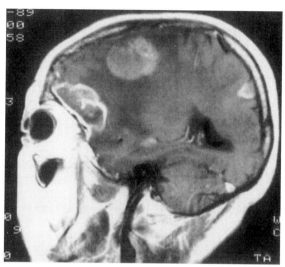

Figure 15–22
MRI scan with enhancement. There are multiple metastatic tumors.

sion in the brain suggests the tumor is metastatic in origin.

Treatment

1. Edema can be controlled by corticosteroids such as dexamethasone (Decadron) 12 mg initially followed by 4 mg q6h. A more rapid reduction of ICP using intravenous mannitol is indicated when there is marked shift of the midline structures with the possibility of herniation.

2. Solitary metastasis can be excised when the primary lesion can be successfully treated or when the symptoms produced by the lesion are incapacitating.[90]

3. Stereotactic radiosurgery is the treatment of choice in asymptomatic or mildly symptomatic patients with small, solitary lesions.[91] This should be followed by whole brain radiation.[92]

4. Whole brain radiation therapy is the treatment of choice for multiple metastases because many are sensitive to radiation. Symptoms usually improve after radiation therapy and survival time may increase.

5. Chemotherapy will frequently produce re-

gression of brain metastasis in chemosensitive tumors.

Prognosis Current available treatments produce effective palliation of neurological symptoms and extension of life and most patients do not die of their brain metastases.[93]

MENINGEAL CARCINOMATOSIS

Meningeal carcinomatosis is the least common form of intracranial metastatic disease and is usually associated with a well-differentiated primary carcinoma of breast or lung. The remaining cases are usually associated with carcinoma of the lung, stomach, and pancreas and malignant melanoma.

The meninges appear dull, gray, and hazy and show the presence of numerous tumor cells and an inflammatory reaction.

Clinical Features The disorder is uncommon but not rare. Symptoms include headache, changes in mentation, signs of meningeal irritation, and cranial nerve palsies, particularly paralysis of the ocular, motor, and facial nerves. Spinal cord involvement with radicular pain or paresthesias is an occasional presentation.

Diagnostic Procedures

1. Lumbar puncture usually reveals a clear CSF under increased pressure with a slight lymphocytic pleocytosis, moderately elevated protein content, and a marked reduction of glucose content. The presence of tumor cells can be demonstrated by a filter technique. The CEA level in the CSF is elevated in patients with meningeal carcinomatosis due to cancer of the breast, lung, alimentary tract, and genitourinary tract. The CEA level may be of value in monitoring response to treatment and relapse.

2. The CSF lactate dehydrogenase levels often show marked elevation in meningeal carcinomatosis. Similar elevation can occur in bacterial meningitis, but the test may be useful in suspected cases of meningeal carcinomatosis.

3. The MRI scan is usually normal but may

show some enhancement of the meninges in some cases and is probably more useful for detecting the presence of unsuspected metastatic lesions elsewhere in the neuraxis.

Differential Diagnosis Meningeal carcinomatosis must be differentiated from all forms of chronic meningitis, including tuberculous meningitis, fungal meningitis, syphilis, sarcoidosis, and lymphoma involving the CNS.

Treatment Irradiation and intrathecal methotrexate are the only available means of treating meningeal carcinomatosis. Most patients show progressive deterioration, but adequate treatment may provide a period of useful remission. Corticosteroids may provide some symptomatic improvement.

TUMORS OF THE SPINAL CORD AND SPINAL CANAL

Tumors of the spinal cord and spinal canal are uncommon, with an annual incidence of between 0.9 to 2.5/100,000 population. The most common tumor is the neuroma,[94] followed by meningioma,[95] glioma, and arteriovenous malformation. Approximately 25 percent of tumors arise in the cervical canal, 55 percent originate in the area of the thoracic canal, and 25 percent arise in the lumbosacral area. Twenty percent are extradural, 50 percent are extradural and intradural, and 30 percent are intradural. Tumors occur at all ages, but congenital tumors tend to occur with increasing frequency in infants and children.

Clinical Features

1. Pain. Most patients with spinal cord tumor present with pain caused by nerve root irritation. This is particularly common in extradural tumors and is frequently misdiagnosed as cervical spondylosis or herniated intravertebral disc. The pain is frequently exacerbated by coughing, sneezing, or straining. Root pains are less common with intramedullary tumors but have been reported. The association of root pain with asymmetry of reflexes and insidious onset is strongly suggestive of spinal cord tumor.

2. Motor weakness. Root pains may be followed by the development of weakness and wasting of the muscles supplied by the affected nerve root. Extension of an extramedullary tumor may produce pressure on the anterior horn cells at several segments in the spinal cord, with gradual increase in focal muscle weakness, wasting, and fasciculations. Compression of the corticospinal tracts produces weakness and spasticity below the level of the lesion. This usually takes the form of progressive spastic paraparesis. However, tumors of the cervical medullary junction may present with an ascending flaccid paralysis resembling the Guillain-Barré syndrome.[96]

3. Sensory change. Many patients experience a dysesthesia in the limbs below the level of the lesion. This is often described as a feeling of temperature change, particularly a feeling of cold. Examination shows a dissociated sense of loss in about one-third of cases. This type of sensory loss is likely to occur in intramedullary tumors but is not confined to this type and can be seen with extramedullary tumors.

4. Sphincter disturbances. Tumors affecting the cervical, thoracic, and upper lumbar spinal cord produce early symptoms of sphincter dysfunction with increasing frequency and urgency of micturition. Rectal disturbances tend to occur somewhat later in most cases. Tumors of the lower lumbar cord and the conus medullaris destroy the parasympathetic neurons responsible for bladder control. This results in retention of urine with overflow incontinence. The development of sphincter disturbances is frequently followed by impotence in men.

5. Syringomyelia. Some intramedullary tumors, particularly ependymomas and hemangioblastomas, are associated with syringomyelia. Astrocytomas are less likely to present in this fashion. Intramedullary spinal cord metastases are a relatively rare cause of syringomyelia.[97] The tumor is likely to lie above rather than below the syrinx and the higher the spinal cord level of involvement, the more likely the presence of the syrinx.[98] The tumor or syrinx may produce destruction of the decussating lateral spinal thalamic fibers in the center of the spinal cord, with loss of pain and temperature sensation below the level

of the lesion on one or both sides of the body. This is often coupled with pressure on the descending corticospinal tracts and progressive spastic paraparesis. Anterior extension of the tumor involves the anterior horn cells at the level of the lesion and results in muscle weakness, wasting, and fasciculations in the muscles supplied by the anterior horn cells.

6. Brown-Sequard-like symptoms. Involvement of one-half of the spinal cord produces a characteristic constellation of symptoms known as the Brown-Sequard syndrome. This consists of progressive weakness, increased tone, clonus, increased reflexes, and an extensor plantar response on the same side below the level of the lesion. Dissociated sensory loss occurs on the contralateral side with impairment of pain and temperature sensations. Posterior common involvement produces ipsilateral loss of vibration and position sense. The Brown-Sequard syndrome is much more common in extramedullary tumors, which are usually benign and operable.

7. Papilledema. Some cases of spinal cord tumor are associated with papilledema. The reason for this development is not clear. It has been postulated that the high protein content of the CSF stimulates increased production of CSF, resulting in papilledema, but this cannot be the sole explanation for this phenomenon. Papilledema is more likely to occur in spinal cord ependymomas but has been described with both intramedullary and extramedullary tumors of other types. The occurrence of papilledema is much more common with tumors of the thoracic and lumbosacral regions.

8. Subarachnoid hemorrhage. Most cases of spinal subarachnoid hemorrhage are secondary to an arteriovenous malformation. The second most likely cause is bleeding from an ependymoma. Spinal hemangioblastomas are a rare cause of subarachnoid hemorrhage because hemangioblastoma is rarely encountered in the spinal cord, but 50 percent can cause subarachnoid hemorrhage.[99]

9. Intramedullary hemorrhage. Intramedullary hemorrhage is usually a complication of an arteriovenous malformation and is a rare event in spinal cord tumors, including astrocytomas, ependymomas, and hemangioblastomas. The majority present as a subarachnoid hemorrhage, but intramedullary hemor-

rhage from a hemangioblastoma may present with acute paraplegia.[100]

The clinical features of spinal cord tumors at different levels include:

1. Upper cervical cord. There is usually involvement of the lower cranial nerves if the tumor extends up through the foramen magnum. A progressive spastic quadriparesis and a positive Lhermitte's sign may be seen. Nystagmus is not unusual, due to involvement of the medial longitudinal fasciculus, which descends from the medulla into the upper cervical cord. Pressure on the vertebral arteries as they ascend over the ventral surface of the medulla may lead to intermittent symptoms of vertebral basilar insufficiency. Patients may experience pain and stiffness of the neck with an abnormal posture of the head. Obstruction of the flow of the CSF at the level of the foramen magnum can lead to hydrocephalus and raised ICP with papilledema.

2. The lower cervical cord. Atrophy of the small muscles of the hand caused by an anteriorly placed meningioma has been reported in tumors at the level of the foramen magnum, due to pressure on the anterior spinal artery, with ischemia of the anterior horn cells in the lower cervical cord. Intramedullary and extramedullary tumors of the lower cervical area produce weakness and increased tone below the level of the tumor, often presenting with progressive spastic paraparesis associated with increased sphincter disturbances. Sensory examination may show the presence of abnormal sensation up to the level of the tumor on both sides of the body. Extramedullary tumors tend to produce a Brown-Sequard syndrome and unilateral Horner syndrome due to involvement of the sympathetic outflow from the lower cervical and upper thoracic cord.

3. Thoracic cord lesions. Most thoracic cord tumors produce severe root pain that radiates in a girdle fashion around the chest or upper abdomen. This is associated with progressive spastic paraparesis and bladder dysfunction. Examination may show a sensory level and Horner syndrome with lesions of the upper thoracic cord.

4. Lumbosacral tumors. Tumors in this area usually present with severe root pain followed by

sphincter disturbances of the bladder and rectum. Men are impotent. Examination shows the presence of flaccid paralysis in the lower extremities with loss of tendon reflexes. There may be sensory loss in the "saddle" area. Tumors in the lumbosacral area can mimic a herniated lumbar disc with production of typical sciatic pain. This occurs with neuromas, meningiomas, and gliomas in the lower lumbosacral cord. Intramedullary lesions of the lumbar portion of the cord may produce flaccid paralysis on one side and evidence of spasticity with increased tendon reflexes and an extensor plantar response on the opposite side.

Diagnostic Procedures

1. The MRI scan is the method of choice in the diagnosis of tumors involving the spinal cord and spinal canal. The extraordinary detail obtained in the sagittal axial or coronal sections of the spinal canal and spinal cord has replaced other procedures or relegated them to second choice (Fig. 15–23). Both unenhanced and enhanced scans should be obtained in all patients with spinal cord tumor. Intramedullary ependymomas and hemangioblastomas show isodense or slightly hyperintense T1-weighted images, but T2-weighted images are hyperintense for hemangioblastoma; ependymomas do not exhibit enhancement. High-resolution imaging of the spinal cord in multiple planes, using T1- and T2-weighted images and gadolinium enhancement, clearly defines intradural extramedullary lesions. Neuromas appear isointense on T1-weighted images, hyperintense on T2-weighted images, and give an intense homogenous signal after gadolinium infusion. Meningiomas appear isointense to the spinal cord on T1- and T2-weighted images but show increased intensity after gadolinium fusion. Axial MRI scans are essential in determining the relationship of the tumor to the spinal cord.[101]

2. Radiography of the cervical spine. The presence of spinal cord tumor may lead to widening of the spinal canal and extramedullary tumors may erode the posterior aspect of the vertebral bodies. Neuromas may produce unilateral enlargement of the intravertebral foramina; neuromas, meningiomas, and metastatic tumors frequently erode the pedicles and

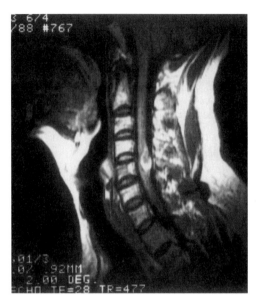

Figure 15–23
MRI scan of the spinal cord, which shows widening of the spinal cord at the fifth cervical segment containing an area of increased signal intensity in a patient with a spinal cord glioma.

laminae. Congenital tumors in children are frequently accompanied by abnormal curvature of the spine. Calcification is unusual but may occasionally occur in some spinal cord tumors. Malignant extradural tumors frequently produce bone destruction, but more benign tumors, such as meningioma, rarely produce new bone formation, unlike meningiomas in the cranial cavity.

3. Myelography. In most cases, a myelogram will locate a spinal cord tumor and differentiate between an intramedullary and extramedullary tumor. The combination of CT and myelography using a water-soluble contrast material is particularly helpful in the diagnosis of spinal cord tumors.

4. Electromyography. Extramedullary tumors tend to be associated with unilateral denervation, which can be detected by electromyography. Bilateral denervation at the same level suggests the presence of an intramedullary tumor.

5. Angiography. Selective angiography of the spinal arteries is particularly useful in the diagnosis

of arteriovenous malformations. Arteriography is not usually required for the diagnosis of other tumors.

6. Lumbar puncture. This procedure has become redundant in most cases because of MRI scanning but is used for the introduction of contrast material for myelography when the following observations can be made. Extramedullary and intramedullary tumors are likely to produce some change in pressure dynamics, ranging from a slow rise in pressure following insertion of the needle to a failure to register any increase in pressure, and a negative Queckenstedt test (see Chap. 16) indicating a block in the spinal subarachnoid space. In these cases, the fluid is likely to be xanthochromic and the protein content markedly elevated. It is usual, however, to find some increase in the protein content of the CSF even when there is no obstruction of the spinal subarachnoid space.

Differential Diagnosis There are no clinical signs exclusively found with intramedullary tumors rather than extramedullary tumors. The presence of root pain and ascending segmental sensory loss occurs more often with extramedullary tumors than with intramedullary tumors. Fasciculations and descending dissociate sensory loss are more characteristic of an intramedullary tumor.

The association of root pain with hyperesthesia to pinprick and weakness of muscles supplied by the same nerve root is strongly suggestive of a neuroma. Meningiomas tend to produce bilateral root pain and paresthesias, followed by unilateral then bilateral motor disturbances.

Treatment Extramedullary tumors should be removed surgically with total excision, if possible. Patients with intramedullary astrocytomas have a 10-year survival rate of 50 percent, whether treated by gross total resection or subtotal resection, or biopsy followed by postoperative radiation therapy in each category.[102] Pilocytic astrocytomas have a better prognosis than nonpilocytic astrocytomas.[103] Spinal ependymomas are usually tumors of low malignancy that can be totally removed. Malignant spinal ependymomas are unusual but carry a poor prognosis. Recurrent low-grade ependymomas should be treated by further surgical ex-

cision and radiotherapy, but recurrence carries a poor prognosis. Surgery has little impact on the course and poor prognosis for anaplastic gliomas.[104] Hemangioblastomas should be removed totally whenever possible, using microsurgical techniques.[105]

Prognosis The prognosis of spinal cord tumors varies according to the histologic type and the degree of malignancy. If all spinal cord tumors are considered, approximately 66 percent of the patients survive 5 years following diagnosis and treatment. Most neuromas and meningiomas can be excised, and patients have a life expectancy corresponding to that of the general population.[106] However, 80 percent of patients have residual complaints following excision of a neuroma, including local pain, radiating pain, paraparesis, sensory deficits, and impaired bladder function. Congenital tumors in children, including dermoids, epidermoids, lipomas, and teratomas, have a good prognosis, although residual neurological deficits, including muscle wasting and weakness of lower limbs and urinary incontinence, persist.

REFERENCES

1. Grabb PA, Kelly DR, Fulmer BB, et al: Radiation-induced glioma of the spinal cord. *Pediatr Neurosurg* 25:214, 1996.
2. Starshak RJ: Radiation-induced meningioma in children: report of two cases and review of the literature. *Pediatr Radiol* 26:537, 1996.
3. Harrison MJ, Wolfe DE, Lau TS, et al: Radiation induced meningiomas: experiences at the Mount Sinai Hospital and review of the literature. *J Neurosurg* 75:564, 1991.
4. Newton HB: Primary brain tumors: review of etiology, diagnosis and treatment. *Am Family Physician* 49:787, 1994.
5. Detta A, Kenny BG, Smith C, et al: Correlation of proto-oncogene expression and proliferation in meningiomas. *Neurosurgery* 33:1065, 1993.
6. Ng HK, Lam PY: The molecular genetics of central nervous system tumors. *Pathology* 30:196, 1998
7. Biegel JA: Genetics of pediatric central nervous system tumors. *J Pediatr Hematol/Oncol* 19:492, 1997.
8. Linskey ME, Gilbert MR: Glial differentiation: a review with implications for new directions in neuro-oncology. *Neurosurgery* 36:1, 1995.

9. Bruner JM: Neuropathology of malignant gliomas. *Semin Oncol* 21:126, 1994.
10. Packer RJ, Vezina G: Pediatric glial neoplasms including brain-stem gliomas. *Semin Oncol* 21:260, 1994.
11. Krouwer HG, Davis RL, Silver R, et al: Gemistocytic astrocytomas: a reappraisal. *J Neurosurg* 79:399, 1991.
12. Campbell JW, Pollack IF: Cerebellar astrocytomas in children. *J Neuro-Oncol* 28:223, 1996.
13. MacDonald DR: Low-grade gliomas, mixed gliomas, and oligodendrogliomas. *Semin Oncol* 21:236, 1994.
14. Fernandez PM, Brem S: Malignant brain tumors in the elderly. *Clin Geriatr Med* 13:327, 1997.
15. Vezina LG: Diagnostic imaging in neuro-oncology. *Pediatr Clin N Am* 44:701, 1997.
16. Byrd SE, Tomita T, Palka PS, et al: Magnetic resonance spectroscopy (MRS) in the evaluation of pediatric brain tumors, Part 1: introduction to MRS. *J Natl Med Assoc* 88:649, 1996.
17. Chaudhuri K-R, Jager R, Bridger J, et al: Hemiplegia in pregnancy due to metastatic angiosarcoma. *Eur Neurol* 34:295, 1994.
18. Sawaya R, Hammoud M, Schoppa D, et al: Neurosurgical outcome in a modern series of 400 craniotomies for treatment of parenchymal tumors. *Neurosurgery* 42:1044, 1998.
19. Haglund MM, Berger MS, Hochman DW: Enhanced optical imaging of human gliomas and tumor margins. *Neurosurgery* 38:308, 1996.
20. Albert FK, Forsting M, Sartor K, et al: Early postoperative magnetic resonance imaging after resection of malignant glioma: objective evaluation of residual tumor and its influence on regrowth and prognosis. *Neurosurgery* 34:45, 1994.
21. Landy HJ, Feun L, Schwade JG, et al: Retreatment of intracranial gliomas. *South Med J* 87:211, 1994.
22. Larson DA, Gutin PH, Leibel SA, et al: Stereotactic irradiation of brain tumors. *Cancer* 65:792, 1990.
23. Lesser, GJ, Grossman S: The chemotherapy of high-grade astrocytomas. *Semin Oncol* 21:220, 1994.
24. Fine HA, Dear KB, Loeffler JS, et al: Meta-analysis of radiation therapy with and without adjuvant chemotherapy for malignant gliomas in adults. *Cancer* 71:2585, 1993.
25. Pech IV, Peterson K, Cairncross JG: Chemotherapy for brain tumors. *Oncology* 12:537, 1998.
26. Sipos EP, Brem H: New delivery system for brain tumor therapy. *Neurol Clin* 13:813, 1995.
27. Kroll RA, Neuwelt EA: Outwitting the blood-brain barrier for therapeutic purposes: osmotic openings and other means. *Neurosurg* 42: 1083, 1998.
28. Laperriere NJ, Bernstein M: Radiotherapy for brain tumors. *CA Cancer J Clin* 44:96, 1994.
29. Lamb SA: Radiation therapy options for management of the brain tumor patient. *Crit Care Nurs Clin North Am* 7:103, 1995.
30. Leibel, SA, Scott CB, Loeffler JS: Contemporary approaches to the treatment of malignant gliomas with radiation therapy. *Semin Oncol* 21:198, 1994.
31. Kalapurakal JA, Thomas PR: Pediatric radiotherapy An overview. *Radiol Clin North Am* 35:1265, 1997.
32. Young RF: The role of the gamma knife in the treatment of malignant primary and metastatic brain tumors. *CA Cancer J Clin* 48:177, 1998.
33. Roman DD, Sperduto PW: Neuropsychological effects of cranial radiation: current knowledge and future directions. *Int J Radiol Oncol Biol Phys* 31:983, 1995.
34. Glass J, Hochberg FH, Gruber ML, et al: The treatment of oligodendrogliomas and mixed oligodendroglioma astrocytomas with P.V.C. chemotherapy. *J Neurosurg* 76:741, 1992.
35. Oppenheim JS, Strauss RC, Mormino J, et al: Ependymomas of the third ventricle. *Neurosurgery* 34:350, 1994.
36. McLaughlin MP, Marcus RB Jr, Buatti JM, et al: Ependymoma: results, prognostic factors, and treatment recommendations. *Int J Radiation Oncol Biol Phys* 40:845, 1998.
37. Arico M, Raiteri E, Bossi G, et al: Choroid plexus carcinoma: report of one case with favorable response to treatment. *Med Pediatr Oncol* 22:274, 1994.
38. Aronica PA, Ahdab-Barmada M, Rozin L, et al: Sudden death in an adolescent boy due to a colloid cyst of the third ventricle. *Am J Forensic Med Pathol* 19:119, 1998.
39. Mamourian AC, Cromwell LD, Harbaugh RE: Colloid cyst of the third ventricle: sometimes more conspicuous on CT than MRI. *AJNR Am J Neuroradiol* 19:875, 1998.
40. Rhodes RH, Cole M, Takaoka Y, et al. Intraventricular cerebral neuroblastoma: analysis of subtypes and comparison with hemisphere neuroblastoma. *Arch Path Lab Med* 118:897, 1994.
41. Rorke LB: Experimental production of primitive neuroectodermal tumors and its relevance to human neuro-oncology. *Am J Pathol* 144:444, 1994.
42. Gusnard DA: Cerebellar neoplasms in children. *Semin Roentgenol* 25:263, 1990.
43. Tait DM, Thornton-Jones H, Bloom HJG, et al: Adjuvant chemotherapy for medulloblastoma: the first multicenter control trial of the International Society of Pediatric Oncology (SIOPI). *Eur J Cancer* 26:464, 1990.
44. Scheurlen W, Kuhl J: Current diagnostic and thera-

peutic management of CNS metastasis in childhood primitive neuroectodermal tumors and ependymomas. *J Neuro-Oncol* 38:181, 1998.

45. Shiminski-Maher T, Wisoff JH: Pediatric brain tumors. *Crit Care Nurs Clin North Am* 7:159, 1995.

46. Balter-Seri J, Mor C, Shuper A, et al: Cure of recurrent medulloblastoma: the contribution of surgical resection at relapse. *Cancer* 79:1241, 1997.

47. Raisanen JM, Davis RL: Congenital brain tumors. *Pathology* 2:103, 1993.

48. Fuller BG, Kapp DL, Lox R: Radiation therapy of pineal region tumors: 25 new cases with review of 208 previously reported cases. *Int J Radiat Oncol Biol Phys* 28:229, 1994.

49. Kirikac M, Arai H, Hidaka T, et al: Pineal yolk sac tumor in a 65-year-old man. *Surg Neurol* 42:253, 1994.

50. Donahue B, Allen J, Siffert J, et al: Patterns of recurrence in brainstem gliomas: evidence for craniospinal dissemination. *Int J Radiat Oncol Biol Phys* 40:677, 1998.

51. Pollack IF, Hurtt M, Pang D, et al: Dissemination of low grade intracranial astrocytomas in children. *Cancer* 73:2869, 1994.

52. Pollack IF: Brain tumors in children. *N Engl J Med* 331:1500, 1994.

53. Hildebrand J, Dewitte O, Dietrich PY, et al: Management of malignant brain tumors. *Euro Neurol* 38:238, 1997.

54. Aron DC, Tyrell JB, Wilson CB: Pituitary tumors. Current concepts in diagnosis and management. *West Med J* 162:340, 1995.

55. Mercado-Asis, Oldfield EH, Cutler GB: Pituitary tumor hemorrhage in Cushing disease. *Ann Intern Med* 122:189, 1995.

56. Della Casa S, Corsello SM, Satta MA, et al: Intracranial and spinal dissemination of an ACTH secreting pituitary neoplasia. Case report and review of the literature. *Ann Endocrinol (Paris)* 58:503, 1997.

57. Samuels MH: Advances in diagnosing and managing pituitary adenomas. *West J Med* 162:371, 1995.

58. Colombo N, Loli P, Vignati F, et al: MR of corticotrophin-secreting pituitary microadenomas. *AJNR Am J Neuroradiol* 15:1591, 1994.

59. Girard N, Brue T, Chambert-Orsini V, et al: 3D-FT thin section MRI of prolactin secreting pituitary microadenomas. *Neuroradiology* 36:376, 1994.

60. Molitch ME: Evaluation and treatment of the patient with a pituitary incidentaloma. *J Clin Endocrinol Metab* 80:3, 1995.

61. Kovacs K, Stephaneanu L, Horvath E, et al: Prolactin-producing pituitary tumor: resistance to dopamine agonist therapy. Case report. *J Neurosurg* 82:886, 1995.

62. Osman IA, James RA, Chatterjee S, et al: Factors determining the long-term outcome of surgery for acromegaly. *Q J Med* 87:617, 1994.

63. Donovan LE, Corenblum B: The natural history of pituitary incidentaloma. *Arch Intern Med* 155:181, 1995.

64. Pulst SM, Rouleau GA, Marineau C, et al: Familial meningioma is not allelic to neurofibromatosis 2. *Neurology* 43:2096, 1993.

65. Markopoulos C, Sampalis F, Givalos N, et al: Association of breast cancer with meningioma. *Eur J Surg Oncol* 24:332, 1998.

66. Carpeggiani P, Crisi G, Trevisan C: MRI of intracranial meningiomas: correlations with histology and physical consistency. *Neuroradiology* 35:532, 1993.

67. Goldsmith BJ, Wara WM, Wilson CB, et al: Postoperative irradiation for subtotally resected meningiomas. A retrospective analysis of 140 patients treated from 1967 to 1990. *J Neurosurg* 80:195, 1994.

68. Gillman GS, Parnes LS: Acoustic neuroma management. A six-year review. *J Otolaryngol* 24:191, 1995.

69. Samii M, Matthies C: Management of 1000 vestibular schwannomas (acoustic neuromas): surgical management and results with an emphasis on complications and how to avoid them. *Neurosurgery* 40:11, 1997.

70. Pollock BE, Lunsford LD, Kondziolka D, et al: Outcome analysis of acoustic neuroma management: a comparison of microsurgery and stereotactic radiosurgery. *Neurosurgery* 36:215, 1995.

71. Haddad GF, al-Mefty O: The road less travelled: transtemporal access to the CPA. *Clin Neurosurg* 41:150, 1994.

72. Leonetii JP: The diagnosis and management of acoustic neuromas: contemporary practice guidelines. *Comp Ther* 21:68, 1995.

73. Hald JK, Eldevik OP, Brunberg JA, et al: Craniopharyngiomas. The utility of contrast medium enhancement for MR imaging at 1.5 T. *Acta Radiol* 35:520, 1994.

74. Weiner HL, Wisoff JH, Rosenberg ME, et al: Craniopharyngiomas: a clinicopathological analysis of factors predictive of recurrence and functional outcome. *Neurosurgery* 35:1001, 1994.

75. Meacham LR, Ghim TT, Crocker IR, et al: Systematic approach for detection of endocrine disorders in children treated for brain tumors. *Med Pediatr Oncol* 29:86, 1997.

76. Oka M, Kawano N, Suwa T, et al: Radiological study of symptomatic Rathke's cleft cysts. *Neurosurgery* 35:632, 1994.

77. Wizigmann-Voos S, Plate KH: Pathology, genetics, and cell biology of hemangioblastomas. *Histol Histopathol* 11:1049, 1996.

78. Minami M, Hanakita J, Suwa H, et al: Cervical hemangioblastoma with past history of subarachnoid hemorrhage. *Surg Neurol* 49:278, 1998.

79. Chandler HC, Friedman WA: Radiosurgical treatment of a hemangioblastoma: case report. *Neurosurgery* 34:353, 1994.

80. Nassar SI, Haddad FS, Abdo A: Epidermoid tumors of the fourth ventricle. *Surg Neurol* 43:246, 1995.

81. Tashiro T, Fukuda T, Nemoto Y, et al: Intradural chordoma: case report and review of the literature. *Neuroradiology* 36:313, 1994.

82. Tai P, Craighead P, Bagdon F: Optimization of radiotherapy for patients with cranial chordoma. A review of dose-response ratios for photon techniques. *Cancer* 75:749, 1995.

83. Habrand IL, Austin-Seymour M, Birnbaum S, et al: Neurovisual outcome following proton radiation therapy. *Int J Radiat Oncol Biol Phys* 29:647, 1989.

84. Miller DC: Hochberg FH, Harris NL, et al: Pathology with clinical correlations of primary central nervous system non-Hodgkin lymphoma. *Cancer* 74:1383, 1994.

85. Goldstein H, Dickson DW, Rubinstein A, et al: Primary CNS lymphoma in a pediatric patient with acquired immunodeficiency syndrome. Treatment with radiation. *Cancer* 66:2503, 1990.

86. Schild SE, Wharen RE Jr., Menke DM, et al: Primary lymphoma of the spinal cord. *Mayo Clin Proc* 70:256, 1995.

87. Balmaceda C, Gaynor JJ, Sun M, et al: Leptomeningeal tumor in primary central nervous system lymphoma: recognition, significance and implications. *Ann Neurol* 38:202, 1995.

88. Brada M, Hjiyiannakis D, Hines F, et al: Short intensive primary chemotherapy and radiotherapy in sporadic primary CNS lymphoma (PCL). *Int J Radiat Oncol Biol Phys* 40:1157, 1998.

89. Routh A, Khansur T, Hickman BT, et al: Management of brain metastases: past, present and future. *South Med J* 87:1218, 1994.

90. Nakagawa H, Miyawaki Y, Fujita T, et al: Surgical treatment of brain metastases of lung cancer: retrospective study analysis of 89 cases. *J Neurol Neurosurg Psychiatry* 57:950, 1994.

91. Loeffler JS, Shrieve DC: What is appropriate therapy for a patient with a single brain metastasis? *Int J Radiat Oncol Biol Phys* 29:915, 1994.

92. O'Neill BP, Buckner JC, Coffey RJ, et al: Subspecial-ity clinics: neurology. Brain metastatic lesions. *Mayo Clin Proc* 69:1062, 1994.

93. Patchell RA: Metastatic brain tumors. *Neurol Clin* 13:915, 1995.

94. Newton HB, Newton CL, Gatens C, et al: Spinal cord tumors: review of etiology, diagnosis, and multidisciplinary approaches to treatment. *Cancer Practice* 3:207, 1995.

95. Roux FX, Nataf F, Pinaudeau M, et al: Intraspinal meningiomas: review of 54 cases with discussion of poor prognosis factors and modern therapeutic management. *Surg Neurol* 46:458, 1996.

96. Beards SC, Robertson LJ, Jackson A, et al: Malignant astrocytoma of the cervico-medullary junction masquerading as Guillain-Barré syndrome. *Postgrad Med J* 70:499, 1994.

97. Keung YK, Cobos E, Whitehead RP, et al: Secondary syringomyelia due to intramedullary spinal cord metastases. Case report and review of literature. *Am J Clin Oncol* 20:577, 1997.

98. Samii M, Klekamp J: Surgical results of 100 intramedullary tumors in relation to accompanying syringomyelia. *Neurosurgery* 35:865, 1994.

99. Neumann HP, Eggert HR, Weigel K, et al: Hemangioblastomas of the central nervous system. A 10-year study with special reference to von Hippel-Lindau syndrome. *J Neurosurg* 70:24, 1989.

100. Yu JS, Short MP, Schumacher J, et al: Intramedullary hemorrhage in spinal hemangioblastoma. *J Neurosurg* 81:937, 1994.

101. Souweidane MM, Benjamin V: Spinal cord meningiomas. *Neurosurg Clin North Am* 5:283, 1994.

102. Cristante L, Herrman HD: Surgical management of intramedullary spinal cord tumors: functional outcome and sources of morbidity. *Neurosurgery* 35:69, 1994.

103. Minehan KJ, Shaw EG, Scheithauer BW, et al: Spinal cord astrocytoma: pathological and treatment considerations. *J Neurosurg* 83:590, 1995.

104. Batra SK, Rasheed BKA, Bigner SH, et al: Oncogenes and anti-oncogenes in human nervous system tumors. *Lab Invest* 71:621, 1994.

105. Xu QW, Bao WM, Mao RL, et al: Magnetic resonance imaging and microsurgical treatment of intramedullary hemangioblastoma of the spinal cord. *Neurosurgery* 35:671, 1994.

106. Seppala MT, Haltia MJJ, Sankila RJ, et al: Long-term outcome after removal of spinal Schwannoma: a clinicopathological study of 187 cases. *J Neurosurg* 83:621, 1995.

Chapter 16

INFECTIOUS DISEASES

Infectious diseases of the nervous system may result from a wide variety of agents. These include bacteria, rickettsiae, fungi, protozoa, viruses, and slow viruses. Early recognition of infection and identification of the source are necessary for effective management. The lumbar puncture and analysis of cerebrospinal fluid (CSF) are the most objective means of identifying the etiologic agent.

LUMBAR PUNCTURE—INDICATIONS, CONTRAINDICATIONS, TECHNIQUE, AND COMPLICATIONS

Indications

Lumbar puncture is indicated to:

1. Confirm a diagnosis. This is particularly important when the computed tomography (CT) scan is negative for subarachnoid hemorrhage (SAH) but clinical signs are indicative of meningeal irritation. The accuracy of CT in documenting SAH diminishes after 24 h and diagnosis is often dependent on lumbar puncture.[1]

2. Identify an organism

3. Test for antibiotic sensitivity

4. Establish the need for treatment of children who are contacts in the case of meningococcal or haemophilus meningitis

Contraindications

Lumbar puncture is contraindicated when there is suspicion of increased intracranial pressure (ICP) caused by an intracranial mass lesion. Papilledema should be excluded. Other contraindications include serious cardiorespiratory disease or when the area through which the spinal needle must pass is infected.

If available, a CT scan or magnetic resonance imaging (MRI) scan should be obtained before lumbar puncture. Contraindications to lumbar puncture, because of increased risk of herniation, include lateral shift of the midline structures, loss of suprachiasmatic and basilar cisterns, obliteration of the fourth ventricle, or obliteration of the superior cerebellar and quadrigeminal cisterns with sparing of the ambiens cisterns.[2]

There is no evidence to recommend CT scan of the brain before lumbar puncture for suspected acute meningitis, unless any of the following features are present: unconsciousness, focal findings, papilledema, other atypical features (e.g., immune compromise, sinusitis, otitis media).[3]

The risk of complications associated with a lumbar puncture, even in patients with papilledema, is 10 to 20 times lower than the risks associated with acute bacterial meningitis alone.

Treatment without lumbar puncture can be considered in cases where there is unequivocal diagnosis of meningitis in a seriously ill individual with a positive blood culture, who has impaired consciousness, raised ICP, and signs of brainstem involvement by uncal herniation or central pressure.

Technique

The patient should be near the edge of the bed in the lateral decubitus position with neck, trunk, hips, and knees flexed (Fig. 16-1). The shoulders and hips must be perpendicular to the bed, and it may be necessary to place a small pillow beneath the head and trunk. The site of puncture is most commonly the L4–L5 interspace, which is located at the level of an imaginary line drawn between the highest points of the iliac crests.

The area should be cleansed with povidone-iodine solution and then wiped with alcohol to remove all traces of the antiseptic solution. The puncture site should be located and the patient draped. It is necessary to change gloves to avoid contaminating the lumber puncture with povidone-iodine. The lum-

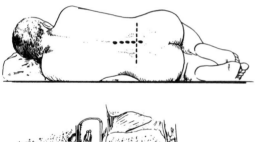

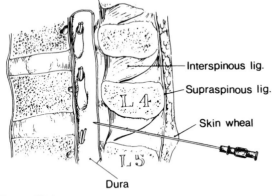

Interspinous lig.

Supraspinous lig.

Skin wheal

L 4

L 5

Dura

Figure 16-1
Technique of lumbar puncture.

Table 16-1
Normal CSF indices

Appearance: clear, colorless, does not clot in tube

Opening pressure: 70–200 mmH$_2$O

Cells: 0–5/mm^3 (mononuclear)

Na$^+$: 142–150 mEq/L; K$^+$: 2.2–3.3 mEq/L; Cl: 120–130 mEq/L

CO$_2$: 25 mEq/L; pH: 7.35–7.40

Glucose:45–80 mg/100 dL

Protein: 5–15 mg/dL (ventricular), 10–25 mg/dL (cisternal), 15–45 mg/dL (lumbar)

Gamma globulin: 5–12% of total protein

Transaminase (GOT): 7–49 U; LDH: 15–71 U; CPK: 0–3 IU

BUN: 5–25 mg/dL; bilirubin: 0

Amino acids: 30% of blood level

Lactic acid 0.8–2.8 mmol/L

BUN, blood urea nitrogen; CPK, creatine phosphokinase; GOT, glutamic oxaloacetic transaminase; LDH, lactate dehydrogenase

bar puncture site is infiltrated with 1% lidocaine hydrochloride for local anesthesia. When a standard cutting tip needle is used, it is inserted at an angle of 10° to 20° cephalad with the bevel of the needle parallel to the long axis of the spine. The needle should be advanced until a "pop" is felt, indicating penetration of the meninges. When the needle has been advanced to the appropriate depth without the sensation of a "give" or "pop," the stilette should be removed every 2 to 3 mm, as the needle is advanced to check for CSF return. If the needle fails to enter the subarachnoid space, it may be necessary to try again in a different interspace.

Once the needle is in place, the manometer should be attached, using the three-way stopcock, and the patient's lower limbs extended before recording the opening pressure. Approximately 3 mL of CSF is collected into each of four tubes, and the closing pressure is measured. The manometer is then detached, the stilette replaced, and the needle removed. Blood should be drawn for glucose determination to allow comparison with the CSF glucose level and to test for the presence of oligoclonal bands for comparison with oligoclonal bands in the CSF. Table 16-1 lists the normal CSF indices. Table 16-2 compares

CSF findings in various central nervous system (CNS) disorders.

If there is suspicion of spinal subarachnoid block, the Queckenstedt test may be performed after the opening pressure is recorded. To perform the test, the jugular veins are compressed, usually manually, with enough force to occlude the veins but without interfering with carotid flow or respiration. Compression should be followed by a prompt rise in recorded pressure on the manometer followed by a fall to the original pressure when compression ceases. If compression with enough force to occlude the jugular veins does not result in a rise in recorded pressure, the Queckenstedt test is negative, and it is presumed that a spinal subarachnoid block is present. It should be noted that this test should never be performed if there is increased ICP or suspicion of a mass lesion above the level of the foramen magnum.

Complications

1. Post-lumbar puncture headache is probably caused by continued leakage of CSF through the

Table 16-2

Cerebrospinal fluid findings in various central nervous system disorders

	Pressure	Appearance	Glucose	Protein	Cells
Viral encephalitis	Normal or mildly increased	Clear, colorless	Normal	Normal or slightly increased	Increased lymphocytes
Aseptic meningitis	Normal	Usually clear, colorless	Normal	Normal or slightly increased	Lymphocytes occasionally normal early or increased to >500 cells/mm
Acute pyogenic meningitis	Increased	Cloudy	Decreased	Increased	Polymorpho-nuclears, usually >500 cells/mm
Tuberculous meningitis, syphilis	Increased	Usually clear, may be cloudy	Decreased	Increased	Increased lymphocytes
Fungal infections	Increased	Varies with organism	Varies with organism	Increased	Increased lymphocytes
Abscess	Increased	Clear, colorless	Normal	Increased	Increased poly-morphonuclears
Cerebral infarction	Normal or mildly increased	Clear, colorless	Normal	Normal or mildly increased	Normal or very mild increase in poly-morphonuclear cells <50/mm
Subarachnoid hemorrhage	Increased	Bloody, does not clot, supernatant—xanthochromic	Normal	Increased	Red cells maximal at onset decreasing and disappearing in about 5 days; mild to moderate polymorphonu-clear and later lymphocytic pleocytosis occur as fluid clears
Traumatic lumbar puncture	Normal	Bloody, clots spontaneously, supernatant—not xanthochromic	Normal	4 mg/dL increase per 5000 red blood cells	Same as peripheral blood; fewer red cells last speci-men than first specimen
Spinal cord tumor	Decreased	Cloudy, may be xanthochromic	Normal	Increased, may clot spon-taneously (Froin syndrome)	May be mildly increased lymphocytes
Frequent seizures	Normal	Clear, colorless	Normal	Normal	<80/mm^3 mostly polymorphonu-clear

puncture hole in the dura created by the needle. This causes a reduction in ICP and traction on the intra-cerebral dura. Other causes include decreased pro-duction of CSF and reduced CSF pressure.[4] Headache can be avoided by the use of a 20-gauge Sprotte atraumatic needle, removing the smallest volume of CSF necessary for chemical and bacteriological stud-ies, and by replacing the stylet and rotating the needle 90° before withdrawing the needle.[5]

2. Labyrinthine disturbances. Complaints of vertigo associated with a change in posture often ac-company headache and should be treated with rest, sedation, and adequate fluid intake.

3. Ocular motor disturbances producing diplopia are the result of downward movement of the brainstem following removal of CSF and traction on the third or sixth nerves, usually the latter.

4. Postlumbar puncture backache is usually the result of multiple unsuccessful attempts to place the needle in the subarachnoid space. The resultant muscle spasm produces pain. This may be avoided by allowing no more than two attempts to enter the sub-arachnoid space. The patient should be referred for needle insertion under fluoroscopy after a second at-tempt has failed. Intravenous and oral caffeine are of-ten effective in the treatment of post-lumbar puncture headache.[6] An epidural blood patch is indicated when noninvasive treatment is unsuccessful and is often ef-fective in relieving symptoms.[7]

5. Intracranial subdural hematoma can occur in patients with brain atrophy who have tension on the perforating veins crossing the subdural space. A sudden decrease in pressure produces further traction and rupture of these veins. This complication should always be considered in elderly patients who have be-come less responsive or develop hemiplegia follow-ing lumbar puncture.

6. Infection, including meningitis or subdural empyema, may result from a break in sterile tech-nique during lumbar puncture. The alpha-hemolytic streptococcus is a major pathogen of iatrogenic meningitis following lumbar puncture indicating the need to wear a face mask when performing this pro-cedure.[8]

7. Uncal herniation is the most devastating complication of lumbar puncture and is due to sudden change in ICP. Lumbar puncture should not be per-formed if there is any suspicion of an intracranial mass lesion.

8. A traumatic tap results from the laceration of vessels in the venous plexus of the spinal canal. Bleeding can be avoided by keeping the needle in the midline and not penetrating to the anterior wall of the spinal canal.

BACTERIAL INFECTIONS

Acute Pyogenic Meningitis

Definition *Acute pyogenic meningitis* is an inflam-matory response to bacterial infection involving the pia and arachnoid membranes covering the brain and spinal cord. Many microorganisms can produce pyo-genic meningitis, which is classified according to the specific etiological agent.

Etiology and Pathology The three most com-mon organisms causing acute pyogenic meningitis are *Streptococcus pneumoniae*, *Neisseria meningi-tidis*, and *Haemophilus influenzae* (Table 16-3 for dis-tinguishing characteristics of the etiologic agents). There is a considerable change in the incidence of bacterial types with age (Table 16-4).

The upper respiratory tract or the umbilical cord are the most common sources of infection in neonates; colonization of the respiratory tract followed by inva-sion and bacteremia is the usual course in children. Extension from an adjacent area such as the middle ear, paranasal sinuses or scalp, direct infection after head trauma, or introduction of infection after a neu-rosurgical procedure or lumbar puncture are occa-sional but rare causes of meningitis. Once the organ-isms cross the blood-brain barrier, they flourish with an outpouring of polymorphonuclear cells into the CSF, which becomes cloudy or milky in appearance. The bacteria release endotoxins that stimulate the re-lease of the cytokines including tissue necrosis factor alpha, and interleukin-1b from microphages and astro-cytes, enhancing the inflammatory response.[9] The in-flammatory reaction is particularly intense in the basal cisterns and over the convexities of the brain. The pia and arachnoid become congested and opaque, and the exudate rapidly becomes fibropurulent. The inflammation extends into layers one and two of the cortex, leading to vasogenic edema, but also involves cerebral veins producing cortical thrombophlebitis, which produces additional edema, venous thrombosis, and infarction. Cytotoxic edema occurs secondary to swelling of the cellular elements of the brain parenchyma, most likely the result of the release of toxic factors from neutrophils or bacteria and secretion of antidiuretic hormone (ADH) with resultant hypotonicity of extracellular fluid, and increased permeability of the brain to water.[10] Interstitial edema is the result of impaired absorption of the CSF through arachnoid granulations, resulting in increased CSF outflow resistance. All three types of edema contribute to cerebral edema in bacterial meningitis.[11] In addition, there is a loss of autoregulation in bacterial meningitis, and cerebral blood flow becomes dependent on perfusion pressure. The brain is then at risk for hypo- or hyperperfusion.[12] The acute inflammatory response may be followed by thickening and fibrosis, and adhesions occur between the meninges and the brain, impairing the circulation of CSF and forming a scar around the cranial nerves at the base of the brain.

Clinical Features The incidence of acute pyogenic meningitis is approximately 5/100,000. The condition occurs equally in both sexes, and the majority of cases occur in the winter months. Children aged 6 months to 1 year are at the greatest risk, and children under 15 years of age comprise 75 percent of all cases. There are many predisposing factors, including upper respiratory tract infection, infection of the lungs, middle ear, paranasal sinuses, skull bones, throat, nasopharynx or mastoids; a history of recent head trauma, a neurosurgical procedure,[13] myelography[9] or spinal anesthesia; contact with a patient who has a meningococcal infection; and debilitating conditions such as sickle cell anemia, alcoholism, leukemia, acquired immunodeficiency syndrome (AIDS), or chronic immunosuppressive therapy. The cardinal signs of meningitis consist of fever, vomiting, and nuchal rigidity, which are the most common presenting symptoms in children 1 to 4 years of age.[14]

Symptoms and signs of meningitis show marked variation with age.

Neonates In the newborn, the symptoms and signs of acute bacterial meningitis are not distinct from those of sepsis or other serious illnesses.[15] The infant shows altered temperature control, bradycardia, respiratory distress, cyanosis, disinterest in feeding, jaundice, and diarrhea.[16] Signs and symptoms of involvement of the CNS are vague, and the infant may only show lethargy and irritability. Seizures occur in 40 percent of newborn infants with meningitis. A bulging fontanelle and meningismus are present in less than 20 percent of cases. Thus, the evaluation of a febrile or hypothermic ill neonate requires a lumbar puncture.

Infants Infants with acute bacterial meningitis present with fever in the afternoon and evening, poor feeding, vomiting, lethargy, and lack of motor response on stimulation, whether visual, auditory, or tactile, and nuchal rigidity.

Children There is rapid onset of fever, headaches, vomiting, nuchal rigidity, and progressive changes in mental status, from irritability and confusion to drowsiness and stupor. Cerebral infarction with hemiparesis and seizures may be present, or seizures can occur secondary to hyponatremia associated with a syndrome of inappropriate secretion of ADH (SIADH).[17]

Adults Most patients present to the emergency center less than 24 h after the onset of symptoms, which consist of headache, fever, and nuchal rigidity,[18] followed by nausea and vomiting, clouding of consciousness, seizures, myoclonus, respiratory difficulties that often require intubation, hemiparesis, or focal cranial nerve deficits. Kernig and Brudzinski signs are elicited in 50 percent of adults with meningitis, and their absence never rules out the diagnosis.[19]

A positive Kernig sign is indicated by the presence of pain in the lumbar area and the posterior aspect of the thigh, when attempting to extend the patient's lower limb when the hip is flexed. The Brudzinski sign is positive if flexion of the patient's neck produces flexion of both legs and thighs. Papilledema is rare in meningitis and suggests the presence of brain abscess, subdural empyema, or venous sinus thrombosis.

Table 16-3

Distinguishing characteristics of etiological agents producing acute pyogenic meningitis

Etiological agent	Microbiologic characteristics	Distinguishing epidemiologic characteristics	Distinguishing clinical features	Mortality	Complications	Therapeutic drug of choice*	Alternative therapy*
Streptococcus pneumoniae (pneumococcus)	Gram-positive, lancet-shaped diplococcus, encapsulated	Adult, head trauma, sickle cell disease, anemic or alcoholic	Cough, positive blood culture (56%)	20–60% depends on population	May be recurrent, subdural effusions, endocarditis	Ceftriaxone 2g IVPB q 12 h 21 days	Vancomycin (pharmacy kinetic dosing 21 days)
Neisseria meningitidis serotypes A, B, C, D, Y	Gram-negative, kidney-shaped diplococcus, intracellular, encapsulated	Youth (6–20 years), epidemics, occurs in early spring or winter	Sore throat, petechiae, and purpura	6–7%	Disseminated intravascular coagulation, endocarditis, adrenal hemorrhage (rare)	Penicillin G 2 million units IVPB q 4 h 14 days	Ceftriazone 2 g IVPB q 12 h 14 days
Haemophilus influenzae serotype B	Gram-negative, pleomorphic rod, encapsulated	Child (2 months–6 years), occurs in late fall or winter	Earache, positive blood culture (79%)	7–8%	Subdural effusions, hydrocephalus	Ceftriaxone 2 g IVPB q 12 h 10 days	Ampicillin 2 g q 4h IVPB 10 days
Streptococcus group B	Gram-positive, cocci in chains	Neonates, premature rupture of membranes		1–2 day old: 80%; 7–14 day old: 40–50%	Endocarditis	Penicillin G as above 14 days	Vancomycin as above 14 days
Escherichia coli	Gram-negative, rod	Neonates, head trauma or neurosurgery	Urinary tract infection 40%	50%	Endocarditis	Ceftriaxone 2 g IVPB q 12 h 21 days	

Organism	Morphology	Clinical setting	Clinical clue		Treatment
Klebsiella pneumoniae	Gram-negative, encapsulated rod	Immunosuppressed or alcoholic patients			Ceftriaxone 2 g IVPB q 12 h 21 days
Pseudomonas aeruginosa	Gram-negative, rod, motile	Head trauma, immunosuppressed, neurosurgery	Greenish CSF		Ceftiazidime plus tobramycin 21 days
Staphylococcus aureus	Gram-positive, cocci in clusters	Neonates, elderly; head trauma or neurosurgery			Vancomycin 21–30 days / Nafcillin (susceptible strains) 2g q 6 h 21–30 days
Listeria monocytogenes	Gram-positive, rod, often mistaken for diphtheroids	Renal transplant patient or neonate	Absence of nuchal rigidity		Ampicillin (as above) 21 days
Neisseria gonorrhoeae	Gram-negative, kidney-shaped diplococcus, intracellular	Pregnant	Gonorrhea joint involvement	Endocarditis	Ceftriaxone 21 days
Clostridium perfringens	Gram-positive, rods	Recent head trauma or neurosurgery		33%	Penicillin G as above 21 days

*Dosages for adult (70 kg) with normal renal function.

Vancomycin and Tobramycin require pharmacy kinetic dosing.

Table 16-4

Age relationship to etiology of acute pyogenic meningitis

Age	Microorganism
Neonate (0–2 months)	*Streptococcus,* group B *E. coli*—coliforms *Listeria* *Staph. aureus* *Enterobacter* *Pseudomonas* *Haemophilus* (non-typeable)
Child	*S. pneumoniae* *N. meningitidis* *H. influenzae*
Youth (6–20 years)	*N. meningitidis* *S. pneumoniae* *H. influenzae*
Adult (>20 years)	*S. pneumoniae* *N. meningitidis* *Streptococcus* *Staphylococcus*

*Rare in countries with universal infant *Haemophilus influenzae* type b immunization.

Older Patients Presentation of meningitis in patients aged 60 and older may be atypical. Fever is not a consistent finding and changes in mentation labelled "confusion" are not infrequent. Nuchal rigidity is an inconsistent finding. Definitive diagnosis relies on examination and culture of the CSF.[20]

Course The disease may run a fulminant course in which the patient's condition reaches maximal severity within 24 h. In other patients, there is an insidious progression of symptoms over several days to weeks. In general, patients with rapid progression of symptoms carry a poorer prognosis. Once proper treatment is begun, the fever should diminish and the CSF should contain a preponderance of mononuclear cells within 72 h. The most common residual deficit following acute pyogenic meningitis is deafness.

Complications The causes of fever after 7 days of proper antibiotic therapy are listed in Table 16-5.

1. Inappropriate secretion of ADH is a common complication of bacterial meningitis and occurs in approximately 80 percent of cases. It is characterized by a serum sodium concentration of less than 130 mEq/L, elevated urine sodium, elevated urine osmolality, and a normal or low blood urea nitrogen. It is managed by fluid restriction (see below).

2. Subdural effusion occurs in as many as 32 percent of infants and children with bacterial meningitis. It should be suspected if there is recurrent vomiting, fever, failure to improve, bulging of the fontanelle, and increased head circumference or seizures. The diagnosis is made by transillumination of the skull, CT scanning, and tapping of the effusion. If the protein content of the fluid is less than 100 mg/dL, it is not a subdural effusion. Repeated taps are not usually necessary.

3. Disseminated intervascular coagulation (DIC) is most commonly associated with meningococcal and gram-negative meningitis and is characterized by petechiae, purpurae, and hypotension. Neurological symptoms are varied, with persistent confusion, disorientation, delirium, lethargy, stupor, or coma. Hemiparesis, aphasia, visual field defects, focal or generalized seizures, and signs of brainstem involvement are encountered occasionally. The spinal cord may also be affected.

The diagnosis is established by demonstration of low fibrinogen levels and the presence of elevated levels of fibrin degradation products in the blood. In addition, the prothrombin time is prolonged and the

Table 16-5

Causes of fever after 7 days of proper antibiotic therapy

1. Phlebitis due to intravenous administration of antibiotics.
2. Intercurrent, hospital-acquired infection or persistence of particular foci of infection (e.g., otitis media).
3. Developing cerebral abscess.
4. Drug fever.
5. Subdural effusion.
6. Subdural empyema.
7. Ventriculitis.

platelet count is reduced. The condition is treated with heparin.

4. Hydrocephalus. Adhesions between the meninges and the brain may impede the circulation of CSF or the arachnoid granulations may be blocked by exudate, resulting in hydrocephalus or a subarachnoid cyst. This should be considered if the CSF glucose level remains depressed and the head continues to enlarge in infants and young children. Hydrocephalus may resolve as the infection is controlled. Refractory cases require placement of a ventriculoperitoneal shunt.

5. Subdural empyema. The spread of inflammatory process and infection to the subdural space can result in the development of a subdural empyema. This is a rare complication and can be diagnosed by MRI or CT scanning.

6. Ventriculitis should be considered in the pediatric patient who does not respond promptly to appropriate antibiotic therapy. It occurs most often in the neonatal age group, with gram-negative meningitis, and the diagnosis is made by CSF cultures or tapping of the ventricles followed by culture of the fluid. Treatment requires administration of antibiotics intravenously after testing for sensitivity, repeated ventricular taps to relieve the pressure of hydrocephalus, and introduction of a ventriculoperitoneal shunt.[21]

Differential Diagnosis There are four considerations in the differential diagnosis of meningitis. These are bacterial, viral, tuberculous, or fungal infections. Table 16-6 illustrates the distinguishing characteristics of these conditions. There is always a possibility that bacterial meningitis not due to *H. influenzae, N. meningitidis,* or *S. pneumoniae* may be secondary to a ruptured brain abscess.

Diagnostic Procedures

1. Lumbar puncture is the only absolute means of substantiating a diagnosis of meningitis. In acute pyogenic meningitis, the opening pressure is elevated, usually greater than 200 mmH$_2$O, and in 85 percent of adults with meningitis, the opening pressure is elevated and averages more than 300 mmH$_2$O.[22] The CSF is cloudy and organisms are present on a direct smear in 40 percent of cases. There is a marked pleocytosis with a preponderance of polymorphonuclear cells in the early stages, followed by a gradual increase of mononuclear cells. The CSF glucose is usually less than 40 mg/dL, and less than 50 percent of the level in a blood sample taken at the time of lumbar puncture. The CSF protein is elevated and varies from 100 to 2000 mg/dL. The CSF should be examined using Gram's stain and the fluid sent for culture.

2. Blood should be drawn for blood cultures before administration of antibiotics in all cases. This is particularly important when lumbar puncture has not been performed, when the blood culture will be positive in 90 percent of children with *H. influenzae,* type B meningitis, and 80 percent of children with meningitis caused by *Streptococcus pneumoniae.*[14]

3. Bacterial antigen detection in blood, urine, or CSF using counterimmunoelectrophoresis (CIE), latex particle agglutination tests, or enzyme-linked

Table 16-6
Differential diagnosis of meningitis

Type of meningitis	Cells	Glucose	Protein	Smear	CSF lactic acid
Bacterial	>500 polymorphonuclear leukocytes/mm³	<½ blood glucose	>45 mg/dL	Organisms	>35 mg/dL
Viral	<500 mononuclear cells/mm³	Normal	Mild increase	No organisms	<35 mg/dL
Tuberculous, fungal	<500 mononuclear cells/mm³	Moderate or marked decrease	Marked increase	+, −	>35 mg/dL

immunosorbant assay (ELISA) are useful in determining the bacterial species and the serotype of encapsulated bacteria.

4.   Chest, skull, mastoid, and paranasal sinus x-rays will rule out fracture, sinusitis, or mastoiditis, which may be a focus of infection.

5.   Elevated CSF lactate acid dehydrogenase isoenzymes 4 and 5 and elevated glutamic-oxaloacetic transaminase have been reported in bacterial meningitis. C-reactive protein is present in the CSF and acute bacterial and tuberculous meningitis but is reported to be absent in viral (aseptic) meningitis.

6.   The MRI or CT scan may reveal evidence of subdural empyema, brain abscess, or cerebral infarction. The T1-weighted MRI scan may show diffuse meningeal enhancement after administration of contrast material in bacterial meningitis (Fig. 16-2).[23]

Treatment

1.   Patients with acute meningitis require complete bed rest with noise and other extraneous stimuli kept to a minimum. Known or suspected meningococcal disease requires isolation until the patient has received several days of appropriate antibiotic therapy. The most serious complications requiring urgent treatment include airway obstruction, respiratory insufficiency, septic or hypovolemic shock, cerebral edema, electrolyte imbalance, seizures, and SIADH.

2.   The airway requires constant attention and excess secretions must be removed by frequent suctioning. Intubation may be necessary and assisted ventilation required in patients who develop seizures or shock.

3.   Fluid balance and electrolytes must be carefully monitored because of the possibility of SIADH and shock. However, treatment of a hypovolemic state is of primary importance and requires initial fluid infusion to maintain blood pressure and tissue perfusion. Pediatric shock resuscitation requires a fluid bolus of 20 mL/kg, 0.9% saline intravenously, or Ringer's lactate solution and should be followed by frequent assessments and rebolusing if needed.[24] A central venous pressure line aids in the maintenance of adequate hydration.

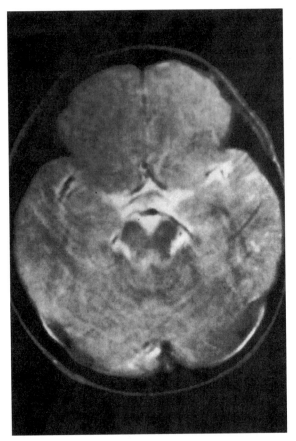

Figure 16-2
MRI scan—T1-weighted image. Young child. High signal intensity indicating pus in the subarachnoid space and suprasellar cistern—purulent meningitis.

4.   Antibiotic therapy as outlined in Tables 16-3 and 16-7 should be administered. A minimum of 2 weeks of therapy is recommended. The CSF should be reexamined if there is any doubt regarding clinical improvement. It is not necessary to re-evaluate the CSF when antibiotics are discontinued in an individual who has had an uninterrupted and uncomplicated course.

Empiric antibiotic therapy should be initiated in patients in whom bacterial meningitis is suspected within 30 min following lumbar puncture and examination of the CSF (see Table 16-7). When cultures become available, treatment may be modified appropriately.[24]

Table 16-7
Initial antibiotic therapy before results of culture are available

Type of patient	Drug of choice
Neonatal	Ampicillin + gentamicin*
Children	Vancomycin or Meropenem + Ceftriaxone/ Cefotaxime** Chloramphenicol
Adult	Ceftriaxone
Postneurosurgical	Ceftriaxone plus Vancomycin
Immunosuppressed or *Pseudomonas* suspect	Ceftazidime plus Vancomycin

*Until organism and susceptibility are identified

**Vancomycin can be discontinued if isolate is a penicillin-susceptible pneumococcus or *N. meningitidis.*

5. Cerebral edema. If there is papilledema or evidence of herniation, the patient should receive intravenous mannitol (see Chap. 2).

6. Seizures can be controlled with intravenous diazepam (Valium) 5 to 10 mg followed by a diazepam drip of 5 mg/h in adolescents and adults. An appropriately smaller dose should be used in younger children or infants who have received phosphenytoin IV or by the rectal route. Diazepam therapy can be augmented by intravenous phenytoin when phosphenytoin is not available (see Chap. 4). Seizures usually resolve as the infection is controlled and a protracted course of anticonvulsants is unnecessary.

7. The administration of corticosteroids as adjunctive therapy in acute bacterial meningitis is controversial, but evidence suggests that mortality, morbidity, and sensorineural hearing loss may be reduced by the use of dexamethasone in children with bacterial meningitis, especially *H. influenzae* type b meningitis.[25] The American Academy of Pediatrics recommends dexamethasone in cases of *H. influenzae* meningitis in previously healthy infants and children over the age of 2 months. Dexamethasone is given q6h intravenously in four divided doses of 0.6 mg/kg per day for the first 4 days of antibiotic therapy.[26]

Prophylactic Treatment

1. Haemophilus conjugate vaccines and meningococcal polysaccharide conjugate vaccines are being introduced into vaccination programs in some countries and should reduce mortality and morbidity in children.[27]
2. Chemoprophylaxis should be considered to eliminate nasopharyngeal carriers in household contacts of patients with *H. influenzae* and *N. meningitidis* meningitis.[28]

Prognosis More than 90 percent of patients with bacterial meningitis died in the preantibiotic era. Currently, 10 to 20 percent of patients die from the infection or its complications. The majority are in the neonatal age group. There is a poorer prognosis for those who are very young or very old, when there is delayed or inadequate therapy, or if the patient has an associated systemic illness. Absence of marked leukocytosis ($< 15,000$ polymorphonuclear leukocytes/mm^3), marked hyperpyrexia ($> 40°C$ rectally), hypotension (blood pressure, <100 mmHg systolic, adult; <70 mmHg systolic, child), seizures, coma, and thrombocytopenia are also associated with a poorer outcome. *S. pneumoniae* meningitis carries the highest mortality, followed by meningococcal infection, then *H. influenzae* meningitis. Relapsing bacterial meningitis is rare in children and adults and is usually associated with subdural empyema, subdural effusions, ventriculitis, brain abscess, mastoiditis, and the presence of a ventricular shunt system.[29]

Brain Abscess

Definition *Brain abscess* is a circumscribed collection of pyogenic material located within the brain parenchyma.

Etiology and Pathology Brain abscesses occur when pyogenic bacteria gain access to the CNS by direct extension of infection from otitis media, mastoiditis, or paranasal sinusitis in most cases.

Occasionally an infection may spread from an osteomyelitis of a cranial bone or may be introduced by head trauma or neurosurgical procedure through an infected area. Brain abscess is a rare complication of pyogenic meningitis. Hematogenous spread of infection from a septic focus, particularly from an infected lung with lung abscess, bronchiectasis, or empyema, is an additional, if less frequent, cause of brain abscess. Acute or subacute bacterial endocarditis or right-to-left intracardiac shunts can give rise to multiple septic emboli and are more likely to cause multiple abscesses, usually located in the area of the white-gray matter junction in the distribution of the middle cerebral artery.

Table 16-8 lists the most common etiological factors, their distinguishing characteristics, and the type of organism usually encountered.

The evolution of a brain abscess proceeds through four stages.

1. Cerebritis. Infection of the brain with surrounding white matter edema.
2. The core of the cerebritis becomes necrotic and enlarges and capsular fibroblasts begin to form.
3. The capsule is well developed, with proliferation of fibroblasts, a surrounding astrocytic proliferation, and edema.
4. A mature, thick capsule surrounds the central cavity containing debris and polymorphonuclear cells. There is usually marked cerebral edema in the surrounding brain tissue in the presence of a mature abscess.

Clinical Features Brain abscesses occur in all age groups. The overall incidence is approximately

Table 16-8

Epidemiologic characteristics in brain abscess

Common etiologic factors in descending frequency	Distinguishing characteristics	Microorganisms typically involved	
		Aerobes	Anaerobes
Middle ear, paranasal sinus, or mastoid infection	Ear infection: temporal lobe abscess. Sinus infection: frontal lobe abscess. Mastoid infection: cerebellar abscess.	Aerobic streptococci *Staph. aureus*	Anaerobic streptococci *Bacterioides*
Metastatic emboli from lung, pulmonary abscess, bronchiectasis, or chronic empyema	Multiple abscesses	*Staph. aureus* *Klebsiella* *S. pneumoniae*	Anaerobic streptococci Fusobacteria
Head trauma or neurosurgery	Gunshot wounds are the most common head trauma associated with abscess	*Staph. aureus* *Pseudomonas*	Anaerobic streptococci
Endocarditis	Drug abuser	*Staph. aureus*	—
Rare causes: Dental procedures Metastatic emboli from abdominal infections or pelvic inflammatory disease Osteomyelitis of skull	—	—	—

1/100,000, and brain abscess is twice as likely to occur in males as in females. The frontoparietal and temporal lobes are more frequently involved, and 13 percent of cases have multiple abscesses (Fig. 16-3).[30]

The patient with a brain abscess usually presents with fever, chills, headache, and progressive focal neurological signs. However, evidence of infection may be absent, and the patient may present with symptoms suggesting brain tumor, including increased ICP, nausea, vomiting, papilledema, bradycardia, and focal signs such as hemiparesis or homonymous hemianopia (see page 394). A history

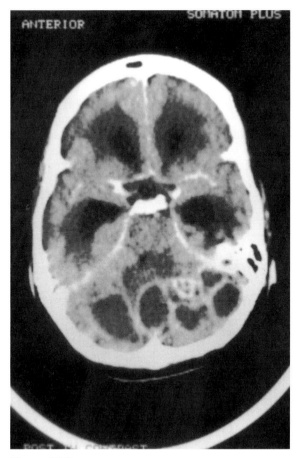

Figure 16-3
Contrast-enhanced CT scan demonstrating multilocular abscesses in the cerebellum with compression of the fourth ventricle and acute hydrocephalus.

of predisposing factors should lead to consideration of brain abscess in such cases.

The neurological examination may reveal papilledema and focal neurological signs, depending on the localization of the abscess. Patients with multiple cerebral abscesses have a more rapid increase in ICP, with headache, drowsiness progressing to stupor, and increasing signs of neurological dysfunction.

Course A brain abscess may follow one of several courses. The abscess may resemble a low-grade astrocytoma or meningioma with a slow progression of symptoms. Others present with a more rapid course and deteriorate over a relatively short period of time. An untreated abscess will continue to extend, with increasing edema leading to herniation, secondary brainstem compression, and death. Rupture of a cerebral abscess into the subarachnoid space or into the ventricles is a rare occurrence.

Complications The complications of brain abscess include herniation, seizures, and rupture of the abscess into the subarachnoid space or into a ventricle. Herniation can be recognized by progressive brainstem compression (see Chap. 2). This condition requires emergency treatment with intravenous mannitol and immediate surgery. Rupture of the abscess is followed by development of acute pyogenic meningitis due to contamination of the subarachnoid space. Rupture of an abscess into a ventricle is rapidly fatal.

Differential Diagnosis

1. Intracranial tumor. The brain abscess may resemble a tumor in that both show progression and focal neurological signs. However, a history of infection and the appearance on CT or MRI scan will usually differentiate the two conditions.

2. Meningitis. An early brain infection producing focal cerebritis may resemble meningitis, with fever, headache, and meningismus, but a fully developed abscess usually presents as a mass lesion with focal signs and papilledema.

3. Chronic subdural hematoma. The history of trauma, lack of infection, and the appearance of MRI or CT scans establishes the diagnosis of subdural hematoma.

4. A subdural empyema is usually a complication of paranasal sinusitis[31] and may closely resemble a cerebral abscess. An MRI or CT scan will distinguish the two conditions.

5. Cerebral infarction is more sudden in onset and the wedge-shaped appearance on the CT scan differs from the typical "ring" appearance of an abscess (Fig. 16-4).

6. Tuberculoma. The history of tuberculosis and the appearance on the CT scan helps to differentiate abscess and tuberculoma.

Diagnostic Procedures

1. There is evidence of infection, with an elevated white blood cell count and an elevated sedimentation rate.

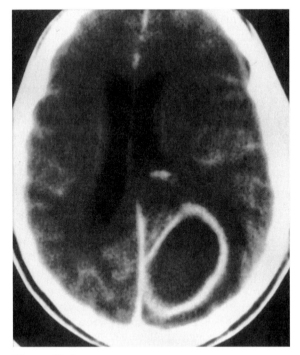

Figure 16-4
Contrast-enhanced CT scan. Typical appearance of a brain abscess with well-defined smooth inner wall. The medial wall is thinner than the lateral wall and there is mass effect on the ventricular system.

2. A lumbar puncture should not be performed in suspected cases of cerebral abscess. The procedure rarely adds any significant information and has been associated with herniation in a significant number of cases. Patients with suspected meningitis and focal neurological signs should have an MRI or CT scan.

3. The MRI scan is more sensitive than the CT scan in the evaluation of suspected parenchymal brain infection. In brain abscess, the T1-weighted image shows a markedly hyperintense lesion with a mass effect. Contrast administration produces marked enhancement of the abscess wall. The T2-weighted scans show hyperintensity of abscess contents surrounded by an area of increased signal intensity, indicating edema.

4. The CT scan demonstrates an abscess as a central area of hypodensity surrounded by a ring of increased density that shows marked enhancement after injection of intravenous contrast material (Fig. 16-5).

5. Bacterial culture should be obtained from any site that may have served as a focus of infection, although antibiotic coverage should not be based entirely on the results of these cultures.

Treatment   A brain abscess should be treated with antibiotic therapy and surgical excision or drainage. The patient should be placed on an appropriate antibiotic (Table 16-9). Early treatment with intravenous antibiotics when the infection is at the stage of a cerebritis may result in total resolution without surgical intervention. Others with a well-formed capsule require total excision when the abscess is sterile. However, when the patient is debilitated, or when the abscess has a thin capsule, treatment by repeated aspiration or fractional drainage is preferable. Antibiotics should be continued for at least 2 to 3 weeks after surgery.

Seizures require an immediate loading dose of phosphenytoin or phenytoin (see page 115) and continuing phenytoin therapy. Status epilepticus should be treated as outlined on page 117. Persistent hydrocephalus requires a ventriculoperitoneal shunt procedure.

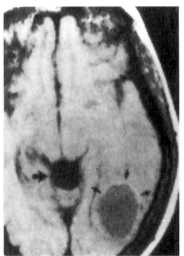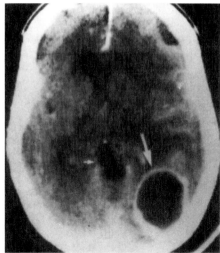

Figure 16-5
MRI scan (left) showing ring-enhanced mass with well-defined wall and necrotic center of a brain abscess.
Enhanced CT scan (right) showing ring enhancement of wall of the abscess. There is an incidental finding of a pineal cyst.

Prognosis The mortality rate for brain abscess has remained at approximately 40 percent since World War II. The mortality is increased in multiple abscesses and in those located in the brainstem or occipital lobes. Coma, deeply located abscesses, ruptured abscesses, and the presence of anaerobic streptococci are poor prognostic factors.

Table 16-9
Choice of antibiotics based on suspected etiology

Suspected etiology	First choice
Sinus infection	Ceftriaxone
Ear infection	Ceftriaxone + metronidazole
Trauma	Vancomycin + ceftazidime

Cranial Subdural Empyema

Definition *Cranial subdural empyma* is a collection of purulent material in the cranial subdural space.

Etiology and Pathology The spread of infection from the paranasal sinuses, especially the frontal sinuses, is the most common etiological factor, followed by infection originating in the mastoid air cells.[32] Other factors include trauma, craniotomy, and spread from a brain abscess. In many cases, there are no identifiable changes in the bone or dura, which suggests that the infection must result from a spread of bacteria through venous channels into the subdural space. A subdural empyema spreads rapidly because there is little resistance to the passage of infection through the subdural space.

Clinical Features An acute subdural empyema runs a fulminating course with a high mortality unless recognized at an early stage.[33] Symptoms consist of severe headache, fever, nausea, vomiting, and meningismus, followed by focal signs of hemiparesis, dysphasia, visual field defects and focal or generalized seizures. Empyema of the falx can cause bilateral lower limb weakness. Signs of increased ICP, including headache, vomiting, and papilledema, are often followed by rapid deterioration, signs of progressive brainstem dysfunction, and death.

Subdural empyema of infancy is usually a complication of a subdural effusion following *H. influenzae* meningitis. This condition presents with fever, seizures, vomiting, lethargy, bulging fontanelles, nuchal rigidity with a rapid deterioration, and death, unless treated promptly.

Diagnostic Procedures

1. The CT scan demonstrates the presence of fluid with increased attenuation compared to the CSF in the subdural space and there is underlying brain edema. There may be associated paranasal sinusitis, mastoiditis, or osteomyelitis demonstrated by scanning.

2. The MRI scan is probably the diagnostic method of choice in demonstrating the empyema with underlying brain edema[34] and in some cases an associated paranasal sinusitis, mastoiditis, or osteomyelitis.[35]

Treatment

1. Prophylactic anticonvulsants should be given as soon as the diagnosis is established because of the high risk of seizure activity. Anticonvulsants should be continued for 2 years after recovery.

2. The airway should be established by intubation in patients who are stuporous or comatose.

3. Measures to reduce elevated intracranial pressure and empirical use of broad-spectrum antibiotics should be instituted emergently.[36]

4. Surgical drainage and placement of drains through burr holes is the standard method of treatment. A bone flap is recommended in patients with osteomyelitis.

5. Appropriate antibiotic therapy should be instituted following culture of the empyema contents and continued for 6 weeks.

Prognosis The condition carries a significant mortality of 9 percent, but permanent neurological deficits occur in more than 50 percent of survivors.[37]

Cranial Epidural Abscess

Definition *Cranial epidural abscess* is a collection of purulent material in the cranial epidural space.

Etiology and Pathology A cranial epidural abscess is often the result of spread of infection from osteomyelitis of the skull by staphylococci or streptococci, or the presence of a foreign body secondary to trauma. Infection of the epidural space has been described in paranasal sinusitis, otitis media, mastoiditis, orbital infection, venous sinus phlebitis, and the presence of a congenital dermal cyst.

The infection remains localized because of the limited space available owing to the firm application of the dura to the inner table of the cranium. The spread of the infection into the subdural space is a dangerous complication with significant mortality.

Clinical Features There is a history of trauma or infection involving the paranasal sinuses, middle ear or inner ear, or a recent otolaryngological procedure. The patient complains of a constant dull headache, often localized to the site of the infection. Additional symptoms such as seizures or focal neurological deficit suggest spread to the subdural space.

Diagnostic Procedures A CT scan with contrast infusion will demonstrate an osteomyelitis or the presence of a localized fluid collection in the epidural space. The CT scan should include views of the paranasal sinuses and mastoid region. An MRI scan T1-weighted image with ganolinium enhancement is equally effective in demonstrating an epidural abscess (Fig. 16-6).

Treatment

1. Antibiotic therapy should be started as soon as possible and continued for 6 weeks.
2. Surgical drainage with removal of any foreign material is necessary because of the risk of spread into the subdural space.

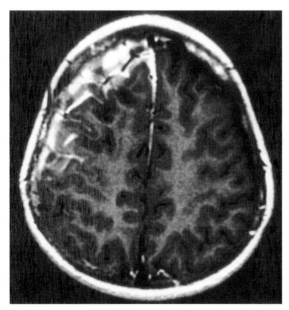

Figure 16-6
MRI T1-weighted image with gadolinium enhancement in a patient with an epidural abscess accompanied by a small area of subdural involvement alongside the falx.

3. Consultation with an otolaryngologist is necessary when there is evidence of paranasal, sinus, middle ear, or mastoid infection.

Spinal Epidural Abscess

Definition *Spinal epidural abscess* is a collection of purulent material in the spinal epidural space.

Etiology and Pathology Most cases of spinal epidural abscess occur in patients with diabetes mellitus. Other casual factors include use of illicit drugs intravenously, recent blunt spinal trauma, recent spinal surgery complicated by infection, spinal nerve block injections, and end-stage renal disease. An associated infection such as furunculosis, dental abscess, or a decubitus ulcer is present in some cases. The predominant bacterial pathogen is the *Staph. aureus*.[38]

Clinical Features The majority of patients present with an acute onset of severe back pain. There is marked limitation of movement and spasm of the erector spinae muscles, with tenderness to palpation over the affected area. The back pain is followed by the development of root pains on the site of the abscess and progressive cord compression, with rapid onset of paraparesis progressing to paraplegia. Bladder function is paralyzed. There is a sensory loss below the level of the lesion. Tendon reflexes are increased in the lower limbs, and there is a bilateral extensor plantar response. The blood shows a raised white cell count with a polymorphonucleocytosis and there is an elevated sedimentation rate.

Approximately 30 percent of cases present with a more chronic course, suggesting a progressive myelopathy.[39]

Differential Diagnosis

1. Acute transverse myelitis may be easily confused but is usually associated with less pain.
2. Guillain-Barré syndrome (acute inflammatory demyelinating polyneuropathy) presents as an ascending flaccid paralysis without pain and usually without but occasionally with an ill-defined sensory loss.
3. In poliomyelitis the paralysis is usually asymmetrical and flaccid, and there are no sensory findings.
4. Cord compression may result from other causes, including tumor, hematoma, and disc herniation.

Diagnostic Procedures

1. Radiography of the spine may reveal osteomyelitis of the vertebrae.
2. A gadolinium-enhanced MRI scan is the procedure of choice. A myelogram followed by a CT scan of the spine will reveal complete obstruction of the spinal subarachnoid space.
3. If lumbar puncture is performed, the needle may enter the abscess with aspiration of pus. If the needle enters the subarachnoid space, the CSF is often xanthochromic, with a polymorphonuclear pleocytosis and elevated protein content. The opening pressure is often low, and the Queckenstedt test indicates the presence of a spinal block.

Treatment

1.   The abscess should be drained or excised as soon as possible to relieve cord compression.[40]

2.   An appropriate antibiotic should be administered. Unasyn 3 g by intravenous piggyback (IVPB) q6h and gentamycin 80 mg IVPB q12h may be given until culture and sensitivity results are available. Antibiotic therapy should be continued for 6 weeks.

Prognosis   Paraparesis secondary to cord compression is a surgical emergency and the compression must be relieved before paraplegia occurs. There is little chance of recovery of function once the patient is paraplegic.[41]

Chronic Spinal Epidural Abscess

Chronic spinal epidural abscesses are usually secondary to tuberculous osteomyelitis of the vertebral body. A "cold" abscess develops and spreads to involve the spinal epidural space. Other causes of infection of the spinal epidural space include syphilis, which can produce granulomatous inflammation and thickening of the meninges, or coccidioidomycosis, brucellosis, and cryptococcosis. A tuberculous abscess usually occurs in the upper or midthoracic region. The abscess may extend around the thoracic or abdominal wall external to the pleura or peritoneum and present anteriorly as a fluctuating mass or the abscess may extend through the psoas sheath and present in the inguinal area as a psoas abscess. Cord damage has a number of causes including direct pressure from a cold abscess, pressure on spinal arteries producing cord ischemia, arteritis of the spinal arteries passing through the abscess, or angulation of the spinal canal due to collapse of the diseased vertebral bodies.

The condition usually presents with root pains radiating in segmental fashion around the chest or abdomen. This is followed by slowly progressive spastic paraparesis, hyperreflexia, and bilateral extensor plantar responses, urgency of micturition followed by incontinence, and development of a sensory level. Spinal deformity is a late complication. The diagnostic procedures are discussed under spinal epidural abscess. Tuberculous infections require prolonged treatment with antituberculous drugs. Patients with syphilitic pachymeningitis may respond to penicillin. The condition must be relieved before paraplegia occurs.

Spinal Subdural Empyema

Definition   A spinal subdural empyema or abscess is a rare condition with infection and pus formation in the spinal subdural space.

Etiology and Pathology   The infection is usually hematogenous, occurring predominantly in patients with diabetes mellitus. Other causes include trauma, spread from an epidermal infection, or introduction of organisms by lumbar puncture or through a congenital dermal cyst tract. Infection, inflammation, and the presence of pus is followed by the development of granulation tissue, which may compress extra- and intramedullary vessels, leading to vascular occlusion and cord infarction. Emerging nerve roots are also involved in a granulomatous reaction.

Clinical Features   The patient experiences fever, back pain, and radiating root pains with signs of spinal cord involvement.

Diagnostic Procedures   The MRI scan shows a localized area of cord compression.

Treatment

1. The cord pressure must be relieved surgically as soon as possible, with removal of as much granulomatous tissue as possible.
2. Appropriate antibiotic therapy should be given following culture and testing for sensitivity, and the therapy should be continued over a 6-week period.

Acute Intramedullary Abscess of the Spinal Cord

Definition   An acute abscess of the spinal cord is a rare condition in which abscess formation occurs within the spinal cord substance.

Etiology and Pathology Abscess formation often follows septicemia in patients who are debilitated or who have a chronic disease such as diabetes mellitus or alcoholism. The infection is usually caused by either staphylococcus or streptococcus, which can reach the spinal cord by direct introduction secondary to trauma, a stab wound, lumbar puncture, or through a dermal cyst or by the hematogenous route from an upper respiratory infection, pneumonia, infected heart valves, urinary tract infection, or a chronic skin infection such as a decubitus ulcer. Intramedullary abscesses tend to occur in the pediatric population when they are associated with lumbosacral dermal sinuses.[42]

The spinal cord is swollen, and the abscess is surrounded by a considerable edema but lacks the venous infarction seen in epidural abscess.

Clinical Features Acute cases present with fever and symptoms and signs resembling an acute transverse myelitis. Pain occurs at the site of abscess formation and there is rapid onset of motor and sensory loss, urinary incontinence, and progressive paraparesis. Cases with a more chronic cause simulate a spinal cord tumor.

Diagnostic Procedures

1. There is evidence of severe systemic infection.
2. The MRI scan is the procedure of choice and readily identifies the presence of a mass lesion and a swollen spinal cord, and clearly delineates a spinal block.

Treatment

1. The cord compression should be relieved urgently by laminectomy and drainage of the abscess.
2. The patient should be treated with high-dose, broad-spectrum antibiotics pending the results of culture and sensitivity, at which time antibiotic therapy can be changed. Antibiotic treatment is continued for 6 to 8 weeks.[43]

Chronic Spinal Subdural and Intramedullary Abscess

Most chronic subdural and intramedullary abscesses are due to tuberculous infection. Syphilis, schistosomiasis, fungal, and yeast infections may occasionally give rise to chronic abscesses. Rarely, a chronic abscess may complicate acute pyogenic meningitis.

The clinical course suggests the presence of a slowly expanding lesion resembling an intramedullary tumor[44] with progressive paraparesis and impairment of bladder function. The diagnosis is established by MRI scanning, the T1-weighted image showing decreased signal intensity with peripheral enhancement following gadolinium infusion. The condition should be treated by appropriate antibiotic therapy and surgical relief of cord compression, if this is indicated by progression of the paraparesis.

Tetanus

Definition Tetanus is an acute toxemia caused by the elaboration of a neurotoxin from the bacillus *Clostridium tetani*. The disorder is characterized by periodic severe muscle spasms.

Etiology and Pathology *Clostridium tetani* is a gram-positive spore-bearing bacillus. The most important factor in the pathogenesis of tetanus is the necessity of an anaerobic environment because the organism is an obligatory anaerobe. Consequently, infection usually occurs by introduction of organisms in deep puncture wounds or soil-contaminated injuries. Under suitable conditions, spores germinate and the organism elaborates an extremely toxic neurotoxin which has two functions: to bind to neurons and to block release of neurotransmitters. The toxin tetanospasmin reaches the CNS by intra-axonal transport, moving at the rate of 75 to 250 mm/day.[45] Once it reaches the brainstem or spinal cord, the toxin produces presynaptic blockade of the synapsis of the inhibitory Renshaw cells and the 1A fibers of the alpha motor neurons, inhibiting the release of γ-aminobutyric acid (GABA) and the GABA precursor, glycine. However, the toxin does not inhibit the synapsis of the Renshaw cells that release acetylcholine. Toxin binding is irreversible. Ultimately, the effect of the toxin spreads throughout the CNS and autopsy reveals swelling of neurons, which show chromatolysis, particularly in the motor cortex and brainstem.

Clinical Features The occurrence of tetanus is sporadic and worldwide because of the ubiquitous nature of the organism. The condition favoring development of tetanus is a deep puncture wound, with introduction of infected soil. However, tetanus has been reported after trivial scratches, insect bites, vaccination, and in intravenous drug addicts using contaminated needles.[46] In some cases, there is no evidence of any kind of wound.

The incubation period is usually 4 to 10 days after infection, but symptoms have been recorded hours to weeks after injury. Initially, the patient may complain of chills, fever, pain, and swelling of the wound site. There are four clinical types of tetanus:[47] generalized tetanus (most common), local tetanus, cephalic tetanus, and tetanus neonatorum.

In the generalized form of tetanus, the toxin has been disseminated throughout the CNS. Tetanospasmin has a specific affinity for motor neurons supplying the face and jaw, and this results in the early signs of lockjaw (trismus), and risus sardonicus (sardonic smile). Eventually, more and more muscle groups become involved, and spasmodic contortions of the body are determined by contraction of the strongest muscles affected. The spasms are intensely painful, accompanied by perfuse perspiration, and gradually increase in severity. The patient is conscious, alert, showing extreme anxiety and terror at the thought of the next agonizing spasm. Severe spasms can result in cyanosis or even asphyxia and death. Eventually the spasms can be precipitated by a sudden noise or by touching patient, or may occur spontaneously. After several days, there is generalized hypertonicity of muscle, producing opisthotonus, and board-like rigidity of the abdomen.

Autonomic dysfunction is a common complication of tetanus and may be the result of the effect of the toxin on brainstem autonomic neurons. This causes sustained tachycardia, profuse sweating, labile blood pressure, hyperpyrexia, and cardiac arrhythmias, and may be followed by sudden cardiac arrest following refractory hypotension. The disease may continue for several weeks.

In a few rare cases, the disease may remain in a localized form, with pain and rigidity restricted to muscles close to a puncture wound. However, such cases have the potential to progress to generalized tetanus. Cephalic tetanus is rare and the symptoms are associated with head wounds and otitis media, and manifested by cranial nerve palsies. Tetanus neonatorum usually presents within 10 days of birth, when the infant shows difficulty, sucking irritability, peculiar grimacing, and intense rigidity of arms, legs and toes. The condition occurs from contamination of the umbilical cord by the *C. tetani*.

Complications

1. The spasms may be of sufficient strength and duration to fracture bones.
2. Asphyxia may occur if there is involvement of the diaphragm and intercostal muscles with rigidity or involvement of the glottis.

Diagnostic Procedures The diagnosis of tetanus is based on the clinical picture because laboratory studies are of little value in this disease. The blood count is usually normal, and lumbar puncture reveals a normal CSF. *Clostridium tetani* can only be recovered from wounds in about 30 percent of cases.

Treatment

1. Early intubation and ventilator support should be instituted in all but minor cases and may prevent death from apnea, laryngospasm, or respiratory arrest. Tracheotomy may be necessary in those with severe disease who require prolonged assisted ventilation.

2. Muscle spasms can be controlled by diazepam, phenobarbital, pentobarbital, or chlorpromazine in the early stages. When these drugs become ineffective, paralysis with Pavulon may be necessary. Intravenous dantrolene sodium has been recommended, and a continuous infusion of intrathecal baclofen has been used to prevent muscle spasms.[48]

3. Human tetanus immune globulin should be administered 3000 to 6000 IU intramuscularly into three sites simultaneously, to neutralize all unbound toxin.

4. The patient should be adequately sedated and kept in a quiet, dark room. Care should be taken to keep all stimuli to a minimum. Good nursing care is essential.

5. Intravenous metronidazole 0.5 g g6h or 1.0 g q12h is believed to be better than penicillin for antibiotic treatment of *C. tetani*.

6. Pronounced autonomic nervous system instability, with the release of large amounts of catecholamines, can be controlled by heavy sedation and infusion of magnesium sulfate 2 to 3 g/h and clonidine.[49]

7. All patients who recover should be immunized with 0.5 mg tetanus toxoid each month for three doses, beginning 6 to 8 weeks after the last antitoxin dose, because the disease does not confer immunity.

8. All children should be immunized. Children 6 weeks to 6 years of age should be given one dose of diphtheria, pertussis, tetanus toxoid on four occasions. The risk of serious acute neurological illness following immunization by this vaccine is minimal.[50] Persons older than 7 years of age should receive three doses of diphtheria, pertussis, tetanus toxoid with a booster dose every 10 years. However, although there is excellent protection for children under 6 years of age, antibody levels decline over time, and one-fifth of older children and the majority of older adults do not have protective antibody levels.[51]

Cerebral Brucellosis

Brucellosis infection by the organisms *Brucella abortus, Brucella melitensis,* and *Brucella suis* may affect the nervous system. The infection is usually acquired from infected farm animals by ingestion of unpasteurized infected milk. The patient may present with an acute febrile illness, with severe headache, myalgia, and weakness. The course of the illness may be intermittent, giving rise to the term undulant fever. Meningomyelitis, mycotic aneurysms, peripheral neuritis, or spondylitis may develop. Meningoencephalitis can result in cranial nerve palsies, hemiplegia, paraplegia, and transient parkinsonism.[52]

Patients with untreated infections or those who relapse after therapy may progress to the chronic form of the disease, which may mimic multiple sclerosis. Serological tests are the most reliable means of identifying the organism, but titers may be low. The patient with acute brucellosis should be treated with a combination of 2 or 3 of the following drugs: doxycycline, streptomycin, trimethoprim/sulfamethoxazole, and rifampin orally for 4 weeks[53]. Chloramphenicol or trimethoprim/sulfamethoxazole may be substituted for tetracycline in children under 8 years of age.

Psittacosis (Chlamydiosis)

Psittacosis is an infection by the organism *Chlamydia psittaci*, which may be acquired by contact with infected wild or domestic birds or contracted during poultry processing.[54] Meningitis or encephalitis may occur. Minor symptoms are usual and consist of persistent headache. More severe symptoms occur in less than 10 percent of cases and consist of headache, photophobia, mental changes, and nuchal rigidity.[55] Respiratory symptoms tend to be a later occurrence. Cerebellar ataxia, papilledema, and cranial neuropathies have been reported. Severe respiratory failure is an uncommon complication requiring ventilator support. Severe hypoxemia or renal impairment are associated with a poor prognosis.[56]

Diagnostic Procedures

1. The CSF is often normal, but elevated protein is present in about 50 percent of cases. A lymphocytic pleocytosis is unusual.
2. Serological tests show a fourfold or greater rise in chlamydial antibodies over a 2-week period.
3. A positive complement fixation test is confirmatory.
4. Rapid diagnosis can be established by the polymerase chain reaction (PCR).

Treatment The infection responds to tetracycline.

Lyme Disease

Definition Lyme disease is the result of infection by the tick-borne spirochete *Borrelia burgdorferi*.

Etiology and Pathology The spirochete is transmitted by the bite of the deer tick with a 1 percent chance of illness following tick bite and is extremely rare if ticks are removed within 48 hours.

Clinical Features Stage 1 or the acute phase is characterized by the development of an enlarged, target-like rash, erythema migrans, associated with a flu-like illness, including acute arthritis, myositis of cardiac and skeletal muscle, and hepatitis in some cases.

Stage 2 occurs a few weeks to several months or even years later, with subacute basilar meningitis. The latter presents with headache, photophobia, and neck stiffness suggesting aseptic meningitis, and is associated with poor memory, emotional lability, difficulty in concentration, and irritability. Cranial nerve involvement, particularly unilateral or bilateral facial nerve palsy, may be the earliest clinical presentation of Lyme disease in stage 2. Diffuse peripheral neuropathies, painful radiculoneuropathies, and unilateral or bilateral brachial or lumbosacral plexopathies have been described. These painful neuropathic conditions are more common in the European than the North American form of the disease.

Encephalopathies with altered levels of consciousness, focal neurological abnormalities, and, rarely, seizures, are uncommon.

Stage 3 occurs months to years after infection with Lyme disease and includes arthralgias, paresthesias, dysesthesias, and numbness of the extremities, fatigue, memory impairment on neuropsychological testing,[57] poor concentration, emotional lability, and difficulty sleeping.[58] The MRI scans and CSF examination are normal in this stage. Neuropsychological examination may show reversal of memory problems after therapy.

Diagnostic Procedures

1. Analysis of CSF shows a mild lymphocytic pleocytosis, up to 100 cells per cubic millimeter, a mild protein elevation, and a normal glucose level in cases with stage 2 meningitis and encephalitis.[59]

2. The MRI scan of the head is normal in aseptic meningitis but shows white matter involvement in the rare encephalitis.

3. Serum ELISA is limited by cross-reactivity with other illnesses, including syphilis, infectious mononucleosis, collagen vascular diseases, and human immunodeficiency (HIV) infection. A rising antibody titer by ELISA on serum and CSF is a strong indicator of lyme disease. Western blotting is useful in distinguishing false-positive cases. A demonstration of *B. burgdorferi* DNA in serum and by polymerase chain reaction CSF is the most sensitive method available.[60]

Treatment Early cases should be treated with doxycycline 100 mg q12h for 1 month, or amoxicillin 1 g q8h orally for 1 month. The recommendation for CNS infection is intravenous ceftriaxone 2 g q12h for 2 weeks, which may be increased to 4 weeks of therapy in severe cases.

GRANULOMATOUS INFLAMMATIONS

Syphilis

Syphilis is the result of infection with *Treponema pallidum* and tends to occur in cycles, with peaks approximately every 10 years. Rates in 1990 were 20.3 per 100,000 and 10.4 per 100,000 by 1993. Primary syphilis is, however, treated effectively in most cases and late symptomatic disease is now unusual, probably because of widespread use of antibiotics with intent to treat syphilis, or inadvertently in treating other infections.[61] This fact should not lead to a complacent attitude toward syphilis. Late symptomatic disease has not been eradicated and may increase once more because there has been a significant increase in syphilis associated with HIV infection.[62] These patients experience less serological improvement after treatment than do patients with syphilis who are HIV negative. In addition, the combination of syphilis and HIV infection leads to a more rapid development of neurosyphilis.[63]

The syndrome of neurosyphilis includes a number of conditions: syphilitic meningitis, chronic basal meningitis, syphilitic arteritis, gumma formation, general paresis, syphilitic optic atrophy, congenital neurosyphilis, syphilis of the spinal cord, and tabes dorsalis.

Syphilitic Meningitis A mild meningeal reaction has been described during the primary stage of syphilis, when *T. pallidum* is disseminated throughout the body. Acute syphilitic meningitis is an occasional feature of the secondary and tertiary stages of syphilis.

Pathology The presence of *T. pallidum* leads to an inflammatory response involving the meninges and the superficial areas of the brain and spinal cord. Marked lymphocytic infiltration of the meninges and perivascular cuffing of the blood vessels occur in the superficial areas of the CNS. These vessels are also the site of an endarteritis.

Clinical Features The patient presents with typical signs of acute meningitis, including headache, fever, nuchal rigidity, nausea, vomiting, and cranial nerve palsies.

Diagnostic Procedures

1. The CSF is under increased pressure and is clear, cloudy, or occasionally xanthochromic. Examination shows a pleocytosis with the presence of 50 to 2000 lymphocytes per cubic millimeter. The protein content is increased and the glucose content is occasionally depressed.
2. There is a positive serological test for syphilitis in the blood and CSF.

Treatment See Table 16-10.

Chronic Basal Meningitis

Chronic basal meningitis is a chronic granulomatous change in the meninges at the base of the brain that occurs in tertiary syphilis.

Pathology The meninges show thickening due to the presence of granulomatous inflammation, particularly around the base of the brain and brainstem. This inflammatory process involves the circle of Willis, the basilar artery, and the upper cranial nerves. There is an extension onto the floor of the fourth ventricle, and obstruction of the foramina of the fourth ventricle may lead to hydrocephalus. Microscopic examination shows the presence of diffuse fibrosis with infiltration of lymphocytes and plasma cells.

Clinical Features The condition usually presents with progressive involvement of the cranial nerves beginning with paralysis of the third and sixth cranial nerves. Extension of this process may lead to involvement of the optic nerves and optic atrophy.

Diagnostic Procedures

1. There is a lymphocytic pleocytosis in the CSF with elevated protein and marked increase in gamma globulin.
2. Serological tests for syphilis are positive in the blood and CSF.

Treatment See Table 16-10. Hydrocephalus may persist despite adequate treatment and may require placement of a ventriculoperitoneal shunt.

Cerebral Syphilitic Arteritis

Syphilitic arteritis is a panarteritis secondary to syphilitic infection involving the cerebral blood vessels.

Pathology Blood vessels in the brainstem and spinal cord show the presence of chronic inflammation, with lymphocytes and plasma cells in all layers of the vessel wall. The internal elastic lamina is preserved but shows reduplication. Endothelial proliferation produces narrowing of the lumina of the affected vessels, with an increased tendency to thrombosis. The penetrating vessels of the brain show a marked perivascular inflammatory response, and there is involvement of the meninges at the base of the brain, with a granulomatous inflammatory change.

Clinical Features Cerebral syphilitic arteritis usually produces symptoms of transient ischemia or cerebral infarction in young individuals. The most common symptom is syphilitic hemiplegia caused by infarction in the distribution of the middle cerebral artery. Vertebral basilar insufficiency or brainstem infarction is probably second in frequency. Involvement of the penetrating vessels of the frontal lobes may produce acute personality change followed by clouding of consciousness, delirium, delusions, and hallucinations. The progressive dementia can be arrested by adequate treatment. Arteritis involving the vessels

Table 16-10
Current treatment of syphilis

A tabular summary of the current recommended treatment schedules from the Centers for Disease Control and Prevention.

Early syphilis (less than 1 year's duration)	Syphilis of more than 1 year's duration (latent syphilis of indeterminate or more than 1 year's duration, cardiovascular, late benign neurosyphilis)
Benzathine penicillin G 2.4 million units IM at a single session, or aqueous procaine penicillin G 4.8 million units. This should be given 600,000 units IM daily for 8 days. If allergic to penicillin: (1) doxycycline 100 mg orally q12h for 2 weeks, (2) tetracycline hydrochloride (HCl) 500 mg qid orally for 14 days. *Note:* Other tetracyclines are not effective. Avoid milk, iron preparations, and antacids with tetracycline because they impair absorption.	Benzathine penicillin G 7.2 million units given as 2.4 million units IM weekly for 3 successive weeks, or aqueous procaine penicillin G 9.0 million units given as 600,000 units IM daily for 15 days. If allergic to penicillin: (1) doxycycline 100 mg orally q12h for 2 weeks, (2) tetracycline HCl 500 mg qid orally for 30 days. Doxycycline or tetracycline should be administered for 4 weeks if infection has been present for more than 1 year.
Syphilis in pregnancy	*Congenital syphilis (infants with abnormal CSF)*
Penicillin in dosage schedules appropriate for the stage of syphilis as recommended for nonpregnant patients. If allergic to penicillin, erythromycin will treat mother only because inadequate doses cross placenta. Tetracyclines are contraindicated in pregnancy. The only acceptable therapy is penicillin. Therefore, skin testing for penicillin allergy is required (<40 percent of patients who believe they have penicillin allergy are confirmed by skin tests). Patients who are skin test negative are treated with penicillin. Patients with confirmed allergy to penicillin require desensitization. This should be carried out by an experienced individual (e.g., an allergist) and should be performed in a health care facility where immediate resuscitative measures are available.	Aqueous penicillin, crystalline penicillin G 100,000–150,000 units/kg IM or IV daily in two divided doses during first 7 days of life and three divided doses thereafter for 10 days or procaine penicillin G 50,000 units/kg IM once daily for 10 days. Infants with normal CSF: benzathine penicillin G 50,000 units/kg IM for one dose. Older infants and children: aqueous penicillin G 50,000 units/kg per day IV or IM q4–6h for 10–14 days.

supplying the brainstem and basal ganglia may result in parkinsonism, dystonia, or ballism.

Diagnostic Procedures

1. Serological tests for syphilis are positive in the blood and CSF.

2. The CSF shows the presence of excessive lymphocytes with increased protein and gamma globulin content.
3. The arteritis can be demonstrated by arteriography. This procedure shows an irregular involvement of blood vessel with segments of narrowing, "beading," and vascular occlusion.

Treatment See Table 16-10. Although the process is promptly arrested by adequate antibiotic treatment, residual neurological deficits due to infarction are often severe.

Syphilitic Gumma

A syphilitic gumma is a tumor-like mass of granulation tissue occurring in the meninges or brain parenchyma of a patient with tertiary syphilis.

Pathology A gumma is a solitary mass of granulation tissue consisting of epithelioid cells, plasma cells, and giant cells surrounding a central area of necrosis.

Clinical Features Gummas of the CNS are extremely rare and behave as expanding mass lesions.

Diagnostic Procedures

1. Serological tests for syphilis are positive in the blood and CSF.
2. The CSF shows the presence of a lymphocytic pleocytosis, elevated protein content, and elevated gamma globulin.
3. There are focal changes on the electroencephalogram (EEG) compatible with a focal structural lesion.
4. Diagnosis of a mass lesion can be made by MRI or CT scanning.

Treatment See Table 16-10. Gummas presenting as an expanding intracranial mass are often excised and a diagnosis is established postoperatively by a histological examination.

General Paresis

General paresis is a chronic syphilitic encephalitis caused by the presence of *T. pallidum* in the brain.

Pathology In advanced cases, the brain shows diffuse cortical atrophy and ventricular dilatation. The ependymal lining of the ventricles is thickened and has a granular appearance. This condition has been termed "granular ependymitis." Histological examination shows thickening of the meninges, which are infiltrated with plasma cells and lymphocytes. The gray matter of the brain shows loss of neurons and proliferation of astrocytes and microglia. The microglia has an atypical rod-shaped appearance often oriented in a perpendicular fashion to the surface of the brain. Blood vessels show the presence of a diffuse syphilitic arteritis. There is marked perivascular cuffing of the vessels penetrating the surface of the brain. Numerous spirochetes may be demonstrated by special staining techniques.

Clinical Features The patient experiences progressive intellectual deterioration beginning with the loss of operational judgment followed by impairment of insight, gradual loss of acceptable social behavior, impairment of recent memory, and personality change. With the passage of time, the affect becomes flat and the patient becomes severely demented and apathetic.

The examination of the patient with established general paresis shows the presence of Argyle Robertson pupils in all cases. A tremor involves the eyelids, lips, tongue, and fingers. The voice is tremulous and rapid alternating movements are impaired because of dyspraxia. Tendon reflexes are symmetrical but diffusely increased. There may be extensor plantar responses.

Diagnostic Procedures

1. Serological tests for syphilis are positive in blood and CSF.
2. The CSF shows the presence of a lymphocytic pleocytosis, increased protein content, and increased gamma globulin.
3. Serial EEGs will show gradual deterioration in the serial records, with a loss of alpha activity and replacement with theta activity and eventually the appearance of delta activity. This activity is symmetrical over both hemispheres. Occasional paroxysmal or epileptic discharges may be recorded.
4. Diffuse cortical atrophy and ventricular dilatation can be demonstrated by MRI or CT scanning of the brain.

Treatment See Table 16-10. Adequate treatment of general paresis in the early stages can arrest the disease before the development of severe dementia. Relapse is rare and requires a second course of treatment.

Syphilitic Optic Atrophy   Syphilitic optic atrophy is optic atrophy caused by, or related to, infection by *T. pallidum*.

Etiology and Pathology   There are two forms of neurosyphilitic optic atrophy. In primary optic atrophy, the condition is a consequence of an inflammatory reaction of the optic nerve. Secondary syphilitic optic atrophy is caused by pressure on the optic nerve due to chronic basal meningitis or increased ICP resulting from hydrocephalus secondary to syphilitic meningitis.

In primary optic atrophy, the optic nerve shows the presence of an inflammatory reaction surrounding the blood vessels that penetrate the nerve (vasa nervorum). This reaction is followed by loss of nerve fibers and demyelination beginning peripherally and gradually involving the center of the optic nerve.

Clinical Features   Syphilitic optic atrophy is characterized by progressive restriction of visual fields beginning peripherally and extending toward the center. The visual loss is usually eccentric and the visual loss is total within a 10-year period. Examination shows marked pallor of the optic discs.

Diagnostic Procedures   The blood serological test for syphilis is positive in most cases but may be negative in patients with optic atrophy and tabes dorsalis.

Treatment   See Table 16-10. Syphilitic optic atrophy is often progressive despite adequate penicillin therapy, and repeated courses of treatment may not prevent the development of blindness.

Congenital Neurosyphilis   Congenital neurosyphilis results when there is transplacental infection of the fetus by *T. pallidum*.

Pathology   The developing fetus is infected during the fourth month of pregnancy; adequate treatment of the mother with active syphilis before the fourth month of pregnancy prevents fetal infection.

The pathological changes are those of syphilis in its early stages.

Clinical Features   The child may be stillborn or show signs of congenital syphilis at birth. Untreated infants with congenital syphilis may develop all of the signs of neurosyphilis at a later stage. The condition includes syphilitic meningitis, chronic basal meningitis, optic atrophy, syphilitic arteritis, and juvenile general paresis. General paresis presents during the second decade as a rapidly progressive dementia. Tabes dorsalis has rarely been described in congenital syphilis.

Diagnostic Procedures[64]

1.   Infants should be evaluated for congenital syphilis if they were born to seropositive women who have untreated syphilis, were treated during pregnancy with erythromycin, were treated less than 1 month before delivery, were treated with penicillin but nontreponemal antibody titers did not decrease sufficiently following treatment, or were treated appropriately but had insufficient serological testing during follow-up.

2.   In evaluation of the infant, a thorough physical examination for congenital syphilis should be performed, and a quantitative serological test for syphilis should be obtained. The CSF should be analyzed for cells, protein, and VDRL. Radiography of the long bones should be performed and pathological examination of the placenta or amniotic cord, using specific antitreponemal antibody staining, should be carried out.

Antibiotic treatment is described in Table 16-10.

Syphilis of the Spinal Cord   Syphilitic involvement of the spinal cord is rare and has been virtually eliminated with penicillin therapy. Acute syphilitic transverse myelitis may occur as an acute infarction of the spinal cord secondary to syphilitic arteritis of the anterior spinal artery or its branches.

Syphilitic meningomyelitis, which is a diffuse granulomatous meningitis involving the spinal cord, may produce progressive paraparesis. Pachymeningitis cervicitis hypertrophica is a condition in which marked thickening of the meninges over the cervical area of the spinal cord occurs. This condition is also associated with a progressive paraparesis. In addition, involvement of the motor nerve roots in the cervical area produces wasting of the muscles of the hand and upper limb girdles. Syphilitic amyotrophy resembles amyotrophic lateral sclerosis and is caused by progressive loss of anterior horn cells secondary to ischemia due to an arteritis involving the penetrating branches from the anterior spinal artery. Spinal gummas are rare and may present as a spinal cord tumor.

Diagnostic Procedures

1. The blood serological tests for syphilis will be positive in all cases.
2. Lumbar puncture may show evidence of occlusion of the subarachnoid space with low opening pressure, positive Queckenstedt test, xanthochromic CSF, lymphocytic pleocytosis, and elevated protein content. The serological tests for syphilis will be positive in the CSF.
3. Areas of spinal cord compression can be demonstrated by MRI scanning or CT scan with myelography.

Treatment Most patients respond to adequate penicillin therapy. Cord compression must be relieved surgically by removal of a gumma or excision of thickened meninges.

Tabes Dorsalis This slowly progressive degenerative condition is a rare complication of syphilis but was common in hospital clinics 40 years ago. The pathological changes, which were the result of *T. pallidum*, began in the posterior nerve roots of the site of penetration of the pia, proximal to the nerve root entry into the spinal cord. Degenerative changes in the nerve root spread into the posterior columns with progressive loss of axons and myelin culminating in total bilateral destruction of the posterior columns.

Clinical Features The earliest symptoms consisted of lightning pains—paroxysmal lancinating pains in the lower limbs eventually spreading to the trunk. Several years later, the patient developed progressive ataxia due to the loss of proprioception with

a typical wide-based, slapping gait. Autonomic involvement resulted in a painless distention of the bladder, with retention of urine, and overflow incontinence. Other autonomic defects produced loss of libido in both sexes and a tendency to postural hypotension.

Loss of joint sensation in the lower limbs resulted in Charcot joints—painless, swollen, hypermobile joints. Syphilitic optic atrophy was not uncommon, often progressing to total blindness. Impaired sensation in the feet resulted in trophic ulcers over the heads of the metatarsal bones or the heels.

Clinical examination showed Argyll Robertson pupils, optic atrophy in some cases, bilateral ptosis, and a prominent nasolabial fold, giving a typical facial appearance. There was generalized hypotonia and a wide-based, ataxic gait with a positive Romberg test.

Diagnostic Procedures

1. The blood serological test for syphilis was positive in about 50 percent of cases of tabes dorsalis.
2. The CSF examination revealed a clear fluid under normal pressure. In some cases, there was a slight increase in lymphocytic content with normal or slightly elevated protein content and an increased gamma globulin.

Treatment The treatment of tabes dorsalis is outlined in Table 16-10. Lightning pains respond to the use of carbamazepine (Tegretol) in some cases, phenytoin (Dilantin), or gabapentin. Charcot joints may require bracing or orthopedic fusion. A patient with bladder involvement should, if possible, use self-catheterization. Men might benefit from transurethral resection of the prostate. Trophic ulcers of the feet should be treated with extra care to avoid infection which leads to bony necrosis.

Syphilis in HIV Infection The manifestation, therapy, and response to treatment of syphilis in patients coinfected with HIV is the subject of controversy. Atypical presentation of syphilis, rapid progression to neurosyphilis, erratic serological findings, and failure of recommended doses of penicillin G benzathine to cure infection have been documented. However, similar problems were described before the advent of HIV infection and have also been described in treatment of syphilis in intravenous drug users in the absence of HIV infection.[64]

A diagnosis of neurosyphilis in HIV-infected patients is complicated by the frequency of abnormalities in the CSF—pleocytosis and elevated protein levels—resulting from HIV infection itself. However, at this time, HIV-infected patients with evidence of syphilis and unexplained CSF pleocytosis or elevated protein levels, as well as those with a positive CSF-VDRL test should be treated with a regimen appropriate for neurosyphilis.[65] Any patient with a lack of decline of nontreponemal antibody titers 6 months after treatment or persistence of symptoms and signs of syphilis requires assessment of the CSF and probably retreatment.[66]

Latent Syphilis   This condition may be defined as periods after acquisition of *T. pallidum* infection when untreated individuals are seroreactive but have no other signs of infection. Data are limited in such cases but suggest that penicillin is effective in preventing progression to clinical neurosyphilis.[67] Lumbar puncture may reveal pleocytosis and elevated protein levels, but these results are nonspecific and unreliable, often representing other comorbidities other than active neurosyphilis.[68] Consequently, treatment of latent syphilis should be instituted in those who show new clinical symptoms or signs of syphilis, particularly neurosyphilis, and in those who show a fourfold increase in serum VDRL titers or a positive serum treponemal antibody absorption test (FTA-ABS).

Tuberculous Meningitis

Definition   Tuberculous meningitis is an infection of the meninges caused by the acid-fast bacillus *Mycobacterium tuberculosis*.

Etiology and Pathology   The bacilli usually enter the body by inhalation. Transmission through the skin or by ingestion are rare causes of infection. Once introduced, the organisms undergo multiplication and

hematogenous dissemination and it is during this stage that the meninges are most likely to become involved. Cell-mediated immunity with migration of macrophages at the site of infection leads to the development of tubercles. When the immune response fails, the subarachnoid space is infected by rupture of meningeal tubercles followed by release of bacilli and the development of meningitis. Rupture of an intracerebral tuberculoma or direct extension from the adjacent focus (e.g., from the spinal or nasal sinuses) into the subarachonoid space is rare.

The presence of bacilli in the subarachnoid space is followed by an intense granulomatous inflammation of the leptomeninges and subjacent cortex. A thick, heavy fibrous and necrotic exudate is produced, which tends to collect at the base of the brain.

The arteries at the base of the brain are involved, and there is inflammation of the adventitia and media, with narrowing and thrombosis of the lumen. Cranial nerves II and III, and occasionally VII and VIII, are subject to compression by the heavy exudate.

Clinical Features   Although the incidence of tuberculous meningitis had decreased in the United States and Western Europe through the 1980s, there has been a disturbing increase in the number of cases worldwide in recent years. This can be attributed to the emergence of drug-resistant bacilli, inadequate disease control programs, and the advent of HIV infection, all of which contribute to the current situation.[69]

The disease occurs in all ages, but the incidence is higher in infants, young children, and the aged. It is more common among the undernourished and in those areas of the world characterized by poor hygiene and overcrowding.

There is a history of contact with an infected individual or a history of previous active tuberculosis in 30 to 50 percent of patients. In the early stages of the disease, the patient experiences anorexia, intermittent headache, lethargy, aching muscles, and low-grade fever. Irritability and poor feeding may be the only evidence of the illness in infants. Some 2 weeks after the initial febrile illness, the patient begins to complain of persistent headache and a stiff neck. This is associated with other signs of meningeal irritation, increased ICP, and focal neurological deficits, including cranial nerve palsies or hemiparesis. Infants may have a tense, bulging fontanelle. There is a slow progression over a period of weeks to months, with increasing drowsiness, evidence of progressive neurological dysfunction, and terminal coma and eventual death. In some cases, the infection is confined to the spinal cord and presents as a radiculomyelopathy. The course of the illness depends on the extent of the meningeal involvement, the immune response of the host, the virulence of the organism, and the stage at which treatment is administered.

Complications

1. Arteritis may be followed by thrombosis of a major artery, resulting in cerebral infarction.

2. Hydrocephalus. The granulomatous exudate or an arachnoiditis may block the aqueduct of Sylvius, the foramina of Luschka and Magendie, or the subarachnoid space, impeding the flow of CSF and causing hydrocephalus.

3. Seizures may occur at any time during the illness and are most common in children less than 2 years of age.

4. Focal motor deficits and impaired cognitive and intellectual functioning can develop during the course of the illness and persist.

5. Hypopituitarism as a sequel to tuberculous meningitis is not infrequent in childhood.[70]

Differential Diagnosis   The differential diagnosis of tuberculous meningitis includes viral encephalitis, partially treated pyogenic meningitis, fungal infections, and other inflammatory disorders that produce progressive neurological dysfunction. The presence of active tuberculosis elsewhere, and the results of CSF examination, are usually sufficient to establish the diagnosis.

Diagnostic Procedures

1. Lumbar puncture. Examination of the CSF is the only definitive procedure in the diagnosis of tuberculous meningitis. The CSF is under increased pressure, is clear or slightly cloudy, and contains a predominance of mononuclear cells (usually >400/mm^3), increased protein (100 to 400 mg/dL), and a decreased glucose content. However, normal glucose levels can occur. It is usually difficult to identify the bacilli in the CSF; examination of the fibrin clot after centrifugation and careful staining by the Ziehl-Neelsen method is necessary. Bacterial culture or guinea pig inoculation requires 4 to 6 weeks' incubation before a positive result might be expected. Consequently, treatment of tuberculous meningitis is often begun on an empiric basis as soon as the diagnosis is suspected. However, the polymerase chain reaction is a sensitive technique for detection of microbacterial and tuberculosis genome in the CSF,[71] giving positive results within a few hours.[72] The inhibition ELISA for *M. tuberculosis* antigen-5 is also a highly selective and reliable method for detecting infected patients within 48 to 72 h.[73] The finding of increasing levels of adenosine deaminase activity in the CSF is highly suggestive of tuberculous meningitis.[74]

2. Protein levels greater than 1000 mg/dL in the CSF and a decreasing opening pressure on serial lumbar punctures suggests a spinal block. The Queckenstedt test usually reveals lack of communication through the spinal subarachnoid space. An MRI scan will confirm the presence of arachnoiditis. More than 50 percent of patients will have an elevated sedimentation rate and a positive tuberculin skin test.

3. A chest x-ray should be obtained to detect pulmonary involvement.

4. A CT scan may reveal enhancement of the basal cisterns. Tuberculomas appear as intense nodular or ring-enhanced masses.[75] The target sign, a central area of calcification and peripheral ring enhancement, is highly suggestive of tuberculoma. Serial CT scans are useful in identifying incipient complications such as hydrocephalus, areas of calcification, encephalomalacia, tuberculous osteitis of the skull, and tuberculous otomastoiditis.[76]

5. The MRI scans are more sensitive than CT scans in detecting basal meningitis cerebral infarction owing to arteritis hydrocephalus and parenchymal tuberculomas often in combination in AIDS patients.[77] T1-weighted gadolinium enhanced images are required to demonstrate basal leptomeningeal involvement.[78]

6. Arteriography may show the presence of arteritis of the circle of Willis or its major branches involved in the basal meningitis process. Affected vessels show irregular areas of narrowing and occlusion.

Treatment

1. Tuberculous meningitis should be treated with a combination of antituberculous drugs. The drugs listed in Table 16-11 are suggested for the initial treatment of tuberculous meningitis lasting 2 months, followed by an alteration in the regimen to complete the course over a 12-month period. The addition of corticosteroids appears to increase survival rates and reduce neurological complications in tuberculous meningitis.[79] Drug-resistant cases require the substitution of more toxic drugs such as ethambutol, cycloserine, streptomycin, kanamycin ciprohexacin, or ethionamide, all of which require careful observation for development of adverse effects. Pyridoxine must be administered in the dosage of 50 mg daily to avoid the development of isoniazid (INH)-induced neuropathy, encephalopathy, or seizures.

2. Spinal arachnoiditis and arteritis may show improvement when treated with corticosteroids.

3. Seizures should be adequately controlled with anticonvulsants. The dosage of phenytoin (Dilantin) may require careful adjustment with frequent monitoring of free plasma phenytoin levels in patients taking INH because this drug inhibits the metabolism of phenytoin.

4. Basal meningitis or a selectively placed tuberculoma can impede or block the flow of CSF out of the ventricular system. Consequently, hydrocephalus associated with deteriorating neurological symptoms should be treated by a ventriculoperitoneal shunting procedure to relieve elevated intraventricular pressure.[80]

5. Paradoxical progression of tuberculosis with the development of tuberculomas during treatment of tuberculous meningitis has been reported. The new lesions progress for some time then regress if the initial antituberculous drug regimen is not changed.[81]

Prognosis The mortality of tuberculous meningitis is still between 10 and 20 percent. The prognosis is poor in infants, the elderly, when treatment is delayed, and in patients with poor nutrition or debilitation from HIV infection or other chronic diseases. The outcome is clearly associated with the stage of the disease at diagnosis and the introduction of early treatment. Those who are conscious and without neurological deficits have a good prognosis; those in coma at the beginning of treatment have a 20 percent mortality and only 20 percent make a complete recovery.[82]

Tuberculoma

A *tuberculoma* is a granulomatous mass resulting from enlargement of a caseous tubercle. Tuberculoma formation is a rare indication of tuberculous infection

Table 16-11
Suggested treatment of tuberculous meningitis

	Drugs	Adult Dosage
Initial treatment (2 months)	oral isoniazid (INH) oral rifampin oral pyrazinamide	300 mg per day 450–600 mg per day 15–30 mg/kg per day
Continued treatment (to 9 months)	oral isoniazid (INH) oral rifampin	

If multi-drug resistance is suspected a 4-drug regimen should be used until susceptibility studies are available. Ethambutol (15–25 mg/kg [800–1600 mg]/day) or capreomycin should be considered as the fourth drug.

in the United States and is more common in Canada, Great Britain, Asia, and Africa. Tuberculomas vary in size and are usually supratentorial and multiple. Most are located in the parietal lobe and may be attached to the dura and predominantly extracerebral or located deep within the brain parenchyma. Signs and symptoms depend on the primary location of the mass, but most cases present with headache, vomiting, and seizures. The diagnosis is usually considered if there is evidence of systemic tuberculosis. A CT or MRI scan will identify a space-occupying mass. A contrast-enhanced CT scan shows an enhancing mass with hypodense central necrosis and hypodense surrounding edema. A T1 gadolinium-enhanced MRI scan shows a strong rim enhancement, whereas a T2 gadolinium-enhanced scan shows hyperintense vasogenic edema, hypointense granuloma ring, and a hyperintense central necrosis.

Tuberculomas are treated with antituberculous drugs (see Table 16-11) and are often excised as a mass lesion before diagnosis. Hydrocephalus requires ventriculoperitoneal shunting. Paradoxical enlargement during antituberculous therapy is encountered occasionally and can be fatal.[83] Adjunctive therapy with steroids may be beneficial and improve the outcome.

Tuberculosis of the Spine

Single or multiple vertebral involvement by tuberculosis is frequently followed by spinal cord compression due to the development of a cold abscess in the epidural space (Pott disease).

The condition presents with pain in the back followed by signs of spinal cord involvement, including spastic paraparesis, urinary frequency and incontinence, and loss of sensation below the level of the cord compression. The site of compression can be localized by MRI scanning.

Treatment consists of antituberculous therapy and surgical decompression using an anterior spinal decompression and fusion.[84]

Tuberculosis or tuberculoma of the meninges or spinal cord without evidence of Pott disease is rare. Most cases present as extradural or arachnoid granulomas and intramedullary tuberculomas are extremely rare. The latter present as spinal cord tumors with progressive paraparesis, loss of bladder control, and back pain. A sensory level may be present with impairment of touch, pinprick, and a temperature below the level of the lesion, and there are increased tendon reflexes in the lower extremities and bilateral extensor plantar responses. Tuberculomas tend to be localized to the thoracic cord. The diagnosis is suggested by the presence of systemic tuberculosis, usually pulmonary disease. Biopsy may be necessary when the diagnosis is in doubt.

Treatment Medical treatment of tuberculosis as outlined in Table 16-11 is indicated. Progressive neurological deficits may require surgical removal of the tuberculoma.[85]

Sarcoidosis

Definition *Sarcoidosis* is an idopathic, noncaseating granulomatous disease that may involve any organ.

Etiology and Pathology The etiology is unknown. Lesions of sarcoidosis are closely related to blood vessels and consist of nodular collections of epithelioid cells without necrosis and caseation. The initial change involves activation of CD4 lymphocytes,[86] which is accentuated in the involved tissue. These cells liberate cytokines, including interleukin-1, interleukin-2, γ-interferon, tumor necrosis factor, and macrophage and granulocyte colony-stimulating factors.[87] The accumulation of macrophages and granulocytes produces granuloma formation followed by fibrosis. The nervous system is involved in about 5 percent of cases[88] but with remarkable diversity.[89]

1. Meningeal involvement produces aseptic meningitis or leptomeningeal granulomas.
2. Meningeal inflammation/fibrosis can obstruct CSF circulation, resulting in hydrocephalus.
3. Spread through the Virchow-Robin spaces results in diffuse or discrete parenchymal involvement.
4. Hypothalamic pituitary involvement may result in endocrine abnormalities, or diabetes insipidus.
5. Optic nerve or optic chiasm lesions result in papilledema, retrobulbar neuritis, optic atrophy, visual field defects, and visual deterioration.

6. Cranial nerve involvement usually encompasses the V, VII, and VIII nerves.
7. Single intracranial lesions can mimic meningiomas, gliomas, or metastases.[90]
8. Spinal cord and cauda equina lesions can also present as single or multiple tumors.[91]
9. Mononeuropathy, polyneuropathy, or symmetrical peripheral neuropathies are occasional complications.
10. Sarcoid myopathy produces proximal muscle weakness and respiratory muscle involvement as a rare complication of sarcoidosis.[92]

Clinical Features Sarcoidosis occurs in both sexes and is most common in the 20 to 40 age group.

Signs of systemic sarcoidosis are not invariably present in patients with involvement of the nervous system and occurs in about 50 percent of patients with neurosarcoidosis. However, when present, systemic involvement includes hilar lymphadenopathy, pulmonary infiltration, parotitis, uveitis, chorioretinitis, papilledema, proximal muscle weakness due to myopathy, and polyarteritis often preceded by bilateral heel pain. Sarcoidosis can damage any cranial nerve[93] but the facial and optic nerves are most commonly involved. Changes in personality and dementia can occur because of space-occupying granulomata, hydrocephalus due to basal meningitis, or metabolic changes secondary to hypothalamic and pituitary involvement. Metabolic encephalopathy may result from hypercalcemia, pulmonary insufficiency and carbon dioxide narcosis, uremia secondary to kidney involvement, or hepatic encephalopathy and severe liver involvement. Meningeal sarcoidosis may present as a chronic meningitis with CSF pleocytosis, normal or reduced glucose, and elevated protein content. Generalized or partial seizures of all types have been described in sarcoidosis.[94] Choreiform movements, parkinsonism, and embolism are rare complications. Sarcoid granulomata may occasionally mimic brain tumors and produce focal signs of brain involvement and increased ICP. Hypothalamic pituitary involvement or diabetes insipidus is probably the most common sign of intracranial sarcoidosis. Diabetes mellitus occurs in about one-third of patients with neurological sarcoidosis. Signs of endocrine deficiency can be demonstrated in many cases. Signs of

brainstem and cerebellar dysfunction are not unusual when there is multiple cranial nerve involvement. Myelopathy is rare but granulomas may occur in the spinal meninges in the nerve roots in the parenchyma of the spinal cord.[95] Transient ischemic attacks may be the only clinical manifestation of intracranial sarcoidosis, and cerebellar or brainstem ischemia can result from granulomatous involvement of the blood vessels. Mononeuropathies and polymononeuropathies result in paresthesias, numbness, pain, muscle weakness, and wasting and frequently have a protracted course.[96]

Diagnostic Procedures

1. Skull and chest x-rays. Sarcoidosis rarely produces radiolucent areas on the skull x-ray. Hilar lymphadenopathy is common and changes in the lung parenchyma are not unusual in this disease.
2. Angiotensin-converting enzyme is elevated in blood or CSF.
3. The sedimentation rate is often elevated; serum calcium and alkaline phosphatase levels are increased, and serum proteins are elevated with increase in the globulin fraction.
4. The EEG may show focal slowing, seizure activity, or generalized slowing.
5. Evoked potentials. Optic nerve and optic chiasm involvement is not uncommon, producing abnormal visual evoked responses. Brainstem auditory evoked responses are abnormal in eighth nerve involvement and somatosensory evoked responses in spinal cord disease.
6. The MRI and CT scans are usually abnormal in intracranial sarcoidosis, with demonstration of granulomatous lesions at the base of the brain, over the convexities in the interhemispheric fissure, occasionally in the periventricular area, or in the cerebellum (Fig. 16-7). Hydrocephalus may be present. Spinal MRI can demonstrate intramedullary disease or tumor-like lesions in the cauda equina.[97]
7. On lumbar puncture, the CSF shows a lymphocytic pleocytosis and elevated protein content. Glucose content is occasionally reduced. Cultures are negative. Oligoclonal bands can be present and the IgG index elevated.

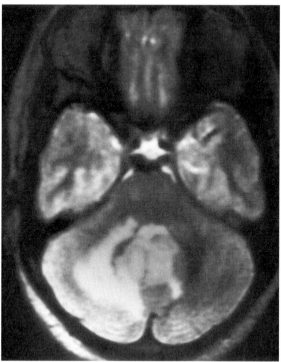

Figure 16-7
MRI T2-weighted image demonstrating a mass involving the floor of the fourth ventricle surrounded by edema of the right cerebellar white matter—sarcoidosis.

8. The arteriogram may show the presence of an arteritis.
9. Nerve conduction studies will demonstrate a peripheral neuropathy.
10. Histological confirmation of sarcoidosis may be obtained with biopsy of muscle, nerve, liver, or scalene lymph node.
11. Endocrine studies are indicated in all cases with intracranial involvement because of the high risk of hypothalamic and pituitary involvement. Tests should include thyroid function tests, prolactin, testosterone, and estrogen levels. Follicle-stimulating hormone, luteinizing hormone, corticotropin, cortisol, and serum sodium determinations should be obtained.
12. Skin tests. A tuberculin test is usually negative. The Kveim test (intracutaneous inoculation of suspension of sarcoid tissue) produces a granulo-

matous papule in about 6 weeks in 80 percent of cases.

Treatment

1. The use of corticosteroids in neurological sarcoidosis (neurosarcoidosis) is often effective and some patients show dramatic improvement when treated with corticosteroid preparations. Dexamethasone (Decadron) 12 mg daily or methylprednisolone (Medrol) 80 mg daily can be reduced to a minimum effective dose once symptoms resolve and can be continued on an alternate-day basis for many months.

   In some cases, a course of corticosteroids can be used and discontinued when symptoms abate, to be reintroduced in the presence of relapse. This method tends to delay the development of adverse effects.
2. When steroids are not effective or absolutely contraindicated because of psychosis or relatively contraindicated in diabetes mellitus or aseptic necrosis of joints, treatment with immunosuppressant drugs is often effective. Methotrexate is an effective alternative therapy in a single dose of 10 mg a week. A complete blood count and renal and hepatic function tests should be performed every month, and a liver biopsy every 2 years.[98]
3. Other alternative therapies include antimalarial drugs such as hydroxycholoroquine, or azathioprine, cyclophosphamide, and chlorambucil. Radiation therapy has been successfully employed for inaccessible sarcoid mass lesions in the brain.[99]
4. Increased ICP due to hydrocephalus can be relieved by a ventriculoperitoneal shunt procedure.
5. Diabetes insipidus and other endocrine deficiencies should be treated with appropriate substitution therapy.
6. Seizures respond to a therapeutic dose of anticonvulsants.
7. Occasionally, large intracranial granulomatous masses can be removed surgically.
8. Sarcoid myopathy responds to corticosteroid therapy.

Prognosis   Many patients show a spontaneous regression and apparent recovery, whereas others have a chronic relapsing, remitting course. The condition can be fatal, but this is unusual. The prognosis is better in patients with involvement of only the peripheral nervous system.

Cat Scratch Disease

Definition   This disease is an infection caused by a gram-negative bacterium transmitted by a cat scratch or bite.

Etiology   The bacterium *Bartonella henselae* is found by serological analysis to be present in 84 percent of cats from households in which patients have had a confirmed diagnosis of cat scratch disease.

Clinical Features   The infection usually results in a benign lymphadenitis involving the lymph nodes draining the area, some 2 weeks after a cat scratch or bite.[100] Encephalitis and cerebral arteritis have been described in about 2 percent of cases and can cause status epilepticus and coma.[101] Patients with cat scratch fever have rising serum antibody titers to *B. henselae* measured by indirect fluorescent antibody assay.[102]

Treatment

1. Although the bacterium is susceptible in vitro to several antibiotics, treatment efficacy is unproven. In severe cases such as encephalitis, treatment with doxycycline, erythromycin, or chloramphenicol is recommended.
2. Seizures should be treated with anticonvulsant medication. Status epilepticus requires emergency treatment (see Chap. 4).

Prognosis   Most patients, including those with encephalitis, recover without sequelae.

Rickettsial Infections

The CNS is frequently affected during epidemic typhus (*Rickettsia prowazekii*), murine typhus (*Rickettsia mooseri*), scrub typhus (*Rickettsia tsutsugamushi*), and Rocky Mountain spotted fever (*Rickettsia rickettsii*).

Etiology and Pathology   A rickettsial infection transmitted by insect vectors including fleas, lice, ticks, and mites.

Pathological changes include swelling of blood vessel endothelial linings and thrombosis. This is followed by a perivascular leukocytosis and inflammation resulting in a typhus nodule. Eventually astrocytosis forms a glial scar.

Clinical Features   Typhus is rare in the United States, but Rocky Mountain spotted fever is increasing in frequency and spreading through the central, southern, and eastern regions of the United States.

Typhus presents as a severe encephalitis, often associated with seizures and focal neurological deficits. In Rocky Mountain spotted fever, nausea, vomiting, headache, and fever are followed by the development of a maculopapular rash on the ankles and wrists, which spreads distally and then proximally. There may be signs of meningeal irritation, seizures, and focal deficits including hemiplegia or hemiparesis.

Diagnostic Procedures

1. There is a progressive rise in serum antibodies to rickettsii.
2. The Weil-Felix reaction is positive in many patients, but false negatives and positives are too frequent to rely on this test.
3. A rapid diagnosis of Rocky Mountain spotted fever or typhus can be established by the polymerase chain reaction.

Treatment   Doxycycline 100 mg q12h is the drug of choice for Rocky Mountain spotted fever. Tetracycline is the second choice, followed by chloramphenicol.[103]

The treatment of Rocky Mountain spotted fever cannot wait for the preparation and transportation of specimens to facilities where rapid diagnostic tests are available. Prompt treatment is essential. Consequently, treatment should be initiated based on clinical symptoms and signs. Delay carries a great risk of complications and death.[104]

FUNGAL INFECTIONS

Definition The systemic fungal infections discussed in this section have the capacity to invade the CNS either directly or through the bloodstream, producing a serious, often fatal disorder that is exceedingly difficult to treat.

Etiology and Pathology There are approximately 20 genera of fungi capable of producing CNS disease. Table 16-12 lists the most common species, tissue characteristics of these fungi, their usual portal of entry into the body, characteristic pathological changes, and treatment.

The majority of fungi gain access to the CNS by hematogenous dissemination from a distant source. Some, such as mucormycosis, may spread directly from an infected orbit or sinus.[105] The fungi spread through the subarachnoid space and produce a chronic basal meningitis with granulomatous lesions composed of epithelioid cells, giant cells, lymphocytes, and plasma cells. Some of the fungi have the capacity to invade the brain parenchyma, and tissue destruction is followed by abscess or cyst formation. Involvement of cerebral vessels may result in thrombosis and ischemic infarction. *Candida* species are the most frequently identified cause of CNS infection.

Clinical Features There has been a steady increase in the number of cases of fungal disease of the CNS due to increasing numbers of immunocompromised hosts,[106] greater physician awareness, and improved diagnostic capability.

The majority of patients present with a history of chronic or subacute relapsing illness. Factors predisposing to fungal infection include hematological malignancies, immunosuppression by cytotoxic drugs and HIV/AIDS.[107] Ventriculoperitoneal shunt recipients, transplant recipients, IV drug abusers, those with debilitating diseases such as diabetes mellitus, alcoholism, narcotic addiction, and those residing in an endemic area are at highest risk for fungal infections. *Candida meningitis* is an emerging problem in neurological patients particularly those who have been treated for an antecedent bacterial meningitis.[108] Initial symptoms of neurological involvement are often nonspecific and consist of headache, anorexia, nausea, vomiting, and insomnia. This may be followed by signs of meningeal irritation and papilledema, or focal signs of cranial nerve involvement or hemiparesis. At the same time, there may be evidence of involvement of other organs, including the liver, spleen, and kidney. Patients who present with chronic sinusitis followed by sudden blindness in one eye, proptosis, a reddish brown nasal discharge, and involvement of the third, fourth, or sixth cranial nerves are usually infected by mucormycosis.

Course Most fungal diseases have a subacute or chronic course, although mucormycosis, which most frequently develops in individuals with poorly controlled diabetes mellitus or immunosuppression,[109] is often rapidly fatal.[110] The mortality approaches 100 percent in untreated fungal disease involving the CNS. Death results from a terminal meningitis, brain herniation, or systemic involvement.

Complications The course of disease may be complicated by hydrocephalus, vertebral body involvement with spinal cord compression, the development of the fungal mycotic aneurysms, or a relapsing course despite adequate chemotherapy.

Diagnostic Procedures

1. Lumbar puncture is the definitive procedure in the diagnosis and determination of the etiology of fungal disease. The CSF is either clear, turbid, or xanthochromic and is usually under an elevated pressure. The fluid has a monocytic pleocytosis and elevated protein content, and a decreased glucose content and elevated lactic acid levels.[111] Occasionally there are organisms in the centrifuged specimen stained with 10 percent potassium hydroxide. India ink is a useful stain in cases of suspected cryptococcosis. A large volume (20 to 50 mL) of CSF may be required to isolate the organism by culture. Cisternal puncture is strongly recommended when there is a high level of suspicion of fungal infection, with repeatedly negative cultures following lumbar puncture.

2. Skin tests, complement fixation tests, fluorescent antibody tests, and latex agglutination tests

Table 16-12
Fungal characteristics

Fungus	Characteristics	Portal of entry	Epidemiology	Persons at risk	Pathology
Cryptococcus neoformans	Yeast-like, budding Large gelatinous capsule Predilection for CNS	Respiratory	Worldwide Found in soil and pigeon droppings	Those who have leukemia, renal transplants, lymphoma, AIDS, or who have undergone chronic corticosteroid therapy	Perivascular cyst formation
Coccidioides immitis	Nonbudding, thick-walled Spherules filled with endospores	Respiratory or skin	Southwestern U.S. Dust-borne	Those who live in an endemic area	
Candida albicans	Yeast-like, budding Small, oval Stains gram-positive	Endocarditis, gastrointestinal, urinary respiratory	Worldwide Skin, gastrointestinal, mucous membrane flora	Drug addicts The elderly Those who are immunosuppressed or have AIDS	Abscess formation
Aspergillus fumigatus	Septate branching, hyphae with small green spores Common laboratory contaminant	Respiratory or skin	Worldwide Soil, water, air Warm, humid climate		Inflammatory granulomas Abscess formation Thrombus formation
Phycomycetes mucor and rhizopus	Large broad nonseptate hyphae Common laboratory contaminant	Nasal sinus or orbit	Worldwide Nasal and throat flora Soil and decaying matter	Diabetes in ketoacidosis Immunosuppressed persons Heroin addicts	Hyphae have affinity for vasculature
Histoplasma capsulatum	Yeast-like, budding Small, oval Predilection for reticuloendothelial system	Respiratory	Central U.S. Soil, bird droppings, bats	Those who live in an endemic area	Inflammatory granulomas

Blastomyces	Yeast-like, single or budding Round, doubly refractile wall	Respiratory or skin	Midwest U.S. Soil	Those who live in an endemic area	Abscess formation
Paracoccidi-oides brasiliensis	Yeast-like Multiple, budding	Oral cavity	South America Central America	Those who live in an endemic area	
Sporothrix schenckii	Budding Round to oval Stains gram-positive	Skin	Gastrointestinal flora		
Cladosporium bantianum	Septate, branching, brown hyphae	Respiratory			Abscess formation
Nocardia asteroides	Anaerobic Stains gram-positive, acid-fast	Respiratory	Soil, water, grass	Those who are immuno-suppressed	Abscess formation, multiloculated, multiple abscesses
Actinomyces	Actinomycotic "granules"—clumps of tangled filaments with radiating terminal "clubs"	Dental abscess Tooth extraction Poor dentition Chronic otitis Chronic sinusitis	Worldwide	Those with poor dentition	Cerebral abscess Subdural empyema Meningitis Actinomycoma

are available for the majority of fungi listed in Table 16-13.

3. The presence of leukocytosis or an abnormal chest x-ray may be evidence of infection elsewhere in the body. Cultures and smears of sputum and skin lesions may be positive for fungi. Bone marrow biopsy and culture are usually positive in disseminated histoplasmosis.

4. Either MRI or CT scans may show the presence of an abscess, granuloma, or hydrocephalus.

5. Skull x-rays may reveal osteomyelitis.

Differential Diagnosis The presence of tuberculous meningitis, bacterial meningitis, brain abscess, or neoplasm should be considered when evidence of fungal infection is lacking.

Treatment

1. Treatment is outlined in Table 16-13. Amphotericin B is frequently used in fungal infections of the CNS and adverse effects from the use of this drug are not uncommon. Consequently, complete blood counts, serum electrolytes, and renal function must be monitored regularly. Intrathecal amphotericin B is recommended for some fungal infections and can be given by intralumbar or intracisternal injections or through an Ommaya reservoir. Adverse effects include headache, fever, nausea, vomiting, and hypotension. There may be disturbance of renal function with azotemia and hyperkalemia and bone marrow suppression producing anemia.

   Penicillin G is the preferred antibiotic for actinomycosis infections. Nocardial infections respond to treatment with trimethoprim/sulfamethoxazole.

2. Symptomatic treatment is required for seizures hydrocephalus, increased ICP, and the toxic effects of antibiotic therapy.

Cryptococcal Meningitis

Cryptococcosis is the most common systemic fungal infection in humans, and cryptococcal meningitis is the most common fungal infection in the CNS in

AIDS,[112] immunocompromised individuals, and in patients with ventriculoperitoneal shunts.[113]

Etiology and Pathology *Cryptococcus neoformans* is present worldwide and is found in soil, wood, bird nests, bird droppings, some fruits, and milk. The yeast is a single budding organism with a prominent gelatinous capsule that grows rapidly in blood agar culture medium at room temperature.

Dissemination is by the airborne route and the organism is believed to gain access to the host by the respiratory route and is contained then by a cell-mediated immune response.[114] An immunodeficiency permits hematogenous spread to other organs, particularly the CNS.

Brain involvement produces a diffuse granulomatous cryptococcal meningitis, or cysts in the cortex, and solid or cystic nodules in the central gray matter (Fig. 16-8). The presence of the organism usually results in a minimal inflammatory reaction in most cases.

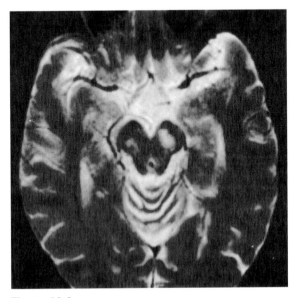

Figure 16-8
MRI T2-weighted image. Well-defined high signal intensity areas bilaterally (gelatinous pseudocysts) and enlarged Virchow-Robin spaces in a case of cryptococcosis.

Table 16-13

Organism	Pathology	Treatment
Actinomycosis	Cervicofacial abscess Pulmonary abscess Chronic meningitis	Penicillin G 10–20 million units qd IV 4–6 weeks, then penicillin V 2–4 g qd po 6–12 months, OR Ampicillin 50 mg/kg/qd IV 4–6 weeks, then 500 mg po q8h 6 months
Aspergillus fumigatus	Meningitis Involvement of arterial walls causing thrombosis and cerebral infarction	Amphotericin B. Rapid increase to 1.0–1.5 mg/kg/qd IV to total dose 2.0–2.5 g OR Itraconazole 600 mg qd po for 4 days, then 200–400 mg qd po for 1 year
Blastomyces	Meningitis (rare)	Itraconazole 200–400 mg qd po at breakfast for 6 months
Candida albicans	Meningitis Meningoencephalitis Cerebral abscess Cerebral granulomas	Amphotericin B 0.6 mg/kg/qd IV for 7 days followed by 0.8 mg/kg qod IV to total dose 0.5–1.0 g OR Fluconazole 400 mg qd IV for 7 days, then po for 14 days after last positive blood culture
Coccidioidomycosis immitis	Meningitis Meningoencephalitis Meningomyelitis	Fluconazole 400–600 mg qd po for 9–12 months OR Amphotericin B 0.6 mg/kg qd × 7 days, then 0.8 mg/kg qod. Total dose 2.5 g plus 0.1–0.3 mg qd intraventricular via reservoir
Cryptococcus neoformans	Meningitis with solid granulomas or cysts in cortex or central gray matter	Amphotericin B 0.5–0.8 mg/kg qd IV plus flucytosine 37.5 mg/kg q6h po until patient afebrile and cultures negative, then stop amphotericin B and flucytosine. Start fluconazole 200 mg qd 8–10 weeks. For HIV positive/AIDS: Amphotericin B 0.5–0.8/kg/qd IV until afebrile without headache, nausea or vomiting. Then discontinue amphotericin B, start fluconazole 500 mg po qd to complete 8–10 weeks course. Maintain on fluconazole 200 mg po qd indefinitely.
Histoplasmosis (*Histoplasma capsulatum*)	Meningoencephalitis particularly in immunosuppressed individuals	Itraconazole 200 mg with breakfast for 9 months. If infection severe, 200 mg tid for 3 days, then 200 mg bid until response, then 200 mg daily. Immunosuppressed patients: Amphotericin B 0.6 mg/kg/day IV for 7 days then 0.8 mg/kg qod for 3 weeks. Total dose 10–15 g. Then begin itraconazole 200 mg/day po.
Mucormycosis	Sinusitis, orbital cellulitis, otitis media, meningitis, meningoencephalitis, cerebrovascular thrombosis, cerebral infarction, cerebral abscess	Amphotericin B increase rapidly to 0.8–1.5 mg/kg/day IV, change to qod when improving. Total dose 2.5–3.0 g. Surgical debridement usually required. Control diabetic ketoacidosis.
Nocardiosis (*Nocardia asteroides*)	Brain abscess	Sulfamethoxazole or trimethoprim/sulfamethoxazole plus ceftriaxone 2.0 g q12h IV plus amikacin 400 mg q12h IV for 4–8 weeks.

Clinical Features The early symptoms are nonspecific, consisting of fever, malaise, headache, nausea and vomiting, with later development of papilledema, other cranial nerve palsies, and seizures. Mild mental changes of irritability and depression ultimately give way to severe psychotic disturbances and severe visual loss in some patients.[115] Relapses and remissions are common, but survival is from 6 months to 1 year in untreated cases. Nuchal rigidity and a positive Kernig's sign can be absent in early infection but are present in all established cases.

Diagnostic Procedures The CSF shows an increased opening pressure and the fluid is usually clear but occasionally xanthochromic. There is usually a pleocytosis with a lymphocytic count up to 1000 cells per cubic millimeter, but absence of a cellular response has been reported. The protein content is elevated and the glucose content reduced. However, CSF abnormalities of a similar composition are not uncommon in AIDS patients with or without cryptococcal infection, indicating the need for additional testing to identify an etiological agent.[116] A CSF cryptococcal antigen titer of more than 1:8 is diagnostic. However, spherical, thick-walled organisms can be identified in the CSF microscopically, using an India ink stain, in many cases, or the diagnosis established by the polymerase chain reaction.

Treatment See Table 16-13. Adverse effects of therapy, including fever, impaired renal function, and leukoencephalopathy, may complicate amphotericin therapy. Flucytosine can cause gastrointestinal, lymphocyte, and bone marrow suppression. Patients with AIDS have a greater than 50 percent relapse rate and require long-term suppression treatment with fluconazole. Itraconazole has been reported to cause reversible hepatitis or hepatotoxicity. This is a rare complication occurring in patients receiving multiple medications. Consequently the causal association with itraconazole is uncertain.

Coccidioidomycosis Meningitis

Coccidioidomycosis is endemic in the Southwestern United States and usually presents as a subclinical infection or a mild pulmonary infection. Disseminated coccidioidomycosis, which usually occurs in immunosuppressed individuals, is occasionally complicated by involvement of the CNS, resulting in considerable morbidity and mortality.[117]

Etiology and Pathology *Coccidioidomycosis immitis* is a dimorphic fungus, which exists in nature as a mycelial form but assumes spherule form in human or animal tissues.

The fungus is disseminated by the airborne route, entering the lungs of the host where it is usually contained by a cell-mediated immune response. When this response fails, the fungus can spread into the CNS, producing meningitis, meningoencephalitis, meningomyelitis, or a vasculitis with extensive parenchymal damage.

Clinical Features Coccidioidomycosis meningitis presents in patients with disseminated coccidioidomycosis in an acute or chronic form. The condition is rare but increasing because of HIV infection and other immunocompromised conditions. Chronic meningitis causes headache, fever, weight loss, and memory loss. Examination shows nuchal rigidity, papilledema, cranial nerve lesions, cerebellar ataxia, and signs of long tract involvement. Meningomyelitis and severe parenchymal damage is rare.

Diagnostic Procedures CSF findings are those of chronic infection with a lymphocytic pleocytosis—mean cell count 260/dL, increased protein, and reduced glucose content. CSF culture is positive in about 50 percent of patients. Modified complement fixation testing of CSF equal to or greater than 1:16 is positive in 95 percent of cases. The diagnosis can be established by the polymerase chain reaction. The MRI scan is compatible with a granulomatous infection of the brain and meninges (Fig. 16-9).

Treatment See Table 16-13.

Histoplasmosis

Definition Histoplasmosis is the most common systemic fungal infection in North America. However, infection is asymptomatic in the great majority of cases, and symptomatic CNS infection is rare.

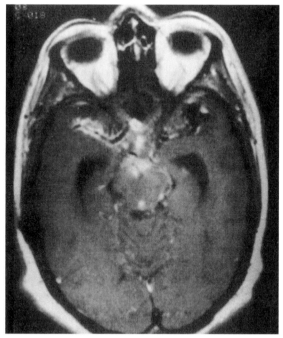

Figure 16-9
MRI T1-weighted image with gadolinium enhancement showing high signal lesions mesencephalic junction with some leptomeningeal enhancement. Compatible with a granulomatous infection—coccidioidomycosis.

Etiology and Pathology   Histoplasmosis is a disease of the Eastern and Southeastern United States, occurring predominantly in the Mississippi, Ohio, and St. Lawrence river valleys, and in North Carolina and Virginia. The majority of adults in these areas have subclinical infections, and overt involvement of the CNS rarely presents as a chronic meningitis, miliary noncaseating granulomas, or larger granulomas containing giant cells and occasionally showing caseation.

Clinical Features   Signs of generalized systemic histoplasmosis include fever, poor appetite, weight loss, and malaise. Neurological symptoms include memory impairment, seizures, hemiparesis, and ataxia with increased tendon reflexes and extensor plantar responses.[118]

Diagnostic Procedures

1.   The CSF usually shows increased protein but normal glucose levels and a variable increase in lymphocytes. Culture for histoplasmosis is often negative.

2.   Detection of histoplasma DNA by polymerase chain reaction is the most sensitive method available for positive diagnosis.

3.   Bone marrow biopsy and culture is usually positive in disseminated histoplasmosis.

Treatment   See Table 16-13.

Aspergillosis

Definition   Aspergillosis is a mold which is usually associated with respiratory or sinus infections with an occasional rare spread to the CNS.

Etiology and Pathology   The mold is found in soil and water, particularly in warm, humid climates. The organism rarely causes infection unless the host is immunosuppressed. The paranasal sinuses, orbit, or lungs are the usual sites of infection, with occasional spread to the CNS, resulting in focal or generalized meningitis or brain abscess. Spread from the paranasal sinuses, orbit, or middle ear results in single or a few abscesses in the frontal or temporal lobes. Hematogenous spread produces multiple small abscesses at the junction of gray and white matter. Involvement of intracerebral arteries results in angiitis with thrombosis and cerebral infarction.

Clinical Features   The most common neurological presentation is cerebral infarction. Headache and seizures can occur. Meningeal irritation is unusual. Meningitis and brain abscess are rare complications of this infection.

Diagnostic Procedures

1.   The CSF pressure can be elevated and the fluid is abnormal, with a lymphocytic pleocytosis, increased protein, and low glucose levels. Culture is usually negative. Normal cerebrospinal fluid has been described.

2. There may be several ring-enhanced lesions on MRI scanning.[119]

3. The sudden onset of a stroke in a young immunocompromised individual should suggest the diagnosis of aspergillosis.[120]

4. The polymerase chain reaction is positive on blood or CSF.

Treatment   See Table 16-13.

PROTOZOAN DISEASES

Toxoplasmosis, amebiasis, and malaria are protozoan organisms that occasionally produce infection in the CNS.

Amebiasis

Primary amebic meningoencephalitis is an acute, severe meningoencephalitis that results from infection by free-living amebae of the genera *Naegleria fowleri*. Infection affects children and young adults and is acquired through the nasal passages while swimming in infected water. There are an acute onset of fever, nausea and vomiting, severe headache, and meningeal irritation, rapidly followed by stupor, seizures, and coma. Lumbar puncture reveals cloudy CSF under increased pressure. There is a polymorphonuclear pleocytosis with a decreased glucose content and elevated protein content. Motile amebae may be evident on wet preparations. Treatment must be administered early and consists of amphotericin B and rifampin. Mortality approaches 100 percent.

Granulomatous amebic encephalitis is a subacute or chronic meningoencephalitis caused by amebae of the *Acanthamoeba* or *Leptomyxa* species.[121] These amebae affect the CNS from the respiratory tract or gastrointestinal tract through the nasal mucosa. The brain shows areas of infarction or abscess formation. There is an angiitis with a blood vessel occlusion. Patients present with personality change, hemiparesis, and seizures. The mortality rate is high.

Malaria

The CNS is involved in approximately 1 to 2 percent of infections in malaria caused by *Plasmodium fal-*

ciparum. Falciparum malaria is one of the most lethal parasitic infections in the world responsible for more than one million deaths in African children per year. Cerebral malaria is the result of a generalized vasculitis[122] aggravated by cytokine production, anemia, and shock.[123] Proinflammatory cytokines including tissue necrosis factor can generate inducible nitric oxide synthase causing nitric oxide to be released in a hypermetabolic state with hyperlactatemia and hypoglycemia.[124] This metabolic abnormality coupled with hypoxia induced by cytoadherence of parasitised erythrocytes in microvascular beds[125] is the probable basis for life-threatening falciparum malaria.[126] There is abrupt onset of confusion and clouding of consciousness in cerebral malaria, with progression to stupor and coma. Partial or generalized seizures, dysphasia, hemianopia, or hemiparesis may occur. Other organs may be involved simultaneously when the vascultitis results in acute tubular necrosis and adult respiratory distress syndrome (ARDS). Additional complications include severe anemia, disseminated intravascular coagulation, and hypoglycemia.[127]

Diagnostic Procedures

1. Peripheral blood smears will reveal the presence of malarial parasites.

2. Blood glucose levels should be monitored frequently because of the risk of hypoglycemia.

3. A CT scan followed by lumbar puncture is necessary to exclude other forms of meningitis.

4. Arterial blood gases, electrolytes, blood urea nitrogen, creatinine, and complete blood counts should be obtained frequently.

Treatment

1. The patient should be given a loading dose of quinine or quinidine intravenously with continuous electrocardiographic monitoring. Quinine sulfate is administered in doses of 600 mg q8h for 7 days. When quinine is not available, quinidine gluconate is of equal potency and should be administered in a 5% glucose solution with electrocardiographic monitoring, in doses of 10 mg quinidine gluconate per kg over 1 to 2 h, followed by a continuous infusion of 0.02 mg quinidine gluconate per kg per

minute. If hypotension occurs, the infusion should be slowed. Treatment should be augmented by the use of tetracycline 500 mg q6h over a 7-day period or doxycycline 100 mg q12h. Cerebral edema may be reduced by the use of mannitol.

2. Exchange transfusion is indicated when the parasite load is very high and blood transfusion may be used for severe anemia.[128]
3. Seizures should be controlled by anticonvulsants.
4. Renal failure requires dialysis.
5. Intravenous glucose is necessary to control hypoglycemia in some cases.
6. Intubation and assisted ventilation is required for ARDS.
7. Gram-negative septicemia is a frequent complication that could be prevented by antibiotics.

Prognosis The mortality of cerebral malaria is high; most untreated patients die within 72 h. Treated patients have a 25 to 50 percent mortality rate.

Cysticercosis

Definition *Cysticercus cellulosae* is the larval stage of development of the cestode *Taenia solium* (pork tapeworm).

Etiology and Pathology Cysticercosis is acquired by the ingestion of the eggs from a gravid adult worm. The covering is dissolved in the stomach and the larvae traverse the mucosal lining of the stomach, enter the bloodstream, and are disseminated throughout the body, including the brain. When mature, the larval stage is known as a cysticercus. It is found in three forms within the CNS: a cystic form involving the ventricles and brain parenchyma, a racemose form involving the meninges, and a miliary form that is common in children. The presence of the parasites results in an intense tissue reaction and the formation of a capsule. The cyst contents and capsule calcify after the larvae die. The cyst then loses osmoregulation and begins to swell. There is a release of parasite antigens and a host immune-inflammatory response with worsening of symptoms including increased intracranial pressure or spinal cord compression at this stage.[129]

Clinical Features Cysticercosis is endemic in Mexico, Latin America, Asia, and the southern United States. The disease accounts for about 30 percent of intracranial mass lesions in Mexico and Latin America. Cysticercosis usually occurs in children and young adults. Symptoms may occur at an early stage following dissemination of the cysticerci, and the patient may present with muscle pain, severe headache, nausea and vomiting, partial or generalized seizures or confusion, delusions, and clouding of consciousness. However, the most frequent clinical manifestation of neurocysticercosis are seizures.[130] Physical examination may reveal subcutaneous nodules and muscle tenderness. There may be papilledema or retinal detachment with visual deterioration or visual field abnormalities, cranial nerve involvement, and focal neurological deficit. In many cases, neurological abnormalities do not appear for many months or years after the parasite is disseminated and matured. The most common symptom at that stage is one of focal or generalized seizures. Cysts blocking the outflow of the ventricular system will cause headache, hydrocephalus, and papilledema. More peripherally located cysts can cause a meningeal reaction with characteristics of a chronic meningitis. The presence of cysts at the base of the brain results in a vasculitis, thrombosis, and cerebral infarction.

Diagnostic Procedures

1. Examination of the stool may reveal the presence of ova in the early stages.
2. The CSF is often abnormal with a mild eosinophilic pleocytosis increased protein, increased gamma globulin, decreased glucose, and a positive complement fixation test (dilution$>$1:16).
3. MRI abnormalities include hydrocephalus or vesicular, colloid vesicular granular nodules or nodular calcified cysts.[131] The MRI scan is superior to CT scan in the evaluation of cysticercosis (Fig. 16-10).
4. An x-ray of muscle often shows the presence of calcified cysts.
5. Biopsy of the organism can be demonstrated by biopsy of a subcutaneous nodule or involved muscle.

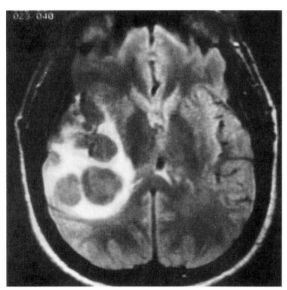

Figure 16-10
MRI—proton density weighted image. There is marked edema surrounding a cystic area in the right hemisphere—racemose cysticercosis.

6. Complement fixation and indirect hemagglutination tests may be positive in blood and CSF. The polymerase chain reaction is the method of choice to confirm the diagnosis.

Treatment Praziquantel 50 mg/kg daily for 2 weeks with dexamethasone coverage will kill the parasite, the steroids limiting the inflammatory response to the foreign substance.[132] Plasma concentrations of the drug are increased by concomitant administration of cimetidine and a high carbohydrate diet.[133] A regimen of praziquantel lasting only 1 day given in 3 doses of 25 mg/Kg at 2-hour intervals exposes the parasite to higher drug concentrations and is considered equally effective. Small single cysts may resolve completely following the use of praziquantel.[134] Albendazole 15 mg/kg daily may be useful in patients who show a partial response to praziquantel therapy.[135] Single cysts should be excised when they are causing hydrocephalus or acting as a mass lesion. Steroid therapy will reduce cerebral edema in the early stages of the disease, but decompression craniotomy may be necessary when elevated ICP and cerebral edema are refractory to treatment. Hydrocephalus may be treated by a shunting procedure, but the shunt is often blocked by debris.[136] Seizures should be controlled with adequate doses of anticonvulsants.[137]

Prognosis The mortality rate is 50 percent in patients with hydrocephalus. Most die within 2 years after shunting. Bacterial meningitis and shunt obstruction are not uncommon. Many cases require multiple surgical procedures.[138]

Hydatid Disease (Echinococcosis)

Echinococcosis is the presence of the larvae of the sheep tapeworm, *Echinococcus granulosus,* in the body tissues. The disease is endemic in sheep- and cattle-rearing countries in Africa, Australia, the Mediterranean countries, the Middle East and the Arctic regions of Asia and North America.

The ova of the tapeworm are transmitted to man who becomes an accidental intermediate host by petting or handling infected dogs. The ova are then ingested in contaminated food and the larvae hatch in the intestinal tract, penetrate the mucosa, and disseminate throughout the body. Children are frequently infected. Rupture of a hydatid cyst in muscle produces an intense focal myositis. Hydatid cysts in the brain or an intraspinal extradural location[139] occur in about 2 percent of cases and often present as slowly developing mass lesions. Rupture of the cyst and liberation of toxic contents results in a severe anaphylactic reaction and disseminated infection.[140] Peripheral eosinophilia is an inconsistent finding. The diagnosis is established by polymerase chain reaction or indirect hemagglutination combined with CIE.[141] An MRI or CT scan will demonstrate the number and positioning of the cysts and allow planning for surgical excision. Hydatid cyst should be included in the differential diagnosis when a cystic brain lesion is found in a patient from an endemic echinococcus area.[142] Cysts should be removed unruptured to prevent spillage of fertile daughter cysts and the high risk of recurrence should this occur.[143]

VIRAL INFECTIONS

Many different viruses have the capacity to invade the CNS. The type of infection depends on the degree of involvement of the CNS. A viral infection that is confined to the meninges results in aseptic meningitis; invasion of the brain parenchyma produces a meningoencephalitis or encephalitis.

In general, a particular family of viruses tends to produce the same type of response. Thus, the enteroviruses are usually associated with aseptic meningitis, whereas arthropod-borne viruses often cause encephalitis (Table 16-14).

Aseptic Meningitis

Definition *Aseptic meningitis* is a syndrome of headache, meningeal irritation, and monocytic pleocytosis and is most commonly caused by the enteroviruses, the mumps virus being the next most common viral agent.

Etiology and Pathology The viruses frequently associated with aseptic meningitis are enteroviruses (Coxsackie A types 7 and 9; Coxsackie B types 1–6; echovirus types 2–6, 9, 11, 14, 16, 18 and 30, poliovirus types 1–3). Other viruses identified with this syndrome include paramyxovirus (mumps), herpes simplex virus type 2, adenovirus, and lymphocytic choriomeningitis. However, the majority of viruses with neurotropic properties are capable of producing this syndrome.

The leptomeninges appear grossly normal in aseptic meningitis but show the presence of a mild inflammatory reaction. There is a predominantly polymorphonuclear response in some cases in the early stages, followed by plasma cell and lymphocytic infiltration within 8 to 12 h. The blood vessels show perivascular cuffing.

Clinical Features Viral meningitis is more common in children and often occurs in epidemics. Enterovirus infections are usually encountered in the summer and fall; mumps-induced aseptic meningitis is more apt to occur in the winter and spring.

The condition is characterized by headache, fever, vomiting, malaise, photophobia, myalgia, irritability, and meningeal irritation, producing a stiff neck and positive Kernig's and Brudzinski's signs. There may be signs of systemic involvement indicating infection by a particular virus such as parotitis in mumps or muscle paralysis in patients with poliovirus infection. However, in general, complications are rare and the patient begins to recover within a few days and the recovery is complete in 2 weeks.[144]

Diagnostic Procedures

1. Lumbar puncture usually reveals an elevated opening pressure and a mild pleocytosis (10 to 1000 cells/mm^3) consisting in some cases of polymorphonuclear cells in the early stages, with early replacement by lymphocytes. However, in most cases, there will be a definite lymphocytic pleocytosis. The protein content is normal or slightly elevated and the glucose content is normal. If the diagnosis is in doubt, the lumbar puncture should be repeated in 8 to 12 h, when there will be a change from polymorphonuclear cells to lymphocytes in questionable cases.

2. The demonstration of a rising antibody titer for a specific virus can be determined in serum samples drawn in the early stages of the illness and after 2 weeks. This means that the diagnosis of a specific viral infection is retrospective.

3. Polymerase chain reaction (PCR) is considered a rapid senstive and relatively simple method for identification of viral DNA or RNA within a few hours.[145]

4. A positive viral culture can be obtained from the CSF in some cases. Counterimmunoelectrophoresis may be of value in identifying the type of virus involved.

5. An oropharyngeal swab and a stool specimen should be obtained for viral culture.

Differential Diagnosis See Table 16-15.

1. Early bacterial meningitis or partially treated bacterial meningitis.

The diagnosis may be difficult in the early stages, because of the presence of polymorphonuclear

Table 16-14

Classification of viruses producing CNS disease

Family	Genus species	Clinical picture
Arenavirus	Lymphocytic choriomeningitis	Meningitis, encephalitis
Bunyavirus	California encephalitis	Encephalitis
Herpesvirus	Group A HSVI, herpes B	Encephalitis
	Group A HSVII	Meningitis, encephalitis
	Group V varicella-zoster	Postinfectious encephalomyelitis, encephalitis (?), herpes zoster, Reye syndrome
	Group B cytomegalovirus (CMV)	Congenital CMV, encephalitis
	Epstein-Barr	Encephalitis
Orthomyxovirus	Influenza B	Reye syndrome, encephalitis
Papovavirus	BK virus, JC virus	Progressive multifocal leukoencephalopathy, Creutzfeldt-Jakob disease
Paramyxovirus	Paramyxovirus mumps	Meningitis, encephalitis
	Pseudomyxovirus measles	Postinfectious encephalomyelitis, encephalitis (?), subacute sclerosing panencephalitis
Picornavirus	Enterovirus—polio, echo, Coxsackie A-B, encephalomyocarditis virus	Meningitis, encephalitis (paralytic disease)
Poxvirus	Orthopoxvirus variola major	Postinfectious encephalomyelitis
	Orthopoxvirus vaccinia	Postvaccine encephalomyelitis
Reovirus	Orbivirus Colorado tick	Encephalitis
Rhabdovirus	Rabies	Encephalitis, postvaccine encephalomyelitis
Togavirus	Alphavirus eastern, western, Venezuelan equine	Encephalitis
	Flavivirus St. Louis, Japanese, Murray-Valley, yellow fever, dengue, West Nile	Encephalitis
	Tick-borne—central European, Louping ill, Powassan	Encephalitis
	Tick-borne—Russian spring-summer	Encephalitis, Russian spring-summer panencephalitis
	Rubella	Postinfectious encephalomyelitis, congenital rubella, progressive rubella panencephalitis

cells in the CSF in both viral meningitis and bacterial meningitis. However, lumbar puncture should be repeated after 12 h and then at 24-h intervals and will demonstrate an early change to a lymphocytic pleocytosis in aseptic meningitis. Bacterial meningitis is usually associated with a polymorphonuclear leukocytosis in the blood, which is not present in the blood in aseptic meningitis. The CSF shows an elevated protein content in both conditions, but there is a normal glucose content in aseptic meningitis and a low

Table 16-15
Differential diagnosis of aseptic meningitis

1. Infectious
   A. Viral
      Enterovirus (Coxsackie, echo, polio);
      Paramyxovirus (mumps, measles);
      Herpes virus (*Herpes simplex* II, *Herpes zoster*);
      Arbovirus (equine, Jap. B, Russian tick, Louping
      ill, Colorado tick); Arenavirus (lymphocytic
      choriomeningitis)
   B. Partially treated bacterial meningitis
   C. Postvaccinal, postinfectious (rabies, vaccinia,
      mumps, etc.), encephalomyelitis
   D. Adjacent area of infection (abscess)
   E. Spirochetal, tuberculosis, fungal, protozoan,
      rickettsial infections
   F. Other: sarcoid, brucellosis, listeria, mycoplasma,
      chlamydial, psittacosis, infectious mononucleosis,
      Behçet's
2. Noninfectious
   A. Irritative: any procedure involving dural puncture
   B. Neoplastic disease
   C. Toxic: lead, arsenic, systemic infection
   D. Vascular: subarachnoid hemorrhage, cerebral
      thrombosis, collagen disease
   E. Demyelinating disease

glucose content in bacterial meningitis, which bacterial culture is positive in 50 percent of cases in the latter condition. The cell count, protein, and glucose levels remain unchanged after 24 h in partially treated bacterial meningitis.[146]

2. Subarachnoid hemorrhage. The presence of red blood cells in the CSF and a xanthochromic supernatant fluid will confirm the presence of subarachnoid hemorrhage.

3. The persistence of symptoms and lymphocytic pleocytosis after 2 weeks suggests an alternative diagnosis such as tuberculosis, a fungal meningitis such as cryptococcosis, syphilis, a rickettsial infection, or HIV infection. Rare causes include sarcoidosis, brucellosis, listeria, mycoplasma or chlamydial infections, psittacosis, Lyme borreliosis, Behçet disease, and Mollaret meningitis, which is believed to be a recurrent infection by herpes simplex 1.

4. Noninfectious conditions producing a lymphocytic pleocytosis include contract myelography, neoplastic infiltration by carcinoma or lymphoma, and multiple sclerosis. Meningeal carcinomatosis usually presents with a very low glucose content in the CSF, and the malignant cells can be identified by filtration and suitable staining.

Treatment The treatment of aseptic meningitis is symptomatic. The prognosis is excellent.

Viral Encephalitis

Definition *Viral encephalitis* is an acute febrile illness with evidence of damage to the parenchymal tissues of the CNS, producing alterations of consciousness, focal neurological signs, and seizures.

Etiology and Pathology The etiology cannot be identified in almost two-thirds of the cases of viral encephalitis but the advent of polymerase chain reaction testing is expanding identification of viral agents or other agents in this disease.[147] The arthropod-borne viruses (arboviruses, Table 16-16) compose the largest category of identified agents in viral encephalitis.[148] Herpes viruses and enteroviruses are also frequently reported. The pathogenicity of each virus varies because some disturb neuronal function temporarily; others are capable of producing widespread neuronal death.

Acute viral encephalitis is characterized by inflammation of and damage to neurons in the gray matter of the CNS. Neuronal inclusion bodies are seen in some encephalitides such as rabies and herpes simplex encephalitis. There is prominent perivascular cuffing by lymphocytes and plasma cells, and the leptomeninges are inflamed. Certain viruses have a predilection for particular areas of the CNS. Herpes simplex produces an intense inflammatory response in the temporal lobes; rabies virus has a predilection for the limbic system, whereas poliovirus infection is mainly confined to the motor neurons, particularly those in the spinal cord and brainstem.

Clinical Features Table 16-16 outlines the epidemiological characteristics of the arthropod-borne encephalitides. These conditions, which constitute the

Table 16-16

Arthropod-borne encephalitis

Virus	Epidemiology	Reservoir	Vector	Clinical features
Eastern equine	Eastern North America Caribbean very young or old summer-fall	Birds	Mosquito	Fulminating course, convulsions, prominent CSF pleocytosis ($>$1000cells/mm^3), high mortality (50–70%), severe sequelae—especially children
Venezuelan equine	South and Central America all ages summer-fall	Small mammals, birds, rodents	Mosquito	Low mortality ($<$1%), moderate sequelae
Western equine	North and South America very young or old summer-fall	Birds	Mosquito	Convulsions Low mortality ($<$5%), severe sequelae—especially children
Japanese B	Asia, Japan, Pacific summer-fall	Birds, pigs	Mosquito	High temperature High mortality, especially in elderly, severe sequelae
St. Louis	West hemisphere, especially central U.S. most common, adults summer-fall	Birds	Mosquito	High mortality, especially in elderly, severe sequelae
California	Midwest, south U.S. male children summer-fall	Small mammals (squirrels and rabbits)	Mosquito	Convulsions Low mortality ($<$5%), few sequelae
Murray-Valley	Australia, New Guinea children February-March	Birds	Mosquito	High temperature, convulsions High mortality
Russia spring-summer	Russia May–September	Birds, mammals	Tick	Bulbospinal paralysis Moderate mortality
Central European	Europe May–September	Birds, mammals	Tick	Resembles Russian spring-summer Low mortality
Colorado tick	Western U.S. May–September	Small rodents	Tick	Extreme myalgia Low mortality
Louping ill	Britain March–May	Birds, mammals	Tick	Bloody CSF Prominent cerebellar signs and symptoms, no reported mortality

most frequent forms of encephalitides, are transmitted by a bloodsucking vector. The insect, usually a mosquito or tick, acquires the virus from an animal that is unaffected by a chronic viremia. The signs and symptoms of viral encephalitis show some variation, depending on the etiological agent. In most cases, there is an acute febrile course with signs of meningeal irritation, headache, nausea, photophobia, vomiting, alteration of consciousness, focal neurological deficits, and seizures. The mortality varies from high in Eastern equine encephalitis[149] to low in Venezuelan equine encephalitis. Residual abnormalities include seizures.[150] Changes in personality, extrapyramidal signs, dementia, and motor sensory impairment may complicate most viral encephalitides. A young age at presentation, presence of semicoma or coma, abnormal oculocephalic responses, and laboratory demonstration of virus infection within the CNS are associated with a poor outcome.[151]

Differential Diagnosis   See Table 16-16.

Diagnostic Procedures

1.   The CSF is clear and the pressure may or may not be elevated There is an early increase in polymorphonuclear cells in some cases, followed by lymphocytic pleocytosis. The glucose content is normal and the protein content normal or mildly elevated.

2.   An MRI or CT scan should be obtained to rule out a space-occupying lesion in an acutely ill individual (Fig. 16-11).

3.   An EEG may reveal focal or widespread slowing and may indicate the possible type of viral infection by EEG pattern, such as bitemporal slowing with 2- to 3-Hz spike and sharp wave complexes in the temporal leads in herpus simplex encephalitis.

4.   The CSF should be examined for virus DNA by polymerase chain reaction.[152] This is a rapid, sensitive, and accurate procedure.

5.   The virus is occasionally cultured from the CSF, stool, urine, nasopharynx, or blood.

6.   Another method in establishing a diagnosis of viral encephalitis is the demonstration of a rise in antibody titers to a particular virus in acute and convalescence sera. Titers are quantitated by hemagglutination-inhibition, complement fixation, or neutralizing methods. This, however, is a delayed and often retrospective method of diagnosis.

Treatment

1.   In the absence of viral identification, the patient should be assumed to be suffering from herpes simplex encephalitis and treated with acyclovir or ganciclovir (see p. 479).

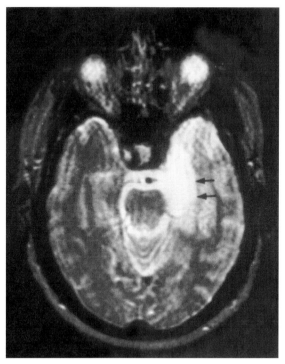

Figure 16-11
MRI T2-weighted image. Area of high signal intensity medial aspect left temporal lobe—viral encephalitis.

2.   The airway must be kept clear, and the semicomatose or comatose patient suctioned frequently. Every effort should be made to avoid pneumonia.

3.   Adequate fluid and electrolyte balance should be maintained at all times.

4.   Seizures should be controlled with initial intravenous phenytoin or phosphenytoin followed by an intravenous diazepem drip (see p. 115).

5.   Increased ICP should be treated with intravenous mannitol to keep the serum osmotic pressure between 300 and 320 mosmol.

Herpes Simplex 1 Encephalitis

Definition   Herpes simplex virus type 1 (HSV-1) encephalitis is an acute, frequently fatal, necrotizing encephalitis with a predilection for the temporal and orbital frontal areas of the brain.

Etiology and Pathology   Herpes simplex type 1 virus is a large, enveloped DNA virus that may possibly spread to the brain from the trigeminal ganglion or other sites where the virus may exist in a latent stage.

The virus exhibits tropism toward neurons in the temporal lobes of the brain and there may be areas of necrosis and hemorrhage, diffuse mononuclear infiltration, neuronal cell loss, and eosinophilic intranuclear inclusions in surviving neurons. There is usually marked cerebral edema, which may affect one temporal lobe or one hemisphere, producing an asymmetrical swelling of the brain (Fig. 16-12).

Clinical Features   The virus is the major cause of herpes labialis (cold sores) and many people have serologic evidence of prior exposure to HSV-1 by the second decade of life.

Herpes simplex encephalitis affects children and adults with no sex preference, and the infection is not enhanced by a compromised immune system. The disease begins with flu-like symptoms, including fever, headache, and malaise, followed by the rapid development of meningeal irritation and disorientation. There may be a prominent psychosis with hallucinations, disorientation, and disturbance of memory, followed by the appearance of focal neurological signs such as aphasia or hemiparesis. The patient is often unable to give a good medical history and rapid deterioration with stupor progressing to coma is not unusual.[153]

An acute necrotizing myelitis with spinal cord necrosis and absence of cerebral involvement has been described. This condition can occur in immunocompromised or nonimmunocompromised individuals and carries a high mortality rate.[154]

Diagnostic Procedures

1.   The CSF is under increased pressure, with a monocytic pleocytosis in the presence and the presence of red blood cells in some cases. There is an elevated protein (60 to 150 mg/dL), and a normal glucose content. The antibody titers to HSV-1 may be elevated.

2.   Serology. There is a rise in anti-HSV complement-fixing antibody titers, but this test is

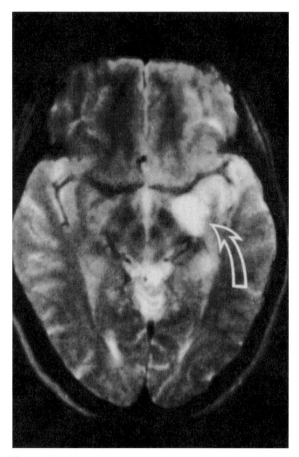

Figure 16-12
MRI scan. T2-weighted image. Area of high signal intensity adjacent to the left middle cerebral artery within the medial and anterior aspect of the left temporal lobe—herpes simplex encephalitis.

unreliable as a rapid diagnostic test and lacks sensitivity. The polymerase chain reaction test is usually positive by the third day, providing a reliable method for determining an etiological diagnosis of HSE,[155] and is highly effective[156] and essential for accurate diagnosis.[157]

3.   The EEG often shows periodic high-voltage, 2- to 3-Hz spike and sharp wave complexes in the temporal leads.

4.   The MRI or CT scan shows the presence of swelling and edema, often more marked in one lobe or one hemisphere (Fig. 16-13).

5. SPECT scans may depict increased perfusion in the characteristically involved temporal lobes.[158]

6. Brain biopsy was the definitive procedure to establish the diagnosis of herpes simplex encephalitis. However, the polymerase chain reaction is so reliable that the need for brain biopsy is questionable.

Differential Diagnosis   The differential diagnosis includes brain abscess, bacterial or fungal meningitis, toxoplasmosis, other viral encephalitides, septic embolization, postinfectious encephalomyelitis, acute necrotizing hemorrhagic encephalitis, and toxic encephalopathies.

Treatment

1. Acyclovir is the antiviral agent of choice for herpes simplex encephalitis.[159] The drug should be administered as early as possible before the onset of coma. Survivors treated after the onset of coma invariably show permanent neurological deficits. Consequently, acyclovir should be administered in all suspected cases without waiting for laboratory confirmation of the diagnosis. An intravenous dose of 10 mg/kg infused over 1 h q8h for 10 days is recommended. Nephrotoxicity due to precipitation of acyclovir crystals in renal tubules can be avoided by adequate hydration to maintain a good urinary output. Toxicity with tremors, hallucinations, agitation, or lethargy is rare. The development of resistance to acyclovir has not been a problem to date in the treatment of immunocompetent individuals. However, acyclovir-resistant HSV strains have emerged in immunocompromised patients. Intravenous foscarnet is the current treatment of choice in such cases.

2. Increased ICP should be treated with an intravenous infusion of mannitol and furosemide. Seizures require aggressive therapy.[160] Surgical decompression may be necessary to avoid herniation in cases with rapidly increasing ICP.

Prognosis   The mortality rate is 30 percent in patients receiving early treatment with acyclovir. Coma is associated with 70 percent mortality and severe neurological deficits in the majority of survivors.

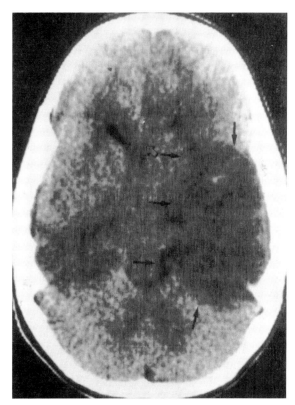

Figure 16-13
CT scan—noncontrast herpes encephalitis. Marked edema of the left temporal lobe.

Herpes Simplex 2 Encephalitis

Infections of the CNS with herpes simplex virus 2 (HSV-2) accounts for 4–6 percent of cases of herpes simplex encephalitis.[161] However, infection by HSV-2 usually presents as an aseptic meningitis occurring in individuals with primary genital HSV-2 infection.[162] Symptoms consist of headache, stiff neck, photophobia, malaise, and fever. The CSF findings consist of a lymphocytic pleocytosis up to 1000 cells per cubic millimeter and normal glucose content. The disease is usually mild and self-limiting, but neurological deficits, including persistent headache, impaired concentration, impaired hearing, and paraparesis, indicate occasional encephalitis. An ascending necrotizing myelitis has been reported. Recurrent infections can occur.

Diagnostic Procedures   As for HSV-1.

Treatment   Intravenous acyclovir is indicated in any patient with signs of parenchymal involvement of the CNS.

Herpes Zoster (Varicella) Encephalitis

Encephalitis is a rare complication of varicella infection and occurs about 7 to 10 days after the appearance of the rash. The encephalitis is usually mild with symptoms of headache, nausea, ataxia, dysarthria, and occasionally seizures. Complete recovery occurs in most cases, but an occasionally life-threatening, more diffuse encephalitis, with cranial nerve palsies, hemiplegia, aphasia, and coma, can occur. Encephalitis has occasionally been reported after shingles. This complication is said to be rare but is probably more common than reported in the past. Many elderly patients report malaise and fatigue and lack of energy after shingles. Careful neurological examination often reveals cerebellar ataxia in such cases, suggesting that a mild rhombencephalitis may have complicated the infection. These patients gradually recover after a period of 6 months or more.

Treatment   See shingles (page 611).

Rabies

Definition   Rabies is an acute, almost invariably fatal infectious illness caused by a neurotropic virus of the rhabdovirus family.

Etiology and Pathology   The rabies virus is a bullet-shaped, enveloped RNA-containing virus that usually gains access to the body by a bite from a rabid animal. The virus then replicates locally in muscle cells, penetrates nerve endings, and travels in retrograde fashion up the nerve axons to the CNS. The virus then replicates once more, spreads throughout the CNS with a higher concentration in the limbic system of the brain and eventually travels out nerve trunks to all parts of the body. The virus is thought to act directly on specific membrane receptors.

The brain and spinal cord show perivascular and perineural mononuclear infiltration, and the leptomeninges are mildly inflamed. The disease is characterized by the presence of intracellular intracytoplasmic eosinophilic inclusion bodies (Negri bodies).

Clinical Features   Human rabies has been identified in all continents except Australia and Antarctica, but approximately 60 countries are reported to be rabies free, owing to geographical isolation, animal control programs, or quarantine regulations. More than 99 percent of cases occur in developing countries, such as China and India, where rates have been reported as high as 3/100,000, although the rate is probably closer to 1/1,000,000 in developing countries at this time. The disease is more common in children aged 5 to 14 years and in adults older than 50 years.[163] Bats,[164] skunks,[165] raccoons, and dogs[166] are implicated in human rabies cases in the United States; the mongoose and jackal in Africa; the fox in Europe and Canada; the wolf in western Asia; and the vampire bat in Central and South America. Occasionally rabies can be transmitted by other means than an animal bite, including inhalation of airborne virus in caves contaminated by bat secretions, or by inhalation in laboratories where the air is contaminated by virus. There are also reports of transmission from a rabid donor to a corneal transplant recipient.[167]

The key to the early diagnosis of rabies is the history of exposure to a rabid or potentially rabid animal. There is an incubation period of 20 to 90 days in the great majority of cases, although longer incubation periods have been reported. This is followed by complaints of pain and paresthesias at the bite site, accompanied by fever, chills, headache, and myalgia in about 50 percent of cases. The majority of patients develop "furious" rabies characterized by a prodromal period of disorientation, bizarre behavior, hallucinations, insomnia, and hyperactivity, followed by cyclic arousal with agitation, associated with pharyngeal and inspiratory muscle spasms on attempted swallowing. Eventually an intense terror develops at the mere thought of water, giving rise to the synonym "hydrophobia" for rabies. Autonomic disturbances are common and the patient may develop hypersalivation, hypotension, hyperpyrexia, and tachycardia. There may be signs of meningeal irritation and cranial and peripheral nerve palsies. Periods of hypersensitivity can be precipitated by tactile, auditory, or visual stimuli. Hyperventilation, fasciculations, and seizures precede the development of stupor and eventual coma. The patient eventually loses consciousness and dies from respiratory arrest or circulatory failure.

Some patients may develop a clinical form of rabies termed "dumb" or "paralytic" rabies. This form of rabies is characterized by an acute ascending symmetrical or asymmetrical paralysis resembling the Guillain-Barré syndrome and occurs in about 15 percent of cases leading to respiratory and bulbar paralysis.

Complications The major complications of rabies include cerebral edema, seizures, SIADH, pneumonia, atelectasis, cardiac arrhythmias, congestive heart failure, cardiac arrest, hypotension, gastrointestinal bleeding, anemia, paralytic ileus, renal failure, and paralsysis of the urinary bladder.

Diagnostic Procedures

1. Immunofluorescent rabies antibody staining of skin biopsies is the most reliable diagnostic procedure.
2. Rapid fluorescent focus inhibition test (RFFIT) measures rabies-neutralizing antibodies from in vitro cell cultures and is positive within 48 h.
3. The CSF is usually under increased pressure with a lymphocytic pleocytosis. CSF antibody levels may not be positive until the seventh day of illness.
4. Serum neutralizing antibodies may be detected by the sixth day of illness.
5. Rabies is rarely seen in the United States and is often not diagnosed until after death.[168] Early diagnosis could be established by detection of rabies RNA by PCR.

Differential Diagnosis

1. Tetanus may be distinguished from furious rabies by the presence of rigidity between muscle spasms and a short incubation period between the bite or wound and onset of symptoms in tetanus. The CSF is normal, and there is lack of hydrophobia in the tetanus patient.
2. Postvaccinal encephalomyelitis is now rare and typically occurs some 2 weeks after the first dose of a vaccine.

Treatment

1. All animal bites should be thoroughly treated. The wound should be vigorously flushed and scrubbed with a 20% soap solution. Tetanus prophylaxis and measures to control bacterial infection may be necessary.[169]
2. Human diploid cell rabies vaccine (HDCV) or rabies vaccine adsorbed (RVA) are currently the treatment of choice.[170]
   a. Pre-exposure dosage. Individuals such as veterinarians who are at high risk of exposure to rabies should receive three 1-mL intramuscular injections of HDCV or RVA, the second dose 1 week after the first, and the third 2 or 3 weeks after the second. Serum antibody levels should be determined 2 to 3 weeks after the last dose of vaccine to be sure of a satisfactory response. A booster dose of 1 mL intramuscularly every 2 years is recommended when there is a continuing risk of exposure to rabies.
   b. Postexposure treatment. The decision whether or not to treat a patient requires consideration of several factors. The algorithm (Fig. 16-14) is a guide to the correct decision in human rabies postexposure prophylaxis.

      When treatment is initiated, human rabies immune globulin (HRIG) should be administered in a dose of 20 μg/kg with half the dose infiltrated at the site of the wound and the rest given intramuscularly. At the same time, a 1-mL dose of HDCV or RVA should be given intramuscularly and repeated on days 3, 7, 14, and 28 after the first dose. A previously immunized person who demonstrated rabies antibodies, who was exposed to rabies, should receive two doses of 1 mL HDCV or RVA, one immediately and one 3 days later. Human rabies immune globulin is not indicated for such patients.
3. Those involved in patient care should be vaccinated and wear face masks, gloves, and gowns when in contact with the patient.
4. Patients with rabies should be treated in an intensive care unit. Patients are acutely ill and require

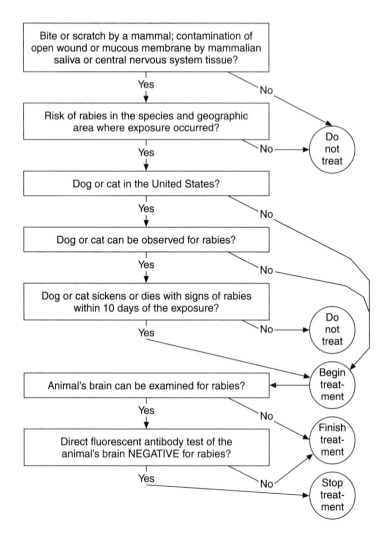

Figure 16-14
Algorithm for human rabies postexposure prophylaxis. With permission from Principles and Practice of Infectious Disease. 4th edition. Gerald L Mondell, John E Bennett, Raphael Dolen eds. Churchill Livingstone. New York 1995.

careful monitoring of cardiovascular and pulmonary function, electrolytes, and parenteral fluids. The intense distress caused by hydrophobia can be reduced by adequate doses of a phenothiazine combined with a benzodiazepine.

Prognosis There are occasional reports of patients who have survived rabies. Unfortunately, the vast majority die of the disease.

HIV Infection and the Nervous System

Infection by HIV can involve the nervous system early in the course of the disease and at multiple

levels from the brain to the peripheral nerve and muscle. Infection may be regarded as primary when the pathological changes are the direct result of HIV alone, or secondary in the case of opportunistic infections. In addition, there are undoubtedly active combinations of primary HIV infection and opportunistic infections or pathological changes that are essentially the toxic effects of anti-HIV therapeutic agents.

The spectrum of HIV infection has gradually widened in the last decade. The early manifestations were the result of immunosuppression, with the development of meningitis and toxoplasmosis in the CNS. However, antibiotic control and prophylactic therapy have improved survival and permitted the development of additional complications such as CNS lymphoma and progressive multifocal encephalopathy or several disorders involving the spinal cord, peripheral nerve, and muscle.

HIV Dementia (AIDS Dementia Complex)

Definition This progressive dementia occurs in AIDS, owing to a direct primary HIV infection of neurons or an indirect neurotoxicity induced by the presence of the virus in the brain.

Etiology and Pathology Although there is ample evidence indicating the presence of HIV in brain in HIV dementia, there is no indication of direct neural infection.[171] In addition, quantitative studies using the polymerase chain reaction show no significant differences in amounts of HIV DNA between brains of demented and nondemented HIV-infected patients.[172] The virus may be transported into the brain by infected peripheral monocytes (Trojan horse theory) and it is believed that something associated with HIV-infected macrophages within the CNS leads to neurological damage.[173] Alternatively, the virus may be transported into the CNS by infected T cells, which penetrate the blood-brain barrier. The virus then infects microglial cells,[174] which may act as a reservoir for persistent infection. The production of gp120, a surface protein of HIV, may lead to the opening of calcium channels, including NMDA-mediated channels in the neuronal membrane, an influx of calcium, and neuronal death. An alternative hypothesis suggests that the presence of HIV in glial cells results in the production of cytokines including tumor necrosis factor alpha,[175] and interleukin-6, and metabolites of the arachidonic acid cascade, resulting in neuronal damage.[176]

The brain shows diffuse atrophic changes, with dilatation of the ventricles and widening of the cortical sulci. There are multiple foci of inflammation, with microglia, macrophages, and multinucleated giant cells.

Clinical Features Dementia is usually a late development in HIV disease when the CD4 lymphocyte count is less than 200 cells per cubic millimeter.

The onset is insidious, and the progression usually slow. The earliest signs can only be established by serial neuropsychologic testing[177] which will reveal early cognitive dysfunction and indicate the need for early treatment with protease inhibitors in triple-drug combinations preventing neuronal cell death.[178] The primary complaint is difficulty with memory, attention, retrieval of information, and planning. This is followed by slowing of higher cognitive functions, including judgment, insight, calculation, and abstraction. Motor signs consist of progressive spasticity and ataxia, with impairment of gait. Later signs include behavioral changes, apathy, frank psychosis and in rare cases, severe generalized chorea.[179] There is progression to paraparesis, incontinence, and seizures, with an inevitable progression to death. Disorders such as toxoplasmosis lymphoma and progressive multifocal leukoencephalopathy can present with similar features and should be excluded.[180]

Diagnostic Procedures

1. Serological tests for HIV infection are positive.
2. The CSF is abnormal, with a mild pleocytosis, elevated protein, increased IgG, intrathecal synthesis of anti-HIV IgG, and oligoclonal bands. The CSF markers include β_2-microglobulin neopterin and quinolinate in HIV infection. Cultures should be obtained to exclude opportunistic infection.
3. An MRI shows cerebral atrophy, ventricular dilatation, and diffuse or multifocal increased signal intensity in the periventricular white matter (Fig. 16-15).
4. Serial PET or SPECT scans will reveal early changes in brain function in HIV-positive patients.[181]

Treatment High doses of zidovudine, 1000 to 2000 mg/day, will produce improvement in some cases. Dideoxyinosine 400 mg/day has been recommended in those who fail to respond to or cannot tolerate zidovudine. Combinations of idinavir, lamivudine, and zidovudine have resulted in remarkable improvement in the treatment of HIV infections.[182] However, optimal treatment of HIV infection has yet to be established.[183]

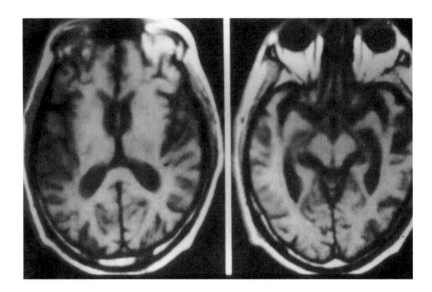

Figure 16-15
MRI T1-weighted image. Diffuse brain atrophy in a patient with AIDS.

Peripheral Neuropathy in HIV Infection Symmetrical peripheral neuropathy associated with HIV infection can present as two distinct pathologic entities. A distal symmetrical axonal neuropathy is a typical dying back phenomenon associated with macrophage infiltration of the peripheral nerves.[184] Direct viral infection of the nerve is unlikely, and it is possible that cytokines such as tumor necrosis factor alpha and other cytokines may interact with nerve growth factors, producing axonal neuropathic changes. Associated conditions such as diabetes mellitus, alcoholism, or vitamin B_{12} deficiency, and the use of antiretroviral nucleosides, may accentuate the neuropathy. Treatment should be directed toward control or diminution of adjunctive factors, withdrawal of putative medications, and the use of amitriptyline, mexiletine, or gabapentin for pain control.

The inflammatory demyelinating polyneuropaty (IDP) of AIDS is similar to the Guillain-Barré syndrome (see p 612). Acute IDP tends to occur early in the disease in patients with negative serum tests, test results for HIV, or at the time of seroconversion. However, cytomegalovirus infection is the likely agent when IDP occurs late in the disease and the CD4 count is low.[185] Some patients respond to immunomodulating therapy with corticosteroids, plasmapheresis or intravenous immunoglobulin.[186] Others should be treated with ganciclovir or foscarnet

therapy, if the PCR-for cytomegalovirus (CMV) is positive. Chronic IDP has also been described and is a slowly progressive disease. Most cases are the result of CMV infection. Less common causes include lymphoma, tuberculosis, and syphilis. Many patients improve when treated with ganciclovir or foscarnet.[187]

Multifocal mononeuropathies are also a feature of HIV infection and can present as a series of asymmetrical polymononeuropathies and acute lumbosacral polyradiculomyelopathy[188] or, rarely, as an asymmetrical multifocal sensorimotor neuropathy.[189] Most cases appear to be related to CMV infection. There may be a good response to ganciclovir or foscarnet therapy.

Primary CNS Lymphoma There has been a marked increase in CNS lymphoma since the beginning of the AIDS epidemic.[190] The increase cannot, however, be entirely attributed to AIDS because the incidence of CNS lymphoma has increased in the non-AIDS population.

The presence of Epstein-Barr virus in AIDS-related lymphoma has been reported in almost 100 percent of cases. Since Epstein-Barr virus DNA can be detected in the CSF it may be of diagnostic value.[191] Thallium 201 brain single photon emission computed tomography is useful in differentiating cerebral lymphoma from toxoplasma encephalitis in AIDS patients.[192]

The clinical features of primary CNS lymphoma are described on page 526.

Treatment Radiation therapy often produces remarkable but temporary improvement and prolonged survival for a median of 4 to 6 months.[193] A combination of radiation therapy and chemotherapy may increase survival time.

Vacuolar Myelopathy Vacuolar myelopathy is often detected at autopsy in AIDS patients and tends to be associated with severe immunosuppression and advanced disease.

Etiology and Pathology Pathological changes consist of vacuolization of myelin sheaths with accumulation of macrophages and microglia; axons are preserved. There is no evidence for direct HIV involvement, and the myelin damage may be attributed to the presence of toxic cytokines such as tumor necrosis factor or vitamin B_{12} deficiency.[194]

Other causes of myelopathy in AIDS include lymphoma, herpes zoster myelitis,[195] CMV infection, and toxoplasmosis.

Clinical Features The condition presents as a slowly progressive spastic ataxic paraparesis with impaired sphincter control and lower extremity sensory symptoms. Examination shows lower limb spasticity, weakness, ataxia, hyperreflexia, extensor plantar responses, and a mild sensory impairment.

Treatment Symptomatic treatment includes measures to decrease spasticity, such as oral baclofen or the use of a baclofen pump, management of sphincter impairment, and physical therapy. There is no reported benefit from antiviral agents. The mean survival after the diagnosis of AIDS is approximately 12 months.[196]

Myopathy Muscle involvement may be detected at any stage of HIV infection.

Etiology and Pathology Myopathy is believed to be the result of an autoimmune response rather than a direct infection by the HIV virus[197]. Affected muscles show inflammation and myofiber degeneration resembling polymyositis. However, nemaline rod bodies,[198] cytoplasm bodies, and mitochondrial abnormalities[199] have been described. These findings have suggested that in some cases, the myopathy in AIDS may be the result of zidovudine therapy.[200] Consequently muscle disorders in HIV infection may be

a) HIV associated myopathies

b) Zidovudine myopathy

c) Opportunistic infections and tumoral infiltration of muscle.[201]

Clinical Features The symptoms are those of a myopathy with proximal muscle weakness, difficulty rising from a chair, and difficulty climbing stairs. Respiratory muscle dysfunction with dyspnea is a late feature.[202] Weight loss is a prominent symptom and myalgia occurs in about 50 percent of cases.

Treatment

1. Zidovudine should be withdrawn temporarily because of the putative association between myopathy and zidovudine therapy.[203] This may result in improvement in some cases, which implies that zidovudine therapy is implicated in the myopathic process, in which case the drug should be withheld permanently. However, the drug can be reintroduced in the face of progressive muscle weakness.

2. Prednisone 60 mg daily improves strength in most patients and can be continued as an alternate-day therapy to minimize adverse effects.[204]

Progressive Multifocal Leukoencephalopathy

Progressive multifocal leukoencephalopathy (PML) is a multifocal demyelinating disease that has been reported as a nonmetastatic complication of neoplasia. It also occurs in immunosuppression therapy in immunocompromised patients with leukemia, lymphoma, tuberculosis, sarcoidosis (following renal transplantation), or AIDS. PML, once an extremely rare disease, has become much more frequent owing to the AIDS pandemic.[205] The disease is the result of infection with JC virus, a human papillomavirus which infects and destroysoligodendrocytes.[206] The pathological changes consist of multiple areas of white matter demyelination, extending through the gray-white matter junction into the cortical gray matter. There are perivascular inflammatory infiltrates and large "balloon" oligodendral glial cells, with nuclear inclusions containing virions.[207]

Clinical features include progressive dementia, visual loss, spastic quadriparesis, and ataxia. Death usually occurs less than a year after the onset of symptoms; HIV-associated progressive multifocal leukoencephalopathy has a median survival time of 2 to 4 months.[208] About 10 percent of patients have a more benign course, with remission and prolonged survival.[209]

Diagnostic Procedures

1. The EEG shows progressive slowing of activity over both hemispheres.
2. The MRI scan reveals extensive white matter lesions bilaterally on T2-weighted imaging (Fig. 16-16).
3. The diagnosis is established by detection of JC virus DNA in the CSF by polymerase chain reaction or by brain biopsy.[210]

Treatment Intravenous cytarabine (ARA-C) improves survival.[211]

Neurological Opportunistic Infections in AIDS

There are three common opportunistic infections in patients with HIV infection.

    a) Toxoplasmosis
    b) Cytomegalovirus
    c) Cryptococcosis (see page 466)

Toxoplasmosis

Definition *Toxoplasma gondii* usually produces an asymptomatic infection in adults but can cause a severe and potentially fatal encephalitis in immunosuppressed persons, particularly following organ transplantation or complicating AIDS. Toxoplasmosis is

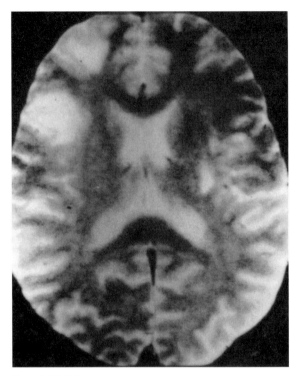

Figure 16-16
MRI scan—T2-weighted image. There are multiple areas of asymmetrical bilateral high signal intensity involving primarily white matter but extending in the gray matter—progressive multifocal leukoencephalopathy.

the most common cerebral mass lesion in patients with AIDS[212] and is believed to represent a reactivation of a previously acquired endogenous infection.[213] Toxoplasmosis can cause severe brain damage when transmitted transplacentally to a developing fetus.

Etiology and Pathology The natural host of *T. gondii* is the cat, but other animals may serve as hosts. Humans are infected by ingesting poorly cooked meat containing encysted trophozoites or more commonly by ingesting the oocyst excreted in cat feces. A parasitemia results and the organisms are distributed throughout the body. The encysted organism is walled off by the body and a granuloma results, which may eventually calcify. Lack of IgM antibodies suggests that cerebral toxoplasmosis represents reactivation of a previously acquired endogenous infection, probably originating in systemic organs and reaching the brain through the choroid plexus[214] by hematogenous dissemination rather than reactivation of latent organisms in the brain. Cerebral toxoplasmosis occurs in advanced HIV with CD4 lymphocyte counts of fewer than 200 cells per cubic millimeter.[215]

Clinical Features Presenting symptoms consist of headache and fever followed by disorientation, lethargy, and seizures. Focal neurological signs include cranial nerve palsies, ataxia, and hemiparesis and are present in the majority of patients, particularly in those with a diffuse encephalitis, who ultimately develop focal signs as the disease progresses.

Congenital infection with toxoplasmosis results in hepatosplenomegaly, jaundice, hydrocephalus, and encephalitis. Surviving children are often microcephalic with chorioretinitis, seizures, and mental retardation.

Diagnostic Procedures

1. On lumbar puncture, CSF analysis reveals lymphocytic pleocytosis, xanthochromia, and an elevated protein content.

2. The CT scan shows single or multiple contrast-enhancing lesions with nodular or ring-enhancing structures.

3. The MRI scans are often more sensitive than CT scanning and reveal additional parenchymal lesions (Fig. 16-17).[216]

4. Serum antitoxoplasma antibodies are usually detected in active disease, but lower or absent titers do not exclude the diagnosis. The use of polymerase chain reaction to detect toxoplasma DNA in the CSF is the most sensitive method of confirming the diagnosis of toxoplasmosis.[217]

5. Brain biopsy may be necessary to establish the diagnosis in some cases.

Treatment

A diagnosis of cerebral toxoplasmosis can be assumed in patients with characteristic CT or MRI

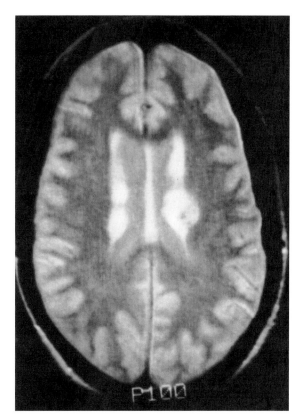

Figure 16-17
MRI—proton density–weighted image. There are several mass-like lesions adjacent to the ventricles—toxoplasmosis in an AIDS patient.

scans and detectable antitoxoplasma antibodies and treated empirically. A combined therapy with pyrimethamine is given in a loading dose of 50 to 200 mg/day for 2 to 6 weeks. This is followed by a maintenance dose of pyrimethamine 25 to 75 mg/day and sulfadiazine 4 to 8 g/day, beginning 2 to 6 weeks after treatment is started, with lifelong continuing therapy to prevent relapse.[150] Adverse effects of sulfadiazine consist of a rash or nephrotoxicity and occur in about 40 percent of cases. Bone marrow suppression by pyrimethamine can be prevented with folinic acid 10 mg daily.

A combination of clindamycin and pyrimethamine is an effective alternative therapy for patients who cannot tolerate sulfadiazine.

Clinical and radiological signs of improvement should appear by the seventh day of therapy. Failure to respond within 2 weeks suggests the need for a stereotactic brain biopsy to establish an alternative brain diagnosis.

Cytomegalovirus Infections

The majority of cases of CMV infection of the central or peripheral nervous system in adults occur in immunocompromised individuals. This group includes patients receiving immunosuppressant therapy for organ transplantation or malignancy and patients with AIDS.

Etiology and Pathology The CMV is a DNA virus of the herpesvirus group, which produces swelling of infected cells that contain large intranuclear inclusions. In infected adults, the brain shows a diffuse or focal encephalitis with microglial nodules in the parenchyma and areas of demyelination in the central white matter of the cerebrum, brainstem, and spinal cord. Cytomegalovirus ventriculoencephalitis with hydrocephalus, vasculitis, and radiculomyelitis is a unique entity in patients with advanced HIV infection.[218]

Clinical Features Encephalitis caused by CMV is a common complication of organ transplantation and AIDS and occasionally occurs in CMV infectious mononucleosis. The infection is probably the result of reactivation of a latent CMV infection because most adults possess antibodies to CMV. However, the ubiquitous nature of the virus is such that infection is easily transferred person to person or by blood transfusion.

Infection by CMV in AIDS usually occurs when the CD4 lymphocyte count falls below 50 cells per cubic milliliter and is often accompanied by infection of other organs,[219] particularly the lungs and adrenal glands.[220]

Symptoms of encephalitis consist of the abrupt onset of headache, fever, and somnolence followed by focal neurological deficits and seizures. Cytomegalovirus polyradiculopathy is often present and can be the initial manifestation of AIDS in some

races.[221] The presence of retinal vasculopathy in AIDS is indicative of CMV infection.[222]

Diagnostic Procedures

1. On lumbar puncture, the CSF shows a mild pleocytosis, increased total protein, and IgG.
2. The MRI scan reveals hydrocephalus and increased signal intensity in periventricular or meningeal structures.
3. Cytomegalovirus DNA can be demonstrated in the CSF using the polymerase chain reaction.[223]
4. Electrolyte abnormalities occur in patients with adrenal insufficiency.
5. Confirmation of polyradiculopathy can be obtained by electromyography (EMG).
6. Liver function tests are abnormal.

Treatment The use of the antiviral agents ganciclovir or foscarnet, alone or in combination, increases survival time for several weeks.[224]

Prognosis Survival is only a matter of weeks in most cases, particularly in those with AIDS.

Infants with CMV encephalitis acquired by transplacental passage from a recently infected mother or at birth develop severe brain damage in many cases. Survivors exhibit signs of multiple neurological abnormalities. Infants with mild or silent infection have some degree of sensorineural hearing loss.

Epstein-Barr Encephalitis

Epstein-Barr virus (EBV) is a DNA virus in the herpes virus group. Infection by EBV results in infectious mononucleosis and is occasionally responsible for Bell's palsy, Guillain-Barré syndrome, transverse myelitis, and acute encephalitis. The encephalitis is usually mild, often presenting as an aseptic meningitis, but occasionally a more severe parenchymal brain infection can occur. The prognosis is good in most cases, but fatalities have been reported. Infection with EBV has been related to primary CNS lymphoma in AIDS patients.

Diagnostic Procedures

1. The blood shows an early leukopenia followed by leukocytosis with atypical lymphocytes.
2. Lumbar puncture. There is a mild pleocytosis, elevated protein and IgG, and the presence of atypical lymphocytes in the CSF.
3. Liver function tests are abnormal.
4. EBV DNA can be demonstrated by PCR.

Treatment   Supportive. Antiviral agents are not effective.

Prognosis   Good, but fatigue, hepatomegaly, and splenomegaly may persist for many months.

Reye Syndrome

Reye syndrome is an acute encephalopathy that occurs predominantly in children and rarely in adults.

Etiology and Pathology   Reye syndrome usually follows infection by influenza A or B, herpes zoster (chickenpox), herpes simplex, and paramyxoviruses. Other possible causes include the combined effect of a virus infection and the use of salicylates. However, the role of salicylates has not been established. There are characteristic pathological changes, including cerebral edema, proliferation of smooth endoplastic reticulum, and morphologically abnormal mitochondria, most marked in the neurons. The abdominal viscera and liver are heavily infiltrated with fat, and mitochondrial damage occurs in the liver cells. It is probable that the mitochondrial abnormalities affecting the brain and liver cells are the crucial pathological changes in Reye syndrome.

Clinical Features   The onset is acute. The syndrome usually presents in a child who is apparently recovering from influenza, varicella, or an upper respiratory infection. There are five stages: (1) onset with lethargy and protracted vomiting; (2) progressive impairment of consciousness with hallucinations, combative behavior, and hyperventilation; seizures may occur; (3) coma with intermittent decerebrate rigidity occurring spontaneously or with minimal stimulation;

brainstem reflexes are intact; (4) coma with decerebrate rigidity, hyperventilation and absence of brainstem reflexes; and (5) coma, respiratory failure, and death.

Diagnostic Procedures

1. Liver function tests are abnormal, with elevation of serum aspartate transaminase (AST) and alanine transaminase (ALT).

2. Serum glucose levels are low, and hypoglycemia occurs in some cases.

3. The plasma prothrombin time is prolonged.

4. Serum ammonia levels are elevated about 50 mg/100 mL.

5. The EEG shows symmetrical slowing. Serial records are useful in assessing the course of the illness.

6. Either MRI or CT scanning shows evidence of cerebral edema with decreased density in the white matter in both hemispheres.

7. There are no abnormalities in the CSF, but the glucose content may be low, in the presence of hypoglycemia. Lumbar puncture should not be performed in cases with suspected increased ICP.

8. The diagnosis can be confirmed by liver biopsy, but this is usually not necessary.

Treatment   When a child is arousable to verbal or painful stimuli, the following measures should be taken:

1. The child should be intubated with a low-pressure nasotracheal tube and placed on a mechanical ventilator.

2. The prothrombin time or partial thromboplastin time should be determined. If these times are prolonged, fresh frozen plasma should be given to reduce the risk of bleeding, should an ICP monitor device be inserted.

3. A ventricular or subdural pressure monitoring device can be inserted, and ICP should be continuously recorded.

4. If ICP exceeds 20 mmHg, mannitol 0.25 g/kg should be given intravenously.

5. The serum osmolality should be maintained between 300 and 320 mosmol/L and it should be measured q2h.

6. A neuromuscular blocking agent such as pancuronium administered under the supervision of an anesthesiologist is required if the ICP remains elevated or the patient cannot tolerate the ventilator. A neurological examination is performed immediately before the use of the neuromuscular blocking agent, which can be discontinued briefly when further neurological assessment is performed.

7. The body temperature is maintained below 30°C, using a refrigerator blanket.

8. A Foley catheter should be inserted and the intake and output monitored.

9. Fluid and electrolyte balance can then be maintained.

10. The central venous pressure and arterial pressure are monitored through a central line.

11. Hypertonic glucose 15% to 20% is infused intravenously to maintain the serum glucose level between 150 and 200 mg/dL.

12. Insulin 1 unit per 10 g glucose should be infused q4h. The dose of insulin is regulated to maintain glucose levels between 150 and 200 mg/dL. Glucose levels should be measured q4h.

13. Neomycin enemas will help to reduce serum ammonia levels.

14. The lungs are checked frequently. Postural drainage and suctioning should be performed q2h or more frequently if necessary.

15. A barbiturate coma should be considered in those rare cases when ICP cannot be controlled (page 140).

Prognosis Children recovering from clinical stages 1, 2 or 3 are usually neurologically normal. Recovery from stages 4 and 5 may be followed by permanent neurological deficits, including spasticity, hemiparesis, dystonia, involuntary movements, and seizures. Recurrence of Reye syndrome is rare.

SLOW VIRAL INFECTIONS

The slow viral infection is a disease process with a long latent period lasting months to years, followed by a protracted clinical course that invariably culminates in death.

There are several slow viral infections of the CNS; the most important are subacute sclerosing panencephalitis (SSPE), progressive multifocal leukoencephalopathy, and Creutzfeldt-Jakob disease.

Measles Virus

Measles virus can cause three distinct syndromes in the CNS: (1) acute measles encephalomyelitis, which presents as a recrudescence of illness during convalescence from measles, with fever, headaches, seizures, and change in mentation; (2) subacute measles inclusion body encephalitis—an encephalitic illness presenting in immunocompromised individuals;[225] and (3) SSPE presenting after a latent period of many years following measles as a slow virus infection.[226]

Subacute Sclerosing Panencephalitis

Definition This chronic progressive panencephalitis occurs in immunocompetent individuals after several years of silent measles virus persistence.

Etiology and Pathology This is a persistent chronic viral infection characterized by lack of viral budding, reduced expression of the viral envelope proteins, and spread of measles virus genomes throughout the CNS, despite a hyperimmune response to measles virus antigens.[227] However, the immune response fails to control the viral infection. The disease is characterized by the presence of viral inclusion bodies in various cell types and white and gray matter. However, neither virus nor viral particles are detectable in autopsy material.[228]

Clinical Features The prevalence of SSPE is 1 per million. It is three times more likely to occur in males than females, and more than 50 percent of those affected give a history of an overt attack of measles before the age of 2 years.

The onset of SSPE usually occurs between 5 and 15 years of age. There are four stages in the progression of the disease: (1) deterioration in school performance, personality change, speech difficulty, seizures, papilledema; (2) myoclonus, ataxia, spasticity, choreoathetosis, and ocular signs including cortical blindness, optic atrophy, and chorioretinitis; (3) marked mental deterioration, coma, decorticate posturing, decerebrate rigidity; and (4) a terminal phase of hypotonia with an exaggerated startle response to noise.

The course is characterized by progressive deterioration, with death occurring 3 months to 3 years after the initial symptoms. Remissions lasting for a few weeks and occasionally for a few years have been reported. The younger the patient, the more likely remissions will occur.

Diagnostic Procedures

1. High antibody titers to measles virus are found in both serum and CSF. There is marked increase in IgG in the CSF with prominent formation of oligoclonal bands in both serum and CSF. Measles virus particles have been demonstrated in the CSF by scanning electron microscopy.

2. A rapid diagnosis can be established by polymerase chain reaction using serum or CSF.

3. An MRI scan shows the presence of high signal intensity in T2-weighted images, which frequently involve the periventricular or subcortical white matter. There is diffuse cerebral atrophy.[229]

4. The EEG shows a characteristic pattern of burst suppression, which consists of bursts of high-amplitude theta activity occurring on a background of low-voltage activity.

5. Brain biopsy reveals involvement of white matter and the presence of inclusion bodies in neurons and glial cells.

Treatment No treatment has proved to be effective. Treatment with ribavirin 20 mg/kg/per day intravenously may be of benefit.

Survivors show moderate to severe intellectual and cognitive deficits.

Rubella Virus

Rubella virus infections usually produce a mild illness with an exanthematous rash in children. However, there may be severe damage to a fetus infected by rubella transmitted transplacentally from an infected mother during the first trimester of pregnancy. The infant may be born with congenital cataracts or other defects, including microcephaly, mental retardation, and deafness. Rubella encephalitis is a rare complication of rubella virus infection in the newborn, producing symptoms and signs similar to congenital rubella infection.

Progressive rubella panencephalitis is a rare disease with clinical signs of infection appearing after a long period following congenital rubella infection. Progressive rubella panencephalitis commonly occurs in the 8- to 21-year-old age group. There are pathological signs of encephalitis and the course is similar to SSPE. Although the age of onset is much older and the course more benign. The main neurological features are dementia, cerebellar ataxia, and seizures. Antirubella antibody titers and lgG are increased in the CSF. The diagnosis can be confirmed by polymerase chain reaction using serum or CSF. MRI scans show diffuse brain atrophy and ventricular dilatation.[230]

Subacute Spongiform Encephalopathy (Creutzfeldt-Jakob Disease)

Definition This is a rapidly progressive spongiform encephalopathy of the CNS.

Etiology and Pathology The disease has an incidence of one new case per million per year[231] and has been transmitted to primates and to man. There appears to be a genetic susceptibility and about 6 to 15 percent of cases have occurred in two or more members of the same family.[232] Iatrogenic spread has been reported in corneal transplant and dural graft recipients, after insertion of depth electrodes in the brain, and injections of pooled human growth hormone prepared from pituitary glands obtained from cadavers. Transmission of the disease to chimpanzees inoculated with brain tissue from affected humans and subsequently transmission to a second generation of chimpanzees has been recorded. The evidence for a transmissible agent is compelling, particularly so following reports of human infection from consumption of beef in Britain. Health care workers carry a low but definite risk of contracting spongiform encephalopathy, with reports of at least 24 such cases to date.[233] However, the long incubation period in the few cases reported in health care workers and the known familial susceptibility suggest that a genetic factor may be present in this disease. The presence of apolipoprotein E in prion protein deposits in spongiform encephalopathy suggests that the apolipoprotein E epsilon 4 allele is a risk factor for this disease.[234]

Pathological changes consist of diffuse brain atrophy with extensive neuronal loss and glial proliferation. The presence of numerous microscopic vacuoles in the cytoplasm of astroglial cells and the dendrites of neurons accounts for the typical spongiform appearance of the brain.

Clinical Features Prodromal symptoms of fatigue, sleep disturbances, weight loss, depression, poor appetite, and emotional lability can occur and last for several weeks. This stage is followed by a rapidly progressive dementia associated with visual symptoms,[235] dysphasia leading to aphasia,[236] cerebellar ataxia, and spasticity. Hallucinations, delusions, and agitation occur in some cases, and stimulus-sensitive myoclonus is a prominent feature. Extrapyramidal signs of rigidity, dystonia, and dysarthria are seen in some patients. Seizures are not infrequent, and there is a rapid decline to a state of akinetic mutism.

Death from infection occurs within 6 months in 75 percent of cases, the minority surviving for up to 2 years.

Diagnostic Procedures

1. The MRI scan shows moderate to severe symmetrical cortical atrophy.

2. Axial fast spin-echo MRI images may reveal marked high signal intensity, which occurs symmetrically or asymmetrically and involves the head and body of the caudate nucleus.[237]

3. The CSF is usually normal or the protein content may be elevated.

4. The EEG shows periodic high-voltage triphasic sharp wave discharges occurring on a background of slow activity.

5. Neuronal-specific enolase (NSE) is elevated in the CSF early in this disease. A positive NSE has a specificity of 92 percent for spongiform encephalopathy in the absence of stroke, brain tumor, and subarachnoid hemorrhage.

6. The presence of 14-3-3 brain protein in the CSF has a high degree of specificity in Creutzfeldt-Jakob disease.[238]

7. The brain biopsy demonstrating spongiform changes in the brain is the definitive diagnostic procedure.

Treatment Treatment is symptomatic. There is no effective therapy for this disease.

Rasmussen Encephalitis

Definition This progressive disorder is characterized by partial seizures, hemiplegia, and dementia.

Etiology and Pathology This cause is unknown. Rasmussen encephalitis may be a focal autoimmune encephalitis or a focal viral infectious process by CMV or HSV-1 confined to one hemisphere.[239]

Clinical Features This progressive, usually childhood, disorder begins with focal seizure activity and progresses relentlessly to hemiplegia and dementia over a period of months or years.[240] Onset in young adults has been described.

Treatment

1. Improvement has been reported following high-dose intravenous immunoglobulin therapy. Improvement may be delayed until after 2 to 4 monthly cycles of high dose IVIG therapy.[241]
2. Plasmapheresis is an effective therapy in some cases.[242]
3. Hemispherectomy is recommended in refractory cases.

Acute Disseminated Encephalomyelitis

This condition is an acute demyelinating disease believed to be an autoimmune response to a systemic viral infection. The illness may begin within a week or as long as 4 weeks after an acute viral infection such as measles, varicella, or rubella, and rarely following mumps or influenza (postinfectious encephalomyelitis). In many cases, the infectious component is unrecorded or may present as a mild upper respiratory tract infection. Acute disseminated encephalomyelitis used to be a recognized complication of vaccination against rabies or smallpox (postvaccinal encephalomyelitis), but this condition has largely been eliminated by the use of modern rabies vaccines and by the eradication of smallpox worldwide. Occasional cases may be seen following injection of tetanus antiserum or earlier forms of rabies vaccine, which are still in use in Third World countries.

Pathology The brain and spinal cord show the presence of perivascular cuffing with lymphocytes and plasma cells and scattered areas of perivascular demyelination. The primary lesion is believed to be a vasculopathy and discrete areas of hemorrhage are seen in some cases. The condition has a similar pathological appearance to experimental allergic encephalomyelitis. In some fulminating cases, the brain is swollen and shows the presence of numerous petechial hemorrhages or hematoma formation. Microscopic changes consist of necrosis of blood vessel walls and the passage of fibrinous exudate into the perivascular spaces. There are marked white matter edema and infiltration of abnormal areas with inflammatory cells. The affected blood vessels may be surrounded by areas of necrosis and demyelination or ball or ring-like hemorrhages (acute hemorrhagic encephalomyelitis).

Clinical Features The decrease in the incidence of acute disseminated encephalomyelitis has been attributed to increased vaccination and immunization against infectious diseases. The onset is usually abrupt, occurring within a week of clinical evidence of infection, but the first symptoms have been reported before any signs of infection, and as long as 2 or 3 months after infection. The early symptoms consist of headache, fever, anorexia, and lethargy. The subsequent course shows considerable variation. The illness may resemble a mild encephalitis with complete recovery, or there may be rapid progression to stupor and coma. Psychiatric symptoms consisting of personality changes, hallucinations, or acute paranoia are not uncommon. Seizures, sensory or motor disturbances, or dysfunction of bladder or bowel may occur.

Differential Diagnosis The disseminated involvement of the CNS in acute disseminated encephalomyelitis produces a clinical picture that mimics acute multiple sclerosis. The development of symptoms following documented infections, however, suggests the diagnosis of acute disseminated encephalomyelitis.

Diagnostic Procedures

1. On lumbar puncture, the CSF is clear, with normal, slightly elevated pressure. There is a lymphocytic pleocytosis and red blood cells are present in some cases. The protein and gamma globulin contents are elevated. The glucose content is normal.

2. The EEG is abnormal in severe cerebral involvement, with diffuse slowing in the theta and delta range.

3. The MRI scan shows the presence of numerous areas of increased signal intensity in the white matter of the brainstem and spinal cord, and in the gray matter of basal ganglia, thalamus, and temporal lobe cortex.[243]

Treatment

1. Plasmapheresis alone[244] or combined with high-dose corticosteroids and cyclophosphamide[245] may produce a successful recovery in some cases.

2. The fulminating acute hemorrhagic form of the disease is associated with rapid increase in ICP and requires ICP monitoring, intravenous mannitol and high-dose barbiturate therapy.

Subacute Herpes Simplex-6 Encephalitis

Involvement of the CNS by herpes simplex virus type 6 (HSV-6) has been reported by several sources and usually occurs in immunocompromised individuals with bone marrow transplants[246] or AIDS.[247] Infection in nonimmunocompromised individuals can occur, however, producing a disease resembling acute disseminated encephalomyelitis in young children or severe acute multiple sclerosis. However, the role of HSV-6 in multiple sclerosis remains to be defined, although the virus has been demonstrated in multiple sclerosis plaques in some cases.[248] A chronic myelopathy with predominantly white matter changes has been described.[249] Thus, HSV-6 may produce an encephalopathy that shares clinical manifestations and demyelinative characteristics with multiple sclerosis but may be etiologically distinct.[250] Alternatively, HSV-6 may have a role in acute multiple sclerosis, which is, as yet, undefined.

Behçet Disease

Definition Behçet disease is a clinical syndrome characterized by recurrent aphthous ulceration of the mouth and genitalia, posterior uveitis, cutaneous vasculitis, synovitis, and meningoencephalitis.[251]

Etiology and Pathology The etiology is unknown, but the condition is believed to be related to a viral infection. The brain shows the presence of perivascular infiltration with neuronal loss and demyelination.

Clinical Features Behçet disease usually occurs in young adults. It is characterized by recurrent aphthous ulceration affecting the mouth and genitalia and at least one of the following: posterior uveitis, cutaneous vasculitis producing skin lesions, and synovitis. Colitis, thrombophlebitis, and large artery aneurysms have been reported.

Involvement of the nervous system is an early feature of the disease, and there are no characteristic clinical findings. Any portion of the neuraxis may be involved. The usual presentation is an aseptic meningitis. However, a severe, frequently fatal meningoencephalomyelitis has been reported. Intracranial hypertension, papilledema, intracerebral hemorrhage, or cerebrovenous thrombosis may occur, and peripheral neuropathy has been reported. Relapses are frequent.

Diagnostic Procedures There is no specific diagnostic test for Behçet disease. The CSF is frequently under increased pressure, with a lymphocytic pleocytosis and elevated protein content. An MRI scan often shows the presence of areas of increased signal intensity involving both gray and subcortical white matter. Gadolinium enhancement of T1-weighted images will reveal abnormal meningeal enhancement.[252] Skin biopsy shows the presence of leukocytoblastic vasculitis or a neutrophilic vascular reaction.

Differential Diagnosis

1.   Mollaret meningitis. There is a history of recurrent meningitis but no history of recurrent aphthous ulceration.

2.   Vogt-Koyanagi-Harada syndrome consists of uveitis, retinal edema, and meningoencephalitis. Alopecia and vitiligo are present, and there is ulceration of the mouth or genitalia.

3.   Inflammatory granulomatous conditions, including tuberculosis, syphilis, and sarcoidosis, must be considered.

4.   Herpes simplex encephalitis can be distinguished by elevated serum antibody titers to herpes simplex and confirmed by the presence of herpes simplex DNA by polymerase chain reaction.

Treatment

1. Corticosteroids. Prednisone 100 mg daily may be effective if given early.
2. Immunosuppression using azathioprine and cyclophosphamide chlorambucil or cyclosporine A have been effective in some patients with severe ocular and meningoencephalitic involvement.

Uveomeningoencephalitic Syndrome (Vogt-Koyanagi-Harada syndrome)

Uveomeningoencephalitic syndrome is a rare disorder characterized by progressive uveitis, meningoencephalitis, and progressive loss of pigment in the skin and hair. The etiology is unknown. The arachnoid over the base of the skull is thickened and infiltrated with lymphocytes and histiocytes. The temporal lobes are frequently affected and show the presence of necrosis and secondary gliosis in severe cases.

The clinical course follows four stages. The prodromal stage presents as a febrile viral-like illness with nausea, headache, photophobia, nuchal rigidity, cranial nerve palsies, tinnitus, impaired hearing, lethargy, disorientation, and delirium. This is followed in a few days by an acute uveitic phase characterized by bilateral chronic iridocyclitis, posterior uveitis including evidence of retinal detachment, papilledema, macular edema, and depigmentation of the retina. The convalescent phase presents with cutaneous involvement several weeks later, consisting of alopecia, vitiligo, and premature graying of the hair (poliosis).[253] This may be followed by a chronic recurrent phase, with recurrent anterior uveitis complicated by cataracts, glaucoma, and subretinal neovascularization.[254] Steroid therapy has been reported to be effective in controlling the condition. Eye involvement should be vigorously treated in an effort to avoid glaucoma and blindness.

Benign Recurrent Aseptic Meningitis (Mollaret Meningitis)

Definition Mollaret meningitis is a rare recurrent meningitis in which the patient shows complete recovery between attacks.

Etiology and Pathology The etiology of Mollaret meningitis is uncertain, but HSV-1 and HSV-2 have been identified as the putative causative agents.[255] Pathological changes have not been reported.

Clinical Features The reported cases of the disorder have occurred in all ages and both sexes. Symptoms consist of brief (2 to 7 day) recurrent attacks of headache and meningeal irritation. The attacks may be accompanied by fever, myalgias, nausea, and vomiting. In a few cases, changes in mentation, focal neurological deficits, seizures, and coma can occur. The attacks are of variable intensity and the patient is symptom free between attacks. The condition resolves completely after a prolonged period of recurrent attacks (1 to 11 years).

Diagnostic Procedures

1. On lumbar puncture, the CSF is clear with a pleocytosis composed initially of large endothelial-like cells that are fragile, have irregular borders, and lyse rapidly. These cells are eventually replaced by lymphocytes. A mild elevation in protein content, elevated gamma globulin and a decrease in glucose content occur.

2. There may be a peripheral eosinophilia.

Differential Diagnosis The differential diagnosis includes posttraumatic relapsing meningitis, meningitis secondary to chronic otitis or sinusitis, Behçet disease, sarcoidosis, granulomatous meningitis, meningitis secondary to parasitic infection, meningeal carcinomatosis, and migrainous headache with severe neurological deficits and CSF lymphocytosis.[256]

Treatment The treatment is symptomatic and there is a rapid and complete recovery. The prognosis is excellent.

Arachnoiditis

Definition *Arachnoiditis* is a chronic inflammation and fibrosis of the leptomeninges, usually occurring in the spinal canal and occasionally in the cranial cavity.

Etiology and Pathology Arachnoiditis has been described following myelography using both water-soluble and oil contrast media. However, there is no doubt that the most common etiological factor in spinal varieties of arachnoiditis is surgical treatment of lumbar disc disease and the use of nonabsorbable oil-based contrast materials for myelography.[257] The association of herniated lumbar intravertebral disc and arachnoiditis has been challenged recently.[258] Chronic inflammation of the leptomeninges is more likely to occur after repeated myelographic studies, and it is possible that the injection of a mixture of contrast media and blood during a traumatic lumbar puncture increases the risk of arachnoiditis. There are also occasional reports of arachnoiditis following injection of antibiotics into the subarachnoid space and following spinal anesthesia. Arachnoiditis has been reported following trauma to the spinal column and spinal canal, and local arachnoiditis is not unusual at the site of a ruptured intravertebral disc. Chronic inflammatory changes in the leptomeninges may follow an acute purulent meningitis or may be related to chronic infections, including syphilis, tuberculosis, sarcoidosis, and fungal meningitis. Localized arachnoiditis may occur at the site of tuberculosis of a vertebral body (Pott disease). Arachnoiditis has also been reported following subarachnoid hemorrhage.

Pathological changes consist of thickening of the leptomeninges and monocytic infiltration or granulomatous inflammation with vascular proliferation. The blood vessels are involved by an arteritis or phlebitis. The presence of thickened leptomeninges may produce constriction of nerve roots or pressure on the spinal cord. This may be compounded by ischemia over the spinal cord, with circumscribed areas of necrosis and fibrosis.

Clinical Features The chief complaint is usually weakness of the lower limbs, which may progress to severe paraparesis or paraplegia. The appearance of weakness is followed by complaints of pain, which may be of two types, a burning pain in the distribution of the affected nerve roots, or a more ill-defined pain below the level of the compression. In addition, patients may complain of numbness, "deadness," and coldness in the lower limbs and trunk below the level of the arachnoiditis. Disturbances of micturition are early symptoms, and many patients develop complete incontinence. Examination shows the presence of spastic paraparesis with increased reflexes and extensor plantar responses. Sensation to pain and temperature is impaired below the level of the cord compression, and posterior column involvement produces impairment of vibration and position sense.

Diagnostic Procedures

1. A CT scan of the spine may show the presence of destruction of the vertebral bodies in cases of tuberculosis.

2. The study of choice is MRI scanning. It is nontraumatic and is as effective as plain film myelography or CT myelography in the demonstration of lumbar arachnoiditis.

3. Lumbar puncture reveals a CSF of reduced pressure with a negative Queckenstedt test in cases of complete spinal block. The CSF is often xanthochromic and the protein content is markedly elevated.

Treatment

1. Prophylactic
   a. Avoid the use of myelography when CT or MRI scans are unequivocally abnormal and indicate the presence of a herniated disc.
   b. If myelography is necessary, the latest type of water-soluble contrast media, which is quickly absorbed with the CSF, should be utilized.

Suspected infection should be effectively treated with antibiotics. Compression of the spinal cord or lumbosacral nerve roots can be relieved surgically in some cases by unroofing the dura mater and separating each nerve root one from the other. Patients with diffuse arachnoiditis may benefit from a course of corticosteroids, which may reduce the inflammatory response. Chronic cases are difficult to treat and may require prolonged use of analgesic drugs. Transcutaneous stimulation may be useful in some cases. Direct cord stimulation using implanted electrodes has had some success.

Prognosis Localized arachnoiditis treated by surgical resection of the leptomeninges usually shows good response to treatment. Patients with severe spinal cord damage can only hope to avoid further deterioration and obtain relief from pain by appropriate use of analgesic medications.

Idiopathic Chronic Hypertrophic Craniocervical Pachymeningitis

Definition This rare condition of chronic inflammatory disease causes hypertrophy of the dura mater.[259]

Etiology and Pathology The etiology is unknown. It is possible that some cases represent occult tuberculous disease.[260] There is diffuse thickening of the dura in the cervical and thoracic spinal cord or in the posterior fossa with involvement of the tentorium cerebelli and occasional extension forward into the middle and anterior cranial fossae with involvement of the falx cerebri. Microscopic examination shows dense fibrous tissue with an intermingled inflammatory exudate composed of lymphocytes, plasma cells, monocytes, and occasional multinucleated giant cells.[261]

Clinical Features The more frequently observed cervical pachymeningitis presents with back and neck pain followed by progressive spastic paraparesis, urgency of micturition and loss of bladder control associated with radicular pain due to progressive involvement of cervical and upper thoracic nerve roots.

The cranial form of the disease causes headache, cranial nerve palsies, cerebellar ataxia, and altered mentation with the development of hydrocephalus.

Differential Diagnosis Other causes of pachymeningitis must be considered, including tuberculosis, sarcoidosis, syphilis, Wegener granulomatosis, fungal or parasitic infections, and rheumatoid arthritis.[262]

Diagnostic Procedures

1. The CT scan shows a diffusely thickened hyperdense dura enhanced in the iodinated contrast study. The gadolinium-enhanced T1-weighted MRI scan shows marked enhancement of the dural edge. The T2-weighted images show relative hypodensity of the thickened meninges with fine hyperintense edges, and there is homogenous enhancement of the thickened dura with gadolinium diethylenetriaminepentaacetic acid.

2. A thorough evaluation should be undertaken to exclude tuberculosis, sarcoidosis, syphilis, and other granulomatous conditions.

3. The CSF is usually under an increased pressure and has an elevated protein content. The glucose content is normal and cultures are negative.

4. Antibodies to herpes simplex may be present.

Treatment

1. There is usually a prompt but temporary response to corticosteroid therapy.[263]

2. Immunosuppression with azathioprine or cyclophosphamide or radiation therapy have inconsistent results.

3. Surgical excision of the hypertrophied dura is mandatory to provide temporary decompression of the cervical cord and prevent paraplegia.

4. A ventricular-atrial shunt procedure may be necessary in patients with hydrocephalus and papilledema.

5. Treatment with acyclovir or famciclovir might benefit patients with elevated herpes simplex antibodies.

REFERENCES

1. Wasserberg J, Barlow P: Lesson of the week. Lumbar puncture still has an important role in diagnosing subarachnoid haemorrhage. *BMJ* 315:1598, 1997.
2. Gower DJ, Baker AL, Bell WO, et al: Contraindications to lumbar puncture as defined by computed cranial tomography. *J Neurol Neurosurg Psychiatry* 50:1071, 1987.
3. Archer BD: Computed tomography before lumbar puncture in acute meningitis: a review of the risks and benefits. *Can Med Assoc J* 148:961, 1993.
4. Wang LP, Schmidt JF: Central nervous side effects after lumbar puncture. A review of the possible pathogenesis of the syndrome of postdural puncture headache and associated symptoms. *Danish Med Bull* 44:79, 1997.
5. Evans RW: Complications of lumbar puncture. *Neurologic Clin* 16:83, 1998.
6. Choi A, Laurito CE, Cunningham FE: Pharmacologic management of postdural puncture headache. *Ann Pharmacotherapy* 30:831, 1996.
7. Peterman SB: Postmyelography headache: a review. *Radiology* 200:765, 1996.
8. Schneeberger PM, Janssen M, Voss A: Alpha-hemolytic streptococci: a major pathogen of iatrogenic meningitis following lumbar puncture. Case reports and a review of the literature. *Infection* 24:29, 1996.
9. Kornelisse RF, de Groot R, Neijens HJ: Bacterial meningitis: mechanisms of disease and therapy. *Eur J Pediatr* 154:85, 1995.

10. Tunkel AR, Scheld WM: Pathogenesis and pathophysiology of bacterial meningitis. *Annu Rev Med* 44:103, 1993.

11. Spellerberg B, Tuomanen EI: The pathophysiology of pneumococcal meningitis. *Ann Med* 26:411, 1994.

12. Brown L, Feigin RD: Bacterial meningitis: fluid balance and therapy. *Pediatr Ann* 23:93, 1994.

13. Haile-Mariam T, Laws E, Tuazon CU: Gram-negative meningitis associated with transsphenoidal surgery: case report and review. *Clin Infect Dis* 18:553, 1994.

14. Ashwal S, Perkin RM, Thompson JR, et al: Bacterial meningitis in children: current concepts of neurologic management. *Curr Prob Pediatr* 24:267, 1994.

15. Smith AL: Bacterial meningitis. *Pediatrics in Rev* 14:11, 1993.

16. Oliver LG, Harwood-Nuss AL: Bacterial meningitis in infants and children: a review. *J Emerg Med* 11:555, 1993.

17. Pohl CA: Practical approach to bacterial meningitis in childhood. *Am Fam Physician* 47:1595, 1993.

18. Dunne DW, Quagliarello V: Group B streptococcal meningitis in adults. *Medicine* 72:1, 1993.

19. Tunkel AR, Scheld WM: Acute bacterial meningitis (review). *Lancet* 346:1675, 1995.

20. Miller LG, Choi C: Meningitis in older patients: how to diagnose and treat deadly infection. *Geriatrics* 52:43–44, 47–50, 55, 1997.

21. Linder N, Dagan R, Kuint J, et al: Ventriculitis caused by *Klebsiella pneumoniae* successfully treated with perfloxacin in a neonate. *Infection* 22:210, 1994.

22. Ashwal S: Neurologic evaluation of the patient with acute bacterial meningitis. *Neurol Clin* 13:549, 1995.

23. Sze G: Diseases of the intracranial meninges: MR imaging features. *AJR* 160:727, 1993.

24. Rockowitz J, Tunkel AR: Bacterial meningitis. Practical guidelines for management. *Drugs* 50:838, 1995.

25. Schaad UB, Kaplan SL, McCracken GH Jr.: Steroid therapy for bacterial meningitis. *Clin Infect Dis* 20:685, 1995.

26. Lauritsen A, Oberg B: Adjunctive corticosteroid therapy in bacterial meningitis. *Scand J Infect Dis* 27:431, 1995.

27. Jones D: Current and future trends in immunization against meningitis. *J Antimicrob Chemother* 31, Suppl B 93, 1993.

28. Cuevas LE, Hart CA: Chemoprophylaxis of bacterial meningitis. *J Antimicrob Chemother* 31, Suppl B 79, 1993.

29. Tang LM, Chen ST: Relapsing bacterial meningitis in adults. *QJM* 87:511, 1994.

30. Ng PY, Seow WT, Ong PL: Brain abscesses: review of 30 cases treated with surgery. *Aust NZ J Surg* 65:664, 1995.

31. Singh B, Van Dellen J, Ramjettan S, et al: Singenic intracranial complications. *J Laryngol Otol* 109:945, 1995.

32. Dolan RW, Chowdhury K: Diagnosis and treatment of intracranial complications of paranasal sinus infections. *J Oral Maxillofacial Surg* 53:1080, 1995.

33. Meeks RB 3rd, Schmidt JH 3rd: The difficult diagnosis of subdural empyema: report of three cases and review of the literature. *West Virginia M J* 92:87, 1996.

34. Brennan MR: Subdural empyema. *Am Fam Physician* 51:157, 1995.

35. Weingarten K, Zimmerman RD, Becker RD, et al: Subdural and epidural empyemas: MR imaging. *AJNR Am J Neuroradiol* 10:81, 1989.

36. Heilpern KL, Lorber B: Focal intracranial infections. *Infect Dis Clin North Am* 10:879, 1996.

37. Dill SR, Cobb CG, McDonald CK: Subdural empyema: analysis of 32 cases and review. *Clin Infect Dis* 20:372, 1995.

38. Darouiche RO, Hamill RJ, Greenberg SB, et al: Bacterial spinal epidural abscess. Review of 43 cases and literature survey. *Medicine* 71:369, 1992.

39. Nussbaum ES, Rigamonti D, Standford H, et al: Spinal epidural abscess: a report of 40 cases and review. *Surg Neurol* 38:225, 1992.

40. Mackenzie AR, Laing RB, Smith CC, et al: Spinal epidural abscess: the importance of early diagnosis and treatment. *J Neurol Neurosurg Psychiatry* 65:209, 1998.

41. Mooney RP, Hockberger RS: Spinal epidural abscess: a rapidly progressive disease. *Ann Emerg Med* 16:1168, 1987.

42. Martin RJ, Yuan HA: Neurosurgical care of spinal epidural, subdural and intramedullary abscesses and arachnoiditis. *Ortho Clin North Am* 27:125, 1996.

43. Byrne RW, von Roenn KA, Whisler WW: Intramedullary abscess: a report of two cases and a review of the literature. *Neurosurgery* 35:321, 1994.

44. Tacconi L, Arulampalam T, Johnston FG, et al: Intramedullary spinal cord abscess: case report. *Neurosurgery* 37:817, 1995.

45. Sanford JP: Tetanus—forgotten but not gone. *N Engl J Med* 332:812, 1995.

46. Sun KO, Chan YW, Cheung RT, et al: Management of tetanus: a review of 18 cases. *J R Soc Med* 87:135, 1994.

47. Loscalzo IL, Ryan J, Loscalzo J, et al: Tetanus: a clinical diagnosis. *Am J Emerg Med* 13:488, 1995.

48. Brock H, Moosbauer W, Gabriel C, et al: Treatment of severe tetanus by continuous intrathecal infusion of baclofen. *J Neurol Neurosurg Psychiatry* 59:193, 1995.

49. Sutton DN, Tremlett MR, Woodcock TE, et al: Management of autonomic dysfunction in severe tetanus, the use of magnesium sulfate and clonidine. *Intensive Care Med* 16:75, 1990.

50. Gale JL, Thapa PB, Wassilak SG, et al: Risk of serious acute neurological illness after immunization with diphtheria-tetanus-pertussis vaccine. A population-based case-control study. *JAMA* 271:37, 1994.

51. Gergen PJ, McQuillan GM, Kiely M, et al: A population-based serologic survey of immunity to tetanus in the United States. New Eng J Med 332:761, 1995.

52. Mousa AR, Koshy TS, Brucella meningitis: presentation, diagnosis and treatment. Aray GF et al: a prospective study of ten cases. *Q J Med* 60:873, 1986.

53. Marzo Sola ME, Calderon Giron C, Ayusa Blanco T, et al: Neurobrucellosis. A report of 13 cases. *Neurologia* 10:375, 1995.

54. Kirchner JT: Psittacosis: Is contact with birds causing your patient's pneumonia? *Postgrad Med* 102:181–2, 187–8, 193–4, 1997.

55. Hughes P, Chidley K, Cowie J: Neurological complications in psittacosis. A report and literature review. *Resp Med* 89:637, 1995.

56. Verweig PE, Meis JF, Eijk R, et al: Severe human psittacosis requiring artificial ventilation: case report and review. *Clin Infect Dis* 20:440, 1995.

57. Logigian EL, Kaplan RF, Steere AC: Chronic neurologic manifestations of Lyme disease. *New Eng J Med* 323:1438, 1990.

58. Kaplan RF, Meadows ME, Vincent LC, et al: Memory impairment and depression in patients with Lyme encephalopathy: comparison with fibromyalgia and nonpsychotically depressed patients. *Neurology* 42:1263, 1992.

59. Shadick NA, Phillips CB, Logigian EL, et al: The long-term clinical outcomes of Lyme disease. A population based retrospective cohort study. *Ann Intern Med* 121:560, 1994.

60. Pachner AR: Early disseminated Lyme disease: Lyme meningitis. *Am J Med* 98:4A30S–4A43S, 1995.

61. Kilmarx PH, St Louis ME: The evolving epidemiology of syphilis. *Am J Public Health* 85:1053, 1995.

62. Yinnon AM, Coury-Doniger P, Polito R, et al: Serologic response to treatment of syphilis in patients with HIV infection. *Arch Intern Med* 156:321, 1996.

63. Musher DM, Hamill RJ, Baughn RE: Effect of human immunodeficiency virus (HIV) infection on the course of syphilis and on the response to treatment. *Ann Intern Med* 113:872, 1990.

64. US Department of Health and Human Services: Sexually transmitted diseases. Treatment and guidelines. MMWR *Morb Mortal Wkly Rep 1993*. 42:RR-14, 1993.

65. Flores JL: Syphilis. A tale of twisted treponemes. *West J Med* 163:552, 1995.

66. Schon B, Maartens G: Treatment of syphilis in HIV-infected individuals—more questions than answers? *SAMJ* 84:320, 1994.

67. Rolfs RJ: Treatment of syphilis 1993. *Clin Infect Dis* 20(Suppl 1):S23, 1995.

68. Carey LA, Glesby MJ, Mundy LM, et al: Lumbar puncture for evaluation of latent syphilis in hospitalized patients. High prevalence of cerbrospinal fluid abnormalities unrelated to syphilis. *Arch Intern Med* 155:1657, 1995.

69. Lipton JD, Schafermeyer RW: Central nervous system infections. The usual and the unusual. *Emerg Med Clin North Am* 13:417, 1995.

70. Lam KS, Sham MM, Tam SC, et al: Hypopituitarism after tuberculous meningitis in childhood. *Ann Intern Med* 118:701, 1993.

71. Monteyne P, Sindic CJ: The diagnosis of tuberculous meningitis. *Acta Neurol Bel* 95:80, 1995.

72. Kaneko K, Onodera O, Miyatake T, et al: Rapid diagnosis of tuberculous meningitis by polymerase chain reaction (PCR). *Neurology* 40:1617, 1990.

73. Radhakrishnan VV, Mathai A: Detection of Mycobacterium tuberculosis antigen 5 in cerebrospinal fluid by inhibition ELISA and its diagnostic potential in tuberculous meningitis. *J Infect Dis* 163:650, 1991.

74. Segura RM, Pascual C, Ocana I, et al: Adenosine deaminase in body fluids: a useful diagnostic tool in tuberculosis. *Clin Biochem* 22:141, 1989.

75. Tartaglione T, DiLella GM, Cerase A, et al: Diagnostic imaging of neurotuberculosis. *Rays* 23:164, 1998.

76. de Castro CC, de Barros NG, Campos ZM, et al: CT scans of cranial tuberculosis. *Radiol Clin North Am* 33:753, 1995.

77. Villoria MF, Fortea F, Moreno S, et al: MR imaging and CT of central nervous system tuberculosis in the patients with AIDS. *Radiol Clin N Amer* 33:805, 1995.

78. Jamieson DH: Imaging intracranial tuberculosis in childhood. *Pediatr Radiol* 25:165, 1995.

79. Dooley DP, Carpenter JL, Rademacher S: Adjunctive corticosteroid therapy for tuberculosis: a critical reappraisal of the literature. *Clin Infect Dis* 25:872, 1997.

80. Gropper MR, Schulder M, Sharan AD, et al: Central nervous system tuberculous: medical management and surgical indications. *Surg Neurol* 44:378, 1995.

81. Rao GP, Nadh BR, Hemaratnan A, et al: Paradoxical progression of tuberculous lesions during chemotherapy of central nervous system tuberculosis. Report of four cases. *J Neurosurg* 83:359, 1995.

82. Newton RW: Tuberculous meningitis. *Arch Dis Child* 70:364, 1994.

83. Afghani B, Lieberman JM: Paradoxical enlargement or development of intracranial tuberculomas during therapy: case report and review. *Clin Infect Dis* 19:1092, 1994.

84. Adendorff JJ, Boeke EJ, Lazarus C. Tuberculosis of the spine: results of management of 300 patients. *JR Coll Surg Edinburg* 32:152, 1987.

85. Citow JS, Ammirati M: Intramedullary tuberculoma of the spinal cord: case report. *Neurosurgery* 35:327, 1994.

86. Stern BJ, Griffin DE, Luke RA, et al: Neurosarcoidosis cerebrospinal fluid lymphocyte subpopulations. *Neurology* 37:878, 1987.

87. Asano M, Minagawa T, Ohmischi M, et al: Detection of endogenous cytokines in sera or in lymph nodes obtained from patients with sarcoidosis. *Clin Ex Immunol* 84:92, 1991.

88. Stern BJ, Krumholz A, Johns C, et al: Sarcoidosis and its neurological manifestations. *Arch Neurol* 42:909, 1985.

89. Briner VA, Muller A, Gebbers JO: Neurosarcoidosis. Schweiz Med Wochen. *J Suisse Med* 128:799, 1998.

90. Jackson RJ, Goodman JC, Huston DP, et al: Parafalcine and bilateral convexity neurosarcoidosis mimicking meningioma: case report and review of the literature. *Neurosurgery* 42:635, 1998.

91. Chitoku S, Kawai S, Watabe Y, et al: Multiple intramedullary spinal sarcoidosis: case report. *Surg Neurol* 48:522, 1997.

92. Ost D, Yeldandi A, Cugell D: Acute sarcoid myositis with respiratory muscle involvement. Case report and review of the literature. *Chest* 107:879, 1995.

93. Chen RC, McLeod JG: Neurological complications of sarcoidosis. *Clin Exp Neurol* 26:99, 1989.

94. Krumholz A, Stern BJ, Stern EG: Clinical implications of seizures in neurosarcoidosis. *Arch Neurol* 48:842, 1991.

95. Jallo GI, Zagzag D, Lee M, et al: Intraspinal sarcoidosis: diagnosis and management. *Surg Neurol* 48:514, 1997.

96. Zuniga G, Ropper AH, Frank J: Sarcoid peripheral neuropathy. *Neurology* 41:1558, 1991.

97. Sherman JL, Stern BJ: Sarcoidosis of the CNS: comparison of unenhanced and enhanced MR images. *AJNR Am J Neuroradiol* 11:915, 1990.

98. Lower EE, Baughman RP: Prolonged use of methotrexate for sarcoidosis. *Arch Intern Med* 155:846, 1995.

99. Stelzer KJ, Thomas CR Jr, Berger MS, et al: Radiation therapy for sarcoid of the thalamus/posterior third ventricle: case report. *Neurosurgery* 36:1188, 1995.

100. Klein JD: Cat scratch disease. *Pediatr Rev* 15:348, 1994.

101. Hadley S, Albrecht MA, Tarsy D: Cat-scratch encephalopathy: a cause of status epilepticus and coma in a healthy young adult. *Neurology* 45:196, 1995.

102. Dalton MJ, Robinson LE, Cooper J, et al: Use of Bartonella antigens for serologic diagnosis of cat-scratch disease at a national referral center. *Arch Intern Med* 155:1670, 1995.

103. Fishbein DB, Dennis DT: Tick-borne diseases—a growing risk. *N Engl J Med* 333:452, 1995.

104. Dalton MJ, Clarke MJ, Holman RC, et al: National surveillance for Rocky Mountain spotted fever 1981–1992: epidemiologic summary and evaluation of risk factors for fatal outcome. *Am J Trop Med Hyg* 52:405, 1995.

105. MacDonell RA, Donnan GA; Kalmins RM, et al: Otocerebral mucormycosis—a case report. *Clin Exp Neurol* 23:225, 1987.

106. Slavoski LA, Tunkel AR: Therapy of fungal meningitis. *Clin Neuropharmacol* 18:95, 1995.

107. Casado JL, Quereda C, Oliva J, et al: Candida meningitis in HIV-infected patients: analysis of 14 cases. *Clin Infect Dis* 25:673, 1997.

108. Nguyen MH, Yu VL: Meningitis caused by Candida species: an emerging problem in neurosurgical patients. *Clin Infect Dis* 21:323, 1995.

109. Harril WC, Stewart MG, Lee AG, et al: Chronic rhinocerebral mucormycosis. *Laryngoscope* 106:1292, 1996.

110. Weprin BE, Hall WA, Goodman J, et al: Long-term survival in rhinocerebral mucormycosis. Case report. *J Neurosurg* 88:570, 1998.

111. Body BA, Oneson RH, Herold DA: Use of cerebrospinal fluid lactic acid concentration in the diagnosis of fungal meningitis. *Ann Clin Lab Sci* 17:429, 1987.

112. Ennis DM, Saag MS: Cryptococcal meningitis in AIDS. *Hosp Pract* 28:99, 1993.

113. Ingram CW, Haywood HB 3rd, Morris VM et al: Cryptococcal ventricular-peritoneal shunt infection: clinical and epidemiological evaluation of two closely associated cases. *Infect Cont Hosp Epidemiol* 14:719, 1993.

114. Powderly WG: Cryptococcal meningitis and AIDS. *Clin Infect Dis* 17:837, 1993.

115. Rex JH, Larsen RA, Dismukes WE, et al: Catastrophic visual loss due to Cryptococcus neoformans meningitis. *Medicine* 72:207, 1993.

116. Garlipp CR, Rossi CL, Bottini PV: Cerebrospinal fluid profiles in acquired immunodeficiency syndrome with and without neurocryptococcosis. *Rev Inst Med Trop San Paulo* 39:323, 1997.

117. Mischel PS, Vinters HV: Coccidioidomycosis of the central nervous system: neuropathological and vasculopathic manifestations and clinical correlates. *Clin Infect Dis* 20:400, 1995.

118. Conces DJ Jr: Histoplasmosis. *Semin Roentgenol* 31:14, 1996.

119. Miaux Y, Ribaud P, Williams M, et al: MR of cerebral aspergillosis in patients who have had bone marrow transplantation. *AJNR Am J Neuroradiol* 16:55, 1995.

120. Denning DW: Invasive aspergillosis. *Clin Infect Dis* 26:781, 1998.

121. Schumacher DJ, Tien RD, Lane K: Neuroimaging findings in rare amebic infections of the central nervous system. *AJNR Am J Neuroradiol* 16(Suppl 4): 930, 1995.

122. Newton CR, Krishna S: Severe falciparum malaria in children: current understanding of pathophysiology and supportive treatment. *Pharm Therapeut* 79:1, 1998.

123. Warrell DA: Cerebral malaria: clinical features, pathophysiology, and treatment. *Ann Trop Med Parasit* 91:875, 1997.

124. Clark IA, al Yaman FM, Jacobson LS: The biological basis of malarial disease. *Int J Parasitol* 27:1237, 1997.

125. Warrell DA: The 1996 Runme Shaw Memorial Lecture: malaria—past, present and future. *Ann Acad Med Singapore* 26:380, 1997.

126. Turner G: Cerebral malaria. *Brain Path* 7:569, 1997.

127. Marsh K, English M, Crawley J, et al: The pathogenesis of severe malaria in African children. *Ann Trop Med Parasitol* 90:395, 1996.

128. Wyler DJ: Malaria: overview and update. *Clin Infect Dis* 16:449, 1996.

129. Pittella JE: Neurocysticercosis. *Brain Pathol* 7:681, 1997.

130. Carpio A, Escobar A, Hauser WA: Cysticercosis and epilepsy: a critical review. *Epilepsia* 39:1025, 1998.

131. Chang KH, Han MH: MRI of CNS parasitic diseases. *J Mag Resonance Imaging* 8:297, 1998.

132. Garg RK: Drug treatment of neurocysticercosis. *Nat Med J India* 10:173, 1997.

133. Sotelo J, Jung H: Pharmacokinetic optimisation of the treatment of neurocysticercosis. *Clin Pharmacokinetics* 34:503, 1998.

134. Rawlings D, Ferriero DM, Messing RO: Early CT reevaluation after empiric praziquantel therapy in neurocysticercosis. *Neurology* 39:739, 1989.

135. Venkatesan P: Albendazole. *J Antimicrobial Chemotherapy* 41:145, 1998.

136. Sotelo J, Marin C: Hydrocephalus secondary to cysticercotic arachnoiditis. A long-term follow-up of 92 cases. *J Neurosurg* 66:686, 1987.

137. Earnest MP, Reller LB, Filley CM, et al: Neurocysticercosis in the United States: 35 cases and a review. *Rev Infect Dis* 9:961, 1987.

138. Colli BO, Martelli N, Assirati JA Jr, et al: Results of surgical treatment of neurocysticercosis in 69 cases. *J Neurosurg* 65:309, 1986.

139. Berk C, Cifrci E, Erdogan A: MRI in primary intraspinal extradural hydatid disease: case report. *Neuroradiology* 40:390, 1998.

140. Taratuto AL, Venturiello S M: Echinococcosis. *Brain Path* 7:673, 1997.

141. Hira PR, Shweiki HM, Siboo R, et al: Counterimmunoelectrophoresis using an ARC 5 antigen for the rapid diagnosis of hydatidosis and comparison with the indirect hemagglutination test. *Am J Trop Med Hyg* 36:592, 1987.

142. Popli MB, Khudale B: Primary multiple hydatid cysts of the brain. *Australas Radiol* 42:90, 1998.

143. Pau A, Brambilla M, Cossu M, et al: Long term follow-up of the surgical treatment of the intracranial hydatid disease. *Acta Neurochir (Wien)* 88:116, 1987.

144. Anderson M: Management of cerebral infection. *J Neurol Neurosurg Psychiatry* 56:1243, 1993.

145. Querol JM, Farga A, Alonso C, et al: Applications of the polymerase chain reaction (PCR) to the diagnosis of central nervous system infections. *An Med Interna* 13:235, 1996.

146. Maxson S, Jacobs RF: Viral meningitis. Tips to rapidly diagnose treatable causes. *Postgrad Med* 93:153, 1993.

147. O'Meara M, Ouvrier R: Viral encephalitis in children. *Current Opin Pediatr* 8:11, 1996.

148. Lowry PW: Arbovirus encephalitis in the United States and Asia. *J Lab Clin Med* 129:405, 1997.

149. Komar N, Spielman A: Emergence of eastern encephalitis in Massachusetts. *Ann NY Acad Sci* 740:157, 1994.

150. Oran B, Ceri A, Yilmaz H, et al: Hydrocephalus in mumps meningoencephalitis: case report. *Pediatr Inf Dis J* 14:724, 1995.

151. Kennedy CR, Duffy SW, Smith R, et al: Clinical predictors of outcome in encephalitis. *Arch Dis Child* 62:1156, 1987.

152. Rowley AH, Whitley RJ, Lakeman FD, et al: Rapid detection of herpes-simplex-virus DNA in cerebrospinal fluid of patients with herpes simplex encephalitis. *Lancet* 335:440, 1990.

153. Levitz RE: Herpes simplex encephalitis: a review. *Heart Lung* 27:209, 1998.

154. Folpe A, Lapham LW, Smith HC: Herpes simplex myelitis as a cause of acute necrotizing myelitis syndrome. *Neurology* 44:1955, 1994.

155. Cinque P, Cleator GM, Weber T, et al: The role of laboratory investigation in the diagnosis and management of patients with suspected herpes simplex encephalitis: a consensus report. The EU Concerted Action on Viral Meningitis and Encephalitis. *J Neurol Neurosurg Psychiatry* 61:339, 1996.

156. Revello MG, Manservigi R: Molecular diagnosis of herpes simplex encephalitis. *Intervirology* 39:185, 1996.

157. Gutierrez KM, Prober CG: Encephalitis. Identifying the specific cause is key to effective management. *Postgrad Med* 103:123–5, 129–130, 140–143, 1998.

158. Masdeu JC, Van Heertum RL, Abdel-Dayem H: Viral infections of the brain. *J Neuroimaging* 5(Suppl 1):S40, 1995.

159. Wutzler P: Antiviral therapy of herpes simplex and varicella-zoster virus infections. *Intervirology* 40:343, 1997.

160. Bertram M, Schwarz S, Hacke W: Acute and critical care in neurology. *Eur Neurol* 38:155, 1997.

161. Skoldenberg B: Herpes simplex encephalitis. *Scand J Inf Dis Suppl* 100:8, 1996.

162. Sasadeusz JJ, Sacks SL: Herpes latency meningitis radiculomyelopathy and disseminated infection. *Genitourinary Med* 70:369, 1994.

163. Fisher DJ: Resurgence of rabies. A historical perspective on rabies in children. *Arch Pediatr Adolesc Med* 149:306, 1995.

164. Warrell MJ: Human deaths from cryptic bat rabies in the USA *Lancet* 346:65, 1995.

165. Rhoades BL: Tennessee rabies update. *J Tenn Med Assoc* 88:356, 1995.

166. Noah DL, Drenzek CL, Smith JS, et al: Epidemiology of human rabies in the United States 1980 to 1996. *Ann Intern Med* 128:922, 1998.

167. Houff SA, Burton RC, Wilson RW, et al: Human-to-human transmission of rabies virus by corneal transplant. *N Engl J Med* 300:603, 1979.

168. Sang E, Farr RW, Fisher MA, et al: Antemortem diagnosis of human rabies. *J Fam Pract* 43:83, 1996.

169. Presutti RJ: Bite wounds. Early treatment and prophylaxis against infectious complications. *Postgrad Med* 101:243–4, 246–52, 254, 1997.

170. Dreesen DW, Hanlon CA: Current recommendations for the prophylaxis and treatment of rabies. *Drugs* 56:801, 1998.

171. Simpson DM, Tagliati M: Neurologic manifestations of HIV infection. *Ann Intern Med* 121:769, 1994.

172. Johnson RT, Glass JD, McArthur JC, et al: Quantitation of human immunodeficiency virus in brains of demented and nondemented patients with acquired immunodeficiency syndrome. *Ann Neurol* 39:392, 1996.

173. Wiley CA, Achim CL: Human Immunodeficiency virus encephalitis and dementia. *Ann Neurol* 38:559, 1995.

174. Epstein LG, Gendelman HE: Human immunodeficiency virus type 1 infection of the nervous system: pathogenetic mechanisms. *Ann Neurol* 33:429, 1993.

175. Wilt SG, Milward E, Zhou JM, et al: In vitro evidence for a dual role of tumor necrosis factor α in human immunodeficiency virus type 1 encephalopathy. *Ann Neurol* 37:381, 1995.

176. Brew BJ, Rosenblum M, Cronin K, et al: AIDS dementia complex and HIV 1 brain infection: clinical virological correlations. *Ann Neurol* 38:563, 1995.

177. Albert SM, Marder K, Dooneief G, et al: Neuropsychologic impairment in early HIV infection. A risk factor for work disability. *Arch Neurol* 52:525, 1995.

178. Goodkin K, Wilkie FL, Concha M, et al: Subtle neuropsychological impairment and minor cognitive-motor disorder in HIV-1 infection. Neuroradiological, neurophysiological, neuroimmunological, and virological correlates. *Neuroimaging Clin North Am* 7:561, 1997.

179. Gallo BV, Shulman LM, Weiner WJ, et al: HIV encephalitis presenting as severe generalized chorea. *Neurology* 46:1163, 1996.

180. Navia BA: Clinical and biologic features of the AIDS dementia complex. *Neuroimaging Clin North Am* 7:581, 1997.

181. Ruiz A, Post JD, Ganz WI, et al: Nuclear medicine applications to the neuroimaging of AIDS. A neuroradiologist's perspective. *Neuroimaging Clin North Am* 7:499, 1997.

182. Havlir DV, Lange JM: New antiretrovirals and new combinations. *AIDS* 12(Suppl A):S165, 1998.

183. Carpenter CC, Fischl MA, Hammer SM, et al: Antiretroviral therapy for HIV infection in 1998: updated recommendations of the International AIDS Society-USA Panel. *JAMA* 280:78, 1998.

184. Griffin JW, Crawford TO, Tyor WR, et al: Predominantly sensory neuropathy in AIDS: distal axonal degrneration and unmyelinated fiber loss. *Neurology* 41(Suppl 1):374, 1991.

185. Morgello S, Simpson DM: Multifocal cytomegalovirus demyelinative polyneuropathy associated with AIDS. *Muscle Nerve* 17:176, 1994.

186. Malamut RI, Leopold N, Chester PA, et al: The treatment of HIV-associated chronic inflammatory demyelinating polyneuropathy (HIV-CIDP) with intravenous immunoglobulin (IVIG). *Neurology* 42(Suppl 3):335, 1992.

187. Kim YS, Hollander H: Polyradiculopathy due to cytomegalovirus: report of two cases in which improvement occurred after prolonged therapy and review of the literature. *Clin Infect Dis* 17:32, 1993.

188. So YT, Olney RK: Acute lumbosacral polyradiculopathy in acquired immunodeficiency syndrome: experience in 23 patients. *Ann Neurol* 35:53, 1994.

189. Roullet E, Assuerus V, Gozlan J, et al: Cytomegalovirus multifocal neuropathy in AIDS: analysis of 15 consecutive cases. *Neurology* 44:2174, 1994.

190. Galetto G, Levine A: AIDS-associated primary central nervous system lymphoma. Oncology Core Committee, AIDS Clinical Trials Group. *JAMA* 269:92, 1993.

191. Cinque P, Brytting M, Vago L, et al: Epstein-Barr virus DNA in cerebrospinal fluid from patients with AIDS-related primary lymphoma of the central nervous system. *Lancet* 342:398, 1993.

192. Ruiz A, Ganz WI, Post MJ, et al: Use of thallium-201 brain SPECT to differentiate cerebral lymphoma from toxoplasma encephalitis in AIDS patients. *AJNR Am J Neuroradiol* 15:1885, 1994.

193. Baumgartner JE, Rachlin JR, Beckstead JH, et al: Primary central nervous system lymphomas: natural history and response to radiation therapy in 55 patients with acquired immunodeficiency syndrome. *J Neurosurg* 73:206, 1990.

194. Tyor WR, Glass JD, Baumrind N, et al: Cytokine expression of macrophages in HIV-1-associated vacuolar myelopathy. *Neurology* 43:1002, 1993.

195. Gray F, Belec L, Lescs MC et al: Varicella-zoster virus infection of the central nervous system in the acquired immune deficiency syndrome. *Brain* 117:987, 1994.

196. Dal Pan GJ, Glass JD, McArthur JC: Clinicopathologic correlations of HIV-1-associated vacuolar myelopathy: an autopsy-based case control study. *Neurology* 44:2159, 1994.

197. Simpson DM, Bender AN: Human immunodeficiency virus associated myelopathy: analysis of 11 patients. *Ann Neurol* 24;79, 1988.

198. Simpson DM, Wolfe DE: Neuromuscular complications of HIV infection and its treatment. *AIDS* 5:917, 1991.

199. Arnaudo E, Dalakas M, Shanske S, et al: Depletion of muscle mitochondrial DNA in AIDS patients with zidovudine-induced myopathy. *Lancet* 337:508, 1991.

200. Morgello S, Wolfe D, Godfrey E, et al: Mitochondrial abnormalities in human immunodeficiency virus-associated myopathy. *Acta Neuropathol (Berl)* 90:366, 1995.

201. Chariot P, Gherardi R: Myopathy and HIV infection. *Curr Opin Rheumatol* 7:497, 1995.

202. Schulz L, Nagaraja HN, Rague N, et al: Respiratory muscle dysfunction associated with human immunodeficiency virus infection. *Am J Resp Crit Care Med* 155:1080, 1997.

203. Simpson DM, Citak KA, Godfrey E, et al: Myopathies associated with human immunodeficiency virus and zidovudine: Can their effects be distinguished? *Neurology* 43:971, 1993.

204. Manji H, Harrison MJ, Round JM, et al: Muscle disease, HIV and zidovudine: the spectrum of muscle disease in HIV-infected individuals treated with zidovudine. *J Neurol* 240:479, 1993.

205. Weber T, Major EO: Progressive multifocal leukoencephalopathy: molecular biology, pathogenesis and clinical impact. *Intervirology* 40:98, 1997.

206. Gallia GL, Houff SA, Major EO, et al: Review: JC virus infection of lymphocytes—revisited. *J Infect Dis* 176:1603, 1997.

207. von Einsiedel RW, Fife TD, Aksamit AJ, et al: Progressive multifocal leukoencephalopathy in AIDS: a clinicopathologic study and review of the literature. *J Neurol* 240:391, 1993.

208. Karahalios D, Breit R, Dal Canto MC, et al: Progressive multifocal leukoencephalopathy in patients with HIV infection: lack of impact of early diagnosis by stereotactic brain biopsy. *J Acquir Immune Defic Syndr Hum Retrovirol* 5:1030, 1992.

209. Berger JR, Mucke L: Prolonged survival and partial recovery in AIDS-associated progressive multifocal leukoencephalopathy. *Neurology* 38:1060, 1988.

210. Sadler M, Nelson MR: Progressive multifocal leukoencephalopathy in HIV. *Inter J STD and AIDS* 8:351, 1997.

211. Nicoli F, Chave B, Peragut JC, et al: Efficacy of cytarabine in progressive multifocal leucoencephalopathy in AIDS. *Lancet* 339:306, 1992.

212. Porter SB, Sande MR: Toxoplasmosis of the central nervous system in the acquired immunodeficiency syndrome. *N Engl J Med* 327:1643, 1992.

213. Luft BJ, Remington JS: Toxoplasmic encephalitis in AIDS. *Clin Infect Dis* 15:211, 1992.

214. Falangola MF, Petito CK: Choroid plexus infection in cerebral toxoplasmosis in AIDS patients. *Neurology* 43:2035, 1993.

215. Jung AC, Paauw DS: Diagnosing HIV-related disease: using the CD4 count as a guide. *J Gen Intern Med* 13:131, 1998.

216. Smirniotopoulos JG, Koeller KK, Nelson AM, et al: Neuroimaging-autopsy correlations in AIDS. *Neuroimaging Clin North Am* 7:615, 1997.

217. Johnson JD, Butcher PD, Savva D, et al: Application of the polymerase chain reaction to the diagnosis of human toxoplasmosis. *J Infect* 26:147, 1993.

218. Arribas JR, Storch GA, Clifford DB, et al: Cytomegalovirus encephalitis. *Ann Intern Med* 125:577, 1996.

219. Morgello S, Cho ES, Nielsen S, et al: Cytomegalovirus encephalitis in patients with acquired immuno-deficiency syndrome: an autopsy study of 30 cases and a review of the literature. *Hum Pathol* 18:298, 1987.

220. Holland NR, Power C, Mathews VP, et al: Cytomegalovirus encephalitis in acquired immunodeficiency syndrome (AIDS). *Neurology* 44(3 Pt 1):507, 1994.

221. Anders HJ, Goebel FD: Cytomegalovirus polyradiculopathy in patients with AIDS. *Clin Infect Dis* 27:345, 1998.

222. Faber DW, Wiley CA, Lynn GB, et al: Role of HIV and CMV in the pathogenesis of retinitis and retinal vasculopathy in AIDS patients. *Invest Oph Vis Sci* 33:2345, 1992.

223. Wolf DG, Spector SA: Diagnosis of human cytomegalovirus central nervous system disease in AIDS patients by DNA amplification from cerebrospinal fluid. *J Infect Dis* 166:1412, 1992.

224. Anders HJ, Weiss N, Bogner JR, et al: Ganciclovir and foscarnet efficacy in AIDS-related CMV polyradiculopathy. *J Infect* 36:29, 1998.

225. Mustafa MM, Weitman SD, Winick NJ, et al: Subacute measles encephalitis in the young immunocompromised host: report of two cases diagnosed by polymerase chain reaction and treated with ribavirin and review of the literature. *Clin Infect Dis* 16:654, 1993.

226. Liebert UG: Measles virus infections of the central nervous system. *Intervirology* 40:176, 1997.

227. Mehta PD, Thormar H, Kulczycki J, et al: Immune response in subacute sclerosing panencephalitis. *Ann NY Acad Sci* 724:378, 1994.

228. Billeter MA, Cattaneo R, Spielhofer P, et al: Generation and properties of measles virus mutations typically associated with subacute sclerosing panencephalitis. *Ann NY Acad Sci* 724:367, 1994.

229. Anlar B, Saatci I, Kose G, et al: MRI findings in subacute sclerosing panencephalitis. *Neurology* 47:1278, 1996.

230. Kuroda Y, Matsui M: Progressive rubella panencephalitis. *Nippon Rinsho-Japanese J Clin Med* 55:922, 1997.

231. Chipps E, Paulson G: Creutzfeldt-Jakob disease: a review. *J Neurosci Nurs* 26:219, 1994.

232. Nicholl D, Windl O, de Silva R, et al: Inherited Creutzfeldt-Jakob disease in a British family associated with a novel 144 base pair insertion of the prion protein gene. *J Neurol Neurosurg Psychiatry* 58:65, 1995.

233. Berger JR, David NJ: Creutzfeldt-Jakob disease in a physician: a review of the disorder in health care workers. *Neurology* 43:205, 1993.

234. Amouyel P, Vidal O, Launay JM, et al: The apolipoprotein E alleles as major susceptibility factors for Creutzfeldt-Jakob disease. The French Research Group on Epidemiology of Human Spongiform Encephalopathies. *Lancet* 344:1315, 1994.

235. Vargas ME, Kupersmith MJ, Savino PJ, et al: Homonymous field defect as the first manifestation of Creutzfeldt-Jakob disease. *Am J Ophthalmol* 119:497, 1995.

236. Kirk A, Ang LC: Unilateral Creutzfeldt-Jakob disease presenting as rapidly progressive aphasia. *Can J Neurol Sci* 21:350, 1994.

237. Yoon SS, Chan S, Chin S, et al: MRI of Creutzfeldt-Jakob disease: asymmetric high signal intensity of the basal ganglia. *Neurology* 45:1932, 1995.

238. Takeoka T: Cerebrospinal fluid examination in the infectious meningitis and encephalitis. *Nippon Rinsho-Japanese J Clin Med* 55:809, 1997.

239. Jay V, Becker LE, Otsubo H, et al: Chronic encephalitis and epilepsy (Rasmussen's encephalitis): detection of cytomegalovirus and herpes simplex virus 1 by the polymerase chain reaction and in situ hybridization. *Neurology* 45:108, 1995.

240. Antel JP, Rasmussen T: Rasmussen's encephalitis and the new hat. *Neurology* 46:9, 1996.

241. Leach JP, Chadwick DW, Miles JB, et al: Improvement in adult-onset Rasmussen's encephalitis with long-term immunomodulatory therapy. *Neurology* 52:738, 1999.

242. Andrews PI, Dichter MA, Berkovic SF, et al: Plasmapheresis in Rasmussen's encephalitis. *Neurology* 46:242, 1996.

243. Caldemeyer KS, Smith RR, Harris TM, et al: MRI in acute disseminated encephalomyelitis. *Neuroradiology* 36:216, 1994.

244. Kanter DS, Horensky D, Sperling RA, et al: Plasmapheresis in fulminating acute disseminated encephalomyelitis. *Neurology* 45:824, 1995.

245. Seales D, Greer M: Acute hemorrhagic leukoencephalitis: A successful recovery. *Arch Neurol* 48:1086, 1991.

246. Drobyski WR, Knox KK, Majewski D, et al. Brief report: fatal encephalitis due to a variant B human herpesvirus 6 infection in a bone marrow transplant recipient. *N Engl J Med* 330:1356, 1994.

247. Saito Y, Sharer LR, Dewhurst S, et al: Cellular localization of human herpesvirus-6 in the brains of children with AIDS encephalopathy. *J Neurovirol* 1:30, 1995.

248. Challoner PB, Smith KT, Parker JD, et al: Plaque-associated expression of human herpesvirus 6 in multiple sclerosis. *Proc Natl Acad Sci USA* 92:7440, 1995.

249. MacKenzie IR, Carrigan DR, Wiley CA: Chronic myelopathy associated with human herpesvirus-6. *Neurology* 45:2015, 1995.

250. Carrigan DR, Harrington D, Knox KK: Subacute leukoencephalitis caused by CNS infection with herpesvirus-6 manifesting as acute multiple sclerosis. *Neurology* 47:145, 1996.

251. Devlin T, Gray L, Allen NB, et al: Neuro-Behcet's disease: factors hampering proper diagnosis. *Neurology* 45:1754, 1995.

252. Banna M, el-Ramahi K: Neurologic involvement in Behcet's disease: imaging findings in 16 patients. *AJNR Am J Neuroradiol* 12:791, 1991.

253. Gilbert JA, Pollack ES, Pollack CCV Jr: Vogt-Koyanagi-Harada syndrome: case report and review. *J Emerg Med* 12:615, 1994.

254. Moorthy RS, Inomata H, Rao NA: Vogt-Koyanagi-Harada syndrome. *Survey Ophthalmol* 39:265, 1995.

255. Picard FJ, Dekaban GA, Silva J, et al: Mollaret's meningitis associated with herpes simplex type 2 infection. *Neurology* 43:1722, 1993.

256. Berg MJ, Williams LS: The transient syndrome of headache with neurologic deficits and CSF lymphocytosis. *Neurology* 45:1648, 1995.

257. Dolan RA: Spinal adhesive arachnoiditis. *Surg Neurol* 39:379, 1993.

258. Jackson A, Isherwood I: Does degenerative disease of the lumbar spine cause arachnoiditis? A magnetic resonance study and review of the literature. *Br J Radiol* 67:840, 1994.

259. Botella C, Orozco M, Navarro J, et al: Idiopathic chronic hypertrophic craniocervical pachymeningitis: case report. *Neurosurgery* 35:1144, 1994.

260. Parney IF, Johnson ES, Allen PB: "Idiopathic" cranial hypertrophic pachymeningitis responsive to antituberculous therapy: case report. *Neurosurgery* 41:965, 1997.

261. Mamelak AN, Kelly WM, Davis RL, et al: Idiopathic hypertrophic cranial pachymeningitis. Report of three cases. *J Neurosurg* 79:270, 1993.

262. Masson C, Henin D, Hauw JJ, et al: Cranial pachymeningitis of unknown origin: a study of seven cases. *Neurology* 43:1329, 1993.

263. Mikawa Y, Watanabe R, Hino Y, et al: Hypertrophic spinal pachymeningitis. *Spine* 19:620, 1994.

Chapter 17

TOXIC AND METABOLIC DISORDERS

CEREBRAL ANOXIA

Cerebral metabolism is almost totally dependent on an adequate supply of oxygen and glucose. When glucose is unavailable, the high energy needs of the brain are met by anaerobic metabolism. This is less efficient, but neurological impairment does not occur. However, as the oxygen content of arterial blood decreases, there is a progressive decline in cerebral function. Higher cortical functions, particularly those associated with the frontal lobes of the brain, are the first to be affected. Vegetative functions are not involved until much later. The rate of onset of hypoxia is also important because slower rates found, for example, in chronic progressive pulmonary disease, are better tolerated.

Etiology and Pathology The most frequent causes of cerebral anoxia are listed in Table 17-1. Most patients have suffered cardiac arrest or traumatic injury with an associated anoxia. The gray matter of the brain, due to its high metabolic rate, is the first to be affected. The pathological changes depend on the length of time the patient survives after the anoxic episode. If the patient dies immediately, the brain shows acute congestion, dilated blood vessels, and petechial hemorrhages. Survival for 2 or 3 days produces additional changes, including neuronal loss in the basal ganglia, particularly the globus pallidus and substantia nigra. Longer survival permits the development of cortical degeneration and gliosis. Delayed postanoxic encephalopathy, in which the patient appears to recover and later shows progressive neurological deterioration, is characterized by diffuse demyelination.

Clinical Features In acute hypoxia of rapid onset, the decline in neurological function is proportional to the decline in arterial oxygen content. A Pao$_2$ of 50 mmHg is associated with decreased mental acuity, impairment of visual acuity, emotional lability, and loss of fine muscle coordination. A further decrease to 40 mmHg produces faulty judgment, analgesia, and a marked lack of coordination. A fall in the Pao$_2$ below 32 mmHg produces loss of consciousness followed by decortication, decerebration, and respiratory arrest.

Patients who survive the initial anoxic episode may recover completely or partially, with permanent neurological deficits, including intellectual difficulties and posthypoxic and intention myoclonus. Those who have experienced severe hypoxia remain comatosed for a prolonged period of time and eventually develop a persistent vegetative state. This

Table 17-1
Causes of cerebral anoxia

1. Ischemia: any condition that prevents adequate blood flow to the brain—cardiac arrest, trauma, or massive blood loss.

2. Decreased inspiration of oxygen: high altitudes, strangulation, drowning.

3. Alveolar hypoventilation: anesthesia; Guillain-Barré syndrome; myasthenic crisis; poliomyelitis; encephalitis; barbiturate poisoning; heroin, cocaine, or other illegal drug overdose, trauma.

4. Impaired ventilation-perfusion relationship: pneumonia, chronic obstructive pulmonary disease, pulmonary embolism.

5. Alveolar capillary block: hyaline membrane disease, interstitial infiltrates.

6. Anemia.

7. Impaired oxygen dissociation: carbon monoxide poisoning.

8. Interference with cellular utilization of oxygen: cyanide poisoning.

condition can be defined as a state of severe brain damage persisting for longer than 3 months in a patient who is mute, lacks recognizable mental function, and has responses limited to primitive postural and reflex limb movements.[1] The majority die within 6 months, but a few survive in a persistent, totally dependent state. Occasional improvement has been reported after a year or more in less than 1 percent of patients, and the extent of recovery is limited. Some patients who survive an anoxic episode appear to make a complete recovery followed by a delayed progressive deterioration. The recovery is abruptly interrupted by the onset of irritability, apathy, and withdrawal 7 to 21 days after the anoxic episode. This is followed by the development of rigidity and psychomotor retardation, and there may be a steady progression to decerebration and death.[2]

Diagnostic Procedures   The cause of the anoxia must be determined to permit appropriate therapy. If the cause is uncertain, carbon monoxide poisoning, barbiturate poisoning, and drug overdose should be excluded by determination of carboxyhemoglobin and serum barbiturate levels and a drug screen. A hemoglobin level, chest film, and arterial blood gases will also provide useful information.

1. In patients who survive, the electroencephalogram (EEG) shows generalized slowing of the background activity to the lower theta and delta range, followed by a gradual increase in theta activity and the appearance of alpha activity in the posterior head regions. Fatal cases show progressive slowing of the EEG. In some cases, however, there may be preservation of diffuse theta activity in deep coma (theta coma) or the development of bifrontal or generalized alpha activity (alpha coma). A burst suppression pattern with periodic medium or high voltage, 4 to 6 Hz activity, interrupted by episodes of low voltage background activity, is usually indicative of severe and fatal anoxic encephalopathy.[3] Focal seizure activity is not unusual in severe hypoxia.

2. Magnetic resonance imaging (MRI) and computed tomography (CT) scans will show the presence of cerebral edema in severe anoxic encephalopathy. Diffuse white matter lesions are present in both hemispheres in postanoxic delayed encephalopathy.

Treatment

1. Any condition contributing to hypoxia should be treated.
2. Increased intracranial pressure (ICP) should be treated with hyperosmolar agents such as mannitol and glycerol.
3. Patients suffering from carbon monoxide poisoning should be given pure oxygen by mask. If a hyperbaric oxygen chamber is available, the patient should be treated with hyperbaric oxygen at 2 atmospheres.[4]
4. Posthypoxic intention myoclonus may respond to treatment with L-5 hydroxytryptophan or clonazepam.

BRAIN DEATH

The availability of mechanical ventilators and their remarkable efficiency are leading to the increased use of mechanical respiratory assistance in the treatment of acute respiratory disease. Although this procedure is usually lifesaving, it is inevitable that a number of patients, given mechanical ventilation assistance, have already suffered irreversible brain damage. Other patients suffer further brain damage or "brain death." Modern methods of treatment ensure that vital function, particularly respiratory and cardiac function, and water and electrolyte balance, are under adequate control. In essence, this means that many body functions can continue for weeks or even months in a controlled situation, despite the presence of brain death. This problem has led to the establishment of criteria to diagnose irreversible brain damage or "brain death" to permit the withdrawal of life support systems when these criteria are met. However, there are no universally accepted criteria for the establishment of brain death. Many institutions or committees have considered the problem and have developed proposals for use in a single institution or, in some cases, nationwide. Although each proposal has some difference in detail, all accept certain criteria that should form the basic content of any document concerned with brain death and withdrawal of life support. The following is modified from the report of the Quality Standards Subcommittee of the American Academy of Neurology, Practice Parameters for Determining Brain Death in Adults (Summary Statement).

Diagnostic Criteria for Clinical Diagnosis of Brain Death

A. Prerequisites. *Brain death* is the absence of clinical brain function when the proximate cause is known and demonstrably irreversible.
   1. Clinical or neuroimaging evidence of an acute process affecting the brain and brainstem that is compatible with the clinical diagnosis of brain death.
   2. Exclusion of any associated medical condition that may complicate clinical assessment. There should be no history of drug ingestion or measurable levels of sedatives (barbiturates, benzodiazepines, or hypnotics) in the blood.
   3. There should be no evidence of significant metabolic derangement (no severe electrolyte, acid-base, or endocrine disturbance).
   4. Brain death determination cannot be established if there is hypothermia. The core temperature should be equal to or greater than 32°C (90°F).
B. The three cardinal findings in brain death are coma, absence of brainstem reflexes, and apnea.
   1. Coma. Absence of cerebral and brainstem response to pain in all extremities (nail bed pressure and supraorbital pressure). Decerebrate and decorticate responses are absent.
   2. Absence of brainstem function.
      a. Pupils. Absence of response to bright light with pupil size 4 mm or dilated up to 9 mm.
      b. Ocular movements.
         i. Absent ocular cephalic reflex on head turning (doll's-eye movements). Testing performed only when there is no evidence of fracture or instability of the cervical spine.
         ii. No deviation of the eyes to irrigation of each ear with 50 mL of iced water, allowing 1 min after injection.
      c. Facial sensation and facial motor response.
         i. No corneal reflex.
         ii. No jaw reflex.
         iii. Absence of grimacing to sustained

pressure on nail bed, supraorbital ridge, or temporomandibular joint.
      d. Pharyngeal and truncal responses.
         i. Absence of reflex movements on stimulation of pharynx with a tongue blade.
         ii. No cough reflex or bradyarrhythmia to bronchial suctioning.
C. Apnea—the test for apnea is the most critical of all tests of brainstem function.[5]
   1. Prerequisites.
      a. Core temperature greater than or equal to 36.5°C (97°F).
      b. Systolic blood pressure greater than or equal to 90 mmHg.
      c. Positive fluid balance in the past 6 h.
      d. Normal P_{CO_2} or P_{CO_2} equal to or greater than 40 mmHg.
      e. Normal P_{O_2} or P_{O_2} greater than or equal to 200 mmHg.
      f. Ventilate patient with pure oxygen for 10 min.
   2. Testing.
      a. Connect pulse oximeter, then withdraw ventilator. Deliver 100% oxygen at 6 L/min through endotracheal tube.
      b. Pa_{CO_2} will rise without hazardous hypoxia.
      c. Look closely for respiratory movements.
      d. Allow a 10-min period of apnea.
      e. Draw blood for P_{O_2} and P_{CO_2}, then reconnect ventilator.
      f. If respiratory movements are absent and Pa_{CO_2} is equal to or greater than 60 mmHg or, if apnea persists when there is a 20 mmHg increase in Pa_{CO_2} over a baseline normal P_{CO_2}, the apnea test is positive and compatible with the diagnosis of brain death.
      g. If respiratory movements are observed, the apnea test is negative and does not support the diagnosis of brain death.
      h. Maintaining a minimal systolic blood pressure of 90 mmHg ensures adequate perfusion of all vital organs.[6] Consequently, should the systolic blood pressure fall to a level equal to or below 90 mmHg, or the pulse oximetry indicate desaturation and cardiac arrhythmias are present, immediately reconnect the ventilator and draw

arterial blood gases. If P_{CO_2} is equal to or greater than 60 mmHg, or the P_{CO_2} increase is equal to or greater than 20 mmHg over a normal baseline, the apnea test is positive.

Aberrant Clinical Observations

Aberrant clinical observations compatible with brain death are encountered occasionally. These responses include spontaneous movements of limbs from spinal reflex activity, including flexion of limbs, raising limbs off the bed, jerking movements of a limb, and grasping movements.

Respiratory-like movements, characterized by shoulder elevation and adduction, back arching, and intercostal expansion, without any significant tidal volume, may occur.

Other responses include profuse sweating, flushing, tachycardia, and sudden increase in blood pressure. Tendon reflexes and extensor plantar responses can be elicited in some cases.

Additional Laboratory Tests

Certain optional tests, include an EEG with a 16- to 18-channel machine operated according to the guidelines established by the American Electroencephalographic Society for recording brain death. Other procedures such as isotope angiography, an enhanced CT scan using technetium 99 hexamethylpropyleneamineoxamine, transcranial Doppler ultrasonography, and somatosensory evoked potentials are used in some centers. These tests are optional rather than mandatory, because abnormal results can be recorded in patients with severe brain damage who do not meet the criteria for brain death.[7]

NEUROLOGICAL COMPLICATIONS OF ELECTROLYTE DISORDERS

Hyponatremia

Definition   *Hyponatremia* is an abnormal decrease in serum sodium content.

Etiology and Pathology   Hyponatremia may be characterized by:

1. Increased extracellular fluid volume and edema.
   a. Renal failure (nephrotic syndrome).
   b. Congestive heart failure.
   c. Hepatic cirrhosis.
2. Normal extracellular fluid volume.
   a. The syndrome of inappropriate antidiuretic hormone secretion (SIADH) following trauma, central nervous system (CNS) infection, subarachnoid hemorrhage.
   b. Water intoxication. Psychiatric disorders: fluid replacement with sodium-free fluids.
   c. Therapeutic use of oxytocin or carbamazepine.
3. Decreased extracellular fluid volume.
   a. Renal origin. Chronic diuretic use: resumption of antihypertensive therapy using diuretics; salt-losing nephritis; hypoaldosteronism; gram-negative urinary tract infections.
   b. Extrarenal origin. Burns, vomiting, diarrhea, fever, and excessive sweating; excess antacids containing magnesium.

The lowering of serum sodium content results in passage of fluid into cells and lowering of the intracellular sodium content. Swelling of cells and some degree of cerebral edema are present.

Clinical Features   Acute hyponatremia is often caused by postoperative fluid overload in general surgical patients who show a postoperative hyponatremia of less than 129 mEq/L. The condition presents as an encephalopathy, beginning with extreme fatigue and progressing through nausea, vomiting, hypotension, and seizures to coma. This acute encephalopathy is more likely to be associated with permanent brain damage or death in premenopausal women than in men.[8]

Chronic hyponatremia may cause extreme fatigue, weakness, muscle cramps, nausea and vomiting, seizures, and also confusion and delirium that may be mistaken for a psychiatric illness.

Injury to the brain by trauma, infection, or subarachnoid hemorrhage can be associated with continued secretion of antidiuretic hormone, despite low plasma sodium values. In addition, depletion of intracellular potassium by excessive fluid loading without potassium supplements, excessive use of diuretics, potassium loss by diarrhea, or sustained alkalosis caused by hyperventilation, leads to the passage of sodium into cells to restore electrolyte balance and an extracellular hyponatremia. This type of chronic hyponatremia will persist until intracellular potassium is replaced.[9]

Diagnostic Procedures

1. The serum sodium level is abnormally low. The serum osmolality is usually low.
2. In the 24-h urine for sodium content, a level less than 20 mEq/L confirms sodium depletion.
3. See page 521 for the characteristics of SIADH.
4. Pseudohyponatremia occurs in hyperlipidemia and hyperproteinemia and is identified by elevated serum lipid or protein levels.
5. In acute cases, the EEG shows diffuse slowing over both hemispheres with irregular high-amplitude activity in the theta range.

Treatment

1. Hyponatremia with increased extracellular fluid should be managed by fluid restriction.

2. Severe hyponatremia with coma and seizures should be treated with 3% sodium chloride to increase sodium at the rate of 1 to 2 mEq/L per h, until severe symptoms improve. The increase in sodium should be kept below 12 mEq/L on the first day. Administration of 1 to 2 mEq/kg per h of 3% sodium chloride will raise the serum sodium by 1 to 2 mEq/L per h.[10]

3. Hyponatremia with normal extracellular fluid volume usually responds to water restriction and the infusion of hypertonic saline solution is rarely needed. Under these circumstances replacement should consist of a basic normal intake of 100 mEq in 24 h, plus one-third of the calculated sodium deficit, until a level of 130 mEq/L is reached. Serum sodium levels should be monitored every 2 to 3 h.

4. Hyponatremia associated with decreased extracellular fluid volume should be managed by treating the cause of the problem and by replacement with normal saline at a rate of no more than 2 mEq/L per h, to a level of 128 to 130 mEq/L. A more rapid correction to normal or hypernatremic levels may result in central pontine myelinolysis.

5. In chronic hyponatremia, lowered serum potassium levels should be restored gradually, infusing 200 mEq potassium chloride per milliequivalent

of serum potassium reduction. Sodium should be replaced slowly at rates that raise serum sodium values by less than 10 mEq/L in the first 24 h, and less than 21 mEq/L in the first 48 h, to a level of 128 to 130 mEq/L. A more rapid correction to normal or hypernatremic levels may result in central pontine and extrapontine (subcortical white matter, basal ganglia, thalamus) myelinolysis.[11,12]

Hypernatremia

Definition *Hypernatremia* is an abnormal increase in serum sodium content.

Etiology and Pathology Hypernatremia may be caused by:

1. Decreased water intake. Severe dehydration may lead to hypernatremia. This is usually seen in children but can occur in elderly individuals who have significant reduction in maximal urinary concentration and an inadequate thirst response to dehydration.[13]

2. Excess sodium intake. This may occur during the postoperative administration of parenteral fluids with high saline content, following treatment of shock, or during administration of sodium bicarbonate after cardiac arrest, particularly in children.

3. Excess water loss in children with vomiting and diarrhea.

4. Enteral tube feeding or parenteral supplementation, using supplements with a high sodium content.

5. Diabetes mellitus with diabetic or nonketotic hyperosmolar coma.

6. Hypothalamic damage and consequent hypernatremia occasionally complicates intracranial surgical procedures; intracranial tumors including pituitary adenoma and craniopharyngioma; Hand-Schüller-Christian disease; and inflammatory conditions involving the neurohypophysis, resulting in impairment of antidiuretic hormone release.

7. Following head trauma and therapeutic measures to prevent cerebral edema.

8. Diabetes insipidus (see p. 521).

Increased serum osmolality results in fluid shift from the intracellular to the extracellular compartment. This may cause tearing of intracranial vessels and hemorrhage.

Clinical Features   Early somnolence and apathy are followed by stupor, meningismus, and eventually decerebrate rigidity and coma. The course may be punctuated by chorea, myoclonus, or seizure activity. Proximal muscle weakness has been associated with hypernatremia, possibly the result of depletion of muscle energy stores due to overworking of the sodium potassium pump in an attempt to correct intracellular electrolyte imbalance.[14]

Diagnostic Procedures

1. The serum sodium level is abnormally high.
2. A high urinary volume with a low specific gravity and low sodium content is seen in diabetes insipidus.
3. A low urinary volume with high specific gravity, over 1.020, occurs in inadequate fluid intake.

Treatment   Rapid correction of hypovolemia may lead to water intoxication, shift of fluid into the intracellular space, and subsequent cerebral edema. This can be avoided by replacing half the calculated water deficit within the first 24 h and the remainder over the next 2 days.[15]

Chronic hyponatremia due to hypothalamic dysfunction may respond to the administration of cortisone acetate.

Prognosis   Severe, acute hypernatremia has a 40 percent mortality rate. Approximately 50 percent of the survivors will show neurological sequelae such as transient choreoathetosis, hemiparesis, dementia, or seizures.

Hypokalemia

Definition   *Hypokalemia* is an abnormal decrease in serum potassium content with a serum potassium level less than 3.5 mEq/L.

Etiology and Pathology

1. Hypokalemia may result from an inadequate potassium intake due to infusion of potassium-free intravenous fluids postoperatively or in any patient who cannot take potassium by mouth.
2. Alkalosis, which causes a shift of serum potassium into the cells.
3. Gastrointestinal loss, which occurs with vomiting, diarrhea, and nasogastric suction.
4. Renal loss. Osmotic diuresis, aldosteronism, renal tubular disease, therapeutic use of diuretics or corticosteroids, and licorice ingestion may result in excessive renal loss of potassium.
5. Drug-induced: epinephrine, isoproterenol, salbutamol, terbutaline, barium, insulin.[16]

Clinical Features   Symptoms do not usually develop until the serum potassium level falls below 3.0 mEq/L. Generalized muscle weakness may be followed by paresthesias, hyporeflexia, confusion, delirium, and tetany. Muscle weakness may be followed by actual paralysis in severe hypokalemia, complicating renal disease, or intractable vomiting, and acute quadriplegia may occur in diabetic ketoacidosis with hypokalemia. Cardiac arrhythmias, such as extra systoles, are not unusual; ventricular tachycardia or fibrillation may occur with rapid onset of hypokalemia.[17]

Diagnostic Procedures

1. Serum potassium levels are abnormally low.
2. Electrocardiographic (ECG) abnormalities, including depression of the ST segment, prolongation of the QT interval, and inverted T waves, followed by the appearance of U waves, and fusion of T and U waves.
3. Primary aldosteronism is characterized by low serum potassium and elevated serum sodium levels. Urinary aldosterone exceeds 14 mg in 24 h. There is a marked fall in urinary potassium clearance following the administration of spironolactone, with a rise in serum potassium levels.
4. Diagnosis of secondary aldosteronism may be established by demonstrating elevated plasma renin and angiotensin levels and the presence of impaired renal function.

Treatment   The cause of hypokalemia should be corrected whenever possible. Potassium should be replaced orally in doses of 20 to 60 mEq/day. This reduces the risk of hyperkalemia. When intravenous potassium is given, the doses should not exceed 20 mEq/h, to a total of less than 100 mEq in 24 h. Administration should always be monitored by serial ECGs and serial serum potassium levels. Primarily aldosteronism will respond to resection of the adrenal adenoma.

Hyperkalemia

Definition   *Hyperkalemia* is an abnormally high serum level of potassium.

Etiology and Pathology   Hyperkalemia may be caused by:

1.   Acidosis. Acidosis causes a shift of potassium from the intracellular to the extracellular compartment.

2.   Decreased excretion. Acute renal failure owing to renal tubular necrosis produces a rising potassium level with other signs of renal insufficiency. Acute adrenal insufficiency produces high potassium levels coupled with low serum sodium concentration and hypotension.

3.   Endogenous and exogenous sources of potassium. Rhabdomyolysis and hemolysis serve as endogenous sources of potassium resulting in hyperkalemia; ingestion of foods high in potassium is an exogenous source.

4.   Acute fluoride intoxication causes potassium efflux from cells.[18]

Clinical Features   Hyperkalemia results in weakness and paresthesias, eventually paralysis and cardiac and respiratory arrest.

Diagnostic Procedures   The serum potassium level is abnormally high. The ECG may reveal depressed ST segments, peaked T waves, prolonged PR intervals, and widening of the QRS complexes.

Treatment   Severe hyperkalemia may be treated with calcium gluconate, sodium bicarbonate, or cation-exchange resin therapy. Dialysis is also an effective method of treatment.

Hypomagnesemia

Definition   *Hypomagnesemia* is an abnormal decrease in serum magnesium content.

Etiology and Pathology   Hypomagnesemia may be caused by:

1.   Inadequate intake of magnesium. This occurs with the prolonged use of intravenous fluid therapy without magnesium replacement.

2.   Excessive gastrointestinal loss due to prolonged diarrhea, vomiting, or continuous nasogastric suction.

3.   Failure of absorption of magnesium due to intestinal obstruction, steatorrhea, or any of the malabsorptive syndromes. Bowel resection may be followed by hypomagnesemia.

4.   Excess loss of magnesium through the kidney, due to prolonged use of mercurial diuretics, or withdrawal from alcohol in the chronic alcoholic. This may be followed by excessive magnesium excretion and hypomagnesemia.

5.   Metabolic causes of hypomagnesemia include diabetic acidosis, porphyria, and pancreatitis. Hyperaldosteronism, hypoparathyroidism, and hyperthyroidism are often associated with hypomagnesemia.

Hypocalcemia and hypomagnesemia often occur together in conditions such as alcoholic liver disease, where hypomagnesemia induces hypoparathyroidism and hypocalcemia. Magnesium is necessary for intracellular enzymatic activity. Hypomagnesemia increases cellular membrane excitability and enhances synaptic transmission.

Clinical Features   Weakness, progressive confusion, irritability, agitation with lack of sleep, muscle twitchings, and myoclonus may be present and may be followed by seizures. Other patients show the presence of tremors, generalized hyperreflexia, personality changes, and choreoathetoid movements. There is often marked tachycardia, and Chvostek and Trousseau signs are present.

Diagnostic Procedures Serum magnesium levels are abnormally low.

Treatment

1.   The causes of hypomagnesemia should be eliminated. If intravenous therapy is required, the patient should be treated with magnesium sulfate 1 g in 100-mL solution over a 1-h period. Oral therapy consists of 1 or 2 10-grain (35 mEq) tablets per day.

2.   Serial serum magnesium levels should be obtained to avoid the development of hypermagnesemia.

Hypermagnesemia

Hypermagnesemia is an abnormally high serum level of magnesium. It is most commonly the result if injudicious use of magnesium-containing pharmaceuticals (e.g., laxatives) in a patient with renal failure. The patient develops nausea and vomiting followed by muscular weakness, drowsiness, and eventually coma. Treatment consisting of intravenous calcium gluconate may be required in severe cases.

NEUROLOGICAL COMPLICATIONS OF RENAL DYSFUNCTION

The neurological manifestations of renal disorders consists of uremic encephalopathy, uremic neuropathy, and neurological complications of chronic hemodialysis and renal transplantation.

Uremic Encephalopathy

Definition *Uremic encephalopathy* results from the effects of the metabolic changes accompanying kidney failure.

Etiology and Pathology The etiology of the uremic encephalopathy is unknown. Although it is possible that uremia is associated with an imbalance of neurotransmitters, this has not been demonstrated consistently in uremic encephalopathy. However, considerable evidence indicates that during uremia, increased concentrations of parathyroid hormone in the brain produce neurotoxicity; this factor may contribute to uremic encephalopathy.[19]

There are no characteristic pathological changes. Cerebral neuronal degeneration and necrosis of the granulocellular layer of the cerebellar cortex have been described but are likely to be the result of preterminal hypoxia.

Clinical Features The earliest signs of uremic encephalopathy are decreased alertness and awareness associated with apathy, fatigue, poor concentration, and insomnia, followed by the development of asterixis, dysarthria, tremors, and restless legs. Defective cognition, hallucinations, and agitation appear later. Release phenomena, consisting of paratonia, sucking, rooting, and grasp reflexes, appear later in the course of the disease, and meningismus may be present. Progressive visual loss with papilledema can occur in patients with uremic anemia and elevated blood pressure. As the disorder progresses, the patient becomes stuporous, then comatosed, with myoclonus and tetany in some cases. Anemia is a significant problem occurring in more than 90 percent of patients. Generalized tonic-clonic seizures are a late feature and are more characteristic of uremic encephalopathy than any of the other metabolic encephalopathies.

Diagnostic Procedures

1.   The standard indices of renal function, such as blood urea nitrogen and serum creatinine, are not reliable predictors of the clinical course in uremic encephalopathy.

2.   The EEG shows progressive, symmetrical slowing of the background activity and paroxysmal bursts of slow wave activity in the anterior head regions. The deterioration in the EEG runs parallel to the deterioration in renal function.

3.   The cerebrospinal fluid (CSF) is clear and under normal pressure. There are a mild lymphocytic pleocytosis and an elevated protein content.

Differential Diagnosis

1. Acute water intoxication. This is often coexistent and is characterized by low serum osmolality (less

than 260 mosmol/L) and low serum sodium levels (less than 120 mEq/L).

2. Hypertensive encephalopathy. A history of hypertension, papilledema, and normal or minimally elevated blood urea nitrogen and serum creatinine suggests hypertensive encephalopathy.

Treatment

1. Seizures should be controlled with phenytoin (Dilantin). Serum levels of phenytoin are depressed in uremia and seizures may be controlled with low serum phenytoin levels.
2. Slow dialysis. This is the definitive treatment for uremic encephalopathy. The procedure requires careful monitoring because the blood-brain barrier is slowly permeable to urea and rapid dialysis may result in water intoxication.
3. Recombinant human erythropoietin is effective in the treatment of renal anemia.[20]

Uremic Neuropathy

Definition   *Uremic neuropathy* is characterized by distal symmetrical sensorimotor loss that occurs predominantly in the lower limbs and affects the majority of patients with chronic renal failure.

Etiology and Pathology   The etiology of uremic neuropathy is uncertain. The condition may be due to retention of toxins or high levels of parathormone. Pathological changes in uremic neuropathy consist of primary axonal degeneration with secondary demyelination.

Clinical Features   One of the most common symptom complexes occurring in uremic neuropathy is the "restless legs" syndrome. Eventually distal symmetrical sensorimotor neuropathy develops. Autonomic involvement may occur. The course may vary and is slowly progressive in the majority of cases. Flaccid quadriplegia is a rare complication in untreated cases.

Diagnostic Procedures   Electrophysiological studies reveal reduced sensory and motor nerve conduction velocities and increased distal latencies. A measure of uremic polyneuropathy is determination of the H reflex, which shows significant delay in uremic polyneuropathy and improves with dialysis.[21] Visual evoked potentials show decreased amplitude, secondary peaks, and increased latency.

Differential Diagnosis   The differential diagnosis of uremic neuropathy is that of a distal symmetrical sensorimotor neuropathy.

Treatment

1. The treatment of choice is hemodialysis. Adequate dialysis may stabilize or slowly improve the clinical condition temporarily.
2. Cholestyramine 5 mg bid or qid may reduce constant irritation in the restless legs syndrome. Carbidopa/levodopa (Sinemet), gabapentin, primipexole and clonidine are also effective in some cases of restless legs syndrome. Codeine 30 mg orally will usually abolish the abnormal sensation.

NEUROLOGICAL COMPLICATIONS OF DIALYSIS

The neurological complications of dialysis consist of disequilibrium syndrome, an increased incidence of intracranial bleeding, and dialysis encephalopathy.

Disequilibrium Syndrome

The disequilibrium syndrome is believed to occur as a result of shift of water into the brain during dialysis. The syndrome occurs toward the end of dialysis.[22] The patient appears restless and complains of severe headache followed by nausea, vomiting, disorientation, and tremors. Seizures and loss of consciousness indicate the presence of increased ICP.

Patients with pre-existing neurological conditions such as head trauma, recent stroke, brain tumor, subdural hematoma, or cerebral edema are at particular risk for development of dialysis disequilibrium.[23] Consequently, deterioration in neurological symptoms at the end of dialysis requires a CT scan of the head to detect focal abnormalities or cerebral edema.

Treatment

1. Correct any serum electrolyte imbalance.
2. Control seizures.
3. Treat cerebral edema by ventricular drainage if necessary. Continuous ventricular drainage and ICP monitoring will avoid uncal herniation during dialysis in such cases.

Cardiac and Cerebrovascular Disease in Uremia

There is a high risk of cardiovascular and cerebrovascular disease in uremia, and 40 percent of dialysis patients die from cardiovascular disease.

The background in the chronic uremic patient is one of chronic hypertension, atherosclerosis, diabetes, left ventricular hypertrophy, cardiomyopathy, coronary artery disease, congestive heart failure, cardiac dysrrhythmias, and myocardial infarction, all of which predispose to heart disease and cardiac mortality. Similarly, patients with end-stage renal disease have increased risk of cerebral infarction and intracerebral hemorrhage, owing to the presence of the same risk factors.[24]

Carpal Tunnel Syndrome

Carpal tunnel syndrome (see p. 600) is an increasingly recognized problem in long-term hemodialysis.[25] The syndrome is usually associated with uremic polyneuropathy but may also be associated with edema of the transverse carpal ligament.

Dialysis Encephalopathy Syndrome (Dialysis Dementia)

Dialysis encephalopathy syndrome is a progressive, invariably fatal encephalopathy that occurs in patients undergoing chronic hemodialysis.

Etiology and Pathology Aluminum is believed to be the principal pathological agent responsible for dialysis encephalopathy syndrome.[26] Pathological findings are nonspecific.

Clinical Features The disorder was first described in 1972 and accounts for approximately 20 percent of deaths in patients who have been on dialysis longer than 3 years. Initially, symptoms consist of speech difficulties characterized by stammering and hesitancy. Personality changes with paranoid thinking, and visual and auditory hallucinations, and movement disorders such as asterixis, twitching, and motor apraxia are also seen. Eventually the patient becomes dysphasic. A global dementia develops, myoclonic jerks may be seen, and finally, coma and death occur.

In the early course of the disorder, the symptoms develop only during dialysis and clear within 24 h. However, as the disorder progresses, the patient becomes more and more incapacitated. The typical course lasts from 6 to 12 months.

Diagnostic Procedures

1. The EEG findings in dialysis encephalopathy syndrome are characteristic and may precede the clinical findings by 6 to 8 months. There are paroxysmal bursts of bilateral synchronous delta and theta waves admixed with spike and sharp wave discharges.
2. An MRI or CT scan may reveal mild to moderate hydrocephalus ex vacuo.
3. On lumbar puncture, the CSF is normal.

Treatment Treatment of dialysis encephalopathy syndrome is entirely symptomatic. Diazepam (Valium) is effective in decreasing symptoms and EEG abnormalities in the early stages of the disease. Chelating with deferoxamine has reversed the neurological symptoms in some patients.

The elimination of aluminum from dialysate has virtually eliminated the dialysis encephalopathy syndrome, but sporadic cases are occasionally encountered, suggesting other sources for aluminum toxicity, such as parenteral nutritional solutions and enhanced gastrointestinal absorption in conjunction with decreased renal excretion.[27]

Muscle Cramps During Dialysis

Some patients develop painful muscle cramps during dialysis, often preceded by hypotension. Various mechanisms have been considered, including vasoconstriction, tissue hypoxia, and carnitine deficiency.

Quinine 325 mg q.h.s. or vitamin E 400 IU q.h.s. usually reduces the frequency and severity of the leg cramps.[28]

Wernicke Encephalopathy

This condition is a rare complication of dialysis[29] (see p. 539).

NEUROLOGICAL COMPLICATIONS OF RENAL TRANSPLANTATION

There is an increased incidence of CNS infections, neoplasia, especially primary lymphoma of the brain, and progressive multifocal leukoencephalopathy in patients who receive chronic immunosuppressive therapy after kidney transplantation.

NEUROLOGICAL COMPLICATIONS OF HEPATIC DYSFUNCTION

Hepatic Encephalopathy

Definition *Hepatic encephalopathy* is a metabolic encephalopathy associated with hepatic dysfunction.

Etiology and Pathology Hepatic encephalopathy is believed to be related to the inability of the liver to clear potentially toxic substances, particularly intestinal-derived toxins of nitrogenous origin, primarily ammonia from the blood. This leads to changes in neurotransmitters in the central and peripheral nervous system, with particular involvement of dopaminergic and γ-aminobutyric acid (GABA)-ergic systems.[30]

Fulminant hepatic encephalopathy is characterized by the presence of diffuse cerebral edema. Chronic hepatic encephalopathy is characterized by brain atrophy involving white and gray matter, with a neuronal loss and proliferation of astrocytes (Alzheimer type II astrocytes) and focal areas of demyelination.

Fulminant Hepatic Encephalopathy

Clinical Features Acute encephalopathy with fulminant hepatic failure develops within 8 weeks of the onset of illness.[31] Viral hepatitis, particularly hepatitis B viral infection, is the most common cause, but several drugs, particularly acetaminophen, anticonvulsants,[32] and isoniazid,[33] and toxic substances are recognized etiological agents. The patient develops increased muscle tone, hyperactive deep tendon reflexes, and extensor plantar responses. Fetor hepaticus, a sweet, musty odor of the breath, may be present. Asterixis, a sudden loss and recovery of posture, may be present in the hands, feet, lips, and eyelids. There is evidence of increased ICP and seizures occur in most cases. The patient becomes progressively confused, obtunded, and eventually comatosed. The morality rate is high, and complications such as renal failure, infection, cerebral edema, and coagulopathies are not uncommon.

Chronic Hepatic Encephalopathy

Chronic hepatic encephalopathy is most commonly seen in patients with cirrhosis of the liver, often caused by chronic alcoholism. The early stages present with a mild dementia with impaired short-term memory. The systemic manifestations of liver disease, such as palmar erythema, spider nevi, icterus, hepatosplenomegaly, and ascites, may or may not be present, depending on the chronicity of the illness. The patient is tremulous; there are increased tendon reflexes and positive grasp reflexes. This stage is followed by lethargy and the appearance of a flapping tremor (asterixis) in the outstretched upper extremities. Further depression of the level of consciousness is associated with spastic paraparesis, hyperreflexia, and bilateral extensor plantar responses. Hyperventilation and respiratory alkalosis are not uncommon.

Complications

1. Electrolyte and acid-base disturbances are common, including hyponatremia, hypokalemia, respiratory alkalosis, and metabolic alkalosis. It is especially important to avoid alkalosis because it promotes diffusion of the nonionized ammonia across the blood-brain barrier.
2. Renal failure may occur as the result of hepatorenal syndrome or acute tubular necrosis.
3. Hyperglycemia may occur but is more common in acute hepatic failure.

Diagnostic Procedures

1. There is evidence of hepatic dysfunction, with an elevated ammonia level. It should be noted that ammonia determination should always be done on arterial blood. Other abnormalities include elevation of serum aspartate aminotransferase (AST), serum alanine aminotransferase (ALT), alkaline phosphatase, and abnormal coagulation studies. Hypoglycemia may be present.

2. In chronic encephalopathy, serum levels of aromatic amino acids and buthionine are elevated, whereas levels of branch-chain amino acids are depressed. In acute encephalopathy, all amino acids are markedly elevated, except branch-chain amino acids, which are normal.

3. Electrolyte and acid-base abnormalities may be present. Blood urea nitrogen and serum creatinine may be elevated in renal dysfunction.

4. Lumbar puncture. In chronic cases, the CSF pressure and protein content are usually normal. The fluid may be xanthochromic and contain bilirubin, glutamine, and α-ketoglutarate. The CSF pressure is often elevated in acute encephalopathy.

5. An EEG is valuable in identifying early dysfunction. There is slowed activity wtith predominant delta and theta waves. The EEG shows marked slowing in hepatic coma with diffuse delta activity associated with high voltage, triphasic sharp waves.

Treatment

1. Gastrointestinal bleeding, infection, and constipation are important precipitating and aggravating factors and should be controlled. Excessive diuresis should be avoided.

2. Liver transplantation may be lifesaving in fulminating hepatic encephalopathy.[34,35]

3. In medically treated patients with less acute or chronic encephalopathy, dietary protein intake should be stopped and then gradually increased by 10 to 20 g/day every 2 to 5 days, depending on the clinical response. Protein derived from milk, eggs, and vegetables is better tolerated than animal protein. Adequate calories and vitamins should be provided.

4. The bowel should be kept as empty as possible. Neomycin 2 to 4 g daily by mouth, or nasogastric tube, or a 1% solution by enema, daily or twice a day, and lactulose 50 to 150 mL daily with the dose adjusted to produce two or three soft stools per day, will help to reduce ammonia levels.

5. Cerebral edema occurring with acute encephalopathy shows a disappointing response to therapy.

6. The nonabsorbable dye saccharide lactitol (β-galactosidase-sorbitol), and lactulose, are both effective in the treatment of chronic hepatic encephalopathy. The mode of action of these substances is unknown, but the benefit is established.

Prognosis The mortality rate in acute fulminant hepatic encephalopathy was as high as 80 percent until recently but has shown some decline following the use of liver transplantation.[34,35] However, this still remains a disease with a high mortality rate.

Patients with chronic encephalopathy usually recover when other factors such as renal failure and infection are controlled.

NEUROLOGICAL COMPLICATIONS OF THYROID DYSFUNCTION

Hyperthyroidism

Definition *Hyperthyroidism* is a condition caused by overproduction of thyroid hormone.

Etiology Hyperthyroidism is usually associated with a diffuse toxic goiter (Graves disease), an autoimmune condition. Single or multiple nodular goiters may begin to secrete thyroxine (T_4) in patients with long-standing goiter, resulting in hyperthyroidism. Other causes include thyroiditis, functioning metastatic thyroid carcinoma, choriocarcinoma, testicular tumors, struma ovarii, and some trophoblastic tumors.

Clinical Features Hyperthyroidism is characterized by weight loss, excessive fatigue, nervousness, palpitations, heat intolerance, increased perspiration, oexistent adrenal insufficiency. Hypothermia requires gentle rewarming to avoid vasodilatation and hypotension. Hyponatremia usually responds to fluid restriction. Hypoglycemia suggests an associated pituitary or adrenal insufficiency and will respond to intravenous glucose administration. Hypoxemia due to hyperventilation and pneumonia may require intubation and mechanical ventilator support.[37]

NEUROLOGICAL COMPLICATIONS OF PARATHYROID DYSFUNCTION

Hyperparathyroidism

Definition   *Hyperparathyroidism* is the result of excessive secretion of parathormone.

Etiology and Pathology   Hyperparathyroidism is caused by an adenoma of the parathyroid gland, with excess production of parathyroid hormone, resulting in hypercalcemia. The disease is not rare, and it has been estimated that there are 100,000 new cases of hyperparathyroidism each year.[38]

The four parathyroid glands are closely related to the posterior aspect of the thyroid gland. However, ectopic parathyroid glands are occasionally located in the mediastinum, thymus, retropharyngeal area, tracheoesophageal groove, or carotid bifurcation.

Clinical Features   Primary hyperparathyroidism has become a common endocrine disorder following the widespread use of multichannel autoanalyzers in medicine.[39] Classical signs of the disease are unusual—osteitis fibrosa cystica is rare; peptic ulceration, cholelithiasis, and renal calculi are uncommon. Many patients are asymptomatic or complain of non-specific symptoms such as easy fatigue, chronic headache, poor concentration, memory impairment, arthralgias, myalgias, and depression. Sustained high levels of serum calcium, greater than 15 mg/dL, can present with agitation, tremor, rigidity, and psychosis followed by coma or death, unless prompt treatment is instituted.[39]

Diagnostic Procedures

1. The serum calcium is elevated and should be tested on three separate occasions.
2. Serum phosphorus is low.
3. Elevated alkaline phosphatase in the absence of liver disease indicates bone involvement.
4. Elevated parathyroid hormone levels can be demonstrated by immunoassay techniques.
5. Adenomas can be localized using ultrasonography, thallium 201/technetium 99m pertechnetate subtraction scintillography or MRI scanning.

Treatment   Patients who are asymptomatic or who have mild symptoms with mild elevation of serum calcium, absence of any episodes of severe hypercalcemia, normal renal function and absence of kidney stones, and normal bone densitometry can be followed and monitored regularly.

Surgery, with removal of the parathyroid adenoma, is indicated in symptomatic patients or in those with sustained high serum calcium levels, increased urinary excretion of calcium, decline in renal function, and decline in skeletal mass.

Hypoparathyroidism

Definition   *Hypoparathyroidism* is caused by deficient production of parathormone.

Etiology   Hypoparathyroidism is usually the result of surgical treatment of hyperparathyroidism. Hypoparathyroidism results in hypocalcemia, which causes hyperexcitability of the central and peripheral nervous system. A number of pseudoparathyroid conditions, in which there is peripheral resistance to the parathyroid hormone by circulating antibodies, abnormal receptors, or abnormal receptor-linked enzymatic activity, have been recognized. Transient hypoparathyroidism with hypocalcemia may be induced by magnesium deficiency in patients with liver disease.[40]

Clinical Features   The patient with hypoparathyroidism or pseudohypoparathyroidism may present with seizures, paresthesias, muscle cramps, headache, or dementia. Chvostek and Trousseau signs are usually present. Papilledema occurs in 20 percent of and diarrhea in an individual with goiter, tachycardia, and fine distal tremor. Exophthalmos with or without ophthalmoplegia and pretibial myxedema are seen in Graves disease.

Neurological complications of hyperthyroidism include a symmetrical primary motor peripheral neuropathy; proximal muscle weakness due to myopathy; ophthalmoplegia; and rarely, optic neuritis, corticospinal tract signs, chorea, and seizures.

Diagnostic Procedures. Levels of triiodothyronine (T_3), thyroxine (T_4), thyroxine-binding globulin (TBG), and thyroid-stimulating hormone (TSH) should be obtained in all suspected cases of hyperthyroidism.

Treatment Antithyroid drug therapy includes radioactive iodine therapy and thyroidectomy, all of which have a place in the treatment of hyperthyroidism. Propanolol (Inderal) is effective in reducing sympathetic overactivity and controlling tremor.

Hypothyroidism

Definition *Hypothyroidism* is a condition caused by deficient production of thyroid hormone.

Etiology Hypothyroidism may be due to a failure of the hypothalamus to secrete thyroid-releasing hormone, a failure of the pituitary to produce TSH, or thyroid gland failure associated with chronic thyroiditis, surgical excision, or an iodine-deficient diet.

Clinical Features The patient with hypothyroidism presents with dry skin, vocal hoarseness, cold intolerance, bradycardia, constipation, and weight gain. Neurological complications include mental dullness, psychomotor retardation, headache, proximal muscle weakness, slow tendon reflexes, and carpal tunnel syndrome. Mononeuropathies due to mucinous deposits that cause nerve damage, or a symmetrical sensorimotor peripheral neuropathy or cranial nerve abnormalities, can occur.[36] Hypothyroid dementia may develop. Chronic cerebellar degeneration with progressive limb and truncal ataxia has been described.

Myxedema Coma

Myxedema coma is a rare but severe and potentia fatal form of hypothyroidism in which there marked decrease in cellular metabolism, with fail to stimulate the sodium pump and a decrease in r tochrondrial metabolism.

The condition usually occurs in women wit long-standing history of hypothyroidism due to toimmune thyroiditis, thyroidectomy for Graves d ease, neck irradiation for cancer, hypopituitarism, use of antithyroid medication. There is a history progressive decline in mental status and dement apathy, neglect, and, in some cases, psychosis culr nating in a stuporous or comatosed state. Examir tion shows the presence of pneumonia or a urin tract infection, which has precipitated the episo Hypoventilation, hypothermia, and bradycardia noted, and the skin is cold and dry. The hair is spar and the face and extremities show a nonpitti edema. There is a marked delayed relaxation of t tendon reflexes.

Diagnostic Procedures

1. The serum T_4 is low and the TSH elevated; cre tine kinase is high with elevation of the MM fr tion in myxedema coma. Hyponatremia, hyp glycemia, and pericardial infusions are r uncommon in myxedema coma. The TSH level occasionally normal, but the typical clinical p ture of myxedema coma establishes the diagnos
2. The EEG reveals diffuse low-voltage slowing the theta range in severe hypothyroidism myxedema coma.

Treatment

1. The neurological complications of I pothyroidism are resolved with replacement thera

2. Treatment of myxedema coma requires broad-spectrum intravenous antibiotic for control infection and the administration of intraveno T_4 300 to 500 μg in a bolus followed by 50 intravenously daily, until the patient can t T_4 orally. Hydrocortisone 200 mg intravenou daily will avoid adrenal crisis in patients w

patients; optic neuritis is rare. Calcification of the basal ganglia is usually asymptomatic but may be associated with parkinsonism. Progressive hearing loss due to altered calcium content in the inner ear occurs in patients with long-standing hypoparathyroidism.[41]

Diagnostic Procedures

1. The serum parathormone level is abnormally low. Serum calcium levels are depressed.
2. A CT scan may demonstrate calcification of the choroid plexus, meninges, or basal ganglia.
3. The ECG shows changes of prolonged QT interval and T-wave abnormalities said to be characteristic of hypoparathyroidism.[42]

Treatment   In most cases, the symptomatology responds to calcium administration. Chronic cases, with evidence of dementia or parkinsonism, may show some signs of improvement with levodopa (see Chap. 6).

Hypercalcemia

Although hyperparathyroidism is a major cause of hypercalcemia, hypercalcemia of malignancy is not uncommon, and these two causes account for 90 percent of cases of hypercalcemia.[43] Elevation of parathyroid hormone is the hallmark of parathyroid disease, whereas elevation of parathyroid hormone-related protein accounts for hypercalcemia of malignancy. In addition, 10 percent of patients with hypercalcemia of malignancy have elevated parathyroid hormone levels. Both parathyroid hormone levels and parathyroid hormone-related protein levels should be measured, in case of hypercalcemia and suspected malignancy.

NEUROLOGICAL COMPLICATIONS OF HYPOTHALAMIC-PITUITARY DYSFUNCTION

Diabetes Insipidus

Diabetes insipidus results from inadequate production of antidiuretic hormone (ADH). The condition can occur following trauma, meningitis, tumor, or neurosurgical procedures producing damage to the supraoptic nucleus of the hypothalamus, the supraoptical-hypophyseal tract, or the posterior pituitary gland by an inflammatory process or tumor. The patient presents with excessive thirst associated with an increased volume of urine of low specific gravity. L-Desamino-8-D-argine (vasopressin) nasal spray produces 8 to 20 h of antidiuresis. Minor cases can be treated with oral medication that enhances the action of ADH. Chlorpropamide 250 to 500 mg daily increases water retention, and chlorothiazide 500 to 1000 mg daily may also be effective, despite its diuretic properties.

Acromegaly

Acromegaly results from the excessive secretion of human growth hormone by a pituitary tumor.

There is peripheral nerve hypertrophy with unilateral or bilateral carpal tunnel syndrome occurring in 50 percent of cases. A symmetrical, predominantly sensory peripheral neuropathy has been described in acromegaly.[44]

Inappropriate Secretion of Antidiuretic Hormone

Etiology and Pathology   The syndrome has resulted from trauma, neurosurgical procedures, intracerebral and subarachnoid hemorrhage, cerebral infarction, acute meningitis, acute encephalitis, acute inflammatory demyelinating polyneuropathy, hydrocephalus, and such extracranial conditions as tuberculosis, staphylococcal pneumonia, lung abscess, and porphyria. Approximately 70 percent of the cases of SIADH are related to malignancy, and 70 percent of the malignancies are small-cell carcinoma of the lung. Other malignant conditions occasionally associated with SIADH include pancreatic carcinoma, Hodgkin lymphoma, lymphosarcoma, and thymoma. Drugs inducing SIADH include chlorpropamide, carbamazepine, cyclophosphamide, vincristine, antidepressant agents, antipsychotic agents, narcotics, barbiturates, and general anesthetics.

Clinical Features   The clinical features are those of hyponatremia (see above).

Diagnostic Procedures   The criteria for the diagnosis of SIADH are:

1. Low serum sodium (< 135 mEq/L).
2. Low serum osmolality (< 280 mOsmol/L).
3. High urine sodium (> 18 mEq/L).
4. Urine osmolality greater than serum osmolality.
5. Normal thyroid adrenal and renal function.
6. Absence of peripheral edema or dehydration.

Treatment

1. The symptomatic patient with serum sodium less than 125 mEq/L should be given furosemide 1 mg/kg intravenously followed by hourly replacement of urinary sodium loss using 3% sodium chloride intravenously. Furosemide should be repeated as needed to maintain a negative fluid balance.[45] When the serum sodium is below 120 mEq/L in the seizure-free conscious patient, water intake is restricted to 500 mL per 24 h. Allow 1000 mL per 24 h for serum sodium 120 to 130 mEq/L. The intake may be increased to 1500 mL per 24 h once serum sodium exceeds 130 mEq/L but should not exceed 1500 mL per 24 h until normal sodium levels are achieved.[46]

2. The asymptomatic patient usually responds to water restriction.

3. Chronic SIADH of unknown etiology often responds to Declomycin 1200 mg daily, decreasing to a maintenance dose of 300 to 900 mg daily.

Panhypopituitarism

Definition   *Panhypopituitarism* is caused by failure of the pituitary gland to secrete stimulating hormones.

Etiology and Pathology   Panhypopituitarism may result from infarction of the pituitary gland during pregnancy (Sheehan syndrome)[47] or from lesions involving the pituitary and hypothalamus, including head injury, gunshot wounds, pituitary tumors, meningioma, chordoma, glioma, and pinealoma. Other causes include internal carotid or anterior communicating artery aneurysms,[48] chronic meningitis, sarcoidosis, and postradiation therapy.

Clinical Features   The patient develops signs of hypothyroidism, hypogonadism, and hypoadrenalism. Patients report loss of axillary and pubic hair, cold intolerance, impotence in men, and amenorrhea in women. Adrenal insufficiency results in low blood pressure and hypoglycemia.

Diagnostic Procedures

1. Evidence of pituitary, parapituitary, or hypothalamic tumor may be seen with MRI or CT scanning.
2. Hormonal levels of follicle-stimulating hormone, luteinizing hormone, prolactin, TSH, T_4, free T_4, cortisol, testosterone in men, and estradiol in women are all low.

Treatment   Surgical excision of tumors and clipping of aneurysms are indicated but are unlikely to alter the hypo- or panhypopituitarism in the immediate postoperative period. Similarly, treatment of chronic meningitis or sarcoidosis will be protracted and require ongoing treatment for pituitary dysfunction.

   Urgent therapy is directed toward replacement of thyroid and adrenal deficiency. Gonadotropic hormone replacement can be instituted at a later date.

Benign Intracranial Hypertension (Pseudotumor Cerebri)

Definition   Benign intracranial hypertension is a syndrome of suspected toxic or metabolic etiology, characterized by the presence of increased ICP, which usually resolves spontaneously.

Etiology and Pathology   The disorder has been associated with otitis media, Behçet disease, cerebral venous obstruction, dural sinus thrombosis, lateral sinus thrombosis, hypovitaminosis and hypervitaminosis A, carbon dioxide retention, endocrine disorders, particularly hypoparathyroidism, hypothyroidism, hypocalcemia, hyperthyroidism, polycythemia, adrenal insufficiency, and estrogen imbalance. Benign intracranial hypertension has also occurred following therapy with tetracyclines, amoxicillin, ampicillin, minocycline, T_4, nitrofurantoin, and amiodarone.

There are no characteristic pathological changes. The brain appears edematous and the ventricles are small in size.

Clinical Features   The patient is usually a child or young adult, typically an obese adolescent girl with menstrual abnormalities and evidence of increased ICP (i.e., headache, nausea and vomiting, visual difficulties, and papilledema). Minor symptoms of neck stiffness, tinnitus, distal extremity paresthesias, joint pains, and low back pain are not uncommon.[49]

Diagnostic Procedures

1. Visual field perimetry may reveal constrictions of the visual fields and enlargement of the blind spot.
2. On lumbar puncture, the only abnormality is elevation of the CSF pressure.
3. The MRI and CT scans are normal, and the ventricles are usually small in size.

Differential Diagnosis   Other causes of increased ICP must be excluded. Meningeal carcinomatosis may present as benign intracranial hypertension.[50]

Treatment   Identifiable causes such as tetracycline therapy should be discontinued. Chronic causes may benefit from corticosteroid therapy using methylprednisolone (Medrol) 64 mg every other day with gradual tapering of the dosage as improvement occurs.

Lumboperitoneal or ventriculoperitoneal shunting procedures are indicated when significant loss of visual acuity or intractable headaches occur.[51] Shunt failure occurs in about 50 percent of cases and requires shunt replacement. Progressive visual failure, despite a successful shunt procedure, requires optic nerve sheath fenestration.

NEUROLOGICAL COMPLICATIONS OF SYSTEMIC DISEASE

Diabetes Mellitus

Diabetes mellitus is a common condition and neurological complications occur in a significant number of patients with this disease.

Diabetic Neuropathy

Diabetic neuropathy is a disease of peripheral nerves that occurs in at least 50 percent of patients who have had diabetes for 25 years. The syndrome includes symmetrical distal polyneuropathy, asymmetrical proximal motor neuropathy, focal asymmetrical mono- or polymononeuropathies, or autonomic neuropathy. These conditions may coexist.

Etiology and Pathology   The etiology is uncertain. There are four hypotheses, which are not necessarily exclusive.

1. Hyperglycemia-polyol-myoinositol hypothesis. Under normal conditions, glucose is phosphorylated by hexokinase to glucose-6-phosphate, which enters the Krebs cycle. Hyperglycemia saturates hexokinase activity and glucose is shunted to the polyol pathway by the action of aldolase reductase with an excess production of sorbitol, which is associated with a decrease in intracellular myoinositol, a precursor of phosphoinositide metabolism. This results in defective Na^+/K^+ adenosine triphosphatase (ATPase) activity, defects in axon transport, and slowing of nerve conduction velocities.[52]

2. Microvascular hypothesis. There are thickening of capillary basement membrane and an increase in the size and number of capillary endothelial cells in diabetes mellitus, the microangiopathy resulting in an increasing number of closed capillaries in peripheral nerves with progressive hypoxia and secondary changes in axons and Schwann cells.[53]

3. Structural changes at the node of Ranvier. The Na^+/K^+ ATPase deficiency leads to increased intra-axonal Na^+ and nodal axonal swelling. This is followed by detachment of myelin and myelin retraction from the nodal area, producing slowing of axonal

conduction. The exposure of paranodal K^+ channels permits leakage of K^+ and further impairment of axonal conduction. There is impairment of axonal transport of essential factors from the axonal body to the periphery and a gradual dying back of axons starting at the distal axon and progressing proximally.

4. Vasculitic neuropathy. Some cases of non–insulin-dependent diabetes mellitus and proximal diabetic neuropathy have an inflammatory vasculopathy with perivascular collections of lymphocytes and axonal neuropathy.[54]

Clinical Features

1. Symmetrical distal polyneuropathies.
   a. Predominantly small fiber type with pain and paresthesias, usually in the lower extremities.
   b. Predominantly large fiber type with decreased vibration and position sense, sensory ataxia, and loss of ankle jerks. Painful or painless foot ulceration can occur.
   c. Mixed small and large fiber types plus autonomic involvement with dissociated sensory loss of pain and temperature sensation; development of Charcot joints in the lower extremities; painless distention of the bladder and Argyll Robertson pupils (diabetic pseudotabes). The combination of diabetic peripheral and autonomic neuropathy, peripheral vascular disease, and trauma results in foot ulceration.[55]

      An acute axonal degeneration involving fibers of all sizes has been termed diabetic neuropathic cachexia. This condition is more prevalent in men.
2. Asymmetrical proximal motor neuropathies (diabetic amyotrophy).
   a. Acute ischemic mononeuropathy multiplex, which is believed to result from asymmetrical small infarcts of proximal motor nerve trunks, results in a sudden asymmetrical weakness of the pelvic musculature, frequently associated with pain. A number of these cases are examples of a vasculitic neuropathy.
   b. Subacute proximal neuropathy results in a slowly progressive weakness of the proximal limb-girdle musculature and may suggest a myopathic rather than a neuropathic process.

3. Focal asymmetrical mono- or polymononeuropathies.
   a. Cranial neuropathies resulting in paralysis of extraocular muscles due to involvement of the third or sixth cranial nerves usually occur in patients over age 50 with long-standing diabetes. The onset of the paralysis is usually preceded by retro-orbital pain of several days' duration. Pupillary sparing is not unusual, even when loss of third nerve function is complete. Resolution usually occurs within a 3-month period.
   b. Painful diabetic thoracolumbar neuropathy presents with gradual onset of painful dysesthesias involving the lower thorax or upper abdominal wall. There may be some weakness of intercostal abdominal muscles. The condition resolves over a period of several months. The correct diagnosis is important because there is usually an immediate suspicion of intrathoracic or intra-abdominal problems at the onset of pain.
   c. Peripheral mononeuropathies in the limbs tend to involve nerves at risk for compression, such as the median nerve at the wrist, the ulnar nerve at the elbow, the radial nerve in the upper arm, the lateral cutaneous nerve of the thigh (meralgia paresthetica), and the common peroneal nerve at the neck of the fibula.
4. Autonomic neuropathies.
   a. Postural hypotension is probably the most common manifestation of diabetic autonomic neuropathy. The patient experiences a sharp drop in both systolic and diastolic blood pressure, without compensatory tachycardia on standing.
   b. Resting tachycardia and wide fluctuations in blood pressure are not unusual in diabetics.
   c. Silent myocardial infarction can occur in cardiac autonomic neuropathy with a loss of pain conduction fibers in the cardiac sympathetic system.
   d. Involvement of the genitourinary autonomic system results in the development of an atonic, painless distended bladder with overflow incontinence, male impotence with failure of ejaculation, and reduced vaginal lubrication and dyspareunia in the female.
   e. Gastrointestinal autonomic neuropathy results

in incoordination of esophageal peristalsis, gastric hypomotility, pylorospasm, intestinal hypomotility and constipation, intestinal incoordination and diarrhea, and anorectal dysfunction with incontinence.

f. Pupillary autonomic disturbances result in meiosis and failure of reaction to light—an Argyll Robertson-like pupil.

Diagnostic Procedures

1. The diagnosis of diabetes mellitus is established in a nonpregnant adult with a fasting blood glucose level greater than 140 mg/dL on two occasions or when the peak random blood glucose level is greater than 200 mg/dL and the 2-h blood glucose level is greater than 200 mg/dL in an individual with fasting blood glucose concentration of less than 140 mg/dL.[56]

2. Motor nerve conduction velocities are slowed and are believed to reflect nerve fiber density. Progressive nerve degeneration is reflected in reduction in amplitude of compound muscle action potentials and a progressive slowing of conduction velocity in multiple nerves.[57] Serial testing should include temperature control, calibration of equipment, and averaging of sensory responses to demonstrate meaningful change in electrophysiological data.

Treatment

1. Intensive diabetic therapy markedly delays or prevents the clinical manifestation of diabetic neuropathy.[58]

2. The patient should maintain ideal body weight.

3. Painful neuropathy usually responds to tricyclics such as amitriptyline 25 mg q.h.s., increasing by 25-mg increments each week to as high as 150 mg q.h.s. if necessary.

4. Carbamazepine and gabapentin are also effective in painful neuropathy.

5. Intravenous lidocaine 5 mg per kg body weight over 30 min, under continuous ECG monitoring, should be reserved for patients with intractable pain.

6. Autonomic dysfunction and postural hypotension require elastic stockings, increased dietary sodium, and fluorohydrocortisone 0.1 to 0.3 mg daily in some cases. Indomethacin 25 to 50 mg tid is also effective, as is a combination of diphenhydramine and cimetidine. Licorice in doses containing 3 g glycyrrhizic acid a day is also effective in ameliorating postural hypotension.[59] An antigravity suit may be necessary in extreme cases.

7. Genitourinary problems require voiding every 3 h and use of self-catheterization. Bethanechol 10 to 25 mg tid will promote detrusor contraction. Imipramine 25 mg tid may prevent retrograde ejaculation. Impotence may be treated with Sildenafil citrate tablets 25 mg, 50 mg, or 100 mg taken 1 hour before sexual activity.

8. Foot ulceration can be prevented by identification of diabetics at risk, education in foot care, prevention of infection, and the development of a multidisciplinary diabetic foot service.

9. Delayed esophageal emptying can be accelerated by bethanechol.

10. Delayed gastric emptying will respond to metoclopramide.

11. Diarrhea in diabetic patients often responds to tetracycline.

Leukemia

An increasing number of patients with leukemia are surviving after treatment and a number are developing neurological complications. These include:

1. Cerebral involvement. The CNS may be infiltrated by leukemic cells, which produce a progressive encephalopathy. Patients with leukemia also have an increased risk of superior sagittal sinus thrombosis. Signs and symptoms include intellectual deterioration, personality change, and the development of dysphasia, hemiparesis, hemisensory loss, and hemianopia. Involvement of the ventromedial thalamus may result in voracious appetite and weight gain. Patients with acute leukemia have an increased incidence of intracerebral hemorrhage, subarachnoid hemorrhage, and subdural hematoma[60] when the platelet count falls below 20,000 per cubic millimeter. Disseminated

intravascular coagulation is a feature of leukemia, appearing with high white blood cell counts soon after the institution of chemotherapy.

2. Meningeal involvement. Meningeal infiltration by leukemic cells has been reported at autopsy in about 20 percent of patients with leukemia.[61] The meningeal infiltration results in acute hydrocephalus with headache, vomiting, papilledema, and separation of sutures in children. Involvement of the meninges at the base of the brain produces progressive cranial nerve palsies. Cranial motor nerves are particularly susceptible to this complication. The CSF is under increased pressure and may show the presence of leukemic cells. The glucose content is decreased and the protein content is elevated.

3. Brainstem involvement. Invasion of the brainstem by leukemic cells results in progressive involvement of brainstem nuclei, progressive ataxia, and disturbance of respiration, including hypopnea and Cheyne-Stokes respiration.

4. Spinal cord involvement. Leukemic infiltration of the spinal epidural space produces spinal cord compression with progressive paraparesis, a sensory level, and sphincter involvement.

5. Peripheral nerve involvement. Infiltration of the posterior root ganglia, proximal nerve roots, or distal peripheral nerves can occur. A progressive polyneuropathy that resembles acute inflammatory demyelinating polyneuropathy (Guillain-Barré syndrome) may occur.

6. Infection. Patients with leukemia have an increased susceptibility to infection. There is an increased incidence of herpes zoster, which may result in neuritis or encephalitis. Leukemic patients have an increased risk of acute pyogenic meningitis, subacute fungal meningitis, and brain abscess. Progressive multifocal leukoencephalopathy is a complication that arises after chemotherapy or radiation.

7. Complications from chemotherapy and radiation. Chemotherapy and radiation may result in neurological complications, including leukoencephalopathy. Methotrexate can produce a diffuse arachnoiditis and a disseminated encephalopathy, with progressive dementia, spasticity, ataxia, and seizures.

Hodgkin Disease and Lymphoma

The neurological complications for Hodgkin disease and lymphoma may be due to either the direct effect of the disease on the nervous system or the remote effect of a neoplastic condition.

The complications include:

1. Cerebral involvement. A progressive encephalopathy with dementia has been described in lymphoma and Hodgkin disease. Direct primary involvement of the CNS has occasionally been reported with lymphoma and Hodgkin disease but is rare.

2. Meningeal involvement. Compression of cranial nerves, particularly of the optic chiasm, has been reported. Hypothalamic compression may result in diabetes insipidus. Subarachnoid hemorrhage is an occasional complication of Hodgkin disease and lymphoma.

3. Spinal cord lymphoma. Cord compression may result from epidural deposits in Hodgkin disease.[62] Involvement of the cord in lymphoma may be followed by the development of syringomyelia.[63]

4. Peripheral nerve involvement is probably the most common complication of Hodgkin disease and lymphoma. Most cases show compression of the brachial plexus or individual nerves arising from the brachial or lumbosacral plexus. An acute symmetrical peripheral neuropathy, resembling acute inflammatory demyelinating neuropathy, has been reported in Hodgkin disease.

5. Remote effects of Hodgkin disease and lymphoma. Most of the conditions described under metastatic effects of carcinoma occur in Hodgkin disease, including progressive multifocal leukoencephalopathy, cerebellar degeneration, and peripheral neuropathy (see p. 534).

6. Increased incidence of CNS infection. Alteration and suppression of immune mechanisms in Hodgkin disease and lymphoma lead to an increased risk of infection, including herpes zoster and chronic fungal infections.

Treatment Space-occupying lesions should be excised whenever possible. This is particularly important in paraparesis secondary to epidural deposits.

Primary CNS lymphoma and Hodgkin disease of the CNS show improved response to combined therapy, which includes chemotherapy and radiation therapy. The survival is significantly extended in patients with primary CNS lymphoma.[64]

Multiple Myeloma

Neoplastic transformation of plasma cells results in multiple myeloma. This condition may present as a single tumor (plasmacytoma) or a disseminated condition with metastatic involvement of multiple sites. Multiple myeloma may produce osteosclerotic or osteolytic lesions in bone or extradural deposits or may directly involve the CNS. In addition, the abnormal plasma cells have the capacity to synthesize abnormal globulins, resulting in IgG or IgM monoclonal gammopathies, macroglobulinemia, or cryoglobulinemia. Amyloidosis may occur in some patients. Involvement of bone produces hypercalcemia and hyperuricemia. Interference with coagulation mechanisms increases the risk of a hemorrhagic diathesis, with hemorrhage into the brain or subarachnoid space.

The complications include:

1. Cerebral involvement. Compression of the brain by an extradural mass or infiltration of the parenchyma, with production of focal signs and progressive encephalopathy, has been described.

2. Meningeal involvement may lead to cranial nerve palsies.

3. Spinal cord involvement. Extradural plasma cell tumors may produce spinal cord compression and progressive paraparesis.

4. Peripheral neuropathy. A sensorimotor neuropathy is found in 50 percent of osteosclerotic myeloma and a condition resembling acute inflammatory demyelinating neuropathy has been reported. Both conditions respond to chemotherapy and plasmapheresis. Median nerve involvement results in carpal tunnel syndrome. A syndrome of polyneuropathy (axonal type), organomegaly, endocrinopathies, myeloma, and skin lesions (POEMS) has been described. The neuropathy is accompanied by hepatosplenomegaly, hypogonadism, hypothyroidism, hyperpigmentation of the skin, edema, excessive hair growth, papilledema, and increased CSF protein.

5. Metabolic effects. Hypercalcemia due to the increased bone destruction leads to mental changes, weakness, and increased disability.

6. There is an increased risk of infection by herpes zoster.

Amyloidosis

Definition   *Amyloidosis* is a syndrome characterized by the extracellular deposition of an amyloid or fibrillary protein in one or more sites in the body.

Etiology and Pathology   Amyloidosis may be inherited, primary, or secondary. Familial amyloidosis is characterized by the deposition of the amyloid protein transthyretin in a peripheral nerve. Primary amyloidosis is associated with deposits of immunoglobulin light chains in the nerve. These are the result of a plasma cell dyscrasia in which clones of plasma cells produce the amyloid, which consists of amino acid terminal regions of the variable fragments of an immunoglobulin light chain.

Secondary amyloidosis is associated with chronic disease such as tuberculosis, chronic osteomyelitis, leprosy, rheumatoid arthritis, systemic lupus erythematosus, polymyositis, scleroderma, tumors including Hodgkin disease, renal cell carcinoma, medullary carcinoma of the thyroid, and familial Mediterranean fever. The amyloid is derived from virtual lysis of the amino terminal fragments of serum amyloid-associated protein.

Clinical Features

1. Familial amyloidosis. Several familial forms of amyloidosis have been described. All are inherited as an autosomal dominant trait and are usually identified by country or geographic area or origin, that is, Portugal, Sweden, Texas, Illinois, Indiana, Maryland, West Virginia, and Denmark.

Symptoms consist of symmetrical peripheral neuropathy, autonomic neuropathy, and multiorgan involvement.

2. Primary systemic amyloidosis. Peripheral neuropathy is an occasional feature of primary amyloidosis. Amyloid is deposited in peripheral nerves, with cuffing of endoneural microvessels and axonal

degeneration. Patients present with cardiac, renal, hepatic, and gastrointestinal symptoms. Pseudohypertrophy of muscle and myopathy result in muscle weakness. Macroglossia indicates tongue involvement. Systemic peripheral neuropathy produces a symmetrical sensory loss and dysesthesias involving the limbs. Carpal tunnel syndrome occurs in about 25 percent of cases. Autonomic involvement results in orthostatic hypotension. The prognosis is poor.

Treatment Prednisone, melphalan, or colchicine have limited value.

Macroglobulinemia

Etiology and Pathology Macroglobulinemia may occur as a primary condition or as a secondary phenomenon in multiple myeloma, leukemia, and lymphoma. The presence of macroglobulins leads to an increased serum viscosity, aggregation of the cellular elements of the blood, and thrombosis of small blood vessels.

Macroglobulinemia is usually associated with diffuse proliferation of leukocytes and plasma cells that infiltrate the subarachnoid space of the brain and spinal cord. This infiltration is often associated with scattered areas of hemorrhage or infarction. Peripheral nerves may contain deposits of IgG and IgM in the myelin sheath.

Clinical Features Increased viscosity produces decreased cerebral blood flow and hypoxia. This results in intellectual deterioration and diffuse headache. Focal signs of cerebrovascular insufficiency, including dysphasia, hemiparesis, and brainstem signs, with cranial nerve palsies, can occur. Increasing tinnitus and decreasing auditory acuity may be the result of involvement of the acoustic division of the eighth nerve or hemorrhage into the cochlea. Subarachnoid hemorrhage is an occasional complication owing to disturbed blood coagulation. Visual deterioration may result from increased ICP or retinal and vitreous hemorrhages. Extradural compression or vascular occlusive disease of the spinal cord will produce a progressive spastic paraparesis with bladder involvement. A condition similar to amyotrophic lateral sclerosis can result from infarction of the spinal cord. A progressive sensory peripheral neuropathy occurs in about 40 percent of cases.

Diagnostic Procedures

1. Abnormal macroglobulins can be demonstrated by serum protein electrophoresis. Antimyelin-associated glycoprotein (MAG) antibodies occur in 50 percent of cases.[65]
2. The CSF shows marked elevation of protein content with the presence of macroglobulins.
3. Decreased circulation and sludging in conjunctival vessels can be demonstrated by slit lamp examination and fluorescein angiography.
4. Serum viscosity levels are elevated.
5. Sural nerve biopsy shows a demyelinating neuropathy with IgM deposits in the myelin sheath or bound to the endoneurium.

Treatment Macroglobulinemia responds to plasmapheresis, which should be repeated biweekly to keep the serum viscosity level below the threshold of symptom recurrence. The polyneuropathy improves following monthly plasma exchange and intravenous cyclophosphamide.[66]

Plasma Cell Dyscrasias

Plasma cell dyscrasias with IgG or IgM monoclonal gammopathy are associated with peripheral neuropathy of a mixed sensorimotor type. The polyneuropathy is slowly progressive, with weakness, sensory loss, and an abnormal gait. There may be elevated IgG or IgM in the serum and the presence of anti-MAG antibodies.

Diagnostic Procedures

1. Motor and sensory nerve conduction velocities are slow.
2. Sural nerve biopsy may reveal a demyelinating or axonal degeneration.
3. Serum IgM antibodies binding to MAG is significantly increased.

Treatment A combination of plasmapheresis and intravenous cyclophosphamide produces improvement lasting up to 24 months in some patients. The treatment can be repeated when relapse occurs.

Cryoglobulinemia

Cyroglobulins are immunoglobulins that precipitate at temperatures below 37°F.

Three major types have been recognized:

1. Monoclonal immunoglobulins, usually IgG only.
2. Mixed type with polyclonal IgG, monoclonal IgM, rheumatoid factor.
3. Mixed type with polyclonal immunoglobulins and polyclonal IgM rheumatoid factor.

Type 2 cryoglobulinemia is probably related to chronic hepatitis C infection.[67]

Patients with cryoglobulinemia experience sludging or thrombosis of vessels on exposure to cold. Raynaud phenomenon is marked. Thrombosis of skin vessels produces purpura and ecchymosis. Hemoptysis and abdominal pain, hematemesis, and hematochezia may occur. Involvement of the kidneys results in albuminuria and eventual development of hypertension and uremia. Neurological complications include a sensorimotor neuropathy.[68] Treatment with interferon-alpha, 3 million units, three times a week, plus methylprednisolone 16 mg daily over a period of 6 months produces remission in the majority of cases.[69]

Polycythemia

Etiology and Pathology   Polycythemia vera is a condition characterized by an elevated erythrocyte count, elevated hemoglobin content, increased circulating blood volume, increased blood viscosity, and marked reduction in cerebral blood flow. The cause is unknown.

Secondary polycythemia occurs as a physiological response to living at high altitudes, in chronic heart disease with right-left shunt, chronic pulmonary disease, chronic renal disease, and renal carcinoma with excess secretion of erythropoietin.

Clinical Features   The patient presents with headache, blurred vision, and lethargy. There is an in-creased incidence of transient ischemic attacks and cerebral thrombosis. Those who develop hypertension have an increased risk of intracerebral hemorrhage and spontaneous subarachnoid hemorrhage. Development of symptoms suggesting a posterior fossa tumor suggests the presence of an erythropoietin-secreting hemangioblastoma.

Diagnostic Procedures   Criteria for diagnosis of polycythemia vera are divided into two categories to facilitate diagnosis.[70]

Category A

1. Increased red cell mass.
2. Splenomegaly.
3. Normal oxygen saturation.

Category B

1. White cell count $> 12,000$ mm^3.
2. Platelet count $> 650,000$ mm^3.
3. Increased leukocyte alkaline phosphatase score.
4. Increased serum vitamin B_{12} level and B_{12} binding capacity.

Diagnosis established if three A criteria are present or A1 plus either A2 or A3 and two of Category B.

Treatment   Patients with mild polycythemia vera or secondary polycythemia respond to repeated vene-section and removal of small volumes of blood. Replacement with low molecular weight dextran reduces the danger of cerebral thrombosis due to a sudden increase in platelets following venesection.

Refractory cases of polycythemia vera should be treated with hydroxyurea. Other agents such as chlorambucil or phosphorus 32 are leukemogenic and should be reserved for patients over 65 years of age.

Porphyria

Definition   The porphyrias consist of four inherited enzymatic disorders, each of which involves biosynthesis of heme with the accumulation of excessive porphyrins or porphyrin precursors.

Etiology and Pathology Porphyrins are produced along the heme synthesis pathway. The end result, heme, consists of protoporphyrin and iron, an essential component of hemoglobin, myoglobin, and heme-requiring enzymes in the cytochrome oxidase system.[71] (Figure 17–1).

An enzymatic defect on any step can, in theory, result in the accumulation of a substrate porphyrin and porphyria.

Excessive early precursors in heme biosynthesis are associated with the neuroporphyrias. A defect in porphobilinogen (PBG) deaminase results in accumulation of porphobilinogen and δ-aminolevulinic acid (ALA) and acute intermittent porphyria. Phlegmboporphyria, a very rare disease, results from a defect in ALA dehydratase.

Abnormalities in the metabolism of the later substrates of the heme pathway result in cutaneous or neurocutaneous forms of porphyria. The cutaneous forms of the disease, with prominent skin lesions but no involvement of the nervous system, consist of porphyria cutanea tarda, congenital erythropoietic porphyria, and erythropoietic protoporphyria.

Neurocutaneous porphyrias are either congenital coproporphyria or variegate porphyria. All porphyrias with neurological complications are inherited as an autosomal dominant trait.

The essential factor in all neuroporphyrias and neurocutaneous porphyrias is the sharp decline in the production of heme, which is essential for the synthesis of cytochrome oxidase in the mitochondria. Lack of cytochrome oxidase results in inhibition of the mitochondrial electron transport system and impaired cellular energy production.

Neuropathological changes consist of degenerative changes in the anterior horn cells of the spinal cord and neurons of autonomic ganglia. Degeneration of axons with areas of demyelination are found in the cerebellum and cerebral white matter.

Clinical Features An attack of acute intermittent porphyria may be precipitated by infection, hypoglycemia, sulfonamides, anticonvulsants, barbiturates, alcohol, griseofulvin, or exposure to industrial solvents. Most patients experience abdominal pain as the initial symptom. This is believed to result from autonomic neuropathy, which also causes tachycardia, urinary retention, sweating, and hypertension. Involvement of peripheral nerves produces a predominantly motor neuropathy that may progress to quadriparesis and respiratory failure. Muscle weakness is believed to result from failure of release of acetylcholine at the motor end plate. Cranial nerve involvement may result in dysarthria, dysphagia, facial diplegia, and external ophthalmoplegia. Optic atrophy has been described. Many patients have a history of mental disturbance, including depression, paranoia, and emotional instability. An acute attack may present with mania, restlessness, visual hallucinations, and delirium. This may be followed by seizures and coma. The attacks vary in duration, frequency, and severity.

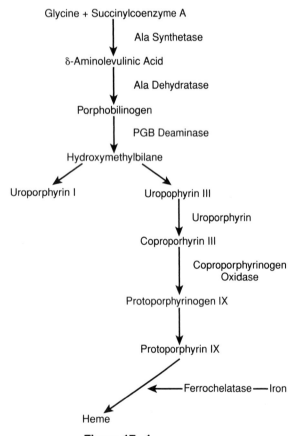

Figure 17–1
Heme synthesis pathway.

Attacks of hereditary coproporphyria or variegate porphyria may present as acute intermittent porphyria but are usually less acute and consist of sensorimotor neuropathies associated with cutaneous involvement.

Diagnostic Procedures

1. Urinary ALA and porphobilinogen levels are increased during acute attacks of porphyria to twice normal levels or higher.

2. The urine may be brown-red in color during an acute attack. In most cases, the urine will darken on standing.

3. In acute intermittent porphyria, urinary porphobilinogen is increased, and erythrocyte porphobilinogen deaminase is low.

4. In both neurocutaneous porphyrias, stool porphyrins are increased.

5. Electromyography shows evidence of fibrillation potentials in the acute phase, followed by the appearance of polyphasic motor unit potentials of reinnervation 6 to 8 weeks later. Near normal nerve conduction velocities with low-amplitude compound muscle action potentials are indicative of axonal neuropathy.

Treatment

1. Known precipitating agents should be avoided.

2. Pain control should be achieved using intramuscular morphine 10 to 15 mg q4h. Anxiety, agitation, and psychotic symptoms respond to chlorpromazine 25 to 50 mg intramuscularly or orally q6h. Hypertension and tachycardia can be treated with propranolol 20 to 40 mg q6h. Diazepam 5 to 10 mg intravenously followed by Valium drip 5 mg/h will control seizure activity.

In some cases, acute attacks can be aborted by administration of intravenous glucose 10 g/h or hematin 4 mg/kg q12h for 3 days.

Cimetidine 800 mg/day may abort attacks.

3. A sudden respiratory failure can occur at any time during an attack. Facilities for endotracheal intubation and mechanical respiration should be available for emergency use.

Whipple Disease

Whipple disease is an inflammatory disease involving the small intestine, owing to infection by *Tropheryma whippelii,* an intracellular pathogen found within macrophages. Involvement of the CNS is common and may be enhanced in immunosuppressed individuals.

Pathological changes consist of inflammation of the hypothalamus, thalamus, and mammillary bodies with the presence of periodic acid-Schiff (PAS)-positive bacillary-like structures within macrophages, microglial nodules, and scattered throughout the neuropil.[72]

Electron microscopic examination reveals intracellular rod-shaped bacilli. Evidence of intestinal involvement, including malabsorption, diarrhea, and steatorrhea, are not always present in patients with cerebral involvement. The disease produces progressive dementia, somnolence, supranuclear ophthalmoplegia, headache, seizures, myoclonus, and ataxia. An unusual feature is the presence of rhythmic convergence movements of the eyes, associated with rhythmic movements of the tongue and masticatory muscles, producing a rhythmic mandibular movement. This finding has been termed oculomasticatory myokymia and may be pathognomonic of Whipple disease of the CNS.[73] Hypothalamic symptoms consisting of disturbed sleep-wake cycle, polydipsia, and hyperphagia have been reported. The examination of the small intestinal mucosa in chronic fatigue syndrome may reveal PAS-positive bacillary structures in the inflammatory cells. The MRI scan shows areas of increased T2-weighted signal intensity in the white matter of the hypothalamus, uncus and medial temporal lobes, which do not enhance with gadolinium.

Trimethoprim-sulfamethoxazole, which can penetrate noninflamed meninges, should be the first choice of therapeutic agent. If relapse occurs, treatment with a third-generation cephalosporin such as cefixime is recommended.[74]

Hypoglycemia

Hypoglycemia is a potent cause of neurological symptoms in infants, children, and adults. Under aerobic conditions, glucose and oxygen are the sole source of energy in the CNS. There is little storage of glycogen or glucose in the brain, and available glucose supplies are exhausted within 30 min when hypoglycemia occurs.

Etiology and Pathology   The main causes of hypoglycemia are outlined in Table 17–2.

Pathological changes include neuronal loss and degeneration. This may be intense in areas with a high rate of metabolism, including the visual cortex and an Ammon's horn in the hippocampus. The subcortical gray matter and Purkinje cells of the cerebellum are also particularly susceptible to hypoglycemia. White matter is relatively resistant.

Clinical Features   Mild cases of hypoglycemia present with ataxia, hemiparesis, dysphasia, profuse perspiration, pallor, confusion, and a feeling of faintness. These symptoms are the result of sympathetic overactivity. Repeated attacks of this type may result in persistent cerebellar ataxia in some cases. Hypoglycemia occasionally causes seizures, and all

Table 17-2
Causes of hypoglycemia

1. Deficient glucose intake: starvation, anorexia nervosa.

2. Deficient absorption of glucose: malabsorption, chronic diarrhea.

3. Excessive glucose utilization: fever, hyperthyroidism, malignancy.

4. Excessive insulin secretion: insulinoma, leucine sensitivity, idiopathic postprandial hypoglycemia.

5. Deficient glycogen synthesis: liver disease, glycogen synthetase deficiency.

6. Deficient conversion of glycogen to glucose, glycogen storage diseases, prediabetic hypoglycemia.

7. Diabetes mellitus: poor control, excessive insulin dose, late onset postexercise hypoglycemia.

8. Drugs: alcohol, biguanides, hydrazine, propoxyphene, pyribenzamine, salicylates, sulfonylureas.

patients with recent onset of seizures should have appropriate tests for hypoglycemia.

In severe hypoglycemia, the symptoms of mild hypoglycemia are followed by confusion, psychosis, stupor, loss of consciousness, and coma. Patients may develop irreversible brain damage unless the blood glucose is restored to normal levels. The encephalopathy of hypoglycemia resembles that of anoxic encephalopathy. Chronic repetitive episodes of hypoglycemia may result in an axonal type of peripheral neuropathy.[75]

Diagnostic Procedures

1.   The diagnosis is established by demonstration of a relationship between symptoms and low serum glucose levels. Symptoms can usually be provoked by fasting 12 to 24 h in most cases.

2.   Elevated serum insulin levels can be demonstrated in patients with hyperplasia of the beta cells, insulinoma, leucine-sensitive hypoglycemia, and idiopathic postprandial or alimentary hypoglycemia.

3.   Liver function tests should be performed in all obscure cases of hypoglycemia. Tests for malabsorption may be required in some cases.

4.   Both MRI and CT scans are usually normal in early cases but may show evidence of cerebral atrophy and ventricular dilatation in patients who have suffered severe encephalopathy.

5.   The EEG shows progressive slowing during an attack of hypoglycemia, with the appearance of symmetrical theta activity followed by the appearance of symmetrical delta activity over both hemispheres. In the early stages, slowing is accentuated by hyperventilation.

Treatment   Every effort should be made to identify the causes of hypoglycemia and to administer appropriate therapy. Persistent hypoglycemia will inevitably lead to brain damage.

Nonmetastatic Effects of Cancer

Definition   Nonmetastatic effects of cancer are the result of damage or dysfunction of the nervous system that occurs without evidence of direct involvement by cancer cells.

Etiology and Pathology

Most cases result from an autoimmune response directed at the nervous system or muscle. Autoantibodies reacting with specific structures can be identified in some cases, and there is increased IgG in the CSF. Inflammatory infiltrates are present in affected tissue in some cases.

Pathological changes are described in Table 17–3.

Clinical Features

Nonmetastatic effects of cancer may involve the brain, brainstem, cerebellum, spinal cord, dorsal root ganglia, peripheral autonomic nervous systems, or muscle. Any of the conditions listed in Table 17–3 may affect the patient before the cancer is evident. The presence of anti-HU antibodies is a strong indicator of occult neoplasia.

In most cases, the patient presents with evidence of involvement of more than one area of the nervous system. Characteristic epidemiological features and signs and symptoms are listed in Table 17–3.

Table 17-3
Nonmetastatic effects of cancer

Syndromes	Pathologic features	Type of carcinoma most frequently associated	Characteristic signs and symptoms
Limbic encephalopathy	Extensive loss of neurons, hippocampus, cingulate gyrus, amygdala, orbital surface frontal lobes, perivascular cuffing	Small-cell carcinoma, lung; Hodgkin disease	Severe impairment, memory. Anxiety, depression, hallucinations, hypersomnia
Brainstem encephalitis	As above; changes mainly in medulla	Small-cell carcinoma, lung; carcinoma uterus	Dementia, bulbar involvement with dysphagia, dysarthria, vertigo, deafness, and/or external ophthalmoplegia
Subacute cerebellar degeneration	Diffuse loss of Purkinje cells	Small-cell carcinoma, lung; ovarian and breast carcinoma, Hodgkin disease	Gait ataxia followed by truncal and upper limb ataxia; vertigo, nystagmus
Opsoclonus-myoclonus	Diffuse loss of Purkinje cells and granular layer cells in cerebellum	Primitive neural ectodermal tumor in children; carcinoma, lung	Continuous arrhythmic multidirectional conjugate eye movements; ataxia, myoclonus head, trunk, and limbs
Subacute motor neuropathy	Degeneration anterior horn cells, demyelination anterior nerve roots, neurogenic atrophy, muscles	Lymphoma, Hodgkin disease	Slow progressive weakness, lower limbs, mild sensory loss
Necrotizing myelopathy	Necrosis, spinal cord; usually thoracic cord but white matter more than gray matter	Carcinoma, lung; lymphoma, leukemia	Sudden onset pain in back. Rapidly progressive weakness, lower extremities ascending to respiratory failure and death
Sensory neuronopathy	Loss of neurons and inflammation in dorsal root ganglia	Carcinoma, lung; Hodgkin disease	Pain, paresthesias numbness, distal limbs extending proximally, mild muscle weakness

Table 17-3 *(continued)*
Nonmetastatic effects of cancer

Syndromes	Pathologic features	Type of carcinoma most frequently associated	Characteristic signs and symptoms
Sensorimotor neuropathy	Peripheral axonal degeneration	Carcinoma, lung; prostate, ovary, lymphoma	Symmetrical weakness and sensory loss, distal lower extremities
Acute inflammatory demyelinating polyneuropathy	Acute demyelination, peripheral nerves	Hodgkin disease	See Guillain-Barré syndrome (see Chap. 19)
Autonomic neuropathy	Axonal degeneration, autonomic nerves	Carcinoma, lung	Orthostatic hypotension, bladder dysfunction, impotence, pupillary abnormalities
Lambert-Eaton syndrome	See page 649	Carcinoma, lung and other sites	See page 649
Carcinomatous polymyositis or dermatomyositis	See page 655	Carcinoma breast, lung, ovaries, stomach, colon	See page 655
Necrotizing myopathy	Widespread necrosis of muscle	Carcinoma lung, breast, colon, stomach	Symmetrical muscle weakness, pain, rapidly progressive respiratory involvement
Myotonia	Polymyositis	Carcinoma lung	Muscle stiffness, cramps, often before detection of tumor

Diagnostic Procedures

1. There is elevation of CSF, protein, and IgG in sensory neuropathy[76] when the CNS is involved.
2. Antibodies indicating an autoimmune reaction, including anti-HU in paraneoplastic sensory neuropathy,[77] may be present in serum and CSF and should indicate the need to search for a small-cell carcinoma of the lung.
3. Somatosensory evoked potentials will be delayed in patients with spinal cord involvement.
4. Nerve conduction velocities are abnormal when peripheral nerves are affected.
5. Electromyography will be abnormal in myopathy, dermatomyositis/polymyositis, or the myasthenic syndrome.

Treatment The neoplasm should be removed whenever possible, although successful removal may not prevent progression of neurological deficits. Treatment with plasmapheresis, immunoglobulin, or corticosteroids has been beneficial in some cases.

VITAMIN DEFICIENCIES AND INTOXICATIONS

Vitamin A Deficiency

Vitamin A is a polyunsaturated, fat-soluble vitamin that is ingested in animal foods and is derived from beta carotene in plant foods.

Dietary vitamin A deficiency is rare in the United States, but malabsorption syndromes and biliary tract or pancreatic duct obstruction may result in a deficiency syndrome. Night blindness is usually the presenting symptom and is due to lack of retinol, the aldehyde form of vitamin A, which is necessary for phototransduction in the retina. Prolonged deficiency may result in keratinization of the epithelium, with corneal necrosis and extrusion of the lens. Cranial nerve palsies, hydrocephalus, and mental retardation have been reported.

Vitamin A Intoxication

Vitamin A intoxication is most often associated with excessive vitamin supplementation. Signs of acute intoxication include nausea, vomiting, irritability, vertigo, drowsiness, weakness, bone pain, blurred vision, dry and flaking skin, and severe bifrontal headaches. Papilledema, headache, mild exophthalmos, hair loss, dry skin, bone thickening, weakness, enlargement of liver and spleen, anemia, joint pains, and menstrual irregularities are associated with chronic vitamin A intoxication. Benign intracranial hypertension may be associated with hypo- and hypervitaminosis A.

Treatment The signs and symptoms of Vitamin A deficiency and intoxication resolve with replacement or discontinuation of vitamin A supplementation.

Vitamin B$_1$ (Thiamine) Deficiency

(See Wernicke encephalopathy, page 539.)

Vitamin B$_6$ (Pyridoxine) Deficiency

Pyridoxal phosphate, the active form of pyridoxine, is a cofactor for a variety of enzymatic reactions. It is important for the conversion of tryptophan to nicotinic acid and for the conversion of glutamic acid to GABA. A deficiency of pyridoxine is associated with generalized seizures in children. Pyridoxine deficiency–induces seizures may be related to pyridoxine's role in the synthesis of the inhibitory neurotransmitter, GABA.

Seizures develop between the ages of 1 and 4 months. The interictal EEG is normal, and there is an excessive xanthurenic acid on administration of tryptophan. Children with pyridoxine-deficiency seizures respond well to anticonvulsants or to oral doses of pyridoxine.

Chronic ingestion of pyridoxine or ingestion of large doses in megavitamin therapy has resulted in a sensory peripheral neuropathy that can be reversed by cessation of vitamin B$_6$ supplementation. Daily intake should not exceed 200 mg.

Niacin (Nicotinic Acid) Deficiency—Pellagra

Derivatives of niacin serve as cofactors in many of the vital biological oxidation-reduction reactions and are indispensable components of the energy transfer process of cellular metabolism. Niacin deficiency is one of the major factors contributing to pellagra, a disease that occurs in populations who consume large quantities of corn-derived food.

Etiology and Pathology Although niacin deficiency is a major factor in the etiology of pellagra, multiple nutritional deficiencies are usually present. Thiamine, pyridoxine, and riboflavin, compounds that act as cofactors in the synthesis of niacin, are also deficient, thus magnifying the problem. The nature of the biochemical lesion in niacin deficiency is uncertain, but it probably involves impairment of respiratory chain function.

Neurons at many levels of the neuraxis are affected. Cells in the cerebral cortex, basal ganglia, brainstem, and occasionally, the anterior horn cells of the spinal cord become swollen and undergo chromatolysis.

Clinical Features In the United States, pellagra is now largely confined to chronic alcoholics. The initial symptoms of pellagra include anorexia, ataxia, insomnia, headache, muscle weakness, nervousness, and burning dysesthesias in the arms, hands, and feet.

Treatment Patients with pellagra respond to a high-protein, low-fat diet that is high in niacinamide, thiamine, riboflavin, and pyridoxine.

Vitamin B$_{12}$ Deficiency

Vitamin B$_{12}$ deficiency has a profound effect on the nervous system, due to the important role the vitamin plays in nervous system metabolism. Vitamin B$_{12}$ serves a cofactor in the synthesis of methionine and tetrahydrofolate. Methionine is metabolized to S-adenosylmethionine, necessary for the methylation of myelin sheath phospholipids. Tetrahydrofolate is a precursor for purine and pyrimidine synthesis.

Etiology and Pathology   Vitamin B_{12} deficiency results in pernicious anemia, which is usually the result of lack of intrinsic factor, a product of the gastric mucosa, which is necessary for the absorption of vitamin B_{12}. Other causes of vitamin B_{12} deficiency include exposure to nitrous oxide during a surgical procedure, intestinal malabsorption, chronic pancreatic disease, Crohn disease, and fish tapeworm infestation. Nutritional deficiency of vitamin B_{12} is rare but has been described in strict vegetarians, pregnancy, and in infants breast fed by vegan mothers.

Vitamin B_{12} deficiency results in pernicious anemia and in subacute degeneration of the spinal cord, characterized by demyelination involving the posterior columns, the pyramidal tracts, the ascending cerebellar tracts, and the anterior columns. Demyelination is followed by loss of axon cylinders and wallerian degeneration. As the disease progresses, more proximal areas of the CNS are affected. Demyelination and degeneration appear in the internal capsule and in the centrum semiovale and may also occur in the papillomacular bundle of the optic nerve. Cranial nerve involvement and segmental demyelination of the peripheral nerves have been reported.

Clinical Features   Patients with subacute combined degeneration usually present with numbness and tingling of the extremities. Vibration is diminished or lost, and position sense may be impaired in the toes. The lower extremities are spastic, with hyperactive knee and ankle reflexes and bilateral extensor plantar responses. The patient becomes ataxic and may be unable to walk. Severe anemia and the resultant cerebral anoxia result in depression and other psychological changes. Progressive dementia is a feature of vitamin B_{12} deficiency.

Diagnostic Procedures[78]

1. A complete blood count and bone marrow examination will indicate the presence of anemia.

2. Serum B_{12} (cobalamin) levels are usually decreased.

3. If serum B_{12} levels are low, intrinsic factor antibodies should be measured. If this test is positive, a Schilling test is not necessary.

4. If serum B_{12} levels are in the low normal range, but B_{12} deficiency is still suspected, homocystine and methylmalonic acid levels should be measured. If positive, this should be followed by measurements of intrinsic factor antibodies.

5. If intrinsic factor antibodies are positive, patients have pernicious anemia. If these antibodies are negative, a part I Schilling test should be performed. If this test is abnormal, the response indicates pernicious anemia, and the abnormality is corrected when the test is repeated with intrinsic factor (Schilling test part II).

6. Failure to absorb vitamin B_{12} after intrinsic factor administration indicates an intestinal cause for the malabsorption of the vitamin.

Treatment   Treatment consists of B_{12} replacement with intramuscular injections of 100 to 1000 μg of B_{12} daily for 5 days, followed by 1000 μg intramuscularly each month for life.

Vitamin D

Long-term injection of high doses of vitamin D can result in calcium deposits in soft tissues and damage to the kidneys. High toxic doses of vitamin D cause nausea, constipation, and muscle weakness. A myopathy has been described in vitamin D deficiency, with prompt response to administration of vitamin D up to 15 mg daily.

Vitamin E

High doses of vitamin E decrease platelet levels and act synergistically with anticoagulants. Consequently, patients receiving anticoagulant therapy should not take high-dose vitamin E supplements.

Vitamin E deficiency can be caused by fat malabsorption disorders, β-lipoproteinemia, or long-term parenteral nutrition in children and adults, leading to the development of neurological symptoms. A few cases of idiopathic vitamin E deficiency without fat malabsorption have been reported. Spinocerebellar degeneration and a symmetrical sensorimotor peripheral neuropathy have been described.[79] Spinocerebellar degeneration presents with ophthalmoplegia, proximal muscle weakness, truncal and limb ataxia, decreased vibration and position sense, and hyporeflexia.[80]

Treatment Vitamin E, 1000 IU, supplemented by desiccated ox bile, will elevate serum vitamin E levels and alleviate symptoms.

NEUROLOGICAL COMPLICATIONS OF ETHANOL

Fetal Alcohol Syndrome

Definition The *fetal alcohol syndrome* is a congenital condition caused by chronic ethanol usage during pregnancy.

Etiology and Pathology Alcohol has a teratogenic effect on the development of the fetus, and chronic ethanol abuse affects fetal development during early embryogenesis.

Clinical Features Affected children exhibit growth retardation and cerebellar ataxia and have an abnormal facial appearance, with short, palpebral fissures, micrognathia, depressed nasal bridge, long convex upper lips (fish mouth), and epicanthic folds. Microcephaly, mental retardation, attention deficit disorder, spasticity, cerebellar ataxia, seizures, strabismus, cleft palate, and congenital heart disease can occur.[81] The neonate may show signs of acute withdrawal characterized by irritability, increased muscle tone, tremors, and tonic seizures, often accompanied by abdominal distention and vomiting.

Treatment Neonatal irritability should be treated with chlorpromazine (Thorazine) 2 mg/kg daily. Phenobarbital 5 mg/kg daily is effective in reducing symptoms and should be used to control seizures.

In adults, neurological complications of ethanol may occur because of the:

1. Direct effect of alcohol on the CNS.
2. Effect of concomitant nutritional deficiencies.
3. Indirect effect of alcohol damage to other organs.
4. Increased prevalence of certain diseases in alcoholics.

Acute Alcohol Intoxication and Coma

Etiology and Pathology An ingestion of large quantities of ethanol over a short period of time may lead to respiratory depression, coma, and death. In addition, there is a risk of vomiting and subsequent aspiration. Some alcoholics are prone to hypoglycemia, particularly if they ingest alcohol in association with other drugs. The combination of ethanol and depressant drugs increases the risk of coma and death.

Diagnostic Procedures and Treatment

1. Acute intoxication with coma is a neurological emergency. One should never assume that a patient who is in a coma and smells of alcohol is simply suffering from alcoholic intoxication. A full neurological examination should be performed.

2. Blood should be drawn and tested for glucose level, alcohol level, and the presence of other drugs (drug screen).

3. The vital signs are recorded every 15 min. The patient should be catheterized and a nasogastric tube inserted and aspirated to remove any ethanol not yet absorbed from the stomach.

4. The airway should be cleared by suction if necessary, and the patient turned from side to side to drain secretions from the oropharynx.

5. An intravenous infusion will be necessary to correct any electrolyte imbalance.

6. On recovery, the patient requires adequate rest, light nourishment, adequate fluid intake, and aspirin for headache.

Alcoholic Ketoacidosis

Definition *Alcoholic ketoacidosis* is a metabolic disturbance resulting from a prolonged intake of alcohol.

Etiology and Pathology The condition arises from a combination of metabolic abnormalities that occur in a fasting volume-depleted alcoholic after abrupt cessation of drinking.[82]

Clinical Features The condition is preceded by heavy alcohol intake of several days' or weeks' duration, followed by abrupt cessation and starvation for 24 to 72 h. This is followed by abdominal pain and vomiting. Examination shows tachypnea or Kussmaul breathing, tachycardia, orthostatic hypotension, and signs of chronic alcoholism, such as spider angiomata and an enlarged, tender liver.

Diagnostic Procedures

1. Blood alcohol levels are low or absent.
2. There is a metabolic acidosis with an elevated ion gap.
3. Hypokalemia, hypochloremia, and bicarbonate depletion are present.
4. Serum glucose level is normal or slightly elevated.
5. Urinalysis shows ketonuria without glycosuria.
6. Serum amylase and liver enzyme levels may be abnormal.

Treatment

1. Correct volume depletion by infusion of normal saline with dextrose.
2. Give potassium supplements to correct hypokalemia.
3. Treat intercurrent processes such as pneumonia, acute pancreatitis, gastritis, or gastric hemorrhage.

Delirium Tremens

Definition *Delirium tremens* is a condition that occurs in chronic alcoholics 72 to 96 h after withdrawal of alcohol. It is characterized by an acute psychosis that may result in death.

Etiology Delirium tremens follows the sudden withdrawal of ethanol in a chronic alcoholic and may be precipitated by infection, trauma, pancreatitis, or malnutrition.

Sudden withdrawal of alcohol produces a rebound sensitivity to carbon dioxide, with hyperventilation and subsequent respiratory alkalosis. Severe dehydration and electrolyte imbalance occur. There is impairment of calcium channel function and excess calcium influx into neurons, producing neuronal dysfunction.

Clinical Features The patient presents with a prodromal phase of tremulousness, irritability, and restlessness. There is an aversion to food, sleep is disturbed, and the patient has nightmares and fragmentary illusions. The patient then passes into an acute psychotic state with hallucinations that may be visual, auditory or, rarely, olfactory or tactile. During this phase, consciousness is clouded, the patient is disoriented, speech is incoherent, and there is extreme restlessness with free vocalizing. Seizures may occur and are usually preceded by the delirium. Autonomic overactivity occurs, with elevated temperature, tachycardia, and profuse perspiration. Severe dehydration occurs if fluids are not replaced.

On examination, there is a coarse tremor involving the tongue, lips, face, limbs, and fingers. The tendon reflexes are hyperreflexic, and the muscles may be tender on palpation.

Treatment

1. Alcohol should be withheld. The belief that alcohol should be given prophylactically in incipient delirium tremens is fallacious.

2. The patient will require rehydration. The patient's water loss may be between 5000 and 6000 mL/day. Any electrolyte imbalance, especially calcium, magnesium, and potassium, should be corrected.

3. The patient will need to be adequately sedated.

The following are recommended:

1. Chlorpromazine (Thorazine) up to 1 g daily in divided doses.
2. Chlordiazepoxide (Librium) 80 to 100 mg q6h.
3. Diazepam (Valium) 5 to 10 mg intramuscularly q4h p.r.n. Alternatively, diazepam 5 mg/h by intra-

venous drip as a constant infusion may be given in severe cases.

4. Supplementary thiamine hydrochloride 200 mg given daily intramuscularly or intravenously.

5. As improvement occurs, the patient requires an adequate diet with vitamin supplements.

Prognosis Patients with delirium tremens are acutely and severely ill. Mortality was high in the past, but rates are less than 15 percent with aggressive treatment in an intensive care unit.[83]

Wernicke Encephalopathy

Wernicke encephalopathy is caused by thiamine deficiency and presents with ataxia, diplopia due to ocular motor abnormalities, and an acute confusional state.

Etiology and Pathology Although Wernicke encephalopathy occurs predominantly in alcoholics, it is not confined to alcoholism and has been described in starvation, malnutrition, intravenous hyperalimentation, renal dialysis, hyperemesis gravidarum, and pernicious vomiting due to high intestinal obstruction. Dietary thiamine is lacking in the inadequate diet of the alcoholic, but alcohol also causes impaired intestinal absorption of thiamine and decreased liver storage of thiamine. The function of the four enzymes—pyruvate, dehydrogenase, α-ketoglutarate dehydrogenase, transketolase, and branch-chain α-ketoacid dehydrogenase—each of which requires thiamine paraphosphate as a coenzyme, is impaired.[84] This results in a high concentration of pyruvate and lactate in the blood and lactic acidosis with damage to neurons.[85]

Pathological changes occur in the periaqueductal gray matter surrounding the third and fourth ventricles, the mammary bodies, thalamus, and cerebellum. Microscopically, degeneration of neurons, demyelination, petechial hemorrhages, and capillary and astrocytic proliferation occur.

Clinical Features The classical triad of Wernicke encephalopathy consists of ataxia, ophthalmoplegia, and acute dementia. Cerebellar lesions are most severe in the superior vermis, resulting in marked gait ataxia, with few signs of upper limb incoordination. Examination shows ptosis, bilateral sixth nerve paralysis, horizontal gaze palsy, and nystagmus. Vertical gaze palsy can also occur. Complete ophthalmoplegia is unusual. The acute dementia presents as disorientation and drowsiness, apathy, and indifference. Agitation is unusual. Stupor and coma are rare but life-threatening, with a mortality rate of more than 50 percent, particularly if hypothermia and respiratory arrest occur.[86]

Most patients who survive Wernicke encephalopathy show nystagmus, ataxia, and some degree of Korsakoff psychosis, which presents with a loss of retention, recall, and recent memory, and confabulation. Remote memory is intact, but there is a striking inability to learn and retain new information.

Diagnostic Procedures

1. Blood alcohol and blood glucose levels, serum electrolytes, blood urea nitrogen, creatinine, calcium, magnesium, and a liver enzyme profile should be obtained.

2. The MRI scan of the brain shows increased signal intensity on T2-weighted images in the periaqueductal gray matter and median thalamus. Mamillary body enhancement occurs in postcontrast T1-weighted images.[87]

Treatment

1. Thiamine 200 mg intravenously should be given upon suspicion of Wernicke encephalopathy and should be repeated q8h for 2 days, followed by 200 mg intravenously daily until the patient can tolerate oral thiamine. Intravenous thiamine must always be given before intravenous fluids containing glucose. Oral thiamine should be continued 100 mg q12h orally, as long as the patient remains an alcoholic.[88]

2. Electrolyte imbalance should be corrected.

3. An adequate diet with multivitamin supplementation and abstinence from alcohol should be a long-term goal.

Alcohol Seizures

A number of possibilities should be considered when seizures develop in an alcoholic.

1. Generalized tonic-clonic seizures occur 7 to 48 h after cessation of drinking and are the prodromal symptom of delirium tremens in about 30 percent of cases.[89]

2. Alcohol lowers the seizure threshold in a known epileptic.

3. Seizures may develop in chronic alcoholics who have repeated head injuries. Repeated contusions lead to the development of glial scars in the cortical gray matter. Such scars have the capacity to alter neuronal metabolism and create an epileptic focus. Seizures, sometimes called "rum fits," are associated with hypomagnesemia, respiratory alkalosis, low arterial P_{CO_2}, and elevated arterial pH. These patients usually have a normal neurological examination and a normal EEG, which is abnormal only during a seizure or in the postictal period. About 50 percent of the patients show a photoconvulsive response to photic stimulation when the EEG is recorded during the period of alcohol withdrawal.

Other causes of seizures in alcoholics reflect the effect of ethanol in combination with certain drugs. One of the most common associations is the use of propoxyphene (Darvon) with ethanol. Propoxyphene is a commonly used analgesic; the combination of propoxyphene and ethanol in a patient who is not taking an adequate diet can produce hypoglycemia and seizures.

It is important to differentiate between alcohol withdrawal seizures and seizures in a known or assumed epileptic, which are induced by alcohol withdrawal.

Patients with alcohol withdrawal seizures develop generalized tonic-clonic seizures within 6 to 48 h after cessation or decrease in alcohol intake. Alcohol withdrawal seizures often occur in binge drinkers. Seizures occur abruptly, are multiple, but usually less than five in number. The whole episode lasts less than 12 h in 95 percent of cases. The neurological examination and baseline EEG are normal.

Alcohol Dementia

Some chronic alcoholics develop a slowly progressive dementia quite distinct from the dementia of the

Wernicke-Korsakoff syndrome. The following causes of dementia should be considered:

1. Patients suffering from early Alzheimer disease may begin to use increasing amounts of alcohol when judgment and insight become impaired.
2. In chronic alcoholics, repeated head trauma produces small areas of contusion in the cerebral cortex and, eventually, severe neuronal loss and dementia.
3. The chronic alcoholic may suffer repeated seizures that cause cerebral anoxia and neuronal damage.
4. The chronic alcoholic is at risk for a chronic subdural hematoma due to frequent falls.
5. Chronic alcoholics may develop chronic hepatic encephalopathy (see p. 517).
6. Some cases are undoubtedly due to the direct effect of alcohol in susceptible individuals who suffer accelerated neuronal degeneration because of chronic alcohol abuse.[90]

Clinical Features   The patient presents with symptoms of progressive dementia, including loss of operational judgment, failing memory, failing insight, and an inappropriate emotional response.

Diagnostic Procedures

1. The MRI or CT scan shows diffuse cortical atrophy with relatively little enlargement of the lateral ventricles.
2. The EEG shows progressive loss of background activity with the increased presence of excessive theta and eventually delta activity, particularly in the temporal leads bilaterally.
3. Neuropsychological evaluation is useful in measuring the degree of intellectual and cognitive impairment, as well as recording improvement in maintained abstinence.[91]

Treatment

1. Patients suffering from alcohol dementia should be withdrawn from ethanol, receive an adequate diet, and be given thiamine supplements.
2. All cases of dementia should be investigated for

possible treatable causes. This includes a careful screening for chronic subdural hematoma.

3. Lithium therapy is reported to reduce drinking and improve symptons of depression in chronic alcoholics. However, lithium does not have any effect on the dementia.

Many chronic alcoholics who remain abstinent demonstrate a remarkable improvement in mental status.[92]

Central Pontine Myelinolysis

Definition Central pontine myelinolysis is a rare condition that occurs in chronic alcoholism and in certain nutritional deficiencies.

Etiology and Pathology Central pontine myelinolysis has been reported to occur in the following conditions: chronic alcohol abuse, cerebral ischemia, cerebral edema, impaired fat metabolism, neoplasia, chronic infection, liver dysfunction, impaired secretion of ADH and electrolyte abnormalities, particularly the rapid correction of hyponatremia. The common factor in the genesis of central pontine myelinolysis appears to be the chronic and severe hyponatremia.[93]

There is a symmetrical demyelination of the central structures of the pons extending up into the midbrain and down into the medulla. In severe cases, there may be a total demyelination of the center of the pons.

Clinical Features Central pontine myelinolysis is characterized by impairment of consciousness and progressive development of cranial nerve palsy, severe ataxia, and dysarthria. Severe cases may develop a "locked-in syndrome."

Diagnostic Features An MRI scan will demonstrate the area of demyelination in the brainstem.[94]

Treatment The patient may recover if treated in an intensive care unit with careful correction of hyponatremia (page 511) nasogastric feeding, correction of other metabolic abnormalities, and immediate antibiotic therapy for intercurrent infection.

Central Demyelination of the Corpus Callosum (Marchiafava-Bignami Disease)

Definition Marchiafava-Bignami disease seems to occur exclusively in chronic alcoholics and was first described in red wine drinkers. It also occurs following the chronic use of other alcoholic beverages.

Etiology and Pathology The etiology appears to be similar to that of central pontine myelinolysis. Pathological changes are confined to the corpus callosum and there is severe central demyelination of this structure.

Treatment There is no effective treatment.

Alcohol Cerebellar Degeneration

Definition Alcohol cerebellar degeneration is, at present, one of the most common complications of chronic ethanol abuse.

Pathology The appearance of the cerebellum is characteristic, with marked atrophy of the anterior lobes of cerebellum and the superior vermis. Involved areas show almost complete loss of Purkinje cells and loss of the neurons in both granular and molecular layers of the cortex. Advanced cases may show some involvement of the neocerebellum, particularly the dentate nucleus.

Clinical Features The condition is not alcohol-dose dependent and occurs in alcoholics who have an unusual sensitivity to alcohol.[95] The patient with alcohol cerebellar degeneration presents with severe ataxia of the lower limbs and trunk, minor cerebellar signs involving the upper limbs, and absence of nystagmus, dysarthria, and dementia.

Diagnostic Procedures The MRI or CT scan reveals atrophy of the anterior lobes of the cerebellum and the superior vermis.

Treatment The treatment includes abstinence, adequate diet, and thiamine supplements.

Alcohol Myelopathy

Spastic paraparesis is occasionally seen in alcoholics. Most cases are probably due to cervical spondylosis aggravated by repeated falls and trauma to the neck. However, there is a rare degenerative condition involving the spinal cord due to chronic ethanol abuse and nutritional deficiencies. Degenerative changes occur in the lateral and, to some extent, in the posterior columns of the spinal cord. These patients show progressive lower limb spasticity and weakness with the presence of ankle clonus, exaggerated knee jerks and ankle jerks, and extensor plantar responses. The upper limbs and bladder function are spared.

Alcohol Peripheral Neuropathy

Etiology and Pathology The majority of cases of peripheral neuropathy in alcoholics are mild and appear after many years of excessive drinking. Peripheral neuropathy in alcoholics has been attributed to a nutritional deficiency or to the toxic effects of alcohol on the peripheral nerve. Many chronic alcoholics have poor dietary habits and it is reasonable to assume that both factors are involved in the development of peripheral neuropathy. The pathological changes consist of wallerian degeneration with loss of myelin and axis cylinders.

Clinical Features The majority of chronic alcoholics have mild symptoms of peripheral neuropathy with peripheral paresthesias and some loss of muscle bulk in the distal lower extremities. More advanced cases show weakness involving the distal portions of all four limbs, and there may be severe pain in these cases. These patients suffer extremity dysesthesias and are often unable to tolerate contact with clothing. Electromyographic and nerve conduction studies are indicative of axonal degeneration.[96]

Treatment The treatment includes abstinence, adequate diet, and thiamine supplements.

Prognosis Symptoms usually persist for many months after initial treatment, despite withdrawal from alcohol, because axonal regeneration is a slow process and recovery is often incomplete.

Alcohol Myopathy

Alcohol myopathy occurs in three forms. It may present as acute myopathy with severe muscle pain and myoglobinuria, acute myopathy with proximal weakness and painful spasms, or a chronic myopathy. The acute form of alcohol myopathy with myoglobinuria usually occurs after a heavy bout of drinking and it is possible that this condition represents the effect of alcohol in a patient who is already susceptible to paroxysmal myoglobinuria. These patients are profoundly ill and are at risk for the development of acute renal tubular necrosis. They should be treated in an intensive care unit with appropriate restriction of fluids, correction of electrolyte imbalance, and sedation until diuresis occurs. Hemodialysis may be necessary in some cases.

The acute myopathy that follows a heavy bout of drinking is characterized by severe proximal weakness, particularly in the lower limb girdle musculature, with painful spasms of the affected muscles. Treatment consists of rest, sedation, adequate diet, and thiamine supplementation.

Chronic alcohol myopathy is a much more common condition, characterized by selective atrophy of type II nerve fibers.[97] There is wasting of the proximal musculature, particularly in the area of the shoulder girdle. Weakness, however, is uncommon.

The treatment consists of abstinence, adequate diet, and thiamine supplements.

NEUROLOGICAL COMPLICATIONS OF METHANOL

Methanol is most commonly ingested by chronic alcoholics who believe they are drinking ethanol. However, even dermal or respiratory absorption of methanol can lead to death or blindness.[98]

Etiology and Pathology Methanol is found in heating agents (canned heat), solvents, cleaning agents, paints, and rubbing alcohol. Methanol itself is not toxic. It is metabolized by alcohol dehydrogenase to formaldehyde and formic acid, both of which are toxic substances.

When methanol is ingested, it is rapidly absorbed. A severe metabolic acidosis results as methanol is metabolized. Formic acid has a toxic affect on oligodendrocytes due to inhibition of cytochrome oxidase, resulting in cerebral edema and axonal compression. The optic nerve is commonly involved.

Clinical Features   Approximately 12 to 48 h after ingestion, the patient begins to complain of headache, nausea, abdominal pain, and blurred vision. The visual symptoms may progress to blindness. The patient is restless, with a drunken appearance that may progress to delirium or seizures and coma.

Diagnostic Procedures

1.   Methanol and formic acid are present in the blood and urine.

2.   There is evidence of high anion-gap metabolic acidosis.

3.   There may be evidence of increased ICP.

Treatment

1.   The treatment of choice is hemodialysis. It permits removal of metabolites and restoration of pH without threat of fluid overload.

2.   As a competitive inhibitor of alcohol dehydrogenase, ethanol will slow the metabolism of methanol into its toxic metabolites. Ethanol should be administered in a loading dose of 50 mg intravenously or 60 mL orally, followed by 10 mg intravenously or 10 mL orally q1h.

3.   Severe metabolic acidosis should be corrected with intravenous bicarbonate.

Prognosis   Ingestion of more than 100 mL methanol is frequently fatal. Blindness is common and parkinsonism is an occasional complication.

NEUROLOGICAL COMPLICATIONS OF ETHYLENE GLYCOL POISONING

Etiology and Pathology   Ethylene glycol is found in antifreeze, detergents, and paints. It has a slightly sweet taste and may be ingested by children. Ethylene glycol is metabolized by alcohol dehydrogenase into toxic metabolites such as oxalic acid.

Clinical Features   The patient has a drunken appearance and develops confusion and stupor within an hour of ingestion of ethylene glycol. Seizures may occur. Between 12 and 24 h later, the patient becomes hypertensive and develops cardiopulmonary failure, acute oliguric renal failure, and coma.[99]

Diagnostic Procedures

1.   Severe high anion-gap metabolic acidosis and hypocalcemia occur.
2.   Examination of the urine reveals crystalluria and the presence of oxalate or hippurate crystals.
3.   Ethylene glycol is present in the blood.

Treatment   The treatment is the same as for methanol poisoning.

NEUROLOGICAL COMPLICATIONS OF COCAINE ABUSE

A number of potentially serious neurological complications have been identified in cocaine abusers.[100]

Cocaine use results in significant constriction of cerebral vessels and cerebral ischemia. In some cases, the development of a cerebral arteritis may result in ischemic or hemorrhagic cerebral infarction or intracerebral hemorrhage. There is also a high risk of subarachnoid hemorrhage from rupture of an aneurysm or arteriovenous malformation in cocaine abusers.

Headache, often associated with nausea, arthralgia, and abdominal and chest pain, is usually benign but recurrent. Generalized tonic-clonic seizures, tremor, and myoclonus may occur within a few hours of cocaine abuse, followed by restlessness, irritability, combativeness, or psychosis. Temporary focal neurological deficits, including transient visual, motor, or sensory disturbances, have been followed by cerebral infarction in a few cases. Long-term cocaine abuse may result in optic atrophy or permanent cognitive impairment. Regional cerebral blood flow studies have shown hypo-perfusion in the frontal periventricular and the temporoparietal areas.[101]

Treatment   Treatment of acute psychosis requires a potent, dopamine-blocking agent such as haloperidol. Seizures should be controlled by intravenous diazepam and phenytoin followed by oral phenytoin.

NEUROLOGICAL COMPLICATIONS OF HEROIN ABUSE

Heroin, a diacetyl derivative of morphine, is more potent and has a shorter period of action than morphine. Heroin is a popular illicit opiate administered by smoking, sniffing the powder up the nose, or injecting subcutaneously or intravenously. Heroin overdose results in respiratory depression and coma. Neurological complications include hypoxia, hypotension leading to anoxic encephalopathy, cerebral infarction, parkinsonism, or transverse myelitis.

Infection from repeated use of contaminated needles results in bacterial endocarditis and mycotic aneurysms. Meningitis, cerebral abscess, and thromboembolic cerebral infarction may occur. Ruptured mycotic aneurysms on the cerebral vessels result in subarachnoid hemorrhage.

Mononeuropathies can occur from injection of individual nerves. Brachial and lumbosacral plexopathies have been described.

Treatment

1. The acute effects of heroin respond to intravenous naloxone, a specific opiate antagonist. Repeated doses may be required.
2. Addicts should be treated in a withdrawal program followed by substitution with oral methadone to prevent recidivism.

Lead Poisoning

Etiology and Pathology   Lead and all inorganic and organic lead compounds are toxic to humans. Lead is absorbed more readily by inhalation than by ingestion, but either may produce toxicity. A blood lead level of more than 1.93 mmol/L is considered potentially toxic. Although the number of deaths from lead poisoning has decreased dramatically in the United States since the 1960s,[102] evidence suggests that low levels of lead may have subtle adverse effects on the mental development, hearing, and growth of young children.[103]

Absorbed lead enters all tissues but is stored preferentially in bone. Tertiary lead phosphate conversion to soluble secondary lead phosphate is enhanced by a low calcium diet, acidosis, multiple bone metastasis, and excess parathormone. The most common sources of lead poisoning are:

1. Inhalation or ingestion of lead by workers engaged in smelting of lead; demolition workers who cut contaminated steel with oxyacetylene torches; workers exposed to dust, fumes, or spray containing lead; those engaged in automobile radiator repairs; production of lead-containing gasoline; lead shot manufacturing; or burning of batteries. The latter has occurred in conditions of fuel shortage, when batteries are burned as a source of fuel.

2. Ingestion of lead paint found in older buildings by children with pica, or by chewing on or burning lead toys. (Lead paint is no longer available for interior decorating.)

3. The ingestion of soft water delivered through lead pipes or lead-contaminated "moonshine" whiskey distilled in old car radiators.

4. Gasoline sniffing of lead-containing gasoline and exposure to lead poisoning from lead shot embedded in the body.[104]

Lead enters the CNS as its blood concentration rises but is removed slowly when blood levels fall. Thus, intermittent exposure produces a gradual increase of lead in the CNS. In children, acute exposure to lead results in a sharp increase in lead concentration in the brain, with the production of cerebral edema and damage to capillary endothelium, increased capillary permeability, interstitial edema, and scattered hemorrhages.

Chronic exposure to lead at any age results in neuronal damage in the CNS and segmental demyelination followed by axonal damage to peripheral nerves.

Clinical Features

1. Lead encephalopathy. Affected children have a history of pica, vomiting, colic, and constipation. Cerebral edema produces drowsiness, which may proceed to coma. Focal or generalized seizures and status epilepticus may occur. Papilledema and focal neurological deficits are not uncommon. Increasing edema produces uncal herniation and death. Survivors may have chronic seizures, mental retardation, optic atrophy, and focal neurological abnormalities.

2. Chronic exposure in children may lead to mental retardation, learning disabilities, behavior problems, and hyperactivity.

3. Adult exposure to lead is followed by personality changes, dementia, rigidity, seizures, optic atrophy, and visual failure.

4. Chronic exposure to lead may result in the development of a condition resembling amyotrophic lateral sclerosis.

5. Chronic exposure in children and adults produces peripheral neuropathy, often presenting with weakness of the hands and bilateral wrist drop.

6. The practice of chronic gasoline sniffing, using leaded gasoline, leads to an encephalopathic process that may be fatal, and survivors often show residual neurological deficits.[105]

Diagnostic Procedures

1. Skull films may reveal evidence of increased ICP. The long bones may have a "lead line."
2. Examination of peripheral blood smear reveals hypochromic microcytic anemia. Basophilic stippling of the red blood cells is usually present.
3. Nerve conduction velocities are slowed in lead neuropathy.
4. Blood lead levels are elevated above 3.8 μmol/L.
5. Urine lead levels are more than 7.2 μmol/L in a 24-hour specimen. Coproporphyrin levels are elevated.

Treatment

1. Acute encephalopathy with increased ICP should be managed with intravenous infusions of manni-tol, corticosteroids, and ICP monitoring.
2. Chelating agents such as calcium, disodium versenate, British antilewisite (dimercaprol), or dimercaptosuccinic acid should be administered.[105,106] In adults, penicillamine may be added.
3. The source of lead exposure should be removed.

Prognosis The mortality rate of acute encephalopathy is less than 5 percent. However, severely affected children develop retardation, optic atrophy, seizure disorders, and behavior problems. Health education and nutritional counseling is the most effective approach for children with exposures less than 0.97 mmol/L (20 μg/dL). Children with levels greater than 0.97 mmol/L should receive more involved medical and environmental intervention aimed at reducing the absorption of lead by chelating therapy and identifying and removing sources of exposure.[107]

Mercury Poisoning

Etiology and Pathology Mercury is encountered in an inorganic form as metallic mercury or a mercuric salt, or as organic mercury, usually methyl mercury. Inorganic mercury is used in the paper and pulp industry, paint manufacturing, and the electric appliance industry. Organic mercury is used in fungicides and may be concentrated by animals and fish living in a polluted environment.

Mercury is toxic to the neurons of the occipital lobes and the granular cells of the cerebellum. Peripheral nerves show axonal degeneration and demyelination.

Clinical Features Early mercury poisoning is characterized by intermittent feelings of panic associated with fine tremor of the fingers, eyelids, and tongue, with progression to involve the arms, head, and legs.[108] Paresthesias of the extremities, followed by numbness, progressive distal weakness, and cerebellar ataxia, are also seen. Peripheral vision is progressively impaired, leading to blindness, slurring of speech, and impaired hearing. In advanced cases, seizures, mania, dementia, and hallucinations are seen.

Congenital mercury poisoning occurs at lower blood mercury levels than adult poisoning, due to the ability of the fetus and placenta to concentrate the metal. Affected children are small for their age, may have a seizure disorder, and may show psychomotor retardation.

Diagnostic Procedures

1. Mercury analysis of hair showing less than 100 ppm of mercury is usually safe and asymptomatic; levels approaching 500 ppm are always associated with symptoms. In children with congenital mercury poisoning, levels greater than 100 ppm are usually associated with significant damage to the nervous system.

2. The EEG may reveal slowing of background activity and epileptiform discharge.

3. Electromyography and nerve conduction studies show delayed motor and sensory distal latencies, reduced sensory response amplitude, and increased prevalence of abnormal electrical activity in muscle.[108]

4. Neuropsychological evaluation reveals significant deficits of attention and concentration, but no change in the level of intellectual functioning.[109]

Treatment   Chelation with penicillamine and the use of selenium and vitamin E have been effective in reducing the neurotoxic effects of mercury poisoning.

Arsenic Poisoning

Etiology and Pathology   Arsenic is found in paints, insecticides, rodenticides, and contaminated food or beer, and is occasionally used in suicide attempts and homicide.

Arsenic disrupts the tricarboxylic acid cycle by interfering with pyruvate oxidase and α-glutarate oxidase symptoms.

Clinical Features   A single large dose of arsenic produces vomiting followed by tachycardia, hypotension, and, in some cases, death. Survivors develop a peripheral neuropathy 2 or 3 weeks later.[110] This is characterized by a distal numbness and intense paresthesias. Position and vibration sense are severely involved. Muscle weakness is a late development. Recovery is slow and occurs over a period of several

months. Chronic exposure to arsenic produces a multisystem illness with several signs and symptoms, including dermatological, gastrointestinal, neurological and hematological conditions. The salient feature is the development of a slowly progressive peripheral neuropathy associated with leukopenia, anemia, and thrombocytopenia. The anemia is usually normochromic and normocytic but occasionally megaloblastic anemia has been described.[111]

Poisoning by organic arsenic insecticides may be followed by an acute symmetrical ascending polyneuropathy resembling acute inflammatory demyelinating polyneuropathy (Guillain-Barré syndrome).

Diagnostic Procedures

1. Lumbar puncture. The CSF glucose and protein content is normal.
2. The blood level of arsenic is 7 ng/100 ml or greater. The urine contains greater than 1 mg/24 hr.
3. Nerve biopsy reveals demyelination and axonal degeneration.
4. Nerve conduction velocities are slowed.

Treatment   The source of arsenic should be avoided. British antilewisite (BAL) and penicillamine are effective chelating agents.

Manganese Poisoning

Manganese is encountered in mining and industrial processes and enters the body by inhalation. This results in a marked neuronal loss in the basal ganglia, particularly in the globus pallidus.[112]

Manganese is primarily cleared by the liver, so an increased concentration in the brain may be the result of manganese overload in patients with liver disease.[113]

Patients with manganese intoxication present with a psychiatric disorder characterized by nervousness, irritability, and emotional lability. This is followed by generalized weakness, impotence, parkinsonism, increased muscle tone, and exaggerated tendon reflexes. The blood manganese level is greater than 0.075 ppm and the administration of 1 g ethylenediaminetetraacetic acid increases the urine level by 0.03 to 0.05 ppm. L-dopa is effective in relieving some of the symptoms of parkinsonism. However, this may be temporary and many patients fail to respond to this medication.[114]

NEUROLOGICAL MANIFESTATIONS OF INDUSTRIAL TOXINS

Table 17–4 lists the more common industrial toxins, where they are encountered, and the neurological signs and symptoms of toxicity.

NEUROLOGICAL MANIFESTATIONS OF PESTICIDES

Organophosphate Pesticide Poisoning

Organophosphates are compounds used in agriculture as pesticides. They are lipid-soluble compounds related to nerve gas, which was developed as a chemical warfare agent during World War II. The mode of action is an irreversible inhibition of cholinesterases, including acetylcholinesterase, which acts in the degradation of acetylcholine at the neuromuscular junction. Persistence of acetylcholine leads to a

Table 17-4
Industrial toxins and neurological signs and symptoms

Toxin	Exposure	Neurological signs and symptoms of toxicity
Acrylamide	Workers handling acrylamide monomer	Sensorimotor polyneuropathy Truncal ataxia
Allyl chloride	Industrial exposure	Polyneuropathy
Carbamates	Pesticides	Sensorimotor polyneuropathy
Carbon disulfide	Cellophane and textile industry Pesticides	Polyneuropathy Psychosis
Carbon tetrachloride	Fire extinguishers Cleaning agents	Polyneuropathy, optic atrophy Cerebellar ataxia, parkinsonism
Gasoline, lead-based	Gasoline sniffing Inhalant abuse	Tremor, ataxia Euphoria, visual hallucinations Irreversible encephalopathy, polyneuropathy
Methyl bromide	Refrigerants, insecticides Fumigants	Sensorimotor polyneuropathy Diplopia, vertigo Ataxia, nystagmus
Methyl-*n*-butyl	Industrial exposure	Polyneuropathy
N-hexane	Glue sniffing Industrial exposure	Sensorimotor polyneuropathy
Nitrous oxide (laughing gas)	Inhalant abuse	Polyneuropathy
Organophosphates	Insecticides, nerve gas	Early: lacrimation, twitching and convulsions, respiratory failure Delayed: sensorimotor polyneuropathy
Thallium	Rodenticides Industrial use	Motor polyneuropathy, cranial nerve palsies Convulsions, psychosis Dementia
Toluene	Spray paint Inhalant abuse	Acute: euphoria, perceptual disorders Subacute: cerebellar damage, polyneuropathy

cholinergic crisis, with muscle paralysis. Organophosphates (parathion, malathion) are used widely as pesticides and in sheep dip in North America and Europe. Poisoning is often the result of a suicide attempt by ingestion.

The immediate response following poisoning is a cholinergic crisis with respiratory failure. The intermediate phase consists of paralysis of motor cranial nerves, neck muscles, and proximal limb muscles 24 to 96 h after poisoning.[115] Chronic exposure to organophosphate pesticides in sheep dip results in subtle changes in the nervous system when measured by neuropsychological performance.[116]

Clinical Features   In acute cases, muscarinic effects are evident within short periods of exposure or ingestion to organophosphate compounds. These begin with muscle twitching and the appearance of fasciculations, followed by drooling, bronchospasm with wheezing and coughing, and increased bronchial secretions leading to respiratory distress and pulmonary edema. Peripherally there is sweating, anorexia, vomiting, diarrhea, bradycardia, and involuntary incontinence of bowel and bladder. The patient may be hypotensive. Pupils are constricted and there are fasciculations of the eyelids.

This stage is followed by progressive muscle weakness leading to paralysis of the respiratory muscles and respiratory failure, necessitating assisted ventilation.

Diagnostic   Procedures   Acetylcholinesterase activity is reduced, often below 50 percent.

Treatment

1. Assisted ventilation with a mechanical ventilator may be required at any stage.
2. The acute cholinergic phase requires large intravenous doses of atropine beginning at 2 to 4 mg, followed by 2 mg every 5 min, until muscarinic symptoms disappear. This should be supplemented by pralidoxime 1 to 2 g intravenously every 5 min, which reactivates cholinesterase. Obidoxime hydrochloride is an effective alternative to pralidoxime. Obidoxime hydrochloride 200 mg intravenously should be given within 12 h of ingestion

or exposure to organophosphates to be effective.[117] The effect of treatment can be monitored by neuromuscular transmission studies, which are performed during the administration of pralidoxime or obidoxime.

Carbamate Pesticide Poisoning

Carbamic acid esters, which differ structurally from organophosphates, are also used as pesticides. Carbamates inhibit acetylcholinesterase and acute delayed toxic effects are similar to those encountered with organophosphate exposure. The clinical features of severe anticholinesterase poisoning have been described in organophosphate poisoning. A delayed symmetrical polyneuropathy has been described in carbamate poisoning, resembling the neuropathy of triorthocresyl phosphate poisoning, another compound accidentally ingested in the past, which inhibits cholinesterase.[118]

Treatment   Treatment is identical to that described under organophosphate poisoning.

REFERENCES

1. Kaufman DM, Lipton RB: The persistent vegetative state: an analysis of clinical correlates and costs. *NY State J Med* 92:381, 1992.
2. Salama J, Gherardi R, Amiel H, et al: Post anoxic delayed encephalopathy and leukoencephalopathy and non-hemorrhagic cerebral amyloid angiopathy. *Clin Neuropathol* 5:153, 1986.
3. Practice parameters for determining brain death in adults (summary statement). The Quality Standards Subcommittee of the American Academy of Neurology. *Neurology* 45:1012, 1995.
4. Dean BS, Verdile VP, Krenzelok EP: Coma reversal with cerebral dysfunction recovery after repetitive hyperbaric oxygen therapy for severe carbon monoxide poisoning. *Am J Emerg Med* 11:616, 1993.
5. Wijdicks EF: Determining brain death in adults. *Neurology* 45:1003, 1995.
6. Hung TP, Chen ST: Prognosis of deeply comatose patients on ventilators. *J Neurol Neurosurg Psychiatry* 58:75, 1995.
7. Wijdicks EF: In search of a safe apnea test in brain

death: is the procedure really more dangerous than we think? *Arch Neurol* 52:338, 1995.

8. Ayus JC, Wheeler JM, Arieff AI: Postoperative hyponatremic encephalopathy in menstruant women. *Ann Intern Med* 117:891, 1992.

9. Kroll M, Juhler M, Lindholm J: Hyponaetramia in acute brain disease. *J Intern Med* 232:291, 1992.

10. Harris CP, Townsend JJ, Baringer JR: Symptomatic hyponatraemia: can myelinolysis be prevented by treatment? *J Neurol Neurosurg Psychiatry* 56:626, 1993.

11. Karp BI, Laureno R: Pontine and extrapontine myelinolysis: a neurologic disorder following rapid correction of hyponatremia. *Medicine (Baltimore)* 72:359, 1993.

12. Oster JR, Singer I: Hyponatremia: focus on therapy. *South Med J* 87:1195, 1994.

13. Snyder NA, Feigel DW, Arieff AI: Hypernatremia in elderly patients. A heterogeneous, morbid, and iatrogenic entity. *Ann Intern Med* 107:309, 1987.

14. Hiromatsu K, Kobayashi T, Fujii N, et al: Hypernatremic myopathy. *J Neurol Sci* 122:144, 1994.

15. Thomas S, Sainsbury CP: Treatment of hypernatraemic dehydration due to diarrhoea. *Br J Clin Pract* 40:535, 1986.

16. Linshaw MA: Potassium homeostasis and hypokalemia. *Pediatr Clin North Am* 34:649, 1987.

17. Villabona C, Rodriguez P, Joven J, et al: Potassium disturbances as a cause of metabolic neuromyopathy. *Intensive Care Med* 13:208, 1987.

18. McIvor ME: Delayed fatal hyperkalemia in a patient with acute fluoride intoxication. *Ann Emerg Med* 16:1165, 1987.

19. Moe SM, Sprague SM: Uremic encephalopathy. *Clin Nephrol* 42:251, 1994.

20. Beccari M: Seizures in dialysis patients treated with recombinant erythropoietin. Review of the literature and guidelines for prevention. *Int J Artif Org* 17:5, 1994.

21. DeWeerd AW, Nihom J, Rozeman CA, et al: H reflexes as a measure for uremic polyneuropathy. A longitudinal study in patients treated with dialysis or renal transplantation. *Electroencephalogr Clin Neurophysiol* 93:276, 1994.

22. Yoshida S, Tajika T, Yomasaki N, et al: Dialysis disequilibrium syndrome in neurosurgical patients. *Neurosurgery* 20:716, 1987.

23. Arieff AI: Dialysis disequilibrium syndrome: Current concepts on pathogenesis and prevention. *Kidney Int* 45:629, 1994.

24. Parfrey PS: Cardiac and cerebrovascular disease in chronic uremia. *Am J Kidney Dis* 21:77, 1993.

25. Sivri A, Celiker R, Sungar C, et al: Carpal tunnel syndrome: a major complication in hemodialysis patients. *Scand J Rheumatol* 23:287, 1994.

26. Murray JC, Tanner CM, Sprague SM: Aluminum neurotoxicity: a revaluation. *Clin Neuropharmacol* 14:179, 1991.

27. Greger JL, Baier MJ: Excretion and retention of low or moderate levels of aluminum by human subjects. *Food Chem Toxicol* 21:473, 1983.

28. Mujais SK: Muscle cramps during hemodialysis. *Int J Artif Organs* 17:570, 1994.

29. Jagadha V, Deck JH, Halliday WC, et al: Wernicke's encephalopathy in patients on peritoneal dialysis or hemodialysis. *Ann Neurol* 21:78, 1987.

30. Collis I, Lloyd G: Psychiatric aspects of liver disease. *Br J Psychiatry* 161:12, 1992.

31. Kirsh BM, Lam N, Layden TJ, et al: Diagnosis and management of fulminant hepatic failure. *Compr Ther* 21:166, 1995.

32. Decell MK, Gordon JB, Silver K, et al: Fulminant hepatic failure associated with status epilepticus in children: three cases and a review of potential mechanisms. *Intensive Care Med* 20:375, 1994.

33. Farrell FJ, Keeffe EB, Man KM, et al: Treatment of hepatic failure secondary to isoniazid hepatitis with liver transplantation. *Dig Dis Sci* 39:2255, 1994.

34. Lidofsky SD: Fulminant hepatic failure. *Crit Care Clin* 11:415, 1995.

35. Pappas SC: Fulminant viral hepatitis. *Gastroenterol Clin North Am* 24:161, 1995.

36. Nemni R, Bottacchi E, Fazio R, et al: Polyneuropathy in hypothyroidism: clinical electrophysiological and morphological findings in four cases. *J Neurol Neurosurg Psychiatry* 50:1454, 1987.

37. Jordan RM: Myxedema coma. Pathophysiology, therapy, and factors affecting prognosis. *Med Clin North Am* 79:185, 1995.

38. Morrow JS, Miller RH: Diagnosis and management of primary hyperparathyroidism. *J Louisiana State Med Soc* 146:77, 1994.

39. Bilezikian JP, Martin TJ: Parathyroid hormone-related disorders. *Henry Ford Hospital Medical Journal* 36:159, 1988.

40. Chiba T, Okimura Y, Inatome T, et al: Hypocalcemic crisis in alcoholic fatty liver with transient hypoparathyroidism due to magnesium deficiency. *Am J Gastroenterol* 82:1084, 1987.

41. Ikeda K, Kobayashi T, Kusakari J, et al. Sensorineural hearing loss associated with hypoparathyroidism. *Laryngoscope* 97:1075, 1987.

42. Connor TB, Rosen BL, Blaustein MP, et al: Hypocalcemia precipitating congestive heart failure. *N Engl J Med* 307:869, 1982.

43. Walls J, Ratcliffe WA, Howell A, et al: Parathyroid hormone and parathyroid hormone-related protein in the investigation of hypercalcaemia in two hospital populations. *Clin Endocrinol* 41:407, 1994.

44. Jamal GA, Kerr DJ, McLellan AR, et al: Generalized peripheral nerve dysfunction in acromegaly: a study by conventional and novel neurophysiological techniques. *J Neurol Neurosurg Psychiatry* 50:886, 1987.

45. Kinzie BJ: Management of the syndrome of inappropriate secretion of antidiuretic hormone. *Clin Pharm* 6:625, 1987.

46. Harrigan MR: Cerebral salt wasting syndrome: a review. *Neurosurgery* 38:152, 1996.

47. Lakhdar AA, McLaren EH, Davda NS, et al: Pituitary failure from Sheehan's syndrome in the puerperium. Two case reports. *Br J Obstet Gynaecol* 94:998, 1987.

48. Nukta EM, Taylor HC: Panhypopituitarism secondary to an aneurysm of the anterior communicating artery. *Can Med Assoc J* 137:413, 1987.

49. Round R, Keane JR: The minor symptoms of increased intracranial pressure: 101 patients with benign intracranial hypertension. *Neurology* 38:1461, 1988.

50. Allen RS, Sarma PR: Pseudopseudotumor cerebri: Meningeal carcinomatosis presenting as benign intracranial hypertension. *South Med J* 80:1182, 1987.

51. Rosenberg ML, Corbett JJ, Smith C, et al: Cerebrospinal fluid diversion procedures in pseudotumor cerebri. *Neurology* 43:1071, 1993.

52. Sima AA: Pathological definition and evaluation of diabetic neuropathy and clinical correlations. *Can J Neurol Sci* 21(suppl 4):S13, 1994.

53. Vanderpump M, Taylor R: New concepts in diabetes mellitus II: complications. *Postgrad Med J* 70:479, 1994.

54. Krendel DA, Costigan DA, Hopkins LC: Successful treatment of neuropathies in patients with diabetes mellitus. *Arch Neurol* 52:1053, 1995.

55. Boulton AJ: End-stage complications of diabetic neuropathy: foot ulceration. *Can J Neurol Sci* 21(suppl 4):S18, 1994.

56. Fore WW: Noninsulin-dependent diabetes mellitus. The prevention of complications. *Med Clin North Am* 79:287, 1995.

57. Bril V: Role of electrophysiological studies in diabetic neuropathy. *Can J Neurol Sci* 21(suppl 4):S8, 1994.

58. The effect of intensive diabetes therapy on the development and progression of neuropathy. The Diabetes Control and Complications Trial Research Group. *Ann Intern Med* 122:561, 1995.

59. Basso A, Dalla Paola L, Boscaro M, et al: Licorice ameliorates postural hypotension caused by diabetic autonomic neuropathy. *Diabetes Care* 17:1356, 1994.

60. Peterson BA, Brunning RD, Bloomfield CD, et al: Central nervous system involvement in acute nonlymphocytic leukemia. A prospective study of adults in remission. *Am J Med* 83:464, 1987.

61. Hoffman MA, Valderrama E, Fuchs A, et al: Leukemic meningitis in B-cell prolymphocytic leukemia. A clinical, pathologic, and ultrastructural case study and a review of the literature. *Cancer* 75:1100, 1995.

62. Higgins SA, Peschel RE: Hodgkin's disease with spinal cord compression. A case report and a review of the literature. *Cancer* 75:94, 1995.

63. Landan I, Gilroy J, Wolfe DE: Syringomyelia affecting the entire spinal cord secondary to primary spinal intramedullary central nervous system lymphoma. *J Neurol Neurosurg Psychiatry* 50:1533, 1987.

64. DeAngelis LM, Yahalom J, Heinemann MH, et al: Primary CNS lymphoma: combined treatment with chemotherapy and radiotherapy. *Neurology* 40:80, 1990.

65. Nobile-Orazio E, Marmiroli P, Baldini L, et al: Peripheral neuropathy in macroglobulinemia: incidence and antigen-specificity of M proteins. *Neurology* 37:1506, 1987.

66. Blume G, Pestronk A, Goodnough LT: Anti-MAG antibody-associated polyneuropathies: improvement following immunotherapy with monthly plasma exchange and IV cyclophosphamide. *Neurology* 45:1577, 1995.

67. Shakil AO, Di Bisceglie AM: Images in clinical medicine. Vasculitis and cryoglobulinemia related to hepatitis C. *N Engl J Med* 331:1624, 1994.

68. Lippa CF, Chad DA, Smith TW, et al: Neuropathy associated with cryoglobulinemia. *Muscle Nerve* 9:626, 1986.

69. Dammacco F, Sansonno D, Han JH, et al: Natural interferon alpha versus its combination with 6 methyl prednisolone in the therapy of type II mixed cryoglobulinemia: a long-term randomized controlled study. *Blood* 84:3336, 1994.

70. Silverstein MN: Relative and absolute polycythemia. How to tell them apart. *Postgrad Med* 81:285, 1987.

71. Tefferi A, Colgan JP, Solberg LA Jr: Acute porphyrias: diagnosis and management. *Mayo Clin Proc* 69:991, 1994.

72. Adams M, Rhyner PA, Day J, et al: Whipple's disease confined to the central nervous system. *Ann Neurol* 21:104, 1987.

73. Schwartz MA, Selhorst JB, Ochs AL, et al: Oculomasticatory myorhythmia: a unique movement disorder occurring in Whipple's disease. *Ann Neurol* 20:677, 1986.

74. Cooper GS, Blades EW, Remler BF, et al: Central nervous system Whipple's disease: Relapse during therapy with trimethoprim-sulfamethoxazole and remission with cefixime. *Gastroenterology* 106:782, 1994.

75. Tintoré M, Montalban J, Cervera C, et al: Peripheral neuropathy in association with insulinoma: clinical features and neuropathology of a new case. *J Neurol Neurosurg Psychiatry* 57:1009, 1994.

76. Chalk CH, Windebank AJ, Kimmel DW, et al: The distinctive clinical features of paraneoplastic sensory neuronopathy. *Can J Neurol Sci* 19:346, 1992.

77. Vega F, Graus F, Chen QM, et al: Intrathecal synthesis of the anti-Hu antibody in patients with paraneoplastic encephalomyelitis or sensory neuronopathy. clinical-immunologic correlation. *Neurology* 44:2145, 1994.

78. Green R, Kinsella LJ: Current concepts in the diagnosis of cobalamin deficiency. *Neurology* 45:1435, 1995.

79. Traber MG, Sokol RJ, Ringel SP, et al: Lack of tocopherol in peripheral nerves of vitamin E-deficient patients with peripheral neuropathy. *N Engl J Med* 317:262, 1987.

80. Yokota T, Wada Y, Furukawa T, et al: Adult-onset spinocerebellar syndrome with idiopathic vitamin E deficiency. *Ann Neurol* 22:84, 1987.

81. Lipson T: The fetal alcohol syndrome in Australia. *Med J Aust* 161:461, 1994.

82. Duffens K, Marx JA: Alcoholic ketoacidosis—a review. *J Emerg Med* 5:399, 1987.

83. McMicken DB, Freedland ES: Alcohol-related seizures. Pathophysiology, differential diagnosis, evaluation, and treatment. *Emerg Med Clin North Am* 12:1057, 1994.

84. Diamond I, Messing RO: Neurologic effects of alcoholism. *West J Med* 161:279, 1994.

85. Thomson AD, Jeyasingham MD: Nutrition and alcoholic encephalopathies. *Acta Med Scand* 717 (suppl):55, 1987.

86. Pearce SH, Rees CJ: Coma in Wernicke's encephalopathy (letter). *Postgrad Med J* 70:597, 1994.

87. Harter SB, Nokes SR: Gadolinium-enhanced MR findings in a pediatric case of Wernicke encephalopathy. *AJNR Am J Neuroradiol* 16:700, 1995.

88. Chataway J, Hardman E: Thiamine in Wernicke's syndrome—how much and how long? (letter). *Postgrad Med J* 71:249, 1995.

89. Morris JC, Victor M: Alcohol withdrawal seizures. *Emerg Med Clin North Am* 5:827, 1987.

90. Lishman WA, Jacobson RR, Acker C: Brain damage in alcoholism: current concepts. *Acta Med Scand* 717 (suppl):5, 1987.

91. Parsons OA: Intellectual impairment in alcoholics: persistent issues. *Acta Med Scand* 717(suppl):33, 1987.

92. Carlen PL, Wilkinson DA: Reversibility of alcohol-related brain damage: clinical and experimental observations. *Acta Med Scand* 717(suppl):19, 1987.

93. Charness ME, Simon RP, Greenberg DA: Ethanol and the nervous system. *N Engl J Med* 321:442, 1989.

94. Rippe D, Edwards MK, D'Amour PG, et al: MR imaging of central pontine myelinolysis. *J Comput Assist Tomogr* 11:724, 1987.

95. Cavanagh JB, Holton JL, Nolan CC: Selective damage to cerebellar vermis in chronic alcoholism: a contribution from neurotoxicology to an old problem of selective vulnerability. *Neuropath Appl Neurobiol* 23:355, 1997.

96. Shankar K, Maloney FP, Thompson C: An electrodiagnostic study in chronic alcoholic subjects. *Arch Phys Med Rehab* 68:803, 1987.

97. Preedy VR, Salisbury JR, Peters TJ: Alcoholic muscle disease: features and mechanisms. *J Pathol* 173:309, 1994.

98. Haines JD Jr: Methanol poisoning. How to recognize and treat a deadly intoxication. *Postgrad Med* 81:149, 1987.

99. Verrilli MR, Deyling CL, Pippenger CE, et al: Fatal ethylene glycol intoxication. Report of a case and review of the literature. *Cleve Clin J Med* 54:289, 1987.

100. Levine SR, Washington JM, Jefferson MF, et al: "Crack" cocaine-associated stroke. *Neurology* 37:1849, 1987.

101. Strickland TL, Mena I, Villaneuva-Meyer J, et al: Cerebral perfusion and neuropsychological consequences of chronic cocaine use. *J Neuropsychiatry Clin Neurosci* 5:419, 1993.

102. Staes C, Matte T, Staeling N, et al: Lead poisoning deaths in the United States, 1979 through 1988. *JAMA* 273:847, 1995.

103. Jin A, Hertzman C, Peck SH, et al: Blood lead levels in children aged 24 to 36 months in Vancouver. *Can Med Assoc J* 152:1077, 1995.

104. Wu PB, Kingery WS, Date ES: An EMG case report of lead neuropathy 19 years after a shotgun injury. *Muscle Nerve* 18:326, 1995.

105. Burns CB, Currie B: The efficacy of chelation therapy and factors influencing mortality in lead intoxicated petrol sniffers. *Aust N Z J Med* 25:197, 1995.

106. Besunder JB, Anderson RL, Super DM: Short-term efficacy of oral dimercaptosuccinic acid in children with low to moderate lead intoxication. *Pediatrics* 96: 683, 1995.

107. Norman EH, Bordley WC, Hertz-Picciotto I, et al: Rural-urban blood lead differences in North Carolina children. *Pediatrics* 94:59, 1994.

108. Singer R, Valciukas JA, Rosenman KD: Peripheral neurotoxicity in workers exposed to inorganic mercury compounds. *Arch Environ Health* 42:181, 1987.

109. O'Carroll RE, Masterton G, Dougall N, et al: The neuropsychiatric sequelae of mercury poisoning. The Mad Hatter's disease revisited. *Br J Psychiatry* 167:95, 1995.

110. Hay R, McCormack JG: Arsenic poisoning and peripheral neuropathy. *Aust Fam Physician* 16:287, 1987.

111. Heaven R, Duncan M, Vukelja SJ: Arsenic intoxication presenting with macrocytosis and peripheral neuropathy without anemia. *Acta Haematol* 92:142, 1994.

112. Calne DB, Chu NS, Huang CC, et al: Manganism and idiopathic parkinsonism: similarities and differences. *Neurology* 44:1583, 1994.

113. Hauser RA, Zesiewicz TA, Rosemurgy AS, et al: Manganese intoxication and chronic liver failure. *Ann Neurol* 36:871, 1994.

114. Lu CS, Huang CC, Chu NS, et al: Levodopa failure in chronic manganism. *Neurology* 44:1600, 1994.

115. Senanayake N, Karalliedde L: Neurotoxic effects of organophosphorus insecticides: An intermediate syndrome. *N Engl J Med* 316:761, 1987.

116. Stephens R, Spurgeon A, Calvert IA, et al: Neuropsychological effects of long-term exposure to organophosphates in sheep dip. *Lancet* 345:1135, 1995.

117. Besser R, Weilemann LS, Gutmann L: Efficacy of obidoxime in human organophosphorus poisoning: determination by neuromuscular transmission studies. *Muscle Nerve* 18:15, 1995.

118. Dickoff DJ, Gerber O, Turovsky Z: Delayed neurotoxicity after ingestion of carbamate pesticide. *Neurology* 37:1229, 1987.

Chapter 18

TRAUMA

Head injury is a common neurological and neurosurgical condition in the United States. It has been estimated that more than one million persons suffer head injury each year and that one-third of accidental deaths are due to head injury. Although the majority of head injuries are trivial, a small percentage of patients suffer severe handicaps and present a major problem in terms of medical care, economic loss, and human suffering.

Most cases of severe head injury are the result of automobile and motorcycle accidents. The general acceptance of these forms of transportation as a modern "way of life" has resulted in apathetic tolerance of the increased risk of severe head injury.

ETIOLOGY AND PATHOLOGY

Traumatic injury to the brain may be primary or secondary.[1] Primary injury is produced by forces of acceleration and deceleration damaging the intracranial contents because of disproportionate movement of the skull and brain. The anteromedial tips of the frontal lobes may be damaged by contact with the frontal bone and the rough floor of the anterior cranial fossa, while the anterior temporal lobe may be injured by the edges of the sphenoid ridge. Damage to the corpus callosum can occur during head injury through contact with the free edge of the falx cerebri. Contact with the tentorium cerebelli can cause damage to the superior surface of the cerebellum or to the brainstem.

When the head strikes a solid object, there is sudden deceleration of the head with subsequent deformity of the skull, a decrease in volume of the cranial contents, and a rise in cerebrospinal pressure. A pressure wave passes from the point of impact through the cranial contents and exits at the opposite side of the brain. The initial impact and negative pressure wave produces tearing of tissue at the site of injury. The exiting pressure wave is associated with the release of energy at the interface of the brain and cerebrospinal fluid (i.e., the interface of a solid and liquid), which results in damage to the brain producing a contrecoup injury.

However, the most important factor in traumatic brain injury is shearing[2]—rapid recurrent rotational forces applied to the brain immediately following traumatic injury. In the mildest of situations, shearing results in concussion with no more than a brief episode of disorientation or brief loss of consciousness with rapid recovery. This state is the response of shearing forces applied to axons passing from the cortical gray matter through the white matter to other areas of the central nervous system (CNS). The concussion effect of the shearing forces is brief and recovery complete. It follows, therefore, that the more intense or repetitive the shearing forces, the more the axonal damage, the longer the duration of loss of consciousness, and the slower the recovery. In practice, the clinical picture is one of coma followed by posttraumatic amnesia. Consequently, the severity of closed head injury can be measured in the duration of coma and posttraumatic amnesia. However, shearing may be of sufficient magnitude to disrupt axons, which ultimately retract toward the cell body, producing axon retraction balls, glial proliferation, and demyelination in the brain parenchyma. Axonal shearing is then the ultimate and paramount primary event in the closed head injury—the greater the axonal disruption, the longer the coma and posttraumatic amnesia, and the more substantial the permanent brain damage.[3] However, secondary factors add to the ultimate result of brain injury because shearing results in laceration of the brain, tearing of blood vessels, hemorrhage, vascular spasm, cerebral edema, intracranial hypertension, reduction in cerebral blood flow, ischemia, hypoxia, all leading to delayed neuronal damage and neuronal death.[4] More than 50 percent of patients dying of head injury have suffered significant secondary changes in the brain,[5] and ischemia is the most important secondary insult[6] present in 80 percent of fatal cases, despite continuous monitoring in an intensive care unit.[7]

Cerebral Blood Flow After Trauma

Evidence mainly from intracranial Doppler ultrasonography indicates that there is a significant reduction in cerebral blood flow following closed head injury.[8] This may be the first phase of ischemia following head injury and the initial phase of ischemic neuronal damage. A second factor to be considered is the occurrence of systemic hypotension in individuals with severe extracranial injuries. Because brain injury is likely to be associated with loss of cerebral autoregulation, systemic vascular hypotension will result in a precipitous fall in cerebral perfusion and a diffuse cerebral hypoxia. This will be followed by cerebral edema, increasing intracranial hypertension, and an increase in venous pressure and further cerebral ischemia.

Other causes of cerebral edema and intracranial hypertension include vasogenic edema in response to intracerebral hemorrhage and cytotoxic edema owing to hypoxia and metabolic changes in neurons and glial cells. The persistent increase in intracranial pressure (ICP) above 20 mmHg is associated with an increase in neuronal damage and a clinical outcome of severe neurological deficits, vegetative state, or death. Many patients who have a slight increase in initial ICP between 11 and 20 mmHg have a poor outcome compared to individuals with initial ICP of 0 to 10 mmHg.[9]

Neuronal Damage and Death

Cerebral hypoxia following head injury is followed by neuronal dysfunction or neuronal death as described in cerebral infarction.

In summary, the conditions leading to brain damage following trauma include epidural hematoma, subdural hematoma, intracranial hematoma or hemorrhage, subarachnoid hemorrhage, and axonal shearing in closed head injury. Other traumatic events include damage to cranial nerves and traumatic CSF rhinorrhea or otorrhea.

TRAUMATIC INTRACRANIAL HEMORRHAGE

Epidural Hematoma

Definition An *epidural hematoma* is an acute hemorrhage into the epidural space. The condition has a 20 percent mortality rate.

Etiology and Pathology The hemorrhage usually occurs with a temporal parietal skull fracture in which the middle meningeal artery or vein are lacerated. In unusual cases, these vessels may be torn during a severe blow to the head without the occurrence of a fracture. Because the middle meningeal artery is frequently involved, there is rapid accumulation of blood in the epidural space with a rapid rise in ICP, uncal herniation, and brainstem compression.

Clinical Features There is a history of head injury with loss of consciousness. In about 50 percent of cases the patient recovers consciousness and there is a "lucid interval" followed by a gradual decrease in the level of consciousness as ICP increases and rostral cortical deterioration occurs (see Chap. 2). In the remaining cases, the lucid interval does not occur, and loss of consciousness is followed by progressive deterioration. An epidural hematoma occasionally occurs in the posterior fossa in which case sudden death may occur as the result of compression of the cardiorespiratory centers in the medulla. Patients who do not experience a lucid interval and those who are involved in high-speed automobile accidents are expected to have poorer prognoses.

Diagnostic Procedures

1.   A computed tomography (CT) scan taken in the emergency center will demonstrate an acute epidural hematoma (Fig. 18-1). These hematomas cannot always be distinguished from an acute subdural hematoma although the epidural hematoma is almost always lenticular in shape. The scan will also show shift of the midline structures and compression of the ipsilateral ventricular system with dilatation of the contralateral ventricle in about 60 percent of cases indicating obstruction of the ventricular system and hydrocephalus.

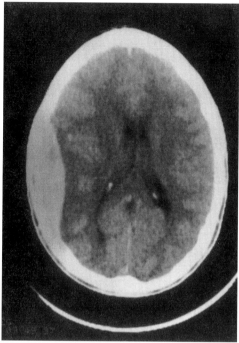

Figure 18-1
Epidural hematoma. The CT scan shows area of increased density in right epidural space. Typical lenticulate structure exerts pressure on the right cerebral hemisphere.

2. Skull films typically show a linear fracture of the temporal parietal area that crosses the middle meningeal vessels. There may be displacement of the calcified pineal gland to the opposite side.

Treatment Emergency neurosurgical evacuation of the hematoma is the treatment of choice. When there are signs of rapidly increasing ICP, the performance of this procedure may be based on the clinical evidence alone. Under these circumstances, the surgical exploration is carried out along the site of the skull fracture.

Acute Subdural Hematoma

Definition An *acute subdural hematoma* is an acute and progressive accumulation of blood in the subdural space. It carries a 50 to 80 percent mortality rate.

Etiology and Pathology Acute subdural hematoma usually follows severe head injury and is associated with considerable damage to the underlying brain.[10] There are a number of rarer causes of acute subdural hematoma including rupture of a saccular aneurysm, bleeding from an arteriovenous malformation, lumbar puncture followed by sudden alteration in ICP, and tearing of bridging veins, or as a rare complication of a bleeding diathesis or anticoagulant therapy.

Head injury causes rupture of the bridging veins that traverse the subdural space to reach the dural sinuses. The brain shows the presence of contusion, hematoma formation, diffuse axonal injury, and edema with displacement of the ventricular system.

Clinical Features There is usually a history of severe head injury with rapid loss of consciousness followed by progressive deterioration with deepening coma and signs of brainstem compression. In some cases, the history suggests the presence of an epidural hematoma because of the occurrence of a lucid interval. Examination may show signs of uncal herniation and rostral-caudal deterioration (see Chap. 2).

Diagnostic Procedures A CT scan taken in the emergency center readily reveals the presence of a subdural hematoma. The inner edge of the hematoma may be concave or convex in relationship to the underlying surface of the brain. A convex lesion suggests the presence of an epidural hematoma or a large subdural hematoma. There are compression of the lateral ventricle on the side of the hematoma and shift of the midline structures. Cerebral edema is not unusual in acute subdural hematoma. A magnetic resonance imaging (MRI) scan is equally effective in demonstrating an acute subdural hematoma but is usually not readily available in the emergency department (Fig. 18-2).

Treatment An acute subdural hematoma is a neurosurgical emergency, and the hematoma must be evacuated as soon as possible. The prognosis is poor when there is diffuse swelling of one hemisphere on the side of the acute hematoma, multiple intracerebral hemorrhages, or hydrocephalus with increased ICP.

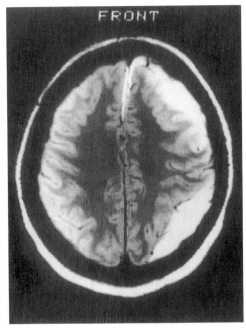

Figure 18-2
An MRI scan T1-weighted image shows an acute sub-dural hematoma after closed head injury.

Subacute Subdural Hematoma

A number of patients with acute head injury have a slow accumulation of blood in the subdural space, which occurs over 1 to 10 days. These patients appear to recover from head injury, which may be quite trivial, and then develop increasing headache, drowsiness, and progressive neurological deterioration. The diagnosis is established by MRI or CT scan. The condition is treated by surgical evacuation of the hematoma.

Chronic Subdural Hematoma

Definition A *chronic subdural hematoma* is an encapsulated accumulation of blood and CSF in the subdural space, which requires at least 10 days to develop.

Etiology and Pathology Chronic subdural hematomas often follow minor head injury. The hematoma develops as a result of tearing of bridging veins with accumulation of blood within the subdural

space. The blood clots and later hemolyzes. The higher osmotic pressure of the hemolyzed blood draws CSF through the arachnoid membrane and increases the volume of the hematoma. This produces tearing of vessels at the periphery of the hematoma and further bleeding into the subdural space, which increases osmotic pressure and attracts more CSF. Proliferation of fibroblasts occurs in the dura and arachnoid, and the collection eventually becomes surrounded by a fibroblastic membrane that thickens over a period of several weeks. Calcification occurs in chronic cases.

Clinical Features The condition most commonly occurs in the elderly and demented or alcoholic patients with atrophied brains. The history of head injury may not be obtained from an elderly debilitated patient or from patients with poor memory. However, younger patients often give a history of quite trivial head injury. Patients with chronic subdural hematomas are conscious but may be confused with a characteristic waxing and waning of symptoms. When alert, the patient complains of generalized headache, and there is impairment of intellectual capacity and recent memory. Dysphasia may occur when the subdural hematoma compresses the dominant hemisphere. There is contralateral hemiparesis with increased tendon reflexes and an extensor plantar response. The gradual increase in ICP may produce uncal herniation and progressive rostral-caudal deterioration. Papilledema is not unusual at this stage.

Diagnostic Procedures

1.   Either MRI or CT scanning is diagnostic with demonstration of a subdural collection, compression of the ipsilateral ventricle, and dilatation of the contralateral ventricular system. The dilution of the blood in the subdural hematoma with the passage of time reduces the density of the hematoma, which eventually becomes isodense with the brain parenchyma when CT scanning is used. In such cases, the displacement of the ventricular system suggests the presence of a mass lesion, and the use of intravenous contrast material increases the chances of outlining the hematoma by enhancing the surrounding membrane. Bilateral isodense hematomas

may present considerable difficulty in diagnosis because of the absence of shift of the midline structures. At the same time, the MRI scan is abnormal (Fig. 18-3).

2. Skull films may show shift of a calcified pineal gland, evidence of a skull fracture, and in long-term cases, calcification of the membranes of the hematoma.

3. The electroencephalogram (EEG) shows the presence of focal slowing and decreased voltage over the subdural collection.

4. Arteriography may be necessary when MRI or CT scanning is not available. The arteriogram will demonstrate an avascular space between the surface of the brain and the inner table of the bone in such cases. This may be particularly useful in patients with bilateral subdural hematomas that have an isodense response on CT scanning.

Treatment Small chronic subdural hematomas that do not produce any neurological deficit may be monitored by repeated neurological examination and serial CT scanning. The presence of any neurological deficit is an indication for surgical drainage. In most cases, a craniotomy is necessary so that thickened membranes may be excised.

Subdural Hygroma

A *subdural hygroma* is an accumulation of CSF in the subdural space. The most likely mechanism of formation involves tearing of the arachnoid membrane during head injury. The torn flap acts as a ball valve, allowing gradual escape of CSF into the subdural space during periods of temporary increase in ICP such as occurs with coughing, sneezing, or straining. Either MRI or CT scanning may reveal an area of abnormality overlying the brain parenchyma. The treatment of choice is surgical drainage.

Traumatic Subarachnoid Hemorrhage

(See Chap. 9.)

Traumatic Intracerebral Hematoma

Definition *Traumatic intracerebral hematoma* is a collection of blood in the substance of the brain following a head injury.

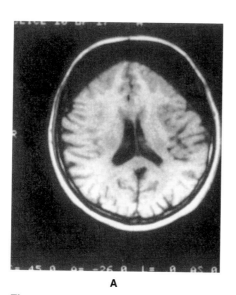
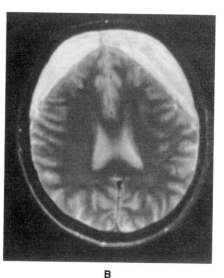

A	B

Figure 18-3
Bilateral large chronic subdural hematomas over the frontal lobes extend to the mid-parietal area bilaterally. T1- (**A**) and T2- (**B**) weighted images.

Etiology and Pathology Intracerebral hematomas are readily demonstrated by CT scanning and are much more common complications of head injury than has been believed in the past. Hemorrhage may occur at any site and results from shearing forces with subsequent rupture of blood vessels within the brain parenchyma.

Clinical Features The level of consciousness and clinical signs and symptoms depend on the size and location of the hematoma (see Chap. 9). A patient who suffers a brief loss of consciousness may have a small hematoma in the frontal temporal lobe, which is asymptomatic following recovery. Large or multiple areas of intracerebral hemorrhage are associated with edema, a rapid rise in ICP, uncal herniation, and downward pressure on the brainstem with rostral-caudal deterioration.

Diagnostic Procedures Intracerebral hematomas present as areas of increased density on CT scanning and are also readily demonstrated by MRI scanning as areas of increased signal intensity on T2-weighted images. Large hematomas are associated with edema, brain swelling, ventricular displacement, and acute hydrocephalus. The hematoma may rupture into the ventricular system.

Treatment Patients with rapidly increasing ICP require emergency treatment to reduce brain edema and swelling. Evacuation of the hematoma or reduction of the hydrocephalus by ventricular drainage may be necessary. In essence, patients should be treated as cases of severe closed head injury as described below.

TRAUMATIC HEAD INJURY

Closed Head Injury

Definition A *closed head injury* is a cranial injury in which the meninges remain intact.

Etiology, Pathology, and Clinical Features A patient with closed head injury may experience no loss of consciousness or a temporary loss of consciousness, or may become comatose.

Closed Head Injury Without Loss of Consciousness The majority of cases of head injury are mild and do not produce loss of consciousness. Skull fractures can occur without loss of consciousness. In general, head injury is considered mild when there is no loss of consciousness and recovery occurs in a short period of time. In most cases, patients report a blow to the head followed by a feeling of confusion, headache, unsteadiness of gait, and rapid recovery. There is no injury to the brain.

The *juvenile head trauma syndrome* is a syndrome occasionally seen in children and adolescents following trivial head injury. There is a history of mild head injury followed by apparent recovery. A few hours later there are complaints of headache, somnolence, and irritability, and the patient may vomit. Confusion may be a prominent symptom and a few patients lapse into coma. Others complain of blindness. The condition is very alarming to parents who urgently seek medical advice. Frequently, many unnecessary laboratory and radiological procedures are performed. The syndrome usually terminates within a few minutes to a few hours. Recovery is complete. The headache resembles a severe migraine. It is most likely due to severe vasoconstriction provoked by head injury. Children who have experienced this condition may develop migraine headaches following minor head trauma later in life.

Closed Head Injury with Loss of Consciousness A *concussion* is an immediate transient impairment of consciousness following head injury and is the result of shearing forces producing temporary impairment of axonal function with rapid recovery. A *contusion* is a more extensive injury to the brain where there is tearing of tissue owing to shearing forces with disruption of axons by axonal shearing and injury to the brain by impact against bony surfaces. The bases, tips, and medial aspects of the frontal lobes and the anterior aspects of the temporal lobes are involved most frequently. The damaged areas are conical in shape with the base at the surface of the brain, predominantly affecting layer one of the cortex. The neurological deficits that most commonly occur with a contusion are changes in behavior, changes in personality, loss of memory, confusion, aphasia, and the development of dementia. Recovery is often accompanied by symptoms of postconcussional syndrome. Most patients make a good recovery.

Postconcussional Syndrome Approximately 30 percent of patients who have suffered mild head trauma with brief loss of consciousness develop a postconcussional syndrome. They present with subjective complaints of headache, loss of energy, fatigue, difficulty concentrating, irritability, anxiety, blurred vision, impaired memory, a feeling of unsteadiness or light-headedness ("dizziness"), depression and deficits in processing information on neuropsychological testing.[11] Unfortunately, many patients are categorized and dismissed as a "hysterical reaction," or the persistence of symptoms is related to secondary gain.[12] However, careful analysis of the headache indicates that the pattern is one of migraine with headache, nausea, photophobia, phonophobia, and a desire to lie in a darkened room and sleep. Neuropsychological testing demonstrates abnormal responses.[13] One explanation is that these cases of minor head injury reflect diffuse bilateral axonal injury in the fornix owing to shearing forces, which act on the brain to produce brief loss of consciousness or occasionally, reported to be of insufficient magnitude to cause loss of consciousness.[14] However, a careful reconstruction of the episode will reveal a significant gap in the details of the head injury. Consequently, a reconstruction of an accident should include second-by-second recollection of events from the patient, others involved, police records, EMS records, and the emergency center records. This careful approach will often reveal amnesia for a period of time immediately after the accident, which is only revealed by careful, methodical questioning and attention to detail. An alternative consideration is that some cases are the result of contusion of the cortex of the tips and medial aspect of the frontal lobes. In either case, the CT scan of the brain will be normal, but abnormalities can be demonstrated by MRI scanning using T2-weighted gradient echo sequences.[15]

Closed Head Injury with Coma Moderate to severe head injury is associated with sudden loss of consciousness and coma with lack of response to painful stimulation. Coma may last for several hours or even several days in severe head injury and is followed by semicoma in which the patient begins to respond to painful stimulation. This stage is followed by stupor, restlessness, and irritability. The patient attempts to avoid all stimuli and prefers to lie curled in a fetal position and to sleep for many hours. The stage of stupor gradually gives way to obtundity, the restlessness increases, and the patient may require sedation. Examination reveals a disoriented patient with defective judgment and insight. There may be extreme irritability and a tendency toward combativeness even with slight frustration. Over a period of hours to days, the patient gradually becomes fully conscious. The severity of head injury is assessed in the emergency center using the Glasgow Coma Scale, which assesses eye, verbal, and motor responses.[16] The total coma score provides a measure of severity of brain injury.[17] Thus, severe head injury is recognized in a patient with a Glasgow coma score of 3 to 8, moderate head injury with a coma scale of 9 to 12, and mild head injury with a score of 13 to 15. However, the definition is problematic for a coma score of 13 to 15. Patients with a score of 15 constitute the overwhelming number of cases of minor head injury and have a low risk of complications in the acute phase[18] and fewer sequelae. A Glasgow coma score of 13 or 14 carries a much higher risk of both acute and chronic complications.

The period of coma or amnesia is generally accepted as a measure of severity of brain injury when a patient is examined months or years after brain injury. However, there are occasions when CT scanning and MRI scanning, in particular, may reveal evidence of severe contusion or shearing in patients who have only a minor episode of loss of consciousness, lasting for a few minutes followed by no record of amnesia who experience memory impairment or posttraumatic seizures.[19]

Diagnostic Procedures Patients with severe head injury should receive diagnostic tests when they can be safely performed during the institution of emergency treatment. The procedures generally used include:

1. A CT scan in the emergency center is indicated in all cases of head injury with a Glasgow coma

score of 14 or less, or in those with documented loss of consciousness and a skull film showing the presence of a fracture (Figs. 18-4 and 18-5). The decision to order a CT scan on an individual with a score of 15 depends on the history and the results of the neurological examination. If there is no history of loss of consciousness and the patient is fully conscious with a normal neurological examination, a CT scan can be omitted and the patient discharged home under observation. A history of loss or impairment of consciousness in an individual who is fully conscious with a normal neurological examination on arrival at the emergency center calls for skull radiographs. If the skull film is negative, the patient can be discharged under observation, but the presence of skull fracture or focal neurological deficits or age greater than 60 years requires an immediate CT scan of the head[20] and admission for observation. All patients discharged for observation at home should be under the care of a responsible individual who is supplied with

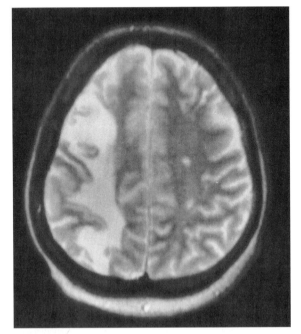

Figure 18-4
A T2-weighted MRI scan shows increased signal in the right hemisphere due to gliosis. The scan was taken more than 3 years after traumatic brain injury following a high-speed head-on collision.

printed instructions covering the period of observation.[21]

Patients with impaired consciousness admitted for observation require neurological assessment every 2 hours by the nursing staff according to a standard protocol.

2. A CT scan of the skull, and x-ray studies of the chest, cervical spine, and pelvis is indicated in all patients with severe head injury. The high incidence of fractures of the cervical spine with severe head injury justifies the taking of cervical spine films in all cases of severe head injury. Patients with upper facial fractures have a high rate of intracranial injuries. In addition to fractures, skull radiography may detect fluid levels in the sphenoid sinus or intracranial areas indicating a risk of infection.

Treatment   The comatose or semicomatose patient:

1. Establish the airway. Clear any obstruction from the upper airways by suction; remove tooth fragments or loose teeth. If secretions or blood accumulate, intubate.

2. Insert a central arterial line and central venous line. Monitor the blood pressure through the arterial line, and use the venous line for continuous monitoring of central venous pressure.

3. Use pulse oximetry for continuous monitoring of oxygen saturation. Blood glucose can be measured intermittently using the arterial line.

4. Continuous monitoring of the electrocardiogram (ECG) is a standard procedure.

5. If shock should occur, it is likely that the patient is bleeding at an extracranial site, such as hemothorax, hemoperitoneum, ruptured spleen, ruptured liver, or fracture dislocation of the hip. Pulmonary artery pressure should be monitored, fluid and blood replacement instituted, and an appropriate consultation obtained on an emergency basis from general surgery, thoracic surgery, and orthopedic surgery.

6. Comatose patients require ICP monitoring using a ventricular catheter or a fiberoptic system in the subarachnoid space.[22] This is particularly important when there are intracranial hematomas that may require urgent neurosurgical treatment. There is no

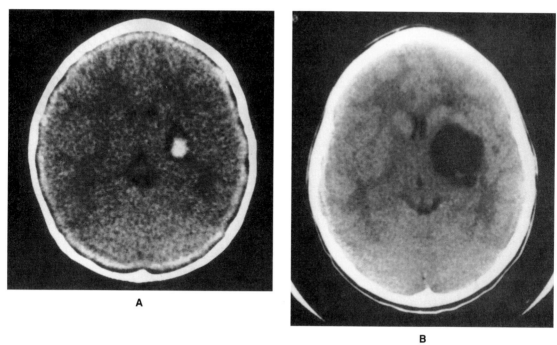

Figure 18-5
*A CT scan shows discrete traumatic hematoma (**A**) following head injury. Condition resolved to a cyst (**B**) containing CSF, indicating a connection with the ventricular system. The patient was treated by a shunting procedure.*

difficulty in making the decision to evacuate a hematoma when there is obvious shift of midline structures, obliteration of the third ventricle, and dilatation of the contralateral ventricle, particularly the temporal horn of the lateral ventricle. However, if there is doubt or when systemic complications require urgent attention, a sustained ICP of above 20 mmHg may hasten the decision to evacuate a subdural or intracerebral hematoma.[23] The treatment of a comatose patient whose initial CT scan of the brain is normal is controversial. Some studies have suggested that these cases are at low risk for the subsequent development of intracranial hypertension.[24] Others disagree and recommend that all comatose, severely head-injured patients, whose CT scan is normal and does not show a mass lesion with midline shift, are at substantial risk for the development of secondary injury due to increased ICP and reduced cerebral perfusion pressure.[25] There seems to be no doubt that intracranial hypertension of 20 mmHg or above calls

for immediate treatment because duration of intracranial hypertension above 20 mmHg is significantly correlated with poor outcome.[26]

7. In patients with evidence of impaired peripheral perfusion, volume expansion is indicated to maintain a positive fluid balance. Fluid therapy consisting of isotonic electrolyte solutions or blood can be used depending on clinical assessment without increasing ICP. Pressure agents such as intravenous dopamine counter hypotension and increase cerebral perfusion, which is reduced by loss of cerebral autoregulation in hypotension following brain injury. Consequently, both fluid replacement and treatment of hypotension increase oxygen transport to the brain without increasing ICP and have a positive effect on outcome.[27]

8. All intubated patients require ventilation to keep P_{CO_2} and P_{O_2} within physiological range and arterial oxygen saturation 100%. The use of

hyperventilation to reduce increased ICP is limited because hyperventilation can increase cerebral hypoxia[28] with adverse effects.[29]

9. Several studies have shown that steroids are not beneficial in the treatment of closed head injury, but there still remains considerable uncertainty regarding the role, if any, of corticosteroids in acute traumatic brain surgery.[30]

10. When ICP develops in patients with adequate ventilation in whom neurosurgical treatment is not indicated, the use of mannitol, an osmotic diuretic, may reduce cerebral edema. Mannitol is given in an initial intravenous dose of 0.5 g/kg body weight and the dose adjusted according to ICP and cerebral perfusion pressure. The addition of furosemide has a synergistic effect, often reducing ICP more effectively. Hyperosmolality, as defined by a serum osmolality greater than 320 mosmol/L must be avoided and a serum osmolality of 300 to 320 mosmol/L maintained. When titration with intravenous mannitol and furosemide is insufficient to maintain ICP below 15 mmHg, barbiturate therapy will reduce cerebral metabolism, cerebral blood flow, and blood volume (see barbiturate coma, Chap. 2). The complication of barbiturate therapy is hypotension, which must be avoided by maintaining a positive fluid balance, cerebral perfusion pressure, and blood pressure.

11. Anticonvulsants (e.g., intravenous phenytoin) are indicated should seizures develop in the acute brain-injured patient. Prophylactic anticonvulsants are used in many centers, but this is controversial.

12. Antibiotics are indicated in patients with open injury, CSF rhinorrhea or otorrhea, the presence of intracranial air, and in the prevention or treatment of pneumonia, an increasing problem in intensive care units.

13. Disseminated intravascular coagulation (DIC) is an occasional complication of acute head injury due to liberation of tissue thromboplastin following trauma. The liberated thromboplastin activates coagulation mechanisms and fibrin thrombi are formed in small blood vessels throughout the body. There is progressive reduction in platelets and clotting factors are depleted resulting in a bleeding diathesis. The bleeding tendency may increase intracranial bleeding and produce hemorrhage in other areas of the body. Disseminated intravascular coagulation should be suspected in patients with severe head injury who show excessive or uncontrolled bleeding following venipuncture or who develop ecchymosis in the skin. Unless surgical procedures are contemplated, DIC should be treated with intravenous heparin. Therapy with fibrinogen, platelet concentrates, or plasma factors is also effective.

14. Patients who are restless or combative may be sedated with phenothiazines, paraldehyde or chlordiazepoxide (Librium).

15. Limb contractures are a common complication in patients who experience prolonged coma. This debilitating complication may inhibit or delay rehabilitation. Limb position and maintenance of joint mobility are an essential part of therapy beginning in the acute stage of injury.

16. Feeding. Head injury is associated with a hypermetabolic and hypercatabolic state suggesting early nutrition may be of benefit. However, feeding by nasogastric tube should be a temporary measure because of the risk of vomiting and aspiration pneumonia, suggesting that nutrition should be parenteral via the jejunum or a percutaneous gastrostomy in comatose or semicomatose patients.[31]

Prognosis Both the Glasgow Coma Scale and pupil reactivity are valuable indicators in predicting outcome in closed head injury. At 6 months, 10 to 20 percent of patients with severe head injury remain severely disabled, 1 to 3 percent in a vegetative state. The presence of coma predicts a poor outcome.[32] Coma with no response at 6 h carries a mortality rate of 50 percent.[33] A Glasgow coma score of 3 when a patient is stabilized in the emergency center predicts a 76 percent mortality; a score of 4 to 5, 49 percent; a score of 6 to 7, 24 percent; and a score greater than 8, a 0.3 percent mortality.[34,35] However, late recovery from a vegetative state lasting more than 6 months, and in some cases more than a year, to one of moderate or severe brain injury has been recorded.[36,37]

The overall mortality rate for patients undergoing craniotomy following head injury is 39 percent. The figures for acute subdural hematoma vary depending on the Glasgow coma score and the time period from injury to craniotomy. Comatosed patients operated on more than 2 h after onset of coma have an 80 percent mortality. This illustrates the need for early surgical intervention in acute subdural hematoma and in epidural hemorrhage, which has a comparable outcome based on time.

The presence or absence of a pupillary light reflex at the initial examination carries important prognostic implications. Absence of response carries a poor prognosis for recovery.[38]

The EEG, which is abnormal with bilateral symmetrical or asymmetrical slowing in severe closed head injury, is of limited value because it is influenced by drugs such as barbiturates. However, the EEG reactivity to external stimuli is valuable in predicting outcome. The appearance of slow waves following external stimulation such as noise or pain carries a better prognosis than a response of temporary flattening, which is, however, better than a nonreactive record. Similarly, a normal central conduction time measured by somatosensory evoked potentials by stimulation of the median nerve indicates a good prognosis, particularly if normal bilaterally.[39] Patients with poor outcome show deterioration in somatosensory evoked potential activity with serial monitoring.[40]

Brainstem auditory evoked potentials and brainstem trigeminal evoked potentials give an accurate assessment of brainstem function and are a good prediction of outcome.[41]

Neuropsychological testing is useful to assess the initial severity of brain damage and serial testing may be used not only to measure improvement in function but also to aid in the design of rehabilitative programs.[42,43]

Traumatic Encephalopathy

Repeated head injury may be followed by the development of traumatic encephalopathy. In the professional boxer this is known as "the punch drunk state." The punch drunk boxer is characterized by evidence of chronic trauma (flattened nose, cauliflower ears); psychomotor retardation; poor judgment; impaired retention, recall, and recent memory; and dysarthria. The mental deterioration is associated with parkin-

sonian-like features, titubation of the head, cerebellar ataxia of limbs, and ataxia of gait.

Posttraumatic Seizures

When traumatic seizures occur, they usually follow severe head injury. Parents have a tendency to ascribe the development of seizures in children to head injury. Most children experience trivial head injuries while at play, and mild head injury rarely leads to the development of seizures.

The incidence of posttraumatic seizures in closed head injury is low (less than 3 percent) in patients with mild injury, defined as a loss of consciousness or amnesia less than 30 min and no skull fracture. Moderate closed head injury with skull fracture or either loss of consciousness or amnesia 30 min to 24 h in duration also carries a low risk of seizures at about a level of 3 percent. The incidence of posttraumatic seizure following severe closed head injury with cerebral contusion, skull fracture, intracerebral hematoma, or more than 24 h of loss of consciousness or amnesia is approximately 20 percent.

Ninety percent of patients who will develop posttraumatic seizures do so within 2 years. The great majority of posttraumatic seizures can be totally controlled with anticonvulsant medication (see Chap. 4). More than 50 percent of cases cease to have seizure activity within 10 years of the head injury. When there is persistence of seizure activity, patients should be fully investigated for the presence of hematoma, cicatrix, or focal areas of atrophy. Many of these conditions are remediable by neurosurgical treatment.

Benign Positional Vertigo

Definition *Episodic vertigo* is caused by dysfunction of the posterior semicircular canal.

Etiology and Pathology Although the majority of cases are categorized as idiopathic, the most common identifiable causes are head trauma, and viral labrynthitis, although the latter is often a matter of conjecture since there is no evidence of infection. Other causes of vertigo are discussed on page 590.

Dense material present in the endolymph falls away from the ampulla, displacing the copula and exciting the posterior ampullary nerve, which transmits excitatory impulses to the brainstem vestibular system.

Clinical Features   The patient experiences brief episodes of vertigo on changing the position of the head. This usually occurs on lying down or sitting up in bed, rolling to one side, bending over, or extending the head to look up. The change of position is accompanied by nystagmus.

The diagnosis can be established by the Hallpike maneuver.

Treatment   A canalith repositioning maneuver is effective in most cases. The maneuver begins with the Hallpike maneuver, with the patient's head at a 45° angle toward the affected ear for 15 s. The head is then turned 45° toward the opposite ear for 20 s. The patient then turns onto the shoulder, and the head is turned 45° parallel to the floor for 20 s, then turned facing the floor for 20 s. The procedure can be repeated if the Hallpike maneuver is still positive. The failure rate is low, but chronic cases may require surgical treatment.[44]

Cranial Nerve Injury

Cranial nerve injury may pass unnoticed in the comatose patient and become apparent only on recovery of consciousness. The optic nerve may be contused in the optic foramen because of sudden movement of the brain during head injury or because of fracture through the optic foramen. The patient may be blind immediately and may recover slowly over the next 4 weeks in some cases. Examination early after the injury reveals a dilated pupil with absence of direct light reflex but preservation of consensual response. Permanent damage results in optic atrophy beginning about 1 month after the injury. Damage to the optic chiasm may result in a bitemporal or binasal, often incongruous, field defect.

The third, fourth, and sixth cranial nerves are vulnerable to injury as they enter the orbit. They may be injured by sudden movement, stretching, or fracture through the superior orbital fissure. Third nerve injury may occur during uncal herniation. Patients who recover may have a persistent third nerve palsy with a dilated pupil, an abducted eye, and ptosis.

Smooth conjugate eye movements may be impaired following brainstem injury.

The fifth cranial nerve may be injured at the foramen ovale by basal skull fractures. Injuries of the face may damage branches of the trigeminal nerve. Occasionally, the superior orbital nerve is compressed at the supraorbital margin, and the inferior orbital nerve may be involved by fractures of the infraorbital foramen or maxilla. Damage to the seventh cranial nerve occurs with head injury in which the petrous portion of the temporal bone is fractured. There is usually an associated ipsilateral hearing loss with hemorrhage into the middle ear. Facial paralysis is occasionally delayed following head injury owing to the gradual development of edema in the facial canal.

Fractures of the middle ear and petrous temporal bone are frequently accompanied by deafness due to destruction of the auditory division of the eighth nerve. This type of injury is often associated with seventh nerve paralysis. Injury to the vestibular division of the nerve results in vertigo, which may persist following the injury. The condition usually responds to treatment, but the patient may have persistent lightheadedness, ataxia, and nausea for many months after injury.

It is unusual for head injuries to involve the lower cranial nerves although this occasionally occurs following fractures of the posterior fossa that involve the jugular foramen. This may produce damage to the ninth, tenth, and eleventh nerves. Similar damage may occur with hematoma formation at the base of the skull.

Traumatic Cerebrospinal Fluid Rhinorrhea or Otorrhea

Definition   *Traumatic CSF rhinorrhea or otorrhea is the abnormal drainage of CSF from the cranial cavity.*

Etiology and Pathology   A fracture through the posterior wall of the frontal sinus may produce a tear of the dura and arachnoid, which allows CSF to leak into the frontal sinus and nasal cavity. Rupture of a cribriform plate or an arachnoid sleeve passing through the cribriform plate is often the result of a sudden wave of increased CSF pressure following head trauma, which results in CSF rhinorrhea. Fracture of the temporal bone may tear the dura and allow CSF to drain from the ear, resulting in otorrhea.

Clinical Features Patients may present with a spectrum of clinical findings indicative of mild to severe brain injury.

The patient who has experienced mild head trauma usually complains of the persistent drainage of clear fluid from the nose, down the posterior pharynx, or from the ear. The drainage increases on head flexion, straining, or coughing. The condition may be complicated by the passage of air into the cranial cavity through the defect, particularly during coughing or sneezing. The air accumulates in the subarachnoid space and often enters the ventricular system causing pneumocephalus. This latter condition is associated with persistent headache and progressive intellectual deterioration.

Those with moderate or severe head injury present with reduced Glasgow coma scores in addition to the complications outlined above.

Diagnostic Procedures For mild head injury in a conscious patient:

1. Glucose and protein are present in the fluid, which distinguishes it from other nasal discharges.

2. Radiographs of the skull and paranasal sinuses may show evidence of fracture involving the cribriform plate, frontal sinus, or temporal bone. A CT scan is a more sensitive procedure for detection of all skull fractures.

3. Radioactive material may be injected into the subarachnoid space and allowed to circulate. Scintillation scanning of pieces of cotton placed in the nose or ear canal will reveal radioactivity.

4. Metrizamide cisternography with CT scanning is the most sensitive method of demonstrating a fistula or tissue deformity at the site of leakage in a dry, nondrop period.[45]

5. Both MRI and CT scanning will demonstrate the presence of air in the ventricular system in cases of pneumocephalus.

6. Lumbar puncture should be performed at the earliest suspicion of meningitis.

Those with moderate to severe head injury should be followed as outlined under diagnostic procedures.

Treatment Most conscious patients with mild head injury respond to conservative treatment with bed rest and instructions forbidding coughing, sneezing, or straining. There is a risk of infection in all cases, and lumbar puncture should be performed if the patient develops fever and nuchal rigidity.

Meningitis after head trauma is rare, occurring in about 1 percent of cases. A CSF culture and sensitivity should be performed in all patients with meningitis and appropriate antibiotics administered. Gram-negative strains resistant to ampicillin and third-generation cephalosporins require imipanem and ciprofloxacin therapy.[46]

Surgical treatment with closure of the fistula is indicated in patients without meningitis who fail to respond to 2 weeks of medical treatment. To prevent recurrence, surgical treatment should always be carried out in patients who have suffered meningitis.

OTHER TRAUMAS

Fat Embolism

Definition *Fat embolism* is the passage of fat emboli into the circulation with consequent respiratory failure and altered levels of consciousness.

Etiology and Pathology The majority of cases of fat embolism follow fracture of long bones. Rarer causes include concussion of long bones, bone marrow transplantation for acute leukemia, alcoholism, systemic lupus erythematosus, acute osteomyelitis, pancreatitis, extracorporeal circulation, steroid therapy in the presence of malignancy and injury to adipose tissue. Fat globules that break loose enter the systemic circulation and are carried to the lungs. The emboli occlude capillaries and are hydrolyzed to highly toxic and unsaturated fatty acids. This causes a leak in the pulmonary capillaries and a hemorrhagic interstitial pneumonitis results. Occasionally, fat emboli pass into the arterial circulation and enter the cerebrovascular system. In these cases, the brain is characterized by numerous petechial hemorrhages and ecchymoses scattered throughout the gray and white matter with generalized edema.

Clinical Features The fulminant form of fat embolism caused by a massive embolism may develop within hours of injury, whereas the classical form of fat embolism appears within 24 to 72 h.[47] Prodromal symptoms consisting of cough, fever, dyspnea, chest pain, and wheezing are followed by agitation, confusion, disorientation, delirium, seizures, and coma. Petechiae may be seen on the upper trunk and head. Focal neurological deficits may develop, and cerebral edema may lead to decerebrate rigidity, progressive brainstem compression and death.[48]

Diagnostic Procedures

1. Blood gas analysis shows a sustained PaO_2 less than 60 mmHg. A sustained $PaCO_2$ of more than 55 mmHg. A pH of less than 7.3.
2. There is a sustained respiratory rate of 35 breaths per minute or more and dyspnea with use of accessory respiratory muscles.
3. Tachycardia is a constant feature.
4. A chest x-ray will reveal a pulmonary infiltration.
5. A CT scan of the brain shows edema and small ischemic lesions. The MRI scan shows ischemic lesions in the cerebral hemispheres and the cerebellum.[49]
6. Serum free fatty acids, triglycerides, and fibrin split products are elevated.
7. Fat droplets may be demonstrated in the blood or urine.
8. The EEG shows loss of normal background activity with generalized slowing. Paroxysmal epileptic activity is present in many cases.

Treatment

1. Prevention is the best treatment. Long bone fractures should be promptly immobilized.
2. Oxygen should be administered. Intubation with mechanical ventilation using positive end expiratory pressure should be initiated as soon as the diagnosis is established.

3. Cerebral vasodilatation may be obtained with inhalation of 5% carbon dioxide and 95% oxygen.
4. Cerebral edema may be controlled with mannitol if necessary. Monitoring of ICP is advantageous.
5. Intravenous methylprednisolone 30 mg/kg, repeated after 4 h, significantly reduces the development of symptomatic fat embolism in patients with long bone fractures.

Air Embolism

Definition *Air embolism* is the passage of air into the general circulation.

Etiology and Pathology The entrance of air into the circulation may occur following injury, cardiac surgery, arterial catheterization, thoracic surgery, transthoracic percutaneous needle biopsy, surgical removal of highly vascular tumors, laparoscopy, and pneumoperitoneum.[50-52] Dysbaric air embolism resulting from pulmonary overpressurization and lung rupture during rapid ascent to the surface is not uncommon in scuba divers.[53] Air bubbles enter the pulmonary veins, left atrium, left ventricle, and systemic circulation causing arterial occlusion and infarction. Large volumes of air that enter the circulation may result in acute cardiac insufficiency and death. When smaller volumes of air enter the circulation, embolization may occur in many organs including the brain.

The brain shows diffuse areas of petechial hemorrhage, generalized edema, and infarction.

Clinical Features The passage of air bubbles into the cerebral circulation results in loss of consciousness, seizures, blurred vision or blindness, dysphasia or aphasia, vertigo, headache, focal weakness, and paresthesias. Conscious patients may complain of chest pain and hemoptysis.

Treatment

1. The source of air embolism must be contained.
2. The patient should be placed in a steep Trendelenburg position and given 5% carbon dioxide and 95% oxygen to increase cerebral blood flow and "wash out" air emboli.

3. If available, treatment in a hyperbaric chamber is indicated. Treatment at 6 atmospheres will reduce the volume size of air emboli and allow their passage out of the cerebral circulation. Longer treatment at 3 atmospheres using 100% oxygen will improve the rate of diffusion of nitrogen from emboli and reduce their volume.

4. Retrograde perfusion of the cerebral circulation through the superior vena cava to remove air bubbles from the cerebral circulation has been performed in massive air embolism following cardiac bypass pump failure.

Near Drowning

Definition *Near drowning* is the survival after submersion of the body in a fluid medium resulting in asphyxia secondary to submersion.

Etiology and Pathology In the majority of cases of near drowning, asphyxia and subsequent hypoxia are due to aspiration of fluid into the lungs resulting in pulmonary edema. It is believed that water destroys pulmonary surfactant, damages pulmonary alveoli, and results in pulmonary edema with the transudation of proteinaceous material into the alveolar spaces. This may be augmented by vomiting and aspiration of gastric contents into the lungs.

In about 10 percent of cases of near drowning, submersion is followed by persistent laryngospasm with little or no water aspiration, and there is no pulmonary edema.

Treatment

1. Clear the airway of vomitus or aspirated material and begin mouth-to-mouth resuscitation as soon as the victim is rescued. Do not wait until the victim is ashore.

2. Once out of the water, institute cardiopulmonary resuscitation, and give oxygen at the highest concentration available.

3. Any near-drowning victim submerged for more than 1 min should be admitted to hospital and observed in an emergency center for 24 h because of the risk of delayed pulmonary edema.

4. Obtain a chest film; levels of arterial blood gases, serum electrolytes, blood urea nitrogen, creatinine, hemoglobin, and a toxin screen for alcohol or drugs.

5. Any patient with abnormal blood gases or chest film should be admitted to an intensive care unit.

6. An arterial line will be required to provide blood for serial gas determinations.

7. Oxygen therapy can be continued by mask or nasal catheter if a Pao_2 of 90 mmHg can be maintained with a forced inspired IO_2 of 0.5 or less. Other patients will require intubation and positive pressure respiratory support using a mechanical ventilator. This is also indicated in cases of apnea or impaired ventilation with $Paco_2$ above 35 mmHg.

8. A nasogastric tube will prevent aspiration of stomach contents, and a Foley catheter is needed to measure urine output.

9. Cerebral edema should be anticipated in those who are deteriorating neurologically and cannot be monitored by ICP monitoring. Measures to counter cerebral edema include hyperventilation to reduce $Paco_2$ to 28 to 32 mmHg and mannitol 0.25 to 0.5 g/kg per dose to reduce ICP to less than 20 mmHg or to maintain serum osmolality between 300 and 320 mosmol/L.

Prognosis Patients with a score of 5 or less on the Glasgow Coma Scale carry a high risk of death or permanent neurological damage. Similarly, patients who are comatose without response or show decerebrate or decorticate state 2 to 6 h after submersion have a poor prognosis. Those who are alert or stuporous 2 to 6 h after submersion usually have normal or near normal recovery.

Electrical Injury to the Nervous System

Definition An electrical injury to the nervous system may be caused by electrocution or lightning strike.

Etiology and Pathology Electrocution is the fifth leading cause of work-related death.[54] Neurological complications in survivors vary from 25 to 67 percent.[55] In most cases, damage to the nervous system following electrocution is the result of anoxia rather than a direct effect of electricity on tissue. Anoxia may result from respiratory arrest due to the electric current passing through the brainstem and affecting the respiratory center or may be caused by cardiac arrest after lightning strike or ventricular fibrillation following high-voltage electrocution.[56] In some cases, however, there is direct damage to the CNS. The passage of the electric current through the nervous system is followed by inflammatory changes in blood vessels leading to thrombosis and infarction; injury to neurons may result in necrosis and gliosis. These changes may occur anywhere in the brain or spinal cord depending on the location of the involved area in the path of the electric current. The passage of an electric current can also produce damage to peripheral nerves, particularly in the limbs.

Clinical Features   Respiratory insufficiency may result in anoxic encephalopathy with loss of consciousness and generalized seizures. Damage to the cerebrum may result in homonymous hemianopia, hemiplegia, impaired memory, headache, dementia, and neuropsychiatric disorders including depression, psychosis, and conversion reaction.[57,58] The passage of an electric current through the brainstem can produce parkinsonism, cranial nerve deficits, or corticospinal tract involvement with spasticity. Spinal cord involvement results in flaccid paralysis, which is often followed by complete recovery. However, in some cases, damage to the anterior horn cells may present as progressive weakness and wasting of muscle associated with a progressive spasticity below the level of the lesion. Passage of an electric current through a limb may be followed by peripheral nerve involvement producing painful neuralgias, causalgias, reflex sympathetic dystrophy,[59] muscle weakness, fasciculations and atrophy, loss of reflexes, and a sensory loss corresponding to the distribution of a particular nerve or nerves such as the median, ulnar, radial, or peroneal nerves[60] or the brachial plexus. Not all neurological sequelae are immediate, and delayed complications of electrical injury may occur days or even years after the event and affect any part of the nervous system.

Treatment   Individuals who have been struck by lightning or electrocuted and show respiratory and cardiac arrest should receive immediate resuscitation. Most of the patients who are resuscitated within 6 min will survive with little or no permanent neurological damage. Patients with electrical injury in which the current passes through the thorax should receive ECG monitoring for at least 24 h because delayed ventricular arrhythmias may develop several hours after the injury.

Radiation Injury to the Brain and Spinal Cord

Definition   Radiation injury may occur inadvertently or during treatment of neoplastic disease. Damage to the CNS from ionizing radiation usually follows radiation therapy for treatment of neoplastic disease. In many cases, the blood vessels of the brain and spinal cord show signs of inflammation with endothelial proliferation and obliteration of the vessel lumen or thrombosis. This suggests that the effects of radiation on the brain and spinal cord are often secondary to ischemia and infarction. Ionizing radiation can also produce direct damage to neurons with neuronal loss and subsequent gliosis.

Clinical Features   Involvement of the circle of Willis by arteritis and thrombosis can result in scattered infarction in both hemispheres. Clinical signs include progressive dementia, spasticity, and rigidity. Involvement of one hemisphere will produce focal signs with hemiparesis and dysphasia if the dominant hemisphere is involved. Seizures are not uncommon. Focal necrosis in the area of an irradiated brain tumor may present as an expanding lesion with increased ICP suggesting tumor recurrence. Damage to the brainstem may result in progressive hemiparesis, paraparesis, quadriparesis, parkinsonism, cranial nerve involvement, dysarthria, and ataxia. Irradiation for nasal pharyngeal carcinoma may be followed by damage to the hypothalamus and symptoms of hypopituitism. Radiation myelopathy has the following features:

1.   Acute transient radiation myelopathy. This is a transient shock-like dysesthesia induced by neck

flexion known as Lhermitte's sign. The neurological examination is normal and full recovery occurs.

2. Acute paraplegia occurring within hours or days of irradiation is presumably due to cord infarction secondary to acute radiation vasculitis.

3. Lower motor neuron disease with muscle atrophy, fasciculations, and loss of tendon reflexes is also rare.

4. Chronic progressive radiation myelitis occurs 9 to 15 months after radiotherapy and presents with progressive paraplegia or quadriplegia, hyperreflexia, extensor plantar responses, sensory loss below the level of the lesion, and progressive impairment of bladder function. The condition may occasionally present as Brown-Sequard syndrome.[61]

The occurrence of pain, sensory disturbance, and weakness in an upper limb in a patient who has previously received radiotherapy for the treatment of carcinoma of breast may be due to metastatic involvement or radiation neuritis.[62] The diagnosis is usually obtained by biopsy because radiation neuritis can be delayed for several years and breast carcinoma metastasis can also present many years after treatment of the primary tumor.

Treatment   The treatment is symptomatic. Surgical decompression is indicated for cord compression following vertebral collapse after irradiation for metastatic disease.

Decompression Damage of the Central Nervous System

Definition   *Decompression damage* of the CNS is a condition in which rapid decompression from a high atmospheric pressure to a lower atmospheric pressure produces damage to the CNS.

Etiology and Pathology   Sudden reduction of atmospheric pressure releases gaseous nitrogen into the circulation. The bubbles of nitrogen alter the rheology of the blood, increasing the viscosity and hematocrit and encouraging erythrocyte aggregation. This results in thrombosis of the smaller vessels and infarction within the CNS involving white matter more

than gray matter. There are often multiple areas of infarction in the white matter of the spinal cord and the cerebral hemispheres, particularly in the areas of marginal supply between the territories of two major cerebral vessels.

Clinical Features   Decompression sickness often presents with joint pains that increase in severity. This is associated with generalized pruritus due to bubbles of nitrogen in the skin capillaries. Involvement of the intercostal muscles and pleura produces dyspnea (the chokes) while impairment of the circulation to the abdominal viscera results in abdominal pain (the bends). When the cerebral hemispheres are involved, there may be a sudden onset of seizures, hemiparesis, aphasia, and visual field defects. Brainstem involvement may cause cranial nerve signs such as acute onset of vertigo, impairment of hearing, facial paralysis or ocular motor palsies. In the spinal cord, the thoracic cord is the more common site of involvement with acute paraplegia, sensory loss below the level of the lesion, and sphincter paralysis.

Treatment

1. Prevention. Deep water divers should be familiar with the regulations governing decompression when diving to depths of more than 40 feet. In general, decompression should never exceed intervals of 1.25 atmospheres.[63]

2. Treatment of decompression sickness. The effective treatment is recompression in the recompression chamber. The affected individual should be placed in the chamber with pressure equal to the previous working depth or 10 to 15 lb higher than the previous working depth. Slow decompression coupled with administration of oxygen and oxygen-helium mixtures is effective in the treatment of decompression sickness.

Injury to the Spinal Canal and Spinal Cord

Etiology and Pathology   There are approximately 30 new cases of spinal cord injuries per million persons in the United States each year. The prevalence rate is approximately 906 per million. The majority of the injuries occur in young adults. About 50 percent result from motor vehicle crashes, 20 percent from falls, and 15 percent from gunshot wounds and stabbings. Injury to the spinal cord may be direct with concussion, laceration, or intermedullary hemorrhage, or indirect due to extramedullary pressure or loss of blood supply and infarction. The mechanisms of spinal cord injuries include:

1.   Fracture of the vertebrae. Fracture of the vertebrae can occur with or without fracture dislocation and may involve the vertebral body, the pedicles, the laminae, transverse processes, or spinal processes. There may be damage to the spinal cord from the concussion effects of the injury or from displaced bony fragments. Fractures have the potential to damage blood vessels such as the vertebral arteries in the neck or the anastomotic vessels to the anterior spinal artery or result in contusion of emerging nerve roots.

2.   Dislocation. Dislocation of vertebrae usually occurs at predictable sites in the spinal column. These are the areas between C1 and C2, C5 and C6, and T11 and T12. Dislocation may be reversible or persistent with marked narrowing of the spinal canal. This may be asymptomatic or result in symptoms varying from a mild concussion of spinal cord to complete severance of the spinal cord. Dislocation with additional narrowing in a spinal canal already affected by cervical spondylosis is often associated with spinal cord compression, and the narrowing may be augmented by disruption and swelling of the anterior and posterior longitudinal ligaments. In addition, dislocation can interrupt blood supply to the spinal cord and also produce damage to emerging nerve roots. Acute dislocation is frequently associated with acute rupture of an intervertebral disc (page 574).

3.   Penetrating wounds. The spinal cord may be injured by a high-velocity missile such as a bullet or by knife wounds with severance or partial severance of the cord.

4.   Epidural hemorrhage. There is a well-defined epidural space in the spinal canal that is often the site of bleeding following trauma. The hemorrhage exerts pressure on emerging nerve roots causing radicular pain and results in progressive paraparesis due to pressure on the cord. The condition is a surgical emergency.[64]

5.   Spinal subdural hematoma. Spinal subdural hematoma is rarer than spinal epidural hematoma. The symptoms are identical, and the condition is a surgical emergency that must be relieved as soon as possible to avoid permanent neurological deficits.

6.   Indirect injury to the spinal cord. The spinal cord may be injured by a pressure wave generated by a blow on the head, a fall on the buttocks, or a fall on the feet, or of when the individual is involved in an explosion. The degree of injury varies from minor concussion to severe cord damage with hemorrhage.

7.   Intermedullary injury. Three stages of change occur following severe spinal cord trauma. The first stage consists of swelling of the cord with contusion and, in some cases, hemorrhage into the cord substance followed by necrosis beginning at 1 h resulting in central cavitation in about 3 h. The second stage begins after several days with absorption of necrotic material leading to a third stage of atrophy, gliosis, and cavity formation over a period of several months.[64]

The earliest changes following traumatic injury are the result of arterial spasm or platelet aggregation in arteries within the spinal cord causing ischemia.[65] Autoregulation is lost and further ischemic changes can occur if there is a fall in systemic blood pressure.[66] Damage to arterioles and gray matter leads to hemorrhage and further ischemia. Loss of endothelial integrity leads to edema of the cord, which is maximal in 2 to 3 days. Release of epinephrine, endorphins, and encephalins produces additional ischemic damage.[67]

Ischemia is associated with increased concentration of the excitatory amino acids, glutamate, and aspartate leading to activation of excitatory amino acid receptors,[68] a depolarization of the membrane, an influx of sodium, and inactivation of the sodium-potassium pump, which prevents repolarization. There is an immediate influx of calcium ions, activation of cellular adenosine triphosphatase (ATPase) and consumption of adenosine triphosphate (ATP) with reduction of energy stores. The decrease in oxygen availability owing to ischemia results in lactic acidosis as metabolism shifts to anaerobic glycolysis and a further loss of ATP production.

The large influx of calcium ions causes activation of phospholipases and release of arachnoidinic acid resulting in lipoperoxidation and free oxidative radical formation. The final result is failure of mitochondrial and endoplasmic reticulum metabolism and neuronal death.

Clinical Features Injury to the spinal canal and spinal cord produces:

1. Injury to the nerve roots. This varies from minor concussion of nerve roots with pain and paresthesias in the appropriate dermatome to complete severance of a nerve root with wasting and fasciculations in the muscles supplied by the affected root and complete sensory loss in the appropriate dermatome.

2. Compression of the spinal cord. An acute compression of the spinal cord produces complete flaccid paralysis and loss of sensation below the level of the lesion. This stage of "spinal shock" resolves after several days or weeks and is followed by the development of radicular pain at the site of the lesion and the gradual development of spastic paraparesis below the level of the lesion. Urine is retained initially with bladder distention and loss of sensation. This is followed by an increased irritability of the bladder and the eventual development after several weeks of a small spastic bladder with reflex emptying. In less severe degrees of spinal cord compression, the patient presents with a slowly progressive spastic paraparesis, urgency, and occasional incontinence of urine and minimal or absence of sensory loss.

3. Complete transection of the spinal cord. In a complete transection, there is a complete paralysis below the level of the lesion immediately after the injury with flaccidity, which changes to progressive spasticity after a period of several weeks. There is initial reflex spasm of the bladder sphincters with painless distention of the bladder. With a gradual return of tone to the paralyzed limbs, the patient develops clonus, increased tendon reflexes and extensor plantar responses. In some cases there are involuntary flexor withdrawal spasm of the lower limbs, which may be associated with a "mass reflex" involving piloerection, sweating, and evacuation of bowel and bladder. Every effort should be made to avoid flexor spasms

by adequate physical therapy and to maintain the state of paraplegia in extension, because paraplegia in flexion encourages the development of decubiti and complicates nursing of paralyzed patients.

4. Hemisection of the cord (the Brown-Sequard syndrome). Hemisection of the cord following gunshot wounds or knife wounds produces a classical picture of ipsilateral spastic monoparesis or hemiparesis with increased tendon reflexes and an extensor plantar response due to involvement of the cortical spinal tracts. There is loss of pain and temperature sensation on the side opposite to the lesion because of the involvement of the lateral spinothalamic tracts and loss of vibration and position sense on the side of the lesion due to involvement of the ipsilateral posterior column.

5. Hematomyelia. Acute hemorrhage into the cerebral gray matter of the spinal cord is an occasional complication of direct or indirect trauma to the cord. The patient experiences sudden pain at the site of the lesion followed by paralysis. There is usually rapid but partial recovery followed by the development of atrophy of muscles supplied by anterior horn cells at the site of the hematomyelia, and spastic paraparesis below the level of the lesion. Sensory examination shows loss of pain and temperature sensation in the dermatomes affected by the hematomyelia, which interrupts the dissection fibers in the lateral spinothalamic tracts (see Chap. 14). Sensation is preserved below the level of the hematomyelia and posterior column function is normal.

6. Posttraumatic syringomyelia. Syringomyelia associated with spinal cord injury is a specific abnormality located in the central gray matter of the cord, dorsal and lateral to the central canal. The cavity arises in the border zone between the area supplied by the anterior and posterior spinal arteries, and may be the result of local infarction, traumatic hemorrhage, or bleeding from an angiomatous malformation.

7. Injury to the upper cervical cord is a complication of the rather unusual fracture dislocation of the atlanto-occipital joint. This occurs with violent hyperextension of the upper cervical cord. There are signs of cord injury and injury to the lower cranial nerves because of the acute downward traction on

these structures. A fracture or dislocation of the odontoid process may follow relatively minor trauma. The symptoms are often mild with persistent neck pain and pain in the distribution of the greater occipital nerves. This fracture usually occurs after traffic accidents, and there is a high incidence of nonunion. This imposes a risk of severe damage to the cord if the patient is involved in further trauma. Fracture dislocation of the second and third cervical vertebrae occurs in acute hyperextension of the neck in automobile accidents. There is bilateral fracture of the pedicles of C2 with avulsion of the lamina arch of C2 and forward dislocation of C2 on C3. The condition can be fatal and is the cause of death in judicial hanging. The fracture is termed "hangman's fracture," and there are relatively few symptoms in survivors who usually complain of stiffness and pain in the neck accompanied by spasm of the cervical muscles.

8. Lesions of the mid and lower cervical cord produce two distinct syndromes:

a. In the central medullary syndrome, there is contusion edema and hemorrhage in the central portion of the cervical cord resulting in quadripatesis, a greater involvement of the upper extremity than the lower, impairment of temperature and pain sensation below the level of the lesion, and impaired sphincter control. The condition tends to show progressive improvement in survivors.

b. Anterior spinal artery occlusion with infarction of the spinal cord is a more severe syndrome producing quadriplegia, loss of sphincter control, and loss of pain and temperature sensation below the level of the lesion. Extension of the infarction into the upper cervical cord is associated with loss of sensation over the face due to involvement of the spinal tract of the trigeminal nerve and Horner syndrome on one or both sides. This condition is often due to an acute protrusion of a cervical disc. Persistent bradycardia is common in severe injuries to the cervical cord due to disruption of the sympathetic pathway located in the cord at this level. Arrhyth-

mias and postural hypotension may also occur during the first 14 days after injury and may be life-threatening.[68]

9. Lesions of the thoracic cord. Injury to the thoracic cord produces a flaccid paraparesis or paresthesia with loss of bladder function and an impaired or complete loss of sensation below the level of the lesion. There may be an associated and temporary paralytic ileus.

10. Injury to the conus medullaris. A compression fracture at the level of the first lumbar vertebra can injure the conus medullaris and damage the sacral segments of the spinal cord. This may produce little or no motor deficit, sensory loss in the sacral dermatomes over the buttocks and perineum, destruction of sensory and motor innervation of the bladder resulting in retention with overflow and impotence in the male.

11. Injury to the cauda equina. Lower spinal injuries involving the cauda equina are associated with flaccid paralysis and wasting of involved muscles; sensory loss in the dermatomes supplied by the involved nerves; retention of urine with distention of the bladder if there is involvement of the nerve roots S2, S3, and S4; and impotence in the male.

Diagnostic Procedures

1. Radiographs of the spine should be taken in anteroposterior lateral and oblique views. If there is any doubt about the presence of a fracture or fracture dislocation, areas of questionable fracture should be examined by CT scanning using bone windows. Radiographs of the cervical spine should be obtained in all patients with closed head injury seen in the emergency room. CT or MRI studies of the whole spine are recommended in cases of multiple injury or closed head injury and coma.

2. An MRI scan produces a clearer image of the spinal cord and surrounding tissues permitting precise localization of cord compression and information concerning damage to surrounding tissues.

3. Myelography or CT scanning following injection of contrast material into the subarachnoid space is indicated if MRI scanning is not available, and if there is residual function below the level of the

lesion and the neurosurgeon wishes to delineate the site of the compression before surgery.

4. Urodynamic studies are indicated in patients who have impaired bladder control following spinal cord injury.

Treatment

ACUTE TREATMENT OF FRACTURES OF THE CERVICAL AND UPPER THORACIC SPINE

There is a risk of increasing damage to the spinal cord when transporting patients who have suffered fracture or fracture dislocation of the spine. There should be as little movement as possible, and all movement should be carried out with great care. A hard cervical collar is fitted by the emergency medical team and the patient transported supine on a board by ambulance to the emergency center. If a cervical collar is not available, lifting should be performed by three people, one who exerts slight traction and extension on the head by grasping the chin and the occiput. The second applies traction to the ankles, and the third lifts the shoulders and hips to maintain the spine in slight hyperextension. The patient should then be placed on a board in a supine position with a roll behind the shoulders to maintain hyperextension. A hard cervical collar is fitted as soon as the patient arrives at the emergency center and any further movement performed with a brace supporting the neck.[69] It is usually necessary to give an analgesic to control pain. This should be given in an adequate dose to produce relief. All patients should be examined for bladder distention and a Foley catheter inserted if necessary.

FRACTURE DISLOCATION OF THE LOWER THORACIC AND LUMBAR SPINE

The lower thoracic and lumbar spine should be maintained in extension with a rolled towel or cushion under the lumbar area. The patient should be transported to the hospital in a prone position that maintains slight extension of the spine.

Management of Cord Injuries in the Emergency Center

The immediate object of emergency treatment is control of pain and prevention of further cord damage. Once this is achieved, further investigation should be carried out as outlined above. Neurosurgical consultation should be obtained as soon as possible, and all patients who do not receive surgical decompression should be treated in an intensive care unit.

Medical management of spinal cord injuries:

1. A 15-min infusion of 1g of methylprednisolone should be given within 8 h of cord injury. This is followed in 45 min by a 23-h infusion of 5.4 mg/kg per hour.[70]

2. Naloxone, which functions as an opiate receptor antagonist, is theoretically beneficial in a restricting spinal cord injury but of questionable benefit in practice.

3. Immediate intubation is necessary in high cord injuries with diaphragmatic paralysis and paralysis of the intercostal muscles. Mechanical ventilation will be required in all C3 level injuries and is often necessary in C4 level injury. Pulse oximetry, frequent estimation of arterial blood gases, and the measurement of pulmonary function are necessary in these patients and in others who may show signs of respiratory deterioration culminating in intubation.

4. Some patients with cervical cord injury develop paradoxical abdominal respiratory movements requiring intubation and mechanical ventilation.

5. Shock can occur for several reasons and further compromise flow to the already ischemic spinal cord. Cervical cord damage interrupts descending sympathetic pathways causing loss of vasoconstriction, peripheral blood pooling, decreased venous return to the heart, decreased cardiac output, and hypotension. This may be compounded by bradycardia induced by uninhibited vagal nerve stimulation of the heart. Consequently, all patients should have constant cardiac monitoring, an indwelling arterial line to monitor blood pressure and arterial blood gases, and a pulmonary artery catheter to measure central venous pressure and pulmonary wedge pressure.[57] Bradycardia responds to intravenous atropine 0.5 to 2.0 mg as needed. Hypotension requires fluid replacement to elevate central venous pressure 12 to 15 cm H_2O. If this fails, dopamine 5 to 10 μkg per minute may be required.

6. Paralytic ileus is an occasional complication of cervical and thoracic spine injuries and should be treated by continuous suction of gastric contents and maintenance of adequate fluid and electrolyte balance with intravenous fluids.

7. The risk of gastric stress ulcer is considerable. Regular guaiac testing of stools and gastric aspirate and estimation of serum hematocrit should be performed. Intravenous histamine H_2-blocking agents are contraindicated because they increase the risk of pneumonia, but sucralfate 1 g q6h by nasogastric tube is effective and has a low risk incidence of pneumonia.[71]

Gastric hemorrhage requires lavage with iced saline solutions, antacids, gastric suction, and transfusion. Endoscopy may be necessary, but laparotomy is rarely required except as a lifesaving measure.

8. Nutritional requirements are high following spinal cord injury and can be met by central total parenteral nutrition until paralytic ileus is resolved. Feeding can then be changed to a continuous infusion through a small bowel feeding tube.

9. An indwelling catheter is required for bladder drainage and replaced by intermittent catheterization at a later date. Urinary tract infection should be treated with appropriate antibiotics. When signs of motor recovery are observed in the lower limbs, removal of the bladder catheter is recommended in an attempt to re-establish bladder control. Persistent bladder paralysis can be treated by the development of reflex bladder emptying or by instructing patients with intact upper limbs the technique of self-catheterization.

10. Prevention of decubiti requires the use of an air mattress, frequent turning, and padding of pressure areas.

11. The development of flexor spasms in the lower limbs is an expected complication of severe paraparesis or paraplegia. This condition often precedes the development of paraplegia in flexion. Flexor spasms may respond to baclofen (Lioresal), tiranidine (Zanaflex), or diazepam (Valium). Any two drugs may be combined if necessary. Patients with flexor spasms benefit from the use of foam rubber or light aluminum splints, which help to preserve extension of the lower limbs. Severe adductor spasms may be treated with an implanted baclofen pump, obturating neurectomy, and intractible flexor spasms will respond to blocking of the anterior nerve roots in the lumbosacral area with intrathecal phenol. This procedure should not be used in patients who have residual voluntary bladder function.

12. Hypertensive crisis is a complication of an overdistention of the bladder, colon distention by impaction, or enemas, disimpaction, catheterization, testicular torsion, or cold air stimulation. The result is a massive autonomic discharge with hypertension, diaphoresis, flushing, headache, anxiety, and piloerection. Treatment with nitroprusside, hydralazine, phenylbenzamine, or phentolamine is effective.

13. Low-dose subcutaneous heparin 5000 units q12h[72] and external pneumatic compression will prevent deep venous thrombosis in the lower extremities and lower the risk of pulmonary embolism.

14. All patients with spinal cord injury require a program of physical therapy as soon as possible after admission to the hospital. The program should be simple at first, consisting of no more than passive movements of the limbs, but can be gradually developed depending on the degree of recovery of the patient. The planned program of rehabilitation should include physical therapy and occupational therapy and should develop into a complete program of vocational rehabilitation at a later date.

Herniated Intervertebral Disc

Definition   A *herniated intervertebral disc* is characterized by protrusion of a portion of the nucleus pulposus into the spinal canal.

Etiology and Pathology   A herniated disc is one of the more common neurological conditions causing signs and symptoms related to the cervical and lumbar areas. The condition can occur at any age but is more frequent in middle-aged and older individuals. Damage to a disc with herniation is a frequent complication of injury to the spinal column but can also be precipitated by unaccustomed lifting or trivial trauma.

Intervertebral discs are fibrocartilaginous joints of the symphysis type situated between the vertebral bodies. There are two parts to the discs. The annulus fibrosis is an outer rim of densely fibrous tissue; the inner nucleus pulposus consists of gelatinous material. The annulus fibrosis is firmly attached to the periosteum of the vertebral bodies and the anterior and posterior longitudinal ligaments. The nucleus pulposus has a high water content, which decreases with age. This loss is accelerated during middle age with a resulting decrease in volume of the disc. At the same time, there is a loss of elasticity of the annulus fibrosis, which facilitates splitting of the annulus under unexpected pressure.

The initial splitting is usually a tear parallel to the circumferential fibers of the annulus fibrosis. This may or may not be associated with some bulging of the disc indicating an area of weakness. After repeated trauma, the annulus tends to rupture posteriorly or posterolaterally, and herniation of the nucleus pulposus occurs into the spinal canal with subsequent pressure on the spinal cord or spinal nerves as they exit through the intervertebral foramina (Fig. 18-6). Occasionally, fragments of the nucleus pulposus are extruded into the spinal canal as isolated cartilaginous bodies and may cause compression of the spinal cord or the spinal nerves. The blood supply to the annulus fibrosis is poor, and healing occurs slowly after herniation and is often incomplete. This enhances the tendency toward recurrence of symptoms of herniated disc in susceptible individuals.

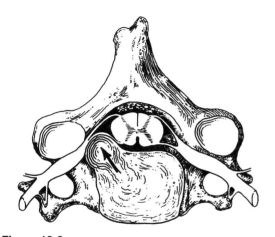

Figure 18-6
Diagrammatic representation of a herniated intervertebral disc.

Clinical Features   Herniated discs most commonly occur in the lumbosacral area, most frequently between L4 and L5 or L5 and S1. Cervical ruptures are one-tenth as common and more commonly involve the disc between C5 and C6. Rupture of thoracic discs is rare.[73]

Fifty percent of patients have a clear cut history of previous injury. In early cases with splitting of the annulus fibrosis rather than herniation, the patient presents with pain in the lumbar area or in the neck. In more advanced cases with disc herniation, numbness and weakness are present while prolonged compression results in wasting and fasciculation of the involved muscles. The localizing signs of herniated disc are summarized in Table 18-1. Spurling's sign can be helpful in herniation of a cervical disc with cervical radiculopathy. In this test, the examiner applies pressure over the vertex with the head in extension or rotation. The production of a radicular pain radiating into the upper limb is likely to be the result of cervical nerve root compression by an osteophyte or disc herniation. In disc rupture involving the L4, L5, or S1 nerve root, straight-leg raising results in low back pain (Lasegue's sign). In both cervical and lumbar ruptures, examination reveals muscle spasm and tenderness in the back or neck and decreased flexion toward the side of the rupture.

The majority of disc rupture in a posterolateral direction. In the cervical and thoracic areas, midline herniation produces pressure on the spinal cord and results in progressive spastic paraparesis and urgency of micturition. A large midline rupture in the lumbar area may compress multiple nerve roots.

Diagnostic Procedures

1.   Radiographs of the spine may show narrowing of the intervertebral space at the level of the suspected disc herniation.

2.   Electromyography will confirm the presence of nerve root involvement in most cases with herniated disc in the cervical or lumbar area. Fibrillations may not appear until 2 or 3 weeks after the onset of nerve compression.

3.   The MRI scan has replaced myelography as the study of choice to demonstrate the presence of a herniated disc. Sagittal and axial scans are neces-

Table 18-1

Localized signs of herniated disc

Level of herniated disc nerve root involved	Location of pain	Location of numbness	Muscular weakness and wasting	Reflex changes
C_4–C_5 C_5	Neck Shoulder	C_5 dermatome	Deltoid Supraspinatus	Depressed biceps reflex
C_5–C_6 C_6	Neck Lateral forearm	C_6 dermatome	Biceps	Depressed biceps and triceps reflex
C_6–C_7 C_7	Neck Middle finger	C_7 dermatome	Triceps	Depressed triceps reflex
L_3–L_4 L_4	Low back, hip Posterolateral thigh Anterior leg	L_4 dermatome	Quadriceps	Depressed Patellar reflex
L_4–L_5 L_5	Sacroiliac joint Posterior thigh Lateral leg to heel	L_5 dermatome	Extensors of the great toe Difficulty walking on the heels	Depressed biceps femoris reflex
L_5–S_1 S_1	Sacroiliac joint Posterior thigh Lateral foot to toes	S_1 dermatome	Plantar flexors of the toes Difficulty walking on the toes	Depressed Achilles reflex

sary to demonstrate disc herniation. If the results of the MRI are ambiguous, a combination of CT scan and iodide contrast myelography should be used.

Treatment

1. Cervical disc disease
   a. Mild pain without muscle wasting
      The affected limb is supported by a hemiplegic sling and the pain controlled by adequate oral analgesics. The patient should be instructed to apply ice packs to the neck for 20 min bid. Some patients prefer to lie on an electric heating pad for half an hour in the morning and half an hour in the evening.
   b. Severe pain without muscle weakness
      The patient is placed on bed rest initially and given sufficient analgesics to abolish pain within 48 h. Ice packs are applied for 20 min bid. The patient should receive adequate sedation to induce sleep at night.

   c. Persistent pain and weakness and wasting
      Patients with these symptoms should be considered surgical candidates and evaluated with an MRI scan in an attempt to accurately delineate the herniated disc. Neurosurgical or orthopedic consultation should be obtained.

2. Lumbar disc disease
   a. Mild pain with absence of muscle weakness or wasting
      The patient should be treated with bed rest on a firm mattress and restricted to one pillow. Once free from pain, the patient is fitted with a lumbosacral belt with posterior steel bars, which should be worn whenever the patient is out of bed during the next 3 months. This serves to prevent sudden flexion movements on ambulation.
   b. Moderately severe pain without muscle weakness or wasting
      Treatment consists of bed rest on a firm mattress with ice packs to the lumbar area for

20 min bid. Adequate analgesics are given to render the patient pain free within 48 h. The patient is then be fitted with a lumbosacral belt before attempting ambulation.

c. Severe pain, muscle weakness and wasting

These patients should be considered surgical candidates and pain controlled with adequate analgesics including morphine 10 to 15 mg q4h p.r.n. Appropriate studies are obtained and if a herniated disc is demonstrated, the patient should be advised to undergo surgical treatment, and a graded program of physical therapy should be started as soon as possible after surgery. Patients are able to ambulate within a short time following surgery, usually within 24 h in a restricted fashion, and should be able to ambulate without difficulty 5 to 7 days after the surgical procedure when they can be fitted with a lumbosacral belt and instructed to refrain from lifting heavy objects for at least 6 months.

Patients who fail to respond to surgical treatment or patients who do not have a herniated disc demonstrated by MRI scan should receive full medical treatment as outlined above.

Hyperextension-Flexion Injuries to the Cervical Spine and Cervical Cord (Whiplash Injury)

Definition A *whiplash injury* is an injury that results in forced hyperextension-flexion of the neck.

Etiology and Pathology This type of injury usually follows a rear end collision that produces a sudden and violent hyperextension movement followed by an equally sudden flexion movement of the head on the neck. This can produce damage to the bony and ligamentous structures of the neck, the nerve roots as they emerge through the intervertebral foramina, the vertebral arteries as they course through the foramina, and the transverse processes of the cervical vertebrae or damage to the cervical cord. Concussion and occasionally contusion of the brainstem may also occur.

Clinical Features Injury to the bony and ligamentous structures of the neck is often a cause of severe pain for many months following this type of injury. There may be damage to nerve roots with pain in the distribution of the dermatomes supplied by the affected nerve root. Pain in the distribution of the greater occipital nerve is not unusual following hyperextension-flexion injury, and is often associated with a persistent dull headache in the occipital area, which radiates forward bitemporally. A careful analysis of the headache will reveal that in many cases, the pattern is one of migraine (headache, nausea, photophobia, phonophobia, and a desire to lie down in a darkened room when the headache is severe). A number of patients experience fatigue, headache, light-headedness, cognitive disturbances, sleep disturbances, and depression. These cases report amnesia or brief loss of consciousness and have experienced shearing of cerebral axons in the accident producing the whiplash injury. Neuropsychological testing has demonstrated cognitive disturbances in some of these individuals.[74]

Injury to the vertebral arteries may result in ischemia to the brainstem. In most cases, recovery occurs without neurological sequelae, but a minority of cases show evidence of brainstem involvement with ataxia and asymmetry of tendon reflexes. Extensor plantar responses are occasionally demonstrated. This tends to occur in older patients with some degree of atherosclerosis, but it can occasionally be demonstrated in younger patients. Concussive effects of injury to the brainstem can also result in permanent neurological deficits.

The cervical spinal cord may be damaged by the excessive movement of the vertebral column or can suffer damage from an acute herniated disc. This can cause hypalgesia to pinprick over one side of the face due to involvement of the spinal tract of the trigeminal nerve. Horner syndrome is often present on one side in such cases. Damage to the vestibulospinal tracts is often associated with vertigo. Involvement of the corticospinal tracts produces a mild degree of spastic paraparesis with inequality of reflexes, which tend to be increased bilaterally.

Diagnostic Procedures

1. Radiography of the cervical spine in the antero-posterior, lateral, and oblique views should be obtained to exclude an unexpected compression fracture of the vertebral body.
2. Electromyography is indicated in patients who have persistent pain in dermatomal distribution with some degree of appropriate muscle weakness.
3. An MRI scan will demonstrate a herniated disc in patients with persistent pain due to nerve root or spinal cord compression.

Treatment   Most patients will respond to bed rest, adequate analgesics, and application of heat or ice packs to the neck. There is a tendency to underrate the damage caused by this type of injury and to send patients back to their occupations while acute symptoms are still present. This often prolongs the discomfort and disability. It is better to allow adequate time for recuperation. Patients with persistent neck pain and persistent headache often respond to amytriptilene beginning 10 mg at bedtime and increasing by 10-mg increments every 5 to 7 days to 100 to 150 mg q.h.s. Migraine headaches usually respond to sumatriptan tablets 50 mg or nasal spray 20 mg.

Cervical Spondylosis

Definition   *Cervical spondylosis* is a degenerative arthritic disease involving the cervical spine with the potential to cause compression of the cervical cord, cervical nerve roots, or vertebral arteries.

Etiology and Pathology   The basic cause of cervical spondylosis is degeneration of the vertebral discs in the cervical spine. There is normally a loss of water content in the vertebral discs with aging, but the narrowing is occasionally associated with posterior herniation of the disc into the spinal canal. Herniation leads to stimulation of osteoblasts in the margin of the vertebral bodies with new bone formation, which protrudes into the spinal canal. This combination of disc protrusion and new bone formation forms a bar of tissue that narrows the diameter of the spinal canal. The normal diameter of the spinal canal (17 mm) is reduced; cord compression occurs when the diameter is less than 12 mm.

Spinal cord damage is enhanced by other degenerative factors including thickening of the dentate ligaments that normally anchor the spinal cord in the spinal canal and thickening of the ligamentum flavum, which protrudes into the posterior aspect of the spinal canal. The spinal cord is thus anchored by the thickened dentate ligaments, making it more susceptible to compression by the spondylytic bars. Narrowing of the disc space produces shortening of the cervical spine and imposes additional stresses on the interpeduncular joints. These joints become the site of osteoarthritic change with formation of osteophytes that encroach on the intervertebral foramina and compress the cervical nerve roots. The lateral extension of the osteophytes around the interpeduncular joints will also encroach on the vertebral arteries as these arteries ascend vertically through the neck in close relationship to the cervical spine. There is also reduction of blood supply to the nerve roots due to compression by osteophytes of segmental radicular arteries. Osteophytic compression of the vertebral arteries, segmental arteries, and nerve roots can be enhanced by head turning, which tends to increase the compression by the osteophytes.

The cervical cord is usually flattened in the anteroposterior diameter in cervical spondylosis, and there are loss of myelin in the posterior columns and loss of neurons in the anterior horn cells occurring in patchy fashion throughout the cervical cord. Such changes are usually due to compression of the cord but can also result from ischemia due to compression of the anterior spinal artery and its branches.

Compression of the cervical nerve roots results in wallerian degeneration.

The kinking and obstruction of the vertebral arteries which is the result of osteophytic formation may be enhanced by arteriosclerotic changes in the vertebral arteries in the elderly. Vertebral basilar insufficiency develops in some cases, and there is an increased risk of infarction of the brainstem and spinal cord.

Clinical Features   There is an increased prevalence of diabetes mellitus in patients with cervical spondylosis. Many patients with cervical spondylosis complain of intermittent pain in the neck and occipital headache. However, it is not unusual to see patients with severe radiographic changes of cervical spondylosis who have not experienced any pain or discomfort in the neck.

Patients with cervical spondylosis may experience sudden onset of nerve root pain due to an increase in disc protrusion at the level of the emergent nerve root. This is often precipitated by trauma. The pain is experienced in the distribution of the dermatome supplied by the compressed nerve root. The onset of pain is often followed by some evidence of weakness and wasting in the muscles supplied by the affected nerve root. Fasciculations are occasionally present and the tendon reflexes innervated through the compressed nerve root are absent or depressed. Subacute or chronic compression of nerve roots produces less pain of dermatomal distribution, but there may be an insidious onset of muscle weakness and wasting with occasional fasciculations and depression of tendon reflexes.

Compression of the cervical cord rarely occurs without evidence of nerve root compression. Compression of the cord is indicated by weakness and wasting of muscles with fasciculations due to compression of anterior horn cells. There may be slow development of spastic paraparesis in the lower limbs characterized by spasticity, ankle clonus, increased tendon reflexes, and bilateral extensor plantar responses due to bilateral involvement of the corticospinal tracts. The patient may develop a spastic or spastic-ataxic gait due to involvement of the corticospinal and spinocerebellar tracts. Increased urgency and frequency of micturition results from involvement of the descending inhibitory fibers to the bladder, but this is often a late complication. Occasionally there is sensory impairment in the lower limbs, usually below the knees, due to involvement of the lateral spinothalamic tracts. There may be sensory loss in the lower limbs with impairment of vibration and position sense when there is involvement of the posterior columns of the spinal cord.

Compression of the vertebral arteries associated with arteriosclerotic changes in these vessels often leads to the appearance of vertebral basilar insufficiency (see Chap. 8). These symptoms can be precipitated by head turning, which increases osteophytic compression of the vertebral arteries. Patients with vertebral basilar insufficiency run an increased risk of infarction of the brainstem.

Diagnostic Procedures

1. Radiographs of the neck with anteroposterior, lateral, and oblique views and extension and flexion should be taken to evaluate fully the extent of cervical spondylosis.
2. Electromyography will demonstrate the extent of nerve root involvement.
3. Somatosensory evoked potentials will show delay in the cervical area of the cervical cord.
4. An MRI scan will demonstrate compression of the spinal cord and nerve roots with exquisite clarity.[75] Use of MRI has superceded myelography and CT as the procedure of choice in cervical spondylosis.

Differential Diagnosis

1. All causes of spinal cord compression should be considered.
2. Amyotrophic lateral sclerosis can be excluded by the presence of sensory change in cervical spondylosis.
3. Patients with prominent signs of posterior column involvement should be examined for subacute combined degeneration of the cord.

Treatment

1. Acute radicular pain can be treated with bed rest, the application of ice packs to the neck for 20 min bid, the adequate use of analgesics, and the use of anti-inflammatory agents such as Naproxen 375 to 500 mg bid.
2. The patient should be placed in a program of physical therapy combined with heat and massage once the pain is under control. This can be followed by neck traction in selected cases.
3. The surgical treatment of cervical spondylosis should always be considered in the presence of:
   a. Persistent severe nerve root pain.
   b. Progressive muscle weakness and wasting.
   c. Evidence of spinal cord compression.
   d. In some cases, when vertebral basilar insufficiency is demonstrably related to cervical

spondylosis by ultrasonography or vertebral arteriography.

Surgical treatment consists of either laminectomy with decompression of the spinal cord or anterior fusion of the vertebral bodies at the affected level. If available, somatosensory evoked potentials should be monitored to evaluate spinal cord function during operative procedures.[76]

Prognosis   Many patients respond well to conservative measures as outlined above, and this can be repeated when indicated. The results of surgical treatment in selected cases are also excellent, but patients with definite myelopathy should be warned that surgery is indicated to prevent further deterioration rather than to produce improvement.

REFERENCES

1. Wald SL: Advances in the early management of patients with head injury. *Surg Clin North Am* 75:225, 1995.
2. Adams JH, Doyle D, Ford I, et al: Diffuse axonal injury in head injury: definition, diagnosis and grading. *Histopathology* 15:49, 1989.
3. Teasdale GM: Head injury. *J Neurol Neurosurg Psychiatry* 58:526, 1995.
4. McIntosh TK, Garde E, Saatman KE, et al: Central nervous system resuscitation. *Emerg Med Clin North Am.* 15:527, 1997.
5. Shackford SR, Mackersie RC, Davis JW, et al: Epidemiology and pathology of traumatic deaths occurring at a level I trauma center in a regionalized system of care: the importance of secondary brain injury. *J Trauma* 29:1392, 1989.
6. Graham DI, Ford I, Adams JH, et al: Ischemic brain damage is still common in fatal non-missile head injury. *J Neurol Neurosurg Psychiatry* 52:346, 1989.
7. Jones PA, Andrews PJ, Midgley S, et al: Measuring the burden of secondary insults in head injured patients during intensive care. *J Neurosurg Anesthesiol* 6:4, 1994.
8. Martin N, Doberstein C, Zane C, et al: Post-traumatic vasospasm: transcranial Doppler ultrasound, cerebral blood flow and angiographic findings. *J Neurosurg* 77:575, 1992.
9. Miller JD, Butterworth JF, Gudeman SK, et al: Further experience in the management of severe head injury. *J Neurosurg* 54:289, 1981.
10. Sahuquillo-Barris J, Lamorea-Cuiro J: Acute subdural hematoma and diffuse axonal injury after severe head trauma. *J Neurosurg* 68:894, 1988.
11. Capruso DX, Levin HS: Cognitive impairment following closed head injury. *Neurol Clin* 10:879, 1992.
12. Evans RW: The postconcussion syndrome and the sequelae of mild head injury. *Neurol Clin* 10:815, 1992.
13. Levin HS, Mattis S, Ruff RM, et al: Neurobehavioral outcome following minor head injury: a three-center study. *J Neurosurg* 66:234, 1987.
14. Blumbergs PC, Scott G, Manavis J, et al: Staining of amyloid precursor protein to study axonal damage in head injury. *Lancet* 334:1055, 1994.
15. Mittl RL, Grossman RI, Hiehle JF, et al: Prevalence of MR evidence of diffuse axonal injury in patients with mild head injury and normal head CT findings. *AJNR Am J Neuroradiol* 15:1583, 1994.
16. Teasdale G, Jennett B: Assessment of coma and impaired consciousness. A practical scale. *Lancet* 2:81, 1974.
17. Williams DH, Levine HS, Eisenberg HM: Mild head injury classification. *Neurosurgery* 27:422, 1990.
18. Teasdale G, Murray G, Anderson E, et al: Risk of traumatic intracranial haematoma in children and adults: implications for management of head injuries. *BMJ* 300:363, 1990.
19. Wilson JT, Teasdale G, Hadley DM, et al: Post-traumatic amnesia: still a valuable yardstick. *J Neurol Neurosurg Psychiatry* 57:198, 1994.
20. Borczuk P: Predictors of intracranial injury in patients with mild head trauma. *Ann Emerg Med* 25:731, 1995.
21. Miller JD, Jones PA, Dearden NM, et al: Progress in the management of head injury. *Br J Surg* 79:60, 1992.
22. Marmarou A, Anderson RL, Ward JD, et al: NINDS traumatic coma data bank: intracranial pressure monitoring methodology. *J Neurosurg* (Suppl) 75:S21, 1991.
23. Eddy VA, Vitsky JL, Rutherford EJ, et al: Aggressive use of ICP monitoring is safe and alters patient care. *Am Surg* 61:24, 1995.
24. Lobato RD, Sarabia R, Rivas JJ, et al: Normal computerized tomography scans in severe head injury. Prognostic and clinical management implications. *J Neurosurg* 65:784, 1986.
25. O'Sullivan MG, Statham PF, Jones PA, et al: Role of intracranial pressure monitoring in severely head injured patients without signs of intracranial hypertension on initial computerized tomography. *J Neurosurg* 80:46, 1994.

26. Marmarou A, Anderson RL, Ward JD, et al: Impact of ICP instability and hypotension on outcome in patients with severe head trauma. *J Neurosurg* (Suppl) 75:S59, 1991.

27. Scalea TM, Maltz S, Yelon J, et al: Resuscitation of multiple trauma and head injury: role of crystalloid fluids and inotropes. *Crit Care Med* 22:1610, 1994.

28. Gopinath SP, Robertson CS, Contant CF, et al: Jugular venous desaturation and outcome after head injury. *J Neurol Neurosurg Psychiatry* 57:717, 1994.

29. Muizelaar JP, Marmarou A, Ward JD: Adverse effects of prolonged hyperventilation in patients with severe head injury: a randomized clinical trial. *J Neurosurg* 75:731, 1991.

30. Alderson P, Roberts I: Corticosteroids in acute brain injury: systematic review of randomized controlled trials. *BMJ* 314:1855, 1997.

31. Saxe JM, Ledgerwood AM, Lucas CE, et al: Lower esophageal sphincter dysfunction precludes safe gastric feeding after head injury. *J Trauma* 37:581, 1994.

32. Snyder JV, Colantonio A: Outcome from central nervous system injury. *Crit Care Clinics* 10:217, 1994.

33. Jennett B, Murray A, Carlin J, et al: Head injuries in three Scottish neurosurgical units: Scottish head injury management study. *BMJ* 2:955, 1979.

34. Jennett B, Teasdale G, Braakman R, et al: Prognosis of patients with severe head injury. *Neurosurgery* 4:283, 1979.

35. Klauber MR, Marshall LF, Barrett-Connor E, et al: Prospective study of patients hospitalized with head injury in San Diego County 1978. *Neurosurgery* 9:236, 1981.

36. Dubroja I, Valent S, Miklu P, et al: Outcome of post-traumatic unawareness persisting for more than a month. *J Neurol Neurosurg Psychiatry* 58:465, 1995.

37. Choi SC, Barnes TY, Bullock R, et al: Temporal profile of outcomes in severe head injury. *J Neurosurg* 81:169, 1994.

38. Marshall LF, Marshall SG, Klauber MR, et al: A new classification of head injury based on computerized tomography. *J Neurosurg* 75:514, 1991.

39. Gutling E, Gonser A, Imtot H-G, et al: EEG reactivity in the prognosis of severe head injury. *Neurology* 45:915, 1995.

40. Konasiewicz SJ, Moulton RJ, Shedden PM: Somatosensory evoked potentials and intracranial pressure in severe head injury. *Can J Neurol Sci* 21:219, 1994.

41. Soustiel JF, Hafner H, Guelburd JN, et al: A physiological coma scale: grading of coma by combined use of brainstem trigeminal and auditory evoked potentials and the Glasgow coma scale. *Electroencephalogr Clin Neurophysiol* 87:277, 1993.

42. Freedman PE, Bluberg J: Anticipatory behavior deficits in closed head injury. *J Neurol Psychiatry* 50:398, 1987.

43. Heinrichs RW, Celinski MJ: Frequency occurrence of a WAIS dementia profile in male head trauma patients. *J Clin Exp Neuropsychology* 9:187, 1987.

44. Epley JM: The canalith repositioning procedure: for treatment of benign paroxysmal positional vertigo. *Otolaryngol Head Neck Surg* 107:399, 1992.

45. Fagerlund M, Wiequist B: Intermittent cerebrospinal fluid liquorrhea: cerebral computed tomography in the non-drop period. *Acta Radiol* 28:189, 1987.

46. Baltas I, Tsoulta S, Sakellariou P, et al: Post-traumatic meningitis: bacteriology hydrocephalus and outcome. *Neurosurgery* 35:422, 1994.

47. Lindique BG, Schoeman HS: Fat embolism and the fat embolism syndrome. A double-blind therapeutic study. *J Bone Joint Surg (Br)* 69:128, 1987.

48. Bell TD, Enderson BL, Frame SB: Fat embolism. *J Tenn Med Assoc* 87:429, 1994.

49. Scopa M, Magatti M, Rossitto P: Neurologic symptoms in fat embolism syndrome: case report. *J Trauma* 36:906, 1994.

50. Robicsek F, Duncan GD: Retrograde arterial embolization in coronary operations. *J Thorac Cardiovasc Surg* 94:110, 1987.

51. Wong RS, Ketai L, Temes RT, et al: Air embolism complicating transthoracic percutaneous needle biopsy. *Ann Thoracic Surg* 59:1010, 1995.

52. Khan AU, Pandya K, Clifton MA: Near fatal gas embolism during laparoscopic cholecystectomy. *Ann R Coll Surg Engl* 77:67, 1995.

53. Kizer KW: Dysbaric cerebral artery embolism in Hawaii. *Ann Emerg Med* 16:535, 1987.

54. Vazquez D, Solano I, Pages E: Thoracic disc herniation, cord compression and paraplegia caused by electrical injury: case report and review of the literature. *J Trauma* 37:328, 1994.

55. Grube BJ, Heimbach DM, Engra LH, et al: Neurologic consequences of electric burns. J Trauma 30:254, 1990.

56. Jensen PJ, Thomsen PEB: Electrical injury causing ventricular arrhythmias. *Br Heart J* 57:279, 1987.

57. Gans M, Glaser JS: Homonymous heminanopia following electrical injury. *J Clin Neuroophthalmol* 6:218, 1986.

58. Kelley KM, Pliskin N, Meyer G, et al: Neuropsychiatric aspects of electric injury. The nature of psychiatric disturbances. *Ann NY Acad Sci* 720:213, 1994.

59. Demun EM, Redd JL, Buchanan KA, et al: Reflex

sympathetic dystrophy after a minor electric shock. *J Emerg Med* 11:393, 1993.

60. Mankani MH, Abramou GS, Boddie A, et al: Detection of peripheral nerve injury in electrical shock patients. *Ann N Y Acad Sci* 720:206, 1994.

61. Goldwein JW: Radiation myelopathy: a review. *Med Pediatr Oncol* 15:89, 1987.

62. Hoang P, Ford DJ, Burke FD: Postmastectomy pain after brachial plexus palsy: metastasis or radiation neuritis. *J Hand Surg (Br)* II:441, 1986.

63. Arthur DC, Margulies RA: A short course in diving medicine. *Ann Emerg Med* 16:689, 1987.

64. McBride DQ, Rodts GE: Intensive care of patients with spinal trauma. *Neurosurg Clin North Am* 5:755, 1994.

65. Nelson E, Gertz SD, Rennels ML, et al: The role of vascular damage in the pathogenesis of central hemorrhagic necrosis. *Arch Neurol* 34:332, 1977.

66. Senter HJ, Venes JL: Loss of autoregulation and post-traumatic ischemia following experimental spinal cord trauma. *J Neurosurg* 50:198, 1979.

67a. Levi L, Wolf A, Belzberg H: Hemodynamic parameters in patients with acute cervical cord trauma: description, intervention and prediction of outcome. *Neurosurgery* 33:1007, 1993.

67b. Simon RP, Swan JH, Griffith T, et al: Blockage of *N*-methyl-*D*-aspartate receptors may protect against ischemic damage in the brain. *Science* 226:850, 1994.

68. Lehmann KH, Lane JG: Cardiovascular abnormalities accompanying acute spinal cord injury in humans: incidence, time course and severity. *J Am Coll Cardiol* 10:46, 1987.

69. Little NE: In case of a broken neck. *Emerg Med* 21:22, 1989.

70. Bracker MJ, Shepard MJ, Collins WF, et al: A randomized controlled trial of methylprednisolone or naloxone in the treatment of acute spinal cord injury. *N Engl J Med* 322:405, 1990.

71. Eddleston JM, Vohra A, Scott P, et al: A comparison of the frequency of stress ulceration and secondary pneumonia in sucrafate or ranitidine treated intensive care patients. *Crit Care Med* 19:1491, 1991.

72. Green D, Hull RD, Mammen EF, et al: Deep vein thrombosis in spinal cord injury. Summary and recommendations. *Chest* 102(6 suppl):633s, 1992.

73. Blumenkopf B: Thoracic intervertebral disk herniations: diagnostic value of magnetic resonance imaging. *Neurosurgery* 23:36, 1988.

74. Kischka U, Ettlin T, Heim S: Cerebral symptoms following whiplash injury. *Eur Neurol* 31:136, 1991.

75. Masaryk TJ, Modic MT: Cervical myelopathy: a comparison of magnetic resonance imaging and myelography. *J Comput Assist Tomogr* 10:184, 1986.

76. Veilleux M, Daube JR, Cuichiaray RF: Monitoring of cortical evoked potentials during surgical procedures on the cervical spine. *Mayo Clin Proc* 62:256, 1987.

Chapter 19

THE PERIPHERAL NEUROPATHIES

ANATOMY OF THE PERIPHERAL NERVES

Motor nerve fibers originate from the anterior horn cells of the spinal cord and leave the cord through the anterior nerve root. The sensory fibers originate from neurons in the posterior root ganglia and enter the spinal cord through the posterior nerve root. The anterior and posterior nerve roots unite distal to the cord to form a mixed spinal nerve (Fig. 19-1). Both anterior and posterior nerve roots are covered by dura as they leave the spinal cord up to the point of exit from the spinal canal where the dura becomes continuous with the epineurium covering the mixed spinal nerve. The mixed spinal nerves unite in the cervical and lumbar areas to form the cervical, brachial, and lumbosacral plexuses. Each plexus gives rise to a number of individual mixed nerves, which are distributed to the periphery to supply muscle, skin, and blood vessels.

Each nerve contains numerous nerve fibers. The central portion of each nerve fiber consists of an axon that contains axoplasm. Axoplasm is a complex structure containing mitochondria, endoplasmic reticulum, Golgi apparatus, neurotubules, and neurofilaments, which are individual nonanastomotic fibrils that extend the entire length of the axon. The surface of the axon is covered by a limiting membrane called the axolemma and by the myelin sheath external to the axolemma. The myelin sheath is derived from the cytoplasm of the Schwann cell and surrounds the axon in concentric layers. Large myelinated axons are either motor axons or sensory axons subserving the modalities of touch, vibration, and proprioception. Small myelinated axons serve pain and temperature, while so-called unmyelinated axons, which are invested by the Schwann cell membrane without sheath

formation, carry pain and deeper ill-defined sensation. The myelin sheath is not a continuous structure but consists of sections, each derived from a single Schwann cell, which are separated by small gaps known as nodes of Ranvier. Electrical impulses are conducted by a series of "jumps" from node to node, a method known as saltatory conduction. This means that the speed of conduction is related to the distance between the nodes. Rapidly conducting axons have relatively few nodes, which are far apart. Axons that conduct more slowly have many nodes, which are close together along the extent of the axon. The so-called unmyelinated nerve fibers are very slow-conducting fibers. Axons are also capable of conducting proteins from the perineurium or cell body to the periphery, and it is known that this conduction is two-directional. There is a functional relationship between the Schwann cells and axons. Schwann cells will not survive without the presence of axons, although axons will survive in the absence of Schwann cells, but their function is markedly altered. Mixed peripheral

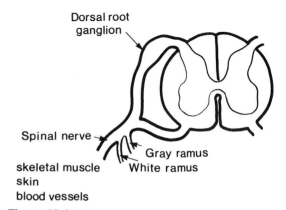

Figure 19-1

Schematic representation of the relationship of a spinal nerve to the spinal cord.

nerves consist of many thousands of axons, each separated by a fine connective tissue called the endoneurium. Axons are collected in bundles or fascicles surrounded by perineurium, and fascicles are separated by a thicker connective tissue known as the epineurium.

Diseases of the peripheral nerves may produce changes in axons or in the myelin sheath. Axonal changes are of two types, axonal (wallerian) degeneration and axonal dystrophy. Axonal degeneration occurs following severance or infarction of a peripheral nerve. The axon dies up to the level of the first internode above the site of trauma, which may be followed by chromatolysis in the perikaryon or cell body of the neuron. The myelin distal to the site of trauma disintegrates and is digested and removed. If the cell body does not die, axonal regeneration occurs by the regrowth of nerve fibrils, which attempt to make contact with the peripheral axolemma and re-establish the previous peripheral connections. If the axolemma is destroyed, degeneration is haphazard and may result in the development of a painful, traumatic neuroma. Once the neurofibrils have regenerated, the Schwann cells reinvest the axon with myelin. A number of nutritional and metabolic disorders are associated with a second type of axonal damage called axonal dystrophy in which there is a gradual dying back of the axons from the periphery. This is commonly seen in diabetic neuropathy but also occurs in alcoholism and in many toxic conditions.[1]

Segmental demyelination occurs when there is primary involvement and death of the Schwann cell. The neuron, including the perikaryon and axon, remains normal, and axonal continuity is maintained. In some cases Schwann cell regeneration occurs, but the nodes of Ranvier are situated closer together than before demyelination. Remyelination is occasionally followed by hypertrophy of the Schwann cells, which surround axons in an "onion ring" fashion. Hypertrophic change occurs in hereditary motor and sensory neuropathies (HMSN) type I-peroneal muscular atrophy, Charcot-Marie-Tooth disease; HMSN type II-Dejerine-Sottas disease; chronic inflammatory demyelinating neuropathy; and occasionally in acromegaly. Demyelination is a feature of some

hereditary neuropathies and the Guillain-Barré syndrome. Mixed types of peripheral neuropathy with both axonal degeneration and demyelination can occur.

Several clinical patterns of peripheral neuropathy are recognized. These include:

1. Mononeuropathy. Mononeuropathy implies involvement of one peripheral nerve. This is commonly the result of trauma but also occurs in diabetes mellitus and in infarction of peripheral nerves (e.g., in polyarteritis nodosa).
2. Polymononeuropathy (mononeuritis multiplex). Polymononeuropathy is a term used to describe involvement of several individual nerves in a haphazard fashion. The etiology is the same as for mononeuropathy.
3. Radiculoneuropathy. A radiculoneuropathy is involvement of the nerve root as it emerges from the spinal cord. This is commonly seen with herniated discs or with epidural masses (e.g., tumor).
4. Plexitis. A plexitis is an inflammation of a plexus such as the brachial plexus (brachial plexitis).
5. Polyneuritis. In polyneuritis or polyneuropathy there is a symmetrical involvement of peripheral nerves. The most common causes are diabetes mellitus and alcoholism. There are, however, numerous causes of peripheral neuropathy and the identification of the etiological agent may be difficult in unusual cases.

Neuropathies, no matter what their cause and type, present with specific signs and symptoms. Involvement of motor axons produces muscle wasting and weakness followed by atrophy and the appearance of fasciculations. The tendon reflexes supplied by the affected nerve are depressed or absent. Involvement of sensory axons produces impairment of sensation with dysethesias or paresthesias. Involvement of axons supplying autonomic function produces loss of sweating, alteration in bladder function, constipation, and impotence in the male. Reflex sympathetic dystrophy, a very painful peripheral dysesthesia, is probably related to disturbance of the autonomic system in the spinal cord and the peripheral nerves.

NEUROPATHIES OF THE CRANIAL NERVES

The Third, Fourth, and Sixth Cranial Nerves

Lesions of the third, fourth, and sixth cranial nerves are conveniently considered together because of the proximity of origin of these nerves in the brainstem and the close relationship in their course through the cranial cavity to supply the extraocular muscles and intrinsic muscles of the eye. Involvement of the third, fourth, and sixth nerve nuclei or the proximal portion of these nerves in the brainstem is usually associated with other signs of brainstem dysfunction. One example is Möbius syndrome, an hereditary condition in which there is dysplasia of the nuclei of the oculomotor and seventh cranial nerves. Other causes of oculomotor palsies include brainstem trauma, encephalitis, syphilis, Wernicke encephalopathy, tumor, infarction, multiple sclerosis, and the spinocerebellar degenerations. Involvement of the oculomotor nerves in the posterior fossa is common with increased intracranial pressure (ICP) associated with herniation of the uncus of the temporal lobe over the free edge of the tentorium. This produces pressure on the third nerve as it crosses the tentorial edge resulting in unilateral dilatation of the pupil, followed by paralysis of the extraocular movements supplied by the third nerve. Other causes of third, fourth, and sixth nerve involvement in the posterior fossa include meningitis, syphilis, polyneuritis, diabetes mellitus, and extra axial tumors. Diabetic mononeuropathy involving the third nerve usually produces paralysis of the extraocular movements supplied by the third nerve with sparing of the pupil. This condition is believed to be due to infarction of the outer layer of the third nerve, which contains the motor fibers supplying extraocular muscles, while the inner core of fibers supplying the constriction of the pupil is preserved.

Isolated sixth nerve palsies are often due to diabetes mellitus or pontine infarction and usually resolve within 3 months. Chronic isolated sixth nerve palsies lasting 6 months or more have been described following lumbar puncture, trauma, raised ICP, and arachnoiditis. Other causes include syphilis, sarcoidosis, and metastatic tumor. Primary tumors include pontine glioma, chordoma, chondrosarcoma, and meningioma in the posterior fossa. The sixth nerve may be compressed by an intracavernous aneurysm, pituitary tumor, or nasopharyngeal carcinoma and is occasionally involved in temporal arteritis.[2]

The third, fourth, and sixth nerves are vulnerable to pressure in the lateral wall of the cavernous sinus. The more common causes include aneurysms of the internal carotid artery and pituitary or parapituitary tumors. Compression of the third nerve has been reported from a persistent trigeminal artery and is occasionally seen as a reversible condition in ophthalmoplegic migraine (see Chap. 5).

The nerves may be involved at the level of the superior orbital fissure, which may be narrowed by inflammation, by Paget disease, or by growth of a nearby tumor, usually a meningioma. Orbital involvement of the third, fourth, and sixth nerves may follow trauma with fracture of the orbital bones. Other causes include orbital cellulitis, abscess, and temporal arteritis. Transient paralysis of the sixth nerve is sometimes seen in infants and children and is a benign condition of unknown etiology. A similar condition is sometimes induced by the use of prochlorperazine (Compazine) in children. Cyclic oculomotor paralysis is a rare condition encountered in children in which there is paralysis of extraocular movements supplied by the third nerve associated with ptosis lasting for a period varying from several seconds to several minutes.

The Fifth Cranial Nerve (Trigeminal Nerve)

Trigeminal Neuralgia (Tic Douloureux)

Definition *Trigeminal neuralgia* is a condition characterized by sudden, severe, lancinating pain occurring in the distribution of the trigeminal nerve.

Etiology and Pathology Trigeminal neuralgia is probably syndromic and may be due to:

1. Degenerative changes in the trigeminal (gasserian) ganglion, producing paroxysmal discharge of neurons.

2. Pressure on the trigeminal nerve root by an aberrant or arteriosclerotic vessel, by a tumor, particularly a meningioma located in the posterior fossa[3] or by displacement of the brainstem by a contralateral tumor with compression of the trigeminal nerve against a bony structure.
3. Increased angulation of the nerve root over the petrous bone caused by demineralization at the base of the skull in the elderly with upward movement of the petrous pyramid.
4. Demyelination of the most proximal portion of the trigeminal nerve root or demyelination affecting the spinal tract in the brainstem in patients with multiple sclerosis. (A similar condition occurs in patients with tabes dorsalis).
5. Familial trigeminal neuropathy has been described in the setting of hereditary peripheral neuropathies, especially HMSN type I, Charcot-Marie-Tooth disease.[4]
6. Paroxysmal discharges of the neurons of the spinal nucleus of the trigeminal nerve. (This concept suggests that trigeminal neuralgia is a form of seizure activity occurring at the brainstem level secondary to degenerative or vascular changes affecting the neurons of the spinal nucleus.)

Clinical Features   The disease predominantly occurs in middle-aged and elderly patients. The occurrence of trigeminal neuralgia in the younger individual suggests the diagnosis of multiple sclerosis, tumor, or aneurysm. The disorder is somewhat more common in women. The condition is characterized by paroxysms of pain occurring in the maxillary or mandibular division of the trigeminal nerve with later spread from one division to involve the other division. Involvement of the ophthalmic division is rare and occurs in less than 5 percent of cases. Trigeminal neuralgia may involve both sides of the face, but paroxysms never occur simultaneously on the two sides. In established cases the pain may be provoked by touching the face, chewing, talking, drinking, brushing the teeth, shaving, or the movement of air across the affected side of the face. Patients recognize certain "trigger points," which will produce a typical paroxysm of pain if stimulated. Established cases exhibit sudden, severe paroxysms of pain with cessation of speech and contortion of the face often accompanied by a cry of distress. The attacks are short-lived with long periods of freedom in the early stages, but the paroxysms gradually become longer and closer together in time. This leads to constant dread of the next attack with depression, suicidal thoughts, and weight loss.

The neurological examination is normal.

Diagnostic Procedures

1. The patient should have radiographs or a CT scan of the base of the skull with visualization of the foramen ovale. Enlargement of the foramen ovale suggests the possibility of intracranial or extracranial tumor.
2. If there is a suspicion of the presence of tumor or aneurysm, a high-resolution computed tomography (CT) scan of the base of the skull and posterior fossa should be performed.

Treatment   Medical treatment using carbamazepine (Tegretol) is successful in most cases. It should be given in small doses initially and gradually increased to effect, beginning with 100 mg at night and increasing by 100 mg every 3 days until the patient is receiving 800 to 1600 mg in three divided doses daily. The slow introduction of carbamazepine will permit the establishment of therapeutic levels of the drug, without the development of unpleasant adverse effects. See Chapter 4 for further information on the use of carbamazepine.

Phenytoin (Dilantin) is less effective than carbamazepine in the control of trigeminal neuralgia but should be used to treat patients who are unable to tolerate carbamazepine. Phenytoin is also useful as an adjunct when carbamazepine produces significant but incomplete control of pain. The dosage of phenytoin should be sufficient to produce therapeutic plasma concentrations of the drug (see Chap. 4).

Baclofen, benzodiazepines, gabapentin, or pimozide 4 to 12 mg daily[5] are occasionally effective when carbamazepine and phenytoin fail to control trigeminal neuralgia.

A number of surgical procedures are currently advocated for the treatment of trigeminal neuralgia. These include alcohol injection of individual nerves or the trigeminal ganglion. This form of treatment relieves pain, but the patient must clearly understand that alcohol injection produces anesthesia, and pain loss is associated with loss of sensation in the affected area of the face. Nerve regeneration often occurs after 6 months with return of the pain in some cases. Other surgical procedures include percutaneous radiofrequency or glycerol trigeminal gangliolysis and suboccipital craniotomy with microvascular decompression of the trigeminal nerve, which has the advantage of relieving pain without producing anesthesia. When the latter is not feasible, partial sensory rhizotomy with sectioning of one-third to one-half of the cross-section area of the sensory root, 2 to 5 mm from the pons, produces complete relief from neuralgic pain in about 50 percent of cases.[6]

Prognosis The majority of cases of trigeminal neuralgia can be controlled medically with carbamazepine but many patients have to continue taking the drug for a prolonged period. An attempt at withdrawal should be made when the patient has been pain free for 6 months. This is successful in some cases.

The Seventh Cranial Nerve

Bell's Palsy

Definition Bell's palsy is the acute onset of an isolated facial paralysis of the peripheral type.

Etiology and Pathology The etiology of Bell's palsy is unknown, but the disease is believed to be the result of a viral infection involving the geniculate ganglion. It is possible that some cases are due to activation of a latent herpes simplex infection.

Pathological changes consist of inflammation and edema of the facial nerve in the facial canal. This produces increasing pressure on the nerve with paralysis of function followed by wallerian degeneration of axons.

Clinical Features Bell's palsy usually occurs in middle-aged and elderly individuals. There is frequently a history of exposure to cold temperatures or drafts preceding the onset of facial paralysis. Most patients give a history of pain or ache in the region of the stylomastoid foramen immediately behind the angle of the mandible some 24 to 48 h before the appearance of the facial paralysis. The paralysis is usually appreciated for the first time on awakening in the morning, and there is a steady progression to severe weakness or total loss of function involving one side of the face. The affected side of the face sags and the eye cannot be closed because of paralysis of the orbicularis occuli. Weakness of the cheek allows food to accumulate between the teeth and the side of the mouth. There is often excess watering of the eye because of inability to move secretions across the cornea to the lacrimal duct. When the edema on the facial nerve extends proximally with involvement of the chorda tympani, there may be loss of taste. Further proximal extension produces hyperacusis because of paralysis of the nerve to the stapedius, and involvement of the geniculate ganglion results in loss of lacrimation and a dry eye. Complaints of numbness or sensory change over the face and the presence of nystagmus suggest involvement of both the trigeminal nerve and the vestibular division of the eighth nerve in some cases of Bell's palsy.[7] The characteristics of seventh nerve paralysis due to lesions at particular sites and common etiologies are listed in Table 19-1.

Diagnostic Procedures Some determination of prognosis can be obtained by observation of evoked responses on stimulating the facial nerve as it emerges from the stylomastoid foramen. The demonstration of a good evoked response on stimulating the facial nerve indicates a good prognosis. Complete loss of excitability on stimulation indicates a poorer prognosis.

Treatment The initial discomfort can be relieved with aspirin or aspirin and codeine compounds. The use of oral corticosteroids in the treatment of Bell's palsy is controversial. However, some studies indicate improvement with corticosteroids, which can be given in a single dose of methylprednisolone (Medrol) 80 mg initially with a gradual reduction of dosage over the 7-day period. Patients who are unable to close the eyelids should be treated with methylcellulose eyedrops q4h, and the eye should be protected by a patch until there is a return of eyelid function.

Table 19-1
Seventh nerve paralysis

Site	Characteristics	Etiology
Supranuclear lesions	Weakness of the contralateral, lower face	Lesion involving corticobulbar tract above pons
Nuclear or pontine lesion	Total facial paralysis on side of lesion Impaired salivary secretion Taste intact Impaired lacrimation same side Associated paralysis of sixth or fifth nerve on same side Eyes may be conjugately deviated toward side of lesion Possible internuclear ophthalmoplegia Possible contralateral hemiparesis	Congenital: Mobius syndrome Infectious: encephalitis, rabies, meningitis Nutritional: Wernicke encephalopathy Neoplastic: pontine glioma Vascular: infarction, hemorrhage Degenerative: multiple sclerosis, syringobulbia, amyotrophic lateral sclerosis
Extracranial in cerebellopontine angle	Total facial paralysis on side of lesion Hearing loss on side of lesion Episodic vertigo Corneal reflex depressed on side of lesion Impaired salivary secretion Impaired lacrimation on side of lesion	Inflammation: meningitis, tuberculosis, syphilis, fungi Neoplastic: acoustic neuroma, meningioma dermoid, chordoma, meningeal carcinomatosis Vascular: aneurysm of basilar artery Degenerative: multiple sclerosis
Extracranial in facial canal		Traumatic: fractures involving petrous temporal bone
a. Between internal auditory meatus and geniculate ganglion	Total facial paralysis same side Hearing loss same side Impaired lacrimation same side Impaired salivary secretion Taste lost anterior two-thirds tongue same side	Infectious: otitis media, mastoiditis, Bell's palsy (see below), herpes zoster of geniculate ganglion (Ramsey-Hunt syndrome) (see Chap. 19–27), sarcoidosis, Guillain-Barré syndrome (bilateral)
b. Between geniculate ganglion and origin of nerve to stapedius	Total facial paralysis same side Impaired salivary secretion Taste lost anterior two-thirds tongue same side Hyperacusis	Metabolic: diabetes mellitus Neoplastic: cholesteatoma, epidermoid temporal bone tumors, parotid gland tumors, leukemic deposits in facial canal
c. Between origin of nerve to stapedius and origin of chorda tympani	Total facial paralysis same side Impaired salivary secretion Taste lost anterior two-thirds tongue same side	
d. Distal to origin of chorda tympani	Total facial paralysis same side only	

Prognosis   The majority of patients with Bell's palsy make a complete recovery over a period of 2 to 3 weeks. The remaining 15 percent show some loss of function, including persistent facial weakness, facial spasm, ectropion, and excess lacrimation some- times called "crocodile tears" caused by regeneration and passage of axons destined for the salivary glands to the lacrimal gland. In the older age group, hyper- acusis, and a very dense paralysis are associated with a poorer prognosis.

Herpes Zoster of the Geniculate Ganglion—Ramsay Hunt Syndrome
(See p. 610).

Geniculate Neuralgia

Definition Geniculate neuralgia is characterized by episodes of severe lancinating pain occurring in the region of the pinna and external auditory canal.

Etiology and Pathology The etiology of this condition is unknown and is believed to be due to a neuralgia affecting the nervus intermedius. The bipolar neurons of the nervus intermedius are located in the geniculate ganglion and the afferent axons enter the spinal tract of the trigeminal nerve. The peripheral fibers are distributed to the external auditory canal and the pinna. There may also be some distribution to deeper structures of the face and hard palate.

Clinical Features Patients experience spasmodic attacks of severe pain in the region of the pinna and external auditory canal. The pain is occasionally felt in the throat, deep in the face, and in the orbit.

Treatment Same as for trigeminal neuralgia. Surgical excision of the geniculate ganglion has been performed in refractory cases.

Facial Myokymia   See Chapter 20, p. 657.

Hemifacial Spasm

Definition Hemifacial spasm is an irregular contraction of the muscles supplied by the facial nerve on one side.

Etiology and Pathology Hemifacial spasm is due to an irritative lesion of the facial nerve and is comparable to trigeminal neuralgia in many ways. The most common cause is believed to be compression of the facial nerve as it emerges from the brainstem by an aberrant or arteriosclerotic vessel. Other causes include multiple sclerosis, an aneurysm of the basilar artery, and tumor or arachnoiditis in the cerebellopontine angle.

Clinical Features Hemifacial spasm usually begins with irregular contractions affecting the orbicularis oculi and gradually spreads to involve all of the muscles supplied by the facial nerve on one side. The condition is always unilateral, and the movements are irregular, lasting for a few seconds to a few minutes with periods of freedom. Hemifacial spasm is increased by tension and emotional upset. Atypical facial pain may occur in some cases and suggests the presence of neoplasm.[8] There are no other abnormalities on neurological examination.

Treatment Carbamazepine (Tegretol) and phenytoin (Dilantin) are rarely successful in controlling hemifacial spasm. Surgical treatment is indicated when hemifacial spasm becomes unacceptable to the patient. This consists of exposure of the facial nerve in the posterior fossa with identification of the compressive lesion, usually a tortuous arteriosclerotic artery.

Loss of Taste   Loss of taste has been described in some cases of Bell's palsy and also occurs in other conditions. Ageusia or dysgeusia, loss or disorder of taste, has been described after an upper respiratory tract infection and is presumably due to a viral neuritis. Other causes include exposure to certain drugs including D-penicillamine, griseofulvin, phenylbutazone, oxyphedrine, and carbamazepine. Loss of taste causes considerable distress to patients and should always be differentiated from loss of smell because most patients confuse these two senses. There is no specific treatment for loss of taste, although the use of oral zinc preparations has been suggested.

The Eighth Cranial Nerve

The majority of eighth nerve neuropathies are due to the toxic effect of drugs. A number of antibiotics, particularly the aminoglycosides, are reported to cause eighth nerve degeneration. Streptomycin and gentamicin affect the vestibular division of the nerve, while neomycin, vancomycin, streptomycin, and kanamycin affect the auditory division of the nerve. Most cases follow parenteral administration of the antibiotic, but toxic neuropathy has been reported following topical application of creams containing kanamycin.

There is a rare, familial degenerative neuropathy affecting the cochlear division of the eighth nerve, which is characterized by progressive deafness. This may be associated with myoclonus and sensory peripheral neuropathy in some cases.

Vertigo

Definition   An illusion of self-motion caused by dysfunction of the vestibular system and its connections.

Etiology and Pathology   In benign positional vertigo, free-floating particles (otoliths) or clumps of otoliths (canaliths) in the endolymphatic compartment of the posterior horizontal or superior semicircular canals displace the cupula and excite ampullary nerves producing benign positional vertigo. Other disorders of vestibular function, such as vestibular neuritis or Meniere's disease, can affect the vestibular system and are associated with intense vertigo. An acoustic neuroma or aberrant artery pressing on the vestibular nerve are recognized causes of vertigo. Migrane or vertebrobasilar insufficiency involving the vestibular nuclei and the brainstem produce recurrent vertigo. Pontine infarction, cerebellar infarction or cerebellar hemorrage are often accompanied by acute vertigo and profound ataxia.

Clinical Features   Benign positional vertigo consists of brief episodes of vertigo on changing the positon of the head. Attacks of vertigo are also brief in vertebrobasilar insufficiency when they are accompanied by signs of brainstem dysfunction. However, vertigo is prolonged in brainstem or cerebellar infarction or cerebellar hemorrage.

Treatment   Treatment should be directed at the underlying cause. Antivertiginous drugs are of limited value.

Disabling Positional Vertigo

Etiology and Pathology   This condition results from vascular compression of the vestibular division of the eighth nerve.

Clinical Features   There is a constant sensation of vertigo, often associated with nausea, which increases in intensity over time. Symptoms are exacerbated by activity and relieved by bed rest; there is little relief from sedation. The patient has a sensation of constant motion and drifts to one side when walking. There is a progressive sensorineural hearing loss.

Treatment   The response to microvascular decompression of the eighth nerve is excellent in most cases.[10]

The Ninth Cranial Nerve

Glossopharyngeal Neuralgia

Definition   *Glossopharyngeal neuralgia* is the occurrence of spasms of pain in the sensory distribution of the ninth and tenth cranial nerves.

Etiology and Pathology   The cause is unknown but is presumed to be pressure on or entrapment of the ninth and tenth cranial nerves. Glossopharyngeal neuralgia has occurred following acute infection of the pharynx but has also been related to compression at many sites, including the cerebellopontine angle, jugular foramen, base of the skull, pharynx, and tonsils.

Clinical Features   The patient experiences spasms of pain in the pharynx, often radiating into the ear. The attacks may be precipitated by swallowing, coughing, chewing, talking, sneezing, turning the head to one side, or touching the tragus of the ear. The attacks are usually brief but may last for several minutes in severe cases. Remissions are common. The neurological examination is normal.

Attacks are occasionally associated with bradycardia, cardiac arrhythmias, hypertension, and syncope due to associated vagal stimulation. Hypersecretion of the parotid gland has been reported.

Diagnostic Procedures   A diligent search should be made for a compressive lesion in the area of the cerebellopontine angle or at the base of the skull using magnetic resonance imaging (MRI) or CT scanning, which provides clear views of the jugular foramen.

Treatment   Most cases respond to carbamazepine (Tegretol) as described under trigeminal neuralgia. Intracranial sectioning of the glossopharyngeal nerve has been performed in intractable cases. This procedure entails a section of the upper two rootlets of the vagus nerve and may be associated with postoperative hypotension and cardiac arrhythmias.

The Tenth Cranial Nerve

Superior Laryngeal Neuralgia This rare condition is associated with episodic lancinating pain radiating over the side of the neck. The disorder is believed to be the result of entrapment of the superior laryngeal nerve as it pierces the hyothyroid membrane. Patients experience pain in the anteromedial aspect of the neck radiating up behind the angle of the mandible on to the face extending as high as the zygoma.

The diagnosis can be established by injection of a local anesthetic into the superior laryngeal nerve as it pierces the hyothyroid membrane. This procedure will produce temporary relief. Most patients respond to carbamazepine (Tegretol). Refractory cases require sectioning of the superior laryngeal nerve at the level of the hyothyroid membrane.

The Eleventh Cranial Nerve

The 11th cranial nerve (accessory nerve) is subject to injury by trauma or surgical procedures or by compression due to tumors or enlarged lymph nodes in the posterior triangle of the neck. The most common cause of injury is lymph node biopsy with accidental damage to the nerve.[11] Involvement of the accessory nerve produces paralysis and wasting of the trapezius with inability to elevate the arm above the horizontal plane without external rotation. There may be pain in the neck and shoulder.

Patients may require analgesics and the use of an arm sling to relieve shoulder pain. Compression may be relieved by surgical procedures.

The Twelfth Cranial Nerve

The hypoglossal nerve is occasionally injured in surgical procedures of the neck. This produces hemiatrophy of the tongue with deviation of the tongue toward the side of the lesion on tongue protrusion.

THE CERVICAL PLEXUS

Anatomy The cervical plexus is formed by looped connections between the anterior primary rami of C1, C2, C3, C4, and C5 on the anterior aspect of the levator scapuli and scalenus medius muscles. Branches from C2 supply the sternocleidomastoid, while C3 and C4 supply the levator scapuli. The phrenic nerve is derived from C3, C4, and C5 and supplies the diaphragm. The most important sensory branch is the greater occipital nerve, which arises from C2. The lesser occipital nerve arises from C2, and the greater auricular nerves arise from C2 and C3. All supply the posterior aspect of the scalp. The transverse cervical and supraclavicular nerves (C2, C3, and C4) supply the neck and the anterior portion of the chest wall down to the level of the T2 dermatome.

Occipital Neuralgia

Definition Occipital neuralgia is characterized by pain occurring in the cutaneous distribution of the greater occipital nerve.

Etiology and Pathology The greater occipital nerve may be compressed in the neck by cervical spondylosis. It is occasionally injured during hyperextension-flexion injuries of the neck, which result in contusion of the nerve root as it passes through the intervertebral foramen.

Clinical Features The patient complains of constant pain in the distribution of the greater occipital nerve over the posterior aspect of the scalp. The nerve is tender to palpation in its course over the occipital bone.

Diagnostic Procedures Occipital neuralgia is frequently misdiagnosed as a "headache." The correct diagnosis can be established by relief of symptoms with local injection of the occipital nerve as it passes over the occipital bone.

Treatment Early cases may respond to the application of ice packs or heat to the upper cervical area and the use of analgesics. Anti-inflammatory agents such as naproxen 500 mg bid may help. When the pain persists, the greater occipital nerve can be injected with local anesthesia and a corticosteroid such as 40 mg methylprednisolone (Medrol), which frequently produces permanent relief of symptoms. Treatment of cervical spondylosis is outlined in Chapter 18.

Lesions of the Phrenic Nerve The phrenic nerve arises from the anterior primary rami of C3, C4, and C5 and passes from the neck into the thorax to supply the diaphragm. The nerve may be damaged during traumatic injury to the cervical spine with contusion or tearing of the anterior primary rami of C3, C4, and C5. The nerve is occasionally involved in chronic meningitis, arachnoiditis, and cervical spondylosis. Compression by tumors of the neck, aneurysms of the major vessels, or enlarged lymph nodes in the neck are additional causes of phrenic paralysis. Compression in the thorax by tumors and enlarged lymph nodes or an aneurysm of the aorta in the mediastinum can also cause phrenic nerve paralysis.

Mononeuropathy of the phrenic nerve has occasionally been reported following viral pneumonia, diphtheria, and exposure to such toxins as alcohol and lead. Unilateral paralysis of the diaphragm usually produces few symptoms and the condition is often diagnosed in the evaluation of patients with tumors or enlarged lymph nodes in the neck or thorax. The sensory fibers of the phrenic nerve can be stimulated by subphrenic conditions such as subphrenic abscess, cholecystitis, pancreatitis, and carcinoma of the pancreas, or by intrathoracic inflammatory conditions producing diaphragmatic pleurisy. This produces referred pain experienced over the shoulder on the same side as the lesion. Peripheral irritation may result in persistent singultus (hiccough). This condition responds to small doses of thorazine.

THE BRACHIAL PLEXUS

Anatomy The brachial plexus is formed by the anterior divisions of C5, C6, C7, C8, and T1 with some variable contribution from C4 and T2. The plexus consists of superior, middle, and inferior trunks, which divide and reunite to form lateral, posterior,

and medial cords, so named because of their relationship to the axillary artery. The trunks and cords give origin to a number of individual nerves supplying motor, sensory, and autonomic fibers to the upper thorax, shoulder, and upper limb (Fig. 19-2).

Birth Injuries to the Brachial Plexus

Etiology and Pathology The brachial plexus may be damaged by excessive lateral traction on the head with the shoulders fixed during a difficult delivery or by excessive downward traction on the shoulders with the head fixed in a breech delivery. Both of these maneuvers produce an increase in the angle between the shoulder and the head and exert pressure on the roots of the brachial plexus.

Clinical Features Three types of injury can occur. These include:

1. Injury to the roots of C5 and C6 (Erb's paralysis).
2. Injury to the roots of C8 and T1 (Klumpke paralysis).
3. Combined upper and lower root injury (Erb-Duchenne-Klumpke paralysis).

ERB'S PARALYSIS Erb's paralysis is characterized by paralysis involving the deltoid (abduction); biceps, brachialis, and supinator (elbow flexion); and supraspinatus and infraspinatus (external rotation). The infant presents with absence of movement of the affected arm. The muscles fail to develop, and the arm and shoulder assume the typical posture of adduction, inward rotation, and pronation of the forearm and hand some months after birth. There are loss of the biceps and brachioradialis reflexes and a small area of sensory loss over the upper lateral aspect of the arm.

TREATMENT

1. All joints of the arm should be moved through a full range of motion several times a day.
2. The upper limb should be splinted in abduction with the elbow flexed to 90° and the forearm in midsupination.

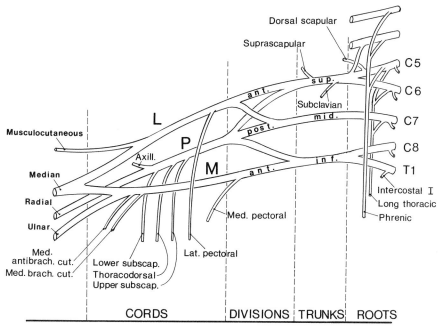

Figure 19-2
The brachial plexus.

3. Orthopedic surgical measures, including partial section of the pectoralis major and pronator teres should be considered in children who do not recover.

PROGNOSIS   Recovery occurs in about 50 percent of cases.

KLUMPKE PARALYSIS   This type of paralysis is rare. Klumpke paralysis is characterized by paresis of the wrist, finger flexion, and small muscles of the hand. The fingers become extended, but the elbow is flexed. There is sensory impairment over the inner aspect of the forearm and hand. Horner syndrome develops when there is avulsion of the cervical nerve roots.

COMBINED PARALYSIS   The combined upper (Erb) and lower (Klumpke) paralysis is extremely rare. It is characterized by paralysis of the shoulder and hand. The arm is wasted and cold, with dependent edema, and Horner syndrome is present.

Traumatic Injury to the Brachial Plexus   Injury to the brachial plexus is common in gunshot wounds, knife wounds, competitive sports, and automotive accidents, particularly motorcycle accidents. The plexus may be stretched and damaged by carrying heavy loads on the shoulders or by prolonged backward displacement of the shoulders during coma and occasionally during general anesthesia. Traumatic injury includes:

1.   A fall onto the apex of the shoulder and the side of the head. This injury abruptly increases the angle between the shoulder and the head and produces stretching or tearing of the nerve roots C5 and C6. This results in loss of abduction of the arm at the shoulder (deltoid, supraspinatus) and weakness of flexion at the elbow (biceps, brachialis). The biceps reflex is depressed.

2.   A blow to the angle between the shoulder and the neck. This may also produce weakness of shoulder movement because of damage to the upper cord of the brachial plexus. This is associated with inability to elevate the shoulder because of damage to

the accessory nerve and paralysis of the trapezius muscle.

3. A fall on the front of the shoulder. This type of injury may cause sudden extension of the shoulder with compression of the lower cord of the brachial plexus, resulting in pain and paresthesias on the medial aspect of the arm, forearm, and hand (C8, T1).

4. A blow to the anterior axilla. This can injure the axillary nerve producing paralysis or paresis of the deltoid muscle. A similar injury damaging the musculocutaneous nerve will result in weakness of the biceps and brachialis muscles with loss of flexion at the elbow and a sensory loss on the lateral aspect of the arm and forearm to the wrist.

5. When the force of an injury is directed upward into the axilla with the arm abducted, the entire contents of the axilla may be severely contused. The posterior cord of the brachial plexus is most vulnerable under these circumstances, resulting in loss of medial rotation of the arm (subscapularis), absence of abduction (deltoid), and paralysis of the triceps and dorsiflexors of the wrist.

6. Dislocation of the shoulder may damage the contents of the axilla, particularly the circumflex nerve, with paralysis of abduction of the arm (deltoid).

7. Gunshot wounds and knife wounds to the axilla or in the supraclavicular area often sever nerves and produce permanent damage to the brachial plexus.

8. Disability may be temporary if the plexus is contused, subjected to pressure by a hematoma, or stretched during coma or general anesthesia.

9. Traction injuries to the brachial plexus may be associated with spinal nerve root avulsions. Prognosis is poor in many of these cases, unless treated by nerve transfer using donor nerves such as the medial pectoral, long thoracic, or subscapular nerves.[12]

10. Traction on the brachial plexus can occur in patients with flaccid hemiplegia following a stroke. This condition can be prevented by early physical therapy and the use of a sling when the patient is out of bed sitting in a chair or walking.

Brachial Neuritis

Definition Brachial neuritis is characterized by a sudden paralysis of muscles supplied through the brachial plexus and is often associated with painful dysesthesia of the arm.

Etiology and Pathology The condition occurs in known viral infections (herpes zoster, Epstein-Barr virus), following injection of tetanus toxoid, in putative viral infections, and as an autoimmune disorder following a surgical procedure.[13] Pathological changes are not well described. In herpes zoster infections the posterior root ganglia are involved.

Clinical Features There is an acute or subacute onset of pain that extends into the shoulder, upper arm, or forearm, followed by weakness, muscle wasting, and sensory loss corresponding to the involved nerves, cords, trunks, or nerve roots. Upper brachial plexus (C5, C6), lower brachial plexus (C8, T1) or whole plexus involvement can occur. The early symptoms are followed by the appearance of the typical rash within a few days in cases associated with herpes zoster. The phrenic and recurrent laryngeal nerves are occasionally involved.[14]

Diagnostic Procedures

1. Other causes of severe pain, such as an acute herniated cervical disc, should be excluded.
2. Electromyography will demonstrate multifocal denervation.

Treatment

1. The condition is often very painful, requiring adequate doses of opioid analgesics for pain control.
2. A short course of oral corticosteroids may reduce the duration of the pain.
3. Cases of herpes zoster infection should be treated with acyclovir, famciclovir, or valacyclovir.
4. Physical therapy should be initiated once the pain is controlled to prevent joint stiffness and adhesions.

Prognosis   Most patients recover completely. Postsurgical cases are often ascribed to stretching or compression of the brachial plexus during the surgical procedure. Many such cases are examples of brachial neuritis following surgery and are not traumatic. This has important medicolegal implications.

Inherited Brachial Plexus Neuropathy   This unusual autosomal dominant neuropathy presents with recurrent episodes of paralysis of an upper limb. Symptoms occur within 7 days of a systemic infection, immunization, or childbirth. There does not appear to be a precipitating factor in many cases. The patient complains of pain in the shoulder and upper limb followed by weakness, then atrophy over a 2-week period. Recovery is satisfactory and often complete. Occasionally an attack can present as a lumbar plexopathy or seventh nerve palsy.

There are no neurological symptoms and no neurological signs, apart from the brachial plexus involvement. Some patients have hypertelorism and prominent epicanthic folds.

Electromyography demonstrates multifocal lesions in the brachial plexus with axonal degeneration. There is no evidence of generalized neuropathy.

Treatment   Treatment includes control of pain and passive therapy to the affected shoulder until recovery occurs.

Inherited Tendency to Pressure Palsy   This rare autosomal dominant condition, also called tomaculous neuropathy, is associated with episodic pressure palsies often precipitated by relatively minor trauma. There is evidence of generalized neuropathy. Nerve conduction studies show slowed conduction and multifocal conduction block compatible with a demyelinating neuropathy. Pathological changes consist of segmental demyelination and hypertrophy. The genetic abnormality and inherited tendency to pressure palsy has been assigned to chromosome 17. Consequently, there is a relationship to HMSN type I, but the two conditions are quite distinct.

Treatment   Physical therapy is recommended. There is no response to corticosteroids.

Neoplastic Involvement of the Brachial Plexus

Etiology and Pathology   Neoplastic involvement of the brachial plexus can occur due to direct extension of a bronchial carcinoma from the apex of the lung, direct extension of a breast carcinoma through the axilla, and with pressure from neoplastic lymph nodes.

Clinical Features   There is usually infiltration of or pressure on the lower trunk or medial cord of the brachial plexus. This produces severe pain in the shoulder and axilla and down the medial aspect of the upper limb with wasting of the small muscles of the hand and Horner syndrome (Pancoast syndrome).

Treatment

1. The condition is very painful and the patient needs adequate doses of opioid analgesics (i.e. morphine sulphate 10 to 15 mg IM q4-6h) to reduce pain.
2. An attempt should be made to control the neoplastic process by irradiation and chemotherapy.

Radiation Damage to the Brachial Plexus   Radiation therapy to the axilla, for the treatment of carcinoma of the breast, may be followed by fibrosis and traction on the brachial plexus. In addition, the vasa nervorum may be damaged producing an ischemic neuropathy. The symptoms are similar to neoplastic involvement of the brachial plexus, and the differential diagnosis can be very difficult.

Treatment   If metastatic recurrence can be ruled out, the patient can be treated with carbamazepine (Tegretol) 200 mg q12h, increasing slowly to 600 mg q12h. Carbamazepine can be combined with phenytoin if this drug produces additional benefit.

Amitriptyline beginning 10 mg q.h.s. and increasing slowly to 200 mg daily if necessary decreases or abolishes pain in some cases. Gabapentin beginning 300 mg q8h and increasing by stages to as high as 3600 mg in 24 hours will control if not abolish pain and can be used in conjunction with analgesics. A fentanyl patch beginning 25 μg and changing every 3 days with an increase in dosage to 50 μg, 75 μg, or 100 μg will relieve pain in many intractable situations. A subcutaneous morphine pump with adjustable delivery system can be installed in selected patients.

Surgical treatment to free the affected nerves from scar tissue may be necessary.

The Thoracic Outlet Syndrome

Definition The *thoracic outlet syndrome* is the result of pressure on the brachial plexus and subclavian artery.

Etiology and Pathology The neurovascular structures of the thoracic outlet, the nerves of the brachial plexus and the subclavian artery, are compressed between the clavicle and the first rib or subjected to pressure from below by a fibrous band, cervical rib, or high first rib.

Clinical Features Pressure on the subclavian artery produces intermittent cyanosis of the hands, which is often associated with painful paresthesias. There may be sudden, extremely painful areas at the fingertips due to emboli that originate in the subclavian artery. Numbness and tingling occur in the ulnar distribution when the medial cord of the brachial plexus is compressed. Pain in the hand may occur, particularly at night, and weakness and wasting develop in the small muscles of the hand. The patient may complain of difficulty in working with the hands elevated above shoulder level because of pain and weakness.

When pressure is exerted on the arm so that the shoulder is pulled downward and backward, the radial pulse is obliterated. A murmur may be heard over the subclavian artery on auscultation.

Diagnostic Procedures Stenosis of the subclavian artery can be demonstrated by real-time ultrasound or retrograde brachial arteriography.

Differential Diagnosis The differential diagnosis includes wasting of the small muscles of the hand (Table 19-2).

Table 19-2
Differential diagnosis of wasting of small muscles of the hand

1. Anterior horn cells (acute): poliomyelitis
2. Anterior horn cells (chronic): amyotrophic lateral sclerosis, syringomyelia, peroneal muscular atrophy
3. Nerve roots: arachnoiditis, pachymeningitis, herniated cervical disc, cervical spondylosis, extramedullary tumors
4. Brachial plexus: trauma, brachial neuritis, metastatic infiltration, post radiation fibrosis
5. Median nerve: trauma, carpal tunnel syndrome
6. Ulnar nerve: trauma, tardy ulnar palsy, cubital tunnel syndrome
7. Muscle: polymyositis, rheumatoid arthritis, distal form of dystrophy

Treatment

1. The shoulder should be elevated on the affected side with a full arm sling to relieve pressure on the subclavian artery and the brachial plexus.
2. Surgical excision of a fibrous band or first rib is indicated in intractable cases.

Prognosis The prognosis is good. This condition has been grossly overdiagnosed in the past and is probably uncommon. Consequently, it is essential to look for other causes that can produce similar symptoms such as cervical spondylosis or the carpal tunnel syndrome.

Neuropathies of Individual Nerves of the Brachial Plexus

Lesions of the Long Thoracic Nerve The long thoracic nerve arises from the anterior nerve roots of C5, C6, and C7 and supplies the serratus anterior muscle. The nerve may be damaged by trauma or by carrying heavy loads. It is occasionally involved by acute (probably viral) neuritis and may be severed during mastectomy. Injury to the nerve results in winging of the scapula. The scapula is medially rotated, and the acromioclavicular joint is displaced posteriorly during pushing or lifting movements of the upper limb.

Lesions of the Suprascapular Nerve

The suprascapular nerve arises from the upper trunk of the brachial plexus (C4, C5, C6) and passes through the suprascapular notch to the posterior aspect of the scapula to supply the supraspinatus and infraspinatus muscles. Entrapment of the nerve as it passes through the suprascapular notch beneath the suprascapular ligament may occur.[15] Injury to the nerve is characterized by pain in the posterolateral aspect of the shoulder and wasting and weakness of the supraspinatus and infraspinatus producing weakness of abduction and external rotation of the arm. The diagnosis is confirmed by electromyography. The nerve may be infiltrated in the suprascapular notch with 2 mL of 1% lidocaine followed by 40 mg methylprednisolone. If the steroid infiltration is not successful after two injections, the suprascapular ligament should be divided surgically.

Lesions of the Musculocutaneous Nerve

The musculocutaneous nerve arises from the lateral cord of the brachial plexus (C5, C6) and supplies the biceps, brachialis, and coracobrachialis muscles. The sensory distribution includes the anterior and posterior aspects of the lateral forearm from the elbow to the wrist. The musculocutaneous nerve may be injured in trauma to the shoulder area or following strenuous exercise such as rowing.[16]

Injury to the nerve is characterized by:

1. Wasting of the flexor muscles of the upper arm and weakness of elbow flexion.
2. Weakness of supination of the forearm.
3. Sensory loss of a small area on the lateral aspect of the forearm.
4. Loss of the biceps reflex.

The patient should wear a full arm sling. Physical therapy should be initiated to maintain range of motion.

Lesions of the Axillary Nerve (Circumflex Nerve)

The axillary nerve arises from the posterior cord of the brachial plexus (C5, C6) and supplies the deltoid and teres minor. The sensory distribution is localized to a small quadrilateral area on the upper lateral aspect of the arm.

The nerve may be injured by direct trauma to the axilla, by penetrating wounds of the axilla, and by fracture of the neck of the humerus. Isolated neuritis is not uncommon, particularly following immunizations or injection of a serum.

The patient develops weakness and wasting of the deltoid with flattening of the contour of the shoulder. There is inability to abduct the arm and weakness of external rotation. Sensory loss occurs over a small area on the upper lateral aspect of the arm.

Lesions of the Radial and Posterior Interosseous Nerves

Anatomy The radial nerve is an extension of the posterior cord of the brachial plexus (C5, C6, C7, C8). It arises in the axilla, enters the spiral groove of the humerus, and terminates at the level of the lateral condyle of the humerus by dividing into a superficial branch and the posterior interosseous nerve. The radial nerve supplies the triceps, anconeus, brachioradialis, and extensor carpi radialis longus in the arm. The nerve also supplies forearm muscles through its posterior interosseous branch including the extensor carpi radialis brevis, supinator, extensor digitorum, extensor digiti minimi, extensor policis brevis, and extensor indices. The sensory distribution includes the lower dorsal forearm, dorsal and lateral aspect of the hand and thumb, and the index and lateral aspect of the middle fingers (except the distal two phalanges).

Etiology The radial nerve is frequently injured by pressure in the axilla when falling asleep with the arm draped over the back of a chair (Saturday night paralysis), by pressure from a crutch, from penetrating injuries of the axilla, or with dislocation of the head of the humerus. A fracture of the humerus can damage the radial nerve in the spiral groove. The nerve is frequently involved in lead neuropathy.

The posterior interosseous nerve is subject to pressure as it passes through the supinator muscle just below the elbow. The nerve is subject to entrapment at the same site in the supinator muscle and may be injured in fractures of the forearm as it lies on the interosseous membrane.

Clinical Features The clinical features depend on the location of the injury and are as follows:

1. Radial nerve. When the radial nerve is injured, wrist drop (paralysis of extensor) associated with paralysis of extension of the elbow (triceps),

weakness of elbow flexion (brachioradialis), weakness of supination (supinator), and paralysis of extension of fingers, thumb, and wrist occur.

2. Interruption of radial nerve just below the branch to the brachioradialis. Same as 1 above, except extension of the elbow remains intact and there is some ability to supinate the forearm.

3. Posterior interosseous nerve. Injury of the posterior interosseous nerve is characterized by progressive atrophy and weakness of the extensor muscles of the forearm. There is loss of extension of the fingers, but wrist drop does not occur because of preservation of the extensor carpi radialis. Entrapment of the nerve is associated with pain and tenderness on the lateral aspect of the elbow and is one of the causes of "tennis elbow."

4. Sensory loss is often restricted to the dorsal surface of the thumb and the adjacent radial half of the dorsal surface of the hand.

Diagnostic Procedures Electromyographic abnormalities of the involved muscles indicate the level of involvement of the radial nerve.

Treatment The wrist should be splinted in extension. Physical therapy is important to prevent contractures of the fingers. Entrapment at the elbow can be treated by injection of 2 mL of 1% lidocaine and 40 mg methylprednisolone (Medrol) or by surgically freeing the nerve in intractable cases.

Lesions of the Ulnar Nerve

Anatomy The ulnar nerve is the largest branch of the medial cord of the brachial plexus (C8, T1). The nerve passes down the medial aspect of the upper arm in close relation to the brachial artery, then inclines backward to enter the ulnar groove at the posterior aspect of the medial epicondyle of the humerus. The ulnar nerve enters the forearm between the two heads of the flexor carpi ulnaris and continues under the cover of that muscle to the wrist, where it crosses the flexor retinaculum and divides into superficial and deep branches, which terminate in the hand.

The ulnar nerve supplies the flexor carpi ulnaris and the medial half of the flexor digitorum profundus in the forearm. The deep branch of the ulnar nerve supplies the adductor pollicis, interossei, third and fourth lumbricals, palmaris brevis, abductor opponens and flexor digiti quinti, and the deep head of the flexor pollicis brevis in the hand.

The sensory distribution through the superficial branch of the ulnar nerve includes the ulnar side of the fourth finger, the whole of the fifth finger on the palmar surface, and the distal two phalanges of the fourth and fifth fingers on the dorsal surface of the hand.

Etiology The ulnar nerve may be injured as follows:

1. At the elbow[17] by:
   a. Fracture of the medial epicondyle of the humerus.
   b. Progressive valgus deformity of the elbow following fracture of the lateral epicondyle, producing stretching of the ulnar nerve behind the medial epicondyle and paralysis occurring many years after the original injury to the elbow (tardy ulnar palsy).
   c. Pressure on the ulnar nerve in the ulnar groove behind the medial epicondyle occurring as an occupational problem (e.g., truck driving or in sedentary occupations where individuals "lean" on the elbow).
   d. Pressure on the ulnar nerve during prolonged surgical operations under general anesthesia.
   e. Entrapment of the ulnar nerve as it passes between the aponeuroses connecting the two heads of the flexor carpi ulnaris muscle just distal to the medial epicondyle (cubital tunnel syndrome).
2. At the wrist by repeated trauma to the wrist in certain industrial occupations, by compression of the ulnar nerve in long distance bicycle[18] or motorcycle riders, or by fracture of the wrist. Rare causes of ulnar nerve involvement at the wrist include arteritis of the ulnar artery, hemorrhage secondary to hemophilia or the use of anticoagulants, and tumors of the wrist.[19]

Clinical Features Ulnar nerve palsy is characterized by:

1. Atrophy of the hypothenar muscles.
2. Atrophy of the interossei.
3. Development of a "claw hand" with extension of the metacarpophalangeal joints and flexion of the interphalangeal joints of the second and third fingers and flexion of the metacarpophalangeal joints (paralysis of the third and fourth lumbosacrals) and the interphalangeal joints of the fourth and fifth digits.
4. Paralysis of the flexor carpi ulnaris, if the ulnar nerve is involved above the middle third of the forearm, producing radial deviation of the hand on flexion of the wrist and weakness of ulnar deviation of the hand.

Diagnostic Procedures

1. Compression of the ulnar nerve at the elbow can be demonstrated by recording delayed nerve conduction in the elbow segment of the nerve.
2. Compression of the ulnar nerve at the wrist produces an increased distal latency recorded in the abductor digiti quinti and the first dorsal interosseous muscle.

Differential Diagnosis The differential diagnosis includes other causes of wasting of the small muscles of the hand (see Table 19-2).

Treatment

1. Splinting is applied to prevent development of a claw hand deformity.
2. Repetitive trauma to the elbow should be prevented by transplanting the ulnar nerve from the ulnar groove to the front of the elbow.
3. Simple surgical decompression of the ulnar nerve in the cubital tunnel is required in cases of cubital tunnel syndrome.
4. Repetitive trauma to the ulnar nerve at the wrist should be avoided. Where appropriate, scar tissue should be excised and other conditions compressing the nerve should be treated.

Prognosis There is usually good restoration of function following adequate treatment of ulnar nerve palsy.

Lesions of the Median Nerve

Anatomy The median nerve arises from the lateral and medial cords of the brachial plexus. The nerve is closely related to the brachial artery as it passes down to the elbow and into the cubital fossa. It continues down the forearm connected to the deep surface of the flexor digitorum sublimis and enters the palm of the hand in close relationship to the palmaris longus tendon by passing beneath the flexor retinaculum.

The median nerve supplies all the flexor muscles of the forearm, except the flexor carpi ulnaris and the medial half of the flexor digitorum profundus.

The abductor pollicis brevis, flexor pollicis brevis, opponens pollicis, and the first two lumbricals are innervated by the median nerve in the hand. A palmar cutaneous branch arises from the median nerve in the lower part of the forearm and pierces the fascia above the transverse carpal ligament to supply sensory fibers to the proximal portion of the palm of the hand. The median nerve then passes beneath the transverse carpal ligament and supplies sensory fibers to the thumb, index, middle, and radial half of the ring finger on the palmar aspect of the hand and to the distal portion of the radial two-thirds of the palm of the hand (Fig. 19-3). The "all median" hand, an anatomical variation in which most of the sensation to the hand is derived from the median nerve, is not uncommon.

Lesions of the Anterior Interosseous Nerve The anterior interosseous nerve arises from the median nerve in the cubital fossa, passes between the two heads of the pronator teres, and descends on the interosseous membrane to the wrist. It supplies the flexor pollicis longus, flexor digitorum profundus, and pronator quadratus.

This nerve is occasionally involved in traumatic injury to the forearm, including extensive lifting, high combined fractures of the ulna and radius, or following cardiac catheterization through the antecubital fossa. Symptoms consist of pain in front of the elbow radiating down the forearm and weakness of the flexor pollicis longus and the flexor digitorum profundus in the index finger. There are no sensory changes because the anterior interosseous nerve does

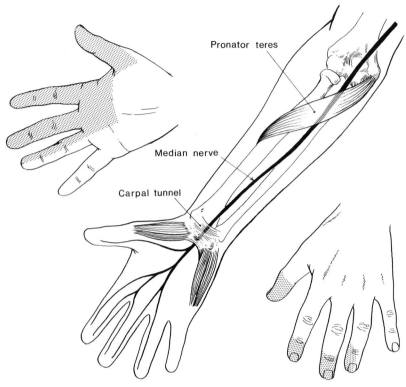

Figure 19-3
The median nerve in the forearm and hand and the cutaneous distribution after passage through the carpal tunnel.

not carry sensory fibers from the skin. Pressure on the median nerve in the cubital fossa exaggerates the pain. This condition is frequently mistaken for "tennis elbow," particularly when there is entrapment of the anterior interosseous nerve between the two heads of the pronator teres. The cubital fossa should be explored with decompression by neurolysis of the nerve from the elbow through the upper third of the forearm.[20]

Carpal Tunnel Syndrome The *carpal tunnel syndrome* is characterized by fluctuating numbness, paresthesia, and pain in the hand due to compression of the median nerve at the wrist. Approximately 80 percent of cases occur in women and the condition is a common temporary phenomenon during pregnancy.

ETIOLOGY AND PATHOLOGY There are many causes of compression of the median nerve at the wrist (Table 19-3).

The median nerve is confined in a relatively limited space as it passes beneath the transverse carpal ligament (flexor retinaculum) to enter the hand. Pressure on the nerve leads to obstruction of the venous circulation and edema. This in turn produces ischemia, increasing pressure on the nerve, and ischemic atrophy of nerve fibers.

CLINICAL FEATURES The earliest symptoms consist of numbness and paresthesias in the sensory distribution of the median nerve in the hand (thumb, index, middle, and lateral half of the ring fingers). Later an ill-defined pain develops, involving the hand and wrist but also extending up into the forearm and

Table 19-3
The carpal tunnel syndrome

1. Hereditary: hereditary neuropathy with liability to pressure palsy: HMSN type III
2. Traumatic: dislocation, fracture, hematoma of forearm, wrist or hand. Wrist sprain. Direct blow to wrist following hand surgery for hand trauma. Occupational causes: repetitive percussion to wrist or repetitive flexion and extension of wrist
3. Infection: tenosynovitis, tuberculosis, sarcoidosis
4. Metabolic: amyloidosis, gout
5. Endocrine: acromegaly, estrogen or androgen therapy, diabetes mellitus, hypothyroidism, pregnancy
6. Neoplastic: ganglion cysts, lipoma, metastatic infiltration, myeloma
7. Collagen vascular diseases: rheumatoid arthritis, polymyalgia rheumatica, scleroderma, systemic lupus erythematosus
8. Degenerative: osteoarthritis
9. Iatrogenic: radial artery puncture, insertion of a vascular shunt for dialysis, hematoma, complications of anticoagulant therapy

often as high as the shoulder. The pain is worse at night, and the patient may hang the hand over the side of the bed or massage the hand in an effort to obtain relief. Complaint of weakness is a late event and is characterized by the inability to unscrew bottle caps or grip properly. Examination may show some wasting of the thenar eminence. Sensory loss is confined to the cutaneous distribution of the median nerve. This area occasionally includes the ring and little fingers if the patient has an anomaly known as the "all median hand," where the cutaneous distribution of the median nerve involves all of the fingers.

DIAGNOSTIC PROCEDURES

1. Electromyography may reveal fibrillations in the muscles of the thenar eminence. Lumbrical sparing can occur in some cases.
2. The distal latency of the median nerve is prolonged, indicating interference with conduction at the wrist.
3. Sensory nerve conduction velocities and the sensory distal latency are prolonged on stimulating the digital nerves of the index finger.
4. Thyroid function tests should be obtained since hypothyroidism is not unusual in carpal tunnel syndrome.

TREATMENT

1. Identified causes should be removed or treated.
2. Temporary and occasionally permanent relief can be obtained by corticosteroid injection around the median nerve in the carpal tunnel. The area around the nerve is infiltrated with 2 to 3 mL of 1% lidocaine followed by an injection of 40 mg methylprednisolone.
3. Patients who fail to respond to injection of corticosteroids performed on two occasions can obtain relief by surgical division of the transverse carpal ligament.
4. A newer technique of endoscopic carpal tunnel release is now available, with less postoperative pain and earlier return to work.[21] The prognosis is excellent if the cause is removed or treated and the affected nerve is released within the carpal tunnel.

Reflex Sympathetic Dystrophy (RSD) (Causalgia, Shoulder-Hand Syndrome, Sudeck's Atrophy)

Definition This results from an augmented response to injury of a body part attributed to sympathetic overactivity owing to uncontrolled stimulation at the spinal cord level.

Pathogenesis Trauma leads to a stimulation of pain fibers (alpha, delta, and C fibers), which synapse in the dorsal horn gray matter (substantia gelatinosa) of the spinal cord. There is a secondary relay through the spinothalamic tract to the thalamus, but there are also axons that synapse with sympathetic efferents. Overstimulation of these efferent fibers leads to a peripheral inflammatory response with liberation of pain, producing peptides such as calcitonin gene-related peptide, neurokinin A and B, substance P, and histamine. This leads to further stimulation of afferent alpha, delta, and C fibers, and reflex activity is established. It is recognized that this is a simplistic description of possible mechanisms in a very complex situation that is currently under intense review.

Clinical Features Trauma is the most common predisposing factor in RSD.[22] However, other conditions have been associated with RSD, including myocardial infarction, cerebral infarction, brainstem infarction, spinal cord injury, spinal cord surgery, cervical spondylosis, lumbar radiculopathy, and neoplasms, particularly of the spinal cord.

There are three signs of RSD:

Stage I: Severe pain, usually following trauma, which may be relatively minor; the pain increases with emotional stress. The presence of allodynia (pain on light touch or contact with clothing) and hyperpathia (increased sensitivity to normal stimuli) are features of the condition.

Dusky mottling or erythematous skin changes can occur. The skin is cool.

Swelling and edema of the affected area, followed by dystrophic skin changes and brittle nails, is usually present. Hyperhidrosis and hypertrichosis are features.

Stage II: Skin changes with a thin skin that is bright and shiny, cool and dusky in appearance. Involuntary tremor, muscle spasms, dystonia, and inability to initiate movements may occur.[23]

Stage III: Progressive skin and subcutaneous tissue atrophy and development of a claw hand occur when that area is affected.

Diagnostic Procedures

1. Radiography of the underlying bone shows patchy osteopenia.

2. Bone scintillography shows increased blood flow, increased blood pooling, and increased periarticular uptake in the affected area.
3. A sympathetic stellate ganglion block will abolish the pain in many cases.
4. Nerve conduction studies are usually normal but may be significantly slowed in damaged nerves when there is an entrapment condition of the digital nerves in the hand, which may mimic the pain of reflex sympathetic dystrophy.

Treatment

1. The patient should be placed in daily physical therapy to improve mobility, and adequate pain medication should be given as needed. Transcutaneous electrical stimulation may be helpful in some cases.
2. When the conservative treatment fails, the use of corticosteroids may be of benefit. This is usually given as prednisone or an equivalent 20 mg q8h decreasing the dose by 5 mg every 4 days.
3. Amitriptyline beginning 10 mg q.h.s. and increasing slowly by 10-mg increments to avoid adverse affects to 150 to 200 mg q.h.s. will control the pain in many intractible cases.
4. When medical treatment of this type has failed, sympathetic nerve interruption should be considered. This can be performed by sympathetic blocking using medications such as phenoxybenzamine, bretylium, and reserpine.
5. If this fails, surgical sympathectomy should be considered.
6. Gabapentin 300 mg q8h increasing by 300-mg increments daily up to 3600 mg per day is effective in producing pain control in some patients.

Prognosis The majority of patients have spontaneous resolution or respond to sympathectomy.

The Lumbar Plexus

The lumbar plexus is a relatively simple plexus formed by the union of the anterior primary rami of L1, L2, L3, and L4 within the substance of the psoas muscle (Fig. 19-4). Lesions of the lumbar plexus are relatively rare because the nerves are well protected within the substance of the psoas muscle. However,

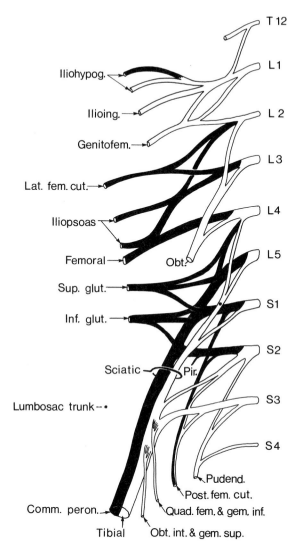

Figure 19-4
The lumbosacral plexus.

iac spine. Entrapment has also been described at this site. The patient presents with pain, paresthesias, and a small area of sensory deficit on the abdominal wall just above the pubic symphysis. Entrapment may be treated by injecting the nerve with a local anesthetic and a corticosteroid at the point where the nerve penetrates the internal oblique muscle.

Lesions of the Ilioinguinal Nerve The ilioinguinal nerve arises from the anterior primary ramus of L1 and traverses the abdominal wall between the transverse and internal oblique muscles to emerge through the superficial inguinal ring. The nerve supplies muscular branches to the abdominal muscles and cutaneous branches to the skin over the canal, the abdominal wall immediately above the pubic symphysis, the root of the penis, the upper part of the scrotum, and a small area on the adjacent medial aspect of the thigh.

The nerve may be compressed by enlarged lymph nodes in the inguinal area and is occasionally cut during herniorrhaphy. Herpes zoster involvement is not uncommon. The patient develops pain or sensory loss in the anatomic distribution of the nerve. Vesicles occur in the same distribution in cases of herpes zoster. Paralysis of the internal oblique muscle may predispose to an indirect inguinal hernia.

Lesions of the Genitofemoral Nerve The genitofemoral nerve is formed within the psoas muscle by the junction of two branches arising from the anterior primary rami of L1 and L2. It accompanies the iliac vessels to the level of the inguinal ligament and divides into a genital branch and a femoral branch. The genital branch enters the deep inguinal ring, traverses the inguinal canal, and supplies the cremasteric muscle, the scrotum, and the skin of the adjacent part of the thigh. The femoral branch enters the thigh beneath the middle of the inguinal ligament and supplies sensation over the femoral triangle. This nerve may also be compressed by enlarged lymph nodes or cut during herniorrhaphy. Pain or sensory loss occur in the anatomical distribution of the genitofemoral nerve.

the plexus may be injured by penetrating wounds or by pressure from a psoas abscess or metastatic neoplasm. Irritation of the rami gives rise to pain in the corresponding dermatome. Destruction of rami leads to muscle weakness and wasting in the appropriate myotome.

Lesions of the Iliohypogastric Nerve The iliohypogastric nerve arises from the anterior primary ramus of L1. The nerve may be injured as it pierces the internal oblique muscle just above the anterior il-

Lesions of the Lateral Cutaneous Nerve of the Thigh The lateral cutaneous nerve of the thigh arises from the anterior primary rami of L2 and L3, penetrates the psoas muscle, and crosses the iliacus to the anterior superior iliac spine. It enters the thigh between the two attachments of the inguinal ligament, penetrates the fascia lata, and divides into two branches about 10 mm below the inguinal ligament. The anterior branch supplies sensation to the lateral part of the anterior aspect of the thigh as far as the knee. The posterior branch supplies the upper two-thirds of the lateral aspect of the thigh and the lateral aspect of the buttock.

Etiology and Pathology The nerve is prone to compression (entrapment) as it passes between the two attachments of the inguinal ligament or where it pierces the fascia lata. This condition seems to occur more frequently in diabetics or in individuals who suddenly gain or lose weight.

Clinical Features Compression of the lateral cutaneous nerve of the thigh results in what is referred to as meralgia paresthetica. The patient complains of pain, paresthesias, and numbness in the distribution of the nerve.

Treatment

1. All constricting items around the waist should be removed and an ice pack applied for 30 min tid, to the site of constriction, where the lateral cutaneous nerve penetrates the fascia lata.
2. Administration of a nonsteroidal anti-inflammatory drug for 7 to 14 days may relieve symptoms.
3. Those who fail to respond should receive infiltration of the area of entrapment with 1% lidocaine and 40 to 80 mg methylprednisolone (Medrol), which produces permanent cure in a majority of patients.
4. Refractory patients require surgical resection of a 4 cm length of the nerve where it exits the pelvis.[24]

Lesions of the Obturator Nerve The obturator nerve is formed by the union of branches from L2, L3, and L4. The nerve emerges from the medial border of the psoas muscle and descends through the obturator foramen to enter the thigh, where it divides into anterior and posterior branches. The obturator nerve sup-

plies muscular branches to the adductor longus, gracilis, adductor brevis, obturator externus, adductor magnus, and (occasionally) pectineus. The cutaneous distribution is to the medial aspect of the thigh.

The obturator nerve may be injured by trauma, including fractures of the femur and gunshot wounds, and following difficult labor. A carcinoma of the cervix, rectum, or bladder may also involve the obturator nerve. The patient presents with weakness of adduction of the thigh with a tendency to abduction of the thigh when walking. Sensory loss occurs in the anatomic distribution of the nerve.

Lesions of the Femoral Nerve The femoral nerve arises within the substance of the psoas muscle from the anterior primary rami of L2, L3, and L4. It passes downward and beneath the inguinal ligament to enter the thigh lateral to the femoral artery where it divides into a number of branches. One of these branches, the saphenous nerve, accompanies the femoral vessels in the femoral canal and continues down the leg on the medial aspect of the knee joint to terminate over the medial malleolus and the medial aspect of the foot.

The femoral nerve supplies muscular branches to the iliacus, pectineus, sartorius, quadriceps femoris, and adductor longus. The cutaneous branches supply the anterior thigh (intermediate and medial cutaneous nerves of thigh) and the medial aspect of the leg and foot (saphenous nerve).

Etiology and Pathology

1. Trauma: fracture of the femur and pelvis, gunshot wounds, hematoma of the psoas muscle from injury or manipulation.
2. Infection: psoas abscess, sarcoidosis, diphtheria, herpes zoster.
3. Neoplasia: compression by pelvic tumor or metastases.
4. Vascular damage: compression by an aortic aneurysm, polyarteritis nodosa.
5. Hemorrhage: spontaneous bleeding with hematoma formation in leukemia, hemophilia, or other bleeding diathesis.
6. Iatrogenic damage: hematoma of the psoas muscle or femoral canal during anticoagulant therapy.

The Sacral Plexus

The sacral plexus is formed by the union of the nerve roots L4, L5, S1, S2, S3, and S4 anterior to the piriformis muscle, which separates it from the lateral part of the sacrum. The most important branches include the superior gluteal nerve (L4, L5, and S1), the inferior gluteal nerve (L5, S1, and S2), the posterior cutaneous nerve of the thigh (S1, S2, and S3), the sciatic nerve (L4, L5, S1, S2, and S3), and the pudendal nerve (S2, S3, and S4).

Lesions of the Superior Gluteal Nerve

The superior gluteal nerve leaves the pelvis through the greater sciatic foramen and supplies the gluteus medius and gluteus minimus. These two muscles act as abductors and medial rotators of the thigh. The nerve may be injured by wounds of the buttocks and is occasionally involved in fractures of the pelvis and by metastatic tumors within the pelvis. Involvement produces paralysis of the gluteus medius and minimus resulting in lateral rotation of the lower limb at rest and flexion of the trunk toward the affected side when walking.

Lesions of the Inferior Gluteal Nerve

The inferior gluteal nerve enters the buttocks below the piriformis muscle and supplies the gluteus maximus. This muscle is responsible for extension of the hip, and paralysis produces difficulty in rising from a sitting position and difficulty in climbing stairs. There is marked atrophy of the affected buttock.

Lesions of the Posterior Cutaneous Nerve of the Thigh

The posterior cutaneous nerve of the thigh leaves the pelvis through the sciatic foramen and passes down the buttock and thigh on the medial aspect of the sciatic nerve. The posterior cutaneous nerve of the thigh supplies sensation to the posterior aspect of the thigh as far as the popliteal fossa. The nerve is often injured in gunshot wounds and penetrating wounds of the thigh and is occasionally injured by injections of irritating material. Damage to the nerve gives rise to a sensory deficit in the back of the thigh, the lateral part of the perineum, and the lower portion of the buttock.

Lesions of the Pudendal Nerve

The pudendal nerve leaves the pelvis through the greater sciatic foramen below the piriformis muscle and passes forward into the ischiorectal fossa. The nerve is occasionally injured in fractures of the pelvis. Damage produces sensory loss in the perineum and scrotum on the side of the lesion. Bilateral lesions produce bladder disturbances with urinary incontinence and overflow.

Lesions of the Sciatic Nerve

The sciatic nerve is the main branch of the sacral plexus and leaves the pelvis through the greater sciatic foramen to enter the buttock. The nerve then passes down the posterior aspect of the thigh to the popliteal fossa, where it divides into the tibial and common peroneal nerves. Compressive lesions of the sciatic nerve produce sciatic pain, which is distributed down the posterior aspect of the thigh, often radiating into the calf and the foot. The most common cause is herniation of a lumbar disc between L4 and L5, or L5 and S1. Other causes of sciatic nerve compression are listed in Table 19-4. The sciatic nerve may be injured by penetrating wounds of the buttocks, thigh, or popliteal fossa. Sciatic nerve paralysis has also been described in association with a fracture of the femur or posterior dislocation of the femoral head. Complete interruption of the sciatic nerve produces a useless lower limb with loss of ability to flex and extend the foot at the ankle, loss of flexion and extension of the toes, and loss of inversion and eversion of the foot. Movement of the lower limb produces a flail-like movement of the foot at the ankle. In addition, there is impairment of flexion at the knee due to paralysis of the biceps femoris, semitendinosus, and semimembranosus, although some movement is still possible by contraction of the sartorius and gracilis muscles supplied by the femoral and obturator nerves, respectively. Extension of the knee is preserved. There is marked sensory loss below the knee with the exception of the medial aspect of the leg and ankle, which is innervated by the saphenous nerve. Wounds of the middle portion of the posterior aspect of the thigh produce loss of function confined to the common peroneal and tibial nerve with preservation of the nerve to the hamstrings. In these cases, flexion of the knee is preserved.

Table 19-4

Causes of sciatic nerve lesions (other than lumbar disc herniation)

1. Nerve root involvement
   a. Cauda equina: herpes zoster, arachnoiditis, tumors of the cauda equina, subarachnoid hemorrhage
   b. Vertebrae and intervertebral foramina: compression fractures or fracture dislocation, spondylosis, lumbosacral stenosis, tuberculosis, Paget disease, metastatic tumors
2. Sacral plexus
   Trauma with fracture of the pelvis, psoas abscess, pelvic abscess, direct extension of pelvic carcinoma, retroperitoneal metastasis, aneurysm of iliac vessels or branches, pregnancy
3. Gluteal area
   Trauma from penetrating wounds, fracture of the pelvis, fracture of the femur, dislocation of the femoral head, traumatic hematoma, traumatic aneurysm of the inferior gluteal artery
4. Thigh
   Penetrating wounds, injection of drugs into sciatic nerve, sciatic nerve entrapment
5. General involvement
   Diabetes mellitus, polyarteritis nodosa

Lesions of the Common Peroneal Nerve The common peroneal nerve arises in the posterior aspect of the thigh as one of the two terminal branches of the sciatic nerve. The common peroneal nerve is injured by penetrating wounds of the lower portion of the posterior aspect of thigh or popliteal fossa. It is occasionally involved in fractures of the lower portion of the femur or the head of the fibula. Symptoms consist of foot drop with a tendency to invert the foot due to unopposed action of the tibialis posterior. There are a high-steppage gait, wasting of the muscles of the anterior compartment of the leg, and a sensory loss extending over the lateral aspect of the leg and dorsum of the foot.

Lesions of the Superficial Peroneal Nerve This nerve arises at the level of the bifurcation of the common peroneal nerve just below the neck of the fibula. The nerve passes down the leg anterior to the fibula between the peroneal and extensor digitorum longus muscles. Lesions of the superficial peroneal nerve produce paralysis of the peroneal muscles with loss of eversion of the foot and a tendency to invert the foot on dorsiflexion. There is a variable sensory loss over the lower lateral aspect of the leg and dorsum of the foot.

Lesions of the Deep Peroneal Nerve The deep peroneal nerve arises just below the head of the fibula as one of the two terminal branches of the common peroneal nerve. The deep peroneal nerve passes onto the interosseous membrane between the tibia and fibula and then courses downward to the ankle supplying the muscles of the anterior compartment of the leg with the exception of the peroneal group. This nerve is commonly affected by pressure over the head of the fibula, often by sitting with the legs crossed for a prolonged period of time. Deep peroneal nerve paralysis produces weakness of the dorsiflexors of the foot and extensors of the toes resulting in foot drop, steppage gait, weakness of the muscles of the anterior compartment of the leg, and a sensory deficit confined to the contiguous surfaces of the first and second toes.

Lesions of the Tibial Nerve Tibial nerve lesions are infrequent, but the nerve is occasionally injured or compressed by cysts or hematomas of the popliteal fossa. There are weakness of plantar flexion and adduction of the foot with a sensory loss involving the sole of the foot.

The Posterior Tibial Nerve (Tarsal Tunnel Syndrome) The posterior tibial nerve is subject to compression as it passes beneath the flexor retinaculum, which forms the roof of the tarsal tunnel at the ankle. The nerve usually divides into medial and lateral plantar nerves in the tarsal tunnel, and symptoms of compression depend on the degree of involvement of these two nerves. Symptoms consist of pain and paresthesias of the sole of the foot, which are aggravated by walking or prolonged standing. There is no weakness, but there may be some wasting of the adductor hallucis. The pain may be aggravated by pressure over the posterior tibial nerve just below the medial malleolus.

Treatment consists of infiltration of the tarsal tunnel with 1% xylocaine followed by 40 mg methylprednisolone (Medrol). Surgical division of the flexor retinaculum is indicated in intractable cases.

Plantar Nerves and Interdigital Nerves   The plantar nerves are occasionally involved by inflammatory conditions such as tenosynovitis. The interdigital nerves are subject to compression as they cross the heads of the metatarsal bones. The interdigital nerve to the third and fourth toes is most commonly involved with the development of a traumatic neuroma. Symptoms consist of severe episodic pain radiating to the contiguous surfaces of the third and fourth toes (Morton's metatarsalgia). The condition may improve following infiltration with local anesthesia and methylprednisolone, but excision of the traumatic neuroma is required in most cases.

HEREDITARY NEUROPATHIES

The hereditary neuropathies are rare or uncommon conditions in which the peripheral neuropathy is the predominant, although not necessarily the sole, abnormality. The neuropathy is genetically determined and is presumably due to a metabolic disorder. Some of the metabolic abnormalities have been identified; others are yet unknown.

Hereditary Motor and Sensory Neuropathies (HMSN)

HMSN Type I or CMT I: Peroneal Muscular Atrophy—Charcot-Marie-Tooth Disease

Definition   This is a genetically determined, chronically symmetrical polyneuropathy.

Etiology and Pathology   The condition is usually inherited as an autosomal dominant trait with microduplication of a segment of chromosome 17 or trisomy of a large region of chromosome 17. In either case, there is an abnormality of the peripheral myelin protein 22 gene (PMP-22 gene)[25,26] and an abnormal expression of PMP-22 protein, producing abnormal function of the Schwann cell, affecting myelination of nerves with hypophosphorylation of neurofilament proteins and axons.[27] There are hypertrophic changes in the myelin with onion bulb formation. Rare autosomal recessive or X-linked recessive forms of the disease have been recognized.[28]

Clinical Features   The disease has a prevalence of 1 per 2500 and usually presents in the first or second decade, with slowly progressive weakness of distal muscles in the lower extremities, leading to foot drop. Weakness and wasting of the small muscles of the hands develop later and spread to the forearm muscles. Sensory impairment to all modalities occurs in the feet and hands. Tendon reflexes are usually absent. The wasting of muscles in the lower extremities may eventually spread to the lower thighs, giving an inverted bottle appearance. However, this appearance is not universally present and calf muscle hypertrophy has been reported in a few cases.[29] Peripheral nerves are palpable in about one-third of cases. All show high arched feet, which may be the only manifestation of the disease in family members who have a forme fruste of the disease. The life span is normal; but there is a wide range in severity of clinical signs.[30] Consequently, a significant number of patients experience impaired respiratory function in the advanced stages of the disease.[31] This carries implications for the management of anesthesia and postoperative monitoring.[32] Tremor, parkinsonism, and dystonia have been reported in some cases.[33] Thus, there is a wide range of signs and symptoms in HMSN type I, but only a minority of patients who have this disease will eventually require wheelchair assistance.

Diagnostic Procedures

1. Nerve conduction velocities are decreased below 40 m/s with velocities uniform between nerves or nerve segments.[34] Compound action potentials are low in amplitude and dispersed.

2. The cerebrospinal fluid (CSF) is normal.

3. Respiratory function tests are indicated in patients who are in the advanced stages of the disease and who are being screened for possible surgical procedures.

4. Electrocardiography (ECG) and cardiac evaluation is advised under similar circumstances.

Mitral valve prolapse occurs in at least 50 percent of patients.

5.   Sural nerve biopsy indicates a hypertrophic neuropathy with frequent onion bulb formation in many cases.

6.   Somatosensory evoked potentials and visual evoked potentials are abnormal in some patients, indicating central nervous system (CNS) involvement.[35]

Treatment   There is no specific treatment for HMSN type I. Patients with foot drop may benefit from ankle-foot orthoses. Orthopedic procedures may be considered in some cases, or tendon transplant in either feet or hands may improve function in those who have severe weakness affecting the extremities.

HMSN Type II, Axonal Type, of Charcot-Marie-Tooth Disease
This condition is usually inherited as an autosomal dominant trait, but it can be inherited as an X-linked dominant or X-linked recessive trait.[36] Linkage to markers on chromosomes Ip has been described.[37] Clinically, onset is later and progression slower than HMSN type I. There is less involvement of upper extremities. A variant HMSN IIE has been described, with diaphragmatic and vocal cord paralysis.[38] Sural nerve biopsies show axonal loss with mild demyelination, compatible with wallerian degeneration. Nerve conduction velocities are normal or slightly slowed, but there is marked diminution of amplitude. Electromyography shows denervation. The CSF is normal.

Treatment   There is no effective treatment for this condition. The measures as described for HMSN type I apply.

HMSN Type III (Dejerine-Sottas)
This autosomal recessive neuropathy is characterized by severe demyelination and early onset.[39] Walking and other milestones are delayed, and the patient is wheelchair dependent in the late teens. There is severe atrophy of distal muscles and a marked sensory ataxia. High arched feet and kyphoscoliosis are prominent. Nerves show thin myelin sheaths with onion bulb formation around small myelinated fibers. Motor nerve conduc-

tion velocities are very slow or unrecordable.[40] Sensory action potentials are absent. The CSF protein is markedly elevated.

Treatment   Treatment is as described for HMSN type I.

HMSN Type IV, Refsum Disease (Heredopathia Atactica Polyneuritiformis)
A rare disorder of inheritance, this autosomal recessive trait results from a deficiency of phytanic acid oxidase.[41] The disease presents in the first or third decades with a slowly progressive polyneuropathy associated with cerebellar ataxia, ichthyosis, cataracts, pigmentary retinopathy, pes cavus, hammer toes, and cardiac conduction defects. Examination shows anosmia, nystagmus, hearing loss, ataxia, and palpable hypertrophic changes in peripheral nerves. The CSF protein is elevated. Motor and sensory nerve conduction velocities are very slow. There is elevation of serum phytanic acid.

Treatment   A diet low in phytanic acid is required.

HMSN Type V
This is an autosomal sensory afferent motor axonal polyneuropathy with steady progression and spastic paraparesis.

HMSN Type VI
As for type I, with optic atrophy.

HMSN Type VII
As for type II, with pigmentary retinopathy and normal phytanic acid metabolism.

HMSN Type VIII
Peripheral neuropathy and spinal cerebellar degeneration.

The syndrome of the hereditary motor and sensory neuropathies is incomplete, with several recent additions to the list of these hereditary diseases. All are rare.

Hereditary Sensory Neuropathies

Type I   This autosomal dominant sensory neuropathy is associated with chronic decrease in small myelinated and unmyelinated fibers. Symptoms begin in the third decade with progressive loss of sensation in the distal lower limbs, slowly extending proximally. Upper extremity involvement is late and mild. There may be painless ulceration of the feet, lightning pains, and mild distal muscle wasting.[42]

Type II (Morvan Disease)   The condition is similar to type I and is inherited as an autosomal recessive trait. There is marked decrease in myelinated axons and a moderate loss of unmyelinated fibers. The condition begins in infancy or childhood, with loss of all sensation distally in the limbs. Severe dystrophic changes and anhidrosis occur in the limbs and tonic pupils, neuropathic joints, and unrecognized fractures can develop in some cases.[43]

Type III (Reilly-Day Syndrome)   This condition is inherited as an autosomal recessive trait with symptoms presenting in infancy. There is episodic cyanosis, vomiting, fever, decreased lacrimation, hyperhidrosis, episodic hypotension, and fluctuating temperature. Examination shows a dissociated sensory impairment with loss of temperature and pain sensation. This results in corneal ulceration, painless skin ulcerations or infection, and Charcot joints. There is generalized areflexia. The prognosis was poor, but use of antibiotics and control of infection has increased survival. There are reports of improvement in adult survivors.[44]

Type IV (Hereditary Anhydrotic Sensory Neuropathy)   This rare autosomal recessive neuropathy is characterized by mental retardation, insensitivity to pain and temperature, anhidrosis, and episodic pyrexia.[45]

Type V   As for type IV, with normal mentation.
Other hereditary sensory neuropathies beginning in childhood or adolescence, associated with spastic paraplegia,[46] or with prominent loss of small myelinated fibers,[47] or associated with hereditary ataxias such as Friedrich's ataxia, have been described.[48]

Familial Amyloid Neuropathy

Amyloidosis may be familial, primary, or secondary. Hereditary (familial) amyloidosis is inherited as an autosomal dominant trait and has been classified into four types based on clinical features and geographical location.[49] Types I and II are characterized by mutations in the transthyretin gene, resulting in an abnormality in the constituent amyloid fiber or protein transthyretin.[50] Type III is associated with a variant form of apolipoprotein A-1 and type IV with an abnormality in gelsolin, an actin-binding protein.

Clinical Features   Type I develops in the third or fourth decade with a progressive, painful sensorimotor neuropathy, affecting lower limbs more than upper limbs, and often associated with carpal tunnel syndrome, autonomic neuropathy, and ulceration of the feet. The type II familial amyloidosis develops in the fourth or fifth decade, with peripheral neuropathy affecting the upper limbs more than the lower limbs, and carpal tunnel syndrome. Type III is characterized by severe sensorimotor neuropathy affecting upper and lower limbs, with severe amyloidosis. Type IV familial amyloidosis presents with cranial nerve palsies and a lattice dystrophy of the cornea.

Diagnostic Procedures

1. Sural nerve biopsy will show deposits of amyloid in the perineurium and endoneurium.
2. Amyloid has an apple green birefringence after staining with Congo red when viewed microscopically under crossed polarized light.
3. Amyloid can be detected in blood using radioimmunoassay and enzyme-linked immunosorbent assay techniques.

Treatment   Liver transplantation has produced regression of amyloid deposits in several patients.[51]

THE INFLAMMATORY NEUROPATHIES

The inflammatory neuropathies are a group of peripheral neuropathies of various etiologies, characterized by an inflammatory response involving the peripheral nerve. The most important inflammatory neuropathies are herpes zoster, diphtheric, infectious mononucleosis, human immunodeficiency virus (HIV) infection, acute inflammatory demyelinating polyneuropathy

(Guillain-Barré syndrome) and chronic inflammatory demyelinating polyneuropathy (CIDP).

Herpes Zoster (Shingles)

Definition   Herpes zoster is an acute, painful mononeuropathy associated with a vesicular eruption in the distribution of the affected nerve.[52]

Etiology and Pathology   The infective agent is the varicella virus. Herpes zoster may represent an infection by recently acquired varicella virus in an individual who has a declining immunity to the virus or a recrudescence of activity by latent varicella virus in the presence of declining immunity.

The viral activity is predominantly located in the dorsal root ganglia or sensory ganglia of the cranial nerves. The ganglia are swollen and show areas of necrosis. There is a marked inflammatory response with necrosis of neurons. The ventral (motor) nerve root is occasionally involved, and inflammatory changes may spread to the spinal cord or brainstem. The vesicles in the skin contain herpes virus, and the surrounding area shows a polymorphonuclear infiltration due to secondary bacterial infection.

Clinical Features   Herpes zoster is a disease of adults and rarely affects children. There is an increased incidence in patients with altered immunity due to such conditions as malignancy, HIV infection, Hodgkin disease, and leukemia. The condition presents with fever followed by pain in the distribution of the involved nerve. Vesicles appear in the affected area within 24 h and are soon involved by secondary bacterial infection, which results in severe regional lymphodermatitis. The pain usually begins to subside after a few days but may persist for months (postherpetic neuralgia). The pustules heal, and crusts separate after about 3 weeks, leaving pigmented scars.

Herpes zoster is not confined to sensory symptoms. Motor weakness from ventral root involvement occurs in 5 to 10 percent of patients.

Complications

1.   Involvement of the ophthalmic division of the fifth cranial nerve is frequently associated with corneal ulceration (Herpes zoster ophthalmicus) and may result in severe damage to the cornea. This condition is occasionally followed by retinal and intracranial arteritis, producing additional visual loss and contralateral hemiparesis.

2.   Herpes zoster involvement of the geniculate ganglion produces a painful vesicular rash involving the pinna, external auditory meatus, and eardrum followed by ipsilateral facial paralysis (Ramsay-Hunt syndrome).

3.   Sacral nerve involvement may be associated with loss of bladder and anal sphincter control.

4.   Herpes zoster encephalitis is probably more common than has been thought in the past. Careful neurological examination may reveal subtle signs of intention tremor or gait ataxia, which should be regarded as encephalitic in origin. However, it is not unusual to find a CSF pleocytosis in the early stages of herpes zoster mononeuropathy.

5.   Retrograde spread of the virus from the posterior root ganglion into the spinal cord occasionally produces an acute transverse myelitis. This may result in permanent cord damage with major neurological deficits. Herpes zoster myelitis usually occurs in immunocompromised individuals.

Differential Diagnosis   It is extremely difficult to diagnose herpes zoster before the characteristic vesicles appear. The pain may mimic many acutely painful conditions such as pleurisy, pericarditis, perforated peptic ulcer, appendicitis, renal colic, and herniated lumbar disc.

Diagnostic Procedures

1.   The white blood cell count is often elevated in the presence of secondary infection.

2.   Lumbar puncture will reveal a lymphocytic pleocytosis in many cases. If there is clinical evidence of CNS involvement, the CSF abnormality is indicative of encephalitis.

Treatment

1.   Herpes zoster is a systemic illness and patients should be treated with bed rest.

2.   Adequate analgesia is mandatory. Narcotics are often required in the early stages.

3. Acyclovir 800 mg q4h orally or famciclovir 500 mg q8h is very effective in aborting an attack of herpes zoster.

4. A course of corticosteroids such as prednisone 80 mg daily for 7 days will produce rapid relief from pain in many cases. However, these antiviral agents must be given within 48 h of onset of herpes zoster.

5. Local application of calamine lotion or calodion, or application of a cream containing acyclovir or capsaicin, and avoidance of contact with clothing or bedclothes help to relieve pain and itching.

6. Herpes zoster encephalitis should be treated with acyclovir or famciclovir intravenously.

7. The rare occurrence of transverse myelitis[53] or vasculitis may respond to intravenous acyclovir or famciclovir.

8. Postherpetic neuralgia is a most debilitating condition, particularly in elderly patients. The condition may persist for many months, but the patient should be informed that it will eventually subside. There is no single effective remedy, but some patients obtain relief from topical capsaicin cream or subcutaneous interferon injections. Carbamazepine (Tegretol), gabapentin 300 mg q8h increasing to 3600 mg per day if necessary for pain control, or phenytoin (Dilantin) may also be effective. These drugs may be used in combination if necessary. Alternatives include amitriptyline (Elavil) beginning 10 mg q.h.s. and slowly increasing by 10-mg increments up to 175–200 mg if necessary. A rapid increase in dosage leads to unacceptable dry mouth, resulting in rejection of the medication, particularly by elderly patients.

Diphtheria   Approximately 10 percent of patients develop signs of neuropathy during diphtheria epidemics. Nerve involvement is the result of the neurotropic properties of the diphtheria toxin.

There are three types of involvement:

1. Early involvement with paralysis of the palate and failure of accommodation occurring within a few days of the onset of the illness.

2. Delayed mononeuropathy or polymononeuropathy in which palatal involvement is followed by paralysis of muscles in any part of the body. (This may occur in a series with recovery of function in one area followed by paralysis of a different muscle group.)

3. A condition resembling Guillain-Barré syndrome (page 612).

Leprosy   This condition is rare in the United States and Europe but is still one of the most common causes of neuropathy worldwide.

The disease is the result of infection by *Mycobacterium leprae* and appears in two forms, the tuberculoid type and the leprous type of leprosy. The form of the disease appears to depend on the immune response of the patient, but in either case, the incubation period may be as long as 10 years before symptoms appear.

In tuberculoid leprosy, there are skin lesions consisting of macules that are relatively few in number, and superficial nerves are affected and may be palpably enlarged. Occasionally, larger nerves such as the median, ulnar, common peroneal, and facial nerves are involved.

In leprous leprosy, the skin lesions are more numerous and the earlobes are affected, as are the dorsal surfaces of the hands, forearms, feet, and anterolateral aspects of the legs. These areas show sensory loss. In addition, there may be a symmetrical peripheral neuropathy.

The condition is diagnosed by muscle biopsy, although the diagnosis can be anticipated in patients with appropriate symptoms in tropical countries.

Treatment

1. Diaminodiphenylsulphone (dapsone) 400 mg/day. Alternatives include rifampin, streptomycin, and isonicotinic acid hydrazide. Chloroquine may also be of benefit.
2. Acute mononeuritis may respond to corticosteroids.

Infectious Mononucleosis   This condition is occasionally complicated by mononeuropathy or by peripheral neuropathy resembling acute inflammatory demyelinating polyneuropathy (Guillain-Barré syndrome) (see below).

Sarcoid Neuropathy   Sarcoidosis is a recognized cause of symmetrical peripheral neuropathy, often associated with cranial nerve involvement, erythema nodosa, lymphadenopathy, relapsing uveitis, parotitis, and hypercalcemia. The peripheral neuropathy may be predominantly motor sensory or mixed in type. Other signs of sarcoidosis may be present.

Diagnostic Procedures

1. Biopsy of the involved site or sural nerve biopsy.
2. Elevated serum angiotensin converting enzyme, abnormal serum immunoglobulin, and elevated alkaline phosphatase are often but not always present.
3. Hypopituitarism, diabetes insipidus, and hypothalamic involvement are occasional complications.
4. The cerebrospinal fluid is often abnormal with a mononuyclear pleocytosis, elevated protein content, presence of oligoclonal bands, and reduced glucose content.

Treatment   Corticosteroid therapy is usually effective. Relapse is not unusual and repeated courses of steroids may be necessary.

Guillain-Barré Syndrome (Acute Inflammatory Demyelinating Polyneuropathy)

Definition   The *Guillain-Barré syndrome* is an acute, symmetrical, ascending polyneuropathy frequently occurring 1 to 3 weeks and occasionally up to 8 weeks after an acute infection.

Etiology and Pathology   The Guillain-Barré syndrome often follows a nonspecific respiratory or gastrointestinal illness but has also been described after a number of specific infections such as cytomegalovirus, Epstein-Barr virus, enterovirus, *Campylobacter jejuni* or mycoplasma, and after immunization. The disease is believed to be due to lymphocytic sensitization to peripheral nerve antigen. There is diffuse, patchy, segmental demyelination of peripheral nerves. Light microscopy reveals an intense lymphocytic, inflammatory infiltrate at the sites of demyelination.

Clinical Features   There is a worldwide incidence of 1.6 to 1.9 cases per 100,000 population per year. More than 50 percent of cases have a clear history of an upper respiratory infection 1 to 3 weeks prior to the onset of neuropathy and an antecedent gastroenteritis is not uncommon. Other antecedent conditions include immunizations, surgical procedures, pneumonia, influenza, tonsillitis, and exanthema of childhood.

The syndrome often begins with myalgia or paresthesias of the lower limbs followed by weakness. About one-third of those affected develop lower limb weakness, which ascends to involve pelvic girdle, abdominal, thoracic, and upper limb muscles. Examination shows symmetrical weakness of muscles with loss of tone and flaccidity. Tendon reflexes are absent. The seventh cranial nerve is frequently involved, and bilateral facial weakness is common. Involvement of the other cranial nerves may result in ptosis or facial myokymia. Dysarthria, dysphagia, and diplopia develop in severe cases. The degree of sensory involvement varies, but this is disproportionately less than the muscle involvement.

The paralysis may progress for about 10 days and then remain relatively unchanged for about 2 weeks. The recovery phase is much slower and may take from 6 months to 2 years for completion.

Complications

1. Respiratory impairment occurs in about 50 percent of patients and respiratory failure in at least 33 percent of patients.

2. Autonomic instability may present as urinary retention in the early stages of the disease. Fluctuations in blood pressure, orthostatic hypotension, and a rare complication of persistent hypertension are late events.

3. Bulbar palsy should always be considered when bilateral facial weakness is present.

4. Pain presenting as myalgia in the lower limbs is an early symptom in some cases, but pain may be a prominent symptom throughout the acute phase of the illness, requiring appropriate and adequate therapy.

5. Secondary infection is a risk with pneumonia complicating respiratory insufficiency and in-

creased risk of urinary tract infection and infected decubitus ulcers.

6. Immobility predisposes to deep venous thrombosis in the lower limbs and pulmonary embolism.

7. Similarly, immobility and failure to change position increase the risk of skin breakdown and decubitus ulcers.

8. Fluid and electrolyte imbalance is not unusual when intake is restricted to parenteral fluids because of bulbar palsy.

9. Papilledema is a rare complication; the cause is unknown.

10. Relapse is uncommon unless treatment is inadequate.

11. Recurrence has been reported, but many of these patients may have had chronic inflammatory demyelinating polyneuropathy presenting with a rather acute onset, rather than the Guillain-Barré syndrome.

Variants Guillain-Barré syndrome may occasionally present with a descending paralysis of pharyngeal cervical brachial muscles rather than the typical ascending paralysis. Other variants include paraparesis with normal strength and reflexes in the upper limbs and an initial severe midline back pain. The Miller-Fisher syndrome of ophthalmoplegia, bilateral facial weakness, severe ataxia, absence of tendon reflexes but only mild limb weakness is believed to be another variant of Guillain-Barré syndrome although optic neuropathy may also occur in this condition.[54]

Diagnostic Procedures

1. The CSF cell count may be normal, or there may be a mild lymphocytic pleocytosis in the early stages of the disease. The protein content begins to rise after the first week of the illness and continues to rise for several weeks to levels above 100 mg/dL.

2. Nerve conduction studies show conduction velocities less than 60 percent of normal in most cases. Distal and motor latencies are prolonged, and proximal stimulation of nerves shows a decrease in amplitude, owing to dispersion of the action potential or conduction block. F-wave responses may be absent or show prolonged latency.

3. About 10 percent of patients show incomplete recovery. A prolonged period (more than 3 weeks) from maximal weakness to initial improvement, associated with reduced motor nerve conduction velocities and evidence of denervation by electromyography, are indicative of a possible incomplete recovery.

Differential Diagnosis

1. Poliomyelitis is characterized by initial fever and severe myalgia followed by asymmetrical flaccid paralysis of muscles. There is an initial CSF pleocytosis, and there is no sensory involvement.

2. Botulism often occurs in a group situation with ingestion of home-canned food. Symptoms begin with diplopia.

3. In heavy metal neuropathy, the onset of weakness is much slower. There is a history of exposure to heavy metals in industry in most cases.

4. Periodic paralysis is characterized by sudden onset of generalized paralysis without respiratory involvement and hypo- or hyperkalemia.

5. Acute polymyositis. There is an acute onset of proximal symmetrical weakness. A rash is often present in dermatomyositis. The sedimentation rate and creatine phosphokinase levels are elevated.

6. Tick paralysis is a flaccid paralysis without respiratory involvement that usually occurs in childhood. Examination will reveal a tick attached to the skin. There is rapid recovery after removing the tick.

7. Acute intermittent porphyria. Acute respiratory paralysis can occur suddenly in this condition. The urine shows the presence of porphobilinogen, and serum delta aminolevulinic acid is elevated.

8. Myasthenia gravis does not present as an ascending paralysis.

9. An acute inflammatory demyelinating polyneuropathy may be associated with HIV zero conversion, acquired immunodeficiency syndrome (AIDS)-related complex (ARC), or AIDS.[55]

Treatment

1.   Good nursing care is essential to prevent the development of pressure sores.

2.   Retention of urine may occur in the early stages and require bladder catheterization.

3.   Respiratory insufficiency should be anticipated in all cases with vital capacity recorded by spirometry q6h. When the readings show a progressive decrease in vital capacity, the procedure should be performed q4h, then every hour when the reading is marginal. In the male patient weighing 70 kg assuming a minimal requirement of 10 mL/kg, a vital capacity of 1 L requires intubation and assisted ventilation. The critical level in a female weighing 50 kg is 750 mL vital capacity. Critical levels are higher in obese and emphysematous patients.

4.   Physical therapy should be given from the initial stages of the disease beginning with passive movements to prevent adhesions around the joints. The program should be increased with more active participation by the patient as soon as there are signs of recovery.

5.   There is no evidence that corticosteroids are beneficial and some evidence shows a detrimental effect in controlled studies.[56]

6.   Plasmapheresis is an effective therapy and treatment consists of exchanging 200 or 250 mL of plasma per kg body weight on alternate days over a 7- to 10-day period.[57] Treatment beginning within a week of onset of weakness is most beneficial, and delay beyond 2 weeks is likely to be ineffective. Because mild cases of Guillain-Barré syndrome do not require plasmapheresis, treatment can be delayed until the patient can no longer walk or shows signs of respiratory or bulbar involvement. However, treatment should begin at an early stage in cases known to be associated with severe deterioration, for example, after rabies vaccination, surgery, or when there is a short interval between antecedent events and onset of symptoms. Limited relapse has been reported from 5 to 42 days after plasmapheresis.[58] Retreatment is effective. Plasmapheresis is occasionally associated with hypotension and cardiac arrhythmias. Thrombosis, hemorrhage, or sepsis are low-risk complications.

7.   Intravenous immunoglobulin (IVIG) has displaced plasmapheresis as the first choice in therapy in many institutions. The IVIG patients have fared better than plasmapheresis-treated patients in controlled studies, and IVIG has fewer adverse effects.[59] However, IVIG has been associated with significant increase in relapse rate, although these episodes are usually mild. Spacing IVIG therapy over a 7- to 10-day period rather than 5 consecutive days reduces the relapse rate.

Prognosis   Complete recovery occurs in 85 percent of cases, but the process is slow, lasting several months or as long as 18 months in some cases. Respiratory insufficiency proposes a life-threatening situation, which can be minimized by the early use of an efficient, modern ventilator. A few patients show partial recovery and then develop prominent signs of peripheral neuropathy. Relapse in the early phase of the illness is not unusual, but relapse weeks or months after recovery suggests that the initial attack may have been a particularly acute episode of recurrent polyneuropathy, such as chronic inflammatory demyelinating polyneuropathy.

Axonal Variant of Guillain-Barré Syndrome

There are occasional examples of cases clinically indistinguishable from Guillain-Barré syndrome that show axonal degeneration rather than demyelination.[60] The CSF protein:cell dissociation is present and the course is often but not invariably benign. The conduction follows a *C. jejuni* or *Legionella* infection in some cases. Diagnosis is established by stool culture for *C. jejuni* and by electromyogram demonstration of primary axonal disease in *Legionella* infections.

Treatment   Treatment is as for classical Guillain-Barré syndrome.

Chronic Inflammatory Demyelinating Polyneuropathy (CIDP)

Definition   *Chronic inflammatory demyelinating polyradiculoneuropathy* is a chronic polyneuropathy in which there is steady progression, intermittent progression, or a relapsing and remitting course over a period of years.

This condition in the past has been described as idiopathic neuritis, nonfamilial hypertrophic neuritis, nonfamilial Dejerine-Sottas disease, relapsing neuritis, and recurrent neuritis.

Etiology and Pathology There is often a history of a preceding infectious process or an injection of a foreign protein, but some cases of CIDP develop in an apparently well individual without a history of prior infection, immunization, or vaccination. Nevertheless, the condition is believed to be an autoimmune response directed against the Schwann cells of the peripheral nerve.

The affected nerves show mononuclear cell infiltration with segmental demyelination and a reactive hyperplasia of Schwann cells producing hypertrophic neuropathy. The involvement is often predominantly proximal involving both sensory and motor nerve roots.

Brainstem involvement has been described in some cases with degeneration of neurons, microglial proliferation, and perivascular lymphocytic infiltration.[61]

Clinical Features Symptoms of sensory involvement and motor weakness occur with equal frequency. Sensory symptoms usually consist of numbness and paresthesias in the hands and feet. Pain is less frequent but occurs in some cases. Motor weakness may be proximal[62] (difficulty in rising from a chair, lifting arms above the head) or distal (poor grip, tripping due to foot drop). Intercostal, diaphragmatic, and bulbar weakness occur in less than 20 percent of cases. The course may be progressive, intermittent, or relapsing and remitting.

Weakness and wasting occur in both proximal and distal muscles and are of equal extent. Sensory loss involving touch, pinprick, vibration, and position sense occurs in symmetrical fashion in upper and lower limbs. Signs of brainstem involvement are not uncommon and include Argyll Robertson pupils, Horner syndrome, diplopia, nystagmus, depressed corneal reflexes, sensory loss over the face, bilateral facial weakness, dysarthria and dysphagia, weakness of the tongue, and intention tremor in the upper limbs. Papilledema occurs in a small number of cases. Hyporeflexia or areflexia are observed in most

patients, but hyperreflexia can occur when brainstem involvement is extensive. The peripheral nerves are palpably enlarged when the demyelinating process extends more peripherally and involves the ulnar or median nerve at the elbow.

The disease may progress to severe disability with confinement to a wheelchair or bed in a minority of cases. Most patients remain ambulatory but handicapped by the disease. Death may occur from intercurrent infection after several years in severely debilitated patients.

Diagnostic Procedures

1. The white blood cell count and erythrocyte sedimentation rate are normal, but there may be an elevation of gamma globulin on serum protein electrophoresis.

2. On lumbar punctures, the CSF has a normal cell content or a mild pleocytosis of less than 75 cells per dL. The cell content is predominantly lymphocytic, but some polymorphonuclear cells are present on occasion. The protein content is usually elevated and may be in excess of 500 mg/dL. The gamma globulin content is elevated in some cases.

3. Nerve conduction velocities of both motor and sensory nerve fibers are usually but not invariably slowed.

4. Sural nerve biopsy shows evidence of demyelination with mononuclear cell infiltration of the epineurium and endoneurium, edema of the endoneurium, and Schwann cell proliferation (onion bulb formation). Teased fibers show evidence of demyelination and remyelination.

5. The MRI scans have demonstrated evidence of demyelination in the brain in some cases of CIDP suggesting that a combined syndrome of central and peripheral demyelination may exist.

Treatment

1. Corticosteroids. There is no doubt that corticosteroids are beneficial in CIDP,[63] but the benefit may be short-lived and long periods of treatment are needed in some cases. This usually results in adverse effects. Tapering to a maintenance dose of steroids to delay the onset of side effects can be attempted, but

long-term treatment at high dose seems to be necessary in some cases.

2. Plasmapheresis is an effective alternative to corticosteroids. This is a safe and effective therapy in children and adults.

3. Intravenous and immunoglobulin therapy is currently recommended as an effective, preferred treatment for CIDP[64,65] in adults and in children.[66] Improvement may be sustained for many months in some cases; others show a short-lived response of 2 weeks to 3 months. However, the response to repeated courses of immunoglobulin therapy is sustained, and in many cases, a hundred courses have been reported without decline in efficacy or the development of adverse reactions.

4. Other immunosuppressive agents have been reported to improve CIDP. There are no controlled studies to date, but the most promising agent appears to be cyclophosphamide, either orally or by pulsed intravenous administration. Cyclosporine A is another immunosuppressant reported to be of benefit when there is a lack of response to steroids, plasmapheresis, or immunoglobulin.[67]

Prognosis Spontaneous recovery has been observed in a small number of cases. Some patients respond to corticosteroids, while others show initial improvement, then apparently fail to respond to further treatment. A number of patients fail to respond to corticosteroids and die from respiratory failure or intercurrent infection several years after the onset of the disease.

Multifocal Motor Neuropathy (MMN)

Definition This is a rare, predominantly motor peripheral neuropathy with a superficial resemblance to motor neuron disease.[68]

Etiology and Pathology It is probably an autoimmune neuropathy. Involved nerves show focal enlargement, occasionally tumor-like swellings. There is chronic demyelination with onion bulb formation.[69]

Clinical Features This is a predominantly motor neuropathy with subtle, patchy sensory loss. Muscle weakness is confined to the distribution of individual affected nerves with motor weakness, atrophy, fasciculations, and cramps. Bulbar involvement is rare, and there are no signs of motor neuron involvement. The disease begins in young adults and involves distal upper limb muscles initially, with slow progression to a more generalized involvement over many years.

Diagnostic Procedures

1. Motor conduction studies show multifocal conduction block confined to motor axons, usually in the forearms and hands[70] with occasionally more widespread, milder conduction changes.
2. Antibodies to GM1 ganglioside occur in 50 to 70 percent of patients.

Treatment There is a good response to long-term immunoglobulin therapy.[71] Relapse can occur. Steroids and plasmapheresis are not effective.

PERIPHERAL NEUROPATHIES IN VASCULAR DISEASE

Although peripheral neuropathy is not unusual in patients with atherosclerotic cerebrovascular disease, such cases are nearly always due to diabetic neuropathy. Peripheral neuropathy of vascular origin is relatively rare and is related almost exclusively to arteritis. The term "arteritis" includes polyarteritis nodosa, Wegener's granulomatosis, giant cell arteritis,[72] rheumatoid arthritis, Sjögren syndrome, and systemic lupus erythematosus (SLE). However, the neuropathy in SLE may be the result of immune complex deposition, antiphospholipid antibodies, or antineural antibodies, rather than an "arteritis." The neuropathies associated with angiopathies may present as a mononeuropathy or diffuse symmetrical peripheral neuropathy.

Diagnosis may require sural nerve biopsy when other signs of disease are lacking and the patient presents with neuropathy alone.

Treatment with corticosteroids is usually effective in giant cell arteritis but may be of less or of no benefit in polyarteritis nodosa and in the other arteritides. The neuropathy of SLE may respond to monthly infusions of intravenous cyclophosphamide.[73]

NEUROPATHIES COMPLICATING HIV INFECTION

Four distinct peripheral neuropathies have been recognized clinically or electrophysiologically in up to 35 percent of patients with HIV infection.[74] However, the incidence is likely to be underestimated because many patients with AIDS have a subclinical peripheral neuropathy.[75]

1. The distal symmetrical peripheral neuropathy is the most frequently encountered neuropathy in AIDS. This condition presents with distal sensory loss consisting of numbness, burning, and paresthesias in the toes, extending up the lower limbs, followed by sensory impairment in the fingers. There is mild weakness of the intrinsic muscles of the feet and marked skin changes distally in the lower limbs, with thinning of the skin, hair loss, and later development of a dusky discoloration and pedal edema. Reflexes are lost at the ankle but preserved at the knees.

2. Chronic inflammatory demyelinating polyneuropathy can develop in AIDS.

3. Mononeuropathy multiplex with abrupt onset, patchy weakness and sensory loss occurs in AIDS. Cranial nerve involvement is often present in these cases. In the early stages of HIV infection, spontaneous resolution can occur. In advanced infection, with CD4 counts below 50 per cubic millimeter, the neuropathy may progress rapidly to quadriparesis.[76]

4. Progressive polyradicular neuropathy involving the lumbosacral nerve roots produces subacute progressive motor and sensory loss, with impairment of bladder and bowel sphincter control. Some cases are the result of cytomegalovirus infection.

Diagnostic Procedures

1. The CSF is normal in distal symmetrical peripheral neuropathy and multineuropathy multiplex but abnormal in CIDP and progressive polyradicular neuropathy.
2. Electrophysiologic studies are abnormal in all four conditions.
3. Sural nerve biopsies are abnormal in CIDP and symmetrical peripheral neuropathy.
4. All patients have antibodies to HIV in the serum.
5. The sedimentation rate is usually elevated.
6. Polyclonal elevation of serum immunoglobulins is present in most cases.

Treatment

1. Patients with CIDP respond to prednisone, plasmapheresis, or intravenous immunoglobulin therapy.
2. Polyradicular neuropathy or mononeuritis multiplex, owing to a cytomegalovirus, requires early treatment with ganciclovir.
3. Treatment of distal symmetrical peripheral neuropathy requires amitryptyline, desipramine, or gabapentin for pain and an ankle-foot orthosis for distal weakness.

TOXIC NEUROPATHIES

Toxins are usually ingested or inhaled and may cause damage to peripheral nerves by attacking neurons, resulting in nerve cell death; by damaging Schwann cells, producing demyelination; or by directly damaging axons, producing distal axonal degeneration. Axonal degeneration is by far the most common reaction and is usually insidious in onset following steady exposure to toxic substances. The lower limbs are affected before the upper limbs, and there is gradual development of sensory loss with a stocking type of hypalgesia. This is associated with loss of the ankle jerk. Muscle wasting and weakness develop later. Recovery is slow once toxic exposure ceases, because axonal regeneration is a slow process, and many patients show residual disabilities for months or years. Examination shows slowing of motor nerve conduction, and the CSF protein is normal. Many substances produce toxic neuropathies. The most common encountered in clinical practice include chloramphenicol, disulfiram, isoniazid, nitrofurantoin, and phenytoin. Industrial or environmental toxins include acrylamide monomer, arsenic, lead, thallium, carbon disulfide, N-hexane, organophosphates, methylbromide, methyl-N-butylketone, triorthocresyl phosphate, polychlorinated biphenyls, and β-amino-propionitrile.

Toxic neuropathies with segmental demyelination or following neuronal death are rare. Demyelinating peripheral neuropathy has been described in buckthorn poisoning, and the neuropathy associated with mercury poisoning is believed to follow destruction of nerve cells in the dorsal root ganglia.

METABOLIC NEUROPATHIES

A considerable number of metabolic abnormalities are associated with peripheral neuropathy. In many cases, the peripheral neuropathy is one of a number of neurological abnormalities related to the metabolic defect. The majority of metabolic conditions and their neurological complications are discussed in chapter 17.

PARANEOPLASTIC NEUROPATHIES

Peripheral neuropathies are not unusual complications in patients suffering from carcinoma. The neuropathy may be directly related to the presence of the carcinoma, may be a nonmetastatic phenomenon, or may be a complication of chemotherapeutic treatment. A number of other conditions—for example, multiple myeloma, macroglobulinemia, cryoglobulinemia—may be accompanied by a progressive and often severe peripheral neuropathy.

Carcinomatous Peripheral Neuropathy Two forms of peripheral neuropathy have been described in association with neoplasia and must be considered to be paraneoplastic effects of cancer in that there is no direct involvement of the peripheral nerve by the neoplastic process. The most common form of carcinomatous peripheral neuropathy is a symmetrical sensorimotor neuropathy that affects the extremities, producing distal weakness and sym-

metrical sensory loss. The condition is slowly progressive. There is a rarer sensory neuropathy occasionally encountered in association with malignancy. This condition begins with sensory loss involving the extremities and progresses in a chronic fashion with involvement of all four limbs. The condition sometimes becomes arrested about 3 months after onset and does not show further progression after that time.

Critical Illness Polyneuropathy

Definition This diffuse polyneuropathy occurs in critically ill patients with a delay in weaning the patient from ventilatory support once the critical illness is under control.

Etiology and Pathology The etiology is obscure. No toxic, metabolic, vascular, or nutritional factors have been identified.

Clinical Features The salient feature is failure to withdraw mechanical ventilatory aid when the systemic illness has improved. Improvement occurs first in the upper limb and proximal limb, followed by the respiratory muscles and later by the distal lower limb musculature.

Diagnostic Procedures The diagnosis can be established by electromyography, which shows widespread denervation and by nerve conduction studies.

Treatment The patient should receive all care necessary for a ventilator-dependent patient until recovery returns.

NUTRITIONAL NEUROPATHIES

Nutritional peripheral neuropathies occur in patients who are subjected to chronic deprivation of essential food constituents. These neuropathies have occurred traditionally during famine or during imprisonment and starvation. Under modern conditions they are more likely to be seen in individuals who follow strict, unbalanced diets, in food faddists, in cases of deliberate starvation to lose weight, in persons who have had alimentary bypass operations, and in alcoholics who obtain the bulk of food calories from alcohol.

Beriberi (Thiamine) Neuropathy

Definition *Beriberi neuropathy* is a symmetrical, distal motor and sensory neuropathy due to chronic vitamin B_1 deficiency.

Etiology and Pathology Vitamin B_1 is essential for the metabolism of carbohydrate, and both the CNS and peripheral nervous system are almost entirely dependent on carbohydrate for energy requirements. Vitamin B_1 deficiency may be due to:

1. Inadequate diet: famine, starvation, food fads, anorexia nervosa, bulimia
2. Poor diet: alcoholism, vegetarians
3. Poor absorption: celiac disease, adult sprue, chronic diarrhea
4. Destruction of thiamine: presence of thiaminosis in fish and certain vegetables, thiaminolytic bacilli in the gastrointestinal tract; prevention of phosphorylation by thiamine antimetabolites such as pyrithiamine

Vitamin B_1 deficiency results in failure of formation thiamine pyrophosphate, which acts as a cocarboxylase in the conversion of pyruvate to active acetate. Thiamine pyrophosphate also acts in the conversion of α-ketoglutarate to succinyl-CoA. Thiamine deficiency interferes with the citric acid cycle, and energy release is severely restricted. There is a failure of breakdown of glycose-y-phosphate into the pentose-phosphate shunt due to a lack of thiamine pyrophosphate, which acts as a coenzyme of transketolase in this cycle.

There is a concomitant loss of myelin sheaths and axonal degeneration with Schwann cell proliferation beginning distally and extending proximally.

Clinical Features Patients complain of distal paresthesias, dysesthesias (burning feet), and muscle cramps beginning 2 to 6 months after the beginning of consistent vitamin B_1 deficiency. These symptoms may be accompanied by lethargy, anorexia, nausea, and vomiting. Early symptoms are followed by development of foot drop and steppage gait leading to paraplegia. There is an ascending glove-and-stocking sensory loss. The patient is severely ataxic and reflexes are absent. Weakness may extend to proximal muscles; muscle atrophy is late. Cranial nerve involvement usually involves the vagus nerve producing tachycardia, hoarseness, and dysphagia, and the facial nerve with bilateral facial weakness.

Acute beriberi is rare and presents with acute vomiting and tachycardia followed by rapidly ascending paralysis involving the lower, then the upper limbs. There is a high risk of death from acute heart failure. "Wet" beriberi is a subacute condition with pericardial, pleural, and peritoneal effusions, severe peripheral edema, and peripheral neuropathy.

Diagnostic Procedures

1. Red blood cell transketolase activity is decreased.
2. Serum pyruvate and lactate levels are elevated.
3. Nerve conduction velocity measurements are slowed. An electromyogram shows evidence of denervation.

Treatment Thiamine 100 mg q12h should be given by intramuscular injection. The prognosis is excellent.

Neuralgia in Pregnancy Pregnancy may be associated with a number of neuralgias, which tend to occur in the later months of pregnancy and resolve after delivery. These neuralgias include meralgia paresthetica, carpal tunnel syndrome, sciatic neuralgia, and intercostal neuralgia.

Intercostal neuralgia may produce severe pain in the chest or upper abdomen, which may lead to an erroneous diagnosis of heart disease or acute intra-abdominal disease. The pain is usually exacerbated by movements that stretch the affected nerves, and there may be an area of sensory change in the affected dermatome. Relief may be obtained by temporary nerve block following an injection of a local anesthetic. The prognosis is excellent. The neuralgias of pregnancy resolve in the immediate postpartum period.

REFERENCES

1. Claus D, Eggers R, Engelhardt A, et al: Ethanol and polyneuropathy. *Acta Neurol Scand* 72:312, 1985.
2. Galetta SL, Smith JL: Chronic isolated sixth nerve palsies. *Arch Neurol* 46:79, 1989.
3. Cheng TM, Cascino TL, Onofrio BM: Comprehensive study of diagnoses and treatment of trigeminal neuralgia secondary to tumors. *Neurology* 43:2298, 1993.
4. Coffey RJ, Fromm GH: Familial trigeminal neuralgia and Charcot-Marie-Tooth neuropathy: report of two families and a review. *Surg Neurol* 35:49, 1991.
5. Lechin F, van der Dijs B, Lechin ME, et al: Pimozide therapy for trigeminal neuralgia. *Arch Neurol* 46:960, 1989.
6. Young JN, Wilkins RH: Partial sensory trigeminal rhizotomy at the pons for trigeminal neuralgia. *J Neurosurg* 79:680, 1993.
7. Uri N, Schuchman G: Vestibular abnormalities in patients with Bell's palsy. *J Laryngology Otol* 100:1125, 1986.
8. Perkin GD, Illingworth RD: The association of hemofacial spasm and facial pain. *J Neurol Neurosurg Psychiatry* 52:663, 1989.
9. Baloh RW: Vertigo. *Lancet* 352:1841, 1998.
10. Moller MB, Moller AR, Janetta PJ, et al: Microvascular decompression of the eighth nerve in patients with disabling positional vertigo: selection criteria and operative results in 207 patients. *Acta Neurocher (Wren)* 125:75, 1993.
11. Donner TR, Kline DG: Extracranial spinal accessory nerve injury. *Neurosurgery* 32:907, 1993.
12. Samardzic M, Grujicic D, Antunovic V: Nerve transfer in brachial plexus traction injuries. *J Neurosurg* 76:191, 1992.
13. Malamut RI, Marques W, England JD, et al: Postsurgical idiopathic brachial neuritis. *Muscle Nerve* 17:320, 1994.
14. Sanders EA, Van der Neste VM, Hoogenroad TU: Brachial plexus neuritis and recurrent laryngeal nerve palsy. *J Neurol* 235:323, 1988.
15. Callahan JD, Scully TB, Shapiro SA, et al: Suprascapular nerve entrapment: a series of 27 cases. *J Neurosurg* 74:893, 1991.
16. Mastaglia FL: Musculocutaneous neuropathy after strenuous physical activity. *Med J Aust* 145:153, 1986.
17. Stewart JD: The variable clinical manifestations of ulnar neuropathies at the elbow. *J Neurol Neurosurg Psychiatry* 50:252, 1987.
18. Hankey GJ, Gubbay SS: Compression mononeuropathy of the deep palmar branch of the ulnar nerve in cyclists. *J Neurol Neurosurg Psychiatry* 51:1588, 1988.
19. Rafecas JC, Daube JR, Ehlman RL: Deep branch ulnar neuropathy due to giant cell tumor: report of a case. *Neurology* 38:327, 1988.
20. Schantz K, Riegels-Nielson P: The anterior interosseus nerve syndrome. *J Hand Surg (Br)* 17:510, 1992.
21. Brown MG, Keyser B, Rothenberg ES: Endoscopic carpal tunnel release. *J Hand Surg (Am)* 17:1009, 1992.
22. Kozin F: Reflex sympathetic dystrophy: a review. *Clin Eur Rheumatol* 10:401, 1992.
23. Schwartzman RJ: Reflex sympathetic dystrophy and causalgia. *Neurol Clin North Am* 10:953, 1992.
24. Williams PH, Trzil KP: Management of meralgia paresthetica. *J Neurosurg* 74:76, 1991.
25. Lupski JR: An inherited DNA rearrangement and gene dosage effect are reponsible for the most common autosomal dominant peripheral neuropathy: Charcot-Marie-Tooth disease type IA. *Clin Res* 40:645, 1992.
26. Chance PF, Pleasure D: Charcot-Marie-Tooth syndrome. *Arch Neurol* 50:1180, 1993.
27. Watson DF, Nachtman FN, Kuncl RW, et al: Altered neurofilament phosphorylation and beta tubular isotypes in Charcot-Marie-Tooth disease type 1. *Neurology* 44:2383, 1994.
28. Malcolm S: Charcot-Marie-Tooth disease, type I. *J Med Gerentol* 29:3, 1992.
29. Uncini A, DiMuzio A, Chiavaroli F, et al: Hereditary motor and sensory neuropathy with calf hypertrophy is associated with 17p11.-2 duplication. *Ann Neurol* 35:552, 1994.
30. Gabreels-Festin A, Gabreels F: Hereditary demyelinating motor and sensory neuropathy. *Brain Pathol* 3:135, 1993.
31. Barry LD, Fluellen J: Charcot-Marie-Tooth disease. Podiatric and systemic considerations. *J Am Pediatr Med Assoc* 81:490, 1991.
32. Greenberg RS, Parker SD: Anesthetic management for the child with Charcot-Marie-Tooth disease. *Anesth Analg* 74:305, 1992.
33a. Rao BB, Garcia CA, Wise CA: Gene dosage as a mechanism for a common autosomal dominant peripheral neuropathy: Charcot-Marie-Tooth disease type IA. *Prog Clin Biol Res* 384:187, 1993.
33b. Cardoso FE, Jankovic J: Hereditary motor-sensory

neuropathy and movement disorders. *Muscle Nerve* 16:904, 1993.

34. Kaku DA, Parry GJ, Malamut R, et al: Uniform slowing of conduction velocities in Charcot-Marie-Tooth polyneuropathy type I. *Neurology* 43:2664, 1993.

35. Ionasescu VV: Charcot-Marie-Tooth neuropathies: from clinical description to molecular genetics. *Muscle Nerve* 18:267, 1995.

36. Hahn AF: Hereditary motor and sensory neuropathy: HMSN type II (neuronal type) and X-marked HMSN. *Brain Pathol* 3:147, 1993.

37a. Verhalle D, Lofgren A, Nelis E, et al: Deletion of the CMT1A locus on chromosome 17p11-2. in hereditary neuropathy with lability to pressure palsies. *Ann Neurol* 35:704, 1994.

37b. Ben Othmane KB, Middleton LT, Loprest LJ, et al: Localization of a gene (CMT2A) for autosomal dominant Charcot-Marie-Tooth disease type 2 to chromosome 1p and evidence of genetic heterogeneity. *Genomes* 17:370, 1993.

38. Dyck PJ, Lichy WJ, Minnerath S, et al: Hereditary motor and sensory neuropathy with diaphragm and vocal cord paresis. *Ann Neurol* 35:608, 1994.

39. Chance PF, Lupski JR: Inherited neuropathies: Charcot-Marie-Tooth disease and related disorders. *Baillieres Clin Neurol* 3:373, 1994.

40. Gabreels-Festen AAWM, Gabreels FJ, Jennekens FGI: Hereditary motor and sensory neuropathies. Present states of types I, II and III. *Clin Neurol Neurosurg* 95:93, 1993.

41. Herbert MA, Clayton PT: Phytanic and alpha oxidase deficiency (Refsum disease) presenting in infancy. *J Inherit Metab Dis* 17:211, 1994.

42. Denny-Brown D: Hereditary sensory radicular neuropathy. *J Neurol Neurosurg Psychiatry* 14:237, 1951.

43. Miller RG, Nielsen SL, Summer AJ: Hereditary sensory neuropathy and tonic pupils. *Neurology* 26:931, 1976.

44a. Chance PF, Fischbeck KH: Molecular genetics of Charcot-Marie-Tooth disease and related neuropathies. *Human Med Genet* 3:1503, 1994.

44b. Dyck PJ, Mollinger JF, Reagan TJ: Not "indifference to pain" but varieties of hereditary sensory and autonomic neuropathy. *Brain* 106:373, 1983.

45. Pinsky L, DiGeorge AM: Congenital familial sensory neuropathy with anhidrosis. *J Pediatr* 68:1, 1966.

46. Schady W, Smith CM: Sensory neuropathy in hereditary spastic paraplegia. *J Neurol Neurosurg Psychiatry* 57:693, 1994.

47. Landrieu P, Said G, Allaire C: Dominantly transmitted congenital indifference to pain. *Ann Neurol* 27:574, 1990.

48. Thomas PK: Hereditary sensory neuropathies. *Brain Pathol* 3:157, 1993.

49. Sunada Y, Shimizu T, Nakase H, et al: Inherited amyloid polyneuropathy type IV (Gelsohn Vorant) in a Japanese family. *Ann Neurol* 33:57, 1993.

50. Chance PF, Reilly M: Inherited neuropathies. *Curr Opin Neurol* 7:372, 1994.

51. Skinner M, Lewis WD, Jones LA, et al: Liver transplantation as a treatment for familial amyloidotic polyneuropathy. *Ann Intern Med* 120:133, 1994.

52. Mayo DR, Booss J: Varicella-zoster-associated neurologic diseases without skin lesions. *Arch Neurol* 46:313, 1989.

53. Devinski O, Cho E-S, Petito CK, et al: Herpes zoster myelitis. *Brain* 114:1181, 1991.

54. Toshniwal P: Demyelinating optic neuropathy with Miller-Fisher syndrome. The case for overlap syndrome with central and peripheral demyelination. *J Neurol* 234:353, 1987.

55a. Thomas PK, Misra VP, King RH, et al: Autosomal recessive hereditary sensory neuropathy with spastic paraplegia. *Brain* 117:651, 1994.

55b. Parry GJ: Peripheral neuropathies associated with human immunodeficiency virus infection. *Ann Neurol* 23(suppl 5):549, 1988.

56. Hughes RA: Ineffectiveness of high dose intravenous methylprednisolone in Guillain-Barré syndrome. *Lancet* 338:1142, 1991.

57. Khatri BO, Flamini JR, Baruah JK, et al: Plasmapheresis with acute inflammatory polyneuropathy. *Pediatr Neurol* 6:17, 1990.

58. Ropper AE, Albert JW, Addison R: Limited relapse in Guillain-Barré syndrome after plasma exchange. *Arch Neurol* 45:341, 1988.

59. VanderMeche FGA, Schmitz PIM and the Dutch Guillain-Barré Study Group: a randomized trial comparing intravenous immunoglobulin and plasma exchange in Guillain-Barré syndrome. *N Engl J Med* 326:1123, 1992.

60. McKhann GN, Cornblath DR, Griffin JW, et al: Acute axonal neuropathies. A frequent cause of flaccid paralysis in China. *Ann Neurol* 33:333, 1993.

61. Mendell JR, Kolkin S, Kissel JT: Evidence for central nervous system demyelination in chronic demyelinating polyradiculopathy. *Neurology* 37:1291, 1987.

62. Bradley WG, Bennett RK, Good P, et al: Proximal inflammatory polyneuropathy with multifocal conduction blocks. *Ann Neurol* 45:451, 1988.

63. Dyck PJ, O'Brien PC, Oviatt KF, et al: Prednisone improves chronic inflammatory polyradiculopathy more than no treatment. *Ann Neurol* 11:136, 1982.

64. Van Dorn PA, Brand A, Strengers PF, et al: High dose intravenous immunoglobulin treatment in chronic inflammatory demyelinating polyneuropathy: a double blind placebo controlled crossover study. *Neurology* 40:209, 1990.

65. Dyck PJ, Litchy WJ, Kratz KM, et al: A plasma exchange versus immunoglobulin infusion trial in chronic inflammatory demyelinating polyradiculoneuropathy. *Ann Neurol* 36:838, 1994.

66. Teasley JE, Parry GJ, Sumner AJ: Chronic inflammatory demyelinating polyradiculoneuropathy in children treated with intravenous immunoglobulin. *Muscle Nerve* 14:921, 1991.

67. Hodgkinson SJ, Pollard LD, McLeod JG: Cyclosporin A in the treatment of chronic demyelinating polyradiculoneuropathy. *J Neurol Neurosurg Psychiatry* 53:327, 1990.

68. Parry GH, Clarke S: Multifocal acquired demyelinating neuropathy masquerading as motor neuron disease. *Muscle Nerve* 11:103, 1988.

69. Lange DJ, Trojaborg W, Latov N, et al: Multifocal motor neuropathy with conduction block: is it a distinct entity? *Neurology* 42:497, 1992.

70. Corse AM, Chaudry V, Crawford TO, et al: Demyelinating pathology in sural nerves in multifocal motor neuropathy. *Muscle Nerve* Suppl 1:S216, 1994.

71. Chaudry V, Corse AM, Cornblath DR, et al: Multifocal motor neuropathy. Response to human immunoglobulin. *Ann Neurol* 33:237, 1993.

72. Caselli RJ, Hunder GG, Whisnant JP: Neurologic diseases in biopsy proven giant cell (temporal) arteritis. *Neurology* 38:352, 1988.

73. Newelt, CM, Lachs S, Kaye BR, et al: Role of intravenous cyclophosphamide in the treatment of severe neuropsychiatric systemic lupus erythematosus. *Am J Med* 98:32, 1995.

74. So YT, Holtzman DM, Abrams DI, et al: Peripheral neuropathy associated with acquired immunodeficiency syndrome. Prevalence and abnormal features from a population-based study. *Arch Neurol* 45:945, 1988.

75. Griffin JW, Crawford TO, Tyor WR, et al: Predominantly sensory neuropathy in AIDS: distal axonal degeneration and unmyelinated fiber loss. *Neurology* 41 (suppl 1):374, 1991.

76. Simpson DM, Tagliati M: Neurologic manifestations of HIV infection. *Ann Intern Med* 121:769, 1994.

Chapter 20

MUSCLE DISEASES

The differential diagnosis of muscle weakness and wasting is a commonly encountered problem in clinical situations. The first step is to determine whether the weakness is episodic, as in periodic paralysis and myasthenia gravis, or nonepisodic. The examiner should then consider the distribution of weakness since this is of value in determining etiology. Proximal weakness is usually encountered in myopathies, whereas distal weakness is more likely to have a neurogenic origin. A myopathy is a disorder of skeletal muscle due to disease of the muscle fiber itself. Muscular dystrophy is a congenital myopathy. A decrease in muscle bulk due to myopathy, dystrophy, or denervation is called muscle wasting. However, the term "muscle atrophy" should be reserved for a decrease in muscle bulk due to denervation of the muscle. Certain investigative procedures, such as serum muscle enzymes, electromyography, and muscle biopsy are invaluable in their ability to differentiate myopathic from neurogenic weakness. The distinguishing characteristics of myopathic and neurological disorders are summarized in Table 20-1. The differential diagnosis of weakness is illustrated in Figure 20-1.

MUSCULAR DYSTROPHIES

The muscular dystrophies are genetically determined myopathies characterized by progressive muscular weakness and degeneration of muscle fibers. The muscular dystrophies are classified according to clinical features.

Duchenne Muscular Dystrophy

Definition Duchenne muscular dystrophy is the most common form of muscular dystrophy and is seen almost exclusively in young males, with a prevalence of 1 in 3500 newborn boys. This type of muscular dystrophy is a result of a mutation of the dystrophin gene located on the short arm of the X chromosome, localized to Xp2. The disease is caused by a new mutation in one-third of the cases.[1]

Table 20-1

Distinguishing Characteristics of Myopathic and Neurogenic Disorders

	Myopathic	*Neurogenic*
Signs and symptoms	Proximal weakness and wasting	Distal weakness and wasting ± Sensory signs and symptoms ± Fasciculations, increased tone, extensor plantar responses
Serum muscle enzymes	Increased	Normal
Nerve condition velocities	Normal	Slowed
Electromyography	Low-amplitude polyphasic motor unit potentials of brief duration	Increased insertion activity Fibrillations, fasciculations Positive sharp waves
Muscle biopsy	Variation in fiber diameter Internal nuclei Degeneration of fibers Increased endomysial connective tissue	Angular fibers, target fibers Pyknotic clumping Type grouping Type I fibers: small Type II fibers: hypertrophied

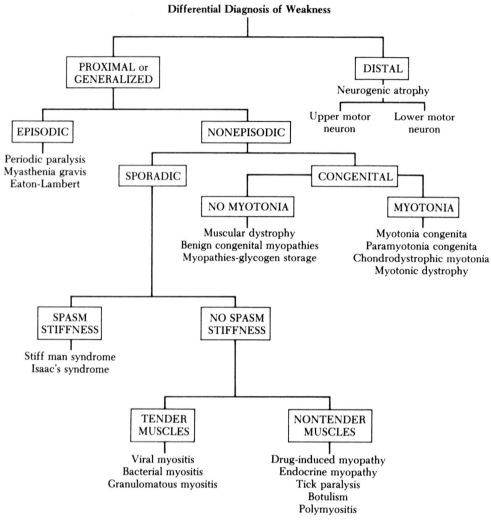

Figure 20-1
Differential diagnosis of weakness.

Etiology and Pathology Duchenne muscular dystrophy is characterized by an absence of the protein dystrophin in the muscle fiber. Dystrophin is normally located in the muscle surface membrane and is part of the membrane cytoskeleton, acting as a stabilizing factor in membrane function.[2] The absence of dystrophin affects the function of dystrophin-associated proteins, which provide a link between dystrophin and the extracellular matrix protein, laminin,[3] the major component of the extracellular matrix. Dystrophin-associated protein dysfunction leads to an increased susceptibility to muscle fiber degradation.[4]

Muscle biopsy shows abnormal variation in muscle fiber size. Other changes include central displacement of nuclei into the muscle fiber, splitting of fibers, fragmentation of the cytoplasm, focal vacuolization, hyalinization and shrinking of the sarcolemmal sheath. There are clusters of necrotic fibers, evidence of regeneration, extensive proliferation of perimysial and endomysial connective tissue, and replacement of muscle fibers by fat.

Clinical Features Affected children appear normal at birth and may be extremely placid. There is normal achievement of early milestones, but there is delay in standing and walking. The child then develops a clumsy, waddling gait and pseudohypertrophy of the calf muscles, associated with difficulty climbing stairs and rising from a chair. Older children have a pronounced lumbar lordosis caused by weakness of the pelvic musculature and the erector spinae. This results in forward tilting of the pelvis, protrusion of the abdomen, and compensatory backward arching of the upper thoracic spine and shoulders. The affected child has difficulty rising to a standing position. He must first roll to a prone position, pull himself to his hands and knees, push with his arms until only his hands and feet are on the floor, and finally, "walk" up his lower extremities until he can extend his trunk and stand. This method of assuming a standing position in the presence of severe proximal weakness has been termed Gower's sign. Eventually the child can no longer ambulate and becomes confined to a wheelchair by the age of 10. Multiple contractures, deformities and severe scoliosis, and distal weakness and wasting are prominent features in the latter stages of the disease. Typically, the patient is bedridden in the teens and dies in the late teens or early twenties. The absence of dystrophin in cardiac muscle results in a primary progressive cardiac dystrophic process.[5] There is a steady decline in cardiac reserve, but heart failure is rare, probably because the patient leads a sedentary life-style. Many develop gastrointestinal hypomotility because dystrophin is absent in smooth muscle. Acute gastric dilatation or fatal intestinal obstruction may occur in advanced cases.[6]

Absence of dystrophin in the brain results in mild impairment of intellectual-cognitive functioning in a subset of patients with Duchenne muscular dystrophy. Lack of dystrophin increases susceptibility to neuronal damage, suggesting that mental impairment may be the result of ischemic insults during fetal life or parturition.[7] Because this is an X-linked, recessive disease, males carrying the abnormal dystrophic mutation express Duchenne muscular dystrophy and females are usually nonexpressing carriers. Occasionally females carrying one copy of the abnormal mutation exhibit a milder form of Duchenne muscular dystrophy, and muscle biopsy demonstrates a mo-saicism of dystrophin expression.[8] The disease may also result from inactivation of the normal X chromosome in some female cases, or an X chromosome translocation, disrupting the dystrophin gene,[9] with selective inactivation of the nontranslocated X chromosome.

Diagnostic Procedures

1. Muscle enzymes. Serum creatine kinase (CK) is elevated and may be abnormal before the onset of clinical signs and symptoms. There are increased serum levels or other muscle enzymes, including aspartate transaminase (AST), alanine transaminase (ALT), lactic dehydrogenase (LDH), and aldolase. The elevation is high in early cases and declines with progression of the disease. Creatinuria and myoglobulinuria may also be present.

2. The electrocardiogram is abnormal at an early age. The initial tachycardia is followed by increased R-wave voltage and eventually development of right bundle branch block and deep Q waves.

3. The electromyogram is abnormal, with myopathic features. Motor unit potentials are reduced in duration and amplitude, and there is increased polyphasic wave activity and early recruitment.

4. Between 2.5 and 10 percent of female carriers of the mutated dystrophin gene have clinical evidence of muscle weakness.[10]

5. In asymptomatic carriers, mutation detection can be performed on lymphocytic genomic DNA obtained from a single blood specimen, using several methods, including Southern blot analysis, field inversion gel electrophoresis, or polymerase chain reaction exon amplification assays. Muscle biopsy can be omitted when mutation detection is positive.

6. Muscle biopsy was the definitive method of diagnosis before the development of genetic diagnostic techniques. Standard light and electron microscopy can be augmented by immunohistochemistry and the use of antidystrophin antisera.

Differential Diagnosis

1. Other forms of dystrophy.
2. Neurogenic muscular atrophy.

3. Polymyositis and dermatomyositis, which are characterized by inflammatory changes on muscle biopsy.
4. Polyneuropathy differentiated by its more rapid onset slow nerve conduction velocities and muscle and nerve biopsy.
5. Benign congenital myopathies (see below).

Treatment

1. There is no specific treatment for Duchenne muscular dystrophy.

2. A physical therapy program will help to delay the development of joint contractures. Obesity should be avoided. Splinting, bracing, and surgical procedures to prevent or treat deformities can prolong the ability to walk.[11]

3. Joint contractures can be relieved by tendon release procedures.

4. Severe scoliosis can be stabilized or reversed by orthopedic surgical techniques.

5. Mild upper respiratory infections are potentially lethal in advanced disease and should be treated with appropriate antibiotics. A decline in respiratory function with difficulty in clearing secretions can be relieved by intermittent continuous positive airway pressure.[12] Nocturnal hypoventilation based on hypoxia hypercapnia measured by blood gas determination requires intermittent noninvasive ventilator support using a nasal mask.[13] Permanent ventilator support usually occurs when forced vital capacity declines below 1.2 L.

6. A lessening of the emotional impact of the disease on the patient and family, and the development of optimal living conditions, can be achieved by a combined effort of the neurologist, physiatrist, psychologist, and social worker.

7. Corticosteroids decrease the rate of muscle loss. Prednisone 0.75/kg daily[14] can be given for as long as 6 months.[15]

8. Newer techniques of gene therapy using myoblast transplantation[16] or gene transfer by reduplication defective retroviruses, adenoviruses, or herpesviruses are currently under investigation.[17] Results have been equivocal.[18]

9. Genetic counseling should be provided. It is important to advise the family regarding the likelihood of involvement in a subsequent pregnancy. Carriers of Duchenne dystrophy may have elevated serum CK levels. Carrier detection or prenatal mutation diagnosis is readily established by DNA diagnostic testing.

Prognosis Duchenne muscular dystrophy is a steadily progressive, incapacitating disease until death in the late teens or early twenties. A better understanding of pulmonary problems and improved treatment of respiratory infections has significantly increased the life span in Duchenne muscular dystrophy and other muscle diseases affecting muscle function.

Becker Muscular Dystrophy

This condition is a milder expression of a disease caused by mutation of the dystrophin gene at Xp21. Patients have an abnormal but functioning dystrophin, reduced in size.[19] There is a wide range of presenting symptoms, varying in severity from a slightly milder form of disease resembling Duchenne muscular dystrophy to asymptomatic elevation of CK.[20]

The affected individual appears to be normal at birth and shows normal developmental milestones; the mean age of onset is 11 years.[21] The initial symptoms often consist of muscle cramps on exercise. Progression is slower than Duchenne muscular dystrophy and patients may walk with bracing until the late twenties or early thirties. Asymptomatic cardiac involvement is not unusual.[22] Symptomatic cardiac involvement is unusual. Hypertrophic cardiomyopathy is rare.[23] Because genetic analysis cannot determine the correct diagnosis in 35 percent of cases, endomyocardial biopsy specimens can be stained by immunostaining techniques in patients with cardiomyopathy suspected to be the result of Becker muscular dystrophy.[24]

Diagnostic Procedures Diagnostic procedures have been discussed under Duchenne muscular dystrophy.

Treatment The most severe cases of Becker muscular dystrophy should be treated as Duchenne muscular dystrophy. Physical therapy measures may maintain ambulation in some cases, up to the age of 30 or more, and many patients survive into their forties. Occasional patients are reported with survival into the seventh decade.[25]

Congenital Muscular Dystrophies

Definition This heterogeneous group of muscular dystrophies is inherited as an autosomal recessive trait characterized by dystrophic changes on muscle biopsy.

Etiology and Pathology The congenital muscular dystrophies are the result of deficient components in the dystrophin-glycoprotein complex. This complex has a structural role in muscle and probably anchors muscle cells to the extracellular matrix. This attachment stabilizes the sarcolemmal membrane and protects it from stressors that develop during muscle contraction. Disruption of this linkage leads to sarcolemmal instability and muscle cell necrosis.[26] Dystrophin, which is localized to the sarcolemma, is completely absent in Duchenne muscular dystrophy. Absence of other proteins in the dystrophin-glycoprotein complex have been identified in other forms of congenital muscular dystrophy. A merosin-negative condition[27] and an adhalin deficiency[28] have been described.

Clinical Features There is profound hypotonia and muscle weakness at birth, with arthrogryposis developing in the first year of life. The clinical course is nonprogressive or slowly progressive. Intellectual development is usually normal, and the condition may stabilize in adolescence. A variant designated as severe childhood autosomal recessive muscular dystrophy, with adhalin deficiency (Fukayama type), in which there are cerebral abnormalities and mental retardation and epilepsy, has been recognized.

Facioscapulohumeral Muscular Dystrophy (FSH)

This is an autosomal dominant form of muscular dystrophy with a frequency of 1 in 20,000.[29] The gene responsible for FSH is localized to chromosome 4q.[30,31] A few families that do not link to chromosome 4 have been reported.[32] Ten percent of cases are the result of mutation.

Pathology The muscle changes are typically those of dystrophy, but inflammatory changes are a common feature.

Clinical Features Symptoms and signs of FSH occur in adolescence, with 95 percent penetrance by age 20.[33] There is initial weakness and atrophy of the facial and shoulder girdle muscles with later progression to the abdominal and pelvic girdle muscles, and foot extensors. Clinical expression shows marked variation, ranging from almost asymptomatic to quadriparesis. Hearing loss occurs in 50 percent of cases and can be severe. Retinal vasculopathy consisting of telangiectasias and microaneurysms has been recognized by fluorescein angiography.[34]

Diagnostic Procedures

1. Serum CK levels are elevated in the active phase of the disease.

2. Electromyographic findings are compatible with a myopathy but may be normal.

3. Muscle biopsy will establish the diagnosis.

Treatment There is no specific treatment for this disease. Supportive measures are indicated as the disease progresses, with emphasis on control of upper respiratory infections in advanced cases.

Scapuloperoneal Muscular Dystrophy and the Scapuloperoneal Syndrome

Definition This is a slowly progressive syndrome of weakness involving the scapuloperoneal musculature.

Etiology and Pathology There are several distinct forms of the disease,[35] a myopathic or neurogenic form inherited as an autosomal dominant trait, and a sex-linked recessive myopathic form in which the affected muscles show dystrophic changes.[36]

Clinical Features   Weakness begins in the peroneal muscles with lesser involvement of the scapula, shoulder, and upper arm musculature, and occasional mild involvement of the facial and laryngeal muscles. The dystrophic form can be accompanied by joint contractures, cardiac conduction abnormalities and cardiomyopathy. The rate of progression varies, and disability can be severe two decades from the time of onset.

The neurogenic condition can occur with or without sensory change, and both axonal and demyelinating variants have been described. The mild facial weakness can lead to an inaccurate diagnosis of facioscapulohumeral dystrophy.

Limb-Girdle Muscular Dystrophy

Definition   This is a heterogenous group of dystrophic muscle diseases, usually sporadic[37] but occasionally inherited as an autosomal recessive trait that maps to chromosome 2p13-16 or inherited as an autosomal dominant trait linked to chromosome 15q.15.1-q21.1[38] with preferential involvement of truncal and proximal limb girdle muscles.

Pathology   There is variation in muscle fiber size, with the presence of small, angular, and hypertrophied fibers showing internally placed nuclei. Fiber necrosis and regeneration are present, with replacement of fibers by fibrous and adipose tissue in advanced cases. Moth-eaten and lobulated fibers occur in most cases. The sarcolemma shows positive staining with antidystrophin antibodies.

Clinical Features   The earliest symptoms consist of weakness of the pelvic girdle or proximal lower limb muscles, which presents at any age from childhood to adulthood, with a mean age of onset of 21 years.[39] The autosomal dominant form of the disease presents in adults and exhibits a slower progression of weakness.[40] The initial symptoms are followed by involvement of upper limb-girdle muscles, then by progressive weakness of truncal or more distal limb muscles, with loss of walking ability 10 to 20 years after onset. Cardiomyopathy is rare and usually asymptomatic, but cardiac failure has been reported.[41]

Diagostic Procedures

1. Serum CK levels are elevated.
2. Electromyography is consistent with an active, chronic myopathy.
3. Dystrophic changes are present in the muscle biopsy.
4. A normal dystrophin staining pattern on muscle biopsy excludes Duchenne and Becker-type muscular dystrophy.

Treatment   Prevention of contractures and bracing to maintain mobility is required in more advanced cases.

Oculopharyngeal Muscular Dystrophy

Definition   This rare muscular dystrophy is inherited as an autosomal dominant trait characterized by late onset of chronically progressive ptosis and dysphagia.

Clinical Features   Most patients are of French Canadian descent,[42] but the condition has been described in other ethnic groups.[43]

Symptoms consist of chronically progressive ptosis and dysphagia beginning in the mid forties or fifties. The ptosis is a result of progressive weakness of the levator palpebrae, and there is preservation of orbicularis oculi function and Bell's phenomenon. There is chronic contraction of the frontalis muscle, and the patient maintains a chin-up head position. Dysphagia is progressive. The patient experiences difficulty with solid food initially and liquids later. The voice has a nasal quality. A late weakness of limb-girdle muscles may occur.

Diagnostic Procedures   Electromyography and muscle biopsy are compatible with a muscular dystrophy, and the muscle biopsy shows granular degeneration of muscle fibers, progressive loss of fibers, and replacement by fibrous tissue. Manometric studies are useful to assess swallowing abnormalities.[44]

Treatment   Surgical treatment of ptosis is successful in most patients. Dysphagia may require myotomy or dilatation of the cricopharyngeal sphincter.

Distal Muscular Dystrophy

There are at least four distinct forms of inherited distal myopathy.[45] Each is characterized by initial weakness in a distal muscle group with progressive involvement of more proximal muscles.

1. Late onset, type 1 (Welander)—autosomal dominant; onset age 40 to 60 years; begins in the small muscles of the hands and spreads proximally. There is late involvement of the anterior tibial and calf muscles.

2. Late adult type 2 (Markesbery)—an autosomal dominant, late onset form beginning with tibialis anterior weakness with slow progression and spread to the calf muscles, and later involvement of the upper limbs.

3. Early adult type 1 (Nonaka)—an autosomal recessive condition with early adult onset, beginning in the tibialis anterior with later spread to the calf muscles, then upper limbs.

4. Early adult type 2 (Miyoshi)—an autosomal recessive type beginning at age 15 to 30 years with involvement of the gastrocnemius and sparing the anterior compartment muscles. There is later involvement of thighs and buttocks and mild involvement of the upper limbs.

MUSCLE DISEASES ASSOCIATED WITH MYOTONIA

Myotonia is a sustained contraction of muscles that may be induced by voluntary contraction, percussion, or electrical stimulation. The primary failure of myotonia is a delayed relaxation due to increased excitability of muscle demonstrated on electromyography, which records discharges of repetitive action potentials following muscle contraction. Myotonia occurs in myotonia congenita, paramyotonia congenita, myotonic dystrophy, and hyperkalemic periodic paralysis.

Myotonia Congenita

Definition *Myotonia congenita* is an hereditary condition characterized by myotonia, a condition of delayed relaxation following voluntary muscle contraction.

Etiology and Pathology Myotonia congenita is caused by a genetically determined abnormality in the voltage gated chloride channel. This results in a blocking of membrane chloride conductance and action potentials can be triggered by a smaller than normal current, resulting in a train of impulses that are self-maintaining, following termination of the stimulating pulse.[46]

Clinical Features Myotonia congenita occurs in a mild form that is inherited as an autosomal dominant trait (Thomsen myotonia) or a more severe form (Becker myotonia) inherited as an autosomal recessive trait. Symptoms of myotonia first appear in infancy or childhood and consist of inability to relax a muscle following contraction. The symptoms tend to increase during childhood and adolescence but may lessen in severity in adult life. Myotonia occurs only in skeletal muscle, and the patient has difficulty initiating movement and making certain movements. Once repetitive movements are initiated, they can be continued without difficulty. Sudden movements may initiate a sustained contraction sufficient to throw the patient off balance. On grasping an object, the patient is often unable to release the object for as long as 60 s. Patients with myotonia congenita have a well-developed musculature and have been described as herculean in appearance. Percussion of an affected muscle produces percussion myotonia, a dimpling of the skin, and sustained contraction. Percussion may also be followed by local swelling of muscle, termed myedema.

Diagnostic Procedures The diagnostic procedure of choice is electromyography. There is marked increased activity after insertion of the needle electrode. Traction or percussion of the muscle produces a series of prolonged potentials that persist when the patient is instructed to relax the contracted muscle. Contraction and relaxation of the muscle produces a typical sound on electromyographic examination, which has been termed the "dive bomber" effect.

Treatment

1. Mexiletine 150 mg q12h, increasing to a maximum of 300 mg q8h, is the drug of choice to reduce myotonia. An electrocardiogram should be obtained before initiating therapy to exclude cardiac conduction abnormalities.

2. Phenytoin (Dilantin) beginning 100 mg q12h and increasing the dose until the serum levels are within therapeutic range is also an effective treatment.

3. A number of other drugs known to be effective in myotonia include procainamide HCl (Pronestyl) 50 mg/kg/day given in divided dosage four times a day and quinine 10 mg/kg/day in divided dosage. Quinine should always be followed by regular visual and audiometric tests because of the risk of optic or otic neuritis.

4. Intractable cases may respond to acetazolamide (Diamox) 8 to 30 mg/kg/day in divided dosage.

Sodium Channel Myotonias

The following conditions are related to sodium channel mutations.[46]

1. Hyperkalemic periodic paralysis.
2. Paramyotonia congenita.
3. Myotonia fluctuans.
4. Myotonia permanens.
5. Acetazolamide-responsive myotonia.

Myotonia Fluctuans   This condition appears in adolescence and is characterized by the appearance of myotonia of delayed onset after exercise.[47] The myotonia increases following potassium loading but is unaffected by cold.

Myotonia Permanens   Symptoms are similar to myotonia fluctuans, but the myotonia is permanent and more severe. There is continuous myotonic activity on electromyography and respiratory exchange may be affected by muscle stiffness.

Acetazolamide-Responsive Myotonia   As suggested by its name, this form of myotonia is dramatically relieved by acetazolamide. The clinical presentation resembles the Thomsen type of myotonia congenita, but the muscle stiffness is painful.[48]

Sodium channel myotonias respond to mexiletine therapy and acetazolamide. Other medications such as phenytoin are less effective.

Chondrodystrophic Myotonia

This condition is inherited as an autosomal recessive trait and is characterized by myotonia, short stature, blepharospasm, muscle hypertrophy, and skeletal deformities. The affected infant presents with hip contractures or dislocation. This is followed by other joint contractures, progressive growth failure, and myotonia. There is a puckering of the mouth, blepharospasm, and small palpebral fissures. Intelligence is normal. Electromyographic findings are typically those of myotonia. Muscular atrophy can occur in older children. The myotonia responds to mexiletine or acetazolamide.

Myotonic Dystrophy

Definition   *Myotonic dystrophy* is a multisystem disorder inherited as an autosomal dominant trait through a locus on chromosome 19.[49] The disease is characterized by progressive muscular weakness, myotonia, cataracts, cardiac abnormalities, hypogonadism, and frontal balding.

Etiology and Pathology   Myotonic dystrophy is the product of an expanded CTG repeat in the 3' untranslated region of a gene that encodes a protein kinase DM-PK on chromosome 19q13.3. There is an expansion of the repeat sequence in myotonic dystrophy and a positive correlation between repeat size and clinical severity.[50] Protein kinases phosphorylate neurotransmitters to achieve a physiological response on specific target cells. Failure of protein kinase activity may cause ion channel dysfunction in myotonia. Expression is maximal in cardiac muscle in myotonic dystrophy but is also present in skeletal muscle and brain.[51]

Affected muscles show evidence of fibronecrosis and degeneration with areas of phagocytosis and increased endomesial connective tissue. Surviving fibers show loss of striations and a characteristic ring fiber has been described. Histochemical studies reveal that degeneration is confined to type 1 muscle fibers and that there may be some increase in the size of type 2 fibers.

Clinical Features   The signs and symptoms appear at any time from birth to age 40 years. Hydrops fetalis has been reported in congenital myotonic dystrophy in a newborn infant who presented with hypertonia, edema, pleural effusion, and respiratory distress.[52] Weakness tends to be nonprogressive in the congenital form of myotonic dystrophy but is slowly progressive in the noncongenital type of the disease.[53] Myotonia is usually the first symptom and affects the hand with later involvement of other muscles, particularly those of the lower limbs. Muscle wasting also affects the hands first then spreads to the facial muscles, muscles of mastication, the sternocleidomastoids, the flexors and extensors of the forearm, the quadriceps, and the dorsiflexors of the feet. The facial appearance is characteristic, with bilateral ptosis and wasting, which has been termed "hatchet face."

Patients with myotonic dystrophy usually have involvement of other organ systems. These include:

1.   Cardiac abnormalities. Prolapsed mitral valve and atrial flutter[54] sometimes occur in the early stages of the disease. More advanced cases with severe cardiac fibrosis suffer cardiac arrhythmias. Syncopal attacks may occur. Subclinical cardiac involvement is not uncommon and may be responsible for sudden death in some cases.[55]

The number of CTG repeats in the myotonic dystrophy gene appears to be a significant predictor of cardiac dysfunction in myotonic dystrophy.[56]

2.   Brain involvement. Neuropsychological testing indicates functional impairment in the majority of patients with myotonic dystrophy.[57] Mental retardation occurs in about 70 percent of cases of congenital myotonic dystrophy but is rarely severe. Progressive dementia occurs in 75 percent of adults with noncongenital disease. Magnetic resonance imaging (MRI) shows cerebral atrophy and areas of increased signal intensity in the white matter in most adults with myotonic dystrophy. However, there is no correlation between the extent of white matter changes and neuropsychological impairment.[58]

3.   Ophthalmic abnormalities. Subcapsular lens opacities, which enlarge and eventually impair vision, are present in most patients.

4.   Endocrine abnormalities. Primary gonadal failure and gonadal atrophy occur in both sexes. Impotence, loss of libido, and testicular atrophy occur in the male. Mild diabetes mellitus may be present in both sexes.

5.   Skin and skeletal abnormalities. Frontal balding occurs at an early stage in the male. A high-arched palate may be present.

6.   Smooth muscle abnormalities. There is impairment of mobility in the gastrointestinal tract, with dilatation of the colon in advanced cases.

7.   Respiratory abnormalities. Respiratory insufficiency, which has been associated with neuronal loss in the medulla, resulting in hypoventilation[59] is a feature in the late stages of the disease when there is an increased risk of aspiration pneumonia.

8.   Hearing loss. There is a high incidence of sensorineural hearing loss in myotonic dystrophy.

9.   Peripheral neuropathy of axonal type is responsible for the areflexia, distal sensory impairment, and fasciculations seen in some cases.

Children born to mothers with myotonic dystrophy may present with congenital myotonic dystrophy in the neonatal period. This condition is characterized by hypotonia, facial diplegia, dysphagia, mental retardation, a high-arched palate, and tented lips. Myotonia develops later in the course of this condition.

Diagnostic Procedures

1.   DNA analysis using a DNA probe allows direct identification of the myotonic dystrophy mutation in DNA extracted from peripheral blood lymphocytes.[60] Southern blot analysis can be used to detect abnormally large DNA fragments with expanded gene repeats. The polymerase chain reaction will detect small expansions of the unstable DNA sequence. DNA testing can also be used for prenatal diagnosis of myotonic dystrophy, as well as detection of carriers.[61]

2. The effect of temperature change. Myotonia may be difficult to demonstrate in some cases. Submersion of the hands in cold water for several minutes may facilitate the appearance of myotonia.

3. The electromyogram is characteristic with an increase in insertional activity and typical myotonic discharges following voluntary contraction of muscle.

4. Cardiac involvement affects predominantly the conduction system in the heart. Atrial fibrillation, atrial flutter, a prolonged PR interval, and various conduction defects may be present.

5. Slit lamp examination reveals the characteristic lens opacities.

6. Serum tests. There are abnormally low levels of IgG, an abnormal glucose tolerance test, and low follicle-stimulating hormone levels in most cases.

7. The MRI and computed tomography (CT) scans and chest and skull x-rays. Thickening of the calvarium and enlargement of the frontal sinuses are often present on skull x-rays. Microcephaly, calcification of the basal ganglia, and cerebral atrophy may be demonstrated by CT scan. The MRI shows the presence of increased signal intensity in the white matter.

8. Pure tone screening and impedance audiometry will detect sensorineural hearing loss.

9. The diagnosis can be established by a muscle biopsy, which shows characteristic findings of a dystrophic process.

Treatment

1. The relief of myotonia is discussed under myotonia congenita. The calcium channel blocking agent, nifedipine, which has no effect on cardiac conduction, decreases myotonia in doses of 10 to 20 mg q8h.

2. In the latter stages, when the risk of aspiration pneumonia increases, respiratory infection should be treated with appropriate antibiotics, postural drainage, and chest percussion.

3. Muscle weakness can be severe in those with marked expansion of CTG repeats. These patients need supportive care, including splinting and use of an electric cart or wheelchair.

4. Cardiac involvement is often the main complication. Patients require regular evaluation of cardiac function and appropriate treatment for arrhythmias.

5. Preoperative and postoperative care and intraoperative monitoring are requred to avoid complications of anesthesia, which carry increased morbidity and may be lethal in myotonic dystrophy.

6. Pregnancy and delivery carry a high risk of complications in mothers with myotonic dystrophy and their offspring. Consequently, mothers should be monitored for increased muscle weakness involving respiratory muscles, reduced fetal movements and hydramnios, and prolonged, often ineffective labor. There is also an increase of spontaneous abortion earlier in pregnancy.

Obstetric complications include retained placenta, placenta previa, and neonatal death.

Prognosis Myotonic dystrophy is a chronic condition with progressive deterioration in most cases. In noncongenital forms of the disease, death occurs between ages 40 and 60 years due to cardiac or respiratory dysfunction.

In congenital muscular dystrophy, there is a 25 percent chance of death before 18 months of age, and a 50 percent chance of survival until the mid-thirties.

Proximal Myotonic Myopathy

This rare variant of myotonic dystrophy is inherited as an autosomal dominant trait in which there is no abnormal enlargement of the CTG repeat in the gene for myotonic dystrophy.

Clinical Features Symptoms are present in adults with complaints of stiffness in the thigh muscles followed by a more generalized myalgia, which can be severe in the thighs. Cataracts can occur at an early stage, and grip myotonia is prominent in most cases. Muscle weakness is often delayed and fluctuates in intensity. Electromyography is abnormal and demonstrates myotonic discharges. The condition is probably compatible with a normal life span because severe cardiac involvement has not been demonstrated.[62]

Benign Congenital Myopathies

The benign congenital myopathies are a heterogenous group of rare disorders. Most congenital myopathies are mild, slowly progressive or nonprogressive, infantile or adolescent conditions associated with specific structural alterations in muscle fiber.

Nemaline myopathy usually presents at birth or in infancy, but symptoms may be delayed until adolescence or adult life.[63] The condition is inherited as an autosomal dominant or recessive trait and presents with generalized muscle hypotonia and weakness from birth or infancy, high-arched palate, long face, pigeon chest, scoliosis, and pes cavus. The severity varies from mild weakness to wheelchair dependency or even use of a mechanical ventilator.[64]

Central core disease is a mild myopathy inherited as an autosomal dominant trait, presenting in infants. The condition is nonprogressive, with proximal muscle weakness and pes cavus. Type I muscle fibers contain central cores of myofilaments lacking mitochondria.

Myotubular myopathy presents as a severe myopathy in infancy, with hypotonia, respiratory failure, and death. Milder cases can occur with survival and these patients present with hypotonia, muscle weakness, delayed psychomotor development, and mental retardation. Muscle biopsies show small myotube-like fibers with central nuclei dispersed between normal-sized fibers.[65]

Vacuolated myopathy is a rare condition of juvenile onset, slow progression, and predominantly proximal muscle weakness. Muscle biopsy shows vacuolated muscle fibers, which probably represent superficial muscle fiber injury associated with sarcolemmal invagination, the result of deposition of complement membrane attack complex on the damaged cell surface membrane.[66]

Diagnostic Procedures   The diagnosis may be established by a muscle biopsy, which indicates a myopathic process. In many cases, a definitive diagnosis requires electron microscopy.

Treatment   Supportive. There is no specific treatment for these conditions.

Prognosis   In the majority of cases, the congenital myopathies are slowly progressive conditions; in some cases, the process appears to become arrested in adolescence or adult life. Other cases show a slow deterioration requiring the eventual use of a wheelchair. There is an increased risk of respiratory infection, which may be fatal unless treated promptly.

Muscle Carnitine Deficiency

This condition is a proximal myopathy with onset in childhood and exhibiting a slowly progressive course. Cardiac muscle involvement and myoglobinuria occur in some cases. Muscle biopsy shows a severe vacuolar myopathy affecting type 1 fibers, with vacuoles staining positive for lipid. The condition results from impaired carnitine transport into muscle; serum carnitine levels are normal or occasionally low, but muscle carnitine content is reduced.

Zidovudine (AZT) therapy may induce a similar myopathy by depletion of mitochondrial DNA, reduced muscle carnitine levels, and lipid storage in muscle fibers.[67]

A systemic form of carnitine deficiency can result from many inborn errors of metabolism. All are associated with deficiency in free carnitine resulting in the limited entry of low-chain fatty acids into mitochondria. Affected children have recurrent attacks of encephalopathy resembling Reye syndrome and later development of myopathy, hepatomegaly, and cardiomyopathy.

TOXIC AND METABOLIC MYOPATHIES

Myopathies Associated with Glycogen Storage Disease

The type, metabolic defect, pathology, clinical features, and diagnostic procedures of glycogen storage diseases associated with neurological symptoms are outlined in Table 20-2.

Table 20-2
Muscle Disorders in Glycogen Storage Diseases

Type	Metabolic defect	Pathology	Clinical features	Diagnostic procedures
Type 2 glycogen storage disease. Acid maltase deficiency	Lack of α-1,4-glycosidase	Excess glycogen in cells of liver, myocardium, muscle, brain, and spinal cord. Prominent vacuolar myopathy	Autosomal recessive condition with genetic defects in gene located in chromosome 17.[68] 1. Infantile. Severe weakness hypotonia, respiratory difficulties, progressive cardiac enlargement. Death within 1 year from congestive heart failure 2. Childhood. Progressive muscle weakness limbs, limb-girdle, neck, pharynx. Hypertrophy calf muscles. Gowers' sign. Waddling gait; kyphoscoliosis 3. Adult. Slowly progressive proximal muscle weakness of limbs and limb-girdle muscles. Benign course	1. Prenatal diagnosis for infantile type by chorionic villi sampling or amniocentesis[69] 2. Marked decrease in acid maltase in urine 3. Normal fasting blood glucose 4. Electromyography — small motor unit potentials; increased short duration polyphasic potentials. Occasional myotonia. Fibrillations and positive waves 5. Muscle biopsy shows presence of glycogen, lysosomes, vacuolar myopathy and lack of 1,4-glucosidase activity
Type 3 glycogen storage disease. Limited dextrinosis	Lack of amylo-1,6-glucosidase	Presence of glycogen inside sarcolemmal membrane and between myofibrils	1. Infantile type. Hypotonia, weakness, hepatomegaly, occasional cardiac involvement. Hypoglycemic episodes 2. Adult type. Chronic progressive generalized myopathy; muscle fatigue marked in hands and forearms	Abnormal glycogen in muscle, liver, red and white cells. Absence of amylo-1,6-glucosidase in muscle and liver biopsy

Table 20-2
Muscle Disorders in Glycogen Storage Diseases

Type	Metabolic defect	Pathology	Clinical features	Diagnostic procedures
Type 4 glycogen storage disease. Amylo-1-4/1-6-transglucosidase deficiency	Lack of amylo-1-4/1-6-transglucosidase	Abnormal glycogen deposits in muscle	Autosomal recessive condition; failure to thrive, hypotonia, muscle weakness, muscle atrophy, hepatomegaly	Deficiency of enzyme in skin fibroblasts in white blood cells
Type 5 glycogen storage disease (McArdle disease)	Lack of muscle phosphorylase	Subsarcolemmal vacuoles containing glycogen in muscle	Autosomal recessive condition. Genetic defect in chromosome 11q13. Exercise intolerance and painful muscle cramps beginning in adolescence. Later rhabdomyolysis and myoglobinuria after exercise. Occasional renal failure. Progressive decline in strength with age-variable muscle wasting.[70] Vitamin B6 may reduce exercise-induced fatigability.	1. Elevated serum aldolase, CK, LDH, AST 2. Electromyography—decreased response on repetitive nerve stimulation 3. No increase in lactic acid on ischemic work test 4. Muscle biopsy—absence of muscle phosphorylase, absence lactate 5. Reliable diagnosis from peripheral blood cells avoids muscle biopsy[71]
Type 7 glycogen storage disease. Phosphofructokinase deficiency	Lack of muscle phosphofructokinase	Increased glycogen in muscle	Autosomal recessive trait. Symptoms similar to phosphorylase deficiency but usually mild.[72] Poor exercise tolerance, muscle weakness, muscle cramps, myoglobinuria. Occasional hemolysis, hyperuricemia, gastric ulcer[73]	1. Elevated serum CK after exercise. 2. Ischemic exercise test shows no increase in lactic acid production. 3. Increased muscle fructose-6-phosphate, decreased fructose-1,6-biphosphate in muscle.[69]

Myopathies Associated with Thyroid Disease

Myopathies have been associated with both hyperthyroidism and hypothyroidism.

Hyperthyroid Myopathy The myopathy of hyperthyroidism consists of a progressive proximal limb-girdle myopathy and exophthalmic ophthalmoplegia. In addition, hyperthyroidism is closely related to myasthenia gravis and hypokalemic periodic paralysis.

Hyperthyroid myopathy is often mild but may be associated with severe atrophy. The myopathy is present in at least 50 percent of patients with hyperthyroidism, but the severity of weakness does not correlate with levels of thyroid hormone. Temporary improvement occurs with beta-adrenergic blockade, using propanolol. There is resolution of symptoms following restoration of the euthyroid state.

Exophthalmic ophthalmoplegia can be regarded as a myopathy of the extraocular muscles associated with an increase in intraorbital fat, edema, and a lymphocytic infiltration. The condition can occur in hyperthyroidism, hypothyroidism, and occasionally in the euthyroid state. The cause is unknown. The MRI scans show enlargement of the extraocular muscles. Treatment with corticosteroids or appropriate therapy for the underlying thyroid dysfunction is often effective. Surgical decompression is indicated when vision is threatened, or the condition becomes disfiguring.

Hypothyroid Myopathy The myopathy associated with hypothyroidism may be congenital or spontaneous, or develop after treatment of hyperthyroidism. The congenital form is associated with cretinism, mental retardation, and muscle hypertrophy, the latter disappearing following replacement therapy.

An asymptomatic delay in relaxation of tendon reflexes can occur in adults with hypothyroidism, as may myoedema, a focal swelling of muscle in response to percussion. Muscle enlargement and cramping is another feature of the hypothyroid state.

Proximal myopathy with muscle weakness and cramping is seen in some cases of hypothyroidism and usually responds to treatment with hormone replacement.

Mitochondrial Myopathies

This heterogenous group contains many disorders that have the common feature of "ragged red fibers," indicating abnormalities of muscle mitochondria. Four groups have been recognized:

A. Defective substrate utilization: pyruvate dehydrogenase deficiency; carnitine palmitoyltransferase deficiency, carnitine deficiency, and defects of B-oxidation enzymes.
B. Defective coupling of oxidation and phosphorylation—control of mitochondrial respiration by adenosine diphosphate is lost with excessive production of energy, which is wasted as heat.
C. Defects of the respiratory chain.
   1. Severe cytochrome C oxidase deficiency resulting in a profound mitochonrdial myopathy, renal failure, and death before the age of 1 year.
   2. Benign reversible muscle cytochrome C oxidase deficiency presenting with severe myopathy at birth, followed by spontaneous improvement and apparent normal function by the age of 3 years.
   3. Subacute necrotizing encephalopathy (Leigh syndrome).
D. Mitochondrial encephalomyopathies.
   The mitochondrial encephalomyopathies are subdivided into three clinical subgroups.
   1. Chronic progressive ophthalmoplegia (Kearns-Sayre syndrome) in which there are large-scale deletions of mitochondrial DNA.[74] This is a degenerative disorder characterized by pigmentary degeneration of the retina (Fig. 20-2), progressive external ophthalmoplegia, heart block, and elevated protein in the cerebrospinal fluid (CSF). Patients are often of short stature and present with mild dementia, cerebral ataxia, hearing loss, and vestibular dysfunction. There is progressive proximal weakness with demonstration of ragged red fibers on muscle biopsy. The condition develops before the age of 20 years and is slowly progressive.

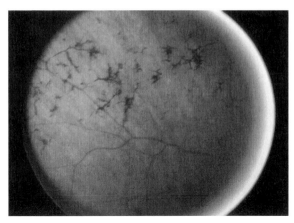

Figure 20-2
Pigmentary degeneration of the retina in chronic progressive ophthalmoplegia (Kearns-Sayre syndrome).

2. Myoclonus epilepsy associated with ragged red fibers (MERRF syndrome), characterized by transitional mutation in the mitochondrial transfer DNA.[75] This condition is characterized by myoclonus, epilepsy, generalized seizures, ataxia, and muscle weakness.

3. Mitochondrial myopathy, encephalopathy, lactic acidosis, stroke-like episodes (MELAS syndrome), in which there are mutations in the mitochondrial transfer RNA.[76] The syndrome occurs in children and adults who exhibit short stature, episodic vomiting, seizures, progressive impairment of hearing, and recurrent strokes causing hemiparesis, hemianopia, or cortical blindness.

Drug-Induced Myopathies

Myopathies produced by drugs are not unusual but are frequently misdiagnosed in seriously ill patients or confused with other myopathies such as polymyositis, dermatomyositis, endocrine myopathies, or paraneoplastic myopathies.[77] This results in delay in discontinuing the offending medication or production of further complications by inappropriate therapy.

A drug-related myopathy should be suspected in individuals who develop or show an increase in proximal muscle weakness during therapy. Corticosteroids are probably the major offender, with production of type 2 fiber atrophy and occasionally rhabdomyolysis. Progressive weakness of the intercostal muscles in the diaphragm can occur in patients with pulmonary disease treated with high doses of steroids. Hypokalemia induced by prolonged use of intranasal steroids may cause muscle weakness.

Colchicine, chloroquine, hydrochloroquine, and cyclosporine are reported to cause proximal myopathy. Muscle biopsy shows a lysosomal vasculopathy that can also occur with cardiac drugs, including amiodarone, labetalol, procainamide, flecainide, and enalapril.

Long-term treatment with D-penicillamine can induce polymyositis and dermatomyositis.

Zidovudine, which inhibits human immunodeficiency virus (HIV) replication, and is used in the treatment of acquired immunodeficiency syndrome (AIDS), causes proximal muscle weakness, which may be difficult to distinguish from HIV-induced myopathy.

Most lipid-lowering drugs have the potential to cause myopathy or myositis[78] associated with rhabdomyolysis in some cases.

Hypokalemic myopathy occurs following regular ingestion of licorice, which may be consumed habitually or ingested in medications or alcoholic beverages. Similarly, chronic diuretic use can cause hypokalemia and myopathy, which also occurs as a complication of aldosteronism, renal tubular acidosis, and potassium depletion.

The hypophosphatemia of sepsis, diabetes mellitus, malignancy, congenital heart failure, chronic obstructive pulmonary disease, diarrhea, and alcoholism can give rise to both rhabdomyolysis and myopathy.

Chronic abuse of cocaine by smoking or intravenous or nasal administration results in myopathy. Heroin, marijuana, amphetamines, barbiturates, and phencyclidine have similar effects.

Alcohol myopathy occurs as an acute process with rhabdomyolysis, a subacute process, or a chronic myopathy, which is much more common in malnourished, chronic alcoholics.

Antibodies rarely cause myopathy, which has been reported following penicillin and sulfonamide therapy. Transient myalgias are a temporary phenomenon during quinolone or cephalosporin therapy.

DISORDERS CHARACTERIZED BY STIFFNESS AND SPASMS

Stiff-Person Syndrome (Stiff-Man Syndrome)

Definition The stiff-person syndrome is a rare disorder characterized by persistent muscle contraction, spasms, and muscle cramps, which disappear during sleep.

Etiology and Pathology The condition is believed to be the result of an autoimmune reaction where antibodies are directed against glutamic acid decarboxylase (GAD), an intracellular enzyme in γ-aminobutyric acid (GABA)-containing neurons.[79] This leads to destruction of these neurons, with a lack of inhibitory influence by the GABA motor neuron system, resulting in continuous motor neuron activity and clinical rigidity.

Clinical Features The patient initially experiences muscle aches and pains followed by stiffness of the muscles of the trunk, limbs, and neck. Voluntary movements are slowed. Emotional or sensory stimuli may exacerbate the stiffness and produce painful spasms. On examination, the muscles are contracted and the patient is unable to relax them. The disorder is progressive and eventually results in considerable disability. Misdiagnosis of a psychogenic movement disorder is not unusual.[80]

A congenital form of the disorder has been reported. In these cases, stiffness is present at birth and gradually resolves, so that by age 3, the tone is almost normal. Later, in adolescence or adulthood, the stiffness reappears in a milder form.

Diagnostic Procedures Electromyography reveals persistent contractions of muscle fibers and bursts of motor unit potentials during spasm.

Treatment The stiffness and spasm improve with diazepam (Valium) 20 to 200 mg/day, or clonazepam, or valproic acid. Baclofen (Lioresal), which reduces spasticity by activating GABA-b receptors in the dorsal horn of the spinal cord, reduces muscle contractions and spasms.[81] The use of the baclofen pump is a most effective form of therapy, but pump failure may be associated with acute autonomic disturbances, a life-threatening situation.[82]

Acquired Neuromyotonia (Isaac Syndrome)

Neuromyotonia is a syndrome associated with a known neuropathic process such as a hereditary neuropathy or an acquired disorder, with or without an associated neuropathy. The syndrome is characterized by myokymia (muscle twitching at rest), cramping of muscle often induced by muscle contraction, impaired muscle relaxation, muscle weakness, increased sweating, and an elevated CK level. Neuromyotonia is believed to be an autoimmune disease where antibodies are directed against potassium channels in motor neurons proximal to the terminal branches.[83] Electromyography reveals neuromyotonic discharges characterized by bursts of motor unit action potentials firing at 150 to 300 Hz for several seconds, or occasionally, myokymic discharges of motor unit action potentials recurring regularly at rates up to 60 Hz. Motor nerve conduction studies may demonstrate a peripheral neuropathy in some cases.[84]

Most patients show excellent response to phenytoin or carbamazepine. Refractory patients should be treated with plasmapheresis.[85]

FAMILIAL PERIODIC PARALYSIS

There are three types of familial periodic paralysis, all of which are inherited as an autosomal dominant trait.

Hypokalemic Periodic Paralysis

Definition *Hypokalemic periodic paralysis* is an inherited condition of episodic muscle paralysis associated with hypokalemia.

Etiology and Pathology Familial hypokalemic periodic paralysis has been linked to a mutation in chromosome 1q31-32.[86] This area is the site of the gene for the alpha$_1$ subunit of the skeletal muscle, DHP-sensitive calcium channel.[87] Mutation in this gene modifies the function of the DHP receptor by altering calcium channel current in hypokalemic periodic paralysis.[88]

Muscle biopsy shows the presence of vacuoles, containing glycogen, in muscle fibers, which are present during an attack, and which may decrease in number immediately after an attack. Other features include tubular aggregates derived from sarcoplasmic reticulum, variations in fiber size, and increased internal nuclei.

Clinical Features Hypokalemic periodic paralysis is more common in men and occurs predominantly during the teens and twenties. Attacks begin at night and the patient awakens with weakness of all skeletal muscles except those involved in respiration and speech. However, there are reports of respiratory involvement and some deaths from respiratory failure, but this is a rare complication. Involved muscles are firm and tender to palpation. The neurological examination is normal, with sparing of muscles supplied by cranial nerves and those involved in respiration and speech. The attacks last from several hours to days. Several factors have been reported to precipitate attacks. These include large meals with a high carbohydrate content; exertion; trauma; heavy alcohol ingestion; upper respiratory tract infection; cold weather; and administration of insulin, thyroid hormone, steroids, epinephrine, thiazides, or licorice. Permanent muscle weakness of the proximal musculature, but spreading later to a more diffuse involvement, can occur.[89]

Diagnostic Procedures

1. The movement of potassium, sodium chloride, phosphate, ions, and water into the muscle fibers during an attack is reflected in decreased serum potassium level below 3.5 mEq/L.

2. Urinary excretion of potassium and sodium is decreased.

3. Electromyography shows decreased amplitude, number, and duration of motor unit potentials or electrical silence during periods of paralysis. Muscle fiber velocity is reduced between attacks.[90]

4. Provocative tests to induce hypokalemia, using glucose and insulin, require close monitoring by electrocardiography because hypokalemia may induce cardiac arrhythmia. A 10-min bicycle exercise test is a safer alternative. Patients with hypokalemic periodic paralysis experience a minimal increase in serum potassium levels 10 and 30 min after exercise, compared to a control population where the increase is significant.[91]

5. Corticotropin 80 to 100 IU intravenously can be used in suspected periodic paralysis of either hypo- or hyperkalemic type. Corticotropin will induce an attack of paralysis with appropriate changes in serum potassium concentration in each condition.[92]

Treatment

1. Attacks may be terminated by oral or parenteral administration of potassium and may be prevented by oral administration of potassium 130 mEq/day.
2. Acetazolamide 125 mg q.o.d., increasing by increments to achieve an optimum dosage, to a maximum of 500 mg q12h orally, is the drug of choice to prevent attacks.
3. Spironolactone 100 mg daily or bid is effective in reducing the number of attacks.
4. Other drugs that may be of benefit include the carbonic anhydrase inhibitor dichlorphenamide, the calcium channel blocking agent, verapamil, or lithium.
5. Predisposing factor should be avoided.

Secondary Hypokalemic Periodic Paralysis

A number of disorders with associated hypokalemia may develop symptoms of periodic paralysis resembling hypokalemic paralysis. This syndrome occurs in thyrotoxic periodic paralysis, which is seen predominantly in men of Asian extraction[93] and is rare in the United States.[94] Other conditions include renal diseases associated with loss of potassium such as renal acidosis types 1 and 2, acute tubular necrosis, and a nephrotic syndrome.[95] Chronic gastrointestinal potassium loss can also cause periodic paralysis in patients with emesis and diarrhea, nasogastric suctioning, fistulae, and malabsorption in celiac disease, tropic sprue[96] and Salmonella enteritis. Other causes include primary hyperaldosteronism, excess licorice ingestion, laxative abuse, and barium toxicity.[97]

Diagnostic Procedures

Primary hypokalemic periodic paralysis and thyrotoxic periodic paralysis may be distinguished from nonthyrotoxic secondary hypokalemic periodic paralysis by a prolonged exercise test.[98]

Treatment

Intravenous propranolol may terminate an attack in patients with thyrotoxic periodic paralysis, who fail to respond to potassium therapy.[99] The underlying cause of secondary hypokalemic periodical paralysis should be identified and treated.

Hyperkalemic Periodic Paralysis

Definition *Hyperkalemic periodic paralysis* is a condition inherited as an autosomal dominant trait, where periodic paralysis is associated with elevation of serum potassium levels.

Etiology and Pathology The disease has been linked to allelic defects in a gene that encodes for the alpha subunit of the tetrodotoxin-sensitive skeletal muscle sodium channel, localized to chromosome 17q23 1-25.3.[100] There is non-inactivation of this channel during an episode of paralysis, with influx of sodium resulting in sustained membrane depolarization.

Muscle biopsy may be normal or may show some nonspecific features, such as large variation in fiber size and central nuclei, increased subsarcolemmal glycogen and the presence of vacuoles in some cases.

Clinical Features Attacks begin in childhood and occur during the day, usually while resting after exercise. Each attack may be preceded by a sensation of heaviness and stiffness in the muscles and paresthesias in the face and extremities. Episodes usually last 1 h. In addition to exercise, paralysis can be precipitated by exposure to cold, hunger, administration of potassium, emotional stress, and pregnancy. Attacks may be prevented by eating a carbohydrate after exercise.

Muscle weakness affects the lower extremities predominantly, but upper extremity and neck muscles can be involved. Mild myotonia can be experienced during muscle weakness. Permanent muscle weakness is an occasional complication. Cardiac arrhythmias have been reported in a few cases.[101]

Diagnostic Procedures

1. Serum potassium levels are increased during an attack, but normal potassium levels have been recorded in some cases, giving rise to so-called normokalemic periodic paralysis.

2. Serum sodium levels decrease as sodium enters muscle fibers.

3. Urinary potassium increases during an attack, resulting in a drop in serum potassium levels and recovery.

4. Electromyography may reveal electrical silence during paralysis or fibrillations, positive sharp waves, and myotonic discharges during paresis. Motor unit potentials are decreased in number and duration.

5. Provocative test with administration of 2 to 10 g potassium chloride will induce an attack within 1 to 2 h. Electrocardiographic monitoring should be performed to detect any abnormalities related to hyperkalemia.

Treatment Attacks can be prevented by thiazide diuretics—hydrochlorothiazide 25 to 75 mg/day. Acetazolamide, albuterol, and metaproterenol are also effective.

Paramyotonia Congenita

Definition This is a familial condition characterized by muscle stiffness induced by exposure to cold or by exercise, followed by muscle weakness. The condition is inherited as an autosomal dominant trait.

Etiology and Pathology Paramyotonia congenita, like hyperkalemic periodic paralysis, is the product of a defect in the skeletal muscle sodium channel. Linkage has been established between paramyotonia congenita and the gene encoding the alpha subunit of the muscle sodium channel localized to chromosome 17q20 231-225.3.[102]

Muscle biopsy may be normal or show nonspecific changes.

Clinical Features The symptoms are present at birth. Babies develop mask-like facies on exposure to a cold environment. This is followed by paradoxical muscle stiffness that increases with exercise. Attacks of weakness are delayed until adolescence and often last several hours or days. The weakness has an upper limb predominance; respiratory muscle involvement is rare. Symptoms can be more severe during pregnancy. Permanent weakness does not occur.

Diagnostic Procedures

1. Muscle cooling results in symptoms of weakness and reduced compound muscle potentials on electromyography.
2. Electromyography demonstrates myotonic discharges at room temperature, enhanced by cooling, but myotonic discharges may decrease or disappear with the onset of paralysis.[103]

Treatment

1. Avoid exposure to a cold environment, which can precipitate an attack.
2. Mexiletine, a cardiac antiarrhythmic drug, is effective in reducing both myotonia and weakness.

DISORDERS OF THE NEUROMUSCULAR JUNCTION

Myasthenia Gravis

Definition *Myasthenia gravis* is characterized by progressive muscular weakness on exertion, followed by recovery of strength after a period of rest. It is an autoimmune condition in which there is an antibody-mediated autoimmune attack directed against acetylcholine receptors at neuromuscular junctions.[104]

The Normal Neuromuscular Junction The neuromuscular junction is illustrated schematically in Figure 20-3. Acetylcholine is contained in synaptic vesicles that fuse with the presynaptic membrane and

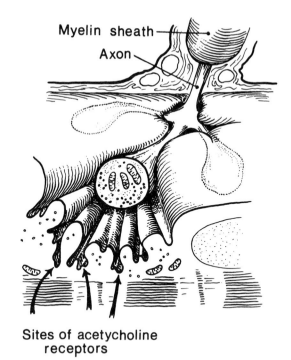

Sites of acetycholine receptors

Figure 20-3
The normal neuromuscular junction.

release a small quantity of acetylcholine into the synaptic cleft. The acetylcholine then diffuses across the cleft and binds to acetylcholine receptors on the postsynaptic membrane. The attachment produces a conformational change that opens the sodium and potassium channels of the postsynaptic membrane. There is a constant and spontaneous release of acetylcholine in small quantities, which is not sufficient to depolarize the membrane but does result in what has been termed "miniature end plate potentials." Bound acetylcholine is removed by diffusion or hydrolyzation by the enzyme acetylcholine esterase, which is concentrated in the postsynaptic membrane. The receptor probably remains refractory for some time after this hydrolysis has occurred.

In physiological muscle contraction, the impulse generated in the motor neuron reaches the presynaptic membrane, causing depolarization, which results in a coordinated release of acetylcholine. The acetylcholine diffuses across the cleft in sufficient quantity to produce a wave of depolarization that is propagated down the muscle fiber. The propagated electrical discharge produces changes in the sarcoplasmic reticulum of the muscle fiber, with release of calcium ions, which promotes fiber contraction. There is an ample reserve of acetylcholine receptors sufficient in number to allow repetitive depolarization of the membrane and repeated muscle fiber contraction.

Etiology and Pathology The postsynaptic membrane is abnormal in myasthenia gravis. There is a loss of secondary folds, which reduces the surface area available for binding of acetylcholine, and there is a decreased number of acetylcholine receptors. The decrease is due, in part, to the blocking of acetylcholine binding sites of the acetylcholine receptor by blocking antibodies. In addition, there is an accelerated degradation of receptors, because antibodies cross-link the receptors, which are drawn together in clusters, internalized by endocytosis, and degraded.[105] The antibodies vary in their capacity to block receptor binding sites or accelerate degradation, but increasing activity of antibodies appears to be associated with increasing severity of the myasthenic response. During repetitive stimulation of the nerve, the available acetylcholine receptors are quickly saturated and remain refractory. This results in a state of receptor insufficiency in which there is not a sufficient number of receptors available to bind acetylcholine and produce depolarization. Therefore, repetitive stimulation will result in a decrease in the number of muscle fibers that are able to respond, as each neuromuscular junction reaches a state of receptor insufficiency. Clinically, this is characterized by a progressive weakness.

The antibodies, which are of the IgG class, are probably produced by B lymphocytes,[106] although T lymphocytes from patients with myasthenia gravis respond to stimulation with acetylcholine receptors, and the production of acetylcholine receptor antibodies. The autoimmune response probably arises in the thymus,[107] because 70 percent of patients with myasthenia gravis have hyperplasia or thymomas,[108] which are of microscopic size in rare cases,[109] and thymectomy is an effective treatment in most cases. The normal and myasthenic thymus contains myoid (muscle-like) cells with surface acetylcholinic receptors.

These cells may be particularly susceptible to an immune reaction, possibly triggered by a viral infection, resulting in changes to the myoid cells and the surrounding lymphocytes within the thymus, and an autoimmune response. One possible mechanism is molecular mimicry, in which there is an immune response to an infectious agent such as herpes simplex virus, which contains a peptide sequence homologous to a sequence on the acetylcholine receptor subunit.

However, not all myasthenics show detectable levels of antibodies to acetylcholine receptors, implying that myasthenia gravis is not a homogenous disorder, and that other, as yet undetected, antibodies may occur in some cases.

Clinical Features Myasthenia gravis is uncommon, with a prevalence of about 1/10,000. The disease is more common among women than men, with a ratio of 2:1. The mean age of onset is 26 years in women and 31 years in men. The incidence in men does not show a smooth distribution. The peak incidence in the early thirties declines through middle age, but there is a second peak between 60 and 78 years of age in men. Why this does not occur in women is unknown. The disease can occur at any age and has been reported in the newborn. There is no significant family occurrence and no genetic pattern has been identified.

Myasthenia gravis can be classified into four groups, or types:

Group 1. Ocular myasthenia.
Group 2. Mild generalized myasthenia.
Group 3. Severe generalized myasthenia.
Group 4. Crisis.

Ocular Myasthenia In this form of myasthenia gravis, the symptoms and signs are confined to the extraocular muscles. The paient develops diplopia and ptosis, usually toward the end of the day. Ocular myasthenia remains localized to the extraocular and eyelid muscles in about 15 percent of cases, but about 85 percent of patients develop generalized myasthenia within a period of 18 months. Nevertheless, ocular myasthenia differs from generalized myasthenia because of male preponderance, low antibody titers, and different histocompatibility and antigen association.[125] Symptoms consist of unilateral or bilateral ptosis and diplopia. The degree of ptosis is variable and may present on one side or the other at different times. There may be quick lid retraction or twitching of the levator palpebrae elicited by having the patient rapidly redirect the gaze from a downward to a neutral position. Eye movements may be saccadic, jerking, or quivering, with gaze-evoked nystagmus.[125]

Mild Generalized Myasthenia Mild generalized myasthenia may be preceded by ocular myasthenia or may present with symptoms of mild weakness involving the extraocular muscles and other muscle groups. There is usually some involvement of the facial muscles, muscles of mastication, and the proximal limb-girdle muscles, while the extraocular muscles are frequently but not invariably involved. This may present with some difficulty in diagosis, particularly when the proximal limb-girdle musculature is the sole site of presentation. When mild generalized myasthenia develops into the severe generalized form of the disease, the transition usually occurs within a period of 18 months.

Severe Generalized Myasthenia In the severe generalized form of myasthenia gravis, there is sufficient weakness of the bulbar and limb girdle musculature to produce marked restriction in activity. Exercise tolerance is reduced, the patient has a sedentary existence, and there is a constant risk of respiratory insufficiency, respiratory infection, or respiratory failure.

Crisis Myasthenic crisis may be defined as myasthenia gravis with respiratory failure. This is a life-threatening situation that develops in patients with severe generalized myasthenia. The onset is often sudden, and crisis is often precipitated by an infection. This usually takes the form of an upper respiratory tract infection that progresses to severe bronchitis or pneumonia.

The stages of myasthenia are not fixed, and it is not unusual for progression to occur from one stage to another within a period of 18 months. Remission can occur in any of the first three stages of myasthenia gravis. However, remission usually occurs within the first 18 months of the disease and is rare at a later stage. Spontaneous remission can be expected in about 25 percent of cases but lasts no longer than 2 years[110] in most cases. Some patients experience several periods of remission.

At the initial interview, the patient with myasthenia gravis should receive a full generalized physical examination, which helps to exclude a number of conditions known to be associated with myasthenia gravis, particularly thyrotoxicosis. This is followed by a full neurological examination, with careful documentation of the degree of muscle involvement. The examiner should attempt to demonstrate progressive weakness of the affected muscles. In the patient with ptosis, the examiner measures the widths of the palpebral fissures, and the patient is then asked to sustain upward gaze. This will produce an increasing degree of ptosis, which can be observed and measured. Similarly, patients with diplopia can be asked to sustain gaze in the direction of the pull of the involved muscle, and the examiner may observe increasing deviation of the ocular axis while the patient complains of progressive diplopia and further separation of the two images. Patients with weakness of the masseters can be asked to bite down on a tongue blade while the examiner attempts to withdraw it. This maneuver will produce fatigue of the masseters, and biting will not be sustained after a short period of time. The patient with a generalized form of the disease may show increasing weakness on stressing any of the muscles involved in the disease process. When the hands are involved, it is possible to obtain a quantitative measure of weakness using a dynamometer.

Diagnostic Procedures

1. Edrophonium (Tensilon) test. Edrophonium is a rapidly acting anticholinesterase inhibitor that blocks the action of acetylcholinesterase. Hydrolysis of acetylcholine is prevented, thus allowing more time for an attachment of acetylcholine molecules to receptor sites. The test is performed as follows:

The examiner selects a weak muscle. For example, if the patient has ptosis, the width of the palpebral fissure can be measured. If the patient has diplopia, the degree of deviation of the ocular axis can be estimated; or if the patient has weakness on chewing, the time that the patient is able to sustain biting of the tongue blade can be recorded. The examiner then draws 10 mg (1 mL) edrophonium into a syringe. The test begins with the intravenous injection of 2 mg (0.2 mL) edrophonium into a vein in the forearm. The examiner then waits 30 s to make sure that the patient does not have any muscarinic reaction to edrophonium. This usually consists of bradycardia, hypertension, lacrimation, sweating, or abdominal colic. If this does not occur, the remaining 8 mg (0.8 mL) edrophonium is injected. If the test is positive, there will be a dramatic response, with increasing strength of the paretic muscle within a period of 30 s. This increasing strength usually lasts about 2 min, then disappears. However, the patient will usually express an appreciation of the increasing strength of the weakened muscle, and the examiner will be able to observe this effect. The test is safe to perform, and adverse effects are unusual. If severe muscarinic adverse effects occur, they can be rapidly resolved by intravenous injection of 0.4 mg atropine.

2. Electromyography and repetitive nerve stimulation. Needle electrode myography is performed in patients with suspected myasthenia gravis or in those who have disorders affecting the neuromuscular junction, which may mimic or coexist with myasthenia gravis, including Lambert-Eaton myasthenic syndrome, drug-induced myasthenic syndrome, peripheral neuropathies, or myopathies, all of which may present with progressive fatigue on exertion. This is particularly valuable when the Tensilon test is equivocal but should also be performed when it is positive. In myasthenia gravis, the electromyogram shows variation in amplitude of motor unit action potentials measured on an oscilloscope on sustained voluntary contraction. This is a result of intermittent failure of synaptic transmission of some of the muscle fibers involved in the motor unit action potential. The abnormality is reversed by administration of edrophonium in patients with myasthenia gravis.

Conventional electromyography should be followed by repetitive nerve stimulation. Cholinesterase inhibitors should be discontinued for at least 12 h before testing. Repetitive nerve stimulation at rates of 3 to 5 Hz, and a supramaximal stimulus of 25 to 50 percent greater than the stimulus intensity necessary to activate all muscle fibers, should be used. In myas-

thenia gravis, the result is a decremental response greater than 10 percent to trains of 3 to 5 Hz stimuli, indicating abnormal neuromuscular transmission.[111] Maximal voluntary contraction for 30 to 60 s may be followed by partial repair of the decremental response, followed by postcontraction exhaustion 3 to 4 min later.

3. Elevated levels of antibodies to acetylcholine receptors occurs in most cases. Titers do not provide a measure of the severity of the disease but can be used to monitor the effect of treatment on an individual basis.

Failure to detect antibody levels occurs in about 10 to 15 percent of cases, with a generalized form of myasthenia in about 50 percent of cases with ocular myasthenia.

Patients with the generalized form of myasthenia gravis and negative serum antibodies, who fail to respond to repetitive nerve stimulation, often have abnormal response to single fiber electromyography. This technique can also be applied to the extraocular muscles for the diagnosis of ocular myasthenia gravis.[112]

4. Muscle biopsy should be performed when the diagnosis is uncertain, and there is a suspicion that there may be an underlying myopathic process with myasthenic features, such as polymyositis. Techniques for immunohistologic study of motor end plates, and quantification of acetylcholine receptors, are available.

After a diagnosis of myasthenia gravis has been established, a series of tests should be performed to rule out associated diseases. These include: (1) a CT scan or MRI scan of the chest should be obtained to eliminate the possibility of a thymic tumor, which occurs in about 18 percent of cases with myasthenia gravis, particularly in elderly men; (2) thyroid function tests should be performed to eliminate the possibility of hyperthyroidism. Thyrotropin-binding inhibitory immunoglobulin determination is indicated in myasthenia gravis patients with exophthalmus and normal thyroid function[113]; (3) an associated collagen vascular disease should be ruled out by appropriate testing, including antinuclear antibodies (ANA), anti-DNA antibodies, anticardiolipin, SSA and SSB antibodies, rheumatoid factor, and complement C3, C4, and CH-50. This will tend to eliminate collagen vascular diseases such as systemic lupus erythematosus,[114] myxedema, thyrotoxicosis, or rheumatoid arthritis[115]; (4) patients with a severe generalized form of the disease should have respiratory function tests performed as soon as the diagnosis is suspected, and every 12 h during treatment, or whenever respiratory insufficiency is suspected. Tests include determination of respiratory muscle strength by testing maximal expiratory pressure (PE_{max}), maximal inspiratory pressure (PI_{max}), and vital capacity. PE_{min} and PE_{max} are more sensitive indicators of early respiratory muscle weakness than vital capacity.[132] However, in general, elective endotracheal intubation is performed when the vital capacity is less than 10 to 15 mL/kg. Although respiratory impairment is usually attributed to weakness of the diaphragm and chest wall muscles, upper airway obstruction should also be considered and can be demonstrated by inspiratory and expiratory flow volume loop determination.[116]

Arterial blood gases are not a reliable method of monitoring patients with myasthenia gravis because the carbon dioxide level can remain deceptively normal until just before respiratory failure.[110]

Differential Diagnosis

1. Polymyositis. The patient with polymyositis may have symmetrical proximal limb-girdle muscle weakness. Some patients show a positive response to edrophonium and the diagnosis can be established only by electromyography and muscle biopsy.

2. Thyrotoxicosis. Thyroid myopathy presents as a proximal limb-girdle muscle weakness. The association of myasthenia gravis and thyrotoxicosis is not unusual, and the presence of myasthenia gravis in a patient with thyrotoxicosis can be suspected if improvement is seen following the edrophonium test. Patients with thyroid myopathy usually do not show improvement following the intravenous administration of edrophonium.

3. Exophthalmic ophthalmoplegia may be progressive and may resemble myasthenia gravis in the early stages. There is progressive weakness of the extraocular muscles, with replacement of muscle by fat and marked fatty infiltration of the orbit, producing exophthalmus. The response to edrophonium is absent, but thyrotropin-binding inhibitory immunoglobulin determination is positive and particularly indicated in myasthenia gravis patients with exophthalmus and normal thyroid function. Exophthalmic ophthalmoplegia and myasthenia gravis can coexist, in which case the response to edrophonium may be positive.

4. Myasthenic syndrome (Lambert-Eaton syndrome). This condition is rare and occurs in association with neoplasia. The muscle weakness involves the proximal limb-girdle muscles and the diagnosis can be established by the characteristic findings on electromyography (see p. 649).

5. Mitrochondrial myopathies (see p. 649) including chronic progressive external ophthalmoplegia, presenting with ptosis and weakness, increasing with exertion, will occasionally respond to anticholinesterase therapy. Such cases have appropriate responses on electrophysiological testing, including single fiber electromyographic studies. However, anti-acetylcholinesterase antibodies are negative. Muscle biopsy will confirm the presence of mitochondrial myopathy in seronegative cases.[117]

6. There may be more than a chance but rare association between myasthenia gravis and sarcoidosis.[118]

7. The association of myasthenia gravis in lymphoma has been reported.[119]

8. Myasthenia gravis might be one of the neuromuscular complications of HIV infection.[120]

9. Periodic paralysis (see p. 638).

10. Botulism (see p. 650).

11. Miscellaneous (penicillamine, acetylcholinesterase agents, particularly organophosphorous compounds).

Treatment Group 1 and group 2 patients may be treated as outpatients. Group 3 patients should be admitted to the hospital. Certain drugs may induce or exacerbate myasthenia gravis (Table 20-3).

1. The anticholinesterase drugs were the first effective treatment for myasthenia gravis and are still widely used. Some evidence suggests that anticholinesterase drugs may increase damage to the postsynaptic membrane, and there is a present trend

Table 20-3

Drugs Which May Induce or Exacerbate Myasthenia Gravis

Antibiotics

ampicillin	kanamycin
ciprofloxacin	lincomycin
clindamycin	neomycin
colistin	polymyxin
erythromycin	streptomycin
imipenem	tobramycin

Anesthetics

ether	ketamine
halothane	methoxyflurane

Anticonvulsants

phenytoin sodium	trimethadione

Antiarrhythmics

beta adrenergic receptor	Other agents
blockade	procainamide
acebutolol	quinidine sulfate
oxprenolol	verapamil
practolol	
propranolol	
timolol	

Anticholinergics

trihexyphenidyl HCl

Antirheumatic

chloroquine	D-penicillamine

Immunosuppressives

corticosteroids	interferon alpha

Psychotropics

amphetamines	bromperidol
amitriptyline	haloperidol
barbiturates	imipramine
chlorpromazine	lithium

Miscellaneous

Anticoagulants

amantadine	procaine
carnitine	radiocontrast media
chlorine gas	a) iothalamic acid
levonorgestrel	b) diatrizoate megulmine
methocarbamol	magnesium citrate
nicotine transdermal	

Modified from Wittbrodt ET: Drugs and myasthenia gravis. An update. *Arch Intern Med* 157:399, 1997.

to restrict the use of anticholinesterase drugs to those with mild disease who show good response.

Patients with mild myasthenia should be given pyridostigmine bromide (Mestinon) 30 mg q4–6 h[108] or neostigmine bromide (Prostigmin) 15 mg over the same time period. Pyridostigmine bromide time-tablets (180 mg) have a longer duration of action and may be used at night. At the next outpatient visit, a Tensilon test should be performed immediately before the next dose of the anticholinesterase preparation. If the test is positive, the physician has the option of increasing the dosage or decreasing the time between administration of the anticholinesterase drugs. In this way, the optimum dose of pyridostigmine or neostigmine can be calculated for each patient. The response to anticholinesterase drugs is good in about 50 percent of patients. Administration of anticholinesterase drugs may be limited by the development of cholinergic side effects, including colic, diarrhea, blurred vision, and bradycardia. Care is needed in administration of anticholinesterase drugs to the elderly because accumulation of acetylcholine at receptor sites in the heart may result in bradycardia, nodal rhythm, atrial fibrillation, or flutter. Hypotensive syncope has also been recorded.

Patients with group 3, or the severe generalized form of myasthenia, should always be admitted to the hospital for treatment. Following admission, an intravenous catheter should be placed; this facilitates the performance of the Tensilon test. The patient is then given 60 mg pyridostigmine orally. The Tensilon test is performed just before the next dose is due, and the dose of medication is increased if the test is positive. Again, this method allows the development of the optimum dose for the patient.

2. Corticosteroids are widely used in the treatment of myasthenia gravis and probably act as an immunosuppressant, suppressing the action of B lymphocytes. All patients scheduled to receive corticosteroids should be screened for tuberculosis, and those with oropharyngeal involvement or respiratory impairment should be treated with plasmapheresis until there is improvement in muscle strength. At that point, prednisone 100 mg/day (methylprednisolone 96 mg/day) is started and maintained for 10 days, followed by alternate-day therapy at the same dose, which is monitored until the maximum benefit is ob-

tained. The dose is gradually decreased until the patient shows signs of weakness, then increased by a small amount. This is the maintenance dose, which can be continued indefinitely in most cases. Anticholinesterase drugs can be reduced or eliminated in many cases, and the morbidity of thymectomy is reduced, particularly following surgery.

Remission or marked improvement can be expected in 75 percent of cases treated with high-dose oral corticosteroids. Nevertheless, about 30 percent of patients show temporary worsening, lasting about 6 days, during the first 3 weeks of high-dose therapy.[108] This complication can usually be managed with anticholinesterase drugs or can be avoided by introducing steroids in low dosage (prednisone 10 to 25 mg/day) and gradually increasing by 10-mg increments every 5 days until maximum improvement occurs. The dose can then be decreased, using an alternate-day regimen, as described above, until the maintenance dose is established.

Adverse effects of corticosteroid therapy are inevitable if high-dose therapy is prolonged. The adverse effects include cushingoid appearance, weight gain, hypertension, cutaneous striae, diabetes mellitus, cataracts, peptic ulcer, osteoporosis, and aseptic necrosis of the femoral head. A weight maintenance diet with low sodium and supplementary calcium is indicated. At the patient's first complaint of gastritis, H_2 antagonists should be used to prevent the development of peptic ulcer.

3. Thymectomy is recommended for patients between the ages of puberty and 60 years or those who have generalized myasthenia gravis. Thymectomy is usually delayed until after puberty because of the significant role of the thymus in the development of the immune system. The results of thymectomy are better in those with nonneoplastic thymic hyperplasia than in those with thymoma, but the latter should always be removed, because of the propensity for local invasion, including spread into the lungs.

The surgical approach to thymectomy involves splitting the sternum and exploring the anterior mediastinum. This permits the removal of the thymus (or thymoma) and any ectopic thymic tissue in the mediastinum or lower cervical area. The alternative methods of cervical thymectomy and transcervical thymectomy carry less morbidity but may fail to detect ectopic thymic tissue. This is less likely with newer fiberoptic technology (thoracoscopy) or visual-assisted thoracoscopy, which provides complete visualization of the thorax.[121, 122] The midline sternotomy is necessary when the thymus is large or when a thymoma is adherent to vascular structures.

Recurrence of thymoma is rare, the reoperative rate reported as 3.6 percent.[123] Thymectomy may be followed by a drug-free remission or by marked reduction in the need for anticholinesterase drugs or other therapies. In some cases, improvement is delayed for months or years after thymectomy, suggesting the presence of residual thymic tissue. This is often ectopic thymic tissue which was not removed during surgery.[121]

4. Immunosuppressant drugs. Azathioprine (Imuran) acts predominantly on T cells and is useful in patients with myasthenia gravis when corticosteroids are ineffective or contraindicated. Treatment begins with a first dose of a 50 mg tablet daily for 1 week. If there are no adverse reactions to the drug, the dose can be increased gradually to 3.0 mg/kg per day if necessary. This is usually effective, but the response is slow, and improvement may not occur for many months.

Adverse effects include an influenza-like reaction in about 10 percent of cases. Other adverse effects include leukopenia, anemia, thrombocytopenia, increase in liver enzyme levels, and gastrointestinal upset.[124] Azathioprine is often used in conjunction with corticosteroids and has a steroid-sparing action, delaying the development of steroid side effects. Many patients require lifelong azathioprine therapy, and any attempt to withdraw the drug without introducing another therapy results in clinical relapse in approximately 50 percent of cases. A short course of corticosteroids or plasmapheresis can be used to control symptoms in such patients, while azathioprine is reintroduced.

5. Plasmapheresis acts by reducing circulating antibodies against acetylcholine receptor and is an accepted method for treating patients with myasthenia gravis when other treatments have been ineffective.[126] Plasmapheresis is effective alone or in combination with azathioprine. The patient will show a good response to plasmapheresis within a short

period of treatment, and this response may be maintained for as long as 6 months. At present, it seems that this form of therapy may have to be repeated at intervals varying from 3 weeks to 6 months.

Plasmapheresis carries a risk of anaphylactic reaction and viral infections, which can be eliminated by immunoadsorption.[127] This technique selectively removes acetylcholine receptor antibodies by adsorption from the plasma, with reinfusion of fluid in the system at the end of the procedure, thus eliminating the need for infusion of plasma proteins used in plasmapheresis.[128]

6. Intravenous immunoglobulin (IVIG). Improvement in myasthenia has been reported following a high dose of intravenous human immunoglobulin 2 g/kg over 2 to 5 days, with increased muscle strength lasting several weeks.[129] Adverse effects including headaches, chills, fever, impaired renal function, cerebral infarction,[130] and aseptic meningitis have been reported.[131] All patients should be screened for impaired renal function before contemplating therapy.

7. Other therapies. Antilymphocytic globulin and antithymocytic globulin have produced improvement in some patients with myasthenia. Aminopyridines, particularly 4-amino pyridine, facilitate transmitter release at central and peripheral synapses, and may be of benefit in refractory cases.

Treatment of Myasthenic Crisis Myasthenic crisis should be regarded as a medical emergency. The condition generally results from gradual failure of response to anticholinesterase drugs. This failure may be precipitated by an upper respiratory tract infection, pneumonia, extreme fatigue, or alcoholic intoxication. The artificial division of patients into myasthenic crisis and cholinergic crisis is no longer tenable. The patient who develops respiratory failure (vital capacity less than 10 to 15 mL/kg) should be diagnosed as crisis and treated as follows.

1. The patient should be intubated, receive mechanical ventilation, and be treated in an intensive care unit.

2. All medications should be discontinued.

3. Because myasthenic crises are precipitated by infection, a diligent search should be made for an infectious process. A chest film should be taken to rule out pneumonia or atelectasis. Infection requires prompt treatment with appropriate antibiotic therapy.

4. The patient should be instructed to suction secretions from the mouth and pharynx using a soft plastic catheter. In cases of extreme weakness, this must be done regularly by those in attendance.

5. The patient should be turned q2h in bed to prevent atelectasis and encourage the flow of secretions from the lungs. This also helps to prevent the development of decubiti.

6. When patients are free from infection, or when infection is controlled by appropriate antibiotics, corticosteroid therapy can be commenced with 100 mg methylprednisolone intravenously piggyback daily. Corticosteroid therapy should be supplemented by antacid therapy. The corticosteroids occasionally produce increasing weakness beginning on the second or third day after therapy is started, reaching a maximum effect on the fifth day. This is followed by rapid recovery of strength. Some patients show an increase in strength immediately following the administration of corticosteroids, and in other patients, there may be no response for as long as 3 weeks. When improvement occurs, the dosage of corticosteroids can be converted to an alternate-day basis and then gradually reduced once the patient shows good response to therapy.

7. The patient should have respiratory function tests performed at the bedside at least twice a day. The determination of vital capacity is often all that is necessary, and the patient should be removed from the mechanical ventilator and placed on a T-bar with oxygen when the vital capacity reaches 10 mL/kg.[132]

8. Once the patient is extubated, treatment should be continued for a severe generalized form of myasthenia gravis.

9. An alternative form of treating patients in crisis is to perform plasmapheresis, which reduces the circulating acetylcholine receptor antibodies and often produces dramatic improvement.

10. The treatment of myasthenia gravis has improved dramatically following the introduction of corticosteroids, immunosuppressants, plasmaphere-

sis, and IVIG. The prognosis of crisis has improved following the widespread use of mechanical ventilators and the wide range of drug therapies available.

DRUG-INDUCED MYASTHENIA SYNDROME

Drug-induced myasthenia is characterized by reversible myasthenic symptoms associated with a particular drug. Several drugs have been reported to cause a reversible myasthenic syndrome (see Table 20-3).

Lambert-Eaton Syndrome (Myasthenic Syndrome)

Definition *Lambert-Eaton syndrome* is believed to represent failure of release of acetylcholine at the neuromuscular junction.

Etiology The syndrome represents an autoimmune condition associated with a number of neoplasms, more than 50 percent of which are small-cell carcinoma of the lung.[133] Noncancerous Lambert-Eaton syndrome occurs in about one-third of cases and is associated with other autoimmune disorders, including multiple sclerosis, rheumatoid arthritis, scleroderma, psoriasis, asthma, and ulcerative colitis. The syndrome is believed to be due to the binding of an IgG antibody to voltage-gated calcium channels in the nerve terminal. These channels fail to function when depolarization occurs, leading to failure of fusion of acetylcholine-containing vesicles within the nerve terminal membrane, and reduction and release of acetylcholine into the synaptic cleft.

Clinical Features The disorder is characterized by proximal muscle weakness, hyporeflexia, and autonomic dysfunction. The weakness affects the proximal lower limb-girdle muscles, with minimal involvement of the upper extremities and the ocular and facial muscles.

Autonomic dysfunction results in sluggish pupillary reaction to light and photophobia, dryness of the mouth and failure of erection in men. Hypohidrosis, orthostatic hypotension, and bladder dys-

function may occur in some cases. Spontaneous respiratory failure has been reported[134] and there may be prolonged apnea or hypoventilation after anesthesia.

Diagnostic Procedures

1. On electromyography, there is a low-amplitude response to single stimulation and further decrease occurs with low rates of stimulation. Higher rates of stimulation, such as 50 evoked potentials per second, produce a marked increase in amplitude of the evoked motor unit potential.

2. Between 50 and 60 percent of patients show antibodies directed at voltage-gated calcium channels in the nerve terminal.

3. Chest MRI and CT scans to reveal small-cell carcinoma of the lung are indicated in all new cases of Lambert-Eaton syndrome.

Treatment

1. Remission will occur in some cases, after removal of the neoplasm, but others remain symptomatic despite tumor removal. Resumption of symptoms after tumor removal indicates tumor recurrence.[135]

2. There may be some improvement in strength with anticholinesterase medication such as pyridostigmine, but the response is usually less effective therapy than in myasthenia gravis.

3. 4-Aminopyridine, a potassium channel-blocking agent, enhances acetylcholine release and improves muscle strength in Lambert-Eaton syndrome. Seizures may occur with doses necessary to produce improved strength. 3-4-Diaminopyridine, with more potent action at the neuromuscular junction and less convulsant properties, can be used alone or in combination with pyridostigmine and anticonvulsant medication, if necessary.

4. Immunosuppressant therapy using prednisone or azathioprine, singly or in combination, is effective in some cases.

5. Plasmapheresis or IVIG may be effective, but the benefits are usually temporary.[136]

6. Guanidine hydrochloride 25 mg tid, increasing slowly up to 35 mg/kg per day, can be used

as a last resort, because of adverse effects including nausea, colic, renal and hematological complications.

Congenital Myasthenic Syndromes

These rare disorders usually present in infancy or childhood, but symptoms may be delayed in mild cases until adult life. There are several conditions included in the syndrome, which should be suspected in individuals showing progressive weakness on exertion, who have a negative intravenous edrophonium test, and absence of acetylcholine receptor antibodies.[137] Electromyography, including single fiber electromyogram, and muscle biopsy with electron microscopy are required to establish the diagnosis.

Botulism

Definition *Botulism* is an acute, potentially fatal toxemia that results from the ingestion of botulinum neurotoxin and is characterized by symmetrical cranial neuropathies followed by descending symmetrical muscle weakness and paralysis.

Etiology and Pathology *Clostridium botulinum* is a strictly anaerobic, gram-positive spore-bearing bacillus that is the source of the most potent toxin known. Botulinum toxin is released on death and autolysis of organisms that have survived in pickled, bottled, or improperly home canned foods. Following ingestion, the toxin is absorbed through the gastrointestinal tract and disseminated throughout the body. The toxin binds to terminal nerve fibers just proximal to the acetylcholine release zone and prevents transmission of impulses that normally release acetylcholine from presynaptic nerve terminals.[138] Cholinergic function is unaffected in the central nervous system.

Clinical Features There are seven known strains of *C. botulinum* (A–G) but only types A, B, E, F and G affect man. Types A and B account for the majority of outbreaks, with type A occurring most commonly in the Pacific coast states, the Rocky Mountains, and the northeastern United States, and type B predominating in the Mississippi River Valley area, the Great Lakes area, and the southeastern United States. Type E, which is usually associated with fish or marine mammal foods,[139] has been reported in the Great Lakes area, Alaska, and Egypt.

There is usually a history of ingestion of home canned foods, and it is rare that a traumatic wound is the source of contamination.[140] Sinus infection with *C. botulinum* can occur in cases of acute sinusitis due to inhalation of contaminated cocaine.[141] Early symptoms occur 12 h to 10 days after ingestion and usually consist of diplopia, ptosis, blurred vision, and photophobia. More caudal cranial nerves may become involved, resulting in dysphonia, dysphagia, and dysarthria. A descending flaccid symmetrical paralysis that threatens respiratory function may develop quite rapidly. Intubation and mechanical ventilation are necessary in approximately 40 percent of patients, particularly in those with type A botulism.[142] Parasympathetic autonomic dysfunction may be manifested by constipation, dry mouth and eyes, and urine retention. The patient remains alert, oriented, and afebrile, and sensation is intact.

Differential Diagnosis Guillain-Barré syndrome, particularly the Miller Fisher variant, myasthenia gravis, brainstem infarction, familial periodic paralysis, diphtheria, tick paralysis, poliomyelitis, and psychiatric disorders may be confused with early or typical cases of botulism. The history, the development of similar symptoms in others, a normal CSF, and the progression of the disorder will differentiate botulism from other conditions.

Diagnostic Procedures

1. The patient's serum, feces, gastric contents, and suspected food should be tested for the presence of botulinum toxin. Similarly, feces, gastric contents, and suspected food should be cultured anaerobically for the presence of *C. botulinum*.

The Centers for Disease Control and Prevention (CDC) provides epidemiologic consultation and laboratory diagnostic services for suspected botulism cases and authorizes release of botulism antitoxin to state health departments and physicians in the United States. These services are available 24 h a day through state health departments.[143]

2. Electrodiagnostic studies should include rapid repetitive stimulation of nerves, which will elicit an incremental response in most cases. Only botulism, the Lambert-Eaton syndrome, aminoglycoside toxicity, and hypermagnesemia are known to produce this electromyographic response.

Treatment

1. The patient should receive a skin test before administration of equine trivalent antitoxin because 20 percent of patients are allergic to the preparation and may require desensitization before treatment. However, the antitoxin should be administered as soon as possible.

Trivalent (ABE) botulinum antitoxin is available on an emergency basis from the CDC in Atlanta, Georgia (404-639-3356 Monday through Friday, 8:00 A.M. to 4:30 P.M.; or 404-639-2888 after hours and on weekends and holidays).

2. If ileus is not present, cathartics and enemas should be administered to remove excess toxin from the intestinal tract.

3. High-dose intravenous penicillin has been recommended by some for treatment of botulism, but the use of antibiotics is questionable and appears to have little effect on the course of the disease.

4. Respiratory care is critical. An adequate airway should be maintained by frequent suctioning. Intubation, tracheotomy, and mechanical ventilation may be necessary.

5. Fluid and electrolyte balance and the nutritional state must be carefully monitored.

Prognosis Although many outbreaks of botulism are mild, type A botulism toxemia has a reported mortality of 50 to 70 percent, followed by type E (30 percent) and type B (20 percent). The length of stay in the hospital among survivors may be protracted, the recovery slow, and the patient may be left with residual ocular paralysis.

Tick Paralysis

Definition Tick paralysis is an acute onset of muscle weakness proceeding to generalized paralysis associated with injection of venom through the skin by a gravid female tick of *Dermacentor andersoni, Dermacentor variabilis,* and *Dermacentor occidentalis* in North America and *Ixodes holocyclus* or *Ixodes cornuatis* in Australia. Although the disease has been described throughout North America, it is usually encountered in the states west of the Rocky Mountains and in British Columbia and Alberta in Canada.

Etiology and Pathology The condition appears to be caused by the absorption of a toxic substance that prevents depolarization of the neuromuscular junction. There are no described pathological changes.

Clinical Features Tick paralysis has been reported in children of both sexes, and there may be a history of exposure to ticks by playing in infested grass or woods. The symptoms appear 3 to 5 days after the tick attaches itself to the skin and are often preceded by malaise, irritability, and diarrhea. Weakness begins in the lower extremities and spreads rapidly, so that the child shows complete symmetrical paralysis of all voluntary muscles within 24 h. Bulbar or respiratory muscle involvement can occur, and assisted ventilation may be necessary. Examination reveals the presence of a tick that is attached to the skin and frequently obscured by hair on the scalp of the patient.

Diagnostic Procedures

1. The history of possible exposure to ticks may be obtained.
2. The diagnosis is established by finding the tick.

Treatment Improvement occurs when the tick is removed. This can be accomplished by the application of petroleum jelly and removal some 20 min later, with forceps pressed down on either side of the mouth parts, to grasp the hypostome of the tick, the gentle detachment by lifting or an upward levering action.

INFLAMMATORY MUSCLE DISEASE

Myositis is an inflammation of muscle characterized pathologically by an inflammatory cell infiltrated in the muscle and clinically by pain, weakness, and occasionally tenderness of the involved muscles.

Viral Myositis

Acute viral myositis is unusual but can occasionally occur in epidemic form (epidemic pleurodynia or Bornholm disease).

Etiology and Pathology   Viral infections associated with acute myositis include Coxsackie (group B), ECHO, influenza types A and B, and HIV.

Muscle biopsy shows evidence of myositis with fiber degeneration and phagocytosis, fiber regeneration, and perivascular inflammation.

Clinical Features   Acute viral myositis presents with sudden onset of severe muscular pain that is exacerbated by movement. The pain may be confined to the intercostal and abdominal muscles (pleurodynia) or involve the neck and limb-girdle muscles. The patient is febrile and restless and suffers from insomnia due to myalgia and headache. Involvement of the intercostal muscles limits respiration and is often associated with severe distress. Myoglobinuria can occur with the risk of renal failure. There may be an associated aseptic meningitis. The condition may be more insidious in some cases in which the patient experiences generalized muscle weakness following a febrile illness.

Diagnostic Procedures

1. There is a polymorphonucleocytosis associated with eosinophilia.
2. The serum CK level is elevated; isoenzyme studies indicate a muscle origin with elevation of the M band. Levels of LDH, AST, ALT, and aldolase are also frequently elevated.
3. The CSF shows a lymphocytic pleocytosis in cases with an associated aseptic meningitis.
4. The virus can be cultured from blood, CSF, nasopharynx, urine, or muscle. A rising titer of viral antibodies can be detected in serum over a 2-week period.
5. Muscle biopsy will show the presence of a myositis.

Treatment   Adequate doses of narcotic drugs are needed to control pain during the first few days of acute viral myositis. The pain is often excruciating and will not respond to simple analgesics. Myoglobinuria may precipitate renal failure; oliguria and anuria should be treated promptly.

Poliomyelitis and the Post-Polio Syndrome

Epidemics of poliomyelitis occurred almost every year in the United States in the first half of the century, until the disease was practically eradicated by effective vaccination.

Etiology and Pathology   Poliomyelitis is caused by a virus that invades motor neurons in the spinal cord and brainstem. Neuronal death results in atrophy of muscle fibers supplied by the affected motor unit, unless there is a compensatory sprouting of new fibers by surviving axons that contact and innervate some of the newly denervated muscle fibers. However, the overall effect is loss of muscle fibers, muscle wasting, and weakness.

Recovery from the acute phase of poliomyelitis is related to the survival of neurons in the spinal cord and brainstem, and improvement could occur for as long as 2 years after the acute episode, with many patients showing residual but stable weakness. However, a number of people who survived acute poliomyelitis have had a further weakness of muscle, a condition of post-polio syndrome.[144] This is believed to be the result of inability of the motor neuron to meet the metabolic demands of the enlarged motor unit and the atrophy of some of the distal nerve terminals.[145] It is not due to reactivation of a latent polio virus infection.[146]

Clinical Features   Post-polio syndrome occurs in approximately 30 percent of patients who survive acute poliomyelitis. The condition tends to occur in patients who had severe, permanent impairment from acute poliomyelitis and is more common in women.[147] Patients report further muscle weakness, muscle pain, and unaccustomed fatigue. However, the deterioration is short-lived, and the condition stabilizes again, with an increased but stable residual weakness.

Diagnostic Procedures Muscle biopsy will show recent and old denervation and reinnervation.

Treatment There is no effective treatment for post-polio syndrome.

Bacterial Myositis

Bacterial myositis is most often the result of infection with Clostridia. Rare examples of infection by *Staphylococcus aureus,*[148] *Streptococcus pyogenes,*[149] *Escherichia coli, Haemophilus influenzae,* and *Leptospira* have been reported. Obligatory anaerobic bacteria may cause myositis in immunocompromised patients.[150]

Etiology and Pathology The organism usually involved is *Clostridium perfringens.*

Clostridial organisms proliferate under anaerobic conditions and infection usually results from the presence of the bacteria in deep puncture wounds, compound fractures, or penetrating gunshot wounds. The clostridial exotoxin produces coagulation necrosis of muscle and breakdown of muscle glycogen with the production of carbon dioxide, which spreads through the muscle and subcutaneous tissues (gas gangrene).

Clinical Features Patients with bacterial myositis and gas gangrene present with high fever, tachycardia, and shock due to the potent effect of the clostridial exotoxin. The affected muscles are swollen, and the presence of gas in the tissues causes crepitus on palpation.

Treatment

1. Affected muscles should be incised, exposed, and drained.
2. Penicillin 40 million units intravenously should be administered q24h until wound cultures are sterile.
3. Hyperbaric oxygen is beneficial if available.
4. Amputation of an affected limb may be necessary in extreme cases.

Prognosis Gas gangrene carries a high mortality rate unless treated immediately. All cases should be regarded as a surgical emergency.

Granulomatous Myositis

Granulomatous lesions have been seen in patients with tertiary syphilis, tuberculosis, sarcoidosis, and toxoplasmosis.

Tuberculous myositis is usually due to extension of infection from bone, synovial lining of joints, infected tendon sheaths, direct inoculation, or hematogenous dissemination.[151] In the case of a psoas abscess, the infection spreads from the spine due to an extension of infection from tuberculous spondylitis (Pott disease). Chest wall abscesses due to spread of *Mycobacterium tuberculosis* from the lung or rib can occur in nonimmunosuppressed or HIV-infected individuals. Cold abscesses are occasionally due to infection by nontuberculous *Mycobacterium* species. Treatment consists of exploration, drainage and resection of the abscess, and therapy with antituberculous antibiotics. The myopathy of sarcoidosis is rare and presents with chronic wasting and proximal muscle weakness. The diagnosis is established by muscle biopsy. Prolonged low-dose prednisone therapy may be necessary to control the disease.[152] Asymptomatic muscle involvement is not unusual in pulmonary sarcoidosis.

Muscle involvement by the yeast *Histoplasma capsulatum* occurs predominantly in immunosuppressed individuals with AIDS but can occur in patients immunosuppressed by cytotoxic drugs or corticosteroids.[153]

Trichinosis

Definition Trichinosis is a myositis caused by the larvae of the nematode *Trichinella spiralis.*

Etiology and Pathology Man is infected by eating undercooked or raw pork products, or bear meat containing larvae of *T. spiralis.* The larvae are liberated in the intestinal tract and develop into adult worms. After 7 days, the fertilized female burrows into the intestinal wall and deposits the larvae in the lymphatics. This process continues for about 4 weeks. The larvae enter the systemic circulation and are carried to all tissues, but survival is limited to skeletal muscle, cardiac muscle, and the CNS. The larvae grow in muscle fibers and assume a spiral form. The presence of the foreign body causes an intense inflammatory reaction, which is sufficient to kill some of the larvae. The survivors develop a connective tissue capsule in about 6 weeks, which begins to calcify after 6 months. Larvae may survive for many years following an infection.

Clinical Features Ingestion of contaminated pork products or bear meat may be followed by a mild gastroenteritis. The entrance of larvae into skeletal muscle is followed by fever, severe myalgia, muscle weakness, and tenderness. Movements of the eyes, face, tongue, jaw, and neck are often painful and restricted, and there may be marked periorbital and facial edema. Intercostal muscle and diaphragmatic involvement restricts respiratory movements, which can be extremely painful. Myocardial involvement is unusual but may result in acute heart failure and death. Trichinella meningoencephalitis is associated with seizures, focal infarction, or hemorrhage. Cerebral edema can lead to brainstem compression, uncal herniation, and death.[154]

Diagnostic Procedures

1. There is a polymorphonucleocytosis with a marked eosinophilia.
2. The diagnosis can be confirmed by muscle biopsy, which reveals the presence of larvae.
3. The CSF examination shows an intense eosinophilic pleocytosis.
4. A positive skin reaction can be obtained after 2 weeks following the intradermal injection of trichinella antigen.
5. An MRI or CT scan will demonstrate multifocal lesions in the brain in patients with neurotrichinosis.
6. Serum complement-fixation precipitin and flocculation tests are positive after 3 weeks.

Treatment

1. The patient should be confined to strict bed rest because of the risk of heart failure. Adequate analgesia is required for pain control.

2. Corticosteroids. Methylprednisolone 100 mg every A.M. should be given and converted to alternate-day therapy as improvement occurs.
3. Flubendazole 40 mg/kg per day prevents larvae production and is toxic to larvae in muscle and brain.[155] Mebendazole 5 mg/kg per day for 10 to 15 days is an effective alternative therapy.
4. Heart failure requires fluid restriction, digitalization, low-salt diet, and diuretics.

Prognosis Recovery occurs in about 6 weeks in untreated cases. Treatment probably shortens the recovery period.

Cysticercosis

Myositis may occur during infection with *Taenia solium.*

Echinococcosis

Myositis may occur during infection with *Echinococcosis granulosis.*

Polymyositis

Definition *Polymyositis* is an inflammatory myopathy of steady progression occurring in adults associated with an autoimmune response; connective tissue disease; viral, bacterial or parasitic infections; or mycotoxic drugs.

Etiology and Pathology The etiology is unknown but polymyositis is believed to be an autoimmune reaction, the result of an antigen-directed cytotoxicity mediated by cytotoxic T cells. These cells, along with macrophages, surround and eventually invade and destroy healthy muscle fibers. These fibers express the class I major histocompatibility complex antigen, which is absent from normal healthy muscle fibers.[156]

Muscle biopsy shows necrosis, phagocytosis, degeneration, and regeneration of muscle fibers with perivascular, perimysial, and endomysial infiltration by inflammatory cells.

Clinical Features Polymyositis is rare in childhood and usually presents after the second decade of life. There is a progressive subacute proximal muscle weakness and distal muscle involvement is a later feature. Myalgia and muscle tenderness occur in some cases early in the disease. Ocular and facial muscles are normal, but pharyngeal muscle and neck muscle involvement is not unusual, causing dysphagia.[157] Respiratory muscle involvement is a late complication. Chronic cases show muscle wasting with normal sensation, preserved tendon reflexes, and plantar flexor responses. Systemic lupus erythematosus is the most common associated connective tissue disease.[158] There is also an association with scleroderma and mixed connective tissue disease. Other conditions include Crohn disease, vasculitis, ulcerative colitis,[159] chronic graft-versus-host disease,[160] HIV,[156] and human T-cell lymphotropic virus type 1 (HTLV-1).[161] Behçet disease, myasthenia gravis, dermatitis herpetiformis, psoriasis, Hashimoto disease,[162] and granulomatous diseases including sarcoidosis are also associated with polymyositis.[156] The relationship between malignancy and polymyositis is controversial.[163]

Diagnostic Procedures

1. The CK levels are elevated in most but not all cases of polymyositis.

2. Serum aldolase or serum myoglobin levels may be elevated in about 80 percent of cases.

3. The muscle biopsy is abnormal (see above).

4. Electromyography is abnormal, with small, short duration, polyphasic motor unit potentials with or without insertional activity and spontaneous potentials.

5. Several cardiac abnormalities, including arrhythmias, bundle branch block, congestive heart failure, and pericarditis have been described.[164]

6. Antibodies consisting of antisynthetases occur in 35 to 40 percent of cases of polymyositis or dermatomyositis.[165] The most common of the antisynthetases is anti-Jo-1 detected as histinyl-1-RNA synthetase.

7. Elevated serum light chain myosin-1 (MLC-1) levels may occur in early cases of polymyositis.[166]

Prognosis Increasing age is an adverse prognostic factor.[167] Patients aged 50 years or more have an adverse prognosis compared to younger patients. Longer duration of symptoms at presentation is also an unfavorable finding.[168] The majority of patients with fatal disease die within 6 months of presentation, and survival beyond 6 months indicates a good prognosis.

Dermatomyositis

Definition *Dermatomyositis* is a progressive myopathy preceding or accompanied by a characteristic rash.

Etiology and Pathology The disease occurs in children and adults and is often associated with lupus erythematosus, mixed connective tissue disease, scleroderma, or malignancy, and there is a strong indirect evidence for an autoimmune process. Dermatomyositis is not familial and infectious agents, including viruses, have not been implicated.

The muscle biopsy shows endomysial, predominantly perivascular inflammation, and the blood vessels exhibit endothelial proliferation, fibrin thrombi, and obliteration of capillaries. There are necrosis, degeneration, and phagocytosis of muscle fibers, usually occurring at the peripheral of the fascicle, due to microinfarction, which is a diagnostic feature of dermatomyositis.

Clinical Features The characteristic skin rash of dermatomyositis is manifested by a heliotrope rash and edema of the upper eyelids, a red rash on the face and upper trunk, with erythema and a raised scaly eruption of the knuckles. This rash may also occur at other sites, including knees, elbows, malleoli, neck, cheek, back, and shoulders, and is exacerbated by exposure to sunlight. Subcutaneous calcifications are common in children and occasionally in adults. Calcium deposits may extrude through the skin, causing ulceration and infection.

Muscle weakness presents initially in the proximal limb-girdle muscles and pharyngeal muscles may be involved, causing dysphagia. Myalgia is an occasional feature early in the disease; fever and weight loss are not uncommon. Cardiac and pulmonary complications, including congestive heart failure or pneumonia, are life-threatening in cases with cardiomyopathy or involvement of respiratory muscles. Gastrointestinal involvement, with ulceration or submucosal dissection due to vasculitis, may result in hematemesis or melena.

Diagnostic Procedures   As for polymyositis.

Treatment of Polymyositis and Dermatomyositis

1. Corticosteroids. It is generally accepted that prednisone or methylprednisolone are the first choice of drugs used in treatment. Prednisone is given 100 mg/day in a single dose at breakfast for 4 weeks, then tapered to 100 mg on alternate days by gradual reduction of the dose on the alternate "off" day by 10 mg/week.[156]

When the patient responds to prednisone, the dose is gradually reduced to 25 mg q.o.d. to maintain improved muscle strength.

However, if there is no benefit from steroid therapy, when the dosage has been reduced to 100 mg q.o.d., the patient is considered to be unresponsive to corticosteroids and prednisone tapering is accelerated, and alternative-day therapy instituted.

The regimen of alternate-day therapy with prednisone minimizes side effects, which include hypertension, diabetes, osteoporosis, avascular necrosis of the hip joints, cushingoid appearance, and obesity.

Corticosteroid therapy should be accompanied by a low-carbohydrate, high-protein, low-salt diet, supplemented by 40 mEq potassium daily. Ranitidine 150 mg q12h orally, or cimetidine 300 mg q8h orally reduce the risk of gastrointestinal upset or peptic ulceration.

The development of steroid myopathy (type 2 muscle fiber atrophy) presents difficulties in deciding whether increased weakness is the result of steroid therapy or resistance to corticosteroids. A temporary increase in prednisone dosage should increase strength when the weakness is the result of polymyositis but will have no effect on steroid myopathy.

2. Intravenous gamma globulin. Several studies have demonstrated significant improvement following intravenous gamma globulin therapy.[169] IVIG is recommended as a secondary choice in therapy for polymyositis/dermatomyositis.[170] The dose of 2 g/kg intravenously can be repeated once a month.[171] Prednisone or other immunosuppressant drugs can be continued during IVIG therapy. Adverse effects are mild.

3. Immunosuppressive therapy. Failure to respond to corticosteroid or IVIG treatment should be followed by immunosuppressive therapy. Available drugs include azathioprine, methotrexate, cyclophosphamide, and cyclosporine.[172] Males with antisynthetase antibodies experience more benefit from methotrexate when there is failure to respond to prednisone.[173] Toxic effects, including anemia, leukopenia, thrombocytopenia, pancytopenia, nausea, liver toxicity, and interstitial cystitis (cyclophosphamide) with remote complications of neoplasia should be considered before using these drugs. However, rapidly progressive, life-threatening disease with respiratory failure is an ample justification for immunosuppressive therapy.

Inclusion Body Myositis

Definition   A myopathy occurring in sporadic and familial forms, which can be differentiated by the presence of inflammation in the sporadic form, and absence of inflammation in the familial or hereditary form of the disease.[174]

Etiology and Pathology   The etiology is unknown. The familial form is inherited as an autosomal dominant trait. The role of viruses, including enteroviruses and mumps virus, appears unlikely.[175,176] There is evidence of antigen-directed toxicity, mediated by cytotoxic T cells because CD8+ cells and macrophages surround healthy muscle fibers and ultimately invade and destroy them. Pathological changes in muscle biopsy consist of basophilic granular inclusions distributed around the edge of slit-like vacuoles situated around the rim of muscle fibers. Groups of small angulated muscle fibers are present, some containing eosinophilic inclusions. Prion protein MRNA, B-amyloid protein, hyperphosphorylated tau, and apolipoprotein E accumulate in vacuolated muscle fibers.[177] This suggests a defect in processing or disposal of certain proteins in this disease, and the cytopathogenesis in Alzheimer disease and inclusion body myositis may share some similar mechanisms.[178]

Clinical Features The disease is probably underdiagnosed[179] because the presentation consists of involvement of distal muscles, especially finger flexors and foot extensors. Weakness of the third, fourth, and fifth finger flexors associated with atrophy of the flexor digitorum sublimis in the forearm is a unique feature of inclusion body myositis. Proximal weakness tends to involve biceps and triceps, quadriceps, femoris, and the iliopsoas muscles. Dysphagia is usually a late and not uncommon complication but may be the presenting symptom in some cases with development of limb weakness later.[180]

Diagnostic Procedures

1. Serum creatinine phosphokinase and serum aldolase levels are elevated.

2. The diagnosis is established by muscle biopsy.

Treatment Most patients with inclusion body myositis are refractory to the various treatments recommended for polymyositis/dermatomyositis.

There have been reports of successful therapy in a few cases following corticosteroid therapy,[181] chlorambucil,[182] and intravenous gamma globulin.[183] This suggests that aggressive therapy, moving from one drug to another after an extended trial, or combining therapies, may be of value in some cases.

Prognosis Inclusion body myositis was a fatal disease until reports of response to treatment began to appear in recent years. The condition is, however, refractory to all treatment in many cases, with progressive weakness and a fatal outcome.

MISCELLANEOUS SIGNS OF MUSCLE DISORDER

Myoglobinuria

Any disorder in which muscle cell membranes are disrupted, allowing leakage of muscle protein, may be characterized by myoglobinuria. Trauma, exercise, myositis, heat stroke, cold, diabetic acidosis, toxins such as alcohol, heroin, cocaine,[184] licorice, amphotericin B, succinylcholine, ϵ-aminocaproic acid, phenylpropanolamine,[185] and intravenous amphetamines, ischemic insults and certain myopathies, including polymyositis, phosphorylase deficiency, phosphofructokinase deficiency, carnitine deficiency, muscle palmitoyl transferase-A deficiency, and amyloidosis may produce myoglobinuria.[186] If myoglobin precipitates in renal tubules, it may produce oliguric or anuric renal failure. An idiopathic form of myoglobinuria occurs and is characterized clinically by muscle weakness, pain, tenderness, cramping, and edema after exertion or exercise.[187]

Facial Myokymia

Definition This condition is characterized by continuous involuntary wave-like undulating, rippling fine movements of facial muscles.

Etiology and Pathology The condition probably results from a change in axonal membrane excitability by several diverse conditions.

Clinical Features Facial myokymia confined to or maximal in the orbicularis oculi is a benign condition occurring in anxiety, fatigue, and ill health. More generalized facial involvement can occur in multiple sclerosis,[188] brainstem tumors in Guillain-Barré syndrome, and rarely in subarachnoid hemorrhage,[189] basilar invagination, syringobulbia, anoxic encephalopathy, brainstem tuberculoma, timber rattlesnake venom induction, radiation, meningeal carcinomatosis, and meningoencephalitis. There may be marked deepening of the nasolabial fold on the affected side.[190] Myokymia usually lasts from 3 weeks to 1 year when the course is benign. Electromyography shows myokymic discharges without fibrillations.

REFERENCES

1. Worton RG: Duchenne muscular dystrophy: gene and gene product; mechanism of mutation in the gene. *J Inherit Metab Dis* 15:539, 1992.

2. Hoffman EP, Wang J: Duchenne-Becker muscular dystrophy and the nondystrophic myotonias. Paradigms for loss of function and changes of function of gene products. *Arch Neurol* 50:1227, 1993.

3. Davies KE, Tinsley JM, Blake DJ: Molecular analysis of Duchenne muscular dystrophy: past, present, and future. *Ann NY Acad Sci* 758:287, 1995.

4. Jimi T, Wakayama Y, Takeda A, et al: Altered distribution of beta-dystroglycan in sarcolemma of human dystrophic muscles: an immunohistochemical study. *Muscle Nerve* 18:910, 1995.

5. Politano L, Nigro V, Nigro G, et al: Development of cardiomyopathy in female carriers of Duchenne and Becker muscular dystrophies. *JAMA* 275:1335, 1996.

6. Miller RG, Hoffman EP: Molecular diagnosis and modern management of Duchenne muscular dystrophy. *Neurol Clin* 12:699, 1994.

7. Bushby KM, Appleton R, Anderson LV, et al: Deletion status and intellectual impairment in Duchenne muscular dystrophy. *Dev Med Child Neurol* 37:260, 1995.

8. Saito K, Ikeya K, Kondo E, et al: Somatic mosaicism for a DMD gene deletion. *Am J Med Genet* 56:80, 1995.

9. van Bakel I, Holt S, Craig I, et al: Sequence analysis of the breakpoint regions on X:5 translocation in a female with Duchenne muscular dystrophy. *Am J Hum Genet* 57:329, 1995.

10. Pegoraro E, Schimke RN, Garcia C, et al: Genetic and biochemical normalization in female carriers of Duchenne muscular dystrophy: evidence for failure of dystrophin production in dystrophin-competent myonuclei. *Neurology* 45:677, 1995.

11. Hsu JD, Furumasu J: Gait and posture changes in the Duchenne muscular dystrophy child. *Clin Orthop Rel Research* 288:122, 1993.

12. Lyager S, Steffensen B, Juhl B: Indicators of need for mechanical ventilation in Duchenne muscular dystrophy and spinal muscular atrophy. *Chest* 108:779, 1995.

13. Robert D, Willig TN, Leger P: Long-term nasal ventilation in neuromuscular disorders: report of a consensus conference. *Eur Respir J* 6:599, 1993.

14. Rifai Z, Welle S, Moxley RT III: Effect of prednisone on protein metabolism in Duchenne dystrophy. *Am J Physiol* 268(PT I):E67, 1995.

15. Khan MA: Corticosteroid therapy in Duchenne muscular dystrophy. *J Neurol Sci* 120:8, 1993.

16. Partridge TA, Davies KE: Myoblast-based gene therapies. *Br Med Bull* 51:123, 1995.

17. Clemens PR, Caskey CT: Gene therapy prospects for Duchenne muscular dystrophy. *Eur Neurol* 34:181, 1994.

18. Mendell JR, Kissel JT, Amato AA, et al: Myoblast transfer in the treatment of Duchenne's muscular dystrophy. *N Engl J Med* 333:832, 1995.

19. Maeda M, Nakao S, Miyazato H, et al: Cardiac dystrophin abnormalities in Becker muscular dystrophy assessed by endomyocardial biopsy. *Am Heart J* 129:702, 1995.

20. Comi GP, Prelle A, Bresoln N, et al: Clinical variability in Becker muscular dystrophy: genetic biochemical and immunohistochemical correlates. *Brain* 117:1, 1994.

21. Bushby KM, Gardner-Medwin D: The clinical genetic, and dystrophin characteristics of Becker muscular dystrophy. I. Natural history. *J Neurol* 240:98, 1993.

22. Nigro G, Comi LI, Politano L, et al: Evaluation of the cardiomyopathy in Becker muscular dystrophy. *Muscle Nerve* 18:283, 1995.

23. Hayashi Y, Ikeda U, Ogawa T, et al: Becker-type muscular dystrophy associated with hypertrophic cardiomyopathy. *Am Heart J* 128:1264, 1994.

24. Nigro, G, Di Somma S, Comi LI, et al: Structural basis of cardiomyopathy in Duchenne/Becker carriers. Endomyocardial biopsy evaluation. *Ann N Y Acad Sci* 752:108, 1995.

25. Heald A, Anderson LV, Bushby KM, et al: Becker muscular dystrophy with onset after 60 years. *Neurology* 44:2388, 1994.

26. Campbell KP: Three muscular dystrophies: loss of cytoskeleton-extracellular matrix linkage. *Cell* 80:675, 1995.

27. Sunada Y, Edgar TS, Lotz BP, et al: Merosin-negative congenital muscular dystrophy associated with extensive brain abnormalities. *Neurology* 45:2084, 1995.

28. Kawai H, Akaike M, Endo T, et al: Adhalin gene mutations in patients with autosomal recessive childhood onset muscular dystrophy with adhalin deficiency. *J Clin Invest* 96:1202, 1995.

29. Padberg GW, Lunt PW, Koch M, et al: Diagnostic criteria for facioscapulohumeral muscular dystrophy. *Neuromuscul Dis* 1:231, 1991.

30. Gilbert JR, Stajich JM, Speer MC, et al: Linkage studies in facioscapulohumeral muscular dystrophy. *Am J Hum Genet* 51:424, 1992.

31. Lee JH, Goto K, Matsuda C, et al: Characterization of a tandemly repeated 3.3-Kb Kpnl unit in the facioscapulohumeral muscular dystrophy (FSHD) gene region on chromosone 4q35. *Muscle Nerve* 2:56, 1995.

32. Gilbert JR, Stajich JM, Wall S, et al: Evidence for heterogeneity in facioscapulohumeral muscular dystrophy (FSHD). *Am J Hum Genet* 53:401, 1993.

33. Upadhyaya M, Maynard J, Osborn M, et al: Germinal mosaicism in facioscapulohumeral muscular dystrophy. FSHD: *Muscle Nerve* Suppl 2:S45, 1995.

34. Padberg GW, Brouwer OF, de Keizer RJ, et al: On the significance of retinal vascular disease and hearing loss in facioscapulohumeral muscular dystrophy. *Muscle Nerve* Suppl 2:S73, 1995.

35. Tawil R, Myers GJ, Weiffenbach B, et al: Scapuloperoneal syndromes. Absence of linkage to the 4q35 FSHD locus. *Arch Neurol* 52:1069, 1995.

36. Wilhelmsen KC, Blake DM, Lynch T, et al: Chromosome 12-linked autosomal dominant scapuloperoneal muscular dystrophy. *Ann Neurol* 39:507, 1996.

37. Yamanouchi Y, Arikawa E, Arahata K, et al: Limb-girdle muscular dystrophy: clinical and pathologic reevaluation. *J Neuro Sci* 129:15, 1995.

38. Richard I, Broux O, Allamand V, et al: Mutations in the proteolytic enzyme calpain 3 cause limb-girdle muscular dystrophy type 2A. *Cell* 81:27, 1995.

39. Stübgen JP: Limb girdle muscular dystrophy: description of a phenotype. *Muscle Nerve* 17:1449, 1994.

40. McDonald CM, Johnson ER, Abresch RT, et al: Profiles of neuromuscular diseases. Limb-girdle syndromes. *Am J Phys Med Rehab* 74(5 suppl):S117, 1995.

41. Mascarenhas DA, Spodick DH, Chad DA, et al: Cardiomyopathy of limb-girdle muscular dystrophy. *J Am Coll Cardiol* 24:1328, 1994.

42. Molgat YM, Rodrigue D: Correction of blepharoptosis in oculopharyngeal muscular dystrophy: review of 91 cases. *Can J Ophthalmol* 28:11, 1993.

43. Chang MH, Chang SP, Cheung SC, et al: Computerized tomography of oropharynx is useful in the diagnosis of oculopharyngeal muscular dystrophy. *Muscle Nerve* 16:325, 1993.

44. Castell JA, Castell DO, Duranceau CA, et al: Manometric characteristics of the pharynx upper esophageal sphincter esophagus and lower esophageal sphincter in patients with oculopharyngeal muscular dystrophy. *Dysphagia* 10:22,1995.

45. Bejaoui K, Hirabayashi K, Hentati F, et al: Linkage of Miyoshi myopathy (distal autosomal recessive muscular dystrophy) locus to chromosome 2p12-14. *Neurology* 45:768, 1995.

46. Hudson AJ, Ebers GC, Bulman DE: The skeletal muscle sodium and chloride channel diseases. *Brain* 118:547, 1995.

47. Ricker K, Moxley RT III, Heine R, et al: Myotonia fluctuans. A third type of muscle sodium channel disease. *Arch Neurol* 51:1095, 1994.

48. Ptacek LJ, Tawil R, Griggs RC, et al: Sodium channel mutations in acetazolamide responsive myotonia congenita, paramyotonia congenita, and hyperkalemic periodic paralysis. *Neurology* 44:1500, 1994.

49. Fu YH, Pizzuti A, Fenwick RG Jr, et al: An unstable triplet repeat in a gene related to myotonic muscular dystrophy. *Science* 255:1256, 1992.

50. Pizzuti A, Friedman DL, Caskey CT: The myotonic dystrophy gene. *Arch Neurol* 50:1173, 1993.

51. Anderson JR: Recent advances in muscular dystrophies and myopathies. *J Clin Pathol* 48:597, 1995.

52. Afifi AM, Bhatia AR, Eyal F: Hydrops fetalis associated with congenital myotonic dystrophy. *Am J Obstet Gynecol* 166:929, 1992.

53. Johnson ER, Abresch RT, Carter GT, et al: Profiles of neuromuscular diseases. Myotonic dystrophy. *Am J Phys Med Rehab* 74(5 suppl):S104, 1995.

54. McLay JS, Norris A, Kerr F: Could it be myotonic dystrophy? Myotonic dystrophy presenting with atrial flutter. *Scot Med J* 37:149, 1992.

55. Melacini P, Villanova C, Menegazzo E, et al: Correlation between cardiac involvement and CTG trinucleotide repeat length in myotonic dystrophy. *J Am Coll Cardiol* 25:239, 1995.

56. Tokgozoglu LS, Ashizawa T, Pacifico A, et al: Cardiac involvement in a large kindred with myotonic dystrophy. Quantitative assessment and relation to size of CTG repeat expansion. *JAMA* 274:813, 1995.

57. Van Spaendonck KP, Ter Bruggen JP, Weyn Banningh EW, et al: Cognitive function in early adult and adult onset myotonic dystrophy. *Acta Neurol Scand* 91:456, 1995.

58. Censori B, Provinciali L, Danni M, et al: Brain involvement in myotonic dystrophy: MRI features and their relationship to clinical and cognitive conditions. *Acta Neurol Scand* 90:211, 1994.

59. Ono S, Kanda F, Takahashi K, et al: Neuronal loss in the medullary reticular formation in myotonic dystrophy: a clinicopathological study. *Neurology* 46:228, 1996.

60. Shelbourne P, Davies J, Buxton J, et al: Direct diagnosis of myotonic dystrophy with a disease-specific DNA marker. *N Engl J Med* 328:471, 1993.

61. Redman JB, Fenwick RG Jr, Fu YH, et al: Relationship between parental trinucleotide GCT repeat length and severity of myotonic dystrophy in offspring. *JAMA* 269:1960, 1993.

62. Reardon W, Newcombe R, Fenton I, et al: The natural history of congenital myotonic dystrophy: mortality and long term clinical aspects. *Arch Dis Child* 68:177, 1993.

63. Pourmond R, Azzarelli B: Adult-onset of nemaline myopathy associated with cores and abnormal mitochondria. *Muscle Nerve* 17:1218, 1994.

64. Wallgren-Pettersson C, Hiilesmaa VK, Paatero H: Pregnancy and delivery in congenital nemaline myopathy. *Acta Obstet Gynecol Scand* 74:659, 1995.

65. Dahl N, Hu LJ, Chery M, et al: Myotubular myopathy in a girl with a deletion of Xq27-q28 and unbalanced X inactivation assigns the MTM1 gene to a 600-kb region. *Am J Hum Genet* 56:1108, 1995.

66. Villanova M, Louboutin JP, Chateau D, et al: X-linked vacuolated myopathy: complement membrane attack complex on surface membrane of injured muscle fibers. *Ann Neurol* 37:637, 1995.

67. Dalakas MC, Leon-Monzon ME, Bernardini I, et al: Zidovudine-induced mitochondrial myopathy is associated with muscle carnitine deficiency and lipid storage. *Ann Neurol* 35:482, 1994.

68. Raben N, Nichols RC, Boerkoel C, et al: Genetic defects in patients with glycogenosis type II (acid maltase deficiency). *Muscle Nerve* Suppl 3:S70, 1995.

69. Reuser AJ, Kroos MA, Hermans MM, et al: Glycogenosis type II (acid maltase deficiency). *Muscle Nerve* Suppl 3:S61, 1995.

70. Beynon RJ, Bartram C, Hopkins P, et al: McArdle's disease: molecular genetics and metabolic consequences of the phenotype. *Muscle Nerve* Suppl 3:S18, 1995.

71. Tsujino S, Shanske S, Nonaka I, et al: The molecular genetic basis of myophosphorylase deficiency (McArdle's disease). *Muscle Nerve* Suppl 3:S23, 1995.

72. Raben N, Sherman JB, Adams E, et al: Various classes of mutations in patients with phosphofructokinase deficiency (Tarui's disease). *Muscle Nerve* Suppl 3:S35, 1995.

73. Nakagawa C, Mineo I, Kaido M, et al: A new variant case of muscle phosphofructokinase deficiency coexisting with gastric ulcer, gouty arthritis and increased hemolysis. *Muscle Nerve* Suppl 3:S39, 1995.

74. Mita S, Tokunaga M, Kumamoto T, et al: Mitochondrial DNA mutation and muscle pathology in mitochondrial myopathy, encephalopathy, lactic acidosis and strokelike episodes. *Muscle Nerve* Suppl 3:S113, 1995.

75. Shoffner JM, Lott MT, Lezza AM, et al: Myoclonic epilepsy and ragged-red fiber disease (MERRF) is associated with a mitochondrial DNA + RNA (Lys) mutation. *Cell* 61:931, 1990.

76. Koga Y, Davidson M, Schon EA, et al: Analysis of cybrids harboring MELAS mutations in the mitochondrial tRNA (Leu(uuR)) gene. *Muscle Nerve* Suppl 3:S119, 1995.

77. Zuckner J: Drug-related myopathies. *Rheum Dis Clin North Am* 20:1017, 1994.

78. Gharavi AG, Diamond JA, Smith DA, et al: Niacin-induced myopathy. *Am J Cardiol* 74:841, 1994.

79. Solimena M, Folli F, Aparisi R, et al: Autoantibodies to GABA-ergic neurons and pancreatic beta cells in stiff-man syndrome. *N Engl J Med* 322:1555, 1990.

80. Henningsen P, Clement U, Kuchenhoff J, et al: Psychological factors in the diagnosis and pathogenesis of stiff-person syndrome. *Neurology* 47:38, 1996.

81. Johnson JO, Miller KA: Anesthetic implications in stiff-man syndrome. *Anesth Analg* 80:612, 1995.

82. Meinck HM, Tronnier V, Rieke K, et al: Intrathecal baclofen treatment for stiff-man syndrome: pump failure may be fatal. *Neurology* 44:2209, 1994.

83. Shillito P, Molenaar PC, Vincent A, et al: Acquired neuromyotonia: evidence for autoantibodies directed against K$^+$ channels in peripheral nerves. *Ann Neurol* 38:714, 1995.

84. Layzer RB: Neuromyotonia: a new autoimmune disease. *Ann Neurol* 38:701, 1995.

85. Sinha S, Newsom-Davis J, Mills K, et al: Autoimmune aetiology for acquired neuromyotonia (Isaacs' syndrome). *Lancet* 338:75, 1991.

86. Fontaine B, Vale-Santos J, Jurkat-Rott K, et al: Mapping of the hypokalaemic periodic paralysis (HypoPP) locus to chromosome 1q31-32 in three European families. *Nat Genet* 6:267, 1994.

87. Gregg RG, Couch F, Hogan K, et al: Assignment of the human gene for the alpha 1 subunit of the skeletal muscle DHP-sensitive Ca^{++} channel (CACNL 1q31-32 1A3) to chromosome 1q31-32. *Genomics* 15:107, 1993.

88. Sipos I, Jurkat-Rott K, Harasztosi C, et al: Skeletal muscle DHP receptor mutations alter calcium currents in human hypokalaemic periodic paralysis microtubules. *J Physiol (Lond)* 483:299, 1995.

89. Links TP, Smit AJ, Molenaar WM, et al: Familial hypokalaemic periodic paralysis. Clinical diagnostic and therapeutic aspects. *J Neurol Sci* 122:33, 1994.

90. van der Hoeven JH, Links TP, Zwarts MJ, et al: Muscle fiber conduction velocity in the diagnosis of familial hypokalemic periodic paralysis—invasive versus surface determination. *Muscle Nerve* 17:898, 1994.

91. Kantola IM, Tarssanen LT: Diagnosis of familial hypokalemic periodic paralysis: role of the potassium exercise test. *Neurology* 42:2158, 1992.

92. Streeten DH, Speller PJ, Fellerman H: Use of corticotropin-induced potassium changes in the diagnosis of both hypo- and hyperkalemic periodic paralysis. *Eur Neurol* 33:103, 1993.

93. Darrow M, Brammer WK, Rowley A: Thyrotoxic periodic paralysis: two case studies. *Arch Phys Med Rehab* 76:685, 1995.

94. Ober KP: Thyrotoxic periodic paralysis in the United States. Report of 7 cases and review of the literature. *Medicine* 71:109, 1992.

95. Koul PA, Saleem SM, Bhat D: Sporadic distal renal tubular acidosis and periodic hypokalaemic paralysis in Kashmir. *J Intern Med* 233:463, 1993.

96. Ghosh D, Dhiman RK, Kohli A, et al: Hypokalemic periodic paralysis in association with tropical sprue: a case report. *Acta Neurol Scand* 90:371, 1994.

97. Stedwell RE, Allen KM, Binder LS: Hypokalemic paralyses: a review of the etiologies, pathophysiology, presentation, and therapy. *Am J Emerg Med* 10:143, 1992.

98. Arimura Y, Arimura K, Suwazono S, et al: Predictive value of the prolonged exercise test in hypokalemic paralytic attacks. *Muscle Nerve* 18:472, 1995.

99. Shayne P, Hart A: Thyrotoxic periodic paralysis terminated with intravenous propranolol. *Ann Emerg Med* 24:736, 1994.

100. Ptacek LJ, Gouw L, Kwiecinski H, et al: Sodium channel mutations in paramyotonia congenita and hyperkalemic periodic paralysis. *Ann Neurol* 33:300, 1993.

101. Baquero JL, Ayala RA, Wang J, et al: Hyperkalemic periodic paralysis with cardiac dysrhythmia: a novel sodium channel mutation? *Ann Neurol* 37:408, 1995.

102. Machkhas H, Ashizawa T, Ptacek L: Familial periodic paralysis, in Appel SH (ed): *Current Neurology,* chap 2 Mosby, St. Louis, 1996, pp 65–92.

103. Borg K, Hovmöller M, Larsson L, et al: Paramyotonia congenita (Eulenburg): clinical, neurophysiological, and muscle biopsy observations in a Swedish family. *Acta Neurol Scand* 87:37, 1993.

104. Drachman DB: Myasthenia gravis. *N Engl J Med* 330:1797, 1994.

105. Kuncl RW, Drachman DB, Adams R, et al: 3-Deazaadenosine: a therapeutic strategy for myasthenia gravis by decreasing the endocytosis of acetylcholine receptors. *J Pharmacol Exp Ther* 267:582, 1993.

106. Hohlfeld R, Wekerle H: The thymus in myasthenia gravis. *Neurol Clin* 12:331, 1994.

107. Levinson AI, Wheatley LM: The thymus and the pathogenesis of myasthenia gravis. *Clin Immunol Immunopathol* 78:1, 1996.

108. Sanders DB, Scoppetta C: The treatment of patients with myasthenia gravis. *Neurol Clin* 12:343, 1994.

109. Puglisi F, Finato N, Mariuzzi L, et al: Microscopic thymoma and myasthenia gravis. *J Clin Pathol* 48:682, 1995.

110. Verma P, Oger J: Treatment of acquired autoimmune myasthenia gravis: a topic review. *Can J Neurol Sci* 19: 360, 1992.

111. Howard JF Jr, Sanders DB, Massey JM: The electrodiagnosis of myasthenia gravis and the Lambert-Eaton myasthenic syndrome. *Neurol Clin* 12:305, 1994.

112. Rivero A, Crovetto L, Lopez L, et al: Single fiber electromyography of extraocular muscles: a sensitive method for the diagnosis of ocular myasthenia gravis. *Muscle Nerve* 18:943, 1995.

113. Okada S, Saito E, Ogawa T, et al: Grades of exophthalmos and thyrotropin-binding inhibitory immunoglobulin in patients with myasthenia gravis. *Eur Neurol* 35:99, 1995.

114. Vaiopoulos G, Sfikakis PP, Kapsimali V, et al: The association of systemic lupus erythematosus and myasthenia gravis. *Postgrad Med J* 70:741, 1994.

115. Christensen PB, Jensen TS, Tsiropoulosi I, et al: Associated autoimmune diseases in myasthenia gravis. A population based study. *Acta Neurol Scand* 91:192, 1995.

116. Putman MT, Wise RA: Myasthenia gravis and upper airway obstruction. *Chest* 109:400, 1996.

117. Le Forestier N, Gherardi RK, Meyrignac C, et al: Myasthenic symptoms in patients with mitochondrial myopathies. *Muscle Nerve* 18:1338, 1995.

118. Takanami I, Imamura T, Kodaira S: Myasthenia gravis complicated by sarcoidosis. *J Thorac Cardiovasc Surg* 109:183, 1995.

119. Abrey LE: Association of myasthenia gravis with extrathymic Hodgkin's lymphoma: complete resolution of myasthenia symptoms following antineoplastic therapy. *Neurology* 45:1019, 1995.

120. Authier FJ, De Grissac N, Degos JD, et al: Transient myasthenia gravis during HIV infection. *Muscle Nerve* 18:914, 1995.

121. Ashour M: Prevalence of ectopic thymic tissue in myasthenia gravis and its clinical significance. *J Thorac Cardiovasc Surg* 109:632, 1995.

122. Yim AP, Kay RL, Ho JK: Video-assisted thoracoscopic thymectomy for myasthenia gravis. *Chest* 108:1440, 1995.

123. Gotti G, Paladini P, Haid MM, et al: Late recurrence thymoma and myasthenia gravis. *Scand J Thorac Cardiovasc Surg* 29:37, 1995.

124. Shah A, Lisak RP: Immunopharmacologic therapy in myasthenia gravis. *Clin Neuropharmacol* 16:97, 1993.

125. March GA Jr, Johnson LN: Ocular myasthenia gravis. *J Nat Med Assoc* 85:681, 1993.

126. Goti P, Spinelli A, Marconi G, et al: Comparative effects of plasma exchange and pyridostigmine on respiratory muscle strength and breathing pattern in patients with myasthenia gravis. *Thorax* 50:1080, 1995.

127. Grob D, Simpson D, Mitsumoto H, et al: Treatment of myasthenia gravis by immunoadsorption of plasma. *Neurology* 45:338, 1995.

128. Shibuya N, Sato T, Osame M, et al: Immunoadsorption therapy for myasthenia gravis. *J Neurol Neurosurg Psychiatry* 57:578, 1994.

129. Edan G, Landgraf F: Experience with intravenous immunoglobulin in myasthenia gravis: a review. *J Neurol Neurosurg Psychiatry* 57 (suppl):55, 1994.

130. Steg RE, Lefkowitz DM: Cerebral infarction following intravenous immunoglobulin therapy for myasthenia gravis. *Neurology* 44:1180, 1994.

131. Ellis RJ, Swendson MR, Bajorek J: Aseptic meningitis as a complication of intravenous immunoglobulin therapy for myasthenia gravis. *Muscle Nerve* 17:683, 1994.

132. Zulueta JJ, Fanburg BL: Respiratory dysfunction in myasthenia gravis. *Clin Chest Med* 15:683, 1994.

133. McEvoy KM: Diagnosis and treatment of Lambert-Eaton myasthenic syndrome. *Neurol Clin* 12:387, 1994.

134. Barr CW, Claussen G, Thomas D, et al: Primary respiratory failure as the presenting symptom in Lambert-Eaton myasthenic syndrome. *Muscle Nerve* 16:712, 1993.

135. Chalk CH, Murray NM, Newsom-Davis J, et al: Response of the Lambert-Eaton syndrome to treatment of associated small-cell lung carcinoma. *Neurology* 40:1552, 1990.

136. Bird SJ: Clinical and electrophysiologic improvement in Lambert-Eaton syndrome with intravenous immunoglobulin therapy. *Neurology* 42:1422, 1992.

137. Engel AG: Congenital myasthenic syndromes. *Neurol Clin* 12:401, 1994.

138. Paterson DL, King MA, Boyle RS, et al: Severe botulism after eating home-preserved asparagus. *Med J Aust* 157:269, 1992.

139. Weber JT, Hibbs RG Jr, Darwish A, et al: A massive outbreak of type E botulism associated with traditional salted fish in Cairo. *J Infect Dis* 167:451, 1993.

140. Burningham MD, Walter FG, Mechem C, et al: Wound botulism. *Ann Emerg Med* 24:1184, 1994.

141. Kudrow DB, Henry DA, Haake DA, et al: Botulism associated with *Clostridium botulinum* sinusitis after intranasel cocaine abuse. *Ann Intern Med* 109:984, 1988.

142. Woodruff BA, Griffin PM, McCroskey LM, et al: Clinical and laboratory comparison of botulism from toxin types A, B, and E in the United States, 1975–1988. *J Infect Dis* 166:1281, 1992.

143. From the Centers for Disease Control and Prevention: Foodborne botulism—Oklahoma 1994. *JAMA* 273:1167, 1994.

144. Windebank AJ, Litchy WJ, Daube JR, et al: Late effects of paralytic poliomyelitis in Olmsted County, Minnesota. *Neurology* 41:501, 1991.

145. Trojan DA, Cashman NR, Shapiro S, et al: Predictive factors for post-poliomyelitis syndrome. *Arch Phys Med Rehab* 75:770, 1994.

146. Melchers W, deVisser M, Jongen P, et al: The post-polio syndrome: no evidence for poliovirus persistence. *Ann Neurol* 32:728, 1992.

147. Ramlow J, Alexander M, Laporte R, et al: Epidemiology of the post-polio syndrome. *Am J Epidemiol* 136:769, 1992.

148. Sato K, Kamata T, Nakayama T, et al: Acute bacterial myositis due to staphylococcus aureus septicemia. *Neurology* 45:390, 1995.

149. Segar A, Binnie NR: Streptococcal myositis and the acute abdomen: a case report. *J R Coll Surg Edinb* 40:328, 1995.

150. Beumont MG, Duncan J, Mitchell SD, et al: Veillonella myositis in an immunocompromised patient. *Clin Infect Dis* 21:678, 1995.

151. Bonomo RA: Tuberculous pyomyositis: an unusual presentation of disseminated *Mycobacterium tuberculosis* infection. *Clin Infect Dis* 20:1576, 1995.

152. al-Saffar ZS, Kelsey CR, Kennet RP, et al: Myositis and eosinophilia in a patient with sarcoidosis. *Postgrad Med J* 70:833, 1994.

153. Voloshin DK, Lacomis D, McMahon D: Disseminated histoplasmosis presenting as myositis and fasciitis in a patient with dermatomyositis. *Muscle Nerve* 18:531, 1995.

154. Ryczak M, Sorber WA, Kandora TF, et al: Difficulties in diagnosing trichinella encephalitis. *Am J Trop Med Hyg* 36:573, 1987.

155. Ellrodt A, Halfon P, Le Bras P, et al: Multifocal cen-

tral nervous system lesions in three patients with trichinosis. *Arch Neurol* 44:432, 1987.

156. Dalakas MC: Clinical, immunopathologic, and therapeutic considerations of inflammatory myopathies. *Clin Neuropharmacol* 15:372, 1992.

157. Palace J, Losseff N, Clough C: Isolated dysphagia due to polymyositis. *Muscle Nerve* 16:680, 1993.

158. Koh ET, Seow A, Ong B, et al: Adult onset polymyositis/dermatomyositis: clinical and laboratory features and treatment response in 75 patients. *Ann Rheum Dis* 52:857, 1993.

159. Chugh S, Dilawari JB, Sawhney IM, et al: Polymyositis associated with ulcerative colitis. *Gut* 34:567, 1993.

160. Hanslik T, Jaccard A, Guillon JM, et al: Polymyositis and chronic graft-versus-host disease: efficacy of intravenous gammaglobulin. *J Am Acad Dermatol* 28:492, 1993.

161. Higuchi I, Montemayor ES, Izumo S, et al: Immunohistochemical characteristics of polymyositis in patients with HTVL-1-associated myelopathy and HTLV-1 carriers. *Muscle Nerve* 16:472, 1993.

162. Fujitake J, Ishikawa Y, Ishimaru S, et al: Localized polymyositis associated with chronic thyroiditis. *J Rheumatol* 21:1147, 1994.

163. Cherin P, Piette JC, Herson S, et al: Dermatomyositis and ovarian cancer: a report of 7 cases and literature review. *J Rheumatol* 20:1897, 1993.

164. Poveda Gomez F, Merino JL, Maté I, et al: Polymyositis associated with anti-Jo I antibodies: severe cardiac involvement as initial manifestation. *Am J Med* 94:110, 1993.

165. Targoff IN: Humoral immunity in polymyositis/dermatomyositis. *J Invest Dermatol* 100:116S, 1993.

166. Mader R, Nicol PD, Turley JJ, et al: Inflammatory myopathy — early diagnosis and management by serum myosin light chains measurements. *Israel J Med Sci* 30:902, 1994.

167. Lilley H, Dennett X, Byrne E: Biopsy proven polymyositis in Victoria 1982–1987: analysis of prognostic factors. *J Roy Soc Med* 87:323, 1994.

168. Fafalak RG, Peterson MG, Kagen LJ: Strength in polymyositis and dermatomyositis: best outcome in patients treated early. *J Rheumatol* 21:643, 1994.

169. Sussman GL, Pruzanski W: The role of intravenous infusions of gamma globulin in the therapy of polymyositis and dermatomyositis. *J Rheumatol* 21:990, 1994.

170. Cherin P, Herson S: Indications for intravenous gammaglobulin therapy in inflammatory myopathies. *J Neurol Neurosurg Psychiatry* 57 (suppl):50, 1994.

171. Dalakas MC, Illa I, Dambrosia JM, et al: A controlled trial of high-dose intravenous immune globulin infusions as treatment for dermatomyositis. *N Engl J Med* 329:1993, 1993.

172. Mehregan DR, Su WP: Cyclosporine treatment for dermatomyositis/polymyositis. *Cutis* 51:59, 1993.

173. Joffe MM, Love LA, Leff RL, et al: Drug therapy of the idiopathic inflammatory myopathies: predictors of response to prednisone, azathioprine and methotrexate and a comparison of their efficacy. *Am J Med* 94:379, 1993.

174. Griggs RC, Askanas V, Di Mauro S, et al: Inclusion body myositis and myopathies. *Ann Neurol* 38:705, 1995.

175. Leon-Monzon M, Dalakas MC: Absence of persistent infection with enteroviruses in muscles of patients with inflammatory myopathies. *Ann Neurol* 32:219, 1992.

176. Fox SA, Ward BK, Robbins PD, et al: Inclusion body myositis: investigation of the mumps virus hypothesis by polymerase chain reaction. *Muscle Nerve* 19:23, 1996.

177. Sarkozi E, Askanas V, Engel WK: Abnormal accumulation of prion protein in mRNA in muscle fibers of patients with sporadic inclusion-body myositis and hereditary inclusion-body myopathy. *Am J Pathol* 145:1280, 1994.

178. Askanas V, Engel WK, Bilak M, et al: Twisted tubulofilaments of inclusion body myositis muscle resemble paired helical filaments of Alzheimer brain and contain hyperphosphorylated tau. *Am J Pathol* 144:177, 1994.

179. Hopkinson ND, Hunt C, Powell RJ, et al: Inclusion body myositis: an underdiagnosed condition? *Ann Rheum Dis* 52:147, 1993.

180. Darrow DH, Hoffman HT, Barnes GJ, et al: Management of dysphagia in inclusion body myositis. *Arch Otolaryngol Head Neck Surgery* 118:313, 1992.

181. Lindberg C, Persson LI, Bjorkander J, et al: Inclusion body myositis: clinical morphological physiological and laboratory findings in 18 cases. *Acta Neurol Scand* 89:123, 1994.

182. Jongen PJ, ter Laak HJ, van de Putte LB: Inclusion body myositis responding to long-term chlorambucil treatment. *J Rheumatol* 22:576, 1995.

183. Adams EM, Plotz PH: The treatment of myositis. How to approach resistant disease. *Rheum Dis Clin North Am* 21:179, 1995.

184. Merigian KS, Roberts JR: Cocaine intoxication: hyperpyrexia rhabdomyolysis and acute renal failure. *J toxicol-Clin Toxicol* 25: 135, 1987.

185. Forwell MA, Hallworth MJ: Nontraumatic rhabdomyolysis and acute renal failure. *Scot Med J* 31:246, 1986.

186. Ross NS, Hoppel CL: Partial muscle carnitine palmitoyltransferase—A deficiency. Rhabdomyolysis associated with transiently decreased muscle carnitine content after ibuprofen therapy. *JAMA* 257:62, 1987.

187. Haverkort-Poels PJ, Joosten EM, Ruitenbeek W: Prevention of recurrent exertional rhabdomyolysis by dantrolene sodium. *Muscle Nerve* 10:45, 1987.

188. Jacobs L, Kaba S, Pullicino P: The lesion causing continuous facial myokymia in multiple sclerosis. *Arch Neurol* 51:1115, 1994.

189. Blumenthal DT, Gutmann L, Sauter K: Subarachnoid hemorrhage induces facial myokymia. *Muscle Nerve* 17:1484, 1994.

190. Gutmann L, Hopf HC: Facial myokymia and contraction persisting 20 years: a case of pontine glioma. *Muscle Nerve* 17:1461, 1994.

INDEX

Page numbers followed by *f* and *t* indicate figures and tables, respectively.